ELSEVIER

W9-BEK-668

evolve

∴ To access your Student Resources, visit the Web address below:

http://evolve.elsevier.com/Potter/Basic/

- **WebLinks**
  Links to places of interest on the Web specific to your classroom needs.

- **Content Updates**

- **Links to Related Products**
  See what Elsevier has to offer in a specific field of interest.

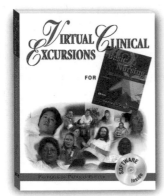
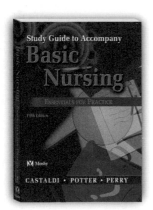

Basic Nursing

ESSENTIALS FOR PRACTICE

Basic Nursing

Fifth Edition
with 700 illustrations

Essentials for Practice

Patricia A. Potter, RN, MSN, EdD, FAAN
Research Scientist
Barnes-Jewish Hospital
St. Louis, Missouri

Anne Griffin Perry, RN, MSN, EdD, FAAN
Professor and Co-Coordinator, Adult Health Specialty
Saint Louis University School of Nursing
Saint Louis University Health Sciences Center
St. Louis, Missouri

Mosby
An Affiliate of Elsevier

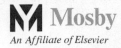
Mosby
An Affiliate of Elsevier

Vice President and Publishing Director, Nursing: Sally Schrefer
Executive Editor: Susan Epstein
Developmental Editor: Linda Stagg
Publication Services Manager: John Rogers
Project Manager: Beth Hayes
Senior Designer: Kathi Gosche

FIFTH EDITION

NOTICE

Permissions may be sought directly from Elsevier's Health Sciences Rights
Department in Philadelphia, USA: phone (+1)215-238-7869, fax: (+1)215-238-2239,
email: healthpermissions@elsevier.com. You may also complete your request on-line
via the Elsevier Science homepage (http://www.elsevier.com), by selecting 'Customer
Support' and then 'Obtaining Permissions'.

Mosby, Inc.
11830 Westline Industrial Drive
St. Louis, MO 63146

Library of Congress Cataloging in Publication Data
Basic nursing: essentials for practice / Patricia A. Potter, Anne Griffin
Perry—1st ed.
    p. cm.
  Includes index.
  ISBN 0-323-01660-X
   1. Nursing. 2. Nursing—Study and teaching. I. Potter, Patricia Ann. II. Perry, Anne
Griffin.

RT71 .B35 2002
610.7'73—dc21

                      2002025077

05 06 07 08   9 8 7 6 5 4

Contributors

MARJORIE BAIER, PhD, APRN, BC
Assistant Professor
Southern Illinois University–Edwardsville, School of
    Nursing
Edwardsville, Illinois

JUDITH C. BROSTRON, RN, BA, JD, LLM
Attorney
Lashly & Baer, P.C.
St. Louis, Missouri

VICTORIA M. BROWN, RN, BSN, MSN, PhD, HNC
Professor of Nursing
Georgia College & State University
Milledgeville, Georgia

GALE CARLI, MSN, MSHed, BSN, RN
Assistant Professor
Ohlone College
Fremont, California

JANICE C. COLWELL, RN, MS, CWOCN
Clinical Nurse Specialist, Wound, Ostomy, and Skin Care
University of Chicago Hospitals
Chicago, Illinois

EILEEN COSTANTINOU, RN, BSN, MSN
Professional Practice Consultant
Barnes-Jewish Hospital
St. Louis, Missouri

MARGARET ECKER, RN, MS
Education Director
Saint John's Health Center
Santa Monica, California

MARTHA KEENE ELKIN, RN, MSN, IBCLC
Lactation Counselor
Stephens Memorial Hospital
Norway, Maine

SUSAN JANE FETZER, RN, BA, BSN, MSN, MBA, PhD
Assistant Professor
University of New Hampshire
Durham, New Hampshire

LEAH W. FREDERICK, RN, MS, CIC
Consultant
Infection Control Consultants
Scottsdale, Arizona

AMY M. HALL, RN, BSN, MS, PhD
Assistant Professor
Saint Francis Medical Center, College of Nursing
Peoria, Illinois

KRISTINE M. L'ECUYER, RN, BSN, MSN
Adjunct Assistant Professor
Saint Louis University, School of Nursing
St. Louis, Missouri

RITA G. MERTIG, RNC, MS, CNS
Professor of Nursing
John Tyler Community College
Chester, Virginia

ELAINE K. NEEL, RN, BSN, MSN
Nursing Instructor
Methodist Medical Center of Illinois
Peoria, Illinois

JULIA BALZER RILEY, RN, MN, HNC
President, Constant Source Seminars
Co-Founder of Holistic Nursing Institute
Faculty, Sarasota Technical Institute
Ellenton, Florida

ELIZABETH SPEAKMAN, RN, EdD
Associate Professor of Nursing
Community College of Philadelphia
Philadelphia, Pennsylvania

PATRICIA A. STOCKERT, RN, BSN, MS, PhD
Associate Professor
Saint Francis Medical Center College of Nursing
Peoria, Illinois

PAMELA BECKER WEILITZ, RN, MSN(R), CS, ANP
Adult Nurse Practitioner
South City Health, LLC
St. Louis, Missouri

RITA WUNDERLICH, RN, MSN(R), PhD(c)
Nurse Manager–Medicine
St. Louis University Hospital–Tenet
St. Louis, Missouri

Clinical Consultants

JANICE C. COLWELL, RN, MS, CWOCN
Clinical Nurse Specialist, Wound, Ostomy and Skin Care
University of Chicago Hospitals
Chicago, Illinois

LOIS C. HAMEL, RN, PhD(c), CS-ANP
Assistant Professor and Adult Nurse Practitioner
University of Vermont
Burlington, Vermont

JUDITH ANN KILPATRICK, RN, DNSc(c)
Lecturer
Widener University School of Nursing
Chester, Pennsylvania

NANCY SEMENZA, RN, PhD(c)
Nursing Faculty
MacMurray College
Jacksonville, Illinois

MARIANNE ADAM, RN, MSN, CRNP
Assistant Professor
St. Luke's School of Nursing–Moravian College
Bethlehem, Pennsylvania

TRACY C. BABCOCK, RN, MSN
Adjunct Assistant Professor
Montana State University, College of Nursing
Bozeman, Montana

SYLVIA K. BAIRD, RN, BSN, MM
Quality Improvement System Coordinator
Spectrum Health
Grand Rapids, Michigan

DORIS BARTLETT, RN, MS
Guest Lecturer
Bethel College
Mishawaka, Indiana

SUSAN BURKETT, RN, MSN, CPN, CPNP
Vice President of TC Thompson Childrens Hospital
Erlanger Medical Center
Chattanooga, Tennesse

JEANIE BURT, RN, MA, MSN
Assistant Professor of Nursing
Harding University
Searcy, Arkansas

DARLENE NEBEL CANTU, RNC, BSN, MSN
Director, Baptist Health System
School of Professional Nursing
Faculty, San Antonio College
San Antonio, Texas

GALE CARLI, MSN, MSHed, BSN, RN
Assistant Professor
Ohlone College
Fremont, California

LAURA CLAYTON, RN, MSN, FNP
Assistant Professor
Shepherd College
Shepherdstown, West Virginia

CAROL A. deBLOIS, BSN, MA, CNOR
Director
Bridgeport Hospital School of Nursing
Bridgeport, Connecticut

H. MICHAEL DREHER, RN, DNSc
Assistant Professor of Nursing
College of Nursing and Health Professions
MCP Hahnemann University
Philadelphia, Pennsylvania

LINDA FASCIANI, RN, MSN
Associate Professor
County College of Morris
Randolph, New Jersey

SUSAN JANE FETZER, RN, BA, BSN, MSN, MBA, PHD
Assistant Professor
University of New Hampshire
Durham, New Hampshire

ROSEMARY FLISZAR, RN, MSN
Curriculum Coordinator
St. Luke's School of Nursing
Bethlehem, Pennsylvania

VICTORIA N. FOLSE, RN, PhD(c), CS, LCPC
Assistant Professor
Bradley University
Peoria, Illinois

MARGARET S. (PEG) FREEL, RN, MSN, CNRN, APN/CS
Instructor, Department of Acute, Chronic, and Long-term
  Nursing
Coordinator, Learning Resource Center
Loyola University–Chicago, Marcella Niehoff School of
  Nursing
Chicago, Illinois

HENRY B. GEITER, JR., RN, CCRN
ICU Nurse
Northside Hospital and Heart Institute
Adjunct Faculty
St. Petersburg College
St. Petersburg, Florida

CARROL GOLD, RN, Phd
Associate Professor, The Graduate Program in Nursing
Barry University
Miami Shores, Florida

THELMA HALBERSTADT, RN, BS, MS, EdD
Professor of Nursing
Northern Essex Community College
Lawrence, Massachusetts

JOHN P. HARPER, RN, MSN, BC
Nurse Educator, Critical Care
Delaware County Memorial Hospital
Drexel Hill, Pennsylvania

LINDA C. HAYNES, RN, BSN, MN, PhD
Assistant Professor
Louise Herrington School of Nursing
Baylor University
Dallas, Texas

ADRIENNE HENTEMANN, BSN, MS
Administrative Associate
Grand Rapids, Michigan

MONICA HENTEMANN, RN, BSN
Staff Nurse
Spectrum Health Downtown Campus
Grand Rapids, Michigan

JANICE J. HOFFMAN, RN, MSN, CCRN
SPRING Program Director
The Johns Hopkins Hospital
Baltimore, Maryland

PATRICIA M. JACOB, BSN, MSN
Nursing Instructor
Bullard Havens Regional Vocational Technical School
Bridgeport, Connecticut

SUSAN JUNAID, MSN, ARNP, WHNP
Assistant Professor
Allen College
Waterloo, Iowa

LINDA L. KERBY, RNC
Educational Consultant
Leawood, Kansas

PATRICIA LANGE-OTSUKA, EdD, MSN, BSN, CCRN
Associate Professor of Nursing
Hawaii Pacific University
Kaneohe, Hawaii

VIRGINIA D. LESTER, RN, BSN, MSN
Clinical Nurse Specialist (Inactive)
Assistant Professor
Angelo State University
San Angelo, Texas

MARY K. MANTESE, RN, MSN
Manager, Regulatory Compliance
Barnes-Jewish West County Hospital
St. Louis, Missouri

MARY JO MATTOCKS, RN, BSN, MN, PhD
Associate Professor
Montana State University Northern
Great Falls, Montana

MARY E. NEWELL, RN, MSN
Director of Nursing
Highline Community College
Des Moines, Washington

RUTH NOVITT-SCHUMACHER, RN, MSN
Instructor
University of Illinois, Chicago
Chicago, Illinois

VERONICA (RONNIE) PETERSON, BA, RN, BSN, MS
Clinical Staff Educator
University of Wisconsin Medical Foundation
Adjunct Clinical Instructor
University of Wisconsin, School of Nursing
Madison, Wisconsin

ELIZABETH PHILLIP, MSN
Instructor
St. Luke's Hospital School of Nursing
Bethlehem, Pennsylvania

MELISSA POWELL, RN, BSN, MSN
Assistant Professor
Eastern Kentucky University
Richmond, Kentucky

ELAINE T. PRINCEVALLI, RN, BSN, MS
Instructor, Practical Nurse Education Program
State of Connecticut, Department of Education
Hamden, Connecticut

MARSHA L. RAY, RN, BSN, MSN
Associate Degree Nursing Faculty
Shasta College
Redding, California

ANITA K. REED, RN, MSN
Instructor of Nursing
St. Elizabeth School of Nursing
Lafayette, Indiana

ROBYN RICE, RNC, MSNR, PhD(c)
Clinical Associate Professor
Barnes College of Nursing
The University of Missouri, St. Louis
St. Louis, Missouri
Home Health Clinical Nurse Specialist
American Nursing Development
Maryville, Illinois

JACQUELINE RAYBUCK SALEEBY, RN, PhD, CS
Associate Professor
Jewish Hospital College of Nursing and Allied Health
Washington University Medical Center
St. Louis, Missouri

SUSAN PARNELL SCHOLTZ, RN, DNSc(c)
Associate Professor of Nursing
St. Luke's School of Nursing
Moravian College
Bethlehem, Pennsylvania

ALICE SEREY, RN, BSN, MSN
Associate Degree Nursing Department Chair
Indian River Community College
Ft. Pierce, Florida

RUTH A. WALGAMUTH SHEARER, RN, MS, MSN
Assistant Professor of Nursing
Bethel College
Mishawaka, Indiana

JULIE S. SNYDER, RNC, MSN
Adjunct Faculty
Christopher Newport University
Newport News, Virginia

SHARON SOUTER, RN, MSN
Director of Nursing Programs
New Mexico State University–Carlsbad
Carlsbad, New Mexico

ROWENA TESSMAN, RN-CS, PhD
Executive Director
Protea Behavioral Health Services
Bangor, Maine

SUSANNE M. TRACY, RN, MN, MA
Associate Professor of Nursing
Rivier College
Nashua, New Hampshire

HEIDI HAHN TYMKEW, PT, MHS, CCS
Physical Therapist
Barnes-Jewish Hosptial
St. Louis, Missouri

ANNE T. FALSONE VAUGHAN, RN, BSN, MSN
Acute Care Nurse Practitioner Student
Indiana University School of Nursing
Indianapolis, Indiana

JOAN DOMIGAN WENTZ, RN, MSN
Assistant Professor
Jewish Hospital College
St. Louis, Missouri

JENNIFER H. WHITLEY, RN, MSN, CNOR
Instructor
Calhoun Community College
Decatur, Alabama

THOMAS WORMS, MSN
Associate Professor
Truman College of Nursing
Chicago, Illinois

ELIZABETH A. AYELLO, RN, BSN, MS, PhD, CS, CETN
Clinical Assistant Professor of Nursing
New York University School of Education, Nursing
Clinical Associate, Enterostomal Therapy Service
New York University Medical Center
New York, New York

PEGGY BRECKINRIDGE, MSN, FNP
Associate Professor of Nursing
College of Health Sciences
Roanoke, Virginia

RICK DANIELS, RN, BSN, MSN, PhD
Professor of Nursing
Oregon Health Sciences University at Southern
Ashland, Oregon

CAROLYN RUPPEL d'AVIS, RN, BSN, MSN
Director, Baccalaureate Program; Adjunct Assistant
  Professor
The Catholic University of America, School of Nursing
Washington, DC

LINDA FASCIANI, RN, BSN, MSN
Assistant Professor of Nursing
County College of Morris
Randolph, New Jersey

CYNTHIA S. GOODWIN, RN, BSN, MSN
Instructor, School of Nursing at Health Professions
University of Southern Indiana
Evansville, Indiana

LOIS C. HAMEL, BS, MS
Assistant Professor of Nursing
Westbrook College–University of New England
Portland, Maine

JUDITH KILPATRICK, MSN, RNC
Lecturer
Widener University
Chester, Pennsylvania

CARL A. KIRTON, RN-C, BSN, MA, ACRN, ANP
Clinical Assistant Professor; Adult Nurse Practitioner
New York University
New York, New York

RUTH LUDWICK, RN, BSN, MSN, PhD, RN-C
Associate Professor
Kent State University, School of Nursing
Kent, Ohio

**MARY KAY KNIGHT MACHECA, RN, BSN, MSN(R),
  CS, CDE**
Certified Adult Nurse Practitioner
The Health Care Group of St. Louis/Unity Medical Group
St. Louis, Missouri

MARY DEE MILLER, RN, BSN, MS, CIC
Regional Director, Epidemiology Services
Mercy Regional Health System
Cincinnati, Ohio

GERALYN A. OCHS, RN, ADN, BSN, MSN
Instructor of Nursing
St. Louis University, School of Nursing
St. Louis, Missouri

MARSHA EVANS ORR, RN, MS, CS, CNSN
Zone Clinical Manager
Apria Healthcare
Phoenix, Arizona

JANICE J. RUMFELT, BSN, MSN, EdD, RNC
Assistant Professor of Nursing
Southern Illinois University–Edwardsville
Edwardsville, Illinois

SHARON SOUTER, RN, BSN, MSN
Nursing Program Director
New Mexico State University–Carlsbad
Carlsbad, New Mexico

RACHEL E. SPECTOR, BS, MS, PhD, CTN, FAAN
Associate Professor
Boston College, School of Nursing
Chestnut Hill, Massachusetts

SUSAN SPERAW, RN, PhD, CNP
Associate Professor of Pediatrics
University of Tennessee, College of Medicine–Chattanooga
  Unit
Chattanooga, Tennessee

To the many friends in my life
for their love, support, and encouragement.
They made my educational adventure
less rocky and more satisfying.

Patricia A. Potter

To professional nurses, nurse educators, and nurse researchers,
who embrace the standards of excellence in education and clinical scholarship
while meeting the diverse needs of their students and clients.

Anne Griffin Perry

Basic Nursing was developed to provide you with all of the fundamental nursing concepts and skills in a visually appealing, easy-to-use format. We know how busy you are and how precious your time is. As you begin your nursing education, it is very important that you have a resource that includes all the information you need to prepare for lectures, classroom activities, clinical rotations, and exams—and nothing more. We've designed this text

to meet all of those needs. This book has been designed to help you succeed in this course, and prepare you for more advanced study. In addition to the readable writing style and abundance of full-color photographs and drawings, we've incorporated numerous features to help you study and learn. We've made it easy for you to pull out important content. **Check out the following special learning aids:**

20

Family Context in Nursing

Objectives

- Define key terms.
- Examine current trends in the American family.
- Examine common family forms and their health implications.
- Evaluate the way family structure and pattern of functioning affect the health of family members and the family as a whole.
- Assess family as context with family as client and explain the way these perspectives influence nursing practice.
- Compare family as context to provide for the health care needs of the family.
- Use the nursing process to provide for the health care needs of the family.
- Interpret both external and internal factors that promote family health.

Learning Objectives begin each chapter to help you focus on the key information that follows.

UNIT IV   Principles for Caring

PATRICK AND MICHELLE O'CONNELL

Patrick and Michelle O'Connell have been married 9 years and live in Auburn, Maine. Patrick is 38 years old, and after being employed by the state in the Department of Public Safety for the past 8 years, he has recently learned that he is in danger of being laid off in the next round of cuts. Patrick has been diagnosed with borderline hypertension and admits his stress level is an 8 on a scale of 1 to 10. He enjoys watching TV, playing war games on the computer, and playing with the family's pet dogs and cats. The family's health insurance is provided through Patrick's job. Michelle is 32 years old, is employed part-time as a receptionist at a building supply company and attends nursing school. They are a child-free couple by choice. Michelle received a diagnosis of cervical cancer 3 months after their wedding, however, and had a vaginal hysterectomy 2 years ago. Michelle has been very worried about their financial problems and her grandmother's health problems, and she fears needing to work full-time. She describes herself as spiritual and attends church occasionally.

Michelle plays the role of keeping the couple connected to their extended families. Because each of their parents divorced and either have since remarried or are cohabitating, they have four sets of parents and 28 step-, half-, and whole brothers and sisters between them. Michelle manages the household duties and finances, works, and goes to school. She is the oldest daughter in her family and is the only one of the siblings to keep in contact with her grandmother, Lois. Michelle has learned from the visiting nurse that Lois's condition is worsened—she is becoming more forgetful and less tolerant of physical activity related to severe cardiac myopathy. Michelle worries about what she can do from 2 hours away geographically. Lois needs continuous support, and for Lois to move in with her, Michelle would have to rid the house of pets, which Lois is allergic to, and her home would require major renovations to accommodate her 80-year-old grandmother.

Bethany, age 28, is the nursing student assigned to Lois in her community health rotation. She sees Lois living alone in a clean mobile home in a nice park. She understands that Lois has been widowed 17 years and that she receives Social Security and has Medicare. However, she receives Social Security insurance to pay for her medications. Bethany is concerned about Lois's financial situation, especially in light of the fact the visiting nurse has said Lois may need different living arrangements.

Major changes have occurred in the concept and structure of the family, but it is clear that the family remains the central institution in American society. The current general assumption is that although the family is in transition and may look very different from the family of the 1950s, the concept of family is here to stay. Although contemporary families have their share of problems and challenges, they are characterized by three important attributes: durability, resiliency, and diversity.

Family durability is the term for the intrafamilial system of support and structure that may extend beyond the walls of the household. The players may change, the parents may remarry, the children may or may not leave home as adults, but the "family" is considered to transcend long periods and inevitable lifestyle changes.

Family resiliency is the ability to cope with expected and unexpected stressors. The family's ability to adapt to role changes, developmental milestones, and crises shows resilience. The goal of the family is not only to survive "the challenge" but also to thrive and grow as a result of the newly gained knowledge.

Family diversity is the attention to uniqueness. Some families will be experiencing marriage for the first time and having children in later life, whereas others are grandparents at the same age. Every person within a familial unit has specific needs, strengths, and important developmental considerations. As nurses it is our job first to understand the make-up, structure, function, and coping capacity of the family and then to see how to design nursing interventions to build on the relative strengths to overcome weaknesses.

SCIENTIFIC KNOWLEDGE BASE
Concept of Family
Family evokes a visual image of adults and children living together in a satisfying, harmonious manner. Families are, however, as diverse as the individuals that compose them, and clients have deeply ingrained values about their families that deserve respect. Thus each individual defines the family. In other words, think of the **family** as a set of relationships that the client identifies as family or as a network of individuals who influence each other's lives whether there are actual biological or legal ties.

Family Forms
Family forms are patterns of people who are considered to be family members. Although all families have some things in common, each family form has unique problems and strengths. Keep an open mind about what constitutes a family so that potential resources and concerns are not overlooked. Several family forms are described in Box 20-1.

CURRENT TRENDS AND NEW FAMILY FORMS. Families are smaller today. People are marrying later, women are delaying childbirth, and couples are choosing to have fewer children or none at all. Divorce rates have tripled since the 1950s, and although the rate appears to have stabilized, it is

---

Progressive Case Studies introduce you to real-life clients, families, and nurses. These engaging scenarios illustrate the nursing process in action and help you develop critical thinking skills.

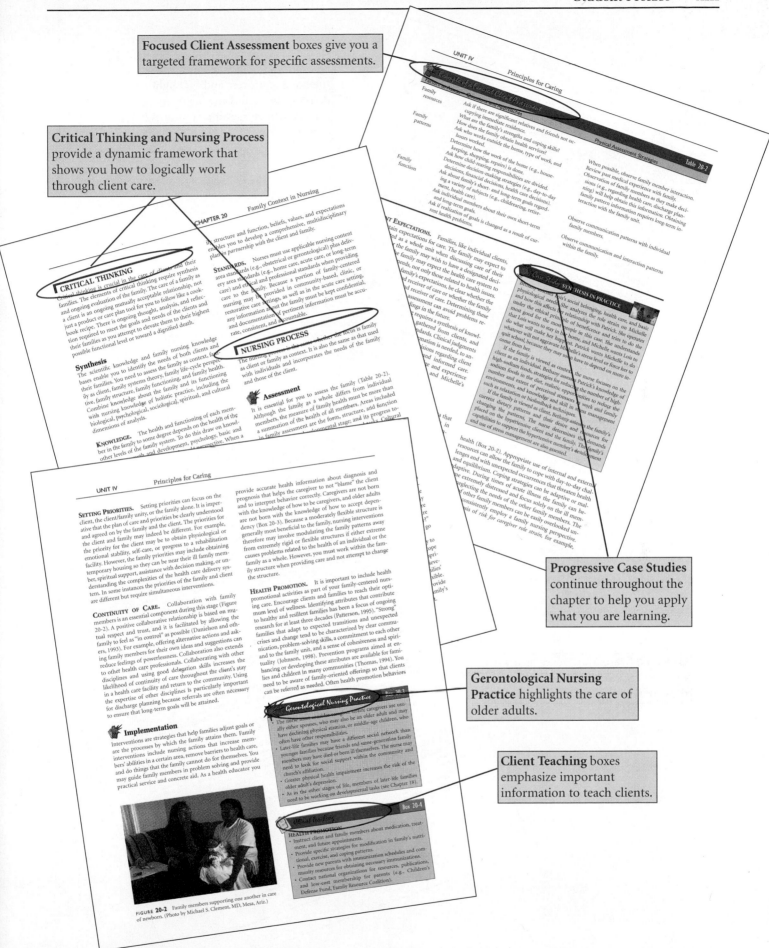

Focused Client Assessment boxes give you a targeted framework for specific assessments.

Critical Thinking and Nursing Process provide a dynamic framework that shows you how to logically work through client care.

Progressive Case Studies continue throughout the chapter to help you apply what you are learning.

Gerontological Nursing Practice highlights the care of older adults.

Client Teaching boxes emphasize important information to teach clients.

FIGURE 20-2 Family members supporting one another in care of newborn. (Photo by Michael S. Clement, MD, Mesa, Ariz.)

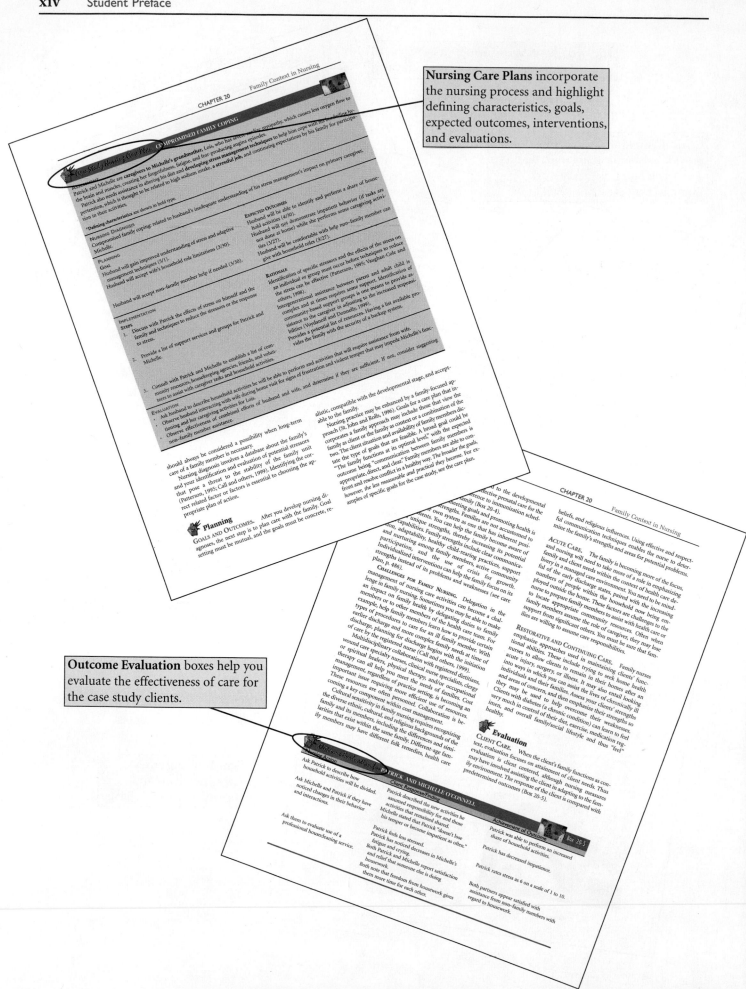

Nursing Care Plans incorporate the nursing process and highlight defining characteristics, goals, expected outcomes, interventions, and evaluations.

Outcome Evaluation boxes help you evaluate the effectiveness of care for the case study clients.

Nursing Skills are presented in a clear, two-column format with steps and rationales so you learn why as well as how.

Delegation Considerations guide you in delegating tasks to assistive personnel.

Equipment lists show specific items needed for each skill.

Critical Decision Points alert you to important information to consider as you perform a skill.

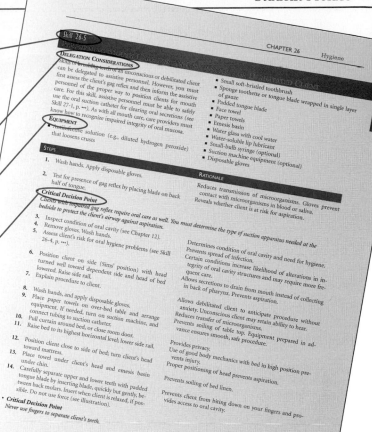

Skill 26-5

CHAPTER 26   Hygiene

DELEGATION CONSIDERATIONS

Skills of brushing teeth of an unconscious or debilitated client can be delegated to assistive personnel. However, you must first assess the client's gag reflex and then inform the assistive personnel of the proper way to position clients for mouth care. For this skill, assistive personnel must be able to safely use the oral suction catheter for clearing oral secretions (see Skill 27-1, p. •••). As with all mouth care, care providers must know how to recognize impaired integrity of oral mucosa.

EQUIPMENT

- Antiinfective solution (e.g., diluted hydrogen peroxide) that loosens crusts
- Small soft-bristled toothbrush
- Sponge toothette or tongue blade wrapped in single layer of gauze
- Padded tongue blade
- Face towel
- Paper towels
- Emesis basin
- Water glass with cool water
- Water-soluble lip lubricant
- Small-bulb syringe (optional)
- Suction machine equipment (optional)
- Disposable gloves

STEPS

1. Wash hands. Apply disposable gloves.

2. Test for presence of gag reflex by placing blade on back half of tongue.

Critical Decision Point
Clients with impaired gag reflex require oral care as well. You must determine the type of suction apparatus needed at the bedside to protect the client's airway against aspiration.

3. Inspect condition of oral cavity (see Chapter 12).
4. Remove gloves. Wash hands.
5. Assess client's risk for oral hygiene problems (see Skill 26-4, p. •••).

6. Position client on side (Sims' position) with head turned well toward dependent side and head of bed lowered. Raise side rail.
7. Explain procedure to client.

8. Wash hands, and apply disposable gloves.
9. Place paper towels on over-bed table and arrange equipment. If needed, turn on suction machine, and connect tubing to suction catheter.
10. Pull curtain around bed, or close room door.
11. Raise bed to its highest horizontal level; lower side rail.

12. Position client close to side of bed; turn client's head toward mattress.
13. Place towel under client's head and emesis basin under chin.
14. Carefully separate upper and lower teeth with padded tongue blade by inserting blade, quickly but gently, between back molars. Insert when client is relaxed, if possible. Do not use force (see illustration).

Critical Decision Point
Never use fingers to separate client's teeth.

RATIONALE

Reduces transmission of microorganisms. Gloves prevent contact with microorganisms in blood or saliva.
Reveals whether client is at risk for aspiration.

Determines condition of oral cavity and need for hygiene.
Prevents spread of infection.
Certain conditions increase likelihood of alterations in integrity of oral cavity structures and may require more frequent care.
Allows secretions to drain from mouth instead of collecting in back of pharynx. Prevents aspiration.

Allows debilitated client to anticipate procedure without anxiety. Unconscious client may retain ability to hear.
Reduces transfer of microorganisms.
Prevents soiling of table top. Equipment prepared in advance ensures smooth, safe procedure.

Provides privacy.
Use of good body mechanics with bed in high position prevents injury.
Proper positioning of head prevents aspiration.

Prevents soiling of bed linen.

Prevents client from biting down on your fingers and provides access to oral cavity.

Clear, close-up **photos** help you learn to perform important techniques.

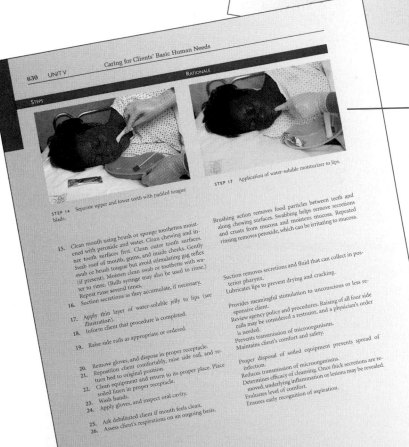

630   UNIT V   Caring for Clients' Basic Human Needs

STEPS

STEP 14 Separate upper and lower teeth with padded tongue blade.

STEP 17 Application of water-soluble moisturizer to lips.

15. Clean mouth using brush or sponge toothettes moistened with peroxide and water. Clean chewing and inner tooth surfaces first. Clean outer tooth surfaces. Swab roof of mouth, gums, and inside cheeks. Gently swab or brush tongue but avoid stimulating gag reflex (if present). Moisten clean swab or toothette with water to rinse. (Bulb syringe may also be used to rinse.) Repeat rinse several times.
16. Suction secretions as they accumulate, if necessary.

17. Apply thin layer of water-soluble jelly to lips (see illustration).
18. Inform client that procedure is completed.

19. Raise side rails as appropriate or ordered.

20. Remove gloves, and dispose in proper receptacle.
21. Reposition client comfortably, raise side rail, and return bed to original position.
22. Clean equipment and return to its proper place. Place soiled linen in proper receptacle.
23. Wash hands.
24. Apply gloves, and inspect oral cavity.

25. Ask debilitated client if mouth feels clean.
26. Assess client's respirations on an ongoing basis.

RATIONALE

Brushing action removes food particles between teeth and along chewing surfaces. Swabbing helps remove secretions and crusts from mucosa and moistens mucosa. Repeated rinsing removes peroxide, which can be irritating to mucosa.

Suction removes secretions and fluid that can collect in posterior pharynx.
Lubricates lips to prevent drying and cracking.

Provides meaningful stimulation to unconscious or less responsive client.
Review agency policy and procedures. Raising of all four side rails may be considered a restraint, and a physician's order is needed.
Prevents transmission of microorganisms.
Maintains client's comfort and safety.

Proper disposal of soiled equipment prevents spread of infection.
Reduces transmission of microorganisms.
Determines efficacy of cleansing. Once thick secretions are removed, underlying inflammation or lesions may be revealed.
Evaluates level of comfort.
Ensures early recognition of aspiration.

Procedural Guidelines provide streamlined, step-by-step instructions for performing basic skills.

Chapters end with a list of **Key Terms,** and the page where each term is introduced.

Key Concepts and Critical Thinking Activities help you review and apply essential content from the chapter.

NCLEX-style multiple-choice **Review Questions** at the end of each chapter help you evaluate learning.

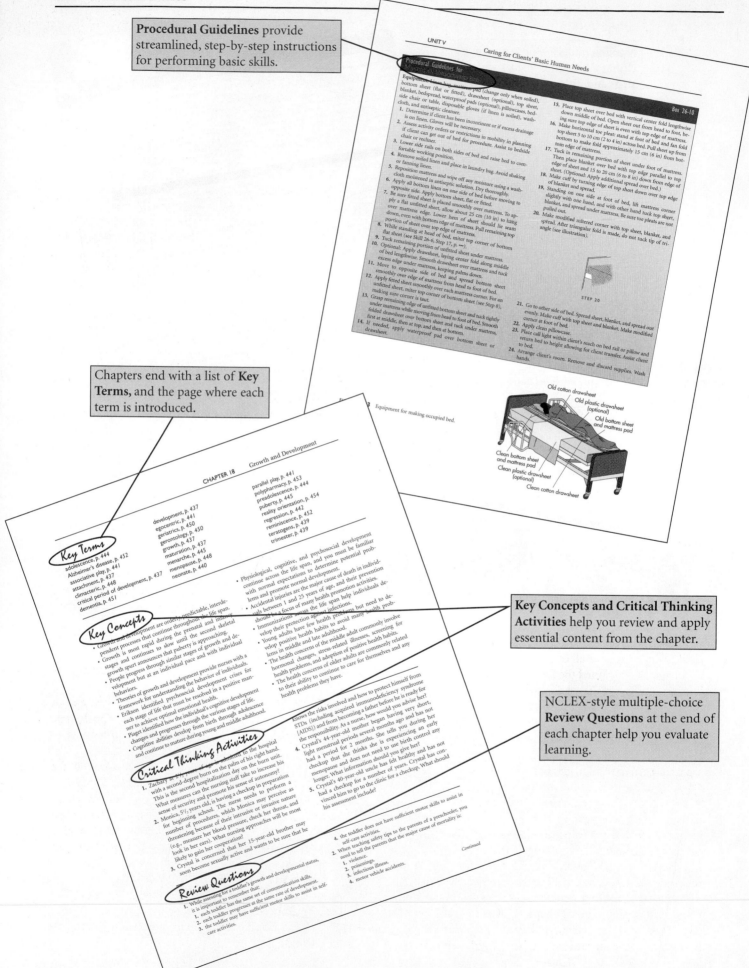

UNIT V   Caring for Clients' Basic Human Needs

Procedural Guidelines for
Making an Unoccupied Bed

Box 26-10

Equipment: Clean linen, mattress pad (change only when soiled), bottom sheet (flat or fitted), drawsheet (optional), top sheet, blanket, bedspread, waterproof pads (optional), disposable gloves (if linen is soiled), bed-side chair or table, disposable gloves (if linen is soiled), bed-cloth, and antiseptic cleaner.

1. Determine if client has been incontinent or if excess drainage is on linen. Gloves will be necessary.
2. Assess activity orders or restrictions in mobility in planning if client can get out of bed for procedure. Assist to bedside chair or recliner.
3. Lower side rails on both sides of bed and raise bed to comfortable working position.
4. Remove soiled linen and place in laundry bag. Avoid shaking or fanning linen.
5. Reposition mattress and wipe off any moisture using a washcloth moistened in antiseptic solution. Dry thoroughly.
6. Apply all bottom linen on one side of bed before moving to opposite side. Apply bottom sheet, flat or fitted.
7. Be sure fitted sheet is placed smoothly over mattress. To apply a flat unfitted sheet, allow about 25 cm (10 in) to hang over mattress edge. Lower hem of sheet should lie seam down, even with bottom edge of mattress. Pull remaining top portion of sheet over top edge of mattress.
8. While standing at head of bed, miter top corner of bottom flat sheet (see Skill 26-6, Step 17, p. ••).
9. Tuck remaining portion of unfitted sheet under mattress.
10. Optional: Apply drawsheet, laying center fold along middle of bed lengthwise. Smooth drawsheet over mattress and tuck excess edge under mattress, keeping palms down.
11. Move to opposite side of bed and spread bottom sheet smoothly over edge of mattress from head to foot of bed.
12. Apply fitted sheet smoothly over each mattress corner. For an unfitted sheet, miter top corner of bottom sheet (see Step 8), making sure corner is taut.
13. Grasp remaining edge of unfitted bottom sheet and tuck tightly under mattress while moving from head to foot of bed. Smooth folded drawsheet over bottom sheet and tuck under mattress, first at middle, then at top, and then at bottom.
14. If needed, apply waterproof pad over bottom sheet or drawsheet.

15. Place top sheet over bed with vertical center fold lengthwise down middle of bed. Open sheet out from head to foot, being sure top edge of sheet is even with top edge of mattress.
16. Make horizontal toe pleat: stand at foot of bed and fan fold top sheet 5 to 10 cm (2 to 4 in) across bed. Pull sheet up from bottom to make fold approximately 15 cm (6 in) from bottom edge of mattress.
17. Tuck in remaining portion of sheet under foot of mattress. Then place blanket over bed with top edge parallel to top edge of sheet and 15 to 20 cm (6 to 8 in) down from top of sheet. (Optional: Apply additional spread over bed.)
18. Make cuff by turning edge of top sheet down over edge of blanket and spread.
19. Standing on one side at foot of bed, lift mattress corner slightly with one hand, and with other hand tuck top sheet, blanket, and spread under mattress. Be sure toe pleats are not pulled out.
20. Make modified mitered corner with top sheet, blanket, and spread. After triangular fold is made, do not tuck tip of triangle (see illustration).

STEP 20

21. Go to other side of bed. Spread sheet, blanket, and spread out evenly. Make cuff with top sheet and blanket. Make modified corner at foot of bed.
22. Apply clean pillowcase.
23. Place call light within client's reach on bed rail or pillow and return bed to height allowing for client transfer. Assist client to bed.
24. Arrange client's room. Remove and discard supplies. Wash hands.

Old cotton drawsheet
Old plastic drawsheet (optional)
Old bottom sheet and mattress pad
Clean bottom sheet and mattress pad
Clean plastic drawsheet (optional)
Clean cotton drawsheet

Equipment for making occupied bed.

CHAPTER 18   Growth and Development

Key Terms

adolescence, p. 444
Alzheimer's disease, p. 452
associative play, p. 437
attachment, p. 437
climacteric, p. 448
critical period of development, p. 437
dementia, p. 451

development, p. 437
egocentric, p. 441
geriatrics, p. 450
gerontology, p. 450
growth, p. 437
maturation, p. 437
menarche, p. 445
menopause, p. 448
neonate, p. 440

parallel play, p. 441
polypharmacy, p. 453
preadolescence, p. 444
puberty, p. 445
reality orientation, p. 454
regression, p. 442
reminiscence, p. 452
teratogens, p. 439
trimester, p. 439

Key Concepts

• Growth and development are orderly, predictable, interdependent processes that continue throughout the life span.
• Growth is most rapid during the prenatal and infancy stages and continues to slow until the second skeletal growth spurt announces that puberty is approaching.
• People progress through similar stages of growth and development but at an individual pace and with individual behaviors.
• Theories of growth and development provide nurses with a framework for understanding the behavior of individuals.
• Erikson identified psychosocial development crises for each stage of life that must be resolved in a positive manner to achieve optimal emotional health.
• Piaget identified how the individual's cognitive development changes and progresses through the various stages of life.
• Cognitive abilities develop from birth through adolescence and continue to mature during young and middle adulthood.

• Physiological, cognitive, and psychosocial development continue across the life span, and you must be familiar with normal expectations to determine potential problems and promote normal development.
• Accidental injuries are the major cause of death in individuals between 1 and 25 years of age, and their prevention should be a focus of many health promotion activities.
• Immunizations across the life span help individuals develop their protection against infections.
• Young adults have few health problems but need to develop positive health habits to avoid many health problems in middle and late adulthood.
• The health concerns of the middle adult commonly involve hormonal changes, stress-related illnesses, screening for health problems, and adoption of positive health habits.
• The health concerns of older adults are commonly related to their ability to continue to care for themselves and any health problems they have.

Critical Thinking Activities

1. Zachary, at 18 months of age, is admitted to the hospital with a second-degree burn on the palm of his right hand. This is the second hospitalization day on the burn unit. What measures can the nursing staff take to increase his sense of security and promote his sense of autonomy?
2. Monica, 5½ years old, is having a checkup in preparation for beginning school. The nurse needs to perform a number of procedures, which Monica may perceive as threatening because of their intrusive or invasive nature (e.g., measure her blood pressure, check her throat, and look in her ears). What nursing approaches will be most likely to gain her cooperation?
3. Crystal is concerned that her 15-year-old brother may soon become sexually active and wants to be sure that he

knows the risks involved and how to protect himself from STDs (including acquired immunodeficiency syndrome [AIDS]) and from becoming a father before he is ready for the responsibility. As a nurse, how would you advise her?
4. Crystal's 44-year-old mother began having very short, light menstrual periods several months ago and has not had a period for 2 months. She tells you during her checkup that she thinks she is experiencing an early menopause and does not need to use birth control any longer. What information should you give her?
5. Crystal's 40-year-old uncle has felt healthy and has not had a checkup for a number of years. Crystal has convinced him to go to the clinic for a checkup. What should his assessment include?

Review Questions

1. While assessing for a toddler's growth and developmental status, it is important to remember that:
   1. each toddler has the same set of communication skills.
   2. each toddler progresses at the same rate of development.
   3. the toddler may have sufficient motor skills to assist in self-care activities.

   4. the toddler does not have sufficient motor skills to assist in self-care activities.
2. When teaching safety tips to the parents of a preschooler, you need to tell the parents that the major cause of mortality is:
   1. violence.
   2. poisonings.
   3. infectious illness.
   4. motor vehicle accidents.

Continued

"Traditional nursing" is a thing of the past. Today's nurses must be prepared to adapt to the continual changes occuring in health care. They play a vital role in the delivery of multidisciplinary health care services. The practice arena is changing—moving more and more to the community setting. The focus of care is changing as well—more emphasis is being placed on health promotion and restorative care. Even the clients are changing—more cultural diversity exists and the percentage of older adult clients continues to increase. Clients are far more involved in and informed about health care.

Despite these changes—perhaps because of these changes—it is essential that the basics of nursing must remain the foundation of practice. Nurses must be knowledgeable and professional. They must be both technically proficient and personally caring. And they must be able to synthesize a broad array of knowledge and experiences when providing care for their clients.

It is this building of the new on the old that serves as the foundation for the fifth edition of **Basic Nursing.** We continue to cover all of the fundamental nursing concepts, skills, and techniques that students must master before moving on to other areas of study. With the addition of a new subtitle— *Essentials for Practice*—we have better focused on the basic content required by the beginning student. We address changes in practice that affect how and where nurses use the skills and knowledge they acquire.

FEATURES

We have designed this text to welcome the new student to nursing, communicate our own love for the profession, and promote learning and understanding. We know that today's students are busy and, too often, overwhelmed by all that they must learn and do. They want their texts to focus on essential content and skills. We want to ensure that these students are ready to continue with their education and will, ultimately, be prepared for all of the challenges of practice. To this end, we have included the following key features:

- Students will appreciate the **clear, engaging writing style.** We have totally revamped the narrative so that it speaks to the reader, making this edition more of an active instructional tool than a passive reference. Students will find that even complex technical and theoretical concepts are presented in a language that is easy to understand.
- The **attractive, functional design** will appeal to today's visual learner. The clear, readable type and bold headings make the content easy to read and follow. Each special element is consistently color-keyed with attractive icons so students can readily identify important information.
- Hundreds of **large, clear, full-color photographs and drawings** reinforce and clarify key concepts and techniques.
- The **five-step nursing process** serves as the organizing framework for all clinical chapters. This logical, consistent framework for narrative discussions is further enhanced by special boxes that highlight assessment,

NANDA diagnoses, care plans, and evaluation of outcome achievement.

- **Critical thinking** is presented in a separate chapter, then incorporated as a consistent partner to the nursing process in each clinical chapter. This application of critical thinking provides a practical, clinical decision-making guide that is easy for even the beginning student to understand.
- **Ongoing case studies** in each clinical chapter introduce "real-world" clients, families, and nurses. The chapter follows the case study through the steps of the nursing process, helping students see how to apply the process, along with critical thinking, to the care of clients. Cases take place in both acute and community settings, and include clients and nurses from a variety of cultural backgrounds.
- **Expected outcomes** are addressed in care plans, special boxes, and narrative to help students understand and apply these key clinical measures.
- Implementation narrative consistently addresses health promotion, acute care, and restorative and continuing care to reflect the current focus on **community-based nursing** and **health promotion.**
- **More than 40 nursing skills** are presented in a clear, two-column format with steps and rationales. Skills include delegation guidelines and critical decision points that alert students to steps requiring special assessment or specific technique for safe and effective administration.
- **Procedural guidelines** provide streamlined step-by-step instructions for performing very basic skills.
- Care of the **older adult** and **client teaching** are stressed throughout the narrative, as well as highlighted in special boxes.
- **Learning aids** to help students identify, review, and apply important content in each chapter include Objectives, Key Terms, Key Concepts, Critical Thinking Activities, and Review Questions.

New to This Edition

- **Active, engaging writing style** speaks to the student, enhancing learning and understanding.
- **Unexpected Outcomes and Interventions** at the end of each nursing skill provides students with appropriate nursing actions for potential undesirable responses to nursing procedures.
- **NCLEX-style multiple-choice review questions** at the end of each chapter help students evaluate learning.
- **Focused Client Assessment boxes** for each clinical chapter provide specific guidelines for factors to assess, questions and approaches, and physical assessment strategies.
- **New chapter on "Caring in Nursing Practice"** and the increased emphasis on caring throughout the text highlight this fundamental principle of nursing.
- **Briefer coverage of higher-level concepts** provides just the right amount of detail on research, theory, professional roles, and management to maintain a strong "essentials" focus.

TEACHING AND LEARNING PACKAGE

In recognition of the incredible challenges faced by both students and educators, we have developed an unsurpassed array of teaching and learning materials.

- The **Electronic Instructor's Resource** on CD-ROM by Gale Carli includes a comprehensive Instructor's Manual, a Test Bank, and an impressive collection of PowerPoint lecture slides and images from the text to enhance classroom lectures. These **Course Resources** are also available online for faculty only.

- **Mosby's Nursing Skills Video Series** provides engaging, action-packed demonstrations of how to perform key nursing procedures in real-life clinical situations. Actual nurses perform each skill as they work through contemporary concepts such as delegation, critical thinking, patient rights, and communication techniques.

- **MERLIN Website** provides content updates and a reliable source of annotated current nursing weblinks for class assignments and independent study.

- **Study Guide** by Patricia A. Castaldi provides students with a wide variety of exercises and activities to enhance learning and comprehension. This study guide features Independent Learning Activities; Chapter Review sections with matching, fill-in-the-blank and NCLEX-style multiple-choice questions; Study Group Questions; Skills Performance Checklists; instructions for creating and using study charts; and Case Studies with related questions.

- **Virtual Clinical Excursions** is a groundbreaking new workbook and CD-ROM experience that brings learning to life in a virtual hospital setting. The workbook guides students as they care for clients, providing ongoing challenges and learning opportunities. Each lesson in *Virtual Clinical Excursions* complements the textbook content and provides the perfect environment for students to practice what they are learning in the text for a true-to-life, hands-on learning experience. This CD/workbook is available separately or packaged at a special price with the textbook.

Acknowledgments

This edition of *Basic Nursing* is the result of an innovative collaborative effort among the authors, nursing editorial, design, production editing, and marketing, each of whom contributed their talents and time to creating what we think is a unique text. The advanced planning and design has ensured our readers a quality textbook.

- We wish to acknowledge Suzi Epstein, Executive Editor, for spearheading the effort to develop a text that offers a new approach to the presentation of *Basic Nursing*. Her enthusiasm, friendship, and support, along with her creativity, attention to detail, and thoughtful editing, enabled us to be innovative while still creating a comprehensive, well-designed textbook.

- Linda Stagg, Developmental Editor, with relentless attention to detail and organization helped to produce a cohesive and well-designed textbook. Her patience and gracious manner was a catalyst in making this project a very enjoyable one. We appreciate her support and professionalism.

- Kathi Gosche, our book designer, contributed a clear, crisp, colorful, and visually distinctive design for *Basic Nursing*. Involved from the beginning, her work helped us to avoid numerous pitfalls and achieve a finished product that is visually appealing.

- Thanks also goes to the production team of Publication Services Manager John Rogers and Project Manager Beth Hayes, who collaborated on the project from the beginning to ensure a well-coordinated and accurate production process.

- To the sales and marketing team of Mary Hamby, Senior District Sales Manager, and Kathy Mantz, Nursing Product Manager, who offered insight into design elements that would enhance the quality of the text.

- To our contributors, excellent clinicians and educators, who share invaluable experiences and knowledge in the chapters they have created. Their attention to detail within their areas of specialization helped us achieve a state-of-the-art textbook. We are fortunate to be associated with excellent nurse authors who are able to convey standards of nursing excellence through the printed word.

- To Rick Brady and Mike DeFilippo for their photographic excellence, and to St. Luke's Hospital for the generous use of their facility for our photo shoot.

- We wish to acknowledge many nursing professionals who influence us every day in our careers. They enable us to envision what excellence in nursing practice truly means. In addition, our reviewers lend us their expertise, candor, and astute comments to assist in developing a text with high standards that reflects professional nursing practice today.

We continue to enjoy and respect our collaborative work as coauthors. However, more important is our rewarding friendship. This friendship encourages each of us to seek new professional challenges and to extend our boundaries. A friendship built on caring, consideration, respect, and compassion is unbeatable, and for that we are truly blessed.

Patricia A. Potter
Anne Griffin Perry

Contents

Basic Nursing

ESSENTIALS FOR PRACTICE

Health and Wellness

Objectives

- Define key terms.
- Discuss the health-illness continuum, and the health belief, health promotion, and holistic health models of health and illness to understand the relationship between clients' attitudes toward health and health practices.
- Discuss the meaning of determinants of health status.
- Describe the variables influencing health beliefs and health practices.
- Describe health promotion and illness prevention activities.
- Discuss the three levels of preventive care.
- Discuss four types of risk factors and the process of risk factor modification.
- Describe the variables influencing illness behavior.
- Discuss the stages of illness behavior.
- Describe the impact of illness on the client and family.
- Discuss the nurse's role in health and illness.

In the past most individuals and societies viewed good health or **wellness** as the opposite or absence of disease. We now understand that some conditions of health may lie between disease and good health. Therefore health should be viewed from a broader perspective. As a nurse, you will use concepts of health, health promotion, wellness, and illness to assist your clients in achieving and maintaining an optimal level of health. Models of health and illness can be used to understand and explain these concepts.

Wellness activities involving health promotion and illness prevention strategies help clients achieve and maintain an optimal level of health. Nurses identify actual and potential risk factors that predispose a person or a group to illness.

People have different attitudes and reactions to illness. Medical sociologists call the reaction to illness *illness behavior*. The nurse who understands how clients react to illness can minimize the effects of illness and assist clients and their families in maintaining or returning to the highest level of functioning.

DEFINITION OF HEALTH

Defining good health is difficult because each person has a personal concept of health. The World Health Organization (WHO) defines health as a "state of complete physical, mental and social well-being, not merely the absence of disease or infirmity" (WHO, 1947). Individual views of health can vary among different age-groups, genders, races, and cultures (Pender, 1996). Pender (1996) explains that "all people free of disease are not equally healthy." **Health** is a state of being that people define in relation to their own values, personality, and lifestyle. Pender (1996) suggests that for many people it is "conditions of life" rather than "pathological states" that define health. Health cannot be measured by simple physiological data such as blood pressure and pulse. Rather, the term *health* reflects all the person is and *wants* to

be (Rice, 2000). Consider the total person, as well as the person's environment, to individualize nursing care and help clients identify and reach their health goals.

MODELS OF HEALTH AND ILLNESS

A model is a theoretical way of understanding a concept or an idea. Models represent various ways of approaching complex issues. Because health and illness are complex concepts, models are used to understand the relationships between these concepts and the client's attitudes toward health and health practices. Nurses have developed the following health models to understand clients' attitudes and values about health and illness so that effective health care can be provided. These nursing models allow you to understand and predict clients' health behavior, including how they use health services, participate in recommended therapy, and care for themselves.

Health-Illness Continuum Model

According to a **health-illness continuum model,** health is a dynamic state that fluctuates as a person adapts to changes in the internal and external environments to maintain a state of well-being. Illness is a process in which the functioning of a person is diminished or impaired when compared with the person's previous condition. In this model, high-level wellness and severe illness are at opposite ends of the continuum (Figure 1-1). Central to the health-illness continuum model are risk factors, which are important in identifying level of health. Risk factors include genetic and physiological, environmental, age, and lifestyle factors. As a person progresses through developmental stages, certain risk factors are more common than others. An adolescent, for example, is more likely than an adult to experience stressors related to body image and self-concept, and an older adult is more likely than a child to develop cardiac illness.

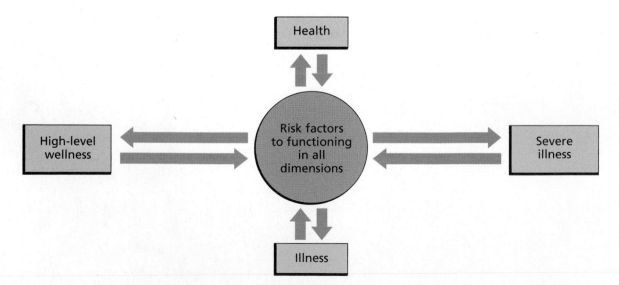

FIGURE 1-1   The health-illness continuum, ranging from high-level wellness to severe illness, provides a method of identifying a client's level of health. Level of health is a reflection of the client's level of functioning in all dimensions.

The way clients view their levels of health depends on their attitudes toward health, values, beliefs, and perceptions of their physical, emotional, intellectual, social, developmental, and spiritual well-being. It is not always easy to describe a client's level of health in terms of one point between two extremes. For example, is a man with a broken leg who has adapted to limited mobility more or less healthy than a physically healthy man experiencing severe depression after the death of his spouse? The health-illness continuum is most effective when used to compare a client's present level of health with his or her own previous level of health. It is useful as you help the client set goals to attain a future level of health.

Health Belief Model

Health beliefs are a person's ideas, convictions, and attitudes about health and illness. They may be based on factual information or misinformation, common sense, or myths. Because health beliefs usually influence health behavior, they can positively or negatively affect a client's level of health. **Positive health behaviors** are activities related to maintaining, attaining, or regaining good health and preventing illness. Common positive health behaviors include immunizations, proper sleep patterns, adequate exercise, and good nutrition. Implementation of positive health behaviors is de-

pendent on an individual's awareness of how to live a healthy life and the person's ability and willingness to carry out such behaviors in a healthy lifestyle. **Negative health behaviors** include activities that are actually or potentially harmful to health, such as smoking, drug or alcohol abuse, poor diet, and refusal to take necessary medications or to care for oneself.

Rosenstoch's (1974) and Becker and Maiman's (1975) **health belief model** (Figure 1-2) addresses the relationship between a person's beliefs and behaviors. It provides a way of understanding and predicting how clients will behave in relation to their health and how they will comply with health care therapies.

The first component of this model involves the individual's perception of susceptibility to an illness. For example, a client needs to recognize the familial link for coronary artery disease. After this link is recognized, the client may perceive a personal risk of heart disease. The second component is the individual's perception of the seriousness of the illness. This perception is influenced and modified by demographic and sociopsychological variables, perceived threats of the illness, and cues to action (e.g., mass media campaigns and advice from family, friends, and medical professionals). The third component, the likelihood that a person will take preventive action, results from the person's perception of the

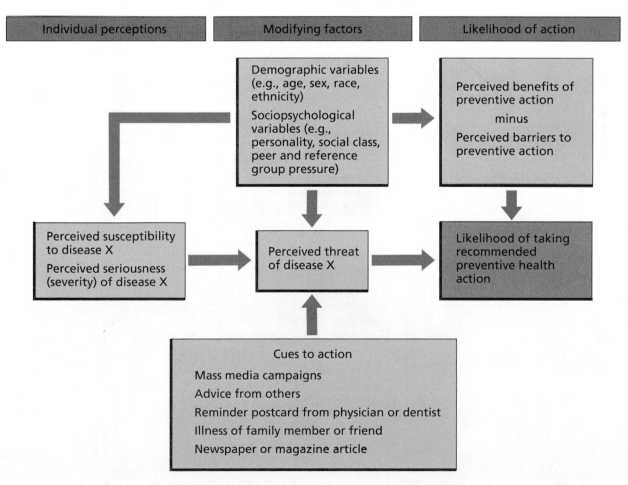

FIGURE **1-2**   Health belief model. (Data from Becker MH, Maiman LA: Sociobehavioral determinants of compliance with health and medical care recommendations, *Med Care* 13[1]:10, 1975.)

benefits of and barriers to taking action. Preventive action may include lifestyle changes, increased participation in recommended medical therapies, or a search for medical advice or treatment.

The health belief model helps you to understand factors influencing clients' perceptions, beliefs, and behavior and to plan care that will most effectively assist clients in maintaining or restoring health and preventing illness.

Health Promotion Model

The **health promotion model** proposed by Pender (1982, 1993, 1996) (Figure 1-3) defines health as a positive, dynamic state, not merely the absence of disease. The health promotion model was designed to be a "complementary counterpart to models of health protection" (Pender, 1993, 1996). Health promotion is directed at increasing a client's level of well-being (Pender, 1993, 1996). The health promotion model describes the multidimensional nature of persons as they interact within their environment to pursue health (Pender, 1996). The model focuses on the three func-

tions of a client's cognitive-perceptual factors (individual perceptions), modifying factors (demographic and social), and participation in health-promoting behaviors (likelihood of action). The model also organizes cues into a pattern to explain the likelihood of a client developing health promotion behaviors (Pender, 1993, 1996). The focus of this model is to explain the reasons that individuals engage in health activities. It is not designed for use with families or communities. Revisions to the health promotion model were made in 1996 to increase its potential use for prediction and intervention of health promotion.

Holistic Health Model

Holistic health is a comprehensive view of the person as a biopsychosocial and spiritual being (Edelman and Mandle, 1998). The intent of the holistic health model is to empower clients to engage in their own healing process (Edelman and Mandle, 1998). The holistic health model involves the use of a variety of techniques that in the past were viewed as "experimental" or "alternative" but have recently gained popu-

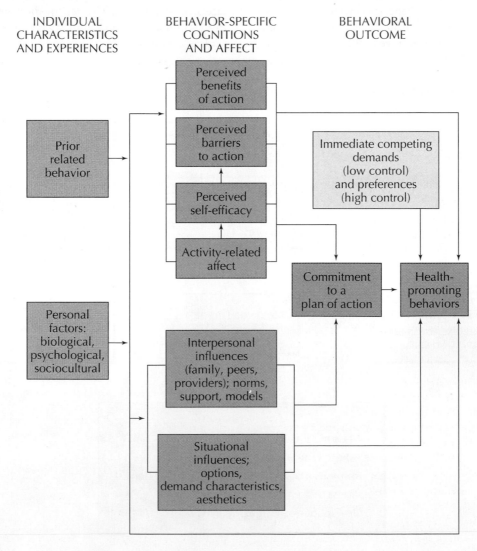

FIGURE **1-3** Health promotion model. (Health promotion in nursing practice, 3/E by Pender, © Reprinted by permission of Pearson Education, Inc., Upper Saddle River, N.J.)

larity among most health care professionals, as we have begun to understand that personal health choices have a powerful impact on an individual's health. Holistic nurses are integrating these therapies into practice to treat physiological, psychological, and spiritual client needs, not to negate but to complement conventional medical therapies (Acee, 1998). Using holistic health interventions allows you to involve your clients in the healing process. Your nursing knowledge, theories, expertise, and intuition will guide you to work with clients and strengthen their responses to the healing process (Acee, 1998).

Some of the most widely used holistic interventions include aroma therapy, biofeedback, breathing exercises, massage therapy, meditation, music therapy, relaxation therapy, therapeutic touch, and guided imagery. Most holistic therapies are easily learned and can be applied to almost any nursing setting and to all stages of health and illness. For example, reminiscence may be used in the geriatric population to help relieve anxiety for a client dealing with memory loss or for a cancer client dealing with the difficult side effects of chemotherapy. Music therapy may be used in the operating room to create a soothing environment. Relaxation training may be useful in any setting to distract a client during a painful procedure, such as a dressing change. Breathing exercises are commonly taught to help clients deal with the shortness of breath that accompanies some chronic respiratory diseases. You can help clients recognize the many options available and assist them in making choices to enhance health.

DETERMINANTS OF HEALTH STATUS: *HEALTHY PEOPLE 2010*

Since the 1970s there has been a nationally focused initiative toward better health for the American people. Three influential documents have been published that outline specific national goals for improving the health of Americans: *Healthy People: The Surgeon General's Report on Health Promotion and Disease Prevention* (U.S. Department of Health and Human Services [USDHHS], 1979); *Healthy People 2000: National Health Promotion and Disease Prevention Objectives* (USDHHS, 1990); and *Healthy People 2010: Understanding and Improving Health* (USDHHS, 2000). These reports are meant to serve as guidelines for government agencies, professional organizations, health care professionals, businesses, and individuals. Widely cited by popular media, in professional journals, and at health conferences, *Healthy People* reports have inspired health promotion programs throughout the country.

In *Healthy People 2010* (USDHHS, 2000), four key elements of goals, objectives, determinants of health, and health status are depicted in a model called a *systematic approach to health improvement* (Figure 1-4). The overall goals for *Healthy People 2010* are to increase the quality and years of life and to eliminate the nation's health disparities (USDHHS, 2000). In the *Healthy People 2010* document, 467 objectives were written in 28 focus areas to provide di-

rection for health care efforts on an individual, community, and national level. These objectives focus either on interventions designed to reduce or eliminate illness, disability, and premature death or on broader issues, such as improving availability and dissemination of health-related information. Each objective has a target for improvements to be achieved by the year 2010 (USDHHS, 2000).

It is necessary to understand that many factors influence or determine the health of individuals and communities. These variables are called **determinants of health.** In the *Healthy People 2010* model (see Figure 1-4), individual biology (genetic make-up and physical and mental health) and individual behavior (responses, actions, and reactions to internal stimuli and external conditions) are able to influence health through their interaction with each other and with the person's social and physical environments. Social and physical environments may include all factors, positive or negative, that affect a person's life. Numerous factors and situations influence the social and physical environment, any of which can affect health. Policies and interventions can also influence health and can be implemented by a variety of agencies. Some examples are disease prevention strategies, such as immunizations, or policies mandating child re-

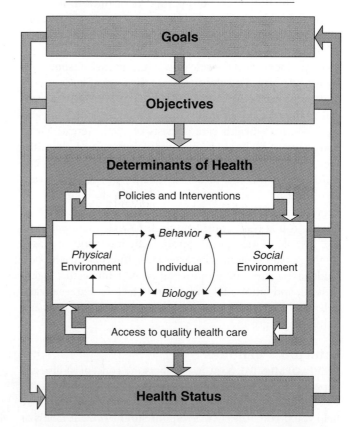

FIGURE **1-4**   A model for a systematic approach to health improvement. (From U.S. Department of Health and Human Services, Public Health Service: *Healthy people 2010: understanding and improving health,* Washington, DC, 2000, U.S. Government Printing Office.)

straints and seat belts. There has been an increased concern regarding the issue of access to health care. The health of individuals and communities depends on access to quality health care services for all individuals (USDHHS, 2000).

Health status is a description of health that can be measured by birth and death rates, life expectancy, quality of life, morbidity from specific diseases, risk factors, and many other factors. The information gathered from monitoring health status measures is used to report on the health of individuals and communities. The understanding that the determinants of health and the knowledge that individual and community health determine the health status of the nation are key aspects to achieving the *Healthy People 2010* goals.

VARIABLES INFLUENCING HEALTH BELIEFS AND HEALTH PRACTICES

Persons' beliefs about their own health, as well as their health practices and the manner in which they care for themselves, will ultimately influence their health status. Health beliefs are a person's ideas and attitudes about health. Health practices are those activities that individuals do to care for themselves. Health practices include activities of daily living, such as bathing and brushing teeth, and formal activities such as taking medications and visiting the doctor for routine checkups. Health practices are related to self-care, or the process of taking care of oneself. It is well known that the manner in which persons care for themselves is an important determinant of their health status. In addition, there has been a shift in the approach to health care that focuses on the role of clients and their responsibility for self-care. The ability to care for oneself is as important for healthy living as it is for managing a complex medical regimen of a chronic illness. Self-care as an integral component of health care consists of diet, exercise, stress management techniques, and the cultivation of a healthy lifestyle (Herrick and Ainsworth, 2000). Many variables can influence clients' health beliefs, health practices, and self-care. Internal and external variables can influence how a person thinks and acts and how a person will deal with an illness. You should consider the impact of these variables and be able to incorporate appropriate interventions based on the person's unique characteristics. Internal variables include a person's developmental stage, intellectual background, and emotional and spiritual factors. External variables include family practices, socioeconomic factors, and cultural background.

Internal Variables

DEVELOPMENTAL STAGE.   A person's concept of illness is dependent on the person's developmental stage (see Chapter 18). Knowledge of the stages of growth and development will help you predict the client's response to the present illness or the threat of future illness. Your educational interventions need to be age appropriate to be effective. For example, you would use different techniques of teaching about contraception to an adolescent and to an adult.

INTELLECTUAL BACKGROUND.   A person's beliefs about health are shaped in part by knowledge (or misinformation) about body functions and illnesses, educational background, and past experiences. Cognitive abilities shape the *way* a person thinks, including the ability to understand factors involved in illness and to apply knowledge of health and illness to personal health practices.

EMOTIONAL FACTORS.   A person's degree of calm or stress can influence health beliefs and practices. The manner in which a person handles stress throughout each phase of life will influence the way the person reacts to illness. A person who generally is very calm may have little emotional response during illness, whereas a person normally unable to cope with stress may either overreact to illness or may deny the presence of symptoms and not take therapeutic action (see Chapter 21).

SPIRITUAL FACTORS.   Spirituality is reflected in how a person lives his or her life, including the values and beliefs exercised, the relationships established with family and friends, and the ability to find hope and meaning in life. Spirituality serves as an integrating theme in peoples' lives (Ross, 1995). Religious practices are one way people exercise spirituality. You must understand clients' spiritual dimensions to involve them effectively in nursing care.

External Variables

FAMILY PRACTICES.   The way that families use health care services generally influences their health practices. Their perceptions of the seriousness of diseases and their history of preventive care behaviors (or lack of them) can influence how clients will think about health. A person raised in a family that believed in the importance of preventive care, for example, dental checkups twice a year, is more likely to continue those health practices as an adult.

SOCIOECONOMIC FACTORS.   Social and economic factors can increase the risk for illness and influence the way that a person defines and reacts to illness. Social variables partly determine how the health care system provides medical care. Because the health care system is organized in certain ways, it determines how clients can obtain care, the treatment method, the economic cost to the client, and the potential reimbursement to the health care agency or client. Economic variables may affect a client's level of health by increasing the risk for disease and influencing how or at what point the client enters the health care system. In addition, a person's participation in the treatment that is designed to maintain or improve health is also affected by economic status. A person who has high utility bills, a large family, and a low income tends to give a higher priority to food and shelter than to costly drugs or treatment or expensive foods for special diets.

CULTURAL BACKGROUND.   Cultural background influences beliefs, values, and customs. It influences the approach to the health care system, personal health practices, and the nurse-client relationship. You need to recognize and understand cultural patterns of behavior and beliefs to interact with the client (see Chapter 16).

HEALTH PROMOTION, WELLNESS, AND ILLNESS PREVENTION

Health promotion activities can be passive or active. With **passive strategies of health promotion,** individuals gain from the activities of others without acting themselves. The fluoridation of municipal drinking water and the fortification of homogenized milk with vitamin D are examples of passive health promotion strategies. With **active strategies of health promotion,** individuals are motivated to adopt specific health programs. Weight reduction and smoking cessation programs require clients to be actively involved in measures to improve their present and future levels of wellness while decreasing the risk of disease.

You need to emphasize health promotion, wellness strategies, and illness prevention activities as important forms of health care because they assist clients in maintaining and improving health. **Health promotion** activities such as routine exercise and good nutrition help clients maintain or enhance their present levels of health and reduce their risks of developing certain diseases. **Wellness education** teaches people how to care for themselves in a healthy way and includes topics such as physical awareness, stress management, and self-responsibility. **Illness prevention** activities such as immunization programs protect clients from actual or potential threats to health. The concepts of health promotion, wellness, and illness prevention are closely related and in practice overlap to some extent. All are focused on the future; the differences between them involve motivations and goals. Health promotion activities motivate people to act positively to reach more stable levels of health. Wellness strategies are designed to help persons achieve new understanding and control of their lives. Illness prevention activities motivate people to avoid declines in health or functional levels.

Health care has become increasingly focused on health promotion, wellness, and illness prevention. The rapid rise of health care costs has motivated people to seek ways of decreasing the incidence and minimizing the results of illness or disability. Approximately 70% of the burden of illness and its associated costs is related to preventable illnesses (Fries and others, 1998). Fries and others (1998) suggest that the best way to reduce costs and improve health is to reduce the demand for health care services by improving self-management, preventive services, and curative services. You have an important role in educating clients to improve their ability to manage their health. You do this in part by helping them recognize their responsibility in the health-related choices they make and also by helping them understand the impact this has on disease prevention. Health promotion, wellness activities, and illness prevention are all strategies aimed at decreasing the incidence of illness and minimizing the deleterious results of that illness or disability.

Levels of Preventive Care

Health activities and nursing care occur at the primary, secondary, and tertiary levels of prevention (Table 1-1). Prevention includes all activities that limit the progression of a disease (Edelman and Mandle, 1998).

Primary prevention is true prevention; it precedes disease or dysfunction and is applied to clients considered physically and emotionally healthy. It is not therapeutic,

The Three Levels of Prevention				Table 1-1
Primary Prevention		Secondary Prevention		Tertiary Prevention
Health Promotion	Specific Protection	Early Diagnosis and Prompt Treatment	Disability Limitations	Restoration and Rehabilitation
Health education	Use of specific	Case-finding measures:	Adequate treatment	Provision of hospital
Good standard of	immunizations	individual and mass	to arrest disease	and community
nutrition adjusted	Attention to	Screening surveys	process and	facilities for
to developmental	personal hygiene	Selective	prevent further	training and
phases of life	Use of environ-	examinations	complications	education to
Attention to person-	mental sanitation	Cure and prevention	Provision of facilities	maximize use
ality development	Protection against	of disease process	to limit disability	of remaining
Provision of	occupational	to prevent spread	and prevent death	capacities
adequate housing	hazards	of communicable		Education of the
and recreation and	Protection from	disease, prevent		public and indus-
agreeable working	accidents	complications, and		tries to use reha-
conditions	Use of specific	shorten period of		bilitated persons to
Marriage counseling	nutrients	disability		the fullest possible
and sex education	Protection from			extent
Genetic screening	carcinogens			Selective placement
Periodic selective	Avoidance of			Work therapy in
examinations	allergens			hospitals

Modified from Leavell HR, Clark AE: *Preventive medicine for doctors in the community,* ed 3, New York, 1965, McGraw-Hill.

does not use therapeutic treatments, and does not involve symptom identification (Edelman and Mandle, 1998). The purpose of primary prevention is to decrease the vulnerability of the individual or population to an illness or dysfunction (Edelman and Mandle, 1998). Primary prevention includes passive and active strategies of health promotion. It can be provided to an individual or to a general population, or it can focus on individuals at risk for developing specific diseases. Wellness activities (Edelman and Mandle, 1998) are synonymous with the activities identified for primary prevention by Leavell and Clark (1965) in Table 1-1.

Secondary prevention focuses on persons who are experiencing health problems or illnesses and who are at risk for developing complications or worsening conditions. Activities are directed at diagnosis and prompt intervention, thereby reducing severity and enabling the client to return to a normal level of health as early as possible (Edelman and Mandle, 1998). A large portion of secondary level nursing care is delivered in homes, hospitals, or skilled nursing facilities. It includes screening techniques and treating early stages of disease to limit disability by delaying the consequences of advanced disease.

Tertiary prevention occurs when a defect or disability is permanent and irreversible. It involves minimizing the effects of long-term disease or disability by interventions directed at preventing complications and deterioration (Edelman and Mandle, 1998). Activities are directed at rehabilitation rather than diagnosis and treatment. Care at this level aims to help clients achieve as high a level of functioning as possible, despite the limitations caused by illness or impairment. This level of care is called *preventive care* because it involves preventing further disability or reduced functioning.

RISK FACTORS

A **risk factor** is any situation, habit, environmental condition, physiological condition, or other variable that increases the vulnerability of an individual or group to an illness or accident. The presence of risk factors does not mean that a disease will develop, but risk factors increase the chances that the individual will experience a particular disease. Risk factors play a major role in how you identify a client's health status. Risk factors can also influence health beliefs and practices if a person is aware of their presence. Risk factors can be placed in the following interrelated categories: genetic and physiological factors, age, physical environment, and lifestyle.

Genetic and Physiological Factors

Physiological risk factors involve the physical functioning of the body. Certain physical conditions, such as being pregnant or overweight, place increased stress on physiological systems (e.g., the circulatory system), increasing susceptibility to illness in these areas. Heredity, or genetic predisposition to specific illness, is a major physical risk factor. For example, a person with a family history of diabetes mellitus is

at risk for developing the disease later in life. Other documented genetic risk factors include family histories of cancer, heart disease, or kidney disease.

Age

Age increases susceptibility to certain illnesses (e.g., the risk of heart disease increases with age for both sexes). The risks of birth defects and complications of pregnancy increase in women bearing children after age 35. Many kinds of cancer pose a greater risk for persons over age 45 than for younger persons. Age risk factors are often closely associated with other risk factors such as family history and personal habits. You need to educate clients about the importance of regularly scheduled checkups for their age-group (Figure 1-5).

Environment

The physical environment in which a person works or lives can increase the likelihood that certain illnesses will occur. A person's home environment may include conditions that pose risks, such as unclean, poorly heated or cooled, or overcrowded dwellings. These conditions can increase the likelihood that infections and other diseases will be contracted and spread. Also, some kinds of cancer and other diseases are more likely to develop when industrial workers are exposed to certain chemicals or when people live near toxic waste disposal sites. Screening for these environmentally based risk factors is directed at the short-term effects of the exposure and the potential for long-term effects (Edelman and Mandle, 1998).

Lifestyle

Lifestyle practices and behaviors can have positive or negative effects on health. Practices with potential negative effects are risk factors; these include overeating or poor nutrition, insufficient rest and sleep, and poor personal hygiene. Other habits that put a person at risk for illness include tobacco use, alcohol or drug abuse, and activities involving a threat of injury such as skydiving or mountain climbing. Some habits are risk factors for specific diseases. For example, excessive sunbathing increases the risk of skin cancer, and being overweight increases the risk of cardiovascular disease. These lifestyle risk factors have gained increased attention because it is known that many of the leading causes of death in the United States are related to lifestyle patterns or habits. This represents a huge impact on the economics of the health care system.

The effect of lifestyle behavior on the risk of developing disease has implications across the life span of a person. You should understand that clients of all ages are vulnerable to the influences of unhealthy lifestyle patterns. You are able to influence choices your clients make by preventing unhealthy behaviors and promoting healthy lifestyle patterns. The lifestyle practices of young children are influenced by those of their parents, caretakers, and teachers. Issues of seat belt use, gun possession, alcohol and drug use, and sexual promiscuity are encountered by many adolescents. Fish and Nies (1996) note that college students who may have been

Clinical Preventive Services for Normal-Risk Adults

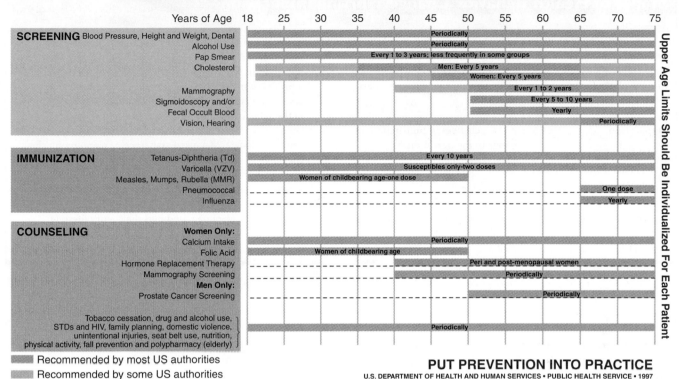

FIGURE **1-5**   Clinical preventive services for normal-risk adults. (From U.S. Department of Health and Human Services: *Put prevention into practice,* 1997, www.ahrq.gov/ppip/pptools.htm.)

taught health promotion behaviors at home are at risk for developing poor health habits in the college years as they establish independence, as a result of either convenience or peer pressure. These habits may affect their health status throughout life. Rowe and Kahn (2000) emphasize that in the older adult population it is often elements of lifestyle and many years of poor health choices, not the aging process alone or the view that disease is inevitable, that is a major risk factor for the development of certain diseases. Therefore it is important to understand the impact of lifestyle behaviors on health status. You can educate your clients and the public on wellness-promoting lifestyle behaviors.

Risk Factor Identification

The goal of risk factor identification is to assist clients in understanding those areas in their lives that can be modified or even eliminated to promote wellness and prevent illness. Comprehensive health risk appraisals, using a variety of available health risk appraisal forms, can be done to estimate a person's specific health threats based on the presence of various risk factors (Edelman and Mandle, 1998). It is important to understand that implementation of a health risk appraisal must be linked with educational programs and other community resources to result in necessary lifestyle changes and risk reduction (Pender, 1996). You are in a prime position to assist clients in examining their lifestyles and identifying the modifiable risk factors that may cause

them to have health problems in the future (Donaldson, 2000). Clients should not be "victimized" by relating all of their health problems to risky behaviors they have followed (Donaldson, 2000).

RISK FACTOR MODIFICATION AND CHANGING HEALTH BEHAVIORS

Identifying risk factors is the first step in health promotion, wellness education, and illness prevention activities. Once risk factors have been identified, you can implement health education programs that may lead a person to change a risky health behavior. This is called *risk factor modification*. Risk factor modification, health promotion, or any program that attempts to change unhealthy lifestyle behaviors can be considered a wellness strategy in that it teaches clients to care for themselves in a healthier way. Wellness strategies need to be emphasized because they have the ability to decrease the potential high costs of unmanaged health problems.

Attempts to change may be aimed at the cessation of a health-damaging behavior (e.g., tobacco use or alcohol misuse) or the adoption of a healthy behavior (e.g., healthy diet or exercise) (Pender, 1996). When engaging an individual into health behavior change, you will use what you have learned from the health belief model to analyze the probability that a person will make changes for improving health or preventing disease (Edelman and Mandle, 1998).

Stages of Health Behavior Change: Nursing Implications   Table 1-2

	Definition	Nursing Implications
Precontemplation	Not intending to make changes within the next 6 months.	Client will not be interested in information about the behavior, and may be defensive when confronted with the information.
Contemplation	Considering a change within the next 6 months.	Ambivalence may be present, but clients will more likely accept information as they are developing more belief in the value of change.
Preparation	Make small changes in preparation for a change in the next month.	Client believes advantages outweigh disadvantages of behavior change. May need assistance in planning for the change.
Action	Actively engaged in strategies to change behavior. This stage may last up to 6 months.	Be aware of previous habits that may prevent action on new behaviors. Identify barriers to and facilitators of change.
Maintenance Stage	Sustained change over time. This stage begins 6 months after action has started and continues indefinitely.	Changes need to be integrated into the client's lifestyle.

Modified from Prochaska JO, DiClemente CC: Stages of change in the modification of problem behaviors, *Prog Behav Modif* 28:184, 1992; and Conn VS: A staged-based approach to helping people change health behaviors, *Clin Nurs Spec* 8(4):187, 1994.

An understanding of the process of changing behaviors can help you support difficult health behavior change in your clients. It is believed that change involves movement through a series of stages. Five stages of change, ranging from no intention to change (precontemplation) to maintaining a changed behavior (maintenance stage), have been identified (Prochaska and DiClemente, 1992; Prochaska and Velicer, 1997). As individuals attempt change in behavior, relapse and recycling through the stages occur frequently. When relapse occurs, the person will return to the contemplation or precontemplation stage before attempting change again. Relapse can be viewed as a learning process, and what is learned from relapse can be applied to the next attempt to change. You need to be able to identify your client's stage of change to implement appropriate care. Health promotion activities can have a greater impact if they are timed appropriately to match a specific stage of change (Prochaska and Velicer, 1997). Nursing implications for each stage are discussed in Table 1-2.

Further work needs to be done to design interventions and wellness strategies for people in all stages of health behavior change. Changes will be maintained over time only if the health behavior changes are integrated into an individual's overall lifestyle. In addition, it should be understood that true change comes from the client's desire to change. Maintenance of healthy lifestyles can prevent hospitalizations and potentially lower the cost of health care. You can assist your clients in adapting to a changed and healthier lifestyle.

▌ILLNESS

Illness is a state in which a person's physical, emotional, intellectual, social, developmental, or spiritual functioning is diminished or impaired compared with previous experience. Cancer is a disease process, but one client with leukemia who

is responding to treatment may continue to function as usual, whereas another client with breast cancer who is preparing for surgery may be affected in dimensions other than the physical. Interestingly, many clients find health within illness. An experience with illness can motivate an individual to adopt more positive health behaviors. For example, a person who experiences a heart attack is now considered to have cardiovascular disease. When advised by health care professionals that a change in diet and an increase in exercise may prevent further problems, the individual may be motivated to adopt the needed health behaviors.

Illness therefore is not synonymous with disease; although nurses must be familiar with different kinds of diseases and their treatments, they are concerned more with illness, which may include not only disease but also the effects on functioning and well-being in all dimensions.

Acute and Chronic Illness

Acute and chronic illness are two general classifications of illness used in this chapter. An **acute illness** is usually short term and severe. The symptoms appear abruptly, are intense, and often subside after a relatively short period. An acute illness may affect functioning in any dimension. A **chronic illness** persists, usually longer than 6 months, and can also affect functioning in any dimension. The client may fluctuate between maximal functioning and serious health relapses that may be life threatening.

Because of successes in public health, medicine, and biomedical technology, acute and infectious diseases are no longer major causes of death, disease, and disability in the United States. Moreover, the heaviest burden of illness today is due to chronic diseases that are largely preventable (Orleans and others, 1999). Beyond the prevention of these diseases as previously discussed, a major role for nursing is to provide client education aimed at helping your clients manage their illness or disability to reduce the occurrence of symptoms and improve the tolerance of symptoms. You can also enhance wellness and improve quality of life for clients living with chronic illnesses or disabilities.

ILLNESS BEHAVIOR

People who are ill generally act in a way medical sociologists call **illness behavior.** It involves how people monitor their bodies, define and interpret their symptoms, take remedial actions, and use the health care system (Mechanic, 1982). Personal history, social situations, social norms, and the opportunities and constraints of community institutions can all affect illness behavior (Mechanic, 1995). Although there is a large variability in the way people react to an illness, illness behavior displayed in sickness can be used to manage life adversities (Mechanic, 1995). If people perceive themselves to be ill, illness behaviors can be coping mechanisms. For example, illness behavior can result in clients being released from roles, social expectations, or responsibilities. For a homemaker, for example, the "flu" may be viewed as an added stressor or it may be a temporary release from child care and household responsibilities.

Variables Influencing Illness Behavior

Just as health behavior is affected by internal and external variables, so is illness behavior. The influences of these variables may affect the likelihood of seeking health care, the participation in therapy, and therefore health outcomes. Based on an understanding of these variables and behaviors, you can individualize care to assist clients in coping with their illness at various stages. The goal of nursing is to promote optimal functioning in all dimensions throughout an illness.

INTERNAL VARIABLES.   Internal variables influence the way clients behave when they are ill. These are the client's perceptions of symptoms and the nature of the illness. If clients believe that the symptoms of their illnesses disrupt their normal routine, they are more likely to seek health care assistance than if they do not perceive the symptoms to be disruptive. If clients believe that the symptoms are serious or perhaps life threatening, they are also more likely to seek assistance. Persons awakened by crushing chest pains in the middle of the night generally view this symptom as potentially serious and life threatening and will probably be motivated to seek assistance. However, such a perception can also have the opposite effect. Individuals may fear serious illness, react by denying it, and not seek medical assistance.

The nature of the illness, either acute or chronic, can also affect a client's illness behavior. Clients with acute illnesses are likely to seek health care and comply readily with therapy. On the other hand, a client with a chronic illness, in which the symptoms may not be cured but only partially relieved, may not be motivated to comply with the therapy plan. Chronically ill clients may become less actively involved in their care, may experience greater frustration, and may comply less readily with care. You will generally spend more time than other health care professionals with chronically ill clients, and you are in the unique position of being able to assist these clients in overcoming problems related to illness behavior.

EXTERNAL VARIABLES.   External variables influencing a client's illness behavior include the visibility of symptoms, social group, cultural background, economic variables, accessibility of the health care system, and social support. The visibility of the symptoms of an illness can affect body image and illness behavior. A client with a visible symptom may be more likely to seek assistance than a client without such a visible symptom.

Clients' social groups may assist them in recognizing the threat of illness or support the denial of potential illness. Families, friends, and co-workers all may influence clients' illness behavior. Clients often react positively to social support while practicing positive health behaviors. Cultural and ethnic background teaches a person how to be healthy, how to recognize illness, and how to be ill. The effects of disease and its interpretation vary according to cultural circumstances.

Economic variables influence the way a client reacts to illness. Because of economic constraints, a client may delay treatment and in many cases may continue to carry out daily activities. Clients' access to the health care system is closely related to economic factors. The health care system is a socioeconomic system that clients must enter, interact within, and exit. For many clients, entry into the system is complex or confusing, and some clients may seek nonemergency medical care in an emergency department because they do not know how to obtain health services otherwise. The physical proximity of clients to a health care agency often influences how soon they enter the system after deciding to seek care.

IMPACT OF ILLNESS ON CLIENT AND FAMILY

An illness of a family member affects the function of the entire family unit. The client and family commonly experience behavioral and emotional changes and changes in body image, self-concept, family roles, and family dynamics.

Behavioral and Emotional Changes

Individual behavioral and emotional reactions depend on the nature of the illness, the client's attitude toward it, the reaction of others to it, and the variables of illness behavior. Short-term, non–life-threatening illnesses evoke few behavioral changes in the functioning of the client or family. A husband and father who has a cold, for example, may lack the energy and patience to spend time in family activities and may be irritable and prefer not to interact with his family. This is a behavioral change, but the change is subtle and does not last long. Some may even consider such a change a normal response to illness.

Severe illness, particularly one that is life threatening, can lead to more extensive emotional and behavioral changes, such as anxiety, shock, denial, anger, and withdrawal. These are common responses to the stress of illness. You can develop interventions to assist the client and the family in coping with and adapting to this stress, because the stressor itself cannot usually be changed.

Impact on Body Image

Body image is the subjective concept of physical appearance. Some illnesses result in changes in physical appearance, and clients and families react differently to these changes. These reactions of clients and families to changes in body image depend on the type of changes (e.g., the loss of a limb or an organ), the adaptive capacity of the family, the rate at which changes take place, and the support services available.

When a change in body image occurs, such as results from a leg amputation, the client generally adjusts by experiencing phases of the grief process (see Chapter 22). Initially the client may be shocked by the change or impending change. As the client and family recognize the reality of the change, they become anxious and may withdraw. As the client and family acknowledge the change, they gradually move toward accepting their loss. At the end of the acknowledgment phase, they accept the loss. During rehabilitation, the client is ready to learn how to adapt to the change in body image.

Impact on Self-Concept

Self-concept is a mental self-image of strengths and weaknesses in all aspects of personality. Self-concept depends in part on body image and roles but also includes other aspects of psychology and spirituality.

Self-concept is important in relationships with other family members. A client whose self-concept changes because of illness may no longer meet family expectations, leading to tension or conflict. As a result, family members may change their interactions with the client. In the course of providing care, a nurse is able to observe changes in the client's self-concept (or in the self-concepts of family members) and develop a care plan to help the client adjust to the changes resulting from the illness (see Chapter 19).

Impact on Family Roles and Family Dynamics

People have many roles in life, such as wage earner, decision maker, professional, and parent. When an illness occurs, the roles of the client and family may change (see Chapter 20). Such a change may be subtle and short term or drastic and long term. An individual and family generally adjust more easily to subtle, short-term changes. Long-term changes, however, require an adjustment process similar to the grief process (see Chapter 22). The client and family often require specific counseling and guidance to assist them in coping with the role changes.

Family dynamics is the process by which the family functions, makes decisions, gives support to individual members, and copes with everyday changes and challenges. Because of the effects of illness, family dynamics often change. Role functions may be halted or delayed. The ill person's usual roles and responsibilities may need to be assumed by another family member. This may create tension or anxiety in the family. Role reversal is also common. If a parent of an adult becomes ill and cannot carry out usual activities, the adult child often assumes many of the parent's responsibilities. Such a reversal can lead to conflicting responsibilities for the adult child or direct conflict over decision making. You must view the whole family and plan care to help the family regain the maximal level of functioning and well-being (see Chapter 20).

Key Terms

active strategies of health promotion, p. 7
acute illness, p. 10
chronic illness, p. 10
determinants of health, p. 5
health, p. 2
health belief model, p.3
health beliefs, p. 3

health-illness continuum model, p. 2
health promotion, p. 7
health promotion model, p. 4
health status, p. 6
holistic health model, p. 4
illness, p. 10
illness behavior, p. 11
illness prevention, p. 7
negative health behaviors, p. 3

passive strategies of health promotion, p. 7
positive health behaviors, p. 3
primary prevention, p. 7
risk factor, p. 8
secondary prevention, p. 8
tertiary prevention, p. 8
wellness, p. 1
wellness education, p. 7

Key Concepts

- Health and wellness are not merely the absence of disease and illness.
- A person's state of health, wellness, or illness depends on individual values, personality, and lifestyle.
- According to the health-illness continuum model, health and illness are in a dynamic, relative relationship.
- The health belief model considers factors influencing health beliefs.
- The health promotion model increases individual well-being and self-actualization.
- Holistic health models of nursing promote optimal health by incorporating active participation of the client in improving the health state.
- Holistic nursing interventions can be used to complement standard medical therapy.
- Many variables determine the health status of an individual or community.
- Health beliefs and practices are influenced by internal and external variables and should be considered when planning care.
- Health promotion activities help maintain or enhance health.
- Wellness education teaches clients how to care for themselves.
- Illness prevention activities protect against health threats and thus maintain an optimal level of health.
- Nursing incorporates health promotion, wellness, and illness prevention activities rather than simply treating illness.
- The three levels of preventive care are primary, secondary, and tertiary.
- Risk factors threaten health, influence health practices, and are important considerations in illness prevention activities.
- Risk factors involve genetic or physiological variables, age, environment, and lifestyle.
- Improvement in health may involve a change in health behaviors.
- Illness behavior, like health practices, is influenced by many variables and must be considered when you are planning care.
- Illness can have many effects on the client and family, including changes in behavior and emotions, family roles and dynamics, body image, and self-concept.

Critical Thinking Activities

1. List the current health promotion, wellness, and illness prevention activities in which you regularly engage. Are there any areas that need to be improved or changed? What will influence your ability to adopt any needed changes?
2. Have you ever tried to modify a lifestyle pattern? What led you to the awareness that you needed to make a change? Describe the process you underwent, and correlate your experiences with the stages of change discussed in this chapter.
3. Assess the lifestyle patterns of someone you know. Identify risk factors that increase the person's vulnerability to illness or susceptibility to disease. Are there risk factors present that could be modified?
4. Think of one group in your community in which you could implement a wellness activity. How would you identify the problem? What strategies would you use to implement the plan? How would you evaluate the effectiveness of your teaching?

Review Questions

1. Health is:
   1. the absence of illness.
   2. the opposite of disease.
   3. a condition between disease and good health.
   4. a state of complete physical, mental, and social well-being.
2. A person's state of health, wellness, or illness depends on an individual's:
   1. self-concept.
   2. lifestyle only.
   3. known risk factors.
   4. values, personality, and lifestyle.
3. The relationship between health and illness in the health-illness continuum model is:
   1. stable.
   2. stagnant.
   3. dynamic.
   4. developing.
4. According to the health belief model, health beliefs usually influence:
   1. health status.
   2. health outcomes.
   3. health behaviors.
   4. health determinants.
5. The health promotion model attempts to explain the:
   1. effect of environment on an individual.
   2. effect of health activities on an individual.
   3. reasons individuals avoid health activities.
   4. reasons individuals engage in health activities.
6. Holistic health interventions are used to:
   1. replace standard medical therapy.
   2. improve standard medical therapy.
   3. complement standard medical therapy.
   4. compete with standard medical therapy.
7. The health status of an individual or community is:
   1. multifactorial.
   2. one dimensional.
   3. determined by genetics.
   4. determined by environment.

Review Questions—cont'd

8. The internal variables that can influence a client's health beliefs and health practices are:
   1. family practices, developmental stage, intellectual background, emotional factors.
   2. cultural background, emotional factors, spiritual factors, developmental stage.
   3. socioeconomic factors, intellectual background, spiritual factors, family practices.
   4. developmental stage, intellectual background, emotional factors, spiritual factors.
9. Health promotion activities are activities that:
   1. treat disease.
   2. prevent illness.
   3. help maintain or enhance health.
   4. aim at protecting against health threats.
10. Primary prevention strategies:
    1. identify disease problems.
    2. treat chronic disease states.
    3. reduce the severity of an illness.
    4. decrease vulnerability to an illness.
11. The presence of certain risk factors:
    1. has no role in health practices.
    2. suggests that a disease will definitely develop.

3. increases the chance that disease will develop.
4. decreases the chance that disease will progress.

12. Changing health behaviors:
    1. is easier for health care professionals.
    2. is difficult without guidance from a health care professional.
    3. may be initiated regardless of the client's stage in the change process.
    4. may be either a cessation of health-damaging behavior or the adoption of a healthy behavior.
13. External variables that influence a client's illness behavior are:
    1. the nature of the illness and the perception of symptoms.
    2. the perception of symptoms and the visibility of the symptoms.
    3. the visibility of symptoms, social group, economics, and social support.
    4. dependent on the degree to which they disrupt the client's normal routine.
14. An illness in a family member affects the function of the:
    1. siblings.
    2. parental dyad.
    3. individual only.
    4. entire family unit.

References

Acee A: Applying holistic nursing, *Am J Nurs* 98(8):36, 1998.

Becker MH, Maiman LA: Sociobehavioral determinants of compliance with health and medical care recommendations, *Med Care* 13(1):10, 1975.

Conn VS: A staged-based approach to helping people change health behaviors, *Clin Nurs Spec* 8(4):187, 1994.

Donaldson L: President's report: the role nurses play, *The Lamp* 57(3):9, 2000.

Edelman CL, Mandle CL: *Health promotion throughout the life span,* ed 4, St. Louis, 1998, Mosby.

Fish C, Nies MA: Health promotion needs of students in a college environment, *Public Health Nurs* 13(2):104, 1996.

Fries JF and others: Beyond health promotion: reducing need and demand for medical care, *Health Aff* 17(2):70, 1998.

Herrick CM, Ainsworth AD: Invest in yourself: yoga as a self-care strategy, *Nurs Forum* 35(2):32, 2000.

Leavell HR, Clark AE: *Preventive medicine for doctors in the community,* ed 3, New York, 1965, McGraw-Hill.

Mechanic D: The epidemiology of illness behavior and its relationship to physical and psychological distress. In Mechanic D: *Symptoms, illness behavior, and help seeking,* New York, 1982, Prodist.

Mechanic D: Sociological dimensions of illness behavior, *Soc Sci Med* 41(9):1207, 1995.

Orleans CT and others: Rating our progress in population health promotion: report card on six behaviors, *Am J Health Promot* 14(2):75, 1999.

Pender NJ: *Health promotion and nursing practice,* Norwalk, Conn, 1982, Appleton-Century-Crofts.

Pender NJ: Health promotion and illness prevention. In Werley HH, Fitzpatrick JJ, editors: *Annual review of nursing research,* New York, 1993, Springer.

Pender NJ: *Health promotion and nursing practice,* ed 3, Stamford, Conn, 1996, Appleton & Lange.

Prochaska JO, DiClemente CC: Stages of change in the modification of problem behaviors, *Prog Behav Modif* 28:184, 1992.

Prochaska JO, Velicer WF: The transtheoretical model of health behavior change, *Am J Health Promot* 12(1):38, 1997.

Rice R: *Home care nursing practice: concepts and applications,* ed 3, St. Louis, 2000, Mosby.

Rosenstoch I: Historical origin of the health belief model, *Health Educ Monogr* 2:334, 1974.

Ross (nee Waugh) L: The spiritual dimension: its importance to clients' health, well-being and quality of life and its implications for nursing practice, *Soc Sci Med* 32(5):457, 1995.

Rowe JW, Kahn RL: Successful aging and disease prevention, *Adv Ren Replace Ther* 7(1):70, 2000.

U.S. Department of Health and Human Services, Public Health Service: *Healthy people: the Surgeon General's report on health promotion and disease prevention,* Washington, DC, 1979, U.S. Government Printing Office.

U.S. Department of Health and Human Services, Public Health Service: *Healthy people 2000: national health promotion and disease prevention objectives,* Washington, DC, 1990, U.S. Government Printing Office.

U.S. Department of Health and Human Services: *Put prevention into practice,* 1997, www.ahrq.gov/ppip/pptools.htm.

U.S. Department of Health and Human Services, Public Health Service: *Healthy people 2010: understanding and improving health,* Washington, DC, 2000, U.S. Government Printing Office.

World Health Organization Interim Commission: *Chronicle of WHO,* Geneva, 1947, The Organization.

The Health Care Delivery System

Objectives

- Define the key terms listed.
- Describe the six levels of health care.
- Explain the relationship between levels of care and levels of prevention.
- Discuss the types of settings where various levels of health care are provided.
- Discuss the role of nurses in different health care delivery settings.
- Differentiate community health nursing from community-based nursing.
- Explain the advantages and disadvantages of managed health care.
- Compare the various methods for financing health care.
- Discuss the implications that changes in the health care system have on nursing.
- Discuss opportunities for nursing within the changing health care delivery system.

As you begin your career in nursing you will quickly realize that the U.S. health care system is very complex. Although a broad variety of services are offered to the public by health professionals from varied disciplines, gaining access to services can be very difficult for those with limited health care insurance. The continuing emergence of new technologies and pharmaceuticals causes the costs of health care to skyrocket. Pressures to reduce costs come from declining reimbursement by third-party payers and from health care institutions being managed more as businesses than as service organizations. The challenges faced in reducing the costs of health care make it difficult for health care providers to maintain high-quality care for their clients. Many clients who would have been hospitalized for their condition 7 years ago are now treated in outpatient facilities, in part to reduce the costs resulting from lengthy hospitalization. As a result, hospitalized clients truly require acute care; they are sicker and their treatment involves a higher level of technological care. Clients are discharged from hospitals sooner, often leaving families with the burden of providing care in the home setting. Nurses also face significant challenges of keeping individuals healthy and well within their own homes and communities.

Nursing is a caring discipline. The values of our profession are rooted in helping persons to regain, maintain, or improve their health, prevent illness, and find comfort and dignity. The health care system of the new millennium has become less service oriented and much more business oriented because of cost-saving initiatives. As a result, the practice of nursing is changing. Nursing must lead the way in change and retain its values for client care while meeting the challenges of new roles and new responsibilities.

HEALTH CARE REGULATION AND COMPETITION

Through most of the twentieth century there were few incentives for controlling health care costs. If a client needed to be in the hospital a few extra days for a wound to heal or for the family to prepare to take care of him at home, there were few obstacles. Whatever a physician chose to order for a client's care and treatment, insurers (third-party payers) paid for. However, as health care costs continued to rise out of control, regulatory and competitive approaches have attempted to control health care spending. For example, **professional standards review organizations (PSROs)** were created to review the quality, quantity, and cost of hospital care provided through Medicare (Garg and others, 1997). Medicare-qualified hospitals have been required to have physician-supervised **utilization review (UR) committees** to review admissions, diagnostic testing, and treatments provided by physicians to clients. The aim was to identify and eliminate overuse of diagnostic and treatment services. Controlling physician habits and influencing their preferences is very difficult and has met with limited success.

One of the most significant factors to influence how health care was paid for and thus affect competition was the **prospective payment system (PPS).** Established by Congress

in 1983, the PPS eliminated cost-based reimbursement. Hospitals serving Medicare clients were no longer paid for all costs incurred to deliver care to a client. Instead, inpatient hospital services for Medicare clients were bundled into 468 **diagnosis-related groups (DRGs).** Each group has a fixed reimbursement amount with adjustments for case severity, rural/urban/regional costs, and teaching costs. Hospitals receive a set dollar amount for each client based on the assigned DRG, regardless of the client's length of stay or use of services in the hospital. Box 2-1 provides a hypothetical scenario, showing how reimbursement for a client's care is determined under the DRG PPS. Most health care providers (e.g., health care networks or managed care organizations) now receive **capitated** payments. Capitation is the payment mechanism in which providers receive a fixed amount per client or enrollee of a health care plan (Appleby, 1996). The aim of capitation is to build a payment plan for select diagnoses or surgical procedures that includes the best standards of care, including essential diagnostic and treatment procedures at the lowest cost.

Capitation and prospective payment have influenced the way care is delivered in all types of health care settings. DRGs are now used in the rehabilitation setting and **resource utilization groups (RUGs)** are used in long-term care. In all settings, efforts are made to manage costs so that the organizations can remain profitable. For example, when clients are hospitalized for lengthy periods, hospitals must absorb the portion of costs not reimbursed. This simply adds more pressure to ensure that clients are managed effectively and discharged as soon as is reasonably possible. Soon after prospective payment was implemented hospitals began to

---

Clinical Scenario of a DRG Example   Box 2-1

Mr. Truman was admitted to the hospital on November 1 after experiencing chest pain and shortness of breath. He had undergone cardiac surgery almost 10 years before but was beginning to have recurrent chest pain, even at rest. He was scheduled for a cardiac catheterization, but it was delayed until November 3. The physician also referred Mr. Truman for diet counseling for a low-cholesterol diet. The cardiac catheterization proceeded without complications, and surgery was unnecessary. Mr. Truman remained hospitalized overnight to ensure that no problems developed. He was discharged on November 4.

Principal diagnosis: Heart ischemia
Secondary diagnosis: Disturbances of heart, functional, long-term effect of cardiac surgery
DRG assigned: DRG 125: Circulatory disorders except acute myocardial infarction with cardiac catheterization without complex diagnosis
Assigned or allowed length of stay: 2.2 days
Actual length of stay: 3.1 days
Payment calculation (based on 2.2 days): payment per discharge × DRG weight = $3400 × 0.7015 = $2385
Actual hospital costs for Mr. Truman: $2960
Loss for hospital: $575

increase discharge planning activities and hospital lengths of stay began to shorten. Because clients are discharged home as soon as possible, home care agencies must now provide complex technological care including intravenous therapy, mechanical ventilation, and long-term parenteral nutrition.

The term **managed care** describes health care systems in which there is administrative control over primary health care services for a defined client population. The provider or health care system receives a predetermined capitated payment for each client enrolled in the program. In this case the managed care organization bears financial risk in addition to providing client care. The organization's focus of care shifts from individual illness care to concern for the health of its covered population. If people stay healthy, the cost of medical care declines. Systems of managed care focus on three values: the capacity to contain or reduce costs, the ability to increase client satisfaction, and the ability to improve the health or functional status of the individual (Pew Health Professions Commission, 1995).

You do not have to be a health care financing expert in your role as a nurse. However, it is important for you to understand the basics of health care financing to recognize the effects on employers and clients. Table 2-1 summarizes the most common types of health care plans.

Health Care Plans   Table 2-1

Type	Definition	Characteristics
Managed care organization (MCO)	Provides comprehensive, preventive, and treatment services to a specific group of voluntarily enrolled persons. Structures include a variety of models: *Staff model:* Physicians are salaried employees of the MCI. *Group model:* MCO contracts with single group practice *Network model:* MCO contracts with multiple group practices and/or integrated organizations. **Independent practice association (IPA):** MCO contracts with physicians who usually are not members of groups and whose practices include fee-for-service and capitated clients.	Focus on health maintenance, primary care. All care provided by a primary care physician. Referral needed for access to specialist and hospitalization.
Medicare MCO	Program same as MCO but designed to cover health care costs of senior citizens.	Premium generally less than supplemental plans.
Preferred provider organization (PPO)	One that limits an enrollee's choice to a list of "preferred" hospitals, physicians, and providers. An enrollee pays more out-of-pocket expenses for using a provider not on the list.	Contractual agreement exists between a set of providers and one or more purchasers (self-insured employers or insurance plans). Comprehensive health services at a discount to companies under contract. Focus on health maintenance.
Exclusive provider organization (EPO)	One that limits an enrollee's choice to providers belonging to one organization. May or may not be able to use outside providers at additional expense.	Limited contractual agreement. Less access to select specialists.
Medicare	Federally funded national health insurance program in the United States for people over age 65. Part A provides basic protection for medical, surgical, and psychiatric care costs based on diagnosis-related groups (DRGs). Part B is a voluntary medical insurance; covers physician and certain outpatient services.	Payment for plan deducted from monthly individual Social Security check. Covers services of nurse practitioners. Does not pay full cost of certain services. Supplemental insurance is encourged.
Medicaid	Federally funded, state-operated program of medical assistance to people with low incomes. Individual states determine eligibility and benefits.	Finances a large portion of maternal and child care for the poor. Reimburses for nurse midwifery and other advanced practice nurses (varies by state). Reimburses nursing home funding.
Private insurance	Traditional fee-for-service plan. Payment computed after services are provided on basis of number of services used.	Policies typically expensive. Most policies have deductibles that clients must meet before insurance pays.
Long-term care insurance	Supplemental insurance for coverage of long-term care services. Policies provide a set amount of dollars for an unlimited time or for as little as 2 years.	Very expensive. Good policy has a minimum waiting period for eligibililty, payment for skilled nursing, intermediate or custodial care, and home care.

LEVELS OF HEALTH CARE

The health care industry is moving toward health care practices that emphasize managing health rather than managing illness. The premise is that in the long term, health promotion reduces health care costs. A wellness perspective focuses on the health of populations and the communities in which they

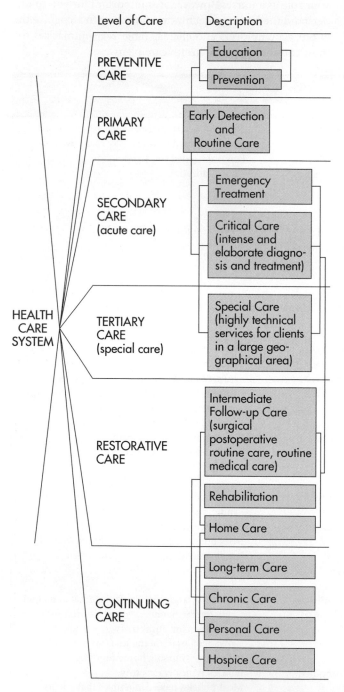

FIGURE **2-1** Spectrum of health services delivery. (Modified from Cambridge Research Institute: *Trends affecting the U.S. health care system,* 262, Health Planning Information Series, Human Resources Administration, Public Health Service, Department of Health, Education, and Welfare, Washington, DC, 1976, revised and updated 1992, U.S. Government Printing Office.)

live rather than just on finding a cure for an individual's disease. Larger health care systems have attempted to develop **integrated delivery networks (IDNs)** that include a set of providers and services organized to deliver a coordinated continuum of care to the population of clients served at a capitated cost. An integrated system can reduce duplication of services, coordinate care across settings, and ensure that clients receive care in the most appropriate setting (Curran, 1997).

The health care system provides six levels of care (Figure 2-1): preventive, primary, secondary, tertiary, restorative, and continuing care. Levels of care describe the scope of services and settings where health care is offered to clients in all stages of health and illness. For example, the secondary level of care is the traditional **acute care** setting where clients who have signs and symptoms of disease are diagnosed and treated. **Restorative care** includes those settings and services where clients who are recovering from illness or disability receive rehabilitation and supportive care. Levels of care are not the same as levels of prevention (see Chapter 1). Levels of prevention describe the focus of health-related activities: avoiding disease (health promotion and disease prevention), curing disease (secondary prevention), and diminishing complications (tertiary prevention). At any level of care, nurses and other health care providers offer a variety of levels of prevention. The nurse working in an acute care, tertiary setting, for example, monitors the recovery of a post-

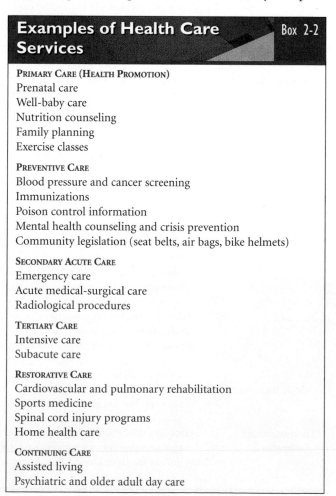

Examples of Health Care Services   Box 2-2

PRIMARY CARE (HEALTH PROMOTION)
Prenatal care
Well-baby care
Nutrition counseling
Family planning
Exercise classes

PREVENTIVE CARE
Blood pressure and cancer screening
Immunizations
Poison control information
Mental health counseling and crisis prevention
Community legislation (seat belts, air bags, bike helmets)

SECONDARY ACUTE CARE
Emergency care
Acute medical-surgical care
Radiological procedures

TERTIARY CARE
Intensive care
Subacute care

RESTORATIVE CARE
Cardiovascular and pulmonary rehabilitation
Sports medicine
Spinal cord injury programs
Home health care

CONTINUING CARE
Assisted living
Psychiatric and older adult day care

operative open heart surgery client while also providing health promotion information to the family concerning diet and exercise.

It is important for you to understand how levels of care are organized and delivered. Each level creates different requirements and opportunities for your role as a nurse. Box 2-2 highlights the types of services available to clients and families at each level of care. Changes unique to each level of care have developed as a result of health care reform. For example, greater emphasis is now placed on wellness; thus more resources are directed toward primary and preventive care. Nursing has the chance to provide leadership to communities and health care systems that are aligning resources to better serve their populations. Critical to the success of improving health care delivery will be the ability to find strategies that better address client needs at all levels of care.

Preventive and Primary Health Care Services

In the settings where preventive and **primary care** are delivered, such as schools, physician offices, occupational health clinics, and nursing centers, health promotion is a major theme (Table 2-2). Health promotion is a key to quality health care. Successful programs help clients acquire healthier lifestyles and achieve a decent standard of living. The focus of health promotion is to keep people healthy through personal hygiene, good nutrition, clean living environments, regular exercise, rest, and the adoption of positive health at-

titudes. Health promotion programs can lower the overall costs of health care by reducing the incidence of disease, minimizing complications, and thus reducing the need to use more expensive health care resources. In contrast, preventive care is more disease oriented and focused on reducing and controlling risk factors for disease through activities such as immunization and occupational health programs.

Community health nursing is an approach that merges knowledge from public health sciences with professional nursing theory to safeguard and improve the health of populations in a community (Ayers and others, 1999). The focus of community health nursing is an emphasis on the health of a community and the subpopulations that inhabit the community (Figure 2-2). An expert community health nurse comes to understand the needs of a population or community through experience with individual families and working through their social and health care issues. Critical thinking (see Chapter 5) becomes important for the nurse to apply knowledge of public health principles, community health nursing, family theory, and communication in finding the best approaches in partnering with families. A successful community health nursing practice involves building relationships with a community and being responsive to changes within the community (Diekemper and others, 1999).

The environment of the community in which a person lives significantly influences the person's health. The health problems that commonly affect members of a low socioeconomic level can often be traced to poor community services,

Preventive and Primary Care Services		Table 2-2
Type of Service	Purpose	Available Programs/Services
School health	Comprehensive programs that integrate health promotion principles throughout a school's curriculum. Program management, interdisciplinary collaboration, and community health principles are stressed.	Positive life skills Nutritional planning Health screening Counseling Communicable disease prevention Crisis intervention
Occupational health	A comprehensive program geared to health promotion and accident or illness prevention. Aim is to increase worker productivity, decrease absenteeism, and reduce use of expensive medical care.	Environmental surveillance Physical assessment Health screening Health education Communicable disease control Counseling
Physicians' offices	Provide primary health care (diagnosis and treatment). Beginning to focus more on health promotion practices. Advanced nurse practitioners often partner with a physician in managing patient population.	Routine physical examination Health screening Diagnostics Treatment of acute and chronic ailments
Nursing centers	Nurse-managed clinics provide nursing services with a focus on health promotion and health education, chronic disease assessment management, and support for self-care and caregivers.	Day care Physical and developmental Health risk appraisal Wellness counseling Employment readiness Acute and chronic care management
Block and parish nursing	Nurses living within a neighborhood provide services to older clients or those unable to leave their home. Fills in gaps not available in traditional health care system.	Running errands Transportation Respite care Homemaker aides

PUBLIC HEALTH IN AMERICA

Vision:
Healthy people in healthy communities

Mission:
*Promote physical and mental health and
prevent disease, injury, and disability*

Public health

- Prevents epidemics and the spread of disease
- Protects against environmental hazards
- Prevents injuries
- Promotes and encourages healthy behaviors
- Responds to disasters and assists communities in recovery
- Assures the quality and accessibility of health services

Essential public health services

- Monitors health status to identify community health problems
- Diagnoses and investigates health problems and health hazards in the community
- Informs, educates, and empowers people about health issues
- Mobilizes community partnerships to identify and solve health problems
- Develops policies and plans that support individual and community health efforts
- Enforces laws and regulations that protect health and ensure safety
- Links people to needed personal health services and assures the provision of health care when otherwise unavailable
- Assures a competent public health and personal health care workforce
- Evaluates effectiveness, accessibility, and quality of personal and population-based health services
- Researches for new insights and innovative solutions to health problems

Source: Essential Public Health Services Work Group of the Core
Public Health Functions Steering Committee

Membership: American Public Health Association
Association of State and Territorial Health Officials
National Association of County and City Health Officials
Institute of Medicine, National Academy of Sciences
Association of Schools of Public Health
Public Health Foundation
National Association of State Alcohol and Drug Abuse Directors
National Association of State Mental Health Program Directors
U.S. Public Health Service
Centers for Disease Control and Prevention
Health Resources and Services Administration
Office of the Assistant Secretary for Health
Substance Abuse and Mental Health Services Administration
Agency for Health Care Policy and Research
Indian Health Service
Food and Drug Administration

FIGURE **2-2**   Public health in America. (From U.S. Public Health Service: *The core functions project, 1993,*
Rockville, Md, 1993, Office of Disease Prevention and Health Promotion.)

such as water treatment, waste disposal, air quality, and transportation services. Pender (1996) notes that communitywide collaboration in health care delivery is a key to developing a system of health promotion services that is user-friendly, well integrated, and responsive to the needs of citizens. Nurses in occupational and school health roles, as well as nurses in business, education, and public policy, influence the conditions of their community at large.

Making a community healthy requires the work of many people. Individual citizens, community organizations, the media, schools, churches, and businesses must all collaborate to meet the needs of the whole community. Community-based intervention enhances opportunities for information exchange and social support. Costs of health promotion programming are reduced because large groups rather than small ones are the recipients of services. A community-based health promotion program offers comprehensive instead of fragmented approaches to health promotion and illness prevention (Weiss, 1984).

Secondary and Tertiary Care

The diagnosis and treatment of illness are traditionally the most commonly used services of the health care delivery system. With the arrival of managed care, these services are now often delivered in primary care settings. For example, more physicians are performing simple surgeries in office surgical suites. However, once a client develops a more complicated problem, the physician is often not able to care for a particular condition. As a result, a medical specialist is often needed, which may require hospitalization of the client. Typically secondary and tertiary care (also called *acute care*) are quite costly, particularly if clients wait to seek health care until after symptoms have developed.

Hospital emergency departments, urgent care centers, critical care units, and inpatient medical-surgical units are the sites that provide secondary and tertiary levels of care. When you work in these settings, you will be challenged to work closely with all members of the health care team. Your ability to think critically and to identify clients' changing problems quickly and accurately will be essential. Planning and coordination of care are necessary to deliver services in a competent and timely manner. Your application of nursing research findings to the selection of nursing interventions will improve client outcomes. As a nurse you will constantly evaluate whether care is effective and how it can be improved.

Client satisfaction becomes a priority in a busy, stressful location such as an inpatient nursing unit. Clients expect you to treat them courteously and respectfully and to involve them in daily care decisions. Acute care nurses must be responsive to learning client needs and expectations early to form effective partnerships that ultimately enhance the level of nursing care given.

HOSPITALS.   Hospitals traditionally have been the major agency of the health care system. Typically, a client came to a hospital for diagnosis and treatment and stayed there until almost fully recovered. This has changed with the arrival of prospective payment and DRGs. Hospitals now offer better public access to outpatient treatment services, and many have redesigned nursing units. Now more services are available on nursing units, thus minimizing the need to transfer and transport clients across multiple diagnostic and treatment areas. Customer service is the philosophy of most acute care organizations.

Hospitalized clients are acutely ill and need comprehensive and specialized tertiary health care. The services provided by hospitals vary considerably. Small rural hospitals may only offer limited emergency and diagnostic services, as well as general inpatient services. In comparison, large urban medical centers offer comprehensive, state-of-the-art diagnostic services, trauma and emergency care, surgical intervention, intensive care units, inpatient services, and rehabilitation facilities. Larger hospitals also offer professional staff from a variety of specialties such as social service, respiratory therapy, physical and occupational therapy, and speech therapy. The focus in hospitals is to provide the highest quality of care possible so that clients can be discharged early but safely to the home or a facility that can adequately manage remaining health care needs.

If you choose to work within a hospital you will have the opportunity to work in a variety of roles and different departments outside of direct client care on a nursing unit. The care of hospitalized clients requires you to have the knowledge and skills for using critical thinking and applying the nursing process (see Unit 2) to deliver appropriate nursing therapies, provide client education, facilitate family support, and coordinate health care services and discharge planning. As your depth of nursing knowledge increases you may choose to specialize in an area of practice. This allows you to become expert in the care of select client populations such as clients with oncologic, orthopedic, pulmonary, or cardiac problems. Other opportunities for nurses within a hospital setting may include the role of client educator, staff educator, nurse manager, clinical nurse specialist, or infection control coordinator.

INTENSIVE CARE.   An intensive care unit (ICU) or critical care unit is a hospital unit in which clients receive close monitoring and intensive medical care. The units are equipped with the most advanced technologies, such as computerized cardiac monitors, intravenous infusion devices, and mechanical ventilators. Although many of these devices can be found on regular nursing units, the clients hospitalized within ICUs are monitored and maintained on multiple devices. Nursing and medical staff within an ICU are educated on critical care principles and techniques. An ICU is the most expensive delivery site for medical care because of the staffing pattern required to deliver care and the related volume of treatments and procedures the clients must undergo.

SUBACUTE CARE.   **Subacute care** units are designated sites that provide medical specialty care for clients who need a greater intensity of care than generally provided in a skilled nursing facility but who no longer require acute care (Stahl, 1994). Generally clients who have suffered an acute illness, injury, or worsening of a disease and require continued hospitalization are candidates for subacute care. The clients require a transitional phase of stabilization and often still have intensive medical, social, and familial needs. Clients receive goal-oriented treatment given immediately after or instead of acute hospitalization to treat one or more specific active, complex medical conditions or to administer technically complex treatments (Stahl, 1994). Many of the clients who require subacute care are **outliers** (clients with extended lengths of stay, well beyond allowed inpatient DRG days). Thus a hospital can transfer a client to a subacute unit and reduce its financial burden, because the stay on the unit meets different reimbursement guidelines. In addition, physicians worry less over releasing clients to an outside setting when a hospital-based subacute unit is available. Subacute units are located in hospitals and in skilled nursing and rehabilitation facilities. The typical clients seen on subacute units include those being rehabilitated after cerebrovascular accidents, trauma, and respiratory failure.

PSYCHIATRIC FACILITIES.　Clients who suffer emotional and behavioral problems such as depression, violent behavior, and eating disorders often require special counseling and treatment in psychiatric facilities. Located in hospitals, independent outpatient clinics, or private mental health hospitals, psychiatric facilities offer inpatient and outpatient services, depending on the seriousness of the problem. Clients may enter these facilities voluntarily or involuntarily. Hospitalization involves relatively short stays with the purpose of stabilizing clients before transfer to outpatient treatment centers. Psychiatric clients receive a comprehensive multidisciplinary treatment plan involving them and their families. Medicine, nursing, social work, and activity therapy collaborate to develop a plan of care that will enable clients to return to functional states within the community. At discharge from inpatient facilities, clients are usually referred for follow-up care at clinics or with counselors.

RURAL HOSPITALS.　Access to health care in rural areas has been a serious problem. Most rural hospitals have had a severe shortage of primary care providers. Many have been forced to close because of economic failure. In 1989 the Omnibus Budget Reconciliation Act (OBRA) directed the U.S. Department of Health and Human Services (USDHHS) to create a new health care entity, rural primary care hospitals (RPCHs). An RPCH provides 24-hour emergency care, with no more than six inpatient beds for providing temporary care for 72 hours or less to clients needing stabilization before transfer to a larger hospital. Physicians, nurse practitioners, or physician assistants staff the RPCH. The RPCH provides inpatient care to acutely ill or injured persons before they are transferred to better-equipped facilities. Basic radiological and laboratory services are also available.

With health care reform, more big-city health care systems are branching out and establishing affiliations or merg-

ers with rural hospitals. The rural hospitals provide a referral base to the larger tertiary care medical centers. Nurses who work in rural hospitals or clinics often function independently in the absence of a physician. Competence in physical assessment, clinical decision making, and emergency care are essential. Nurse practitioners use medical protocols or work under collaborative agreements with staff physicians.

Restorative Care

Clients recovering from acute illnesses or who have chronic illnesses or disabilities usually require services designed to restore the client's level of health. Care is necessary until clients return to their previous level of function or reach a new level of function limited by their illness or disability. The goal of restorative care is to assist an individual to regain maximal functional status, thereby enhancing the individual's quality of life. The intent is to promote client independence and self-care. With the emphasis on early discharge from hospitals, there are few clients who do not require some level of restorative care. For example, surgical clients require ongoing wound care, activity and exercise management, and sometimes diet interventions until they have recovered to a point at which they can independently resume normal activities of daily living.

The intensity of care has increased in restorative care settings, because clients leave hospitals earlier. It is not uncommon to have clients in a home or rehabilitation setting still receiving intravenous fluids (see Chapter 14), enteral nutrition (see Chapter 30), and pain control therapy (see Chapter 29). The restorative health care team is an interdisciplinary group of health professionals and includes the client and family or significant others. In restorative settings, nurses recognize early that success is dependent on effective partnering with clients and their families. Clients and families require a clear understanding of goals for physical recovery, the rationale for any physical limitations, and the purpose and potential risks associated with therapies. The more clients and families are involved in restorative care, the more likely that they will be motivated to follow treatment plans and that clients will be able to achieve optimal functioning.

Community-based nursing involves the acute and chronic care of individuals and families that enhances their capacity for self-care and promotes autonomy in decision making (Ayers and others, 1999). Although care takes place in community settings such as the home, the focus is nursing care of the individual or family. Because clients receive direct care services where they live, work, and play, it is important for community-based nursing to remain individual and family oriented and to appreciate the values of a community (Zotti and others, 1996). As a nurse working in a community-based practice you must understand the interaction of all social units while caring for the client and family in their natural environment. The human ecology model seen in Figure 2-3 reveals the units you will interact with as a nurse. You will become involved in the first three circles (individual and immediate family, extended family, and local

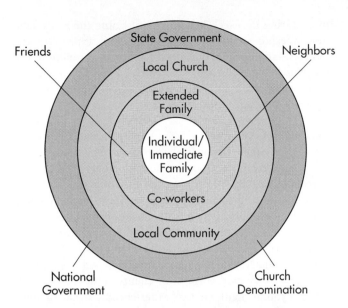

FIGURE **2-3** These concentric circles represent the social interaction units of the human ecology model. (From Ayers M, Bruno AA, Langford RW: *Community-based nursing care: making the transition,* St. Louis, 1999, Mosby.)

community) when you provide health care. For example, as a home health nurse working with a diabetic client attempting to control blood sugar levels, you will work closely with the client and family to establish a comprehensive plan for the client's health. You may become involved in knowing the habits or lifestyle patterns when the client is with friends and co-workers to anticipate ways to plan an exercise schedule and meal routines. You will work closely with family members or friends, educating them on signs and symptoms of hypoglycemia and what to do should the client have a crisis. Knowing available community resources (e.g., medical supply shops, local diabetes association support groups) will enable you to provide the client comprehensive support.

Although community-based nursing cares for clients from diverse cultures and backgrounds, and with various health conditions, changes in the health care delivery system have made a nurse's principal clients those from high-risk groups. **Vulnerable populations** of clients are those who are more likely to develop health problems as a result of excess risks, who have limits in access to health care services, or who are dependent on others for care. Individuals living in poverty, older adults, homeless persons, individuals in abusive relationships, mentally ill persons, and new immigrants to this country are examples of vulnerable populations. Vulnerable individuals and families often belong to more than one of these groups. Frequently these clients come from varied cultures, have different beliefs and values, face language barriers, and have few sources of social support (Chalmers and others, 1998). To become competent in a community-based nursing practice you must have a strong knowledge base in family theory (see Chapter 20), principles of communication (see Chapter 8), and cultural diversity (see Chapter 16).

HOME HEALTH.   **Home health care** is the provision of medically related professional and paraprofessional services and equipment to clients and families in their homes for health maintenance, education, illness prevention, diagnosis and treatment of disease, palliation, and rehabilitation. Nursing is the one service most often used as a result of client needs; however, home health care might also include medical and social services; physical, occupational, speech, and respiratory therapy; and nutritional therapy. A home health service also coordinates the access to and delivery of home health equipment, or durable medical equipment (DME), which is any medically related product adapted for home use.

Home health care agencies provide almost every type of health care service in the client's home. Health promotion and education are traditionally the primary objectives of home care, yet at present, most clients receive professional services on the basis of some medically related need. The focus is on client and family independence. Recovery and stabilization of illness must be addressed in the home, where problems related to lifestyle, safety, environment, family dynamics, and health care practices can be identified.

Home health care agencies provide skilled and intermittent professional services and home health aide services. These services usually are delivered once or twice a day, up to 7 days a week. Box 2-3 summarizes some of the services offered by home health care agencies. Approved home health care agencies usually receive reimbursement for services from the government (such as **Medicare** and **Medicaid** in the United States), private insurance, and private pay. The government has strict, elaborate regulations for governing reimbursement for home health care services. An agency cannot simply charge for a service and expect to receive full reimbursement. Most professional services are reimbursed at the costs for providing the service by government programs. Commercial payers, such as Blue Cross, often negotiate contract rates or provide reimbursement for billed charges.

Home health nurses provide individualized care and have one-on-one contact with clients and families. They are independent and have their own caseloads. The home health nurse helps clients adapt to any permanent or temporary physical limitations so that a more normal daily home routine can be assumed.

REHABILITATION.   **Rehabilitation** is the restoration of a person to the fullest physical, mental, social, vocational, and economic usefulness possible (Clemen-Stone and others, 1995). Clients require rehabilitation after a physical or mental illness, injury, or chemical addiction. Rehabilitation was once available primarily for clients with illnesses or injury to the nervous or musculoskeletal system, but the health care delivery system has expanded its scope of such services. At present, specialized rehabilitation services, such as cardiovascular and pulmonary rehabilitation programs, help clients and families adjust to necessary changes in lifestyle and learn to function with the limitations of their disease. Drug rehabilitation centers help the

---

Home Health Care Services   Box 2-3

WOUND CARE

Sterile dressing changes, debridement and irrigations, packing, and instructing clients and families in wound care techniques

RESPIRATORY CARE

Oxygen therapy, mechanical ventilation, suctioning, and care of tracheotomies

VITAL SIGNS

Monitoring blood pressure and cardiopulmonary status; instructing clients and families in vital sign measurement

ELIMINATION

Ostomy care, appliance application, skin care, and irrigation; insertion of indwelling and intermittent urinary catheters, irrigation, and instructing families in catheter management; home dialysis

NUTRITION

Administration of tube feedings and enternal feedings; assessment of nutrition and hydration status; instructing clients and families in tube feedings

REHABILITATION

Ambulation and gait training, use of assistive devices, range-of-motion exercises, and instructing clients and families on transfer techniques

MEDICATIONS

Monitoring compliance; administering injections; and instructing clients and families on drug information, medication preparation, and steps to take in the event of side effects

INTRAVENOUS THERAPY

Administration of blood products, analgesic and chemotherapeutic agents, and long-term hydration

Instructing clients and families on use of intravenous devices, steps to take in the event of disconnection of accidental fluid infusion, and side effects

LABORATORY STUDIES

Blood glucose monitoring (including client and family instruction) and drawing blood for specific diagnostic purposes

---

client become free from drug dependence and return to the community.

Rehabilitation services include physical, occupational, speech therapy, and social services. Ideally rehabilitation begins the moment a client enters a health care setting for treatment. For example, some orthopedic programs now have clients undergo physical therapy exercises before major joint repair to enhance their recovery postoperatively. Initially rehabilitation may focus on the prevention of complications related to the illness or injury. As the condition stabilizes, rehabilitation helps to maximize the client's functioning and level of independence.

Rehabilitation occurs in many health care settings, including specific rehabilitation institutions, outpatient settings, and the home. Frequently clients needing long-term rehabilitation (e.g., stroke and spinal injury clients) have severe disabilities affecting their ability to carry out the activities of daily living. When rehabilitation services are provided in outpatient settings, clients receive treatment at specified times during the week but remain at home the rest of the time. Specific rehabilitation strategies are applied to the home environment so that maximal levels of function and independence can be achieved. Nurses and other members of the health care team visit homes and help clients and families learn to adapt to illness or injury.

EXTENDED CARE FACILITIES.   An **extended care facility** provides intermediate medical, nursing, or custodial care for clients recovering from acute illness or clients with chronic illnesses or disabilities. Extended care facilities include intermediate care and skilled nursing facilities. Some include long-term care and assisted living facilities (see later discussion of continuing care). At one point, extended care facilities primarily cared for older adults. However, as hospitals manage clients toward early discharge, there is a greater need for intermediate care settings for clients of all ages. For example, a young client who has experienced a stroke or traumatic accident may be transferred to an extended care facility for rehabilitative or supportive care until discharge to the home becomes a safe option. The growth of extended care facilities will increase as the number of older adults grows.

An intermediate care or **skilled nursing facility** offers skilled care from a licensed nursing staff. This may include administration of intravenous fluids, wound care, long-term ventilator management, and physical rehabilitation. Clients receive extensive supportive care until they can move back into the community or into residential care. Extended care facilities provide around-the-clock nursing coverage. Nurses employed in such a setting have expertise similar to that of nurses working in acute care inpatient settings, in addition to a background in gerontological nursing principles (see Chapter18).

Continuing Care

Clients across the life span who have long-term health care needs are the chronically ill and disabled. Continuing care describes a collection of health, personal, and social services provided over a prolonged period to persons who are disabled, who never were functionally independent, or who suffer a terminal disease. The need for continuing health care services is growing in the United States and Canada. People are living longer, and many of those with continuing health care needs have no immediate family members to care for them. A decline in the number of children families choose to have, the aging of care providers, and the increasing rates of divorce and remarriage complicate this problem. Continuing care is available within institutional settings (e.g., nursing centers or nursing homes, group homes, and retirement communities), communities (e.g., adult day care and senior centers), or the home (e.g., home health, home-delivered meals, and hospice) (Lueckenotte, 2000).

NURSING CENTERS OR FACILITIES.   The language of long-term care is confusing and constantly changing. The nursing home has been the dominant setting for long-term care (Lueckenotte, 2000). With the Omnibus Budget

---

The Major Regulatory Level A Requirements Defined by OBRA 1987
Box 2-4

Resident rights
Admission, transfer, and discharge rights
Resident behavior and facility practices
Quality of life
Resident assessment
Quality of care
Nursing services
Dietary services
Physician services
Specialized rehabilitative services
Dental services
Pharmacy services
Infection control
Physical environment
Administration

From Leuckenotte A: *Gerontologic nursing,* ed 2, St. Louis, 2000, Mosby.

Minimum Data Set and Examples of Resident Assessment Protocols
Box 2-5

MINIMUM DATA SET
Resident's background
Cognitive, communication/hearing, and vision patterns
Physical functioning and structural problems
Mood, behavior, and activity pursuit patterns
Psychosocial well-being
Bowel and bladder continence
Health conditions
Disease diagnoses
Oral/nutritional and dental status
Skin condition
Medication use
Special treatments and procedures

RESIDENT ASSESSMENT PROTOCOLS (EXAMPLES)
Delirium
Falls
Pressure ulcers
Psychotropic drug use

Reconciliation Act of 1987, the term *nursing facility* became the term for nursing homes and other facilities where long-term care is provided. Now, *nursing center* is the most appropriate term. A nursing center typically provides 24-hour intermediate and custodial care such as nursing, rehabilitation, dietary, recreational, social, and religious services for residents of any age with chronic or debilitating illnesses. In some cases clients stay in nursing centers for room, food, and laundry services only. The majority of persons living in nursing centers are older adults. A nursing center is a resident's temporary or permanent home with surroundings made to be as homelike as possible (Sorrentino, 2000).

The number of people over the age of 65 in the United States who live in nursing centers or nursing facilities is estimated at over 1.4 million (AARP, 1998). Nursing centers have been under attack for years because of claims regarding inadequate care and abuse. Many of the claims have been justified. However, the nursing center industry has become one of the most highly regulated industries in the United States. These regulations have raised the standard of services provided. One regulatory area that deserves special mention is that of resident rights. Nursing facilities must recognize residents as active participants and decision makers in their care and life in institutional settings (Lueckenotte, 2000). This also means that family members are active partners in the planning of residents' care. Box 2-4 summarizes the types of standards currently established for nursing centers.

Interdisciplinary functional assessment of residents is the cornerstone of clinical practice within nursing centers (Lueckenotte, 2000). Government regulations require that each resident be comprehensively assessed, with care planning decisions made within a prescribed period. A resident's functional ability (e.g., ability to perform activities of daily living

and instrumental activities of daily living) and long-term physical and psychosocial well-being are the focus. The Resident Assessment Instrument (RAI) must be completed on all residents. The RAI consists of the **Minimum Data Set (MDS)** (Box 2-5), Resident Assessment Protocols (RAPs), and utilization guidelines of each state. The RAI ultimately can provide a national database for nursing facilities so that policy makers can better understand the health care needs of this long-term care population. In addition the MDS is a rich resource for nurses in determining the best type of interventions to support the health care needs of this growing population.

ASSISTED LIVING. **Assisted living** is one of the fastest growing industries within the United States (Meyer, 1998). Assisted living offers an attractive long-term care setting with a homier environment and greater resident autonomy. Clients require some assistance with activities of daily living but remain relatively independent within a partially protective setting. A group of residents live together but each resident has his or her own room and shares dining and social activity areas. Usually people keep all of their personal possessions in their residences. Facilities range from hotel-like buildings with hundreds of units to modest group homes that house a handful of seniors. Services in an assisted living facility include laundry, assistance with meals and personal care, 24-hour oversight, and housekeeping (Sorrentino, 2000). Some facilities provide assistance with medication administration. Nursing care services are not directly provided, although a home care nurse can visit an assisted living facility after a client is discharged home.

Unfortunately most residents of assisted living facilities pay privately (Meyer, 1998). With no government fee caps and little regulation, assisted living may not be an option for individuals with limited financial resources. Many states are under pressure to provide financial help through Medicaid. Assisted living is seen as a viable and cheaper alternative to nursing centers.

RESPITE CARE.   The need to care for family members within the home can create great physical and emotional burdens for adult caregivers, especially when the family member is physically or cognitively limited in function. The caregiver is usually an adult who not only has the responsibility for providing care to a loved one (e.g., spouse, parent, sibling) but often must maintain a full-time job, raise a family, and manage the routines of daily living as well. **Respite care** is a service that provides short-term relief or time off for persons providing home care to an ill, disabled, or frail older adult (Lueckenotte, 2000). Adult day care is one form of respite care. Respite care can also be provided by trained volunteers in the home. The family caregiver is able to leave the home for errands or just some social time while a responsible person stays in the home to care for the loved one. Alternatively, a client may be temporarily placed in a nursing center to provide the family relief.

ADULT DAY CARE CENTERS.   **Adult day care centers** provide a variety of health and social services to specific client populations who live alone or with family in the community. Services offered during the day allow family members to maintain their lifestyles and employment and still provide home care for their relatives (Lueckenotte, 2000). Day care centers may be associated with a hospital or nursing home or exist as independent centers. Frequently the clients of such centers do not require hospitalization but need continuous health care services while their families or support persons work. These clients include older adults needing daily physical rehabilitation, individuals with emotional illnesses needing daily counseling, and individuals with chemical dependence problems who are involved in rehabilitation programs. The centers usually operate 5 days per week during typical business hours and usually charge on a per diem basis. Adult day care centers allow clients to retain more independence by living at home, thus potentially reducing the costs of health care by avoiding or delaying an older adult's admission to a nursing center.

Services offered in day care settings include transportation to and from the facility, assistance with personal care, nursing and therapeutic services (e.g., counseling, rehabilitation), meals, and recreational activities (Lueckenotte, 2000). Nurses working in day care centers provide continuity between care delivered in the home and in the center. For example, nurses ensure that clients continue to take prescribed medication and administer specific treatments. Knowledge of community needs and resources is essential in providing adequate support of clients, who often spend only a few hours a week in the day care setting (Ebersole and Hess, 1998).

HOSPICE.   A **hospice** is a system of family-centered care that allows clients to live and remain at home with comfort, independence, and dignity while alleviating the strains caused by terminal illness. The focus of hospice care is palliative care, not curative treatment (see Chapter 29). A hospice can benefit a client in the terminal phases of any disease, such as cardiomyopathy, multiple sclerosis, AIDS, or cancer.

A client entering a hospice is at the terminal phase of illness, and the client, family, and physician agree that no further treatment can reverse the disease process. Staff collaborate to provide care that ensures death with dignity in the client's home. Hospice care is available 24 hours a day, 7 days a week, and services continue without interruption if the client's care setting changes. Occasionally a client must be admitted to a hospice unit within a hospital. The client and family must accept the fact that the hospice will not use emergency measures such as cardiopulmonary resuscitation to prolong life. The focus is on symptom management and ensuring the client's comfort. The hospice multidisciplinary team collaborates continuously with the client's physician to develop and maintain a client-directed individualized plan of care.

Hospice nurses work in institutional and community settings. They are committed to the philosophy and objectives of the facilities for which they work. They provide care and support for the client and family during the terminal phase and at the time of death and continue to offer bereavement counseling and follow-up to the family after the client's death. Many hospice programs provide respite care, which is important in maintaining the health of the primary caregiver and family.

ISSUES IN HEALTH CARE DELIVERY

The climate in health care today influences health care professionals as well as consumers. In the midst of an evolving health care system, you as a nurse must be prepared to participate fully and effectively within the managed care environment. Berwick (1994) suggests "only those who provide care can in the end change care." As you face issues of how to maintain health care quality while reducing costs, you will need to acquire the knowledge, skills, and values necessary to practice competently and effectively. It will also become more important than ever before to collaborate with your colleagues in health care in designing new approaches for client care delivery.

Competency

The Pew Health Professions Commission (1991), in response to the *Healthy People 2000* initiative, recommended competencies for health care professionals that included the practice of prevention and caring for the community's health (Box 2-6). A close look at these competencies suggests they can be applied to institutional settings as well. The health care practitioner competencies offer an excellent yardstick for gauging how well you practice nursing and the type of professional you become. A consumer of health care should expect that the standards of nursing care and practice in any health care setting are appropriate, safe, and efficacious. Ongoing competency is your responsibility. Health care organizations ensure quality care by establishing policies, procedures, and protocols that are scientifically sound

Pew Commission Competencies for Health Care Practitioners   Box 2-6

CARE FOR THE COMMUNITY HEALTH

Broad understanding of health determinants (environmental, socioeconomic, behavioral, genetic, medical)

Ability to work with others in the community to integrate services to prevent illness and promote and protect health

EXPAND ACCESS TO EFFECTIVE CARE

Participation in efforts that promote health care access for individuals, families, and communities

PROVIDE CONTEMPORARY CLINICAL CARE

Possession of up-to-date clinical skills that meet the public's health care needs

EMPHASIZE PRIMARY CARE

Ability and willingness to function in new health care settings

Participation in interdisciplinary arrangements designed to meet primary health care needs

TAKE PART IN COORDINATED CARE

Ability to work as effective team member in organized settings

Emphasis on quality, cost-effective, and integrated services

ENSURE COST-EFFECTIVE, APPROPRIATE CARE

Ability to balance cost and quality in decision-making processes

PRACTICE PREVENTION

Emphasis on primary and secondary preventive strategies with all people

INVOLVE CLIENTS AND FAMILIES IN DECISION-MAKING PROCESS

Expectation of active participation in health care decisions by individuals and their families

Active involvement of client and family in evaluation of quality and acceptability of care received

PROMOTE HEALTHY LIFESTYLES

Ability to assist individuals, families, and communities in maintaining healthy behaviors

ASSESS AND USE TECHNOLOGY APPROPRIATELY

Understanding of, and ability to use, increasingly complex technology

IMPROVE THE HEALTH CARE SYSTEM

Understanding of determinants and operations of health care system from political, economic, social, and legal perspectives

Ability to improve the operations and accountability of the health care system

MANAGE INFORMATION

Ability to manage and use large volumes of scientific, technological, and client information

UNDERSTAND THE ROLE OF THE PHYSICAL ENVIRONMENT

Ability to assess, prevent, and mitigate impact of environmental hazards on the public

PROVIDE COUNSELING ON ETHICAL ISSUES

Participation in discussions of ethical issues in health care that affect the public and the health care system

Provision of counseling to clients about pertinent ethical issues

ACCOMMODATE EXPANDED ACCOUNTABILITY

Responsiveness to increasing levels of public, governmental, and third-party participation in, and scrutiny of, the shape and direction of the health care system

PARTICIPATE IN A RACIALLY AND CULTURALLY DIVERSE SOCIETY

Appreciation of growing diversity of the population

Understanding of health status and care needs from different cultural perspectives

CONTINUE TO LEARN

Anticipation of changes in health care and maintenance of professional competency throughout practice life

Data from Pew Health Professions Commission: *Health America: practitioners for 2005,* Durham, NC, 1991, The Commission.

and follow national accrediting standards. Your responsibility is to follow policies and procedures and to know the most current practice standards. As you progress in your career it becomes your responsibility to obtain necessary continued education and to earn certifications when you choose to practice in specialty areas.

Patient-Centered Care

Hospitals across the country have made changes based on **patient-centered care** concepts to improve work efficiency by changing the way client care is delivered. Ultimately the goal of patient-centered care is to improve the quality of health care while reducing costs. Guiding principles of patient-centered care include the appropriate grouping of clients, restructuring of organizational services for improved responsiveness, decentralization of services, empowerment of employees, and continuity of care. Clients with similar medical or surgical conditions requiring similar services are grouped together on a hospital unit. Redesign of services may include changes such as revising numbers of work stations and supply areas or placing computers or chart stations closer

to client rooms. State-of-the-art technologies such as computerized medical record systems, paging devices, and even wireless phones for medical house staff may be added to improve communication between professional staff members and to help them perform their duties more quickly.

An organization often takes steps to reduce the duplication of tasks and reduce the overall size of the workforce. **Work redesign** is a concept that refers to changing the actual structure and ultimately the responsibilities of the jobs people perform (Tonges, 1992). Specifically, health care institutions look at how care is delivered to clients. Hundreds of work processes make up the work of client care. In work redesign, staff look for ways to work more efficiently, help care providers become more productive, and improve clients' satisfaction with the level of care delivered. Most hospitals can point to inefficiencies in services as a source of increasing costs. The work of client care involves a variety of care providers, often resulting in duplication of work. In work redesign, the staff who are involved in a work process collaborate to determine how the process is being performed (e.g., the admission of clients). Each task or activity (e.g., nursing history, delivering supplies, gathering specimens) associated with the process is reviewed to determine if it is necessary or appropriate. Then the analysis asks who is performing the task and whether that person should be doing it (Tonges, 1992).

In many work redesign efforts it becomes obvious that indirect or nonnursing care activities (e.g., gathering supplies, delivering meals, cleaning client units) take up some of the nurses' time. Work redesign on a client care unit involves identifying care activities that can be safely and appropriately assigned to nonlicensed staff. Many hospitals have developed positions such as the patient service representative. This multiskilled staff member provides no direct client care but assumes a role that combines the elements of housekeeping, dietary, supply clerk, and unit maintenance aspects of a nurse's aide role (Tonges, 1992). Services formerly centralized in hospital departments are often redistributed to client units. Frequently redesign efforts lead to enhanced telecommunication systems and improved support service processes. Well-planned work redesign can improve efficiency, client outcomes, and staff and client satisfaction.

Another important aspect of patient-centered care is continuity of care. As a staff nurse, you will be responsible for contributing to the **discharge planning** process. Discharge planning is a centralized, coordinated, multidisciplinary process that ensures that the client has a plan for continuing care after leaving a health care agency. The process helps in the transition of the client's care from one environment to another (e.g., from hospital to home, from hospital to a rehabilitation facility). Because clients leave hospitals as soon as their physical conditions allow, they often have continuing health care needs when they go home or to another facility. For example, a surgical client may still require wound care. A stroke client may still require ambulation training. Client and family worry about how they will care for the client's needs and manage his or her illness over the long term. As the nurse, you can help by anticipating and identifying clients' continuing needs before the actual time of discharge and by coordinating health team members in achieving an appropriate discharge plan.

Discharge planning begins the moment a client is admitted to a health care facility. The process can occur with any nursing delivery of care model. However, **case management** is particularly focused on discharge planning. In the case management model there is a case manager (usually a nurse or social worker) whose primary responsibility is to coordinate the efforts of all disciplines to achieve the most efficient and appropriate plan of care for the client. The case manager advises nursing staff on specific nursing care issues, coordinates the referral of clients to services provided by other disciplines, ensures that client education has been implemented, and monitors the client's progress through discharge. In many settings a case manager continues caring for clients after discharge from acute care facilities.

Certain clients are more in need of discharge planning because of the risks they present (e.g., clients with limited financial resources, limited family support, and clients with long-term disabilities or chronic illness). However, any client who is being discharged from a health care facility with remaining functional alterations or who must follow certain restrictions or therapies for recovery needs discharge planning. All caregivers who care for a client with a specific health problem must participate in discharge planning. The process is truly multidisciplinary. For example, the diabetic client visiting an education center requires the collaboration of a nurse educator, dietitian, and physician to ensure that the client returns home with the right information to manage the condition. A client who has experienced a stroke will not be discharged from a hospital until plans have been established with physical and occupational therapists to begin a program of rehabilitation.

Effective discharge planning often requires referrals to various health care disciplines. In many agencies a physician's order is needed for a referral, especially when specific therapies are planned (e.g., physical therapy). It is best to have clients and families participate in referral processes so that they are involved early in any necessary decision making. Some tips on making the referral process successful include the following:

- Make a referral as soon as possible.
- Inform the care provider receiving the referral of as much information about the client as possible. This avoids duplication of effort and exclusion of important information.
- Involve the client and family in the referral process, including selecting the necessary referral. Explain the service to be provided, the reason for the referral, and what to expect from the referral's services.
- Determine what the referral discipline recommends for the client's care, and incorporate this into the treatment plan as soon as possible.

Good discharge planning depends on comprehensive client and family education (see Chapter 9). Clients need to know what to do when they get home, how to do it, and what to observe for when problems develop. The Joint Commission on Accreditation of Healthcare Organizations (JCAHO) (2000) requires the following instruction before clients leave health care facilities:

- Safe and effective use of medications and medical equipment
- Instruction on potential food-drug interactions and counseling on nutrition and modified diets
- Rehabilitation techniques to support adaptation to and/or functional independence in the environment
- Access to available community resources as needed
- When and how to obtain further treatment
- The client's and family's responsibilities in the client's ongoing health care needs and the knowledge and skills needed to carry out those responsibilities
- Maintenance of good standards for personal hygiene and grooming

Good discharge planning involves the client from the beginning, uses the strengths of the client in planning, provides resources to meet the client's limitations, and is focused on improving the client's long-term outcomes.

Quality Health Care

Quality health care is difficult to define. Research shows that what clients define as quality health care may not necessarily be the same as what health professionals define as quality (Gerteis and others, 1993). Unless health care providers can define quality, the purchasers of health care (e.g., employers, insurers, HMOs) will buy services based on price alone. The health care system that can deliver a given service (e.g., delivery of a baby and mother-infant care) for the cheapest price will become the primary provider of that service. Health care providers are trying to define how their services are better than their competitors', by measuring health care outcomes. An outcome is a measure of what actually does or does not happen as a result of a process of care; it is the end result (desirable or undesirable) of care delivered (Donabedian, 1966). Examples of outcomes are the readmission rates for surgical clients, functional health status of clients after discharge (e.g., ability and time frame for returning to work), and the rate of infection after surgery. Nursing staff play an important role in gathering and analyzing quality outcome data.

Health plans throughout the United States rely on the Health Plan Employer Data and Information Set (HEDIS) as a quality measure (Greene, 1998). Participating health plans provide vital statistics on more than 70 quality indicators, allowing employers to check on the performance of different health plans. HEDIS is the database of choice for the Health Care Financing Administration (HCFA). One of the most common quality outcome measures is client satisfaction. The JCAHO (2000) requires health care organizations to determine how well an organization meets client needs and expectations. Organizations are using outcomes such as client satisfaction as a basis to redesign how care is managed and delivered in hopes of improving quality in the long term.

CLIENT SATISFACTION.   Almost every major health care organization measures certain aspects of client satisfaction. The Picker/Commonwealth Program for Patient-Centered Care has identified seven dimensions of client-centered care (Box 2-7) that most affect clients' experiences with health care (Gerteis and others, 1993). The seven dimensions cover much of what is the scope of nursing practice. This should be no surprise because nurses are involved in almost every aspect of a client's care in a hospital. A close look shows that most of the dimensions that can be reflected in client satisfaction can be applied to almost any health care setting.

The Picker/Commonwealth Program has a survey tool that measures client satisfaction along the seven dimensions. The survey looks globally at client perceptions of care in an attempt to understand how all hospital departments influence client satisfaction. The survey is conducted through telephone interviews after the client is discharged from the health care setting. Many other companies have developed similar client satisfaction surveys that are distributed in the mail to clients. Staff involved in client care receive the satisfaction scores as feedback regarding their success in meeting client expecta-

The Dimensions of Client-Centered Care   Box 2-7

RESPECT FOR CLIENT'S VALUES, PREFERENCES, AND EXPRESSED NEEDS
Clients expect to be treated with dignity and respect.
Clients want to be informed and involved in decisions about their care.
Clients' perception of needs should not be completely different from those identified by a care provider.

COORDINATION AND INTEGRATION OF CARE
Clients' feelings of powerlessness can be reduced by a competent and caring staff.
Clients look for someone to be in charge of care and to communicate clearly with other health team members.
Clients look to have services and procedures well coordinated.
Clients need to know at all times whom to call for help.

INFORMATION, COMMUNICATION, AND EDUCATION
Clients expect to receive accurate and timely information about their clinical status, progress, or prognosis.
Clients and families need to be informed of major changes in therapies or status.
Tests and procedures must be explained clearly in language clients understand.
Clients and family members want to know how to manage care on their own to the extent they desire or are able.

PHYSICAL COMFORT
Physical care that comforts clients is one of the most elemental services caregivers can provide.
Nurses should respond in a timely and effective way to any request for pain medication, explain the extent of pain clients can expect, and offer alternatives for pain management.

Clients expect privacy and to have their cultural values respected. The health care setting environment should be clean and comfortable.

EMOTIONAL SUPPORT AND RELIEF OF FEAR AND ANXIETY
Clients look to care providers to share their fears and concerns.
Clients need to understand the impact illness will have on their ability to care for themselves and their family.
Clients worry about their ability to pay for their medical care. Are there staff who can help with those worries?

INVOLVEMENT OF FAMILY AND FRIENDS
Care providers must recognize and respect the family and friends on whom clients rely for support.
Clients have the right to determine if family members are to be involved in decisions about their care.
Clients expect those family or friends who will provide physical support and care after discharge to be properly informed.

TRANSITION AND CONTINUITY
Clients want information about medications to take, dietary or treatment plans to follow, and danger signals to look for after hospitalization or treatment.
Clients expect to have their continuing health care needs met after discharge with well-coordinated services.
Clients and family members expect access to any necessary health care resources after discharge.

Data from Gerteis M and others: *Through the patient's eyes*, San Francisco, 1993, Jossey-Bass.

tions. It is the responsibility of staff to identify the unique issues that influence client satisfaction for their area. For example, nurses working on an oncology unit will have different client satisfaction issues around physical comfort than nurses caring for new mothers. Client satisfaction findings become the basis for many quality improvement studies.

It is important for nurses to recognize the need to identify client expectations. The seven dimensions of care provide a useful guide. By learning early what a client expects with regard to information, comfort, and availability of family and friends, you can better plan client care. When should you ask about a client's expectations? It should become a routine question when the client first enters a health care setting, episodically as care continues, and when a client is ultimately discharged from your care. Client expectations are an important measure of the evaluation of nursing care.

Technology in Health Care

Technological advances are influencing where and how nurses provide care to clients. Sophisticated equipment such as computerized intravenous (IV) infusion devices, cardiac telemetry (a device that can monitor a client's heart rate wherever the client is located on a nursing unit), and electronic clinical information systems are just a few examples changing the way health care is delivered. In many ways technological systems make nurses' work easier but they do not replace a nurse's judgment. For example, it is your responsibility when managing a client's intravenous therapy to monitor the infusion to be sure it infuses on time and without complications. An electronic infusion device can provide a constant rate of infusion but you must be sure you calculate the rate correctly. The device will set off an alarm if the infusion slows, making it important for you to respond to the alarm and to troubleshoot the problem. Technology does not replace a nurse's astute, critical eye and clinical judgment.

Electronic clinical information systems have replaced the traditional printed medical record. A comprehensive electronic record of a client's medical problems, treatment, diagnostic procedures, and nursing care offers a rich source of information to clinicians who provide client care. An electronic database also provides valuable information for research and quality improvement activities. For example, a nurse researcher who wishes to track a nursing staff's progress in timely assessment of clients' pain can examine a database to review actual client assessments and the time they occurred.

Documentation on a clinical information system minimizes free text entries and instead allows you to enter information quickly on specially designed flow sheets, pop-up screens, and nursing care plans. The computer displays important data in a way that allows you to follow your client's progress and course easily. An electronic system does not minimize your responsibility for ensuring that clinical information about a client is documented accurately and completely in a timely manner. All members of the health care team usually are able to gain access to the electronic record, thus information must be made accessible as soon as possible. Many hospitals have placed computers at the client's bedside so that the nurse can document care as soon as it is provided. It is important to remember not to depersonalize your care when you use a bedside computer system. As you enter data it can often become easy to avoid interacting with the client, who likely is interested in the type of information you are recording. The use of electronic information systems also requires rigorous confidentiality protocols. It is now easier for anyone to visit a nursing unit and try to gain access to a computer to obtain client information. You will play a role in protecting client rights and ensuring that information is only accessible to those directly involved in a client's care. Chapter 7 reviews principles of nursing documentation.

▌ THE FUTURE OF HEALTH CARE

This discussion on the health care delivery system began with the issue of change. Change threatens many of us, but it also opens up opportunities for improvement. The issue in designing and delivering health care is ultimately the health and welfare of our population. Health care services are not perfect. Many clients fail to obtain a continuum of care when they require multiple health care providers. Many clients are uninsured or underinsured and are unable to gain access to necessary services. However, health care organizations are striving to become better prepared to deal with the challenges in health care. In a survey conducted by *Hospitals and Health Networks,* a health care management journal, hospital executives were asked to rate the importance of 27 issues (Thrall and Hoppszallern, 2001). Box 2-8 lists the top 10 issues executives identified. As you look at these issues it is easy to find nursing right in the middle, strategically positioned to make a difference. Professional nursing is an important player in the future of health care delivery. The solutions necessary to improve the quality of health care will likely not be found without nursing's active participation.

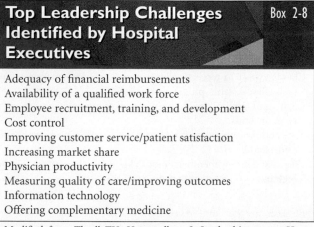

Top Leadership Challenges Identified by Hospital Executives   Box 2-8

Adequacy of financial reimbursements
Availability of a qualified work force
Employee recruitment, training, and development
Cost control
Improving customer service/patient satisfaction
Increasing market share
Physician productivity
Measuring quality of care/improving outcomes
Information technology
Offering complementary medicine

Modified from Thrall TH, Hoppszallern S: Leadership survey, *Hosp Health Netw* 75(3):33, 2001.

Key Terms

acute care, *p. 18*
adult day care centers, *p. 26*
assisted living, *p. 25*
capitation, *p. 16*
case management, *p. 28*
community-based nursing, *p. 22*
community health nursing, *p. 19*
diagnosis-related groups (DRG), *p. 16*
discharge planning, *p. 28*
extended care facility, *p. 24*
home health care, *p. 23*

hospice, *p. 26*
independent practice association (IPA), *p. 17*
integrated delivery networks (IDN), *p. 18*
managed care, *p. 17*
Medicaid, *p. 23*
Medicare, *p. 23*
Minimum Data Set (MDS), *p. 25*
outliers, *p. 22*
patient-centered care, *p. 27*
primary care, *p. 19*
professional standards review organizations (PSRO), *p. 16*

prospective payment system (PPS), *p. 16*
rehabilitation, *p. 23*
respite care, *p. 26*
restorative care, *p. 18*
resource utilization groups (RUG), *p. 16*
skilled nursing facility, *p. 24*
subacute care, *p. 21*
utilization review (UR) committees, *p. 16*
vulnerable population, *p. 23*
work redesign, *p. 27*

Key Concepts

- Changes in health care are being driven by increasing costs and decreasing reimbursement, forcing health care institutions to deliver care more efficiently without sacrificing quality.
- In a managed care system the provider of care receives a predetermined capitated payment regardless of services used by a client.
- The Medicare prospective reimbursement system is based on payment calculated on the basis of DRG assignment.
- Levels of health care describe the scope of services and settings where health care is offered to clients in all stages of health and illness.
- Health promotion occurs in home, work, and community settings.
- Occupational health nursing includes reducing exposure to environmental hazards, health education, and helping workers return to work safely.
- Nurses are facing the challenge of keeping individuals healthy and well within their own homes and communities.
- A successful community health nursing practice involves building relationships with the community.

- Hospitalized clients are more acutely ill than in the past, requiring better coordination of services before discharge.
- Rehabilitation allows an individual to return to a level of normal or near-normal function after a physical or mental illness, injury, or chemical dependency.
- Nurse-managed clinics offer primary care delivered by advanced practice nurses with a focus on helping clients assume more responsibility for their health.
- Home health care agencies provide almost every type of health care service with an emphasis on client and family independence.
- The redesign of care delivery can involve identifying aspects of traditional nursing care that can be safely and appropriately assigned to unlicensed staff.
- Discharge planning helps in the transition of a client's care from one environment to another.
- Health care organizations are being evaluated on the basis of outcomes such as prevention of complications, clients' functional outcomes, and client satisfaction.
- Consumers of health care should be guaranteed competent health care professionals.

Critical Thinking Activities

1. Mrs. Ramirez is a 42-year-old woman who is employed as an advertising agent for a large corporation. She travels 65% of the time. Her company requires her to have a physical examination every 2 years. During a recent "checkup," Mrs. Ramirez was found to have an elevated cholesterol and triglyceride level. Her blood pressure was 134/84 mm Hg, up from 2 years ago. The nurse who conducted the health history learned that Mrs. Ramirez eats "on the go" and only exercises when at home. She also smokes two packs of cigarettes a day. What level of health care did Mrs. Ramirez pursue?

2. When entering Mr. Pierce's room, the nurse notices that he is anxious to speak with her. Mr. Pierce explains, "I am concerned about going home. My doctor wants me to go home tomorrow. My neighbor was in the hospital last year, and he felt like they threw him out before he was ready. I live by myself and I would like to stay here a few more days." Is Mr. Pierce's concern justified? What might the nurse say?

3. Ms. Yim is a 65-year-old married woman who experienced a stroke 4 days ago. She has lost movement on her left side but is able to speak clearly. Explain how she would benefit from case management and why?

Review Questions

1. A client who is concerned about a family history of breast cancer makes an appointment for a routine screening mammography. This is an example of:
   1. tertiary care.
   2. restorative care.
   3. secondary care.
   4. primary care.

2. The greatest amount of health care resources will likely be used when a client receives care in a:
   1. secondary care setting.
   2. continuing care setting.
   3. restorative care setting.
   4. preventive care setting.

3. An example of a nurse providing community health nursing would include:
   1. helping a client obtain resources to pay her electric bill.
   2. providing education to assist a client in managing migraine headache attacks.
   3. setting up a health center to provide respite care services to families of older adults.
   4. assisting a homeless person to acquire medical equipment for insulin injections.

4. A client who is most likely to use the services of a subacute care unit is:
   1. an outlier.
   2. a homeless person.
   3. an acutely ill and unstable client.
   4. a client assigned to a critical pathway.

5. A client who is most likely to be considered a member of a vulnerable patient population is:
   1. a single mother who is raising two children.
   2. an older adult who is unable to pay for monthly drug prescription costs.
   3. a client who has suffered a traumatic spinal cord injury and is unable to walk.
   4. a cancer client who has decided to undergo experimental treatment for his tumor.

6. Respite care is best described as:
   1. a transitional level of care provided between tertiary and restorative care.
   2. a health promotion clinic designed to screen for health problems experienced by the homeless.
   3. a service that offers short-term relief for persons who provide home care to ill family members.
   4. medical specialty care for clients with chronic illness and who require continued hospitalization.

7. An example of a health care outcome is:
   1. the number of times clients seek health screening services.
   2. the ability of clients to return to work following hip replacement.
   3. the average length of time it takes to admit a client to a hospital unit.
   4. the total number of immunizations administered to well babies in a community.

References

American Association of Retired Persons: *A profile of older Americans: 1998,* Washington, DC, 1998, The Association.

Appleby C: Managed care's true values, *Hosp Health Netw* 70(8): 20, 1996.

Ayers M and others: *Community-based nursing care: making the transition,* St. Louis, 1999, Mosby.

Berwick DM: Eleven worthy aims for clinical leadership of health system reform, *JAMA* 272:797, 1994.

Cambridge Research Institute: *Trends affecting the U.S. health care system, 262,* Health Planning Information Series, Human Resources Administration, Public Health Service, Department of Health, Education, and Welfare, Washington, DC, 1976, revised and updated 1992, U.S. Government Printing Office.

Chalmers KI and others: The changing environment of community health practice and education: perceptions of staff nurses, administrators, and educators, *J Nurs Educ* 37:109, 1998.

Clemen-Stone S and others: *Comprehensive community health nursing,* ed 4, St. Louis, 1995, Mosby.

Curran C: The future of academic health centers in a cost-driven market. In McCloskey JC, Grace HK, editors: *Current issues in nursing,* ed 5, St. Louis, 1997, Mosby.

Diekemper M and others: Bringing the population into focus: a natural development in community health nursing practice, part I, *Public Health Nurs* 16:3, 1999.

Donabedian A: Evaluating the quality of medical care, *Milbank Memorial Fund Q* 44:166, 1966.

Ebersole P, Hess P: *Toward healthy aging: human needs and nursing response,* ed 5, St. Louis, 1998, Mosby.

Garg ML and others: Controlling health care costs: regulation versus competition. In McCloskey JC, Grace HK, editors: *Current issues in nursing,* ed 5, St. Louis, 1997, Mosby.

Gerteis M and others: *Through the patient's eyes,* San Francisco, 1993, Jossey-Bass.

Greene J: Blue skies or black eyes? *Hosp Health Netw* 72(8):27, 1998.

Joint Commission on Accreditation of Healthcare Organizations: *Accreditation manual for hospitals,* Oakbrook Terrace, Ill, 2000, The Commission.

Lueckenotte A: *Gerontologic nursing,* ed 2, St. Louis, 2000, Mosby.

Meyer H: The bottom line on assisted living, *Hosp Health Netw* 72(14):22, 1998.

Pender NJ: *Health promotion in nursing practice,* ed 3, St. Louis, 1996, Mosby.

Pew Health Professions Commission: *Health America: practitioners for 2005,* Durham, NC, 1991, The Commission.

Pew Health Professions Commission: *Health professions education and managed care: challenges and necessary responses,* San Francisco, 1995, UCSF Center for the Health Professions.

Stahl D: Subacute care: the future of health care, *Nurs Manage* 25(10):34, 1994.

Sorrentino S: *Mosby's textbook for nursing assistants,* ed 5, St. Louis, 2000, Mosby.

Thrall TH, Hoppszallern S: Leadership survey, *Hosp Health Netw* 75(3):33, 2001.

Tonges MC: Work designs: sociotechnical systems for patient care delivery, *Nurs Manage* 23(1):27, 1992.

U.S. Public Health Service: *The core functions project, 1993,* Rockville, Md, 1993, Office of Disease Prevention and Health Promotion.

Weiss S: Community health promotion demonstration programs: introduction. In Matarazzo JD and others, editors: *Behavioral health: a handbook of health enhancement and disease prevention,* New York, 1984, John Wiley & Sons.

Zotti ME and others: Community-based nursing versus community health nursing: what does it all mean? *Nurs Outlook* 44(5):211, 1996.

Legal Principles in Nursing

Objectives

- Define key terms.
- Explain the legal concepts that apply to nursing practice.
- Give examples of legal issues that arise in nursing practice.
- Describe the legal responsibilities and obligations of nurses.
- Understand the concept of negligence.
- List sources for standards of care for nurses.
- Define the legal aspects of nurse-client, nurse-physician, and nurse-employer relationships.
- Describe the common legal issues that apply to nursing specialties.

*A*s a nurse it is important to have an understanding of the law and how it affects nursing practice. You will be faced with many legal issues that will require the use of critical thinking abilities to practice safe nursing care. Safe and competent nursing care includes an understanding of the legal boundaries within which you must function.

Laws are changing constantly to reflect changes in society and changes in the delivery of health care. You should be aware that state laws vary widely across the country. It is also important to know the law in your own state and the rules and regulations of your state's **regulatory agencies.** If you have specific questions, consult with your own attorney or with your employing institution's attorney.

LEGAL LIMITS OF NURSING

An understanding of the law coupled with sound judgment helps to ensure safe and appropriate nursing care. You must understand the legal limits or standards that affect nursing practice to know your responsibilities as a nurse and to protect clients from harm.

Sources of Law

Nursing practice is subject to statutory law, regulatory law, and common law. Elected legislative bodies such as the U.S. Congress and state legislatures create **statutory law.** An example of a statute enacted by the U.S. Congress is the Americans With Disabilities Act (ADA), which protects the rights of handicapped individuals (ADA, 1990). An example of statutes enacted by state legislatures are the **Nurse Practice Acts,** which are found in all 50 states and the District of Columbia. Administrative bodies such as State Boards of Nursing create regulatory law or administrative law when they pass rules and regulations. An example of regulatory law is the duty to report incompetent or unethical nursing behavior to the state board of nursing. Courts create **common law** when individual legal cases are decided. Examples of common law are informed consent and the client's right to refuse treatment.

Statutes are either criminal or civil. **Criminal law** is classified as a felony or a misdemeanor. A **felony** is a serious offense that has a penalty of imprisonment for greater than a year or possibly even death. A **misdemeanor** is a less serious **crime** that has a penalty of a fine or imprisonment for less than a year. An example of criminal conduct for nurses would be misuse of a controlled substance.

Civil laws protect individual rights. Violation of a **civil law** results in the payment of money to the injured party. A **tort** is a civil wrong or injury for which the court provides a remedy in the form of money damages (Black, 1999). Torts are classified as intentional or unintentional. Intentional torts are willful acts that violate another person's rights. Examples of intentional torts are assault and battery. Unintentional torts include negligence. **Negligence** is conduct that falls below the standard of care. Malpractice is one example of negligence. **Malpractice** is defined as professional misconduct or unreasonable lack of skill (Black, 1999).

INTENTIONAL TORTS

ASSAULT.   **Assault** is any intentional threat to bring about harmful or offensive contact with another individual. No actual contact is necessary. The law protects clients who are afraid of harmful contact. It may be considered an assault to threaten to give a client an injection or to threaten to restrain a client for an x-ray procedure when the client has refused consent.

BATTERY.   **Battery** is any intentional touching without consent. The contact can be harmful to the client and cause an injury, or it can be merely offensive to the client's personal dignity. A battery always includes an assault, which is why the two terms *assault* and *battery* are commonly combined. In the example where you threaten to give a client an injection without the client's consent, if you actually give the injection, it may be considered a battery. Another example of a battery is when the wrong surgical procedure is performed. For example, if a client gives consent for an appendectomy but the surgeon performs a tonsillectomy, a battery has occurred.

UNINTENTIONAL TORTS

NEGLIGENCE AND MALPRACTICE.   Negligence is conduct that falls below the standard of care. The **standard of care** is established by law to protect people from the unreasonable risk of harm (Black, 1999). It is very simply the conduct of a "reasonable person." For example, if you are driving a car and fail to stop at a stop sign, your conduct is negligent. In general, courts define negligence as failure to use that degree of care that a reasonable person would use under the same or similar circumstances.

Malpractice is one type of negligence, called *professional negligence.* To establish the elements of negligence against you, the client must allege the following: (1) you (**defendant**) owed a duty to the client (**plaintiff**), (2) you breached that duty, (3) the client was injured, and (4) the injury occurred as a result of your breach of duty (Showers, 2000; Fiesta, 1999). If you give nursing care that does not meet appropriate standards, a claim for negligence or nursing malpractice may be alleged against you. That negligence may involve your failure to check a client's arm band and administering medication to the wrong client. It may also involve your administering a medication to a client even though it has been documented that the client has an allergy to that medication. In general, the law defines nursing negligence as failure to use that degree of care that a reasonable nurse would use under the same or similar circumstances (Showers, 1999).

Certain common negligent acts have resulted in lawsuits against hospitals and nurses (Box 3-1). All of these acts have something in common. They are generally caused by carelessness or mistakes involving medications, intravenous (IV) therapy, equipment, or client falls. They can also be caused by failure to monitor the client's condition appropriately and communicate that information to the physician.

The best way to avoid being liable for negligence is to follow standards of care; to give competent health care; to com-

Common Sources of Negligence
Box 3-1

You should be aware of the common negligent acts that have resulted in lawsuits against hospitals and nurses:

1. Medication errors that result in injury to clients
2. Intravenous therapy errors resulting in infiltrations or phlebitis
3. Burns to clients caused by equipment, bathing, or spills of hot liquids and foods
4. Falls resulting in injury to clients
5. Failure to use aseptic technique where required
6. Errors in sponge, instrument, or needle counts in surgical cases
7. Failure to give a report, or giving an incomplete report, to an oncoming shift
8. Failure to adequately monitor a client's condition
9. Failure to notify a physician of a significant change in a client's status

municate with other health care providers; to document client assessments, interventions, and evaluations fully; and to develop a caring rapport with the client. A client who believes that you performed your duties correctly and were concerned with his or her welfare is less likely to initiate a lawsuit against you. In addition, if you are brought into a lawsuit, careful, complete, and thorough documentation is one of your best defenses (Showers, 2000). Be sure you know the current nursing literature in your area of practice. You should also know and follow the policies and procedures of the institution in which you work. By being sensitive to common sources of client injury, such as falls and medication errors, you will be in a position to prevent client injury (Fiesta, 1998). Finally, you must communicate with the client, explain the tests and treatment to be performed, and listen to the client's concerns about the treatment. Any significant changes in the client's condition must be reported to the physician and documented in the medical record.

MALPRACTICE INSURANCE.   **Malpractice insurance** usually provides you with an attorney, the payment of attorney's fees, and the payment of any judgment or settlement if you are sued for medical malpractice. If you are employed by a health care institution, you are generally covered by that institution's insurance while working within the scope of your employment. Usually you do not need to purchase any supplemental insurance unless you plan on practicing nursing outside of your employing institution. If you were called on by neighbors and friends to provide nursing care on a volunteer basis, you would not be covered by the hospital's insurance if a neighbor or friend filed suit against you. However, if you volunteered in an emergency, you would be covered by your state's Good Samaritan laws as long as you acted without gross negligence (Higginbotham, 2000).

STANDARDS OF CARE

Nursing standards of care are the legal guidelines for safe nursing practice. The standards of care are defined in the

Nurse Practice Acts of the State Board of Nursing of each state, state and federal hospital licensing laws, professional and specialty organization standards, and the written policies and procedures of the employing institution (Showers, 2000). There is also a body of law referred to as case law or common law, which consists of prior court rulings that affect nursing practice.

The Nurse Practice Acts of each state define the scope of nursing practice and expanded nursing roles, set educational requirements for nurses, and distinguish between nursing practice and medical practice. There are also rules and regulations enacted by the State Boards of Nursing that define the practice of nursing more specifically. For example, a state board may develop a rule regarding the administration of intravenous therapy.

Professional organizations also define standards of nursing care. The American Nurses Association (ANA) has developed standards for nursing practice, policy statements, and similar resolutions (see Chapter 4). The standards delineate the scope, function, and role of the nurse and establish clinical practice standards. The Joint Commission on Accreditation of Healthcare Organizations (JCAHO) requires that accredited hospitals fulfill certain standards with regard to nursing practice, such as having written policies and procedures. Nursing specialty organizations also define the standards of care for nurses to be certified in specialty areas such as the operating room or critical care areas. These standards of care also determine whether a nurse is acting appropriately when performing professional duties.

The written policies and procedures of an employing institution define the standards of care for nurses at that institution. These policies are usually quite specific and are set forth in policy and procedure manuals found on most nursing units. For example, a policy and procedure will outline the steps to take when changing a dressing or administering a medication. Know the policies and procedures of your employing institution because this is one of the standards by which you will be measured if you are involved in a lawsuit.

If you are involved in a malpractice trial, the jury will be told the standards of care and it will determine whether you have acted the way a reasonable nurse would have acted in similar circumstances. If you are a specialized nurse such as a nurse anesthetist, intensive care nurse, certified nurse midwife, or operating room nurse, you may be held to the standards of care and skill exercised by those in the same specialty area. In most cases a nursing expert will testify for the client about the standards of care to establish that you were negligent. You will also most likely have a nursing expert testify on your behalf as to the appropriate standard of care and whether your actions were reasonable.

The best way to stay familiar with the current legal issues affecting your practice is to read the nursing literature in your practice area. Current nursing literature deals with the changing obligations and standards of care for nurses, explains pertinent state and federal laws, and should keep you up-to-date on any new rules, regulations, or case law.

GOOD SAMARITAN LAWS

Good Samaritan laws have been enacted in almost every state to encourage nurses to assist in emergency situations. These laws limit liability and offer legal immunity if a nurse helps at the scene of an accident. For example, if you stop at the scene of an automobile accident and give appropriate emergency care such as applying pressure to stop hemorrhage, you are acting within accepted standards, even though proper equipment was not available. If the client subsequently develops complications as a result of your actions, you are immune from liability as long as you acted without gross negligence (Higginbotham, 2000). The statutes also provide that a nurse can assist a minor in an emergency at the scene of an accident or a competitive sports event before obtaining the parent's consent.

LICENSURE

To practice nursing, you must be licensed by the Board of Nursing of the state in which you practice. All states require registered nurses to have a passing score on the National Council Licensure Examination (NCLEX) to obtain an initial license. Some states require accrual of continuing education credits for relicensure.

A nursing license can be suspended or revoked by the State Board of Nursing if a nurse's conduct violates provisions of the licensing statute. For example, performance of an illegal act such as selling or taking controlled substances could jeopardize your license status. Because your license is considered a property right, due process must be followed before your license can be suspended or revoked. Due process means that you must be notified of the charges against you and a hearing must be conducted so that you can present evidence to defend yourself. The hearing would not be conducted by a judge in a courtroom but would probably be heard by a panel of members of the State Board of Nursing. Some states allow you to file an appeal in court if you have tried and lost all other forms of appeal within the State Board of Nursing.

LEGAL RELATIONSHIPS IN NURSING PRACTICE

In nursing practice, you have a relationship with your clients, with other nurses and health care providers, and with your employer. Liability issues can arise in any of these relationships. *A Patient's Bill of Rights,* adopted by the American Hospital Association, is an unofficial statement of guidelines that provides for collaboration between clients and physicians and other health care professionals (Box 3-2).

Student Nurses

Student nurses are responsible for all of their actions that cause harm to clients. When a client is injured as a direct result of your actions, the liability for the incorrect action may be shared by you, your instructor, the staff nurses working with you, and the hospital or health care facility. Faculty members are responsible for instructing and observing their students, but in some situations staff nurses may also share these responsibilities. As a student nurse you should never be assigned to perform tasks for which you are unprepared. Your instructors should carefully supervise you as you learn new procedures. Every nursing school should provide clear definitions of student responsibility. During the clinical rotation, you as a student nurse are generally covered by the hospital's medical malpractice insurance; however, you should always check with your school as to the specific coverage.

Sometimes you may be employed as a nursing assistant or a nurse's aide when you are not attending classes. During the time when you work as an employee of a health care facility, you should perform only tasks that appear in a job description for a nurse's aide or nursing assistant and the tasks of a licensed nurse should not be delegated to you (Spital, 1999). For example, even if you have learned how to administer intramuscular medications in class, you may not perform this task as a nurse's aide. When you are working at a health care facility, you are probably covered by the institution's insurance. Any time that you are employed, however, you should always inquire about malpractice insurance coverage.

Physician Prescriptions

The physician is responsible for directing the medical treatment of a client. You are responsible for carrying out that medical treatment unless the physician's order or prescription is in error, violates hospital policy, or would be detrimental to the client. Therefore you must assess all physician prescriptions, and if you determine them to be erroneous or harmful, you should obtain further clarification from the physician (Figure 3-1).

If the physician confirms the prescription, but you still believe that it is inappropriate, inform the medical house officer or your supervisor (Warlick, 2000). You should not carry out the physician's prescription if there is a risk that harm will come to your client. Your supervisor should help resolve the questionable prescription. If you carry out the questionable prescription, you may be legally responsible for harm suffered by the client (Fiesta, 1998b).

All physician prescriptions should be in writing and dated and timed appropriately. Make sure that they are transcribed correctly. Verbal prescriptions or telephone prescriptions are not recommended because they leave possibilities for error. If a verbal or telephone prescription is necessary in an emergency, it should be written and signed by the physician as soon as possible, usually within 24 hours (JCAHO, 2001).

In the event that a physician has documented in the progress notes that the client is deteriorating and the decision not to administer cardiopulmonary resuscitation has been made by the physician and the client, the physician should write a "no code" or "do not resuscitate" (DNR) order. Many times the decision regarding lifesaving treatment is in writing in the client's living will or medical directive. If

A Patient's Bill of Rights
Box 3-2

INTRODUCTION

Effective health care requires collaboration between patients and physicians and other health care professionals. Open and honest communication, respect for personal and professional values, and sensitivity to differences are integral to optimal patient care. As the setting for the provision of health services, hospitals must provide a foundation for understanding and respecting the rights and responsibilities of patients, their families, physicians, and other caregivers. Hospitals must ensure a health care ethic that respects the role of patients in decision making about treatment choices and other aspects of their care. Hospitals must be sensitive to cultural, racial, linguistic, religious, age, gender, and other differences, as well as the needs of persons with disabilities.

The American Hospital Association presents *A Patient's Bill of Rights* with the expectation that it will contribute to more effective patient care and be supported by the hospital on behalf of the institution, its medical staff, employees, and patients. The American Hospital Association encourages health care institutions to tailor this bill of rights to their patient community by translating and/or simplifying the language of this bill of rights as may be necessary to ensure that patients and their families understand their rights and responsibilities.

BILL OF RIGHTS*

1. The patient has the right to considerate and respectful care.
2. The patient has the right to and is encouraged to obtain from physicians and other direct caregivers relevant, current, and understandable information concerning diagnosis, treatment and prognosis.

    Except in emergencies when the patient lacks decision-making capacity and the need for treatment is urgent, the patient is entitled to the opportunity to discuss and request information related to the specific procedures and/or treatments, the risks involved, the possible length of recuperation, and the medically reasonable alternatives and their accompanying risks and benefits.

    Patients have the right to know the identity of physicians, nurses, and others involved in their care, as well as when those involved are students, residents, or other trainees. The patient also has the right to know the immediate and long-term financial implications of treatment choices, insofar as they are known.
3. The patient has the right to make decisions about the plan of care prior to and during the course of treatment and to refuse a recommended treatment of plan of care to the extent permitted by law and hospital policy and to be informed of the medical consequences of this action. In case of such refusal, the patient is entitled to other appropriate care and services that the hospital provides or transfer to another hospital. The hospital should notify patients of any policy that might affect patient choice within the institution.
4. The patient has the right to have an advance directive (such as living will, health care proxy, or durable power of attorney for health care) concerning treatment or designating a surrogate decision maker with the expectation that the hospital will honor the intent of that directive to the extent permitted by law and hospital policy.

Health care institutions must advise patients of their rights under state law and hospital policy to make informed medical choices, ask if the patient has an advance directive, and include that information in patient records. The patient has the right to timely information about hospital policy that may limit its ability to implement fully a legally valid advance directive.

5. The patient has the right to every consideration of privacy. Case discussion, consultation, examination, and treatment should be conducted so as to protect each patient's privacy.
6. The patient has the right to expect that all communications and records pertaining to his/her care will be treated as confidential by the hospital, except in cases such as suspected abuse and public health hazards when reporting is permitted or required by law. The patient has the right to expect that the hospital will emphasize the confidentiality of this information when it releases it to any other parties entitled to review information in these records.
7. The patient has the right to review the records pertaining to his/her medication care and to have the information explained or interpreted as necessary, except when restricted by law.
8. The patient has the right to expect that, within its capacity and policies, a hospital will make reasonable response to the request of a patient for appropriate and medically indicated care and services. The hospital must provide evaluation, services and/or referral as indicated by the urgency of the case. When medically appropriate and legally permissible, or when a patient has so requested, a patient may be transferred to another facility. The institution to which the patient is to be transferred must first have accepted the patient for transfer. The patient must also have the benefit of complete information and explanation concerning the need for, risks, benefits, and alternatives to such a transfer.
9. The patient has the right to ask and be informed of the existence of business relationships among the hospital, educational institutions, other health care providers, or payers that may influence the patient's treatment and care.
10. The patient has the right to consent to or decline to participate in proposed research studies or human experimentation affecting care and treatment or requiring direct patient involvement, and to have those studies fully explained prior to consent. A patient who declines to participate in research or experimentation is entitled to the most effective care that the hospital can otherwise provide.
11. The patient has the right to expect reasonable continuity of care when appropriate and to be informed by physicians and other caregivers of available and realistic patient care options when hospital care is no longer appropriate.
12. The patient has the right to be informed of hospital policies and practices that relate to patient care, treatment, and responsibilities. The patient has the right to be informed of available resources for resolving disputes, grievances, and conflicts, such as ethics committees, patient representatives, or other mechanisms available in the institution. The patient has the right to be informed of the hospital's charges for services and available payment methods.

*These rights can be exercised on the patient's behalf by a designated surrogate or proxy decision maker if the patient lacks decision-making capacity, is legally incompetent, or is a minor. (Reprinted with permission of the American Hospital Association, copyright 1992.)

Continued

A Patient's Bill of Rights—cont'd

Box 3-2

The collaborative nature of health care requires that patients, or their families/surrogates, participate in their care. The effectiveness of care and patient satisfaction with the course of treatment depend, in part, on the patient fulfilling certain responsibilities. Patients are responsible for providing information about past illnesses, hospitalizations, medications, and other matters related to health status. To participate effectively in decision making, patients must be encouraged to take responsibility for requesting additional information or clarification about their health status or treatment when they do not fully understand information and instructions. Patients are also responsible for informing their physicians and other caregivers if they anticipate problems in following prescribed treatment.

Patients should also be aware of the hospital's obligation to be reasonably efficient and equitable in providing care to other patients and the community. The hospital's rules and regulations are designed to help the hospital meet this obligation. Patients and their families are responsible for making reasonable accommodations to the needs of the hospital, other patients, medical staff, and hospital employees. Patients are responsible for providing necessary information for insurance claims and for working with the hospital to make payment arrangements, when necessary.

A person's health depends on much more than health care services. Patients are responsible for recognizing the impact of their life-style on their personal health.

CONCLUSION

Hospitals have many functions to perform including the enhancement of health status, health promotion, and the prevention and treatment of injury and disease; the immediate and ongoing care and rehabilitation of patients; the education of health professionals, patients, and the community; and research. All these activities must be conducted with an overriding concern for the values and dignity of patients.

Reprinted with permission of the American Hospital Association, copyright 1992.

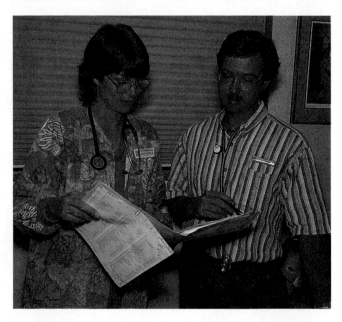

FIGURE **3-1** If an order creates questions, the nurse clarifies it with the physician.

the client is not able to make health care decisions, the order should be discussed with the person designated in the client's durable power of attorney. A "no code" or DNR order should be written, not given verbally. Physicians should regularly review DNR orders in case the client's condition warrants a change. You should be familiar with your institution's policies and procedures concerning DNR orders. Physicians should list all specifics of DNR orders pursuant to the client's living will or durable power of attorney (Eckberg, 1998). For example, a physician may order vasopressor and fluid management to maintain a client's blood pressure but specifically state no chest compression or intubation for cardiac arrhythmias or respiratory arrest.

Consent

A signed consent form from your client is necessary for all routine treatment, hazardous procedures such as surgery, some treatment programs such as chemotherapy, and participation in research studies (JCAHO, 2001). A client will sign a general consent form for treatment when the client is admitted to the hospital or other health care facility. Separate special consent forms must be signed by clients or clients' representatives before specialized procedures may be performed.

State statutes provide the designation of individuals who are legally able to give consent to medical treatment (Austin, 2000). In general, those who may consent to medical treatment include the following:

I. Adults
  A. Any competent individual 18 years of age or older for himself or herself
  B. Any parent for his or her unemancipated minor
  C. Any guardian for his or her ward
  D. Any adult for the treatment of his or her minor brother or sister (if an emergency and parents are not present)
  E. Any grandparent for a minor grandchild (if an emergency and parents are not present)
II. Minors
  A. For his or her child and any child in his or her legal custody
  B. For himself or herself in the following situations:
    1. Lawfully married or a parent (emancipated)
    2. Pregnancy (excluding abortions)
    3. Venereal disease
    4. Drug or substance abuse
  C. Unemancipated minors in some states may not consent to abortions without one of the following:
    1. Consent of one parent
    2. Self-consent being granted by court order
    3. Consent specifically given by a court

If a client is deaf, illiterate, or speaks a foreign language, an interpreter should be available to explain the terms of consent (Austin, 2000). If a client is under the effects of a sedative, the client may not be able to clearly understand the implications of an invasive procedure. As the nurse, you should make every effort to assist your client in making an informed choice.

It is important to be sensitive to the cultural issues of consent and to understand the way in which clients and their families communicate and make important decisions. Also be sure to understand the various cultures with which you will interact. The cultural beliefs and values of your clients may be very different from your own. It is important for you not to impose your own cultural values on your clients.

Informed Consent

Informed consent is a client's agreement to allow something to happen, such as surgery, based on a full disclosure of the risks, benefits, alternatives, and consequences of refusal (Black, 1999). Informed consent requires that the client be given all relevant information required to make a decision, that the client be capable of understanding the relevant information, and that the client actually gives consent. If a procedure is performed on a client without informed consent, the person performing the procedure may be found liable for battery.

The following factors are necessary for consent to be valid (Prosser and Keeton, 1988):

1. The person giving the consent must be mentally and physically competent and be legally an adult (usually over 18 years of age or emancipated).
2. The consent must be given voluntarily; no forceful measures may be used to obtain it.
3. The person giving the consent must thoroughly understand the procedure, its risks and benefits, and alternative procedures.
4. The person giving consent has a right to have all questions answered satisfactorily and confirm his or her understanding of any planned treatment with a health care provider.

Informed consent is part of the physician-client relationship (Fiesta, 1999). Because nurses do not perform surgery or direct medical procedures, obtaining a client's informed consent does not fall within a nurse's responsibility. Even though a nurse may assume the responsibility for witnessing the client's signature on the consent form, the nurse does not legally assume the duty of obtaining informed consent. When you provide consent forms for clients to sign, ask clients if they understand the procedures for which consent is being given. If clients deny understanding, or if you suspect that they do not understand, you must notify the physician or your nursing supervisor. A client refusing surgery or other medical treatment must be informed about any harmful consequences of refusal. If the client persists in refusing the treatment, this rejection should be written, signed, and witnessed (Dunn, 2000).

Parents are usually the legal guardians of pediatric clients, and therefore they are the persons who must sign consent forms for treatment. If the parents are divorced, the parent with legal custody should give consent. Occasionally a parent refuses treatment for a child. In those cases, the court may intervene on the child's behalf.

It may be difficult for you to obtain consent if your client is unconscious. Consent must be obtained from a person legally authorized to give consent on the client's behalf. If the client has executed a durable power of attorney, the document will designate an individual who may give consent for medical treatment. If the client has been declared legally incompetent in a judicial proceeding, consent must be obtained from the client's legal guardian (Austin, 2000; Dunn, 2000). In emergency situations, if it is impossible to obtain consent from the client or an authorized person, treatment may be undertaken. In such cases, the law assumes the client would wish to be treated.

Psychiatric clients must also give consent. They retain the right to refuse treatment until a court has legally determined that they are incompetent to decide for themselves.

Death and Dying

Nurses must know their legal responsibilities concerning death and dying. You must document all events that occur when the dying client is in your care. There are two standards for the determination of death: cardiopulmonary and whole brain (Uniform Determination of Death Act, 1980). The cardiopulmonary standard requires irreversible cessation of a client's circulatory and respiratory functions. The whole brain standard requires irreversible cessation of all functions of the entire brain, including the brain stem. The reason for the development of the different definitions is to facilitate recovery of organs for transplantation. Even though a client may be legally "brain dead," other organs may be healthy for donation. The definitions are also useful when there is a question of whether to continue life support.

An autopsy requires consent by the client before his or her death or by a close family member at the time of the client's death. In many states there is an order of priority for the giving of consent for autopsies, such as (1) decedent (client), in writing before death; (2) durable power of attorney; (3) surviving spouse; and (4) surviving child, parent, brother, or sister in the order named. State statutes provide that when there are reasonable grounds to believe that a client died as a result of violence, homicide, suicide, accident, or death occurring in any unusual or suspicious manner or if a client's death is unforeseen and sudden and a physician has not seen the client in over 36 hours, the coroner should be notified.

You will encounter legal issues associated with caring for clients who are terminally ill, severely debilitated, or in a persistent vegetative state (permanently comatose). One of these legal issues involves the right to refuse medical treatment and the withholding of food and nutrition. The doctrine of informed consent ensures that the client has the right to refuse treatment. The Supreme Court has held that a competent person has the right to refuse medical treatment, including lifesaving food and nutrition (Cruzan, 1990).

You are legally obligated to treat your deceased client's remains with dignity and care. Wrong handling could cause emotional harm to survivors. In one legal case, survivors sued when a mislabeling of bodies led to an Orthodox Jewish person being prepared for a Roman Catholic funeral and a Roman Catholic person being prepared for an Orthodox Jewish burial (In re Schiller, 1977).

Organ and Tissue Donation

A signed consent is necessary before a client's body, tissues, or organs can be donated for medical use. In some states a client can sign the back of his or her driver's license in the presence of witnesses, indicating consent to having his or her body donated. Consent is valid unless the driver's license is revoked, canceled, or suspended, and consent has to be given each time the license is renewed. The hospital will not be liable for honoring the consent of the client even if the family does not give consent. State laws provide whether a nurse may witness the consent of an individual donating his or her body, organs, or tissues for medical use. You should be aware of the policies and procedures of your employing institution and your state's laws when you are asked to serve as a witness for a person who is giving consent for organ donation.

In most states there is a law requiring that at the time of death a qualified health care provider ask the client's family members to consider organ or tissue donation (National Organ Transplant Act, 1984). Individuals can be approached in the following order: (1) the spouse, (2) adult son or daughter, (3) either parent, (4) adult brother or sister, (5) grandparent, and (6) guardian. The person in the highest class can make the donation unless he or she knows of a refusal or contrary indications by the decedent (Uniform Anatomical Gift Act, 1987).

The law also provides that the physician who certifies death shall not be involved in the removal or transplant of organs or tissues. The law also prohibits selling or purchasing of organs and regulates this area of medical and nursing practice. Organ and tissue donation remains voluntary. Consent forms are available for this purpose.

Advance Directives

You will find that many of your clients have living wills or durable powers of attorney (also referred to as medical directives or health care powers of attorney) identifying health care surrogates. A health care surrogate is an individual appointed by the client to make health care decisions. These documents provide written instructions after a client becomes incapacitated (Eckberg, 1998). The Patient Self-Determination Act (1992) requires health care institutions to inquire whether an advance directive such as a living will or durable power of attorney has been created. Be familiar with your employing institution's policies and procedures that comply with the act because you may be asked to provide information about these documents or to inform clients about how they can obtain legal assistance.

Living wills are documents instructing physicians to withhold or withdraw life-sustaining procedures in clients whose death is imminent (Figure 3-2). A **durable power of attorney** is a document that appoints a health care surrogate named by the client to make health care decisions for the client if and when the client becomes incapacitated. Each state providing for living wills has its own requirements for executing them, but generally two witnesses, neither of whom can be a relative or the physician, are needed when the client signs the documents. Durable powers of attorney must be legally prepared with the appropriate witnessing of the client's signature.

MINIMIZING LIABILITY

As a nurse, you will be faced with nursing issues that could become liability concerns. It is important for you to anticipate these issues to be better prepared to deal with any problems that arise.

Short Staffing

You may encounter inadequate staffing during times of nursing shortages, staff downsizing periods, or cost containment. The JCAHO requires institutions to have guidelines for the number of staff needed to care for clients. Legal problems may arise if an institution does not have enough registered nurses to provide competent and safe care. Liability issues occur if a client is injured as a result of negligent care by any personnel (Spital, 1999). Registered nurses (RNs) are always responsible for performing the nursing process. Even though RNs may delegate care to assistive personnel or licensed practical nurses (LPNs), they maintain responsibility for client outcomes (Spital, 1999; Helm, 1998).

If you are assigned to care for more clients than is reasonable for safe care, notify your nursing supervisor. If you are required to accept the assignment, document this information in writing and provide the document to nursing administrators. Although documentation does not relieve you of responsibility if clients suffer harm because of inattention, it shows that you attempted to act appropriately. Whenever you document information about short staffing, keep a copy of the document. Do not walk out when staffing is inadequate because a charge of abandonment could be made. It is important to know your institution's policies and procedures on how to handle inadequate staffing before such a situation arises. The institution may ultimately be held responsible for staffing the hospital so that safe care can be provided (Helm, 1998; Davino, 2000).

Floating

Nurses within acute and long-term care facilities are often required to "float" from the area in which they normally practice to other nursing units. If you float, inform your supervisor of any lack of experience in caring for the types of clients on the new nursing unit. You should also request and be given orientation to the unit. Even if you float to a nursing unit, you will be held to the same standard of care as nurses who regularly work in that area. A supervisor can be

---

LIVING WILL

DECLARATION

I have the primary right to make my own decisions concerning treatment that might unduly prolong the dying process. By this declaration I express to my physician, family and friends my intent. If I should have a terminal condition it is my desire that my dying not be prolonged by administration of death-prolonging procedures. If my condition is terminal and I am unable to participate in decisions regarding my medical treatment, I direct my attending physician to withhold or withdraw medical procedures that merely prolong the dying process and are not necessary to my comfort or to alleviate pain. It is not my intent to authorize affirmative or deliberate acts or omissions to shorten my life rather only to permit the natural process of dying.

Signed this .... day of ....

Signature .... City, County and State of residence ....

....

The declarant is known to me, is eighteen years of age or older, of sound mind and voluntarily signed this document in my presence.

Witness ....

Address ....

Witness ....

Address ....

REVOCATION PROVISION

I hereby revoke the above declaration.

Signed ....
(Signature of Declarant)

Date ....

Missouri Revised Statutes, section 459.015 (1985)

FIGURE **3-2**   Living will form.

---

held liable if a staff nurse is assigned to a client for whom he or she cannot safely care. In one case the court noted that if employers are going to float nurses out of their usual work area of practice, then the employers should provide training and education to prepare the nurses to work in the other areas (*Winkelman v. Beloit Memorial Hospital,* 1992).

Incident Reports

It becomes necessary to complete an **incident report** when anything unusual happens that could potentially cause harm to a client, visitor, or employee or when you make an error. For example, if you administer an incorrect medication to a client or if a client suffers a fall in the hospital, an incident report should be prepared. Most institutions provide specific forms for this purpose (Figure 3-3). You should objectively record the details of the incident and any statements made by the client. An example follows: "Mrs. Jones found lying on floor on right side. Abrasion on right forehead. Client stated, 'I fell

and hit my head.'" At the time of an incident, always contact the physician to examine the client. After examining the client, the physician should document assessment findings and treatment plans in the progress notes. Any untoward effects caused by the incident must also be documented. Subjective assumptions and statements assigning blame or fault should not be included in the chart or the incident report.

Incident reports are not a part of the client's medical record. The reports are generally not admissible in court and in some jurisdictions are considered privileged documents. Know your employing institution's policies and procedures on incident reports. Incident reports are also used by employing institutions for quality improvement and risk management. By reviewing incident reports, administrators can determine areas of client risk. For example, if a certain kind of problem has occurred repeatedly, such as client falls when being transferred to x-ray carts, educational methods can be used to help prevent the problem in the future. In addition,

CONFIDENTIAL INCIDENT REPORT

NOT PART OF MEDICAL RECORD—DO NOT COPY OR RELEASE. This report is prepared in anticipation of litigation for the purpose of securing legal advice on potential claims and to facilitate the prompt intervention and management of such claims by the hospital's attorneys and risk manager. This report and the information contained herein is priviliged.

Dept. #	Incident Date	Incident Time	Person Involved
		____ a.m. ____ p.m.	____ Patient ____ Visitor

Sex	Age	Condition Prior to Incident
____ Male ____ Female		____ Alert & Oriented ____ Other: ____

\# ____
Use addressograph plate or list full name, address and date of birth.

BRIEF DESCRIPTION OF INCIDENT & LOCATION: ____

MEDICATION ☐

____ Dosage
____ Route
____ Omission
____ Duplication
____ Transcription
____ IV Rate
____ IV Infiltration
____ Patient Identification
____ Adverse Reaction to
     Medication/Contrast Media
____ Different Medication/IV Fluid
____ Time Administered
____ Discontinued/Unordered
____ Missing/Stolen
____ Protocol Not Followed
____ Equipment Failure/Malfunction
____ Other ____

Medication(s) Involved:
____
____
____

FALL ☐

____ From Bed With Rails Up Full
____ From Bed With Rails Down x ____
____ From Bedside Commode
____ From Chair/Equipment
____ Going To/From Bathroom
____ While Walking or Standing
____ On Stairs/Ramp
____ Assisted/Lowered to Floor
____ Fainting/Dizziness
____ Slip/Twist (Other than fall)
____ Unknown

Fall Risk Assessment ____

Describe Footwear: ____
____

Describe Surface: ____
____

Other: ____

	YES	NO
Out of Bed Privileges	____	____
Up With Assistance	____	____
Call Light Within Reach	____	____
Call Light Used	____	____
Bed Alarm On	____	____
Sitter on Duty	____	____
Family Notified of Fall	____	____
Protective Device Used	____	____

(Check Type)
____ Posey ____ Wrist
____ Other ____

On Medication ____ ____
(Check Types)
____ Hypnotics
____ Narcotics, I, II
____ Diuretic
____ Antihypertensive
____ Psycotropic
____ Antianxiety
____ Antidepressant

OTHER ☐

NATURE OF INJURY ____ No Apparent Injury ____ Puncture ____ Abrasion ____ Property Other *(describe)*
____ Redness/Edema ____ Contusion/Hematoma ____ Laceration/Skin Tear ____ Burn   Damaged/
____ Numbness ____ Sprain/Strain/Soreness ____ Fracture/Dislocation ____ Hives   Lost ____

ASSESSMENT OF CONDITION   V.S.: B/P____ T.____ P.____ R.____
Other ____

Physician Notified: ____ Yes ____ *(Time/Date)* ____ No   Orders Received: ____ Yes ____ No ____ N/A
To Emergency Department: ____ Yes ____ No ____ Care Refused   **Assessment**
X-Ray Taken: ____ Yes ____ No Results: ____   **Performed By:** ____

WITNESSES
(List Names & Addresses, Unknown or None)
____
____

EQUIPMENT INVOLVED ____ YES ____ NO If **Yes**, list: Type: ____ Manufacturer: ____
Serial No.: ____ Hospital ID No.: ____ Present Location: ____

Report Prepared By *(Name and Title):* ____   **Report Date:** ____

FORM-01

FIGURE **3-3** Confidential Incident Report.

the insurance carrier for a hospital or other institution relies on incident reports to assess liability and possible future claims. Incident reports supplement quality improvement programs to ensure provision of high-quality care.

Risk Management

Risk management is a system of ensuring appropriate nursing care. The steps involved in risk management include identifying possible risks, analyzing them, acting to reduce the risks, and evaluating the steps taken. One tool used in risk management is the incident report.

The underlying rationale for quality improvement and risk management programs is for the organization to achieve the highest possible quality of care. Some insurance companies, medical and nursing organizations, and the JCAHO require the use of quality improvement and risk management procedures (JCAHO, 2001).

Risk management also requires good documentation. Your documentation of nursing care may be your only memory of what actually was done for a client and can serve as proof that you acted reasonably and safely. Documentation should be thorough, accurate, and performed in a timely manner (see Chapter 7). The best way to avoid having to defend yourself in court is to chart factually and defensively. If you chart "physician notified," it may be insufficient when you are questioned about the lawsuit if you do not recall what facts you reported to the physician. When a lawsuit is filed, very often the nurses' notes are the first thing reviewed by an attorney. Your assessments and the reporting of significant changes in the assessments are very important factors in defending a lawsuit.

Reporting Obligations

Health care providers are required to report incidents such as child, spousal, or older adult abuse; rape; gunshot wounds; attempted suicide; or certain communicable diseases. For example, if you examine a sexually abused child in the emergency department, you must report that information to the Division of Family Services. You may also be required to report unsafe or impaired professionals. Because information that must be reported varies among states, you should become familiar with the appropriate statutes in your state and the policies and procedures of your employing institution.

LEGAL ISSUES IN NURSING PRACTICE

It is crucial to be aware of changes in the laws that affect nursing practice and the delivery of the client's care. Certain areas of the law such as the administration of narcotics have remained constant, whereas the issues of abortion and care for clients with the human immunodeficiency virus (HIV) are changing and will change in the future.

Controlled Substances

In 1970 the Comprehensive Drug Abuse Prevention and Control Act was passed in the United States. It controls substances such as narcotics, depressants, stimulants, and hallucinogens. The act regulates hospital drug distribution systems.

Nurses may only administer controlled substances under the direction of a licensed physician. (Some states allow advanced practice nurses to prescribe controlled substances.)

Controlled substances should be kept securely locked, and only authorized personnel should have access to them (see Chapter 13). Precise records must be maintained regarding the dispensing and storage of controlled substances. There are criminal penalties for the misuse of controlled substances. There have been cases in which physicians have illegally prescribed and dispensed controlled substances. If you are employed by such a physician and fail to report these activities, you may be legally accountable for aiding and abetting the physician.

Acquired Immunodeficiency Syndrome

Nurses will care for clients with acquired immunodeficiency syndrome (AIDS) in every segment of their nursing practice, including clients with AIDS on medical-surgical units, mothers and infants in perinatal units, and pediatric clients with hemophilia. Nurses must utilize standard precautions for the control of transmission of the HIV virus when caring for all clients (see Chapter 10). Nurses have the responsibility to safeguard themselves and others from exposure to infectious material. Therefore nurses must appropriately handle, discard, and/or decontaminate items or areas contaminated with body fluids.

The ADA protects the rights of disabled people and is the most extensive law on how employers must treat HIV-infected clients and health care workers (ADA, 1995). Persons with infectious diseases are protected under the handicapped and disabilities laws. Co-workers who refuse to work with HIV-infected people can leave companies open to indirect charges of discrimination if the employer does not monitor the work environment.

Issues of disclosure, privacy, and confidentiality are an important concern when working with HIV- or AIDS-infected clients or peers. Several cases have held that the health care provider may be obligated to disclose the fact that he or she is infected with HIV. The ADA regulations protect the privacy of infected people by giving individuals the opportunity to decide whether to disclose their disability.

As a health care worker, you are not required to be tested for HIV as a condition of employment. If you are contaminated by a client whose HIV status is unknown, you cannot check the client's blood for HIV without the client's consent.

Abortion Issues

In 1973 in the case of *Roe v. Wade,* the U.S. Supreme Court ruled that there is a fundamental right to privacy, which includes a woman's decision to have an abortion. The court ruled that during the first trimester a woman could end her pregnancy without state regulation because the risk of natural mortality from abortion is less than with normal childbirth. During the second trimester the state has an interest in protecting maternal health and the state may enforce regulations regarding the person performing the abortion and the abortion facility. By the third trimester, when the fetus becomes viable, the state's interest is to protect the fetus, so the state can therefore prohibit abortion except when necessary to save the mother. Several subsequent cases have substantially narrowed the *Roe v. Wade* decision primarily in the area of informed consent and the consent of minors.

LEGAL ISSUES IN NURSING SPECIALTIES

Within every specialty of nursing there are legal issues that will affect your nursing practice. Some of the more common legal issues follow.

Psychiatric Nursing

A client can be admitted to a psychiatric unit involuntarily or on a voluntary basis. If a client is admitted involuntarily, a petition for involuntary detention must be filed with the court within 96 hours of the client's initial detention. A hearing must be conducted within 2 days of the filing of the involuntary petition. If the judge determines that the client is a danger to himself or others, the judge will grant the involuntary detention and the client can then be detained for 21 more days for psychiatric treatment.

Many lawsuits occur as a result of suicidal attempts that result in death or disability. The allegations in the lawsuits are usually that the health care provider failed to provide adequate supervision and failed to safeguard the facilities. If the client's history and medical records indicate suicidal tendencies, you must keep the client under supervision. Documentation in the medical record of the frequency of suicide checks and the precautions taken against suicide is essential.

Home Care Nursing

Hospital stays are short due to the expense of inpatient health care, and as a result many clients are being discharged from the acute care setting when they still require nursing care. Nursing care may range from assistance with daily living activities to ventilator care. If you are a home care nurse, you may find that you have greater responsibility and autonomy in the home. Home care, however, differs from the acute care setting because in the hospital setting, hospital personnel and physicians are available to assess client changes. In the home you must know when to call your supervisor or the physician. You must know the policies and procedures of your employer particularly with respect to "chain of command," equipment failure, and informed consent. Chain of command generally means that you must know the hierarchy of supervisors and physicians to report to if problems arise (Warlick, 2000). Be sure to document your assessments and interventions in the client's record so that any claim of inadequate or improper care can be defended.

Key Terms

assault, *p. 34*
battery, *p. 34*
civil law, *p. 34*
common law, *p. 34*
criminal law, *p. 34*
crime, *p. 34*
defendant, *p. 34*

durable power of attorney, *p. 40*
felony, *p. 34*
Good Samaritan laws, *p. 36*
incident report, *p. 41*
informed consent, *p. 39*
living wills, *p. 40*
malpractice, *p. 34*
malpractice insurance, *p. 35*
misdemeanor, *p. 34*

negligence, *p. 34*
Nurse Practice Acts, *p. 34*
plaintiff, *p. 34*
regulatory agencies, *p. 34*
standard of care, *p. 34*
statutory law, *p. 34*
tort, *p. 34*

Key Concepts

- With the increased emphasis on client rights, you must understand legal obligations and responsibilities to clients.
- Under the law you must follow standards of care, which originate in Nurse Practice Acts, the guidelines of professional organizations, and written policies and procedures of employing institutions.
- You are responsible for performing procedures correctly and exercising professional judgment when you carry out physician orders.
- All clients are entitled to confidential health care and freedom from unauthorized release of information.
- You can be found liable for malpractice if the following are established: (1) you (defendant) owed a duty to the client (plaintiff), (2) you did not carry out that duty or breached that duty, (3) the client was injured, and (4) the client's injury was caused by your failure to carry out that duty.

- Informed consent must meet the following criteria: (1) the person giving consent must be competent and of legal age; (2) the consent must be given voluntarily; (3) the person giving consent must thoroughly understand the procedure, its risks and benefits, and alternative procedures; and (4) the person giving consent has a right to have all questions answered satisfactorily.
- You are obligated to follow the physician's prescription unless you believe that it is in error, violates hospital policy, or could be detrimental to the client, in which case you must make a formal report explaining the refusal.
- You must file an incident report in any unusual situation that could potentially cause harm to a client; such reports are also used for quality assurance and risk management.
- A legal definition of death aids in determining when it is appropriate to pursue organ or tissue donation.
- You must be aware of changes in the law that affect nursing practice, including the changing areas of AIDS and abortion.

Critical Thinking Activities

1. You are taking care of Mr. Jones, a confused older adult client with congestive heart failure. You and the orderly from the x-ray department are having a social conversation and not paying attention while transferring Mr. Jones from the bed to the x-ray cart. Mr. Jones falls and fractures his hip. Identify the elements of negligence and how those elements will be applied to this fact situation.
2. At one of your child's school sporting events, Tommy Brown, a 7-year-old, falls from the highest bleacher and stops breathing and is pulseless. What should you do? Should you attempt CPR on the child without his parent's consent? Will your hospital malpractice insurance cover you if you are sued? Will any of your other insurance policies cover you if you do not have your own malpractice insurance?
3. As you are restarting Mr. Smith's intravenous line, it infiltrates and medication leaks into his tissues, causing chemical burns. Subsequently he suffers sloughing of the tissue in his hand, which impairs the use of his hand. Mr. Smith files a lawsuit for negligence against you and the hospital. What definition of negligence will the court use? What standard of care will you be measured by?

Review Questions

1. The most common source of client injury is:
   1. decubitus ulcers.
   2. burns from hot liquids.
   3. transfers from bed to cart.
   4. medication errors and falls.
2. When preparing an incident report:
   1. a copy should be put in the client's record.
   2. subjective information should always be included.
   3. statements made by the client should be included in the report.
   4. if someone was at fault, that person should be blamed in the report.
3. Even though you may obtain the client's signature on a form, obtaining informed consent is the responsibility of the:
   1. client.
   2. physician.
   3. student nurse.
   4. supervising nurse.
4. Your employer's malpractice insurance covers you for:
   1. incidents that occur at your home.
   2. incidents that occur while you are driving to work.
   3. incidents that occur when you are driving home from work.
   4. incidents that occur while you are working within the scope of your employment.
5. When you stop to help in an emergency at the scene of an accident, if the injured party files suit and your employing institution's insurance does not cover you, you will probably be covered by:
   1. your automobile insurance.
   2. your homeowner's insurance.
   3. *A Patient's Bill of Rights,* which may grant immunity from suit if the injured party consents.
   4. the Good Samaritan laws, which grant immunity from suit if there is no gross negligence.
6. You are obligated to follow a physician's order unless:
   1. the order is a verbal order.
   2. the physician's order is illegible.
   3. the order has not been transcribed.
   4. the order is in error, violates hospital policy, or would be detrimental to the client.
7. The legal definition of death that facilitates organ donation is:
   1. cessation of pulse.
   2. cessation of respirations.
   3. cessation of functions of the entire brain.
   4. cessation of circulatory and respiratory functions.

References

American Hospital Association: *A patient's bill of rights,* Chicago, 1992, The Association.

Austin S: Staffing: know your liability, *Nurs Manage* 31(7):19, 2000.

Black HC: *Black's law dictionary,* ed 7, St. Paul, Minn, 1999, West Publishing.

Davino M: What's your risk of liability, *RN* 63(8):80, 2000.

Dunn D: Staff development special: exploring the gray areas of informed consent, *Nurs Manage* 31(7):2025, 2000.

Eckberg E: The continuing ethical dilemma of the do-not-resuscitate order, *AORN J* 67(4):783, 1998.

Fiesta J: Liability for falls, *Nurs Manage* 29(3):24, 1998a.

Fiesta J: Restructuring liability, part I, *Nurs Manage* 29(5):20, 1998b.

Fiesta J: What health care professionals need to know, part I, *Nurs Manage* 30(6):8, 1999.

Helm A: Liability, UAPs, and you, *Nursing* 28(11):52, 1998

Higginbotham E: When the person in danger is not a patient, *RN* 63(8):80, 2000.

Joint Commission on Accreditation of Healthcare Organizations: *Accreditation manual for hospitals,* Chicago, 2001, The Commission.

Prosser W, Keeton W: *Prosser and Keeton on the law of torts,* ed 5, St. Paul, Minn, 1988, West Publishing.

Showers J: Protection from negligence lawsuits, *Nurs Manage* 30(9):23, 1999.

Showers J: What you need to know about negligence lawsuits, *Nursing* 30(2):4549, 2000.

Spital J: Take the anxiety out of working with UAPs, *Nursing* 29(5):32, 1999.

Warlick D: Negligence goes to the top, *Nurs Manage* 31(6):2224, 2000.

Statutes and Cases

Americans With Disabilities Act, 42 USC SS 121.010-12213, 1995.

Cruzan v Director, Missouri Department of Health, 497 U.S. 261 (1990).

Missouri Revised Statutes, section 459.015 (1985).

National Organ Transplant Act, Public Law 98-507, 1984.

Patient Self-Determination Act, 42 CFR 417, 1992.

Roe v Wade, 410 U.S. 113 (1973).

In re Schiller, 148 NJ Super 168 (1977).

Uniform Anatomical Gift Act, 1987.

Uniform Determination of Death Act, 1980.

Winkelman v Beloit Memorial Hospital, 484 NW 2d 211 (Wi 1992).

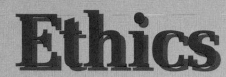

Ethics

Objectives

- Define the key terms listed.
- Discuss accountability and responsibility in nursing practice.
- Discuss client advocacy.
- Describe the role of ethics in nursing practice.
- Discuss the process used to analyze an ethical dilemma.
- Describe ethical conflicts experienced by nurses in different settings.

Nursing practice involves care during all aspects of health, sickness, personal life, and community life. As a nurse, you will play an important and often intimate role in the lives of your clients. Your relationship with clients and with others on the health care team will sometimes require participation in difficult or controversial decisions. Because we live in a nation of many different cultures, you may find yourself faced with complicated situations that arise from these differences. With the support of professional codes of practice and a commitment to critical thinking skills, you will be able to contribute a vital and unique voice to the process of health care delivery.

The study of ethics has occupied the attention of civilization for thousands of years. When human beings gather in community, they turn to concerns about right living. Whether you look to the ancient Chinese philosophers, the dialogues of the ancient Greeks, or traces of Mayan and Aztec culture, you will find evidence of a fundamental human effort to define right and wrong behavior. The term **ethics** refers to the consideration of standards of conduct or the study of philosophical ideals of right and wrong behavior (*American Heritage Dictionary,* 2000).

BASIC DEFINITIONS

Ethical issues differ from legal issues. The content of the **law** is determined by systems of government. Laws are enforced by the same system (Harris, 1998). Breaking a law usually results in a public consequence, such as a ticket for speeding or jail time for stealing. The law guides public behavior that will affect others and that will preserve community. Ethics, on the other hand, has a broader base of interest and includes personal behavior and issues of character, such as kindness, tolerance, and generosity.

A **value** is a personal belief about the worth you hold for an idea, a custom, or an object. The values you hold reflect cultural and social influences. For example, if your family makes a living in a rural place, you may value the environment differently from someone who visits rural areas for recreation. You use your values to shape your own point of view. Systems of ethics usually grow from shared values, negotiated and discussed over time by people who share values, such as religious groups, ethnic groups, or work groups.

As you enter the nursing profession, you will undergo a socialization into the profession. You will learn new values that help to define your role as a nurse and that will influence your point of view. When you have a clear understanding of your values and your point of view, you and the health care team will be able to make effective resolutions regarding difficult ethical issues.

The terms *ethics* and *morals* sometimes are used interchangeably. **Morals** usually refers to judgment about behavior, and ethics is the study of the ideals of right and wrong behavior. Moral codes are more likely to reflect the character of the social setting from which they spring (Davis and Aroskar, 1991).

The study of **bioethics** represents a particular branch of ethics, namely, the study of ethics within the field of health care. Bioethics "narrows ethical inquiry to the moral 'oughts' of those who work in professional clinical practice, basic research, or the education of health professionals. Bioethics affects all health professionals and those who seek their knowledge and skills" (O'Neil, 1998).

The field of bioethics has become a prominent branch of the study of ethics, especially in the last 25 years. When kidney transplant technology was perfected in the early 1970s, the immediate ethical concern became the limited number of kidneys available compared with the greater number of clients in need of a transplant. The advent of advanced medical technologies requires society to face difficult ethical questions. Who should get what resources? What constitutes quality of life? Who should decide? In the study of bioethics, health care professionals agree to negotiate these difficult and important questions.

Nursing professionals play an important role in the practice of bioethics. As O'Neil (1998) explains, "The focus now is a truly interdisciplinary effort by which professionals and society attempt to gain knowledge, guidelines, and agreement on these very complex issues." Nurses participate in bioethical discourse in two distinct ways: As professionals, nurses construct a professional code of ethics that reflects and defines practice; and as colleagues in the practice of health care delivery, nurses develop a specific point of view for contribution to ethical discourse on health care issues.

ETHICAL PRINCIPLES

Practitioners in health care delivery agree to a set of ethical principles that guide professional practice and decision making. These principles are common to all professions in health care. You will find these principles especially useful because they guide our commitment to advocacy, an important concept in caring for others (Table 4-1).

Autonomy refers to a person's independence. As a principle in bioethics, autonomy represents an agreement to respect the client's right to determine a course of action. The agreement to respect autonomy represents the recognition that clients are "in charge of their own destiny in matters of health and illness" (O'Neil, 1998). The purpose of the preoperative consent, for example, is the assurance in writing that the health care team respects the client's independence

Principles of Health Care Ethics		Table 4-1
Principle	Definition	
Autonomy	Independence; self-determination; self-reliance	
Justice	Fairness or equity	
Fidelity	Faithfulness; striving to keep promises	
Beneficence	Actively seeking benefits; promotion of good	
Nonmaleficence	Actively seeking to do no harm	

by obtaining permission to proceed. The consent process implies that a client may refuse treatment, and in most cases, the health care team must agree to abide by the client's refusal.

Justice refers to the principle of fairness. You will often refer to this principle when discussing issues of health care resources. What constitutes a fair distribution of resources may not always be clear. For example, approximately three times more candidates are on a waiting list for liver transplants than there are livers available for transplant in the United States. The just distribution of available organs can be difficult to determine. In the United States, a national multidisciplinary committee strives for fairness by ranking recipients according to need, rather than resorting to selling organs for profit or distributing them by lottery.

Fidelity refers to the agreement to keep promises. The principle of fidelity also promotes your obligation as a nurse to follow through with the care offered to clients. For example, if you assess a client for pain and then offer a plan to manage the pain, the principle of fidelity encourages you to do your best to keep the promise to improve the client's comfort.

The principle of **beneficence** promotes taking positive, active steps to help others. It encourages you to do good for the client. It helps to guide decisions in which the benefits of a treatment may pose a risk to the client's well-being or dignity. A child's immunization may cause discomfort during administration, but the benefits of protection from disease, both for the individual and for society, outweigh the temporary discomforts. The agreement to act with beneficence requires that the best interest of the client remains more important than self-interest. For example, you will not simply practice obedience to medical orders but you will act thoughtfully to understand client needs and then work actively to help meet those needs.

Nonmaleficence refers to the fundamental agreement to do no harm. It is closely related to the principle of beneficence. This principle can be helpful in guiding your discussions about new or controversial technologies. For example, a new bone marrow transplant procedure may promise a chance at cure, but the long-term prognosis may be uncertain, or the procedure may require long periods of pain or suffering. These risks should be considered in relationship to the potential good that may come of the procedure. The principle of nonmaleficence promotes a continuing effort to consider the potential for harm even when it may be necessary to promote health.

CODES OF ETHICS

A **code of ethics** is a set of **ethical principles** that are generally accepted by all members of a profession. A profession's ethical code states the group's expectations and standards of behavior. Codes serve as guidelines to assist nurses and other professional groups when conflict or disagreement arises about correct practice or behavior. The code of ethics for nursing sets forth ideals of nursing conduct and provides a common foundation for nurses' training. The American Nurses Association (ANA) and the International Council of

Nurses (ICN) have established widely accepted codes that you as a nurse should follow. Although these codes differ in specific emphasis, they reflect the same underlying principles (Boxes 4-1 and 4-2), including responsibility, accountability, competency, judgment, and advocacy.

A nurse assumes responsibility and accountability for all nursing care delivered. **Responsibility** refers to the execution of duties associated with a nurse's particular role. The responsible nurse demonstrates characteristics of reliability and dependability. When administering a medication, for example, you are responsible for assessing the client's need for the drug, for giving it safely and correctly, and for evaluating the response to it. By agreeing to responsibility, you will gain trust from clients, colleagues, and society.

When nurses perform care, they must be accountable. **Accountability** refers to the ability to answer for your actions. You are accountable to yourself most of all. You must also balance accountability to the client, the profession, the employing institution, and society (Potter and Perry, 1997). For example, you may know that a client who will be discharged soon re-

---

American Nurses Association Code of Ethics   Box 4-1

1. The nurse, in all professional relationships, practices with compassion and respect for the inherent dignity, worth, and uniqueness of every individual, unrestricted by considerations of social or economic status, personal attributes, or the nature of health problems.
2. The nurse's primary commitment is to the patient, whether an individual, family, group, or community.
3. The nurse promotes, advocates for, and strives to protect the health, safety, and rights of the patient.
4. The nurse is responsible and accountable for individual nursing practice and determines the appropriate delegation of tasks consistent with the nurse's obligation to provide optimum patient care.
5. The nurse owes the same duties to self as to others, including the responsibility to preserve integrity and safety, to maintain competence, and to continue personal and professional growth.
6. The nurse participates in establishing, maintaining, and improving health care environments and conditions of employment conducive to the provision of quality health care and consistent with the values of the profession through individual and collective action.
7. The nurse participates in the advancement of the profession through contributions to practice, education, administration, and knowledge development.
8. The nurse collaborates with other health professionals and the public in promoting community, national, and international efforts to meet health needs.
9. The profession of nursing, as represented by associations and their members, is responsible for articulating nursing values, for maintaining the integrity of the profession and its practice, and for shaping social policy.

The ICN Code of Ethics for Nurses

Box 4-2

PREAMBLE

Nurses have four fundamental responsibilities: to promote health, to prevent illness, to restore health and to alleviate suffering. The need for nursing is universal.

Inherent in nursing is respect for human life, including the right to life, to dignity, and to be treated with respect. Nursing care is unrestricted by considerations of age, color, creed, culture, disability or illness, gender, nationality, politics, race, or social status.

Nurses render health services to the individual, the family and the community and co-ordinate their services with those of related groups.

THE CODE

The *ICN Code of Ethics for Nurses* has four principal elements that outline the standards of ethical conduct.

ELEMENTS OF THE CODE

1. Nurses and People

The nurse's primary professional responsibility is to people requiring nursing care.

In providing care, the nurse promotes an environment in which the human rights, values, customs and spiritual beliefs of the individual, family and community are respected.

The nurse ensures that the individual receives sufficient information on which to base consent for care and related treatment.

The nurse holds in confidence personal information and uses judgement in sharing this information.

The nurse shares with society the responsibility for initiating and supporting action to meet the health and social needs of the public, in particular those of vulnerable populations.

The nurse also shares responsibility to sustain and protect the natural environment from depletion, pollution, degradation and destruction.

2. Nurses and Practice

The nurse carries personal responsibility and accountability for nursing practice, and for maintaining competence by continual learning.

The nurse maintains a standard of personal health such that the ability to provide care is not compromised.

The nurse uses judgement regarding individual competence when accepting and delegating responsibility.

The nurse at all times maintains standards of personal conduct which reflect well on the profession and enhance public confidence.

The nurse, in providing care, ensures that use of technology and scientific advances are compatible with the safety, dignity and rights of people.

3. Nurses and the Profession

The nurse assumes the major role in determining and implementing acceptable standards of clinical nursing practice, management, research and education.

The nurse is active in developing a core of research-based professional knowledge.

The nurse, acting through the professional organization, participates in creating and maintaining equitable social and economic working conditions in nursing.

4. Nurses and Co-Workers

The nurses sustains a co-operative relationship with co-workers in nursing and other fields.

The nurse takes appropriate action to safeguard individuals when their care is endangered by a co-worker or any other person.

Modified from International Council of Nurses: *ICN code of ethics for nurses,* Geneva, 2000, 3, place Jean-Marteau, CH-1201, The Association.

mains confused about how to self-administer insulin. The action that you take in response to this situation will be guided by the professional commitment to accountability. You might request more hospitalization or arrange home care to continue teaching at home. The goal is the prevention of injury to the client. The principle that guides you is accountability.

A responsible nurse is competent in knowledge and skills. **Competence** refers to specific skills necessary to perform a task (*American Heritage Dictionary,* 2000). Regulations that guide the documentation of competence vary from state to state, but the agreement to practice with competence is contained in the nursing code of ethics. For example, you make sure you know all about a drug before you administer it. You understand a client's expected response to the medication. Because you are competent, the client can trust that medications you offer are safe.

Judgment refers to the ability to form an opinion or draw sound conclusions (*American Heritage Dictionary,* 2000). You begin to learn good judgment in nursing school. You will improve your judgment skills continuously over your career.

Advocacy involves giving clients the information they need to make decisions and then supporting those decisions. It also implies that caretakers will strive to understand and then to articulate a client's point of view. Within the health care sys-

tem, a multidisciplinary team participates in the delivery of care. All members strive to advocate for the client. You will become an important and unique part of that team. You will know your clients through your assessments, while administering difficult or uncomfortable procedures, while teaching new skills, and preparing for discharge or home care. These activities allow you to witness important aspects of a client's ability to cope, learn, and heal. Your ability to document, articulate, and contribute forms a key aspect of client advocacy.

DEVELOPING A PERSONAL POINT OF VIEW

The ability to clarify and articulate your own **point of view** and then to assess and speak for the point of view of clients provides the foundation for your ability to adhere to the professional code of ethics. An individual's point of view reflects cultural and societal influences. It is influenced by relationships with others and by personal values. Values vary among people and develop and change over time. Understanding your own values and recognizing the value systems of others may help reduce conflict during decision making.

An **ethical dilemma** exists when the right thing to do is not clear or when members of the health care team cannot agree on the right thing to do. Many ethical dilemmas require the negotiation of differing points of view. Once you have come to understand and clarify your own point of view, you can turn to the client and begin to clarify the client's point of view. Your goal with a client is effective nurse-client communication. As the client becomes more willing to express problems and feelings, you can better establish an individualized plan of care. If ethical problems arise, your clear understanding of the client's point of view will help you to speak for the client even if your own point of view differs.

When the topic concerns issues of health, personal habits, and quality of life, all participants in a discussion will benefit by a clarity of personal values and personal points of view. Your respect for client differences and your skills in helping a client to clarify a point of view will promote your ability to teach and to heal.

Ethics concerns itself with what people see as good and in that sense flows from values and personal points of view. Ethics is a disciplined reflection on good conduct, character, and motives that seeks to settle claims of what constitutes the "good" or valuable among people with differences. The use of ethics in decision making strives to go beyond personal preferences and to establish standards on which individuals, professions, and societies agree.

ETHICAL SYSTEMS

Traditional study of ethics tends to be highly abstract and theoretical (O'Neil, 1998; Beauchamp and Childress, 2001). When health care providers struggle with ethics, they require concrete strategies. Traditional theories of ethics, however, do provide a foundation for devising strategies. These philosophies overlap in some areas and compete in others. It will be important for you to acquire a basic understanding of these perspectives. For one thing, many health care providers use language from one or another of these philosophies when they discuss ethical issues. In addition, you should be aware of the differences between philosophies. Your point of view will be influenced by these philosophies. Your personal values will probably influence which of these will work best for you as you learn to negotiate difficult ethical situations that arise in your practice.

Deontology

This system of ethics is perhaps most familiar to practitioners in health care. Deontology defines actions as right or wrong based on their "right-making characteristics such as fidelity to promises, truthfulness, and justice" (Beauchamp and Childress, 2001). It locates the essence of right or wrong in these principles, as opposed to looking to consequences of actions to determine rightness or wrongness. The conventional use of ethical principles such as justice, autonomy, and beneficence (see Table 4-1, p. 47) constitutes the practice of deontology.

Deontology proposes that we determine the presence or absence of autonomy, justice, fidelity, beneficence, and nonmaleficence in an individual situation. We then use this determination as a guide for decisions about right action. If an act is just, respects autonomy, and provides good, then the act will be ethical. Difficulty arises when a person must choose between conflicting principles, which is often the case in health care ethical dilemmas. Also, conflict may occur when people do not agree on definitions of the principles.

Utilitarianism

A utilitarian ethic proposes that the value of something is determined by its usefulness. The greatest good for the greatest number of people is the guiding principle for all action in this system. As with deontology, this theory relies on the application of certain principles, namely, measures of "good" and "greatest." The fundamental difference between utilitarianism and deontology is in the focus on consequences or outcomes. Utilitarianism measures the effect that an act will have; deontology looks to the pure presence of principle. Difficulties arise when people have conflicting definitions of "greatest good."

Feminist Ethics

A strong foundation for feminist ethics grew out of the changes in society that occurred as more women entered the workplace during the last century (Sherwin, 1992). For example, until the early 1980s, conventional teaching held that the highest stages of moral development tend to be more commonly reached by men than by women (Kohlberg, 1981). For Kohlberg, moral development occurs in measurable, predictable stages. The most complex stage incorporates a sense of justice, and by Kohlberg's measure, young girls do not reach this stage as often as young boys. Carol Gilligan (1993) argues that Kohlberg's measures of moral development were gender biased. Her theory of moral development attempts to accommodate gender differences without valuing one gender over the other. She maintains that young girls tend to pay attention to community and to individual circumstances, and young boys tend to process dilemmas through ideals or principles determined abstractly.

Feminist ethics proposes that an inequality of attention to women can be remedied by asking, routinely, how ethical decisions will affect women (Sherwin, 1992). For example, in a discussion regarding the ethics of fetal surgery (surgical intervention before birth of the child), feminist ethics would propose that the effect of the intervention on the mother is paramount and would hold the mother's autonomy higher than the autonomy of the fetus.

Ethics of Care

This ethical theory explores issues of nursing, gender, and ethical dilemmas. Its proponents pay special attention to the nursing point of view and nursing practice (Fry, 1989). As Leininger (1988) has written, care is the "central and unifying domain for the body of knowledge and practices in nursing." Its principles apply to all members of a health care community, not just nurses (see Chapter 15).

The word *care* derives from an old English term, *caru,* meaning "sorrow" or "troubled state of mind" (*American Heritage Dictionary,* 2000). Contemporary use generally implies feeling concern or interest in one who has sorrow or perhaps even sharing that concern. It can also mean taking care of in the sense of providing for or protecting against trouble.

Nurses base their work in caring: for the client, for the client's family, and for the maintenance of the institutions that provide the services. **Ethics of care** suggest that ethical dilemmas will be solved by attention to relationships, by attention to particular narratives or stories of the participants, and by the examination and promotion of any fundamental act of caring. This attention to relationship distinguishes the ethics of care from other ethical viewpoints because it does not necessarily apply universal principles that are intellectual or analytical (Watson, 1994).

The ultimate test of an ethical system lies in its ability to guide individuals through dissent or confusion. The technologies of contemporary medicine often create ethical dilemmas, in which competing points of view leave members of the health care team or the team and the client in conflict. You strengthen your ability to advocate for a client when you can identify your personal point of view and then accurately identify the views of the client.

HOW TO PROCESS AN ETHICAL DILEMMA

Ethical problems can be distressing for both clients and caregivers. An ethical outcome, however, is not obtained by considering only what people want and feel. A guide for processing ethical dilemmas serves to protect individual points of view while promoting resolution.

Most health care institutions have an ethics committee by which ethical dilemmas are processed. An ethics committee is generally multidisciplinary, with representatives from nursing, medicine, and other disciplines. Some institutions, especially hospitals, may maintain a council specifically for nurses. Such a council serves to educate nurses and others about the ethical process. A nursing ethics committee can be especially helpful for the nurse who feels powerless or confused in the presence of an ethical dilemma.

Whether an ethical dilemma is resolved in a committee setting, at the bedside, or in a family conference, the nurse applies a careful, critical processing of the dilemma (Box 4-3). Resolving an ethical dilemma is similar to the nursing process because it requires deliberate, systematic thinking (Miller and Babcock, 1996).

Step 1: Is this an ethical dilemma?

The first step guides you to determine if the problem is an ethical one. Not all problems are ethical. You will learn to distinguish ethical problems from questions of procedure, legality, or medical diagnosis. Curtin and Flaherty (1982) suggest that a true ethical dilemma has one or more of the following characteristics:

1. It cannot be resolved solely through a review of scientific data. To make this determination, it is necessary to gather detailed information about the situation from medical records, health care literature, or consultation with colleagues or with the client and family. What at first appears to be a dilemma may resolve on learning, for example, that a review of a diagnostic procedure reveals a different prognosis.

> ### How to Process an Ethical Dilemma   Box 4-3
>
> **Step 1. Is this an ethical dilemma?**
> If a review of scientific data does not resolve the question, the question is perplexing, and the answer will have profound relevance for several areas of human concern, then an ethical dilemma may exist.
>
> **Step 2. Gather all the information relevant to the case.**
> To be sure it is a true dilemma, it will be important to review all pertinent information. Occasionally, an overlooked fact may provide quick resolution. At this point, client, family, institutional, and social perspectives are important sources of relevant information.
>
> **Step 3. Examine and determine your own values on the issues.**
> Values clarification provides a foundation for clarity and for confidence during discussions that will be necessary for resolution of a dilemma.
>
> **Step 4. Articulate the problem.**
> A clear, simple statement of the dilemma may not always be easy, but it is essential for the next step to take place.
>
> **Step 5. Consider possible courses of action.**
> To respect all sides of an issue, it is helpful to list potential actions, especially when the list will reflect opinions that conflict.
>
> **Step 6. Negotiate the outcome.**
> Sometimes courses of action that seem unlikely at the beginning of the process take on new possibility as they are put to rational and respectful consideration. Negotiation requires a confidence in your own point of view and a deep respect for the opinions of others.
>
> **Step 7. Evaluate the action.**

2. It is perplexing. You cannot easily think logically or make a decision about the problem, or you may disagree with a decision that others are making, and the difference of opinion is perplexing.

3. The answer to the problem will have profound relevance for several areas of human concern.

Step 2: Gather all relevant information.

Accurate information and complete information are essential for the ethical process to go forward.

Step 3: Examine and determine your values and opinions on the issues.

A part of gathering information also will include a determination of your own opinion as it relates to the issues. The distinction between personal opinion and the facts of the case or the opinions of others is essential for resolution to proceed. People come to different conclusions about the same situation with no malice intended toward other people. Remembering this will help you to be an effective arbitrator in conversation.

Step 4: Articulate the problem.

After reviewing relevant information, develop a clear statement of the problem in language that all involved in the ethical discussion can understand. The statement lays the groundwork for the negotiations that follow. Discussions are more likely to remain focused and constructive when all parties agree on the statement of the dilemma.

Step 5: Consider possible courses of action.

You can facilitate a discussion of ethical dilemmas by listing possible courses of action as they occur to the group. Possibilities may occur at any time during deliberations.

Step 6: Negotiate the outcome.

After considering all alternatives, have all persons involved in the ethical conflict come to a point of resolution or agreement, and then take action.

Step 7: Evaluate the action.

Make decisions and evaluate them in an ongoing manner.

Documentation of the ethical process can take a variety of forms. Whenever the process involves a family conference or results in a change in the management plan, the process should be documented in the medical record. Some institutions use a formal consultation format whenever a request for discussion comes to the ethics committee. If the ethical dilemma does not directly affect client care, however, documentation may occur by means of minutes from a meeting or in a memorandum to affected parties.

POTENTIAL ETHICAL PROBLEMS IN NURSING

In any practice setting you may be confronted with ethical issues unique to that practice. The following sections describe examples of ethical dilemmas from different practices.

Ambulatory Care Settings

The nurse in the ambulatory care setting is especially concerned with the social and environmental factors in health and wellness. The implementation of an effective plan of care often depends on factors that are difficult or impossible to control, such as personal habits, poverty, or access to care (Gallagher, 1999). For example, you may explain the importance of regular Pap smears, and may even determine from the history that the client is highly motivated to obtain a Pap smear. A lack of community resources to provide the Pap smear or lack of resources to pay for it, however, may prevent the client from following through.

Step 1: Is this an ethical dilemma?

Cancer prevention for female clients depends in part on regular Pap smears. Yet this client cannot obtain one, even though she describes strong motivation to do so. Not only is this situation perplexing for the client and for you, but the solution also has profound relevance.

Step 2: Gather all the information relevant to the case.

An investigation into the client's community resources, a search into other communities for their solutions to similar situations, and perhaps even a review of nursing literature might offer ideas for a solution to this problem. You might also look to the client and her personal resources to see if the client herself is able to contribute to the solution.

Step 3: Examine and determine your own values and opinions on the issues.

What do you feel are the obligations to this client? What do you feel are obligations to the community? Perhaps you are busy with a personal life and other job responsibilities, and the follow-through on this project might diminish time

available for other worthy activities. On the other hand, you may determine that an investment of your expertise into this project would be valuable.

Step 4: Articulate the problem.

What are your obligations to this client and to her community? How can you practice fidelity to the client?

Step 5: Consider possible courses of action.

You may decide to establish better community resources for this client and others like her. You may seek out others, such as community leaders or social workers, who could recruit resources to help this client. The client herself might have ideas on the location for support, such as other family members or civic groups.

Step 6: Negotiate the outcome.

In this case a part of the negotiation would include a determination of the best use of your time, taking into consideration the implications for all parts of your personal and professional life and obligations to this client and her community.

Step 7: Evaluate the action.

The successful resolution of the dilemma will include obtaining the Pap smear for the client.

Acute Care/Managed Care Settings

In the acute care setting, managed care systems place a growing emphasis on decreasing hospitalization days. To safely accomplish a shorter hospitalization, a great deal of teaching and discharge planning falls to the bedside nurse. An ethical dilemma might arise if you determine that the client and the client's family have not mastered a skill needed to provide safe care in the home, yet the client's insurance will not cover further days in the hospital.

Step 1: Is this an ethical dilemma?

The situation is perplexing because it seems that whether the client remains in the hospital or not, the consequences will be dire. A safe and affordable solution to this dilemma has relevance for the client and for the acute care setting.

Step 2: Gather all the information relevant to the case.

Who pays for this client's care, and who in this setting is responsible for negotiating with payers? What is the prognosis for this client, and how long will home care be necessary? What might be the financial impact of unsafe care in the home? How much longer do you estimate the client will need to learn the home care? Can a home care service provide the care and continued teaching?

Step 3: Examine and determine your own values and opinions on the issues.

You may have had very positive or very negative experiences with managed care in the past. It is important to separate personal responses in the past from this situation. The professional evaluation of the client's readiness for discharge will play a critical role in the negotiations, so opinion must be clearheaded.

Step 4: Articulate the problem.

What resources will provide the safest AND most cost-effective care for this client? How can you protect the principle of beneficence for this client and yet remain accountable to the hospital and to the managed care plan?

Step 5: Consider possible courses of action.

You could take time to educate administrators and physicians about the lack of knowledge for this client. You could construct a proposal for solution by investigating the location and quality of home care services. You might learn more from the client about family resources.

Step 6: Negotiate the outcome.

Working with social workers, physicians, and admission and utilization review personnel may help you to devise a safe plan for discharge. Certainly, working within the guidelines of the managed care plan will be essential for success. In addition, the client may respond to the dilemma by identifying other family members or community resources that might facilitate a safe discharge. At the very least, you could ensure that the physician and others become aware of the potential for unsafe conditions after discharge.

Step 7: Evaluate the action.

The nature of the outcome will depend on your ability to pursue an option that protects this client during and after discharge.

Restorative Care Settings

Working with the chronically ill or disabled client places you in contact with decisions about quality of life, such as the client's ability to maintain independence and functional status (Tilden and others, 1996). The determination of measures of quality represents a relatively new field of study. For example, a stroke victim who is profoundly disabled may begin to suffer from aspiration problems during feedings. Would a gastrostomy tube serve to prevent aspiration, or would it represent a surgical intervention that will prolong suffering?

Step 1: Is this an ethical dilemma?

Scientific data could help to predict improved nutrition and improved safety for this client, but they do not help to address the ethical issues about quality of life. You may be perplexed, as is the family, about the right decision. A decision that felt "right" to all parties would have profound relevance for this dilemma and might influence similar clinical situations in a positive way.

Step 2: Gather all the information relevant to the case.

What is the prognosis for this client? What are the surgical risks and benefits from placement of the gastrostomy tube? What is the medical risk of aspiration pneumonia in this client, before and after tube placement? Would pneumonia and the treatment represent an uncomfortable experience for the client?

Step 3: Examine and determine your own values and opinions on the issues.

Begin by exploring your personal feelings about the quality of this client's life. Is the client able to express an opinion? If yes, you will probably have personal opinions about the competence of the client. These opinions are important to articulate. How do you feel about the competence of the family members and significant others? If a decision were made with which you disagree, it might be important to consider whether you could still participate in the care of the

client. Could you advocate for a position that was in conflict with your own values?

Step 4: Articulate the problem.

Will a gastrostomy tube improve the quality of this client's life, or will a gastrostomy tube prolong suffering? How can the team best respect this client's autonomy?

Step 5: Consider possible courses of action.

The gastrostomy tube could be placed. Perhaps a nasogastric tube could be placed temporarily while the more difficult ethical issues are explored with the client and the client's family. The client or the client's significant others could elect to decline a gastrostomy tube.

Step 6: Negotiate the outcome.

If the client is competent and an adult, the client's decision will determine the outcome. If not, then the health care team will have to rely on family members, significant others, or even legal documents that identify legal guardians to make the decision. In this last case the decision may be more difficult to obtain. Your role in the negotiations would include the contribution of the nursing perspective on quality of life for this individual.

Step 7: Evaluate the action.

Regardless of the decision in this case, it would be possible to reverse the decision if conditions or feelings changed. Continuing discussion with the client and the family or significant others would ensure a satisfactory conclusion to this dilemma.

Multidisciplinary Collaboration

As new technologies introduce improved outcomes for many diseases, these technologies may also require collaboration of several disciplines. Not only will different subspecialties be involved but also social workers, psychologists, physical therapists, and others. Disagreement about prognosis or plan of care often evolves (Davis, 2000). Your role may include advocating for the client's point of view or coordinating communication between teams. You may also disagree with a plan of care. For example, a client with a brain tumor may have medical providers from oncology, neurology, neurosurgery, and radiology. You may care for a client for whom conventional therapy has not controlled the tumor growth. The continued ability of the client to think clearly may even be in question. One specialty may wish to proceed with experimental therapy; another specialty may not. You may feel the experimental therapy would prolong suffering.

Step 1: Is this an ethical dilemma?

The client is confused and unable to exercise true autonomy. Because the team that cares for this client is multidisciplinary, a decision must come from consensus, and consensus seems impossible. Further review of the scientific literature will not change the opinion of any of the medical providers. The situation is perplexing because both options seem to have merit. In addition, the client's point of view is difficult to determine because the client has access only to information from the physicians who disagree. The solution will have relevance for this client's condition. It may also provide guidance for similar clinical situations.

Step 2: Gather all the information relevant to the case.

Perhaps the best way to begin would be for you to request a team conference. An important piece of information includes the current clinical condition of the client. Nursing assessment of this condition is critical to the discussion.

Step 3: Examine and determine your own values and opinions on the issues.

What is your opinion on the prognosis of this client? If you were in the condition of the client, what would your personal decision be? How does the answer to this question differ from the client's answer? This last question is perhaps most important. When you present a point of view at a conference, it will be essential to differentiate between your personal point of view and the client's point of view.

Step 4: Articulate the problem.

What plan of care will provide the best quality of life for this client? Who will make this decision?

Step 5: Consider possible courses of action.

The client might decide to receive experimental therapy, even after learning of the possible side effects or complications. The client might decline experimental therapy. The team might determine that the prognosis is poor regardless of further therapy and relieve the client of the need to make a decision.

Step 6: Negotiate the outcome.

Once the team has reached consensus, then the client and the client's family will be better able to make an informed decision. Be an advocate and emphasize the confusion that the client suffers so that the team members will be motivated to negotiate differences. You may also provide a neutral voice that can organize a discussion between medical teams that are in conflict. Your own point of view, however, is equally important. If in your personal opinion further treatment might constitute prolonged suffering, then the conference between caregivers will be an effective place to negotiate and discuss this position.

Step 7: Evaluate the action.

The outcome could be considered successful if the client's autonomy receives respect while the health care team practices nonmaleficence or keeps a commitment to do the least harm. Even if team members continue to disagree about the correct course of action, a general sense of resolution remains the goal.

Cultural and Religious Sensitivity

The professional standards of justice and beneficence require respect for cultural differences in the health care setting, regardless of personal opinion or feeling (Davis and Koenig, 1996). Occasionally, you may face a challenging situation in which cultural differences present an ethical dilemma. For example, a 15-year-old girl is admitted for management of her leukemia. You note that the client's religious beliefs do not allow her to receive blood transfusions, yet her condition will soon require a blood transfusion to prevent dire consequences. Her parents share her religious convictions but would be willing to compromise. The client refuses to compromise.

Step 1: Is this an ethical dilemma?

Further review of the clinical situation will not change the dilemma. Scientific data will not affect the strong feelings of the client or of her parents. The case is perplexing because respecting the client's autonomy will conflict with the health care team's wish to do no harm. The resolution of this dilemma will be difficult and will have profound relevance for several areas of concern, including the life of the client.

Step 2: Gather all the information relevant to the case.

How soon must the transfusion be administered? What are the legal definitions of "minor" in your state? Has the family agreed to transfusions in the past, and if so, what was the mechanism for reaching a compromise? What are the specific religious constraints against blood transfusions that affect this case? Is the client competent? Is she fully aware of the consequences of her decision to refuse the transfusion?

Step 3: Examine and determine your own values and opinions on the issues.

How do you feel about this client's religious beliefs? How close or distant are the client's beliefs from your personal beliefs? What is your personal opinion on the rights of minors to determine their medical course?

Step 4: Articulate the problem.

A client, who is a minor, will refuse a lifesaving transfusion on the grounds of religious belief. If she is forced to receive the transfusion, she will consider herself violated in the eyes of her God. If she does not receive the transfusion, she will probably not survive.

Step 5: Consider possible courses of action.

The client could be forced to receive a transfusion, requiring restraints or use of physical force. The client's wishes could be respected. The client and the client's family could be encouraged to explore this dilemma with the guidance of a religious leader from their faith.

Step 6: Negotiate the outcome.

In this case your contribution could consist of accurate documentation of the client's state of mind. A client care conference with the client and the client's family would be necessary. If the medical team decides to insist on the transfusion, then a court order would be sought. As advocate for the client, even in the face of personal disagreement, you would ensure that the client's voice was fairly represented to the judge.

Step 7: Evaluate the action.

The outcome will depend on the ability of the conference members to reach consensus. The goal will be the balancing of respect for autonomy with the principle of beneficence.

Delegation

Most health care delivery models involve nurse assistants, technicians, and licensed practical nurses. The team includes assistants, licensed and some unlicensed, who work with a registered nurse leader. The registered nurse will use delegation skills and the guidance of legal statutes to determine and assign work to assistants. Occasionally this collaboration may present ethical dilemmas. The dilemmas may be especially troubling because the nurse leader is accountable for clients' care. Furthermore, the issues may not always be associated directly with client care, but with behavior and work habits. For example, an unlicensed assistant who is basically a reliable team member performs her work in a timely and accurate manner. But you notice that the assistant spends most of her time with one client, ignoring the special needs of others.

Step 1: Is this an ethical dilemma?

Technically this situation constitutes a personnel issue rather than an ethical dilemma. However, professional standards of beneficence and justice suggest that care for clients be equally distributed. Because the assistant's behavior is otherwise meeting expectations, the situation is perplexing. A solution could have relevance for her work with others.

Step 2: Gather all information relevant to the situation.

If other nurses work with this assistant, how do they describe their relationship with her? What is her job description officially? What was her training for this position? Who is her supervisor? How do clients describe her care? How does the law hold you accountable for the actions of others on the health care team?

Step 3: Examine and determine your own values and opinions on the issue.

What are your personal opinions about the team approach to nursing? Have you had training in delegation skills or supervision skills? How does the assistant's behavior affect your work responsibilities?

Step 4: Articulate the problem.

Is this assistant working in an inappropriate way? If yes, who is responsible for correcting the behavior?

Step 5: Consider possible courses of action.

You could meet privately with the assistant to confer about the reasons for the assistant's behavior and determine resolutions. You could refer the situation to a supervisor. You could devise classes on caring for all assistants.

Step 6: Negotiate the outcome.

You might first confer with the nursing supervisor. As health care systems move through rapid changes, it is helpful to stay informed about institutional policies, and it is important to seek guidance from colleagues. What does the law dictate in regard to accountability for client care? The ability to advocate for nursing standards, especially an ethic of care, will remain a professional obligation. The recognition and articulation of an ethical dilemma begin the process.

Step 7: Evaluate the action.

The outcome of this dilemma might be measured best by monitoring client satisfaction.

To resolve an ethical problem, you should refer to a systematic process to understand the nature of the problem and to plan a responsible course of action. Although ethical dilemmas may present challenging problems, the nurse offers a unique and valuable voice to the process of resolution.

Key Terms

accountability, *p. 48*
advocacy, *p. 49*
autonomy, *p. 47*
beneficence, *p. 48*
bioethics, *p. 47*
care, *p. 50*
code of ethics, *p. 48*

competence, *p. 49*
deontology, *p. 50*
ethical dilemma, *p. 49*
ethical principles, *p. 48*
ethics, *p. 47*
ethics of care, *p. 51*
feminist ethics, *p. 50*
fidelity, *p. 48*
judgment, *p. 49*

justice, *p. 48*
law, *p. 47*
morals, *p. 47*
nonmaleficence, *p. 48*
point of view, *p. 49*
responsibility, *p. 48*
utilitarianism, *p. 50*
value, *p. 47*

Key Concepts

- Ethics refers to the study of philosophical ideals of right and wrong behavior.
- A code of ethics provides a foundation for professional nursing.
- Professional nursing promotes accountability, responsibility, and advocacy.
- An ethical nurse maintains competence in practice and assumes responsibility for nursing judgments.
- The primary functions of advocacy are to inform and to support.
- Professional nurses have a commitment to clients, the profession, and society to provide high-quality health care.

- Basic principles of ethics in health care include autonomy, justice, fidelity, beneficence, and nonmaleficence.
- Ethical problems arise from differences in values, changing professional roles, technological advances, and uncertainty in decision making.
- A standard process for thinking through ethical dilemmas helps nurses resolve difficult situations.
- Critical thinking is an essential part of processing ethical dilemmas.
- Ethical dilemmas in nursing may occur in any segment of the health care delivery system.
- The nurse's point of view provides a unique and valuable voice in the resolution of ethical dilemmas.

Critical Thinking Activities

1. Medical decisions at the end of life are difficult. Grief, confusion, and ambiguity characterize the experience and challenge our ability to make decisions. For example, a 42-year-old woman is admitted to the intensive care unit (ICU) where you are a staff nurse. She requires a machine to keep her breathing, she is unresponsive, apparently suffering irreversible damage to her brain after a fall in her bathroom. She was found by a neighbor. Her history of alcoholism and substance abuse is well known by the neighbor and by emergency department staff. The client does not have an advance directive.

   The client's father is eventually located, but he describes a strained relationship with his daughter. He has supported her financially off and on throughout her troubled addiction, but recently he has refused her request for financial assistance, a refusal made in an effort to encourage her to seek professional help.

   Should this father participate in decision making for his daughter?

2. Genetics testing now makes possible detection of a gene that causes a rare but aggressive form of breast cancer. A woman who knows she carries this gene might be guided in her decisions about hormone replacement therapy, preventive mastectomy, or other actions. At the same time, she may risk loss of disability or medical insurance coverage.

   If you were a nurse in a mammogram clinic, would you favor counseling patients to obtain this genetic test?

Review Questions

1. Ethical dilemmas often arise over a conflict of opinions. Once you have determined that the dilemma is ethical, a critical first step in negotiating the differences of opinion would be to:
   1. consult a professional ethicist to ensure that the steps of the process occur in full.
   2. gather all relevant information regarding the clinical, social, and spiritual aspects of the dilemma.
   3. list the ethical principles that inform the dilemma so that negotiators agree on the language of the discussion.
   4. ensure that the attending physician has written an order for an ethics consultation to support the ethics process.

2. In the United States, access to health care usually depends on a client's ability to pay for health care, either through insurance or by paying cash. You are caring for a client who needs a liver transplant to survive. This client has been out of work for several months and does not have insurance or enough cash. A discussion about the ethics of this situation would involve predominately the principle of:
   1. accountability, because you as the nurse are accountable for the well-being of this client.
   2. respect for autonomy, because this client's autonomy will be violated if he does not receive the liver transplant.
   3. ethics of care, because the caring thing that a nurse could provide for this patient is resources for a liver transplant.
   4. justice, because the first and greatest question in this situation is how to determine the just distribution of resources.

3. The code of ethics for nurses is composed and published by:
   1. the National League for Nursing.
   2. the American Nurses Association.
   3. the American Medical Association.
   4. the National Institutes of Health, Nursing Division.

4. In most ethical dilemmas, the solution to the dilemma requires negotiation between members of the health care team. As the nurse, your point of view is valuable because:
   1. nurses have a legal license that mandates their presence at ethical discussions.
   2. the principle of autonomy guides all participants to respect their own self-worth.
   3. nurses develop a relationship to the client that is unique among all care providers.
   4. the nurses' code of ethics recommends that a nurse be present at any ethical discussion about client care.

5. Successful ethical discussion depends on participants who have a clear sense of personal values. When many people share the same values, it may be possible to identify a philosophy that these values comprise. For example, the philosophy of utilitarianism proposes that:
   1. the value of something is determined by its usefulness to society.
   2. the value of people is determined solely by leaders in the Unitarian Church.
   3. the decision to perform a liver transplant depends on a measure of the moral life that the client has led so far.
   4. the best way to determine the solution to an ethical dilemma is to refer the case to the attending physician.

6. The philosophy sometimes called the ethics of care suggests that ethical dilemmas can best be solved by attention to:
   1. relationships.
   2. ethical principles.
   3. home care nurses.
   4. code of ethics for nurses.

7. Although it may seem redundant, health care providers, including professional nurses, agree to "do no harm" to their clients. The point of this agreement is to reassure the public that in all ways, the health care team will not only work to heal patients, they agree to do this in the least painful and harmful way possible. The principle that describes this agreement is called:
   1. beneficence.
   2. accountability.
   3. nonmaleficence.
   4. respect for autonomy.

8. Nurses and other providers agree to be advocates for their patients. Practice of advocacy calls for the nurse to:
   1. seek out graduate education as soon as possible.
   2. work to understand the law as it applies to the client's clinical condition.
   3. assess the client's point of view and prepare to articulate this point of view.
   4. document all clinical changes in the medical record in a timely and legible way.

References

American Heritage Dictionary, ed 4, Boston, 2000, Houghton Mifflin.

American Nurses Association: *Code for nurses with interpretative statements,* Kansas City, Mo, 2001, The Association.

Beauchamp T, Childress J: *Principles of biomedical ethics,* ed 5, New York, 2001, Oxford University Press.

Curtin L, Flaherty MJ: *Nursing ethics: theories and pragmatics,* Bowie, Md, 1982, Brady.

Davis A, Aroskar M: *Ethical dilemmas and nursing practice,* Norwalk, Conn, 1991, Appleton & Lange.

Davis AJ: The bioethically constructed ideal dying patient in USA, *Med Law* 19(1):161, 2000.

Davis AJ, Koenig BA: A question of policy: bioethics in a multicultural society, *Nurs Policy Forum* 2(1):7, 1996.

Fry ST: The role of caring in a theory of nursing ethics, *Hypatia* 4(2):88, 1989.

Gallagher SM: Citizenship ethics: a call to action, *Ostomy Wound Manag* 45(2):16, 1999.

Gilligan C: *In a different voice,* Cambridge, Mass, 1993, Harvard University Press.

Harris CH: Legal aspects of nursing. In Deloughery G: *Issues and trends in nursing,* ed 3, St. Louis, 1998, Mosby.

International Council of Nurses: *ICN code of ethics for nurses,* Geneva, 2000, 3, place Jean-Marteau, CH-1201, The Association.

Kohlberg L: *Essays on moral development,* vols I-III, San Francisco, 1981, Harper & Row.

Leininger M: *Caring: an essential human need,* Detroit, 1988, Wayne State University Press.

Miller MA, Babcock DE: *Critical thinking applied to nursing,* St. Louis, 1996, Mosby.

O'Neil J: Ethical decision making and the role of nursing. In Deloughery G: *Issues and trends in nursing,* ed 3, St. Louis, 1998, Mosby.

Potter P, Perry A: *Fundamentals of nursing: concepts, process, and practice,* ed 4, St. Louis, 1997, Mosby.

Sherwin S: *No longer patient: feminist ethics and health care,* Philadelphia, 1992, Temple University Press.

Tilden V and others: Decisions about life-sustaining treatment, *Arch Intern Med* 155:633, 1996.

Watson J, editor: *Applying art and science of human caring,* New York, 1994, National League of Nursing Press.

5

Critical Thinking and Nursing Judgment

Objectives

- Define key terms.
- Discuss the nurse's responsibility in making clinical decisions.
- Describe the components of a critical thinking model for clinical decision making.
- Discuss critical thinking skills used in nursing practice.
- Explain the relationship between clinical experience and critical thinking.
- Discuss the effect attitudes for critical thinking have on clinical decision making.
- Explain how professional standards influence a nurse's clinical decisions.
- Discuss how reflection can improve knowledge of nursing.
- Discuss the relationship of the nursing process to critical thinking.
- Apply elements of a critical thinking model to a case study.

*A*s a professional nurse, you will face a variety of situations involving clients with uniquely different types of health care problems. In every type of situation you will need to think critically so that the client ultimately receives the very best nursing care. You cannot learn critical thinking overnight. It is a process that can only be acquired through hard work, commitment, and an active curiosity about learning. This chapter introduces you to a model for critical thinking. You will learn to apply the elements of the model simultaneously as you face client situations and determine the type of nursing care each client requires.

CLINICAL SCENARIO

Mrs. Bryan is a widowed 78-year-old client who lives alone in a small rural community. Her daughter, Joyce, lives approximately 100 miles away in a large urban city. Mrs. Bryan has always been a very independent woman. She loves music, art, bird-watching, and cooking. Over the last year Mrs. Bryan's health has declined. She was diagnosed with stomach cancer over a year ago. Her condition cannot be treated with surgery. She comes to the community clinic at least monthly to see her physician for follow-up and recommendations for supportive care. As a result of her condition, Mrs. Bryan has had a 10-pound weight loss, and she reports a poor appetite and generalized weakness. She receives Meals on Wheels for lunch from a local church and frequently has dinner with a close friend who lives down the street. Mrs. Bryan's daughter wants her mother to move closer to her so that she can receive the appropriate care and attention she needs. This may mean that Mrs. Bryan will have to live in a nursing home, because Joyce has no room at home to care for her mother herself.

Inez Santiago is a 36-year-old married student nurse assigned to the community clinic Mrs. Bryan visits. Inez has two children and worked part-time as a schoolteacher while raising her children. Now that her children are older, Inez has chosen nursing as a career. When she first meets Mrs. Bryan, she finds the client to be friendly, alert, and happy to have a student. During their discussion, Inez and Mrs. Bryan discuss Mrs. Bryan's feelings about her health and the possibility of having to leave her home. Mrs. Bryan replies, "I love my home. I know Joyce knows what is best for me, but I cannot imagine never seeing my friends again."

CLINICAL DECISIONS IN NURSING PRACTICE

When caring for clients, you have the responsibility for making accurate and appropriate clinical decisions. Clinical decision making is a skill that separates professional nurses from technical and ancillary staff (Hughes and Young, 1992). To assist persons in maintaining, regaining, or improving their health you must be able to think critically to problem solve and find solutions for clients' health problems. Many clients have problems for which there are no textbook solutions. Their clinical symptoms, the information they share about themselves, and the situation in which you meet may not immediately present a clear picture of what actions you should take. Instead you must learn to

question, wonder, and then be self-directed in exploring different interpretations and finding the one that can best help your client (Whiteside, 1997).

Clients have a variety of experiences, behaviors, social perspectives, values, and signs and symptoms related to health problems. These variables can change while caring for a given client. In the presence of such variation you will need to observe the client closely, search for and examine ideas and **inferences** about client problems, consider scientific principles relating to the problems, recognize the problems, and develop an approach to nursing care. You will need to creatively seek new knowledge as needed, act quickly when events change, and make sound decisions that promote the client's well-being. No nursing action or interaction with a client is trivial or ordinary (Fox, 1980). Although the responsibility for making clinical decisions may seem frightening, it helps define what makes nursing a rewarding and challenging profession.

CRITICAL THINKING DEFINED

Thinking and learning are interrelated, lifelong processes. Over time, your knowledge and practical experiences help you to broaden your ability to make thoughtful observations, judgments, and choices. **Critical thinking** is the active, organized, cognitive process used to carefully examine one's thinking and the thinking of others (Chaffee, 1994). It involves use of the mind in forming conclusions, making decisions, drawing inferences, and reflecting (Gordon, 1995). It means taking nothing for granted. A critical thinker identifies and challenges assumptions, considers what is important in a situation, imagines and explores alternatives, considers ethical principles, and thus makes informed decisions. When you care for a client, critical thinking begins by asking these questions: What do I really know about this nursing care situation? How do I know it? What are the options available to me? (Paul and Heaslip, 1995).

You can begin to learn critical thinking early in your practice. For example, as you learn about administering bed baths and other hygiene measures to your clients, take time to read in the nursing literature about the concept of comfort (Brock and Butts, 1998). What are the defining criteria for the concept of comfort? How do clients from other cultures think about the concept of comfort? What are the different factors that contribute to comfort? Thinking critically and then learning about the concept of comfort will prepare you to better anticipate your clients' needs and to provide appropriate care. Critical thinking involves a commitment to think clearly, precisely, and accurately and to act on the basis of what is known. When you as the nurse direct thinking toward understanding and assisting clients in finding solutions to their health problems, the process becomes purposeful and goal oriented.

It is clear that critical thinking requires not only cognitive skills but also a person's disposition, or tendency, to ask questions, to remain well informed, to be honest in facing personal biases, and always to be willing to reconsider and

Critical Thinking Skills		Table 5-1
Skill	Nursing Practice Application	
Interpretation	Be systematic in data collection. Look for patterns to categorize data (e.g., nursing diagnoses [Chapter 6]). Clarify any data you are uncertain about.	
Analysis	Be open minded as you look at information about a client. Do not make careless assumptions. Do the data reveal what you believe is true, or are there other options?	
Evaluation	Look at all situations objectively. Use criteria (e.g., expected outcomes, pain characteristics, learning objectives) to determine results of nursing actions [Chapter 6]. Reflect on your own behavior.	
Inference	Look at the meaning and significance of findings. Are there relationships between findings? Do the data about the client help you in seeing that a problem may exist?	
Explanation	Support your findings and conclusions. Use knowledge to select strategies you use in the care of clients.	
Self-regulation	Reflect on your experiences. Identify in what way you can improve your own performance.	

Modified from Facione P: *Critical thinking: a statement of expert consensus for purposes of educational assessment and instruction. The Delphi report; research findings and recommendations prepared for the American Philosophical Association*, ERIC Doc No. ED 315-423, Washington, DC, 1990, ERIC.

think clearly about issues (Facione, 1990). There are core critical thinking skills that, when applied to nursing, are useful in showing the complex nature of clinical decision making (Table 5-1). Being able to apply all of these skills takes practice, a sound knowledge base, and the thoughtful consideration of the knowledge gained in clinical care of clients.

The nurse who is a good critical thinker faces problems without forming a quick, single solution and instead is focused on the options for what to believe and do (Kataoka-Yahiro and Saylor, 1994). Learning to think critically will help you to care for clients as their advocate and to make better informed choices about their care. Critical thinking is more than just problem solving. It is an attempt to continually improve how you apply yourself when faced with problems in client care. As a nurse, each clinical experience will help you pursue learning opportunities with a focused desire to excel in your practice. Three important aspects of critical thinking—reflection, language, and intuition—enable you to excel in critical thinking.

CLINICAL SCENARIO

Consider the situation involving Mrs. Bryan and Inez Santiago. Mrs. Bryan returns to the clinic with her friend. Inez observes the client's slow, deliberate movements, unsteady gait, and facial expression of fatigue. Drawing the preliminary conclusion that Mrs. Bryan is "tired" may result from Inez's experience with other clients or from having seen Mrs. Bryan the previous visit and witnessing that a change has occurred. When Mrs. Bryan provides more information on "feeling tired," Inez begins to consider the client's health status, observes for subtle signs of how Mrs. Bryan moves about or sits in the chair, and begins to ask the client focused questions. The questions may be direct, such as, "Tell me how you are feeling," "Have you been unable to sleep?" or "Are you having pain?" Measurement of the client's pulse, blood pressure, and respiratory rate may offer further information about Mrs. Bryan's status. The process whereby Inez uses information to reason, to make inferences as to the meaning and significance of findings, and to form a mental picture of what is happening to Mrs. Bryan is called critical thinking.

Reflection

An important aspect of critical thinking is **reflection.** You reflect when you purposefully think back or recall a situation to discover its purpose or meaning. For example, after caring for a client who is suffering chronic pain from a bone tumor, you might reflect on how the client reacted when you discussed nursing approaches to pain management. What did it mean when the client said, "I don't know, I feel like I will never get any relief," or "I just want the pain to be relieved so I can get out of this bed." As a nurse it is very helpful to think back on a client situation to explore the factors that influenced how you handled the situation. Reflection is like the playback function on a videotape. It involves playing back a situation in your head and taking time to honestly review everything you can remember about the situation. Reflection requires adequate knowledge and is necessary for self-evaluation and review of one's successes or opportunities for improvement. O'Neill and Dluhy (1997) caution you not to question or doubt every judgment that you make because too much emphasis on reflection can deter your thinking in a clinical situation as a result of the second-guessing it creates.

The process of reflection helps you to seek and understand the relationships between concepts learned in class and real-life clinical situations. Through reflection you can judge your personal performance while also judging whether you were able to follow standards of nursing practice in your care. Reflection helps make sense out of an experience so that the next time a similar experience arises you can use approaches that were successful or revise an approach to achieve better client outcomes.

Engaging in reflection is very individualized (Miller and Babcock, 1996). Learning to be reflective takes practice. When you choose to reflect on a clinical experience you must be open to new information and be able to look at the client's perspective, as well as your own. Learning from experience with clients can create an "aha" feeling, because reflection reveals an awareness of how well you are performing as a professional. Box 5-1 lists tips on how to use reflection in your practice.

CLINICAL SCENARIO

After spending the day at the clinic, Inez spends some time recalling her experience with Mrs. Bryan. In an attempt to learn more about Mrs. Bryan's feelings toward a nursing home, Inez had discussed the value of a nursing home as a safe environment. Mrs. Bryan immediately became less talkative. Inez reflects on why Mrs. Bryan's response concerned her; the client's willingness to participate in the discussion had changed. Perhaps her explanation was not the best approach if Mrs. Bryan had not yet accepted the idea of going to the nursing home. Asking open questions about Mrs. Bryan's feelings might have been more useful. For example, Inez might have asked, "Tell me what you think about your daughter's concerns for your safety." Inez thinks about how she will approach Mrs. Bryan differently during her next visit. Reflection allows Inez to be proactive and hopefully more effective.

Language

Another important aspect of critical thinking is the use of language. Thinking and language are closely related processes. The ability to use language is closely associated with the ability to think meaningfully (Miller and Babcock, 1996). To become a critical thinker, you must be able to use language precisely and clearly. When language is vague and inaccurate, it reflects sloppy thinking.

As you care for clients, it is important to communicate clearly with clients and families and with health care professionals. When you fail to use correct terminology and use jargon or vague descriptions, communication is ineffective. This may become obvious if the client is unable to cooperate with nursing therapies or if members of the nursing team do not follow through on your recommendations. Critical thinking requires you to carefully frame your thoughts and to send a message that is clear.

Intuition

Intuition is the inner sensing that something is so. In other words, you may walk into a client's room and, by looking at the client's appearance without the benefit of a thorough assessment, sense that he or she is about to deteriorate physically. It is a common experience that many people have when interacting with their environments. Intuition in nursing develops as one's clinical experience increases. For example, an experienced home health nurse may suspect by looking at a client's expression, observing the disarray in the home environment, and making a quick assessment of the client's mood, that a client is depressed. The nurse knows this intuitively without benefit of a detailed assessment of the client's mood or behavior.

What is important to remember is that quality nursing practice does not depend solely on intuition. Just as it is critical for you to know what knowledge you have, it is even more critical to know what you do not know. Trust your intuition as a red flag that something is not quite right, but do not take your intuition as an automatic truth. As soon as intuition strikes be sure to probe further to assess a client's situation (Fowler, 1998). If you do not recognize how much you

Tips on Facilitating Reflection   Box 5-1
Stop and think about what is going on with your client and what your assessment means. When you chart or report on your client, what is the meaning of his or her symptoms? Always ask what could be happening (Fowler, 1998).
Reflect carefully on any critical incidents (e.g., safety episodes, cardiac arrests, pivotal events in the progression of a client's disease, or complex-care clients) (Bittner and Tobin, 1998). What occurred? What actions were taken? How did the client respond? Were there optional actions you might have taken?
Keep a journal of your experiences with clients. Be sure to include the following elements: identification, description, significance, and implications (Baker, 1996). Telling a story and drawing a picture are two ways to identify the situation or experience you wish to reflect on. Describe in detail what you felt, thought, and did. Analyze the significance of the experience by considering feelings, thoughts, and possible meanings. Describe the implications of the experience in terms of your own clinical practice or self-perceptions as a learner. Refer to the journal often when you care for clients in similar situations.
Talk with a close friend who works with you and has observed your clinical work. Ask if the friend's observations are the same as yours.
Keep all written care plans or clinical papers. Use them frequently as a resource for future clients.
Take time to reflect, both after having cared for a client and before caring for new clients with similar conditions. How is your current client similar to or different from previous clients?

do not know about your clients, there is a risk of malpractice and even endangering your clients. Learn to carefully think through each clinical situation. Thoughtful analysis of what you know, plus a review of the most current clinical data, allows you to make an accurate and sound clinical decision.

CRITICAL THINKING COMPETENCIES

Kataoka-Yahiro and Saylor (1994) have described critical thinking competencies as the cognitive processes a nurse uses to make judgments. These include general critical thinking, specific critical thinking in clinical situations, and specific critical thinking in nursing (Kataoka-Yahiro and Saylor, 1994). General critical thinking competencies are not unique to nursing. They are used in other disciplines and in nonclinical situations. General critical thinking processes include the **scientific method, problem solving,** and **decision making.** Specific critical thinking competencies in clinical situations include **diagnostic reasoning,** clinical inferences, and clinical decision making. These competencies are used by physicians, social workers, nurses, and other health care professionals in deciding about the clinical care and support of clients. The specific critical thinking competency used in nursing practice is the **nursing process.**

Scientific Method

The scientific method is one approach to reasoning that is used in nursing, medicine, and a variety of other disciplines. It is an approach to seeking the truth or verifying that a set of facts agrees with reality. Nurse researchers use the scientific method when testing research questions in nursing practice situations. For example, a nurse researcher might observe that clients in a hospice program often have difficulty communicating their feelings to family members. The nurse learns more about what causes this problem and considers the possibility that family members might have ineffective communication skills. The nurse asks the question, "Can family members who receive instruction on communication principles provide support to loved ones with a terminal illness?" The nurse might design a study that involves formal instruction on communication skills and uses a support group to help family members practice and apply the skills. Once the instruction is complete, the nurse may ask clients to interpret their feelings about communication with loved ones. The nurse hopes that results from the study will give other nurses working in hospice settings useful approaches for improving family communication. The scientific method is one formal way to approach a problem, plan a solution, test the solution, and come to a conclusion.

Problem Solving

We all face problems every day, whether it is a computer program that does not function properly even though we know we have used the right sequence of keystrokes or the ever-popular VCR that we cannot program correctly. When a problem arises, we obtain information and then use the information plus what we already know to find a solution. Clients routinely present problems in nursing practice. For example, consider the situation when you enter a client's room and find the client lying in a twisted manner. You know that the client underwent back surgery and is supposed to remain in straight anatomical alignment to avoid stress on the surgical area. You suspect the client is having pain but instead learn through questioning that he or she is uncomfortably cold. You reposition the client and provide an additional blanket for warmth. When returning to the client's room 30 minutes later, you find the client asleep. You obtained information that correctly clarified the client's source of discomfort and tested a solution that was successful.

Effective problem solving also involves evaluating the solution over time to be sure that it is still effective. You return to the client's room to evaluate whether the client remains comfortable. It may become necessary to try different options if the problem recurs. Having solved a problem in one situation adds to your experience in your practice and allows you to apply that knowledge in future client situations.

Decision Making

When you are faced with a problem or situation and must choose a course of action from several options, you are engaging in decision making. Decision making is an end point of critical thinking that is focused on resolving a problem. For example, decision making occurs when you choose an elective course to take in your nursing program. To make a decision you must first recognize and define the problem or situation (need to select a course that meets program requirements), assess all options (consider courses recommended by faculty and colleagues or choose one that is scheduled for a convenient time), weigh each option against a set of criteria (reputation of faculty, value of course as it pertains to your career goals), test possible options (talk directly with the faculty), consider the consequences of the decision (examine pros and cons of selecting one course over another), and then make a final decision. Although the set of criteria seems to follow a sequence of steps, decision making involves moving back and forth in considering all criteria. Utilization of the decision-making process leads to a conclusion that is informed and supported by evidence and by reason (Bandman and Bandman, 1995). Examples of decision making in the clinical area include deciding on a choice of dressings for a client with a surgical wound or deciding on the best approach to teaching a family how to assist a stroke client who is returning home. You learn to make sound decisions by approaching each clinical situation thoughtfully and by applying each component of the decision-making process mentioned above.

Diagnostic Reasoning

As soon as you receive information about a client in a particular clinical situation, diagnostic reasoning begins. It is a process of determining a client's health status when you assign meaning to the behaviors, physical signs, and reported client symptoms that are presented (O'Neill and Dluhy, 1997). An example of diagnostic reasoning is forming a nursing diagnosis (see Chapter 6). Diagnostic reasoning is a series of clinical judgments you make during and after data collection, resulting in an informal judgment or formal diagnosis (Carnevali and Thomas, 1993). The process of diagnostic reasoning provides a clear perspective of a client's health status and whether or not the client is progressing.

CLINICAL SCENARIO

In addition to stomach cancer, Mrs. Bryan had a myocardial infarction, a "heart attack," just 4 months ago. She must periodically be monitored for possible chest pain, shortness of breath, and/or irregularity of vital signs (signs and symptoms of recurrent cardiac problems). If Mrs. Bryan has a regular heart rate, denies discomfort, is breathing normally without difficulty, and has stable laboratory results, Inez can make the diagnostic decision that Mrs. Bryan's cardiac status is currently stable. Inez makes her diagnostic decision based on a thorough and comprehensive assessment. She must critically analyze changing clinical situations so that Mrs. Bryan's status can immediately be determined. This allows Inez to initiate appropriate therapies, such as progressive monitored exercise, so that Mrs. Bryan can develop activity tolerance within her limitations. In addition, any further diagnostic conclusions made by Inez during her visit with Mrs. Bryan help the physician pinpoint the nature of a problem more quickly and select proper medical therapies.

Clinical Decision Making

When you approach a clinical problem, such as a client who has developed a pressure ulcer or who is anxious about having surgery, you make a decision that identifies the problem and then you choose the best nursing interventions that will reach mutually established goals. Nurses make clinical decisions all the time in an attempt to improve a client's health or to maintain ongoing wellness. For example, look at the case scenario at the beginning of this chapter. During a clinic visit Inez observes a bruised area of the skin over Mrs. Bryan's right hip. Mrs. Bryan describes it as a scrape that she received when she fell against the edge of her bathtub. Inez must consider her nursing knowledge and the unique situation of the client when making a decision about the therapies that will promote healing and prevent further injury. Criteria that will help Inez make an appropriate clinical decision include the following (Strader, 1992):

- What needs to be achieved (healing of the skin, a safe home environment)?
- What needs to be preserved (mobility, nutrition, comfort, safety)?
- What needs to be avoided (further tissue injury, infection, further falls)?

Clinical decision-making criteria assist you in setting priorities as they relate to a client's situation (see Chapter 6). Because different clients bring different variables to a situation, an activity may be more of a priority in one situation and less of a priority in another. For example, if a client is physically dependent, unable to eat, and incontinent of urine, skin integrity is a greater priority than if the client was immobile but continent of urine and able to eat a normal diet. Do not assume that a certain condition is an automatic priority. For example, when surgical clients return to a nursing division from surgery, it is expected that they will experience a certain level of pain, which often becomes a priority of nursing care. However, if clients are experiencing severe anxiety that heightens pain perception, it may become necessary to focus on ways to relieve anxiety before pain-relief measures can be effective. New pain research suggests that nurses may erroneously arrive at conclusions about clients' pain postoperatively without asking clients enough about their experience to gain an objective assessment.

After determining a client's nursing care priorities, choose the nursing therapies most likely to relieve each problem. A wide range of choices may be available, from nurse-administered to client self-care therapies. Collaborate with the client and then select, test, and evaluate each approach. Try to anticipate what might go wrong, and consider alternative approaches to minimize or prevent problems. For example, Inez will talk with Mrs. Bryan's daughter about having someone check the condition of Mrs. Bryan's bathroom to see if there are any obstacles creating a risk for falls. Based on the findings, Inez will make recommendations to Mrs. Bryan on ways to minimize any hazards or obstacles in her home so that the risks for further injury are reduced.

You will make decisions about individual clients and about groups of clients. If you work on a busy hospital unit,

Clinical Decision Making for Groups of Clients	Box 5-2

Identify the nursing and collaborative problems of each client.

Analyze clients' problems and decide which problems are most urgent on the basis of basic needs, the client's changing or unstable status, and problem complexity.

Consider how to involve the clients as decision makers and participants in care.

Consider the time it will take to care for clients whose problems are of high priority.

Decide how to combine activities to resolve more than one client problem at a time.

Decide what if any nursing care procedures can be delegated to assistive personnel so that you can devote your time to activities requiring professional nursing knowledge.

you will likely care for several clients. You will need to use criteria such as the clinical condition of the client, Maslow's hierarchy of needs (Chapter 6), risks involved in treatment delays, and the clients' expectations of care to determine which clients have the greatest priorities for care. For example, a client whose blood pressure drops suddenly and faints, requires attention immediately. The client who needs to be assisted for a walk down the hallway will have to wait until you can attend to caring for the patient who has fainted. Visit the client who has had no visitors and has recently been given a diagnosis of cancer before checking on the recovering surgical client whose family has just arrived. To be able to manage the wide variety of problems associated with groups of clients (Box 5-2), skillful, prioritized decision making is critical.

The Nursing Process as a Competency

The **nursing process** is a systematic approach that nurses use to gather client data, critically examine and analyze the client's data, identify the client's response to a health problem, design expected outcomes and interventions, take action, and then evaluate whether the action is effective. The format for the nursing process is unique to the discipline of nursing and provides a common language and process for nurses to "think through" clients' clinical problems (Kataoka-Yahiro and Saylor, 1994). The nursing process is systematic and comprehensive. An overview of the process is provided on p. 67.

THINKING AND LEARNING

Learning is a lifelong process. Our intellectual and emotional growth involve acquiring new knowledge and refining the ability to think, problem solve, and make judgments. To learn, you must be flexible and always open to new information. Learning and thinking are inseparable. Over time, as you have new experiences and apply the knowledge gained, you become better able to form assumptions, present ideas, and make valid conclusions.

As a professional nurse you must learn to think and to anticipate. This involves looking ahead and asking the following questions: What is a client's status? How might it change? How can nursing knowledge be applied to improve the client's condition? You cannot allow your thinking to become routine or standardized. Instead, learn to look beyond the obvious, recognizing that each client is unique. This does not mean that you know nothing about a client until having met him or her. Your experience with other clients aids in recognizing patterns of behavior, seeing commonalities in signs and symptoms, and anticipating reactions to therapies. Thinking about those experiences enables you to better anticipate client needs and recognize problems before or when they develop.

Nursing practice is always changing. As new knowledge becomes available, you must challenge traditional ways of doing things and discover those interventions that are most effective, have scientific relevance, and result in better client outcomes. Your ability to think critically demonstrates a commitment to learning and enhances your ability to positively influence nursing practice.

A CRITICAL THINKING MODEL

Models serve to explain concepts. Because critical thinking is complex, a model can help to explain what is involved as you make clinical decisions and judgments about your clients. Kataoka-Yahiro and Saylor (1994) have developed a model of critical thinking for nursing judgment based in part on previous work by Paul (1993), Glaser (1941), and Miller and Malcolm (1990) (Figure 5-1). The model defines the outcome of critical thinking: nursing judgment that is relevant to nursing problems in a variety of settings. According to the model, when you enter into any clinical experience there are five components of critical thinking that lead you to make the clinical judgments necessary for safe, effective nursing care (Box 5-3). The components occur simultaneously. You learn to apply your specific knowledge base (scientific and nursing), experience, critical thinking competencies, and standards as you conduct the nursing process to provide the very best individualized care for your clients.

Specific Knowledge Base

The first component of critical thinking is a nurse's specific knowledge base. This varies according to your educational experience, including basic nursing education, continuing education courses, and additional college degrees. In addition, it includes the initiative you take in reading the nursing literature so as to remain current in nursing science. Your knowledge base includes information and theory from the basic sciences, humanities, behavioral sciences, and nursing. You will use your knowledge base in a different way from other health care disciplines in regard to how you think about client problems. The broad knowledge base gives you a more holistic view of clients and their health care needs. The depth and extent of knowledge influence your ability to

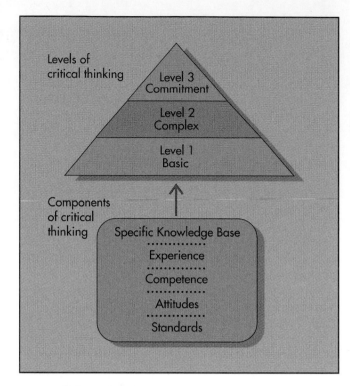

FIGURE **5-1**   Critical thinking model for nursing judgment. (Redrawn from Kataoka-Yahiro M, Saylor C: A critical thinking model for nursing judgment, *J Nurs Educ* 33[8]:351, 1994. Modified from Glaser E: *An experiment in the development of critical thinking,* New York, 1941, Bureau of Publications, Teachers College, Columbia University; Miller M, Malcolm N: Critical thinking in the nursing curriculum, *Nurs Health Care* 11:67, 1990; and Paul R: The art of redesigning instruction. In Willsen J, Blinker AJA, editors: *Critical thinking: how to prepare students for a rapidly changing world,* Santa Rosa, Calif, 1993, Foundation for Critical Thinking.)

think critically about nursing problems (Figure 5-2). Referring to the clinical scenario, Inez Santiago previously earned a degree in education. She is just starting her third year of study in nursing. She has successfully completed courses in anatomy and physiology, introduction to nursing concepts, and communication principles. Although still a novice to nursing, her preparation and knowledge base will help her make the clinical decisions necessary to care for Mrs. Bryan.

CLINICAL SCENARIO

As Inez Santiago thinks about her clinical experiences with clients, she recognizes she still has a lot to learn. However, each client has provided her with valuable learning experiences. Specifically, she has been able to acquire good interviewing skills, she understands the importance of the family in an individual's health, and she has learned the role nurses play as advocates for clients. Her time in the physical assessment laboratory and her first semester in a clinical area helped her to learn to be a watchful observer. Inez also knows that her previous experience as a teacher will help her apply educational principles in her nursing role.

Components of Critical Thinking in Nursing

Box 5-3

I. Specific knowledge base in nursing
II. Experience in nursing
III. Critical thinking competencies
    A. General critical thinking competencies
    B. Specific critical thinking competencies in clinical situations
    C. Specific critical thinking competency in nursing
IV. Attitudes for critical thinking
    A. Confidence   G. Perseverance
    B. Independence   H. Creativity
    C. Fairness   I. Curiosity
    D. Responsibility   J. Integrity
    E. Risk taking   K. Humility
    F. Discipline
V. Standards for critical thinking
    A. Intellectual standards
        1. Clear   9. Deep
        2. Precise   10. Broad
        3. Specific   11. Complete
        4. Accurate   12. Significant
        5. Relevant   13. Adequate
        6. Plausible   (for purpose)
        7. Consistent   14. Fair
        8. Logical
    B. Professional standards
        1. Ethical criteria for nursing judgment
        2. Criteria for evaluation
        3. Professional responsibility

Modified from Kataoka-Yahiro M, Saylor C: A critical thinking model for nursing judgment, *J Nurs Educ* 33(8):351, 1994. Data from Paul R: The art of redesigning instruction. In Willsen J, Blinker AJA, editors: *Critical thinking: how to prepare students for a rapidly changing world*, Santa Rosa, Calif, 1993, Foundation for Critical Thinking.

Experience

The second component of the critical thinking model is experience in nursing. Unless you have the opportunity to practice and make decisions about client care, critical thinking in clinical decision making cannot develop. You will learn from your experiences in observing, sensing, and talking with clients and then reflecting actively on your experiences. Clinical experience is the laboratory for testing nursing knowledge. You will learn that "textbook" approaches lay important groundwork for practice, but you must make adaptations to accommodate the setting, the unique qualities of the client, and the experiences you have gained from caring for previous clients. Benner (1984) notes that the expert nurse understands the context of a clinical situation, recognizes cues suggesting patterns, and interprets them as relevant or irrelevant. This level of competency comes with experience and a lifelong commitment to learning. Perhaps the best lesson you can learn is to value all client experiences. Each clinical experience serves as a stepping stone to building new knowledge and stimulating innovative thinking.

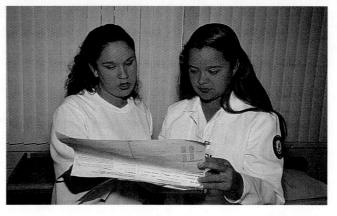

FIGURE **5-2**   Student nurse in conversation with colleague.

Critical Thinking Competencies

The model for critical thinking includes the competencies discussed on pp. 61-63. In your practice, the nursing process is the specific competency you will use to deliver nursing care.

Attitudes for Critical Thinking

The fourth component of the critical thinking model is attitudes. Paul (1993) identifies 11 attitudes that are central features of a critical thinker (see Box 5-3). These attitudes define how you must approach a problem to be a successful critical thinker. For example, when you are faced with determining how to help a client adjust to a permanent loss of speech, you must persevere to understand how the client feels about the loss and think independently to find the interventions that will help the client communicate needs to others. When you use the attitude of integrity, it improves your ability to recognize that problems exist and to accept the need for evidence in support of what you believe is true (Watson and Glaser, 1980). Attitudes provide guidelines for how to approach a problem or decision-making situation. You must have cognitive skills to think critically, but it is also important to ensure that these skills are used fairly and responsibly. Table 5-2 summarizes how critical thinking attitudes can be applied in nursing practice situations. A summary of each critical thinking attitude follows.

CONFIDENCE.   To be confident is to feel certain in your ability to accomplish a task or goal. Confidence grows with experience and a maturity in recognizing your strengths and limitations. Confidence is not arrogance or the feeling of superiority. Instead, confident critical thinkers remain aware of the balance between what they know and what they do not know. When you demonstrate confidence, your clients recognize it in the manner in which you communicate and the way you perform nursing care. Confidence builds trust between you and your clients, conveys a sense of caring, and is often effective in helping to achieve client outcomes.

THINKING INDEPENDENTLY.   As you mature and gain new knowledge, you learn to consider a wide range of ideas and concepts before forming an opinion or making a judg-

Critical Thinking Attitudes and Applications in Nursing Practice Table 5-2

Critical Thinking Attitude	Application in Practice
Confidence	Learn how to introduce yourself to a client. Speak with conviction when you begin a treatment or procedure. Do not lead a client to think that you are uncertain of being able to perform care safely. Always be prepared before performing a nursing activity.
Thinking independently	Read the nursing literature, especially when there are different views on the same subject. Talk with colleagues and share ideas about nursing interventions.
Fairness	Listen to both sides in any discussion. If a client or family member complains about a colleague, listen to the story and then speak with the colleague as well. Weigh all facts.
Responsibility and authority	Ask for help if you are uncertain about an aspect of client care. Report any problems immediately. Follow standards of practice in your care.
Risk taking	If your knowledge causes you to question a physician's order, do so. Offer alternative approaches to nursing care when colleagues are having little success with clients.
Discipline	Be thorough in whatever you do. Use known criteria for activities such as assessment and evaluation. Take time to be thorough.
Perseverance	Be wary of an easy answer. If colleagues give you information about a client and some fact seems to be missing, go clarify information or talk to the client directly. If problems of the same type continue to occur on a nursing division, bring colleagues together, look for a pattern, and find a solution.
Creativity	Look for different approaches if interventions are not working. A client may need a different positioning technique or a different instructional approach that will suit his or her unique needs.
Curiosity	Always ask why. A clinical sign or symptom can indicate a variety of problems. Explore and learn more about the client so as to make the right clinical judgments.
Integrity	Recognize when your opinions may conflict with those of a client; review your position, and decide how best to proceed to reach mutually beneficial outcomes.
Humility	Recognize when you need more information to make a decision. When you are newly assigned to a clinical division and you are unfamiliar with the clients, ask to be oriented to the area. Ask nurses regularly assigned to the area for assistance. Read the professional journals regularly to keep updated on new approaches to care.

ment. This does not mean you ignore other people's ideas. You must learn to consider all sides of a given situation. However, a critical thinker does not accept another person's ideas without question. When thinking independently, you challenge the ways others think and look for rational and logical answers to problems. Independent thinking and reasoning are essential to the improvement and expansion of nursing knowledge and practice.

FAIRNESS. A critical thinker deals with situations in a just manner. This means that bias or prejudice does not enter into a decision. For example, regardless of how you feel about obesity, you should not allow personal attitudes to influence the way you deliver care to clients who are overweight. Fairness helps you to look at a situation objectively, analyzing all viewpoints, to understand the situation completely before arriving at a decision. Developing a sense of imagination aids in the development of fairness. Imagining what it must be like to be in the situation your clients face can help you to see situations with new eyes and appreciate their complexity.

RESPONSIBILITY AND ACCOUNTABILITY. When caring for clients, you have a responsibility to correctly perform nursing care activities based on standards of practice, which are the minimum level of performance accepted to ensure high-quality care. For example, you do not take shortcuts

when you administer medications to a client. Remaining competent in performing nursing therapies is part of your responsibility as a professional nurse and contributes to your growing ability to make clinical decisions about and with clients. When you intervene for a client, you must be answerable or accountable for the results of your nursing actions. As an accountable nurse you are reliable and willing to recognize when nursing care is effective or ineffective. Ultimately you assume accountability for whatever decisions and resultant actions are made on the client's behalf.

RISK TAKING. When a person takes a risk in acting or making a decision, it often is perceived that a potential loss may be at stake. Driving 30 miles an hour over the speed limit is a risk that might result in injury to the driver and an unlucky pedestrian. However, risk taking does not have to cause injury. Risk taking can be desirable, particularly when the result is a positive outcome. A critical thinker is willing to take certain risks in trying different approaches to solving problems. The willingness to take risks often comes from experience with similar problems. In nursing, risk taking frequently results in client care innovations. Nurses in the past have taken risks in trying different approaches to skin and wound care, pulmonary hygiene, and pain management, to name a few. When taking a risk, you considers all options, analyze any potential danger to a client, and then act in a well-reasoned, logical, and thoughtful manner.

DISCIPLINE.   To be a good critical thinker you must use discipline. A disciplined thinker misses few details and follows an orderly approach when making decisions or taking action. For example, by assessing a client's pain thoroughly you are more likely to select the most appropriate nursing interventions. Disciplined thinking does not lessen your creativity but instead ensures that any decision you make is made systematically with a comprehensive approach.

PERSEVERANCE.   As a critical thinker you must become determined to find effective solutions to client care problems. This is especially important when problems remain unresolved or when they reoccur. You must learn as much as possible about a problem, try various approaches to care, and continue to seek additional resources until a successful approach is found. A critical thinker who perseveres is not satisfied with minimal effort, but constantly strives to achieve the highest level of quality care.

CREATIVITY.   Creativity involves original thinking. This means you find solutions outside of the standard routines of care. Miller and Babcock (1996) describe creativity as a great motivator that enables one to generate options and alternative approaches and to see the future. Often clients pose problems that require unique approaches. A client's clinical problems, social support systems, and living environment are just a few examples of factors that can make the simplest nursing procedure more complicated if you do not consider a creative approach for the client's unique situation.

CURIOSITY.   Probably the favorite question of a critical thinker is, "Why?" In any clinical situation you will learn a great deal of information about a client. As you analyze client information, data patterns emerge that are not always clear. Having a sense of curiosity motivates you to inquire further and to investigate a clinical situation so that all the information needed to make a decision is obtained.

INTEGRITY.   Critical thinkers question and test personal knowledge and beliefs as rigorously as they test the knowledge and beliefs of others. Your personal integrity as a nurse builds trust from peers and subordinates. A person of integrity is honest and willing to admit to any mistakes or inconsistencies in his or her own behavior, ideas, and beliefs. There are few of us who have not made mistakes in our practice. To be a strong professional you must strive to adhere to high standards of practice even in the face of adversity.

HUMILITY.   It is important for you to admit to your limitations in knowledge and skill. Critical thinkers admit what they do not know and try to acquire the knowledge needed to make a proper decision. A client's safety and welfare may be at risk if you are unable to admit to your inability to deal with a practice problem. You must rethink a situation, pursue additional knowledge, and then use the information to form an opinion and draw a conclusion.

Standards for Critical Thinking

The fifth component of the critical thinking model developed by Kataoka-Yahiro and Saylor (1994) includes intellectual and professional standards. Paul (1993) identified the 14 intellectual standards (see Box 5-3) universal for critical thinking. When you consider a client problem, it is important to apply standards such as preciseness, accuracy, and consistency to ensure that clinical decisions are sound and just. For example, when Inez tries to look at the extent of Mrs. Bryan's bruise, she seeks information from Mrs. Bryan and clarifies any confusing statements. Any measurements, such as the size of the bruise, and a description of its appearance are precisely made. The wound location is described in Mrs. Bryan's medical record using specific anatomical terms. Inez examines Mrs. Bryan further to ensure that her findings are accurate and that no other signs of injury are present. The use of intellectual standards involves a rigorous approach to clinical practice and demonstrates that critical thinking cannot be done haphazardly.

Professional standards for critical thinking refer to ethical criteria for nursing judgments (see Chapter 4), criteria to be used for evaluation, and criteria for professional responsibility. Application of professional standards requires that nurses use critical thinking for the good of individuals or groups (Kataoka-Yahiro and Saylor, 1994). Professional standards also ensure that the highest level of quality is promoted. For example, Inez Santiago will be facing an ethical decision if Mrs. Bryan's daughter actively considers a nursing home for her mother. The decision must be made with Mrs. Bryan and her daughter involved so that the ethical standard of autonomy is met. This standard ensures client participation in decision making and support of the client's independence. Mrs. Bryan's feelings and ideas must be accepted, and she must have the emotional support to make a well-informed decision about her future.

Critical thinking also requires the use of evaluation criteria when making clinical judgments. These criteria may be based on standards of care or practice developed by clinical agencies or professional organizations. The standards set the minimum requirements necessary to ensure quality of care. For example, critical pathways used in managing the care of clients with designated medical diagnoses include both recommended interventions and outcomes that clinicians use for evaluating clients' clinical progress. The outcomes provide evaluation criteria with which clinical staff can make sound and consistent clinical judgments. Evaluation criteria also include norms established through nursing research that can be applied when determining the clinical status of a client. Box 5-4 summarizes types of evaluation criteria available for use in your daily practice.

▌ NURSING PROCESS OVERVIEW

In the critical thinking model presented in this text, the nursing process is a specific critical thinking competency. It is a cognitive thinking process that consists of five steps: assessment, nursing diagnosis, planning, implementation, and evaluation. Whenever you care for a client, you apply the nursing process while at the same time using critical thinking. This may sound complicated, but if you can learn how to be a critical thinker as you use the nursing process, your clients will benefit and you will become proficient in your professional practice.

The three characteristics of a process are purpose, organization, and creativity (Bevis, 1978). The nursing process features all three. The purpose of the nursing process is to identify, diagnose, and treat actual or potential human responses to health and illness (American Nurses Association, 1995). Organization is the series of five steps in the nursing process you use to achieve the goal of providing effective individualized nursing care. When you use the process, it organizes your approach to delivering nursing care. Creativity is characteristic of the nursing process. It can be applied to individual clients or families and clients of any age and culture, and it can change in response to a client's needs.

The nursing process is often called a blueprint for client care. It is flexible enough to be used in all settings and with all clients. When you use the nursing process you are able to identify a client's health care needs, determine priorities, establish goals and expected outcomes of care, establish and communicate a client-centered plan of care, deliver nursing interventions, and evaluate the effectiveness of your care (Table 5-3). When you become more competent in using the nursing process, you will be able to focus not only on a single client problem but on multiple problems. As a nurse you must always be thinking and recognizing what step of the process is being used. Within each step of the process you will apply critical thinking to provide the very best professional care to your clients.

SYNTHESIS IN PRACTICE

As a beginning student it becomes important for you to see the relationship between the nursing process and critical thinking. Eventually the nursing process and critical thinking are synthesized, meaning the two come together in a manner that allows you to become a competent nurse professional. As you develop professionally you will synthesize all of your knowledge and experience that applies to a clinical situation, reflect on previous experiences, and exercise the right attitudes and standards when using the nursing process to deliver safe and effective nursing care. For students like you who are new to nursing, this text provides a model that reinforces the importance of critical thinking in nursing practice. Throughout the clinical chapters of this text, the components of critical thinking are summarized in a Synthesis in Practice section to help you better understand its relationship to the nursing process. Let's look back to Mrs. Bryan and Inez Santiago one more time to show how synthesis of critical thinking and the nursing process works.

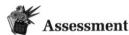 **Assessment**

Inez has scheduled a clinic appointment for Mrs. Bryan on a day when she knows that Mrs. Bryan's daughter is in town visiting. She has previously assessed Mrs. Bryan's physical condition (e.g., nutritional status, activity limitations, coordination and strength, condition of the skin, and respiratory and cardiac function). Although she has not fallen again, Mrs. Bryan is slow and deliberate as she walks into the clinic office. Inez knows how Mrs. Bryan feels about remaining independent and being able to stay in her home. Even though her physical condition has declined, Mrs. Bryan insists she can care for herself. Inez expands the assessment now to learn more about Mrs. Bryan's daughter, her concerns, her relationship with Mrs. Bryan, and the reasons for her wanting Mrs. Bryan to move. Inez learns that Mrs. Bryan and her daughter have a very good relationship. The two initially speak openly and listen to one another's feelings. However, when the topic of moving from home comes up, Mrs. Bryan becomes resentful. She acknowledges her daughter's concern but stresses that going to a nursing home would "kill" her. She instead tells her daughter that she prefers to be able to stay in her hometown, even if it means living with a nearby friend. The daughter is most concerned about her mother's safety, and she questions whether the friend is capable of caring for Mrs. Bryan properly. She seems uncertain about trusting her mother's friend. The friend is younger, reportedly healthy, and has offered to let Mrs. Bryan live with her.

Synthesis of Critical Thinking With the Nursing Process

(Knowledge) Inez has learned that family support is important to a client's well-being. If there is a way to find a solution that both Mrs. Bryan and her daughter can agree to, the outcome will likely be more positive. Inez has also read about home safety. She knows that certain conditions must be in

Summary of Nursing Process		Table 5-3
Component	**Purpose**	**Steps**
Assessment	To gather, verify, and communicate data about client so that database is established	1. Collecting nursing health history 2. Performing physical examination 3. Collecting laboratory data 4. Validating data 5. Clustering data 6. Documenting data
Nursing diagnosis	To examine the data for patients that identify health care needs of client to formulate nursing diagnoses	1. Analyzing and interpreting data 2. Identifying client problems 3. Formulating nursing diagnoses 4. Documenting nursing diagnoses
Planning	To identify client's goals; to determine priorities of care, to determine expected outcomes, to design nursing strategies to achieve goals of care	1. Identifying client goals 2. Establishing expected outcomes 3. Selecting nursing actions 4. Delegating actions 5. Writing nursing care plan 6. Consulting
Implementation	To carry out nursing actions necessary for accomplishing plan	1. Reassessing client 2. Reviewing and modifying existing care plan 3. Performing nursing actions
Evaluation	To determine extent to which interventions helped achieve goals of care	1. Comparing client response to criteria 2. Analyzing reasons for results and conclusions 3. Modifying care plan

place for a person to be able to move about freely within the home with minimal risk of injury. *(Experience)* After having seen Mrs. Bryan several times, Inez knows that Mrs. Bryan fears moving to a nursing home. Inez has also had the experience of caring for clients in a nursing home and has seen clients become depressed when separated from their home and family support. *(Attitudes)* Inez knows she cannot make a decision for Mrs. Bryan and her daughter. She must be fair and listen to the feelings and concerns of both individuals while working toward a creative solution that will meet the needs of both people. *(Standards)* Ethically, it is important to preserve Mrs. Bryan's autonomy. A decision must be made with her input and support.

Nursing Diagnosis

Inez reviews the information she has collected on Mrs. Bryan and her daughter. Mrs. Bryan has verbalized concern about having to leave her home. Joyce, the daughter, has verbalized concern that her mother will be at risk unless she moves to a nursing home. Joyce knows the neighbor is an option but has reservations about how living arrangements can be made. It is clear to Inez that Joyce cares very much for her mother. The daughter's concern over Mrs. Bryan's welfare is conflicting with Mrs. Bryan's desire for independence. After reviewing all assessment data, Inez sees a pattern in the information collected. Based on the guidelines of the North American Nursing Diagnosis Association (NANDA), Inez forms the following nursing diagnosis (see Chapter 6): *Decisional conflict related to threat over loss of independence.*

Planning

For the diagnosis of *decisional conflict* Inez establishes a goal of "Client will make an informed choice regarding client's residence." Outcomes will include the following:

Client will choose place to reside.

Choice will be consistent with client's values.

Client and daughter will understand options for client's continued care.

Planned interventions will include the following:

Plan a meeting with Mrs. Bryan, her daughter, and Mrs. Bryan's friend. Arrange a tour of the friend's home.

Arrange a visit to the city where Mrs. Bryan's daughter lives, and have mother and daughter tour selected nursing homes.

Encourage Mrs. Bryan to identify features she feels are important to have in a living environment.

Arrange times for the daughter and Mrs. Bryan to participate in joint decision making.

Implementation

Inez proceeds to arrange a visit to the clinic for Mrs. Bryan, Joyce, and Mrs. Bryan's neighbor. Inez also has her instructor attend so that some expert assistance is available. The visit is timed in the morning, when Mrs. Bryan feels most alert. Inez acts only as a mediator, being sure all participants discuss the issues most important to them. Before the meeting ends, Joyce agrees to visit the neighbor's home with her mother.

In planning the nursing home visits, Inez helps Mrs. Bryan pick features she believes are important to have in a living environment. Inez and Mrs. Bryan's daughter select two to three nursing homes that have the features Mrs. Bryan prefers. A tour of the nursing homes is scheduled in the morning so that Mrs. Bryan will become less fatigued. Mrs. Bryan and her daughter make plans to discuss Mrs. Bryan's decision.

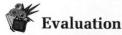 **Evaluation**

Inez meets with Mrs. Bryan and her daughter to discuss their thoughts on the recent visits to the neighbor's home and the nursing homes. Together the three of them identify some criteria necessary for making a decision: safety, cleanliness, ability for Mrs. Bryan to remain independent with self-care, and availability of medical support.

Mrs. Bryan and her daughter agree that the neighbor's home appears safe and very clean. The neighbor is very in-dependent and has offered to let Mrs. Bryan have a first-floor room as her bedroom. A small bath is adjacent to the room. The neighbor agrees to allow Mrs. Bryan's daughter to set up an alarm system in the home that will dial emergency medical services immediately if a problem arises. They decide to have Mrs. Bryan live with her friend for a 3-month trial period.

Inez will continue to care for Mrs. Bryan, assessing her client's situation and deciding when and if modifications are needed. The plan of care will be revised to ensure that Mrs. Bryan and her daughter take time over the next 3 months to evaluate how well things are going. Use of the nursing process coupled with strong critical thinking skills has helped Inez assist the Bryan family in developing a workable and realistic plan of care.

Key Terms

Key Concepts

- Critical thinking is the active, organized, cognitive process used to examine your thinking and the thinking of others.
- Reflection is a form of self-evaluation that involves recalling an experience with a client and exploring the actions, meaning, and purpose of the event.
- The basic level of critical thinking is concrete and based on a set of rules or principles.
- In complex critical thinking you analyze and examine alternatives more independently and take initiative to solve problems.
- In commitment you choose an action that coincides with your knowledge and you remain accountable for it.

- Intuition raises a red flag but should not be accepted as automatic truth.
- Decision making is an end point of critical thinking.
- When making clinical decisions learn to ask what needs to be achieved, preserved, and avoided.
- Critical thinking includes knowledge, experience, critical thinking competencies, attitudes, and standards.
- You learn through experience by observing, sensing, and talking with clients and then reflecting actively.
- Attitudes provide guidelines for how to approach a problem or decision-making situation.

Critical Thinking Activities

1. At 10 AM John went to the medication room to prepare the medications for his four assigned clients on a busy medical nursing unit. Just before John completed preparing the medications, a nurse told him that Mr. Williams in Room 10 was requesting pain medication. John saved some time and prepared the morphine 10 mg ordered for Mr. Williams. He gathered the medications he had prepared and went to Room 10 first, giving Mr. Lazar his ordered medications and then giving Mr. Williams the requested injection of morphine. After administering all of the medications, John gathered Mr. Williams's chart and discovered he had received morphine only 2 hours ago. The medication is to be given no sooner than every 4 hours. Within 15 minutes of giving the morphine, Mr. Williams's vital signs were stable. As a follow-up, John completed an incident report describing the medication error. Reflect on this experience while considering the errors that were made, and describe what John might learn from the experience.

2. Miss Stechmeyer has been hospitalized for 2 days. She has had major abdominal surgery. You are familiar with her past medical history of a myocardial infarction (heart attack) just 2 years ago. When you enter the room, Miss Stechmeyer says, "Nurse, I am having this terrible pain." If you apply critical thinking standards in your assessment of Miss Stechmeyer, explain how you would be specific, accurate, and logical.

Review Questions

1. A client has nursing diagnoses of *anxiety* and *knowledge, deficient concerning impending surgery*. You decide that the client's anxiety must be addressed first in order for the client to be receptive to any formal instruction about surgery. This decision is considered a part of:
   1. planning.
   2. evaluation.
   3. assessment.
   4. implementation.

2. A 72-year-old woman has been a client on the medicine unit for about 4 days. When she was first admitted, she was alert and oriented. For the last 24 hours she has become acutely confused and has repeatedly attempted to get out of bed. The nursing staff have discussed the possibility of using restraints; however, you insist that use of orientation and meaningful diversion should be tried. Your alternative is an example of the critical thinking attitude:
   1. integrity.
   2. risk taking.
   3. thinking independently.
   4. responsibility and authority.

3. During the day you spend time instructing a client in how to self-administer insulin. After discussing the technique and demonstrating an injection, you have the client try it. After two attempts the client obviously does not understand how to prepare the correct dose. When you return to the medication room, you discuss the situation with the charge nurse, reviewing your approach with the client and asking for her suggestions on your technique. This is an example of:
   1. reflection.
   2. risk taking.
   3. client assessment.
   4. care plan evaluation.

4. A client had hip surgery 24 hours ago. When you begin the nursing shift, you refer to the written plan of care, noting that the client has a drainage device collecting wound drainage. The physician's order requires that the physician be notified when drainage in the device exceeds 100 ml for the day. When you enter the room, you look at the device and carefully note the amount of drainage currently in the device. This is an example of:
   1. planning.
   2. assessment.
   3. evaluation.
   4. nursing diagnosis.

5. You ask a client how she feels about her impending surgery for breast cancer. Prior to the discussion you reviewed the description in your textbook of loss and grief in addition to therapeutic communication principles. The critical thinking component involved in your review of the literature is:
   1. experience.
   2. problem solving.
   3. knowledge application.
   4. clinical decision making.

References

American Nurses Association: *Nursing's social policy statement,* Washington, DC, 1995, The Association.

Baker CR: Reflective learning: a teaching strategy for critical thinking, *J Nurs Educ* 35(1):19, 1996.

Bandman EL, Bandman B: *Critical thinking in nursing,* ed 2, Norwalk, Conn, 1995, Appleton & Lange.

Benner P: *From novice to expert,* Menlo Park, Calif, 1984, Addison Wesley.

Bevis EM: *Curriculum building in nursing: a process,* St. Louis, 1978, Mosby.

Bittner NP, Tobin E: Critical thinking: strategies for clinical practice, *J Nurs Staff Dev* 14(6):267, 1998.

Brock A, Butts JB: On target: a model to teach baccalaureate nursing students to apply critical thinking, *Nurs Forum* 33(3):5, 1998.

Carnevali DL, Thomas MD: *Diagnostic reasoning and treatment decision making in nursing,* Philadelphia, 1993, JB Lippincott.

Chaffee J: *Thinking critically,* ed 3, Boston, 1994, Houghton Mifflin.

Facione P: *Critical thinking: a statement of expert consensus for purposes of educational assessment and instruction. The Delphi report: research findings and recommendations prepared for the American Philosophical Association,* ERIC Doc No. ED 315-423, Washington, DC, 1990, ERIC.

Fowler LP: Improving critical thinking in nursing practice, *J Nurs Staff Dev* 14(4):183, 1998.

Fox RC: The evolution of medical uncertainty, *Milbank Mem Fund Q Health Society* 58(1):1, 1980.

Glaser E: *An experiment in the development of critical thinking,* New York, 1941, Bureau of Publications, Teachers College, Columbia University.

Gordon M: *Nursing diagnosis: process and application,* ed 3, St. Louis, 1995, Mosby.

Hughes KK, Young WB: Decision making: stability of clinical decisions, *Nurse Educ* 17(3):12 1992.

Kataoka-Yahiro M, Saylor C: A critical thinking model for nursing judgment, *J Nurs Educ* 33(8):351, 1994.

Miller M, Babcock DE: *Critical thinking applied to nursing,* St. Louis, 1996, Mosby.

Miller M, Malcolm N: Critical thinking in the nursing curriculum, *Nurs Health Care* 11:67, 1990.

O'Neill ES, Dluhy NM: A longitudinal framework for fostering critical thinking and diagnostic reasoning, *J Adv Nurs* 26:825, 1997.

Paul R: The art of redesigning instruction. In Willsen J, Blinker AJA, editors: *Critical thinking: how to prepare students for a rapidly changing world,* Santa Rosa, Calif, 1993, Foundation for Critical Thinking.

Paul RW, Heaslip P: Critical thinking and intuitive nursing practice, *J Adv Nurs* 22: 40, 1995.

Potter PA, Perry AG: *Fundamentals of nursing,* ed 5, St. Louis, 2001, Mosby.

Strader M: Critical thinking. In Sullivan EJ, Decker PJ: *Effective management in nursing,* ed 3, Redwood City, Calif, 1992, Addison-Wesley Nursing.

Watson G, Glaser E: *Watson-Glaser critical thinking appraisal manual,* New York, 1980, Macmillan.

Whiteside C: A model for teaching critical thinking in the clinical setting, *Dimens Crit Care Nurs* 16(3):152, 1997.

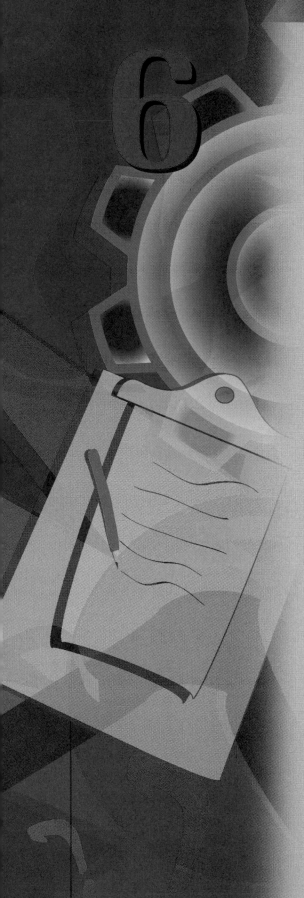

Nursing Process

Objectives

- Define the key terms listed.
- Describe each component of the nursing process.
- Explain the relationship between critical thinking and each component of the nursing process.
- Explain the difference between comprehensive, problem-oriented, and focused assessments.
- Differentiate between subjective and objective data.
- Discuss the necessity for validating assessment data.
- List the steps of the nursing diagnostic process.
- Describe the way in which defining characteristics and the etiological process individualize a nursing diagnosis.
- Demonstrate the ability to prioritize a list of nursing diagnoses.
- Describe goal setting.
- Discuss the difference between a goal and an expected outcome.
- Discuss the process of selecting nursing interventions.
- Develop a plan of care from a nursing assessment.
- Discuss the differences between protocols and standing orders.
- Evaluate nursing actions selected for a client.
- Describe how evaluation can lead to revision or modification of a plan of care.

In Chapter 5 you read about Mrs. Bryan. When you first meet her, you need to determine her health status. You might learn that she has pain. Certainly you and she would agree that pain management is important. You would think about how you could best help to relieve her pain. Perhaps you might decide that a back massage might be helpful. You would then proceed, at the earliest appropriate time, to give Mrs. Bryan a massage. After the massage, you would ask Mrs. Bryan if her pain had been reduced. If it had, you would plan additional massages as part of her care. If not, you would need to think about other ways to manage her pain. Your approach to Mrs. Bryan's care involves use of the nursing process.

As you read this chapter, you will learn more about Mrs. Bryan and her clinical status. The clinical scenarios will be used to guide you in understanding each step of the nursing process. You will see how the critical thinking skills presented in the previous chapter are essential to correctly use each step of the nursing process.

NURSING PROCESS OVERVIEW

The **nursing process** enables you to organize and deliver appropriate nursing care to a client. To successfully apply the nursing process, you need to integrate elements of critical thinking to make judgments and take reasoned actions. The nursing process is used to identify, diagnose, and treat human responses to health and illness (American Nurses Association, 1995). The process includes five steps: assessment, nursing diagnosis, planning, implementation, and evaluation (Figure 6-1). It is a dynamic continuous process, which enables you to modify care as your client's needs change. Using the nursing process promotes individualized

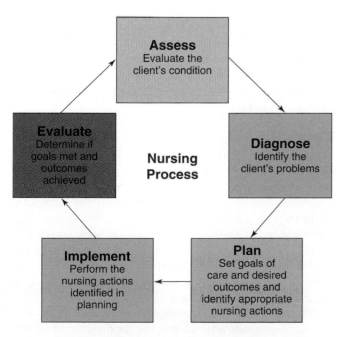

FIGURE **6-1**   Five-step nursing process.

nursing care and assists you in responding to client needs in a timely and consistent manner to improve or maintain the client's level of health.

The nursing process is simply one variation of scientific reasoning that allows you to organize care for your clients, whether the client is an individual, family, or community. It is an approach that allows nurses to differentiate their practice from that of physicians and other health care professionals. Table 6-1 (p. 74) compares each step of the nursing process with problem solving and the scientific method. As you read through each section of the nursing process you will see that during assessment you not only encounter the client's health problems, but you collect information related to the problem and other facets of the client's life and health status. When you formulate the nursing diagnoses, you identify the exact nature of the problem. As you create the individualized plan of care you are specifying an exact plan of action for your client's health care problems. During implementation you carry out the plan. Last, evaluation enables you to determine success, failure, or the need to modify the plan.

Assessment

Nursing **assessment** includes two steps. First, collect and verify data from a primary source (the client) and secondary sources (family, health professionals). Then analyze those data as a basis for developing nursing diagnoses and an individualized plan of nursing care. The purpose of the assessment is to establish a **database** about the client's perceived needs, health problems, and responses to these problems. In addition, the data reveal related experiences, health practices, goals, values, lifestyle, and expectations from the health care system.

An assessment must be relevant to a client's particular health problem. You apply critical thinking to determine what is relevant to include in your client's assessment. For example, if a woman comes to an urgent care setting because of a possible ankle fracture, you consider the implications of a musculoskeletal injury, associated pain, and immobility to focus your assessment. You do not need her childbirth or surgical history. Your assessment will focus on the ankle injury and its effects on the client.

It is important that you learn to think critically about what to assess. Determine when a question or measurement is appropriate based on your clinical knowledge and experience and your client's response. When you first meet a client, make a quick observational overview. Usually an overview is based on the treatment situation. For example, a community health nurse assesses the neighborhood and the community of the client; an emergency department nurse uses the A-B-C (airway-breathing-circulation) approach; and a psychiatric nurse may focus on the client's orientation to reality, anxiety level, and violence potential (Carnevali and Thomas, 1993).

The initial overview of your client's situation allows you to use key assessment data to respond to priorities, such as

Comparison of Steps in Problem Solving, the Scientific Method, and the Nursing Process

Table 6-1

Problem Solving	Copi and Cohen's Seven-Step Scientific Method*	Nursing Process
Encountering problem	The problem	Assessing
	Preliminary hypothesis	
Collecting data	Collecting additional facts	
Identifying exact nature of problem	Formulating hypotheses	Forming a nursing diagnosis
Determining plan of action	Deducing further consequences	Planning (outcome identification)
Carrying out plan	Testing consequences	Implementing
Evaluating plan in new situation	Application	Evaluating
Plan of action		

*Modified from Copi IM, Cohen C: *Introduction to logic,* ed 9, New York, 1994, Macmillan.

Typology of 11 Functional Health Patterns*

Box 6-1

Health perception–health management pattern: Describes the client's perceived pattern of health and well-being and how health is managed

Nutritional-metabolic pattern: Describes the client's pattern of food and fluid consumption relative to metabolic need and pattern indicators of local nutrient supply

Elimination pattern: Describes patterns of excretory function (bowel, bladder, and skin)

Activity-exercise pattern: Describes patterns of exercise, activity, leisure, and recreation

Sleep-rest pattern: Describes patterns of sleep, rest, and relaxation

Cognitive-perceptual pattern: Describes sensory-perceptual and cognitive patterns

Self-perception–self-concept pattern: Describes the client's self-concept pattern and perceptions of self (e.g., self-conception/worth, body image, feeling state)

Role-relationship pattern: Describes the client's pattern of role engagements and relationships

Sexuality-reproductive pattern: Describes the client's patterns of satisfaction and dissatisfaction with sexuality pattern; describes reproductive pattern

Coping–stress-tolerance pattern: Describes the client's general coping pattern and the effectiveness of the pattern in terms of stress tolerance

Value-belief pattern: Describes patterns of values, beliefs (including spiritual), and goals that guide the client's choices or decisions

From Gordon M: *Nursing diagnosis: process and application,* ed 3, St. Louis, 1994, Mosby.

*The pattern areas were identified by the author in the mid-1970s to teach assessment and diagnosis at Boston College School of Nursing. Colleagues have suggested some minor changes in labels and content. Faye E. McCain's and Dorothy Smith's assessment concepts were particularly influential, as were the comments of clinical specialists and students who reviewed and tried out the categories in practice.

the onset of pain. It is important that you recognize that the client's situation can change at any time during assessment and that data collection must be accurate, relevant, and appropriate. You must continually assess and interpret the cues from your client.

There are times when an assessment needs to be more comprehensive. Carnevali and Thomas (1993) suggest two approaches. One is through the use of a comprehensive database framework, for example, Gordon's (1994) functional health patterns (Box 6-1). The **functional health pattern** assessment model provides a holistic framework for assessment and a database for deriving a broad range of nursing diagnoses (Gordon, 1994).

The second model to assessment is a problem-focused approach. The assessment begins with problematic areas, such as headache pain. Then you ask the client follow-up questions to clarify and expand how the problem affects lifestyle, level of health, ability to function, relationships with others, and more (Table 6-2).

Thorough and detailed assessment makes it possible to identify accurate nursing diagnoses and to develop appropriate goals, outcomes, and nursing interventions for your client. Begin by organizing the assessment and determining which data must be collected. For example, during assessment it is important to consider the nurse-client interaction. What approach is likely to build trust with the client? Will others, such as family members be involved? What knowledge do you have about the situation? These factors influence your success in developing a relationship with the client and family, which assists in obtaining a purposeful and comprehensive assessment.

Collecting Data

Data collection includes the gathering of subjective and objective data from or about your client. **Subjective data** are your clients' perceptions about their health problems. Only clients can provide this kind of information. For example, a client's report of headache pain is a subjective finding. Only the client can provide information about its frequency, duration, location, and intensity. Subjective data usually include feelings of anxiety, physical discomfort, or mental stress. Subjective data are more difficult to measure (McNaull and others, 1992).

Objective data are observations or measurements you make during assessment. Identifying the presence of a body rash is an example of observed objective data. The measure-

Example of Focused Client Assessment		Table 6-2
Factors to Assess	Questions and Approaches	Physical Assessment Strategies
Nature of pain	Ask to describe pain Ask client about location of pain Ask client to rate pain	Observe client's nonverbal cues as pain is described. Observe where client points to pain, noting if it radiates or is localized. Use a 0-10 pain scale and ask client to numerically rate his or her pain. Following any pain relief measures, reassess using same 0-10 pain scale.
Precipitating factors	Ask if client notices any activities, time of day, during which pain occurs or gets worse Ask if pain is associated with any food or beverages	Observe client during activity, noting any occurrence or changes in pain associated with change of body position, body posture, or activity.
Relieving factors	Ask client about any measures he or she may use to reduce pain	Observe client during activities to relieve or avoid headaches such as medication, biofeedback, etc.

ment of objective data is based on an accepted standard, such as a thermometer, on which the Fahrenheit or Celsius scale is the standard or unit of measure for body temperature. Data collected during assessment should be descriptive, concise, and complete and should not include interpretive statements.

For efficient data collection use a systematic "branching" technique (Milner and Collins, 1992). In branching, after determining the primary data, you begin to collect additional data in areas in which a dysfunction or abnormality appears to exist and abbreviate the assessment in areas in which no problem is apparent. For example, when assessing headache pain, you further assess your client for areas of stress and lifestyle issues. During the assessment, you obtain data about your client's job-related stressors and lack of exercise that may contribute to frequent headaches. You only minimally assess areas like skin condition or nutrition, because they do not relate to the client's headache.

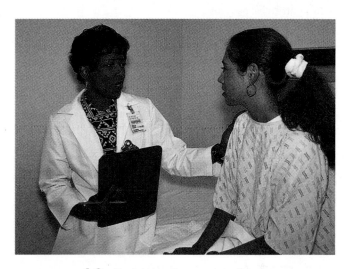

FIGURE **6-2** Explaining the purpose of the interview.

INTERVIEW AND HEALTH HISTORY. The first step in establishing a database is to collect subjective information by interviewing the client. An **interview** is an organized conversation with the client to obtain the client's health history and information about the current illness. During the interview you have the opportunity to:

1. Introduce yourself to the client, explain your role, and the role of others during care
2. Establish a therapeutic relationship with the client
3. Gain insight about the client's concerns and worries
4. Determine the client's goals and expectations of the health care delivery system
5. Obtain cues about which parts of the data collection phase require in-depth investigation

Your interview includes the orientation, working, and termination phases. During the orientation phase of the interview, introduce yourself, your position, and tell the client the purpose of the interview (Figure 6-2).

Explain to the client why the data are being collected and assure the client that any information obtained will remain confidential and will be used only by health care profession-

als who participate in his or her care. These courtesies lessen client anxieties about giving personal information and enlist the client as a partner in health care management. First, collect demographic data, as specified by the facility. Because this information is the least personal, it helps initiate development of the therapeutic relationship and ease transition into the working portion of the interview.

During the working part of the interview you will gather information about the client's health status. Remember to stay focused, orderly, and unhurried. During the working part of the interview investigate the client's current illness, health history, and expectations of care. The general format for a **nursing health history** usually contains several basic components (Box 6-2).

The initial interview is normally the most extensive of all interviews. Major topics that should be covered include biographical data, progress of current illness, and health history. Ongoing interviews, which occur each time you interact with your client, do not need to be as extensive. They update the client's status and are more focused toward changes in previously identified ongoing and new problems.

Basic Components for a Nursing Health History
Box 6-2

Biographical information: Date of birth, sex, address, family members' names and addresses, marital status, religious preference and practices, occupation, source of health care, and insurance

Reasons for seeking health care: Goals of care, expectation of the services and care delivered, and expectations of the health care system

Present illness or health concern: Onset, symptoms, nature of symptoms (e.g., sudden or gradual), duration, precipitating factors, relief measures, and weight loss or gain

Health history: Prior illnesses throughout development, injuries and hospitalizations, surgeries, blood transfusions, allergies, immunizations, habits (e.g., smoking, caffeine intake, alcohol or drug abuse), prescribed and self-prescribed medications, work habits, relaxation activities, and sleep, exercise, and eating or nutritional patterns

Family history: Health status of the immediate family and living relatives, cause of death of relatives, and risk factor analyses for cancer, heart disease, diabetes mellitus, kidney disease, hypertension, or mental disorders

Environmental history: Hazards, pollutants, and physical safety

Psychosocial and cultural history: Primary language, cultural group, community resources, mood, attention span, and developmental stage

Review of systems: Head-to-toe review of all major body systems, as well as the client's knowledge of and compliance with health care (e.g., frequency of breast or testicular self-examination or last visual acuity examination)

-or-

Functional health patterns: Method for organizing assessment data based on function

As in the other phases of the interview, the termination phase requires skill on the part of the interviewer. Ideally your client should be given a clue that the interview is coming to an end. For example, you may say, "There are just two more questions," or "We'll be finished in 5 to 6 minutes." This helps the client maintain direct attention without being distracted by wondering when the interview will end. This approach also gives the client an opportunity to ask questions. When concluding the interview, summarize the important points and ask your client whether the summary was accurate.

INTERVIEWING TECHNIQUES.   The manner in which the interview is conducted is just as important as the questions asked. Attention to the environment, client comfort, and communication techniques (see Chapter 8) often ensures a successful interview. During the interview you are responsible for directing the flow of the interview so that you obtain adequate information and your client has the opportunity to contribute freely.

A good environment provides for privacy by eliminating distractions, unnecessary noise, and interruptions. The client is more likely to be candid if the interview is conducted privately, out of earshot of other clients, visitors, and

staff. Timing is important in avoiding interruptions. If possible, a 15- to 30-minute period should be set aside when no other activities are planned. The client should be made to feel relaxed and unhurried.

Before you begin the interview, be sure the client is comfortable. This includes adequate light, warmth, and positioning. If possible, sit facing the client to facilitate eye contact. During the interview, observe your client for signs of discomfort or fatigue.

Good communication starts with a nonjudgmental, interested, and caring attitude. This is conveyed nonverbally if you and the client are at approximately the same eye level. Initially, open-ended questions such as "Tell me about your pain" or "Describe the symptoms you've noticed" provide the opportunity for the client to indicate major concerns. When more specific information about a topic is needed, closed questions serve best. For example, "Is the pain aggravated by walking?" "Why" questions must be avoided because they are often unanswerable and may make your client feel defensive. Conducting the interview by only asking questions may make the client feel like a subject of interrogation. Other communication techniques such as making observations and clarifying should be interspersed throughout the interview to encourage the exchange of information. If the client is talkative, you may need to refocus the interview when the client strays from the topic. Summarization and validation are always used when concluding an interview. Active listening is important during the entire interview; it makes you alert to unspoken cues and reinforces the therapeutic relationship.

PHYSICAL EXAMINATION.   During **physical examination,** vital signs and other objective measurements are taken, and all body systems are examined. You observe for abnormalities that may yield information about past, present, and future health problems. Physical assessment should be nonthreatening, so begin with the familiar procedure of taking vital signs (see Chapter 11). Then proceed in an orderly sequence, using the four techniques of inspection, auscultation, palpation, and percussion (see Chapter 12).

Actual hands-on physical assessment should be conducted so that your client's anxiety is not aroused. You can minimize anxiety by explaining each step of the exam and continuing throughout the exam to explain and ask about specific functions and discomforts. Be sure you protect the client's privacy, dignity, and warmth.

OBSERVATION OF CLIENT'S BEHAVIOR.   During the interview and physical examination, observe you client's behavior for level of function, consistency, and congruency. This information adds greater depth to the objective database.

The level of function includes physical, developmental, psychological, and social aspects. Observation of the level of function differs from the interview in that it is what you see the client doing, such as self-feeding or making a decision rather than what the client says he or she can do. Level of function differs from the physical assessment in that this is the degree of function at which the client is operating, rather than the greatest extent of function present determined by the hands-on physical examination.

Consistency refers to the degree to which the client operates at the same level of function throughout the assessment and day by day. Any inconsistency is worthy of further data collection.

Congruency is the matching or agreement between two or more things. The client's statements should match mood and behavior. Subjective and objective data should generally agree. Incongruence indicates the need for further data collection.

DIAGNOSTIC AND LABORATORY DATA.   The results of diagnostic and laboratory tests can identify or verify alterations questioned or identified during the nursing health history and physical examination. For example, during the health history the client indicates recurrent upper respiratory tract infections and at present has a productive cough with brown sputum. On physical examination, you note an elevated temperature, increased respirations, and decreased right lower breath sounds. You obtain an ordered complete blood count (CBC) to look for an elevated white blood cell count and a chest x-ray film to determine the presence of a right lower lobe infiltrate. Such findings suggest the client has pneumonia.

Clients may collect and monitor some laboratory data in the home. This is especially true for clients with diabetes mellitus who need blood glucose monitoring. Ask clients about their routine results to determine their response to illness and information about the effects of later treatment measures. Laboratory data are compared with the established norms for a particular test, age-group, and gender.

MEDICAL RECORD.   The **medical record** provides pertinent data about the client's medical history, laboratory tests and diagnostic study results, and the physician's proposed treatment plan. The data contained in the medical record are baseline information about the client's response to illness and information about the effects of later treatment measures. The client's medical record is a resource for additional information and is a tool for checking the consistency and congruency of personal observations.

OTHER SOURCES OF DATA.   Health care team members, families and significant others, and nursing and medical literature are important resources for completing the assessment database. **Health care team** members include physicians, nurses, and ancillary staff (see Chapter 2). Team members can provide data about the way the client interacts within the health care environment, reacts to information about diagnostic tests, and responds to visitors.

The client's family, friends, and significant others know the client from a point of view unavailable to the health care team. They frequently provide background information essential to understanding the client's situation and responses. In cases of severe illness or emergency situations or when the client is an infant, a child, or mentally disabled, the family or

significant others may be the only available source of data about health-illness patterns, current medications, allergies, and onset of illness.

A literature review about the client's illness helps to complete the database. The review increases your knowledge about the symptoms, treatment, and prognosis of a specific illness. A knowledgeable nurse also researches information pertinent to assessment and planning of nursing care.

Interpreting Assessment Data and Making Nursing Judgments

The successful interpretation of assessment data requires critical thinking. When you correctly analyze data you will be able to make necessary clinical decisions in your client's care. Critically think about how to interpret the information to determine the presence of abnormal findings, conduct further observations to clarify information, and then identify the client's problems in the form of nursing diagnoses. You will first interpret the data collected and then validate it. You then cluster and document your findings.

DATA INTERPRETATION AND VALIDATION.   After gathering assessment data, you validate the collected information to ensure its accuracy. **Validation** of assessment data involves comparing the data with another source (Figure 6-3). Ask your client or a family member to validate the information obtained during the interview and health history. Any additions or corrections should be noted and added to the database. Findings concerning physical examination and observation of client behavior can be validated by comparing data in the medical record with consultation from another health team member, family member, or significant other.

When you validate data with both the client and family it opens the door for gathering more information. Thus you are continually analyzing and thinking about your client's data to make concise, accurate, and meaningful interpretations about the client's responses to health care problems. Critically thinking about client data enables you to fully understand the problems, to judge the extent of the problems more carefully, and to discover possible relationships between the problems.

DATA CLUSTERING.   After interpreting and validating the assessment, organize the information into meaningful and usable clusters, keeping in mind your client's response to illness. A cluster is a set of signs or symptoms that are grouped together in a logical order. During **data clustering,** organize data and focus attention on client functions needing support and assistance for recovery. Focused data clustering using a systems approach or functional health pattern approach assists you in correctly classifying and organizing data, which ultimately provides the framework for developing individualized nursing diagnoses for the client (Box 6-3). Clustering also helps make documentation more concise and focused.

DATA DOCUMENTATION.   **Data documentation** is the last part of a complete assessment. A thorough and accurate

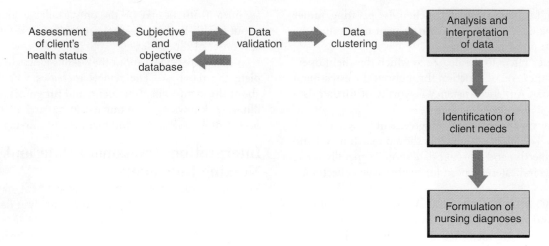

Focused Data Clustering   Box 6-3

SYSTEM-ORIENTED FORMAT
Integumentary System
Intact, flushed skin that is hot and dry to touch
Dry oral mucosa, coated tongue, and cracked lips

Gastrointestinal System
Distended, firm abdomen that is tender to palpation in upper
   quadrants
20-pound weight loss

Medical Record
Hemoglobin: 10 g/dl
Diagnosis of stomach cancer

FUNCTIONAL HEALTH PATTERN FORMAT
Activity and Exercise Pattern
Statement of increased fatigue when walking
Demonstration of ability to perform activities of daily living (ADLs)
Fatigued, dyspneic appearance when performing ADLs

Sleep and Rest Pattern
Report of difficulty in falling and remaining asleep
Denial of use of sleeping aids

Medical Record
Previous history of decreased activity tolerance and poor sleeping
   2 weeks before hospital admission for congestive heart failure
Chest x-ray film showing pulmonary congestion

documentation of facts is necessary when recording client data. If an item is not recorded, it is lost and unavailable to anyone else caring for the client. If specific information is not given, the reader is left with only general impressions.

Being factual is easy after it becomes a habit. The basic rule is to record all observations. When you record data, attention should be paid to facts, and an effort should be made to be as descriptive as possible. Anything heard, seen, touched, or smelled should be reported exactly. Do not generalize or form judgments too early. Conclusions about such observations become nursing diagnoses. As you gain experience and become familiar with patterns of signs and

symptoms, you may correctly conclude the existence of that problem.

Thorough documentation ensures that information is available to those caring for the client's needs. Even information that does not seem to indicate an abnormality should be recorded. It may become important later, serving as baseline data for a change in status. A general rule of thumb is that if it was assessed, it should be recorded.

 Nursing Diagnosis

Nursing diagnosis is the second step of the nursing process. This step of the nursing process gives meaning to the data you collect and organize during assessment. The process of diagnosing is the result of your identification of specific client responses to **health care problems.** Diagnosis means "to distinguish" or "to know." A **nursing diagnosis** is a clinical judgment about individual, family, or community responses to actual and potential health problems or life processes. On the basis of nursing diagnoses you select nursing interventions to achieve desired client outcomes (North American Nursing Diagnosis Association [NANDA], 2001). A nursing diagnosis focuses on the client's actual or potential response to a health problem rather than on the physiological event or complication.

A **medical diagnosis** is the identification of a disease condition based on a specific evaluation of physical signs, symptoms, history, diagnostic tests, and procedures. Physicians are licensed to treat diseases or pathological processes by performing surgery, prescribing medication, and ordering specific invasive and noninvasive therapies. Thus the focus of the medical diagnosis is the identification, treatment, and cure of the disease or pathological process.

A nursing diagnosis is a statement of a client's actual or potential response to a health problem that you are licensed and competent to treat. It reflects your client's level of health or response to a disease or pathological process. Medical and nursing diagnoses are derived from the analysis of physiological, psychological, sociocultural, developmental, and spiritual dimensions of the client database.

The goals and objectives of a nursing diagnosis differ from those of a medical diagnosis. The **goal** of a nursing diagnosis is to identify actual and potential client responses, whereas the goals of a medical diagnosis are to identify the cause of an illness or injury and design a treatment plan.

Identification of nursing diagnoses leads to the development of an individualized plan of care so that your client and family can adapt to changes resulting from health problems. For example, a client with a medical diagnosis of appendicitis requires the physician to remove the infected appendix. After the appendectomy, the client may have a nursing diagnosis of *impaired physical mobility related to painful incision.* Nursing care would be directed at gradually increasing the client's mobility to preoperative levels by decreasing incisional pain.

Critical thinking is necessary in formulating nursing diagnoses so that you can individualize care for your client. During the diagnostic phase you will use scientific and nursing knowledge and previous experience to analyze and interpret data collected about the client, to select the correct diagnosis.

NANDA Diagnoses

The use of standard nursing diagnostic statements endorsed by the North American Nursing Diagnosis Association (**NANDA**) serves several purposes (Box 6-4). Each diagnosis has a precise definition that gives all members of the health care team a common language for understanding the client's needs. Also, because the nursing diagnoses deal with clients' responses to illness or health problems rather than medical diagnoses, they distinguish the nurse's role from the physician's role and help the nurse focus on the scope of nursing practice.

NANDA has identified several types of nursing diagnoses. An **actual nursing diagnosis** describes human response to health conditions or life processes that exist in an individual, family, or community. It is supported by defining characteristics that cluster in patterns of related cues or inferences (NANDA, 2001). For example, a woman who is 2 hours postpartum of a vaginal delivery has a distended bladder, is voiding small frequent amounts, and states she feels continued sensation of the urge to void has an actual nursing diagnosis of *urinary retention related to swelling of the perineum following vaginal birth.*

A **risk nursing diagnosis** describes human responses to health conditions or life processes that may develop in a vulnerable individual, family, or community (NANDA, 2001). For example, an overweight client with a spinal cord injury is at *risk for impaired skin integrity.* The key assessment for this type of diagnosis is the data that support the client's vulnerability. Such data may include physiological, psychosocial, familial, lifestyle, and environmental factors that increase the client's vulnerability to, or likelihood of developing, the condition.

A **wellness nursing diagnosis** describes human responses to levels of wellness in an individual, group, or community that may move from a specific level of wellness to a higher level of wellness (NANDA, 2001). This type of diagnosis is used when the client wishes to or has achieved an optimal level of health. For example, *readiness for enhanced family coping related to unexpected birth of twins.* The nurse and the family unit work together to adapt to the stressors associated with twins and identify the family's strengths, resources, and needs. In doing so, the nurse incorporates the client's strengths into a plan of care, with the outcome directed at an enhanced level of coping.

Diagnostic Process

The **diagnostic process** consists of the decision-making steps used to develop a diagnostic statement (Carnevali and Thomas, 1993). The data validation and clustering derived from assessment serve as the first step, followed by analysis and interpretation of data, identification of client needs, and formulation of nursing diagnoses (see Figure 6-3, p. 78).

Analysis and Interpretation of Data

During assessment, you collected data from a variety of sources, validated, and then sorted the data into clusters. You should continually revise your client's database to include changes in the client's physical and emotional status. It is important for you to eventually identify the client's needs. A health problem does not automatically indicate a certain nursing diagnosis exists. For example, Mrs. Bryan has stomach cancer. She knows her medical diagnosis but needs assistance with pain management, weight loss, and mobility. At present, the client is seeking treatment for headaches. For this client you must perform **data analysis** on the data clusters, recognize patterns or trends, compare them with normal, healthful standards, and come to a reasoned conclusion about the client's response (Box 6-5).

When looking for a pattern or trend, examine the clusters of data carefully. Individual signs or symptoms cannot support a diagnostic label. However, when multiple signs or symptoms are placed or clustered together as a group, you are able to think about the relationship between and among these assessment findings. For example, you assessed Mrs. Bryan, who has stomach cancer and other health problems. Your database included fatigue, decreased nutritional intake, weakness, and fear. Alone, these symptoms could be related to multiple nursing diagnoses, but when analyzing them together, you begin to think about which pattern fits Mrs. Bryan's symptoms.

Taking clusters of data to form a pattern is perhaps best demonstrated through the following example. Gray hair does not necessarily indicate that a person is an older adult. However, if gray hair, wrinkled skin, and age spots are clustered together, these characteristics increase the probability that the person is an older adult. The identified pattern is then compared with data that are consistent with normal, healthful patterns. Use widely accepted norms, such as normal laboratory and diagnostic test values, and professional knowledge as the basis for comparison and judgment. When comparing patterns, be sure to judge whether the grouped signs and symptoms are normal for the client and whether they are within the range of healthful responses. In the case of

NANDA Nursing Diagnoses Taxonomy II

Box 6-4

Activity intolerance
Activity intolerance, risk for
Adjustment, impaired
Airway clearance, ineffective
Allergy response, latex
Allergy response, risk for latex
Anxiety
Anxiety, death
Aspiration, risk for
Attachment, risk for impaired parent/
  infant/child
Autonomic dysreflexia
Autonomic dysreflexia, risk for
Body image, disturbed
Body temperature, risk for imbalanced
Bowel incontinence
Breastfeeding, effective
Breastfeeding, ineffective
Breastfeeding, interrupted
Breathing pattern, ineffective
Cardiac output, decreased
Caregiver role strain
Caregiver role strain, risk for
Comfort, impaired
Communication, impaired verbal
Conflict, decisional
Conflict, parental role
Confusion, acute
Confusion, chronic
Constipation
Constipation, perceived
Constipation, risk for
Coping, compromised family
Coping, defensive
Coping, disabled family
Coping, ineffective
Coping, ineffective community
Coping, readiness for enhanced community
Coping, readiness for enhanced family
Denial, ineffective
Dentition, impaired
Development, risk for delayed
Diarrhea
Disuse syndrome, risk for
Diversional activity, deficient
Energy field, disturbed
Environmental interpretation
  syndrome, impaired
Failure to thrive, adult
Falls, risk for
Family processes, dysfunctional: alcoholism
Family processes, interrupted
Fatigue
Fear
Fluid volume, deficient
Fluid volume, excess
Fluid volume, risk for deficient

Fluid volume, risk for imbalanced
Gas exchange, impaired
Grieving
Grieving, anticipatory
Grieving, dysfunctional
Growth and development, delayed
Growth, risk for disproportionate
Health maintenance, ineffective
Health-seeking behaviors
Home maintenance, impaired
Hopelessness
Hyperthermia
Hypothermia
Identity, disturbed personal
Incontinence, functional
Incontinence, reflex urinary
Incontinence, stress urinary
Incontinence, total urinary
Incontinence, urge urinary
Incontinence, risk for urge urinary
Infant behavior, disorganized
Infant behavior, risk for disorganized
Infant behavior, readiness for enhanced
  organized
Infant feeding pattern, ineffective
Infection, risk for
Injury, risk for
Injury, risk for perioperative-positioning
Intracranial adaptive capacity, decreased
Knowledge, deficient
Loneliness, risk for
Memory, impaired
Mobility, impaired bed
Mobility, impaired physical
Mobility, impaired wheelchair
Nausea
Neglect, unilateral
Noncompliance
Nutrition, imbalanced: less than body
  requirements
Nutrition, imbalanced: more than body
  requirements
Nutrition, risk for imbalanced: more than
  body requirements
Oral mucous membrane, impaired
Pain, acute
Pain, chronic
Parenting, impaired
Parenting, risk for impaired
Peripheral neurovascular dysfunction,
  risk for
Poisoning, risk for
Post-trauma syndrome
Post-trauma syndrome, risk for
Powerlessness
Powerlessness, risk for
Protection, ineffective

Rape-trauma syndrome
Rape-trauma syndrome: compound
  reaction
Rape-trauma syndrome: silent reaction
Relocation stress syndrome
Relocation stress syndrome, risk for
Role performance, ineffective
Self-care deficit, bathing/hygiene
Self-care deficit, dressing/grooming
Self-care deficit, feeding
Self-care deficit, toileting
Self-esteem, chronic low
Self-esteem, situational low
Self-esteem, risk for situational low
Self-mutilation
Self-mutilation, risk for
Sensory perception, disturbed
Sexual dysfunction
Sexuality patterns, ineffective
Skin integrity, impaired
Skin integrity, risk for impaired
Sleep deprivation
Sleep pattern, disturbed
Social interaction, impaired
Social isolation
Sorrow, chronic
Spiritual distress
Spiritual distress, risk for
Spiritual well-being, readiness for
  enhanced
Suffocation, risk for
Suicide, risk for
Surgical recovery, delayed
Swallowing, impaired
Therapeutic regimen management,
  effective
Therapeutic regimen management,
  ineffective
Therapeutic regimen management,
  ineffective community
Therapeutic regimen management,
  ineffective family
Thermoregulation, ineffective
Thought processes, disturbed
Tissue integrity, impaired
Tissue perfusion, ineffective
Transfer ability, impaired
Trauma, risk for
Urinary elimination, impaired
Urinary retention
Ventilation, impaired spontaneous
Ventilatory weaning response,
  dysfunctional
Violence, risk for other-directed
Violence, risk for self-directed
Walking, impaired
Wandering

From North American Nursing Diagnosis Association: *NANDA nursing diagnoses: definitions and classifications, 2001-2002,* Philadelphia, 2001, The Association.

Steps of Data Analysis   Box 6-5

1. Recognize pattern (cluster of defining characteristics).
   20-lb weight loss
   Poor appetite
   Weakness
   Previous falls
2. Compare with normal standards.
   No weight loss
   Adequate nutritional intake
   No falls
3. Make a reasoned conclusion.
   Mobility and stability problems
   Inadequate nutritional intake

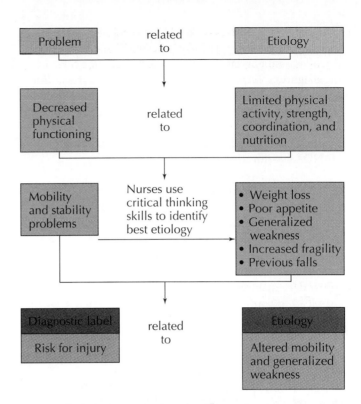

FIGURE **6-4**   Relationship between diagnostic statement and format.

aging these characteristics are a normal response. However, defining characteristics that are not within healthy norms are isolated and form the basis for **problem identification.**

When you identify a pattern or relationship among data clusters, a list of client-centered needs begins to emerge, such as the needs for Mrs. Bryan to have an improved nutritional status and activity tolerance. The patterns of data consist of **defining characteristics,** the clinical criteria that support (validate) the presence of a diagnostic category. **Clinical criteria** are the objective or subjective signs and symptoms or risk factors (Carpenito, 2000). The multiple defining characteristics identified in your analysis support the nursing diagnosis. Absence of these characteristics suggests that the proposed diagnosis should be rejected and you must critically assess further until you identify the correct diagnosis. You achieve accuracy when all characteristics are evaluated, irrelevant ones are eliminated, and relevant ones are confirmed (Collier and others, 1996).

IDENTIFICATION OF CLIENT NEEDS.   As mentioned earlier, you and perhaps the client begin to identify emerging patterns of needs. Identifying client needs enables you to individualize nursing diagnoses, by considering all assessment data and focusing on the more relevant data. It may help you to think of the identification phase as recognizing the general health care need. Then the formulation of the nursing diagnosis involves recognizing the specific health care need. For example, a general health care need is problems with elimination and the specific problem is *constipation.* Thus in describing your client's health care needs, you move from general to specific.

FORMULATION OF NURSING DIAGNOSES.   Once your client's assessment data are analyzed and interpreted and needs are identified, you select an appropriate nursing diagnosis. The diagnostic statement itself follows a specific format that is a result of your individualized assessment.

NURSING DIAGNOSIS FORMAT.   The nursing diagnosis format (i.e., how the actual diagnosis is stated) flows from the diagnostic process. Throughout this text, nursing diagnoses are stated in a two-part format: the diagnostic label followed by a statement of a related factor (Table 6-3) (NANDA, 2001). The

diagnostic labels are categories approved by NANDA (see Box 6-4). The related factor is a condition or etiology identified during your assessment that is associated with the client's actual or potential response to a health problem and can be changed by nursing interventions. For example, the nursing diagnostic statement includes the diagnostic label (e.g., *risk for injury*) and the related factor (e.g., *related to confusion*).

The **related factors** are etiological or contributing conditions that have influenced the client's response to the health problem. The "related to" phrase identifies the etiology or cause of the problem. This is not a cause-and-effect statement; rather it indicates that the etiology contributes to or is associated with the problem (Figure 6-4). The inclusionary phrase "related to" requires you to use critical thinking skills to individualize the nursing diagnosis and subsequent interventions (Table 6-3).

The **etiology** or cause of the nursing diagnosis must be within the domain of nursing practice and a condition that responds to nursing interventions. Sometimes medical diagnoses are recorded as the etiology of the nursing diagnosis. This is incorrect. Nursing interventions cannot change a medical diagnosis. However, nursing interventions can be directed at behavior or conditions that you can treat or manage. For example, the nursing diagnosis *acute pain related to breast cancer* is incorrect. Nursing actions cannot affect the medical diagnosis of breast cancer. Rewording the diagnosis to read *acute pain related to impaired skin integrity secondary to mastectomy incision* results in nursing interventions directed at reducing stress on the suture line and improving the client's comfort.

Table 6-4 demonstrates data clustering, identification of client need, and formulation of nursing diagnoses from pertinent assessment data. Table 6-5 (p. 83) uses the three nursing diagnoses, *ineffective airway clearance, self-esteem disturbance,* and *ineffective individual coping,* to demonstrate the way that the defining characteristics and probable etiologies assist in the development of the total diagnostic label. The defining characteristics and relevant etiologies are from the NANDA classification (NANDA, 2001).

Sources of Diagnostic Errors

Errors can occur in the diagnostic process during data collection, data clustering, data interpretation, and statement of the nursing diagnosis. During data collection, be sure you collect sufficient data. When insufficient data exist, you may fail to identify a problem. On the other hand, too much data may result in disorganized information, which may lead to confusion when identifying problems. During data collection, begin to make judgments regarding data interpretation and selection of the diagnostic label (Collier and others, 1996).

During data interpretation apply critical thinking standards for being accurate, relevant, and complete. When analyzing data, consider conflicting data. Data must be reliable and valid. Therefore determine that equipment used during assessment is functioning properly and that you used appropriate skills to assess your client's problems. Last, it is necessary to consider the client's developmental stage and culture when interpreting data. It is possible to incorrectly interpret a finding as a deficit or abnormal, when that finding may be entirely appropriate for the client's developmental state or cultural heritage.

Errors in data clustering occur when data are clustered prematurely, incorrectly, or not at all. Premature closure of clustering occurs when you make the nursing diagnosis before all data have been grouped. Incorrect clustering occurs when you try to make the nursing diagnosis fit the signs and symptoms obtained. The nursing diagnosis should be derived from the data, not the other way around. An incorrect nursing diagnosis affects quality of care.

The last type of error that can occur is the manner in which the nursing diagnosis is stated. There are some common guidelines to reduce errors in the diagnostic statement itself.

AVOIDING AND CORRECTING ERRORS. Nursing diagnoses are easy to write if you remember that the problem portion of the statement is concerned with your client's response to the illness or condition and that the etiology portion must be within the scope of nursing to diagnose and treat. The following suggestions should help you to avoid the most common errors in formulating nursing diagnoses accurately:

1. Identify the client's response, not the medical diagnosis (Carpenito, 2000). Because the medical diagnosis requires medical interventions, it is legally inadvisable to include it in the nursing diagnosis. The diagnosis *acute*

NANDA Nursing Diagnosis Format	Table 6-3
Diagnostic Statement	**Related Factors**
Constipation	Inadequate dietary fiber
	Effects of medications
	Inadequate fluid intake
	Decreased activity
Fatigue	Discomfort
	Excessive role demands
	Increased energy requirement
Impaired skin integrity	Fluid retention
	Excessive secretions
	Immobilization
	Altered circulation

Formulation of Nursing Diagnoses		Table 6-4
Clustering Data	**Identification of Client Need**	**Nursing Diagnosis Formulation**
Weight loss Poor appetite Decreased hemoglobin	Excessive weight loss	Imbalanced nutrition: less than body requirements related to poor nutritional intake
Decreased mobility Decreased stability Previous falls Weakness	Mobility and stability problems	Risk for injury related to altered mobility and generalized weakness
40 pack-year history of smoking Slight change of emphysema shown on chest x-ray film Crackles auscultated in lung fields	Risk for respiratory complications	Ineffective airway clearance related to generalized weakness
Client's desire to remain independent Client's fear of nursing home placement Daughter's fear for her mother's comfort and safety	Conflict between mother and daughter regarding future care	Decisional conflict related to threat over loss of independence

pain related to myocardial infarction may be changed to *acute pain related to physical exertion.*

2. Identify a NANDA diagnostic statement rather than the symptom. Nursing diagnoses are derived from a cluster of defining characteristics; one symptom is insufficient for problem identification. For example, shortness of breath, pain on inspiration, and productive cough should be written as *ineffective breathing pattern related to increased airway secretions.*

3. Identify a treatable etiology rather than a clinical sign or chronic problem. Nursing interventions are directed toward correcting the etiology of the problem. A diagnostic test or a chronic dysfunction is not an etiology or nursing intervention. Altered respiratory function supported by abnormal arterial blood gases can be correctly stated as *ineffective tissue perfusion related to inadequate oxygen intake.*

4. Identify the problem caused by the treatment or diagnostic study rather than the treatment or study itself. Clients experience many responses to diagnostic tests and medical treatment. These responses are the area of nursing concern. The client who has angina and is scheduled for a cardiac catheterization may have a nursing diagnosis of *anxiety related to lack of knowledge about cardiac catheterization.*

5. Identify the client response to the equipment rather than the equipment itself. Clients are often unfamiliar with medical technology. The diagnosis *anxiety related to cardiac monitor* can be changed to *deficient knowledge regarding the need for cardiac monitoring.*

6. Identify the client's problems rather than your problems. Nursing diagnoses are always client centered and form the basis for goal-directed care. Potential intravenous complications related to poor vascular access indicates a nursing problem in initiating and maintaining intravenous therapy. The diagnosis *risk for infection related to presence of invasive lines* properly centers attention on client needs.

7. Identify the client problem rather than the nursing intervention. Nursing interventions are later planned to alleviate client problems. The statement *offer bedpan frequently because of altered elimination patterns* should be changed to identify the problem and etiology. *Diarrhea related to food intolerance* corrects the misstatement and allows proper implementation of the nursing process.

8. Identify the client problem rather than the goal. Goals are established in terms of client problems. If the problem is not identified, evaluation of problem resolution is difficult. *Client needs high-protein diet related to potential alteration in nutrition* should be changed to *imbalanced nutrition: less than body requirements related to inadequate protein intake* to allow for planning to correct the etiology.

9. Make professional rather than prejudicial judgments. Nursing diagnoses are based on subjective and objec-

Defining Characteristics and Etiologies to Support Nursing Diagnoses		Table 6-5
Defining Characteristics	**Nursing Diagnoses**	**Etiologies ("related to")**
Abnormal breath sounds Changes in rate or depth of respiration Cough Cyanosis Dyspnea Smoking history	Ineffective airway clearance	Decreased energy and/or fatigue Tracheobronchial infection, obstruction, secretion Pain
Verbal or nonverbal response to actual or perceived change in structure or function Missing or impaired body part, not looking at or touching body or body part Trauma to body Refusal to acknowledge change	Situational low self-esteem	Biophysical (e.g., amputation or loss of function of extremity) Cognitive and/or perceptual (e.g., expressions of worthlessness and sorrow) Psychosocial (e.g., withdrawal behavior and excessive crying)
Verbalization of inability to cope Inability to meet role expectations Inability to problem solve Inability to meet basic needs Alteration in societal participation Destructive behavior Inappropriate use of defense mechanisms Verbal manipulation Change in usual communication patterns High rate of illness High rate of accidents	Ineffective coping	Situational crises (e.g., unexpected illness and financial difficulties) Maturational crises (e.g., marriage and parenthood)

tive client data and should not include your personal beliefs and values. Your judgment can be removed from *risk for impaired skin integrity related to poor hygiene habits* by changing the nursing diagnosis to read *risk for impaired skin integrity related to knowledge about perineal care.*

10. Avoid legally inadvisable statements (Carpenito, 2000). Statements that imply blame, negligence, or malpractice can result in litigation. The diagnosis *recurrent angina related to insufficient medication* implies inadequate prescription by the physician. Correct problem identification might read *chronic pain related to improper use of medications.*

11. Identify the problem and etiology. Be careful to avoid a circular statement. Such statements are vague and give no direction to nursing care. *Alteration in comfort related to pain* can be changed to identify the client problem and the cause: *ineffective breathing pattern related to incisional pain.*

12. Identify only one client problem in the diagnostic statement. Every problem has different specific expected outcomes. Confusion during the planning step occurs when multiple problems are included in a nursing diagnosis. It is, however, permissible to include multiple etiologies contributing to one client problem. *Pain and anxiety related to difficulty in ambulating* should be restated as two nursing diagnoses, such as *impaired physical mobility related to pain in right knee* and *anxiety related to difficulty in ambulating.*

Documentation

Once you identify the client's nursing diagnoses, list them on the plan of care. In the clinical facility, nursing diagnoses are usually listed chronologically as they are identified. When initiating the original care plan, always place the highest priority nursing diagnoses first. Thereafter, add additional nursing diagnoses to the list. Date nursing diagnosis at the time of entry. This documentation system and changes in the client's status eventually result in a list of nursing diagnoses that may not be in order of priority. When reviewing

the list, identify those nursing diagnoses with the greatest priority regardless of chronological order.

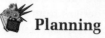 **Planning**

Planning is a category of nursing behavior in which client-centered goals are established and interventions are designed to achieve the goals. Planning requires you to use deliberate decision-making and problem-solving skills to design nursing care for each client (Liukkonen, 1992). During planning you set priorities, determine goals, develop expected outcomes, and formulate a plan of care. In addition to collaborating with the client and family, consult with other members of the health care team, review pertinent literature, modify care, and record relevant information about the client's health care needs and clinical management.

Establishing Priorities

Priority setting involves ranking nursing diagnoses in order of importance. Because clients have multiple nursing diagnoses, you select mutually agreed-on priorities based on the urgency of the problem, the nature of the treatment indicated, and the interaction among the diagnoses. Establishing priorities is not merely a matter of numbering the nursing diagnosis on the basis of severity or physiological importance. Rather, it is a process through which you and the client mutually rank the diagnoses in order of importance based on the client's safety, desires, and needs.

Priorities are classified as high, intermediate, or low (Table 6-6). Nursing diagnoses that, if untreated, could result in harm to the client or others have the highest priorities. High priorities can be both psychological and physiological. Avoid classifying only physiological nursing diagnoses as high priority.

Intermediate-priority nursing diagnoses involve the non-emergent, non–life-threatening needs of the client. Low-priority nursing diagnoses are client needs that may not be directly related to a specific illness or prognosis but may affect the client's future well-being.

Priority Setting	Table 6-6
Nursing Diagnosis	Rationale
High Priority	
Ineffective coping related to anxiety about unknown medical diagnosis	Prompt intervention for anxiety will help client prepare for and cope with a diagnostic test, treatment, or diagnosis.
Ineffective airway clearance after surgery related to abdominal incision pain	Because of the risk of postoperative pulmonary complications, nurse will institute preventive client education early in nursing care.
Intermediate Priority	
Imbalanced nutrition: less than body requirements related to chronic diarrhea for 3 weeks	This nursing diagnosis does not affect client's immediate physiological or emotional status. Possible surgery will also assist nurse in resolving diagnosis.
Low Priority	
Deficient knowledge regarding smoking cessation programs	This nursing diagnosis reflects client's long-term needs.

Whenever possible, involve the client in priority setting. In some situations you and the client may assign different priority rankings to the nursing diagnoses. If you each place a different value on health care needs and treatments, these differences can be resolved through open communication. However, when the client's physiological and emotional needs are at stake, you need to assume primary responsibility for setting priorities.

Goals and Expected Outcomes

Goals and expected outcomes are specific statements of client behavior or responses that you aim to achieve as a result of nursing care. After assessing, diagnosing, and establishing priorities about the client's health care needs, you formulate goals and expected outcomes with the client for each nursing diagnosis (Gordon and others, 1994).

There are two purposes for writing goals and expected outcomes. First, goals and expected outcomes provide direction for the selection and use of nursing interventions. Second, the goals and outcomes provide the focus for evaluation of the effectiveness of your interventions. These goals and expected outcomes indicate anticipated client responses. Each goal and expected outcome statement must have a time frame for evaluation. The time frame depends on the nature of the problem, etiology, overall condition of the client, and treatment setting.

GOALS OF CARE.   A **client-centered goal** is a specific and measurable behavior or response that reflects the client's highest possible level of wellness and independence in function. Whenever possible, client-centered goals are mutually set between the nurse and client.

Goals should not only meet the immediate needs of the client but should also strive toward prevention and rehabilitation. Two types of goals, short-term goals and long-term goals, are developed for the client depending on the nature of the client's need or problems and the nature of the nursing services provided.

A *short-term goal* is an objective behavior or response that is expected to be achieved in a short time, usually less than a week. For example, client will maintain a balanced fluid status within the next 48 hours. A *long-term goal* is an objective behavior or response that is expected to be achieved over a longer period, usually over weeks or months. For example, client will be tobacco free within 90 days.

Goal setting establishes the framework for the nursing care plan. Table 6-7 shows the progression from nursing diagnoses to goals and expected outcomes, which are individualized to meet client needs. These goals may focus on prevention, rehabilitation, discharge, and health education. Through goals the nurse is able to provide continuity of care and promote optimal use of time and resources.

EXPECTED OUTCOMES.   An **expected outcome** is the specific, step-by-step objective that leads to attainment of the goal and the resolution of the etiology for the nursing diagnosis (Table 6-7). An outcome is a measurable change of the client's status in response to nursing care. Expected outcomes are the desired measurable responses of a client's condition, including responses in the physiological, social, emotional, developmental, or spiritual dimensions. The expected outcomes, derived from short- and long-term goals, determine when a specific, client-centered goal has been met.

Expected outcomes have several functions. They provide a direction for selecting nursing activities. They include observable client behavior and measurable criteria for each goal. They also provide a projected time span for goal attainment and an opportunity to state any additional resources that may be required to achieve the goal, including additional equipment, personnel, or knowledge. Finally, expected outcomes serve as criteria to evaluate the effectiveness of nursing activities and resolution of the nursing diagnosis.

GUIDELINES FOR WRITING GOALS AND EXPECTED OUTCOMES.   There are seven factors to consider when writing goals and expected outcomes: client-centered, singular, observable, measurable, time-limited, mutual, and realistic factors.

Focus on the client. Outcomes and goals should reflect the client behavior and responses expected as a result of nursing

Examples of Goal Setting With Expected Outcomes for Mrs. Bryan — Table 6-7

Nursing Diagnoses	Goals	Expected Outcomes
Ineffective coping related to fear of negative prognosis	Mrs. Bryan will openly discuss diagnosis.	Mrs. Bryan will ask pertinent questions about diagnosis by 6/1. Mrs. Bryan will express fears by 6/2. Mrs. Bryan will identify at least two strategies for dealing with fears by 6/4.
Ineffective airway clearance related to incisional pain	Mrs. Bryan's lungs will remain clear throughout postoperative period.	Mrs. Bryan will turn, cough, and deep breathe every hour. Mrs. Bryan achieves incentive spirometer goal of 90% every 2 hours. Mrs. Bryan's pain level remains ≤4 on a scale of 0-10.
Deficient knowledge regarding postoperative care at home related to inexperience	Mrs. Bryan will state four postoperative risks before discharge.	Mrs. Bryan drinks 2 to 3 L of fluid every day by 6/2. Mrs. Bryan will name three signs of wound infection by 6/3. Mrs. Bryan will demonstrate aseptic wound care by 6/3. Mrs. Bryan will state home activity restrictions by 6/5.

interventions. A common error occurs when the goals are written to reflect nursing goals or interventions rather than client-centered goals. A correct statement is, "Client will ambulate in the hall three times a day." A common error is to write, "Ambulate client in the hall three times a day."

Address only one goal or outcome. Be sure to provide a precise method to evaluate client response to a nursing action. If the statement reads, "Client's lungs will be clear to auscultation and respiratory rate will be 22/min by 8/22," but when you evaluate the client after the nursing actions the lungs are clear but the respiratory rate is 28/min, it will be difficult to determine whether the expected outcome has been achieved. By splitting the statement into two parts, "Lungs will be clear to auscultation by 8/22" and "Respiratory rate will be 22/min by 8/22," you can determine specifically if each outcome has been achieved.

Develop outcomes that are observable. Through observation you must be able to determine if change has taken place. Examples include "Lungs will be clear on auscultation by 8/22" and "Wound drainage will be absent by 9/12."

Write outcomes that can be measured. Goals and expected outcomes are written to give you a standard against which to measure the client's response to nursing care. Examples of outcomes are "Body temperature will remain 98.6° F" and "Apical pulse will remain between 60 and 100 beats per minute." A goal or an outcome that is stated in measurable terms allows you to objectively quantify changes in the client's status. Common mistakes are made when using vague qualifiers such as "normal," "acceptable," "stable," or "sufficient" in the expected outcome statement. Vague qualifiers have different meanings to different people.

Clearly state time frame. The time frame for each goal and expected outcome indicates when the expected response should occur. Time frames assist you and the client in determining that progress is being made at a reasonable rate. Time frames also promote accountability in the delivery and management of nursing care.

Consult with the client. Mutual setting of goals and expected outcomes ensures that the client and caregiver agree on the direction and time limits of care. Mutual goal setting can increase the client's motivation and cooperation.

Be realistic. Set goals and expected outcomes that can be achieved. Achievable goals provide a sense of accomplishment. In turn, this sense of accomplishment can further increase the client's motivation and cooperation. When establishing realistic goals, you, through assessment, must know the resources of the health care facility, family, and client; the client's physiological, emotional, cognitive, and sociocultural potential; and the costs associated with treatment and resources available to reach expected outcomes in a timely manner.

Planning Nursing Care

After establishing goals and expected outcomes select the appropriate nursing interventions or actions. All of these elements must be identified before a plan of care can be written. Selecting suitable nursing interventions is a decision-making process. Use critical thinking to select interventions that will successfully meet the client's established goals and expected outcomes (Carnevali and Thomas, 1993). To select interventions you must be competent in three areas. You must (1) have knowledge of the **scientific rationale** for the interventions, (2) possess the necessary psychomotor and interpersonal skills to perform the interventions, and (3) be able to function within a particular setting to use the available health care resources effectively.

TYPES OF INTERVENTIONS. There are three categories of **nursing interventions:** nurse-initiated, physician-initiated, and collaborative interventions. **Nurse-initiated interventions** are those interventions a nurse can independently initiate to manage a client's health care needs. This type of intervention is based on scientific rationale that is performed to benefit the client in a predicted way (McCloskey and Bulechek, 2000).

Each state within the United States has developed nurse practice acts that delineate the legal scope of nursing practice (see Chapter 3). According to the nurse practice acts in a majority of states, nursing actions pertaining to activities of daily living, health education, health promotion, and counseling are in the domain of nursing practice.

Physician-initiated interventions are based on the physician's response to a medical diagnosis. The nurse follows the physician's written and/or verbal orders (McCloskey and Bulechek, 2000). Administering a medication, implementing an invasive procedure, changing a dressing, and preparing a client for diagnostic tests are examples of such interventions.

Each physician-initiated intervention involves specific nursing responsibilities, scientific and nursing knowledge, and technical competence. For example, when administering medications, you are responsible for knowing the classification of the drug, its physiological action, normal dosage, side effects, and nursing interventions related to its action or side effects (see Chapter 13). When diagnostic testing is ordered, you are responsible for scheduling the test, preparing the client, and knowing the normal findings and associated nursing implications.

Collaborative interventions are therapies that require the combined knowledge, skill, and expertise of multiple health care professionals. For example, in the clinical scenario introduced earlier, Mrs. Bryan is a 78-year-old widow, living alone in a rural community. She has inoperable stomach cancer, and has just recently moved into the home of her friend. Mrs. Bryan's overall goal and health care need is to remain independent. Because of poor appetite and subsequent weight loss, she is very weak. She needs interventions developed by multiple health care professionals, as well as community resources. Inez Santiago, Mrs. Bryan's nurse, schedules a visit with a home health aide, an occupational therapist (OT), and a physical therapist (PT). During their visit, the OT and PT evaluate Mrs. Bryan's safety and tolerance for certain activities of daily living, modify the home to remove risks to safety, establish an exercise program, and develop a schedule of interventions to be completed by the home health aide. The weekly plan now includes one visit by the nurse, two visits from the home health aide, and one visit from the OT or PT, on alternating weeks. Thus in addition to Mrs. Bryan living with a friend, there is a total of four visits a week to Mrs. Bryan's home. Her daughter is more accepting of her mother's recent move. The care for this client requires the coordination of collaborative interventions all directed toward the long-term goal of maintaining Mrs. Bryan's independence and safety, as well as supporting her level of health.

Nurse-initiated, physician-initiated, and collaborative interventions require critical nursing judgment and decision making. When encountering physician-initiated or collaborative interventions, you do not automatically implement the therapy but you must determine whether it is appropriate for the client.

You will face an inappropriate or incorrect order at some time. A strong knowledge base will help you recognize the error and seek to correct it. Your ability to recognize incorrect therapies is particularly important when administering medications or implementing procedures. An error can occur in writing the order or transcribing it to the Kardex or medication card. Clarifying an order is competent nursing practice, and it protects the client and members of the health care delivery system. The nurse carrying out an incorrect or inappropriate intervention is as much in error as the person who wrote or transcribed the original order and is liable for any complications resulting from the error. Chapter 3 explains legal issues affecting nursing practice.

SELECTION OF INTERVENTIONS.   Use clinical decision-making skills when selecting nursing interventions. Consider six factors when choosing interventions for a client: (1) characteristics of the nursing diagnosis, (2) expected outcomes and goals, (3) knowledge and research base (nursing knowledge) for the intervention, (4) feasibility of the intervention, (5) acceptability to the client, and (6) competency of the nurse providing care (McCloskey and Bulechek, 1998) (Box 6-6). You may also review standardized care plans, textbooks, and nursing and related health care literature and collaborate with other health care professionals. As you select interventions, review your client's needs, priorities, and previous experiences to select those nursing interventions that have the best potential for achieving the expected outcomes.

Nursing Care Plan

Generally a written nursing care plan includes a nursing diagnostic statement, goals, expected outcomes, and specific nursing activities and interventions. It is a written guideline for client care used by all members of the nursing team. The care plan coordinates nursing care, promotes continuity of care, and lists outcome criteria to be used in the evaluation of nursing care. In addition, the written care plan communicates nursing care priorities to other health care professionals. A written care plan decreases the risk of incomplete, incorrect, or inaccurate care.

The care plan is organized so that you and your colleagues can quickly identify the nursing actions to be delivered. In hospitals, outpatient settings, and community-based

---

Choosing Nursing Interventions

Box 6-6

CHARACTERISTICS OF THE NURSING DIAGNOSIS

Interventions must be directed toward altering the etiological factors or signs and symptoms associated with the diagnostic label.

Interventions may be directed toward altering or eliminating risk factors, which are associated with "*risk for*" nursing diagnoses.

EXPECTED OUTCOMES

Outcomes are stated in measurable terms and used to evaluate the effectiveness of the interventions.

RESEARCH BASE FOR INTERVENTION

Review articles that describe the use of research findings in similar clinical situations and settings.

FEASIBILITY OF THE INTERVENTION

Consider interaction of nursing interventions with treatments being provided by other health professionals.

Cost: Is intervention both clinically effective and cost efficient?

Time: Are time and personnel resources well managed?

ACCEPTABILITY TO THE CLIENT

Treatment plan must match client's goals and health care values.

Mutually decided nursing goals.

Client must have required self-care abilities or have a person who can assist with health care.

COMPETENCY OF THE NURSE

Knowledge of scientific rationale for the intervention.

Possession of necessary psychosocial and psychomotor skills.

Ability to function within setting and effectively and efficiently use health care resources.

Modified from Bulechek GM, McCloskey JC: Nursing interventions: what they are and how to choose them, *Holistic Nurs Pract* 1(3):36, 1987.

---

settings, the client often receives care from more than one nurse, physician, allied health professional, and health technician. The written nursing care plan makes possible the coordination of nursing care, subspecialty consultations, and scheduling of diagnostic tests.

The care plan can also identify and coordinate resources used to deliver nursing care. The listing of specific equipment and supplies necessary for nursing actions is an economically efficient mechanism for selecting equipment. If all equipment and supplies are included in the care plan, the nurse's time is used more effectively in providing care as opposed to determining the supplies needed.

The nursing care plan enhances the continuity of nursing care by listing specific nursing actions necessary to achieve the goals of care. These nursing activities can be carried out throughout the day and from day to day. A correctly formulated nursing care plan facilitates the continuity of care from one nurse to another. As a result, all nurses have the opportunity to deliver the same high-quality care.

Written nursing care plans organize information exchanged by nurses in change-of-shift reports. Nurses focus these reports on nursing care and treatments delineated in care plans. At the end of nursing care, nurses discuss care plans with the next caregivers. Thus all nurses are able to discuss current and pertinent information about the client's care plan.

The written care plan can also be adapted to the discharge needs of the client. Same-day surgeries and earlier discharges from hospitals require you as the nurse to begin planning discharge needs from the moment the client enters a health care agency (see Chapter 2). Incorporating the goals of the care plan into discharge planning is particularly important for a client who will be undergoing long-term rehabilitation in the community. The adaptation of the care plan enhances the continuity of nursing care between nurses working in hospital settings and those working in community agencies.

CRITICAL PATHWAYS.   **Critical pathways** allow staff from all disciplines, such as medicine, nursing, and pharmacy, to develop integrated care plans for a projected length of stay or number of visits for clients with a specific case type. For example, in Figure 6-5 the pathway is for a lung transplant evaluation, which recommends on a day-by-day basis the client's activities, consults, procedures, and discharge planning activities, as well as educational topics expected for the client's progression through the transplantation process. The nurse and other health team members use the pathway to monitor a client's progress and as a documentation tool. Because of the arrival of managed care (see Chapter 2), documentation tools that integrate the standards of care for multiple disciplines are necessary. Critical pathways, also called CareMaps, meet this need, and charting by exception is frequently the method of choice (see Chapter 7). When using critical pathways to plan care, many other forms (e.g., the nursing care plan, flow sheets, nurse's notes) are eliminated, because all the pertinent components are included in the pathway format.

Consulting Other Health Care Professionals

Consultation may occur at any step in the nursing process but is needed most often during planning and intervention, because the nurse is more likely to identify a problem requiring additional knowledge or skills or a need to obtain community or agency resources. **Consultation** is a process in which a specialist's (such as a dietitian or clinical nurse specialist) help is sought to identify ways to handle problems in client management or problems related to the planning and implementation of programs. Consultation is based on the problem-solving approach, and the consultant is the stimulus for change. Through consultation and collaboration you are able to tap the best resources to individualize nursing actions to meet expected outcomes.

WHEN TO CONSULT.   The need for consultation in nursing occurs when you have identified a problem that cannot be solved using personal knowledge, skills, and resources. Consultation increases your knowledge about the problem and helps in learning skills and obtaining the resources needed to solve the problem. After the consultation you may be able to resolve similar problems in the future.

HOW TO CONSULT.   The first step in the consultation process is identification of the general problem area, which provides the consultant with a starting point. Second, the consultation should be made with the appropriate professional, who may be another nurse or another member of the health care team. A consultation requested of the wrong individual delays problem solving and diminishes the quality of care delivered to the client.

Third, provide the consultant with pertinent information about the problem area. You may include a pertinent, brief summary of the problem, methods used to resolve the problem, and outcomes of those methods. Other resources may include the client's medical record and conversations with nurses, other members of the health team, and the client's family.

Fourth, you should not bias consultants. Consultants are in the clinical setting to help identify and resolve a nursing problem, and biasing them can hinder problem resolution. Bias can be avoided by not overloading consultants with subjective and emotional conclusions about the client and problem.

Fifth, be available to discuss the consultant's findings and recommendations. When a consultation is requested, provide a private, comfortable atmosphere in which the consultant and client can meet. However, this does not mean that you leave the environment. A common mistake is turning the whole problem over to the consultant. The consultant is not there to take over the problem but to assist you in resolving the problem. When possible, request the consultation for a day when both you and the consultant are scheduled to work and during a time when distractions are minimal.

Finally, incorporate the consultant's recommendations into the care plan. The success of the advice depends on the implementation of the problem-solving techniques suggested.

 Implementation

Implementation describes the initiation of nursing behavior in which the actions necessary for achieving the goals and expected outcomes of nursing care are initiated and completed. Implementation includes interventions for performing, assisting, or directing the performance of activities of daily living (ADLs); counseling and teaching the client or family; providing direct care; delegating, supervising, and evaluating the work of staff members; and recording and exchanging information relevant to the client's continued health care.

Types of Nursing Interventions

After developing a plan according to client needs and priorities, you perform specific individualized nursing interventions, which include nurse-initiated, physician-initiated, and collaborative interventions (McCloskey and Bulechek, 2000). In addition, nursing interventions may be entirely based on protocols and standing orders. A clear description of protocols and standing orders is necessary for safe nursing practice.

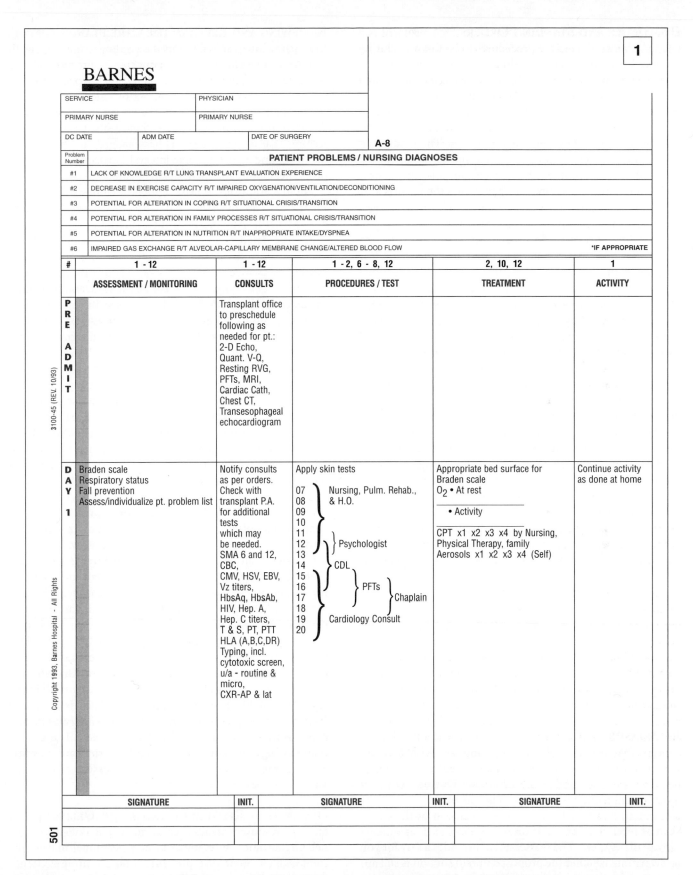

FIGURE **6-5**   Portion of critical pathway. (Courtesy Barnes-Jewish Hospital, St. Louis.)

PROTOCOLS AND STANDING ORDERS.   A **protocol** is a written plan specifying the procedures to be followed during an assessment or when providing treatment for a specific condition or nursing care problem. For example, nurses in a specialty area such as oncology will follow a protocol for administering chemotherapy. In another example, nurses on a general medical unit will follow a protocol to provide wound care for different stages of pressure ulcers. The established protocol delineates the conditions that nurses are permitted to treat, such as controlled hypertension, and the recommended treatment plan, including therapies the nurse is permitted to administer, such as diet counseling, stress management, and prescriptions of antihypertensives.

A **standing order** is a document containing orders for the conduct of routine therapies, monitoring guidelines, and/or diagnostic procedures for specific clients with identified clinical problems. The orders direct the conduct of client care in various clinical settings. Standing orders are approved and signed by the physician in charge of care before their implementation. They are commonly found in critical care settings and other specialized practice settings where clients' needs can change rapidly and require immediate attention. Standing orders are also common in the community health setting, in which the nurse encounters situations that do not permit immediate contact with a physician. Thus protocols and standing orders give you the legal protection to intervene appropriately in the client's best interest.

Before implementing any therapy, including those included in protocols and standing orders, you must use sound judgment in determining whether the intervention is correct and appropriate. Second, before you implement any intervention you have the responsibility to obtain correct theoretical knowledge and develop the clinical competencies necessary to perform the intervention. Nursing responsibility is equally great for all types of interventions.

Implementation Process

Adequate and thorough preparation before implementation ensures efficient and effective nursing care. Follow these five preparatory activities: reassess the client, review and revise the care plan, organize resources and care delivery, anticipate and prevent complications, and implement nursing interventions.

REASSESSING THE CLIENT.   Assessment is a continuous process that occurs each time you interact with a client. When new data are gathered and a new client need is identified, you need to modify the care plan. During the initial phase of implementation, reassess the client. This is a partial assessment and may focus on one dimension of the client, such as level of comfort, or on one system, such as the cardiovascular system. The reassessment provides a way for you to determine whether the proposed nursing action is still appropriate for the client's level of wellness. For example, you planned to ambulate a client following lunch; however, a reassessment reveals shortness of breath and increased fatigue, which require you to assist the client back to bed.

REVIEWING AND REVISING THE CARE PLAN.   Although the nursing care plan is developed according to the nursing diagnoses, changes in the client's status can require modification of the plan. Before beginning care, review the plan and consider current assessment data to verify stated nursing diagnoses and to determine whether the nursing interventions are still the most appropriate for the clinical situation. If you determine that the client's status has changed and the nursing diagnoses and related nursing interventions are no longer appropriate, modify the client's plan of care.

Modification of the existing plan includes several steps. First, revise the assessment database to reflect the client's current status. Any modifications entered on the care plan should be dated to inform the health care team when the change occurred. Second, revise the nursing diagnoses to reflect any change in the client's needs or problems. Some nursing diagnoses may no longer be relevant, and new nursing diagnoses are added. Third, revise specific interventions to correspond to the new nursing diagnoses and goals. The new interventions should indicate the client's greater independence from or dependence on nursing. In addition, the revised interventions can include the client's specific needs for health care resources. In the clinical scenario for Mrs. Bryan, her plan of care required multiple collaborative interventions. As her fatigue and weight loss progressed, she became weaker and her nursing needs changed. Mrs. Bryan moved in with a friend, and more community, friends, and family resources were used to safely maintain Mrs. Bryan's independence.

Revisions to nursing care occur in all types of care settings. Some situations require more quick responsive changes than others. For example, a client in an acute care setting is recovering from abdominal surgery, and as he progresses postoperatively, his nursing care needs change (Table 6-8). The nurse modifies the care plan for one nursing diagnosis: *risk for ineffective airway clearance related to pain of abdominal incision.* On the second postoperative day, the nurse assesses the client and notes decreased chest wall movements, crackles that are auscultated in the right lower lobes, and an elevated temperature (39° C). The client has a standing order for a chest x-ray film, which is taken immediately and reveals the collapse of alveoli in the right lower lobe. The nursing diagnosis is revised to read *ineffective airway clearance related to decreased inspiratory effort secondary to pain of abdominal incision.* The goal of maintaining a patent airway is still appropriate. Specific nursing interventions are developed to assist in achieving a patent airway.

ORGANIZING RESOURCES AND CARE DELIVERY.   A facility's resources include equipment and skilled personnel. Organization of equipment and personnel makes efficient, skilled client care possible. After planning a client's care, prepare the necessary supplies and decide on the time and provider of care. Preparation for care delivery also involves preparing the environment and client for the nursing intervention.

A Revised Nursing Care Plan — Table 6-8

Assessment	Goals	Implementation	Evaluation
Nursing diagnosis: Ineffective airway clearance after surgery related to pain of abdominal incision **Definition:** Ineffective airway clearance after surgery is the state in which an individual is unable to clear secretions or obstructions from the respiratory tract to maintain airway patency.			
Smoked two packs/day 20 years; chest x-ray film showing slight change of emphysema; crackles auscultated in lung field; scheduled for abdominal surgery	Client's airway remains patent by 7/1.	Demonstrate turn, cough, and deep breathing to client. Client demonstrates turning, coughing, and deep breathing exercises.	Productive cough is produced. Airway is clear to auscultation.
Modified 24 Hours After Surgery **Nursing diagnosis:** Ineffective airway clearance related to decreased inspiratory effort secondary to pain of abdominal incision			
Decreased chest wall movements; crackles in base that do not clear with coughing; fever; tachypnea (7/1)	Coughs productively by 7/2.	Administer chest physiotherapy to all lobes of the lung: 8-12-4-8-12-4. Ensure that client coughs and deep breathes every 2 hours around the clock.	Lung fields are clear on auscultation. Client becomes afebrile. Sputum is clear. Chest x-ray film demonstrates atelectasis resolving.
	Lungs are free of abnormal lung sounds by 7/2.	Suction nasotracheal area every 2 hours if client is unable to cough productively. Teach client to splint incision with pillow before and during coughing.	Client does not report increased pain during coughing.

EQUIPMENT. Most nursing procedures, from bed making to client teaching, require some equipment or supplies. Analyze each planned intervention for needed items and gather all supplies, placing them where they will be used. Realistic interventions call for only those items available in the facility.

PERSONNEL. Nursing care delivery systems vary among facilities and must be considered when allocating resources. The system by which nursing is organized determines the way in which personnel are designated for client care delivery. The most common types of nursing care delivery systems are functional, team, total client care, primary nursing, and case management (see Chapter 23).

Three categories of functions are inherent to professional nursing practice: direct care, delegation, and coordination. These functions assume varying levels of importance, depending on the nursing system (see Chapter 23). For example, a total client care system has a registered nurse or licensed practical nurse who is responsible for the total care of several clients throughout a shift. Client care is totally individualized; the nurse assigned to the client is responsible for direct client care, coordination with other departments for services, and contribution to the care plan. Continuity of care is best achieved when the same nurse cares for the same clients over consecutive days. Assistive personnel may work along with the registered nurse or licensed practical nurse to assist with direct care activities.

In another example, in a primary nursing system a primary nurse (registered nurse) is accountable for a client's nursing care from admission to discharge. This includes identifying relevant nursing diagnoses, establishing the plan of care, and coordinating activities such as client education and discharge planning. When the primary nurse is off duty, an associate nurse (registered nurse or licensed practical nurse) assumes care of the client. If a problem arises, the associate nurse confers directly or indirectly with the primary nurse, who retains full authority and responsibility for the client's nursing care plan.

No matter what the nursing care delivery system, continuity of individualized care is a primary consideration when assigning and organizing personnel.

ENVIRONMENT. Environmental factors influence the delivery and reception of care. The surroundings in which nursing activities occur should be safe and conducive to the implementation of therapies. Your client's safety is always the first concern. If the client has sensory deficits or an alteration in level of consciousness, for example, special precautions are needed to arrange the environment to prevent injury. Using special rooms, providing assistive devices (e.g., walkers, eyeglasses), rearranging furniture and equipment, making rooms free of clutter, and providing for additional personnel are examples of creating safe surroundings.

The client benefits most from nursing interventions when surroundings are compatible with activities. Privacy promotes relaxation when body parts are exposed. Reducing distractions enhances learning opportunities. Provision of adequate warmth and lighting prevents intrusion of environmental factors.

CLIENT.   Before you begin to perform interventions, be sure the client is as physically and psychologically comfortable as possible. Symptoms such as nausea, dizziness, or pain, for example, frequently interfere with a client's full concentration and cooperation. Comfort measures or medication for pain before initiating interventions enables the client to participate more fully. If client alertness is needed, the dose of pain medication should be sufficient to relieve discomfort but not impair mental faculties.

Even if symptoms are not a factor, the client should be made physically comfortable during interventions. Controlling environmental factors, positioning, and taking care of other physical needs should precede initiation of interventions. You should also consider the client's level of endurance and plan only the amount of activity the client can comfortably tolerate.

Awareness of the client's psychosocial needs helps you create a favorable emotional climate. Some clients feel reassured by having a significant other present to lend encouragement and moral support. Other strategies include planning sufficient time or multiple opportunities for the client to work through and ventilate feelings and anxieties. Adequate preparation allows the client to obtain maximal benefit from each intervention.

ANTICIPATING AND PREVENTING COMPLICATIONS. Risks to the client arise from both illness and treatment. As the nurse, you must identify these risks, evaluate the relative benefit of the treatment versus the risk, and initiate risk prevention measures.

Many client conditions place the client at risk for additional complications. For example, the client with preexisting chronic lung disease is at risk for developing pneumonia following abdominal surgery. Your knowledge of pathophysiology helps in the early identification of complications that can occur. Scientific rationales for how certain interventions can prevent or minimize complications help you evaluate the usefulness of preventive measures. A confused client, for example, is at risk for pulmonary complications because of extended periods of immobility. You should know that getting the client out of bed will reduce this risk because mobility enables the client to breathe more deeply and expand the bases of the lungs. However, you also realize this activity poses a risk to the client's safety. Preventive safety measures may require remaining with the client while he or she is out of bed or having the family stay with the client to encourage deep breathing.

Some nursing procedures also pose risks for the client. You need to be aware of potential complications and institute precautionary measures. For instance, the client receiving feedings through a nasogastric tube is at risk for aspiration. You should elevate the head of the bed and have pharyngeal suction equipment at the bedside before initiating the feedings.

IDENTIFYING AREAS OF ASSISTANCE.   Some nursing situations require you to acquire assistance by seeking additional personnel, knowledge, and/or nursing skills. Before implementing care, evaluate the plan to determine the need for assistance and the type required.

Situations requiring additional personnel vary. For example, when you are assigned to care for an overweight, immobilized client you may require additional personnel to help to turn, transfer, and position the client. You also need to determine the number of additional personnel and when they are needed. Then discuss the need for assistance with potential resources, such as other nurses or assistive personnel.

Some nursing situations require additional knowledge and skills. You need additional knowledge when administering a new medication or implementing a new procedure. Such information can be obtained from a hospital's formulary or procedure book. If you are still uncertain about the new medication or procedure, other members of the health care team can be consulted.

Because of the continual growth of health care professions and related technology, you may lack the skills needed to perform a new procedure. When this occurs, first locate information about the procedure in the literature and the agency's procedures book. Next, collect all equipment necessary for the procedure. Finally, ask another nurse who has completed the procedure correctly and safely to provide assistance and guidance. The assistance can come from another staff nurse, a supervisor, an educator, or a nurse specialist. Requesting assistance occurs frequently in all types of nursing practice and is a learning process that continues throughout educational experiences and into professional development.

COMMUNICATING NURSING INTERVENTIONS.   Nursing interventions are communicated verbally and in writing. When written, nursing interventions are incorporated into the nursing care plan and client's medical record. After the interventions are implemented, document the interventions and the client's response to the treatment on the appropriate record form (see Chapter 7). If there are any variations to an intervention, such as the number of repetitions of range of joint motion or the type of client education materials provided, document the information to provide continuity of care. This information usually includes a brief description of the nursing assessment, the specific procedure, and the client's response.

Documenting a brief description of pertinent assessment findings and client response in the client's medical record validates the need for a continued nursing intervention. Writing the time and the details of the intervention documents that the procedure was completed.

Nursing interventions are also communicated orally from one nurse to another or to other health professionals. Nurses commonly communicate orally when changing shifts, transferring a client to another unit, or discharging a client to another health agency.

Implementation Skills

Nursing practice is composed of cognitive, interpersonal, and psychomotor (technical) skills. Each type of skill is needed to implement nursing interventions. You are responsible for knowing when one type of implementation skill is preferred over another and for having the necessary knowledge and skill to perform each.

COGNITIVE SKILLS.   Cognitive skills involve application of nursing knowledge. This allows you to anticipate and recognize client needs and know the best nursing approaches. You must know the rationale for therapeutic interventions, understand normal and abnormal physiological and psychological responses, know nursing science, be able to identify client learning and discharge needs, and recognize the client's health promotion and illness prevention needs.

INTERPERSONAL SKILLS.   Interpersonal skills are essential for effective nursing action. You must develop a trusting relationship and communicate clearly with the client, family, and other members of the health care team (see Chapter 8). Client teaching and counseling must be done to the level of the client's understanding. You must also be sensitive to the client's emotional response to the illness and treatment. Proper use of interpersonal skills enables you to be perceptive to the client's verbal and nonverbal communication.

PSYCHOMOTOR SKILLS.   Psychomotor skills require the integration of cognitive and motor activities, such as learning to give an injection. You must understand anatomy and pharmacology (cognitive) and the mechanics of preparing and giving an injection (motor). Psychomotor skills are needed to provide the direct care needs of clients such as changing a dressing, giving an injection, or suctioning a tracheostomy. You have a professional responsibility to correctly complete these skills. Some of these skills may be new. If that is the case, assess your present level of competency and obtain the necessary resources to ensure that the client receives the treatment safely.

Various types of nursing interventions are selected to achieve the goals of care. These interventions include assisting with **activities of daily living (ADLs),** counseling, teaching, providing direct care, delegating and supervising, and recording and exchanging information. The nurse carries out the nursing care plan by using several implementation methods (Table 6-9). For example, the client with the nursing diagnosis *impaired physical mobility related to bilateral arm casts* may require assistance in performing ADLs. The client with *ineffective coping related to fear of medical diagnosis* may require counseling as a method of nursing intervention (see Chapter 21). The client with *deficient knowledge* needs health education focusing on the area of need (see Chapter 9).

Providing Direct Care

To achieve therapeutic goals for the client, you must initiate direct care interventions to compensate for adverse reactions to therapy, use precautionary and preventive measures in providing care, apply correct techniques in administering care and preparing the client for special procedures, and initiate lifesaving measures in emergency situations.

An **adverse reaction** is a harmful or unintended effect of a medication, diagnostic test, or therapeutic intervention. Nursing actions that compensate for adverse reactions reduce or counteract the reaction. For example, a client may have an unknown hypersensitivity to penicillin and may develop hives after the second dose. Record the reaction and stop further administration of the drug. Consult the physician's standing orders and administer diphenhydramine (Benadryl), an antihistamine (reduces allergic response) medication with antipruritic (antiitch) properties.

When caring for a client who is undergoing or who has undergone a particular diagnostic test, you must understand the test and any potential adverse effects. For example, a client has not had a bowel movement in 24 hours after a barium enema. Because a bowel impaction is a potential side effect of a barium enema, you increase fluid intake and instruct the client to let the nursing personnel know when a bowel movement occurs.

Types of Nursing Interventions		Table 6-9
Category of Nursing Interventions	Examples of Nursing Diagnoses	Specific Examples
Activities of daily living	Impaired physical mobility Confusion, acute and chronic Fatigue Self-care deficit	Assistance with feeding, hygiene, ambulation, positioning, elimination
Counseling	Anxiety Coping (all types) Fear Grieving Hopelessness Post-trauma syndrome	Short-term crises intervention, long-term crises intervention, referral to psychiatric or social work professionals, group support
Teaching	Ineffective health maintenance Health-seeking behaviors Noncompliance	Specific education programs for disease management, such as for diabetes mellitus or asthma, behavior changes, such as used for smoking cessation, weight reduction

Preventive nursing actions are directed at promoting health and preventing illness. Prevention includes assessment and promotion of the client's health potential, application of prescribed measures such as immunizations, health teaching, and early diagnosis and treatment. In the case of the client who has a hypersensitivity to penicillin, you must indicate the penicillin allergy in the client's medical record, inform the client and family of the need for a medical alert bracelet or tag, and teach actions they should take if the client is given penicillin again. You also teach the client and family that this is a potentially life-threatening allergy and provide a list of specific drugs to be avoided.

A **lifesaving measure** is implemented when a client's physiological or psychological state is threatened. The purpose of the lifesaving measure is to restore physiological or psychological equilibrium. Such measures include administering emergency medications, instituting cardiopulmonary resuscitation, restraining a violent client, and obtaining immediate counseling from a crisis center for a severely anxious client.

Delegating, Supervising, and Evaluating the Work of Other Staff Members

Depending on the system of health care delivery, the nurse who develops the care plan frequently does not perform all of the nursing interventions. Some activities must be delegated to other members of the health care team and coordinated by the nurse (see Chapter 23). Noninvasive and frequently repetitive interventions such as skin care, range-of-joint-motion exercises, ambulation, grooming, and hygiene measures are examples of care activities that can be assigned to assistive personnel. The nurse assigning tasks is responsible for ensuring that each task is appropriately assigned and is completed according to the standard of care and that indirect care interventions are delegated to those personnel competent to provide the specific type of care (McCloskey and others, 1996).

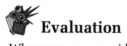 **Evaluation**

Whenever you provide nursing care to a client, you must evaluate two aspects of care. First, evaluate your client's response to nursing care. You need to ask yourself questions about the care, such as: "Was the therapy effective in improving the client's level of health or functional status?" "Did the client benefit?" It is important to evaluate whether each client reaches a level of wellness or recovery that the health care team and client established in the goals of care. Second, you must evaluate if your client's expectations of care have been met. Ask your clients questions relating to their perception, such as "Did you receive the type of pain management you expected?" "Did you get enough information to help you manage your asthma at home?"

The **evaluation** step of the nursing process measures the client's response to nursing actions and the client's progress toward achieving goals. You collect data on an ongoing basis to measure changes in functioning, daily living, or in availability or use of external resources (Carnevali and Thomas, 1993). Evaluation occurs each time you have contact with your client. The emphasis is on client outcomes. You evaluate

whether the client's behavior or responses reflect a reversal or improvement in the client's level of health. During evaluation, you decide if the nursing interventions were effective in minimizing or resolving the client's problems, by examining the client's responses and comparing them with the behavior stated in the previously established expected outcomes.

Critical Thinking Skills and the Evaluation of Nursing Care

While caring for your clients, you compare subjective and objective data gathered from the client, other nurses or caregivers, and family to determine the degree of success in meeting goals and expected outcomes. If outcomes are met, the overall goals for the client are also met. Compare client behavior and responses assessed before nursing interventions are delivered with behavior and responses that occur after administering nursing care. You apply knowledge about the client's condition, consider previous experience with similar clients, and review data from the assessed baseline to critically analyze if the client's condition is changing. Critical thinking directs you to analyze the findings from evaluation. Is the client's condition improved? Can the client improve, or are there physical factors preventing recovery? To what degree does this client's motivation or willingness to pursue healthier behavior influence response to therapies?

In evaluation, you continually redirect nursing care to best meet client needs. For example, when evaluating your client for a change in vital signs, you apply knowledge of disease processes and physiological responses to interpret whether a change has occurred and whether the change is desirable. A client in acute pain may have an increased heart rate and increased muscular tension. You know that this is a sympathetic nervous system response to painful stimuli. After administering a pain medication, helping the client to try a relaxation exercise, and repositioning the client, you return to evaluate if the client's perception of pain has decreased and if the vital signs have returned either to a more acceptable level or to the client's baseline before pain.

Positive evaluations occur when desired results are met, and lead you to conclude that the nursing intervention effectively met the client's goal of improved comfort. Negative evaluations or undesired results indicate that the intervention was not effective in minimizing or resolving the actual problem or avoiding a potential problem, or that new data about the client's condition have altered the client's ability to meet the established outcome. As a result, you must change the care plan and try different therapies or a different approach in administering existing therapies.

This sequence of critically evaluating and revising therapies continues until problems are appropriately resolved. Outcomes must be realistic and adjusted based on the client's prognosis and condition. Remember that evaluation is dynamic and ever changing, depending on the client's nursing diagnoses and condition. A client whose health status continuously changes requires more frequent evaluation. In addition, priority diagnoses are often evaluated first. For example, you evaluate a client's *acute pain* before evaluating the status of *deficient knowledge*.

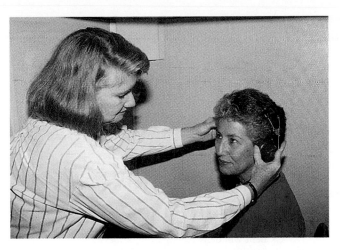

FIGURE **6-6**   Nurse evaluates the client's hearing acuity. (Courtesy Phillip James Acker, Motorola, Inc.)

Evaluative Measures and Sources

Evaluative measures are simply the assessment skills and techniques you use to evaluate a client. For example, auscultation of lung sounds, observation of a client's skill performance, inspection of the skin, and inquiry regarding the severity of pain are all evaluative measures (Figure 6-6). In fact, they are the same as assessment measures, but you perform them after providing care. The intent of evaluation is to determine if the nursing interventions have been effective in minimizing or resolving the problems, if the problems have worsened, or if the list of problems has changed.

The data collected during evaluation are critically analyzed and compared with expected outcomes to determine whether changes occurred. After caring for a client over a long period, you are able to make subtle comparisons of responses and behavior. Your practice and experience along with your scientific knowledge base are keys to critical thinking. The accuracy of evaluation improves when you are familiar with the client's behavior and physiological status. Evaluation is also more accurate after you have seen more than one client with a similar problem.

The primary source of data for evaluation is the client. However, you may also use the family and other caregivers. Documentation and reporting in the evaluation process are critical. Written nursing progress notes, assessment flow sheets, and information shared between nurses during change-of-shift reports (see Chapter 7) should communicate a client's progress toward meeting expected outcomes and goals for the nursing plan of care. If a client is cared for using a critical pathway or CareMap (see Chapter 7), the nurse and team members clearly know what outcomes are to be met for a given day. The CareMap as a documentation tool includes expected outcomes that the care team predicts will be met during the client's projected length of stay.

Evaluation of Goal Achievement

One purpose of nursing care is to assist the client in minimizing or resolving actual health problems, preventing the occurrence of potential problems, and promoting the maintenance of a healthy state. Evaluation of the goals of care de-

termines whether this purpose was accomplished. You match your client's behavior (e.g., self-administration of insulin or anxiety-free behavior) or physiological response (e.g., decrease in size of pressure ulcer or fall in body temperature) with the behavior or response specified in the goal. For example, during an initial assessment, a client may report acute abdominal pain, rate the pain 8 on a scale of 10 (see Chapter 29), and grimace or hold the abdomen during attempts to move in bed. You may have used this data to support the nursing diagnosis of *acute pain* and establish the goal, "client will have reduced pain within 48 hours." Evaluation determines if the outcomes that reflect goal accomplishment were met. Did the interventions of positioning, proper and timely administration of analgesics, and use of relaxation successfully reduce the client's pain? Outcomes may include, "client will verbalize pain at 3 on a scale of 10" and "client will position self without nonverbal signs of discomfort." After providing appropriate comfort measures, evaluate the client by measuring the subjective report of pain, observe facial expressions, and note if the client initiates turning and repositioning. Compare the client responses with outcome criteria to determine whether predicted changes have occurred (Table 6-10). To objectively evaluate the degree of success in achieving a goal, use the following steps:

1. Examine the goal statement to identify the exact desired client behavior or response.
2. Assess the client for the presence of that behavior or response.
3. Compare the established outcome criteria with the behavior or response.
4. Judge the degree of agreement between outcome criteria and the behavior or response.
5. If there is no agreement (or only partial agreement) between the outcome criteria and the behavior or response, what are the barriers? Why did they not agree?

There are different degrees of goal attainment. If the client's response matches or exceeds the outcome criteria, the goal is met. If the client's behavior begins to show changes but does not yet meet criteria set, the goal is partially met. If there is no progress, the goal is not met. A clearly defined goal with specific outcomes is easily measured.

Care Plan Revision and Critical Thinking

As goals are evaluated, adjustments to the care plan are made as indicated. If a goal was successfully met, that portion of the care plan is considered resolved. Unmet and partially met goals require you to reactivate the nursing process sequence. After you reassess your client, nursing diagnoses may be modified or added with appropriate goals, expected outcomes, and interventions established. At this time, you also re-examine priorities. Knowing how the client is progressing and how problems might resolve, stay the same, or worsen are important. Your careful monitoring and early detection of problems are a client's first line of defense (Benner, 1984). Because changes in clients' status may be very subtle, evaluation must be client specific, based on a close familiarity with how clients behave, and take into account the client's physical status and reaction to caregivers.

Evaluation Measures to Determine the Success of Goals and Expected Outcomes

Table 6-10

Goals	Evaluation Measures	Expected Outcomes
Client's pressure ulcer will demonstrate healing within 7 days.	Inspect color, condition, and location of pressure ulcer. Measure diameter of ulcer daily. Note odor and color of drainage from ulcer.	Erythema will be reduced in 2 days. Diameter of ulcer will decrease in 5 days. Ulcer will have no drainage in 2 days. Skin overlying ulcer will begin to close in 7 days.
Client will tolerate ambulation to end of hall by 11/20.	Palpate client's radial pulse before exercise. Palpate client's radial pulse 10 minutes after exercise. Assess respiratory rate during exercise. Observe client for dyspnea or breathlessness during exercise.	Pulse will remain below 110 beats per minute during exercise. Pulse rate will return to resting baseline within 10 minutes after exercise. Respiratory rate will remain within two breaths of client's baseline rate. Client will deny feeling of breathlessness.

Accurate evaluation leads to the appropriate revision of ineffective care plans and discontinuation of therapy that has been successful.

DISCONTINUING A CARE PLAN. After determining that expected outcomes and goals have been achieved, confirm this evaluation with the client. If you both agree that the expected outcomes have been met, discontinue that care plan. For example, a client has the nursing diagnosis *deficient knowledge regarding insulin therapy related to inexperience.* To achieve the ultimate goal of accurate client administration of insulin, you establish outcomes including, "Client will describe the purpose of insulin by 9/20," "Client will correctly prepare insulin in syringe by 9/20," and "Client will administer insulin injection independently by 9/22." Discuss the information with your client and determine whether the client understands explanations and is comfortable with the information provided. In addition, observe the client's preparation of the medication and actual self-injection. Once outcomes are met successfully it is unnecessary to teach additional information about insulin administration. The care plan for this nursing diagnosis can be documented as discontinued. This ensures that other nurses will not unnecessarily continue a care plan. Continuity of care assumes that care provided is relevant to client needs. Significant time is wasted when achieved goals are not communicated.

MODIFYING A CARE PLAN. When goals are not met, you must identify the factors that interfered with goal achievement. Usually a change in the client's condition, needs, or abilities makes alteration of the care plan necessary. For example, when teaching self-administration of insulin, you discover that the client has a literacy problem or a visual impairment that prevents the reading of insulin dosages on the syringe. As a result, original outcomes cannot be met. Thus you develop new interventions and revise outcomes to meet the goal of care.

Lack of goal achievement may also result from an error in nursing judgment or failure to follow each step of the nursing process. Clients frequently have very complex problems.

Always remember the possibility of overlooking or misjudging something. When there is failure to achieve a goal, no matter what the reason, the entire nursing process sequence is repeated.

REASSESSMENT. Evaluate your client's response to care. Collect data about the client's status following the implementation step of the nursing process. During reassessment, use critical thinking skills to compare data collected during evaluation with previously obtained information. Reassessment ensures that the database is accurate and current. You may apply knowledge from previous experiences with other clients to direct the reassessment process. Day-by-day encounters over time with clients and families who have similar health problems give you a library of knowledge to use in anticipating client needs and planning care. For example, consider Mr. Landis, who has the nursing diagnosis *acute pain related to trauma of a surgical incision.* Two days after surgery he continues to have a poor appetite despite the fact that there are no obvious surgical complications. If he continues to have pain, the novice nurse may associate loss of appetite with discomfort. However, the experienced nurse may recall a previous client who became depressed after surgery. After exploring the problem further, the nurse learns that Mr. Landis's family has not been visiting and that he is fearful of losing his job. For these reasons, Mr. Landis simply has lost interest in eating. Although he continues to have pain, a new priority may be *imbalanced nutrition: less than body requirements related to loss of appetite.* As in the original assessment, data are collected from all available sources. Depending on your findings, it often becomes necessary to assess variables that were not covered on the initial assessment.

Assessment may also reveal pieces of information that were previously overlooked and thus interfered with goal achievement.

NURSING DIAGNOSES. After reassessment, determine whether the nursing diagnoses continue to be valid. Revise the list of nursing diagnoses to reflect the client's changed status. Your care is based on an accurate list of nursing diagnoses. Accuracy is more important than the number of diagnoses selected. As the client's condition changes, the diagnoses do too. If a previous diagnosis no longer accurately reflects the problem, it should be discontinued, and a modified statement entered. For example, you find that a client with diabetes has a serious visual impairment, it may be unlikely that the client will be able to self-administer insulin. Assessment reveals that a family member is available as a resource. To develop a plan designed to educate an alternate caregiver about the administration of insulin, establish a new diagnosis, *ineffective health maintenance related to inability to self-administer insulin secondary to visual impairment.*

GOALS AND EXPECTED OUTCOMES.   When care plans are revised, review the goals and expected outcomes for needed changes. Even the goals for unchanged nursing diagnoses should be examined for continued appropriateness. Determining that each goal and expected outcome is realistic for the problem, etiology, and time frame is particularly important. Unrealistic expected outcomes and time frames make goal achievement difficult.

Clearly document goals and expected outcomes for new or revised nursing diagnoses so that all team members are aware of the revised care plan. When the goal is still appropriate but has not yet been met, you may change the evaluation date to allow more time. All goals and expected outcomes should be client centered, with realistic expectations for client achievement.

INTERVENTIONS.   The evaluation of interventions examines two factors: the appropriateness of the interventions selected and the correct application of the implementation process. The appropriateness of an intervention may be based on the **standard of care** for a client's health problem. If the client has a specific nursing diagnosis such as *acute pain,* the standard of care established by a nursing department for this problem includes pain control measures. Review the standard of care

to determine whether the right interventions have been chosen or if additional ones are required.

It may only be necessary to increase or decrease the frequency of interventions. Use clinical judgment based on previous experience and the client's actual response to therapy. For example, if a client continues to have congested lung sounds, you increase the frequency of coughing exercises to remove secretions.

During evaluation, you may determine that some planned interventions are designed for an inappropriate level of nursing care. If the level of care needs to be changed, a different action verb, such as *assist* in place of *provide,* may be substituted. Sometimes the level of care is appropriate, but the interventions are unsuitable because of a change in the expected outcome. In this case the interventions should be discontinued and new ones planned.

Changes in the plan of care should be guided by the nature of the client's response. Consulting with other nurses may yield suggestions for improving the approach to care delivery. Senior nurses are often excellent resources because of their experience. Simply changing the care plan is not enough. You must implement the new plan and reevaluate the client's response to the nursing actions. *Evaluation is continuous.*

Occasionally an error made during care planning and delivery is discovered during evaluation. This should be anticipated. The nursing process is designed to be a systematic, problem-solving approach to individualized client care, but there is a wide array of variables for each client with a health care problem. Clients with the same health care problem are not treated the same. You must consistently incorporate evaluation into practice to minimize error and ensure that the most appropriate interventions are used.

Evaluation is the final step of the nursing process and provides a systematic method for analyzing the results of nursing care. The consistent application of evaluation principles ensures that you determine whether the outcomes of your client's care are beneficial and that the care plan remains current and appropriate.

Key Terms

Key Terms—cont'd

related factor, *p. 81*
risk nursing diagnosis, *p. 79*

scientific rationale, *p. 86*
standard of care, *p. 97*
standing order, *p. 90*
subjective data, *p. 74*

validation, *p. 77*
wellness nursing diagnosis, *p. 79*

Key Concepts

• The purposes of the nursing process are to identify the client's health care needs, establish a nursing care plan, and complete nursing interventions designed to meet the needs.
• The nursing process has five component steps: assessment, nursing diagnosis, planning, implementation, and evaluation.
• Sources of client data are the client interview and health history, physical examination, observation of client behavior, medical records, consultation with health team members and family or significant others, and professional literature.
• Effective communication skills are essential to the client interview.
• Physical examination requires the skills of inspection, auscultation, palpation, and percussion.
• Data validation ensures accuracy of the assessment.
• Data clustering organizes the assessed information into meaningful clusters.
• The diagnostic process includes analysis and interpretation of data, identification of client and family needs, and formulation of the nursing diagnostic statement.
• Nursing diagnoses state actual or potential problems in the client's health status.
• Nursing diagnostic errors may lead to inadequate nursing care.
• A correctly written nursing diagnosis is within the domain of nursing practice and contains a NANDA-approved diagnostic problem statement and a precise statement of the influencing factors contributing to the problem, connected by the phrase *related to*.

• During the planning component, client goals are determined, priorities are established, expected outcomes of nursing care are developed, and a nursing care plan is written.
• The nurse begins the nursing care plan by first addressing the nursing diagnoses that have the highest priority.
• The care plan is a written guideline for client care so that all members of the health care team can quickly understand the care given.
• Critical pathways are multidisciplinary treatment plans that predict the interventions and outcomes to be met for selected clients over a projected length of stay.
• Correctly written nursing interventions include specific information about the actions, frequency, quantity, method, and the person to perform them.
• Preparation for implementation includes reassessing the client; reviewing, setting in order of priority, and modifying the care plan; identifying areas in which assistance is needed; organizing supplies and personnel; and preparing the client, family, and environment.
• Nursing actions to achieve therapeutic goals include preventing adverse reactions, using correct techniques for administering care, preparing the client for procedures, and implementing lifesaving measures.
• Evaluation determines a client's response to nursing actions and the extent to which goals of care have been met.
• The nurse compares the client's response to nursing actions with expected outcomes established during planning.
• Evaluation enables the nurse to determine the reason that the care plan was successful or unsuccessful.

Critical Thinking Activities

1. Develop examples of closed and open questions you would use to determine Mrs. Bryan's health care needs. Practice using them on a classmate, and compare the information you gather.
2. You greet Mrs. Jacob on your first home visit after she has undergone major abdominal surgery. You introduce yourself and explain your role and the physician's postoperative orders. What aspect of the interview has taken place? What will you do next?
3. During an assessment, you note that a client mentions an increase in the number of colds, that sputum is thick and yellow, and an increase in shortness of breath. Which step of the diagnostic process is taking place?
4. What information is necessary to plan nursing interventions for your clients? If you had assisstive personnel, how would you plan those nursing strategies that could be delegated to these persons?

5. Mr. Clark is a 45-year-old man admitted with congestive heart failure. His lung sounds are clear; his blood pressure is 130/88 mm Hg, his pulse is 112 beats per minute, and his respirations are 24 per minute. His nursing history reveals that he does not consistently take all of his medications nor does he follow a low-sodium diet, which was designed to reduce fluid retention. List the specific types of interventions that you may select to assist in resolving Mr. Clark's present illness and prevent further complications. Include the type of intervention (e.g., nurse initiated, physician initiated, collaborative).
6. Mr. Vacaro has been visiting the clinic for over a month. He visits weekly for follow-up care for a chronic venous stasis ulcer of the left leg. The nurse's note at the time of his first visit contained the following information: "Ulcer with irregular margins, 4 cm wide by 5 cm long and approximately 0.5 cm deep, and foul-smelling purulent yellowish drainage. Only subcutaneous tissue visible. Brownish rust-colored skin around ulcer. Zinc oxide and calamine gauze

applied to ulcer. Ace bandage applied to gauze. Client instructed to return in 2 weeks." As the nurse caring for the client on the follow-up visit, what expected outcomes would you anticipate for the goal of "Wound will demonstrate healing within 4 weeks"? What evaluative measures would you use to determine if the wound is healing?

Review Questions

1. The identification of your client's health care needs occurs in the nursing process step of:
   1. planning.
   2. evaluation.
   3. assessment.
   4. implementation.
2. You have just met your client, who complains of abdominal pain that occurs 2 hours following a meal and states that the pain is not aggravated by a specific type of meal. To obtain more information about the client's perceptions of the pain you will first need to:
   1. complete a detailed physical examination.
   2. conduct a detailed nursing history about the pain.
   3. review the related nursing and medical literature about abdominal pain.
   4. consult with other health care professionals regarding the identification and treatment of abdominal pain.
3. The most important skills needed to obtain accurate information from your client are:
   1. teaching skills.
   2. cognitive skills.
   3. psychomotor skills.
   4. interpersonal skills.
4. Before formulating a list of nursing diagnoses you must first:
   1. establish a list of priorities.
   2. document your assessment findings.
   3. review your assessment with other health team members.
   4. validate the interpretation of the data with your client and physical examination findings.
5. Establishing priorities for your client's care occurs in the nursing process step of:
   1. planning.
   2. evaluation.
   3. assessment.
   4. implementation.
6. Expected outcomes are needed in a plan of care to:
   1. identify the anticipated client response to care.
   2. determine that the nursing care was delivered.
   3. provide documentation of the type of care given.
   4. support the need for additional health care personnel.
7. During implementation it may be necessary to delegate portions of a client's care to other personnel. When delegating it is important to remember that:
   1. delegation is a means to reduce the client's cost of care.
   2. the delegated personnel are responsible for the client's care.
   3. the nurse still has primary responsibility for the quality of the client's care.
   4. delegation of care is never within the domain of nursing practice, and the nurse is not responsible for delegation.
8. Evaluation is an important part of nursing care. During this process, you best determine the effectiveness of a specific nursing action by:
   1. reassessing the client for new problems.
   2. determining that the specific nursing action was completed.
   3. comparing the client's response to the nursing action with other clients who received the same nursing action.
   4. comparing the client's response to the nursing action with the expected outcomes established during planning.

References

American Nurses Association: *Nursing: a social policy statement,* Washington, DC, 1995, The Association.

Benner P: *From novice to expert: excellence and power in clinical nursing practice,* Menlo Park, Calif, 1984, Addison-Wesley.

Bulechek GM, McCloskey JC: Nursing interventions: what they are and how to choose them, *Holistic Nurs Pract* 1(3):36, 1987.

Carnevali DL, Thomas MD: *Diagnostic reasoning and treatment decision making in nursing,* Philadelphia, 1993, JB Lippincott.

Carpenito LJ: *Nursing diagnosis application to clinical practice,* ed 8, Philadelphia, 2000, JB Lippincott.

Collier IC and others: *Writing nursing diagnoses: a critical thinking approach,* St. Louis, 1996, Mosby.

Copi IM, Cohen C: *Introduction to logic,* ed 9, New York, 1994, Macmillan.

Gordon M: *Nursing diagnosis: process and application,* ed 3, St. Louis, 1994, Mosby.

Gordon M and others: Clinical judgment: an integrated model, *Adv Nurs Sci* 16:55, 1994.

Liukkonen A: The nurse's decision-making process and the implementation of psychogeriatric nursing in a mental hospital, *J Adv Nurs* 17(3):356, 1992.

McCloskey JC, Bulechek GM: Nursing interventions core to specialty practice, *Nurs Outlook* 46(2):61, 1998.

McCloskey JC, Bulechek GM: *Iowa intervention project: nursing interventions classification,* ed 3, St. Louis, 2000, Mosby.

McCloskey JC and others: Nurses' use and delegation of indirect care interventions, *Nurs Econ* 14(1):22, 1996.

McNaull FW and others: A comparison of education methods to enhance nursing performance in pain assessment, *J Contin Educ Nurs* 23(6):267, 1992.

Milner EM, Collins MB: Tools to improve systematic client assessment in undergraduate nursing education, *J Nurs Educ* 31(4):186, 1992.

Mortensen M, McMullin C: Discharge score for surgical outpatients, *Am J Nurs* 86:1347, 1986.

North American Nursing Diagnosis Association: *NANDA nursing diagnoses: definitions and classifications, 2001-2002,* Philadelphia, 2001, The Association.

Redman BK: *The process of patient education,* ed 7, St. Louis, 1993, Mosby.

Windel PE: Critical pathways: an integrated documentation tool, *Nurs Manage* 25(9):80F, 1994.

Zander K, McGill R: Critical and anticipated recovery paths: only the beginning, *Nurs Manage* 25(8):34, 1994.

7

Documentation and Reporting

Objectives

- Define key terms.
- Describe multidisciplinary communication within the health care team.
- Identify purposes of health care records.
- Discuss legal guidelines for documentation.
- Maintain confidentiality of records and reports.
- Describe six guidelines for quality documentation and reporting.
- Compare different methods used in documentation.
- Discuss case management and critical paths as related to documentation.
- Identify common record-keeping forms.
- Discuss advantages and disadvantages of standardized documentation forms.
- Identify elements to include when documenting discharge plans.
- Discuss advantages of computerized documentation.
- Describe the content and process of change-of-shift reports.
- Explain documentation related to telephone use.

Documentation is a vital aspect of nursing practice. **Documentation** is defined as anything written or printed within a client record. This information reflects the quality of care and provides accountability for each health care team member's care. Expected outcomes and the nursing care you provide for a client are documented in the medical record (e.g., assessments and interventions). The health care environment creates many challenges for accurately documenting and reporting the care delivered to clients. The quality of nursing care depends on your ability to communicate effectively verbally and in writing, and you are held accountable for the accuracy of documentation you enter into the client's record. Regulations require health care institutions to monitor and evaluate the quality and appropriateness of client care (see Chapters 2 and 6).

A **record** is a permanent legal written communication that includes information relevant to a client's health care management. Information about the client's health care is recorded after each client contact. The record is a continuing account of the client's health care status and is available to all members of the health care team.

Reports are oral, written, or audiotape exchanges of information between caregivers. Common reports given by nurses include change-of-shift reports, telephone reports, transfer reports, and incident reports. Incident reports are documented on a record that is not part of the client medical record.

CONFIDENTIALITY

Information about clients' status may not be disclosed to other clients or to staff not involved in their care. Legal and ethical obligations require you to keep information about clients strictly confidential. The Health Insurance Portability and Accountability Act of 1996 (HIPAA) provides national standards for confidentiality (HIPAA, 2001). Nurses, other health care professionals, and students may have reason to use records for data gathering, research, or continuing education. These uses are permitted if the records are used as specified and permission is granted.

STANDARDS

Your documentation must conform to the standards of the Joint Commission on Accreditation of Healthcare Organizations (JCAHO) to maintain institutional **accreditation** and to minimize liability. Current documentation standards require that all clients who are admitted to a health care facility have an assessment of physical, psychosocial, environmental, self-care, knowledge level, and discharge planning needs (JCAHO, 1999). JCAHO standards require that your documentation be within the context of the nursing process, including evidence of client and family teaching and discharge planning. Recently JCAHO standards incorporated a collaborative and interdisciplinary approach to pain management. This includes individualized pain control strategies involving frequent reassessment of pain, use of

both pharmacological and nonpharmacological strategies, and a formalized approach to the implementation of pain management strategies (Phillips, 2000). Evaluation of nursing care communicates the degree of progress and success in meeting expected outcomes of care.

PURPOSE OF RECORDS

Documentation serves multiple purposes: it facilitates communication with health care providers for continuity of client care, it maintains a legal and financial record of care, it aids in clinical research, and it guides professional and organizational performance improvement (Comprehensive Accreditation Manual for Hospitals [CAMH], 2000).

Although each agency may use a different record format, records contain basically the same information. Each page of the record must include the current date and is stamped with client identification including basic demographic data (age, birth date), physician, date admitted, and medical record number. Each client record includes admission data, a signed consent for treatment, physician's orders, medical history and physician's physical examination, and nurses' documentation of ongoing assessments, interventions, and evaluation. The record also contains medication records, physician's progress notes, progress notes from other disciplines such as respiratory therapy and physical therapy, results of laboratory tests, and discharge information.

Communication

The record is a means by which health care team members provide continuity of care and communicate client needs and progress toward meeting desired client outcomes. The record also includes the client's responses to interventions and consequent modifications in the plan of care.

Legal Documentation

Effective documentation is one of the best defenses for legal claims associated with health care (Box 7-1). To limit nursing liability, nursing documentation must clearly indicate that individualized, goal-directed nursing care was provided to clients based on the nursing assessment. This is best accomplished when you chart as you provide care. It is important to avoid recording data that is routine, superficial, or not pertinent, for example, "bath given" or "watching TV." In some settings a registered nurse may be required by agency policy to co-sign documentation completed by licensed practical or vocational nurses or assistive personnel. This indicates that the nurse was aware of the care and client status when care was delivered by others that the nurse was supervising. Problems arise when a record is reviewed in a malpractice suit and time gaps are found, information is squeezed between lines or crossed out, or key facts were omitted (Ladebauche, 1995).

Financial Billing

Diagnosis-related groups (DRGs) have become the basis for establishing reimbursement for client care. Under the prospective payment system, hospitals are reimbursed a set dollar amount by Medicare for each DRG (see Chapter 2). Your nursing documentation provides verification of the specific nursing care provided to support the reimbursement to health care agencies.

Education

A client's record contains a variety of information (e.g., medical and nursing diagnoses, signs and symptoms of disease, successful and unsuccessful therapies, diagnostic findings, client behaviors). Reading the client care record can be an effective way to learn the nature of an illness and the client's response to the illness. Patterns of information can be identified in clients with similar medical problems. Health care team members can learn patterns and be able to anticipate the type of care a client may require.

Nursing Process

The record provides data used to identify and support the nursing plan of care (see Chapter 6). The initial admission nursing assessment usually is comprehensive and provides a baseline of the client's health status. Before caring for any client, refer to the client care record for relevant medical findings in addition to your own nursing assessment. This allows you to anticipate the status of the client and, as you conduct additional assessments, to recognize changes from previous assessment findings. At regular intervals

continuing nursing progress notes detail ongoing assessments as nursing care is provided.

Research

Statistical data can be gathered from client records, including the frequency of clinical disorders, complications, use of specific medical and nursing therapies, recoveries from illness, and mortality. After you obtain formal institutional approvals, you may use clients' records during a research study to collect information on a particular health problem. For example, if you suspect that early ambulation decreases the complications in postsurgery clients, appropriate client records could be examined to evaluate that supposition.

Auditing and Monitoring

The JCAHO requires hospitals to establish quality improvement programs to conduct objective, ongoing reviews of client care and asks institutions to establish standards for quality care. Quality improvement programs keep you informed of standards of nursing practice to maintain excellence in nursing care (see Chapter 2).

GUIDELINES FOR QUALITY DOCUMENTATION AND REPORTING

High-quality recording and reporting are necessary to enhance efficient, individualized client care. Quality documentation and reporting have six important characteristics: they are factual, accurate, complete, current, organized, and confidential.

Factual

A record must contain descriptive, objective information about what you see, hear, feel, and smell. Objective data are defined as data that are measured and observed. Avoid words such as *appears, seems,* or *apparently* because they lead to conclusions that cannot be supported by objective information.

The only subjective data included are what the client says. Write subjective information with quotation marks, using the client's own words. For example, Client states "*My lower back hurts*" is subjective and acceptable documentation. However, in the case of pain you need to further assess and objectively describe pain intensity using a pain scale; for example, the client rates pain as a 6 on a scale of 0 to 10, with 10 the worst pain. Clients can also use the Faces Pain Rating Scale (smile-frown) or the verbal descriptor scale (Platt and Reed, 2001). It is also important for you to include objective findings that further clarify the extent of the client's pain, such as position, limited movement, facial expression, and increased blood pressure and pulse rate. It is acceptable not to use quotation marks when you paraphrase the client's words.

Accurate

The use of precise measurements achieves accuracy. For example, documenting that "Client voided 450 ml clear urine" is more accurate than "Voided an adequate amount."

Accuracy is also maintained by using an institution's accepted abbreviations, symbols, and system of measurement. To avoid misunderstandings, you must write out any abbreviations that may be confusing (e.g., od [once daily] can be misinterpreted to mean O.D. [right eye]). Correct spelling demonstrates a level of competency and attention to detail. Misspelled words can lead to confusion. For example, often words sound the same but have different meanings, such as *accept* and *except* or *dysphagia* and *dysphasia.* Incorrect use of terms can confuse the intended meaning.

JCAHO standards (1999) require that "all entries in medical records be dated and there is a method to identify all authors of entries." Therefore any descriptive entry in a client's record is ended with the caregiver's full name and status. Occasionally you may include observations reported to another caregiver or interventions performed by someone else, for example, "Client suctioned by J. Hill, RN." As a nursing student, you need to enter full name, student nurse abbreviation, and educational institution, such as "Marianne Smith, SN [student nurse], CMTC [Central Maine Technical College]." The abbreviation for *student nurse* may be regionally different, being either *NS,* which stands for *nursing student,* or *SN,* which stands for *student nurse.* The signature holds this person accountable for information recorded.

Complete

The information within a recorded entry needs to be complete and thorough, as in the following example:

> 0845 Reports continuous throbbing pain on lateral aspect of left fractured femur increased with movement of the leg with a severity of 8 (scale 0-10). B/P = 132/74, T = 37°, P = 92, R = 18. Morphine 10 mg IV given for pain. Sue Jacobs, RN.
>
> 0915 Reports pain at 2 (scale 1-10) and able to turn in bed independently. Sue Jacobs, RN.

Routine activities such as daily hygiene measures, vital signs, and pain assessment are often included in flow sheets. These activities are described in greater detail when it is pertinent because of a change in functional ability or status. For example, it could be considered pertinent for you to document that a client who has previously required a total bath improves to the extent that the client can now wash his or her face, hands, and upper body.

Current

Making entries promptly is essential in effective documentation (JCAHO, 1999). Delays in documentation can result in serious omissions and untimely delays in client care. You need to communicate the following nursing care at the time of occurrence:
1. Vital signs
2. Pain assessment
3. Administration of medications and treatments
4. Preparation for diagnostic tests or surgery
5. Change in client status and who was notified

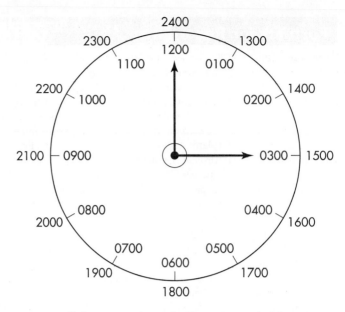

FIGURE **7-1**   Comparison of military time and civilian time.

6. Admission, transfer, discharge, or death of client
7. Treatment for sudden changes in client status
8. Client response to intervention

Many agencies use military time, a 24-hour system that uses four-digit numbers to indicate morning, afternoon, and evening times. Figure 7-1 compares military and corresponding civilian times.

Organized

Written communication is easier to understand when written in a logical order. For example, an organized note describes your assessment, interventions, and client's response in a sequence. It is also more effective when concise, clear, and to the point. To make clear and organized entries it is often helpful to make a list of what needs to be included before beginning to write in the permanent legal record. Once you have identified the pertinent content, you can often delete unnecessary words. This process becomes easier with practice.

METHODS OF RECORDING

The documentation system selected by a nursing service reflects the philosophy of the department. It is a challenge to create a record-keeping system that ensures optimal communication. There are several acceptable formats for recording health care information (Table 7-1).

Narrative Documentation

Narrative documentation is the traditional method for nursing care records; however, in many settings narrative charting has been replaced by other formats. Narrative charting uses a storylike format to document information specific to client conditions and nursing care. Narrative charting is beneficial in emergency situations in which a chronological order of events is needed.

Formats for Recording   Table 7-1

Narrative note	Client stated: "I'm dreading surgery. Last time I had such pain when I got out of bed." Discussed alternatives for pain control and importance of postoperative activity. Encouraged to ask for pain medication before pain is severe. Client stated: "I feel better prepared now." Able to verbalize that activity enhances circulation and healing.
SOAP	S (subjective data): "I'm dreading surgery. Last time I had such pain when I got out of bed." O (objective data): Noted muscle tension and loud voice. A (assessment/analysis): Fear of postoperative pain. P (plan): Assess pain level every 2 hours. Provide comfort measures and give analgesics as needed.
PIE charting	P (problem): Client stated: "I'm dreading surgery. Last time I had such pain when I got out of bed." I (intervention): Discussed alternatives for pain control and importance of postoperative activity. Encouraged to ask for pain medication before pain is severe. E (evaluation): Client stated: "I feel better prepared now." Able to verbalize that activity enhances circulation and healing.
Focus charting	D (data): Client stated: "I'm dreading surgery. Last time I had such pain when I got out of bed." A (action): Discussed alternatives for pain control and importance of postoperative activity. Encouraged to ask for pain medication before pain is severe. R (response): Client stated: "I feel better prepared now." Able to verbalize that activity enhances circulation and healing. Note: Some agencies add P (Plan). Example: P (Plan): Assess pain level every 2 hours. Provide comfort measures and give analgesics as needed.

Problem-Oriented Medical Records

The **problem-oriented medical record (POMR)** is a structured method of documentation that places emphasis on the client's problems. The method corresponds to the nursing process and facilitates communication of client needs. Data are organized by problem or diagnosis. Ideally, each member of the health care team contributes to a single list of identified client problems. The POMR is composed of the following: database, problem list, care plan, and progress notes.

DATABASE. The database contains all available assessment information pertaining to the client. This section is the foundation for identifying client problems and planning care. The database should remain active and current, and revisions should be made as new data are available.

PROBLEM LIST. The problem list is developed after the data are analyzed. The problems are listed in chronological order to serve as an organizing guide for the client's care. New problems are added as they are identified. After a problem has been resolved, the date is recorded, and a line is drawn through the problem and its number.

CARE PLAN. The care plan is developed for each problem by the disciplines involved in the client's care. Nurses document the plan of care in a variety of formats. Generally these plans of care include nursing diagnoses, expected outcomes, and interventions (see Chapter 6).

PROGRESS NOTES. Progress notes are used by health care team members to monitor and record the progress of a client's problems. Narrative notes, flow sheets, and discharge summaries are forms used to document the client's progress.

SOAP DOCUMENTATION. A **SOAP note** is an acronym for the POMR method of documentation as follows:

S: Subjective data (verbalizations of the client)
O: Objective data (data that are measured and observed)
A: Assessment (diagnosis based on the data)
P: Plan (what the caregiver plans to do)

An *I* and *E* are sometimes added (i.e., SOAPIE) in various institutions. The *I* stands for *intervention,* and the *E* represents *evaluation.* The logic for SOAP(IE) notes is similar to that of the nursing process. Collect data about each of your client's problems, draw a conclusion, and develop a plan of care. Number each SOAP note, and title it according to the problem on the list.

PIE DOCUMENTATION. The **PIE note** documentation format is similar to SOAP charting in its problem-oriented nature. However, it differs from the SOAP method in that PIE charting has a nursing origin, whereas SOAP originated from the medical model. PIE is an acronym for *problem, interventions, evaluation* as follows:

P: Problem or nursing diagnosis applicable to client
I: Interventions or actions taken
E: Evaluation of the outcomes of nursing interventions

This format simplifies documentation by unifying the care plan and progress notes into a complete record. The PIE format also differs from SOAP because the narrative note does not include assessment information. Your daily assessment data appear on special flow sheets, thus preventing duplication of information. The PIE notes can be numbered or labeled according to the client's problems. Resolved problems are dropped from daily documentation after the nurse's review.

Components of a Source Record

Table 7-2

Admission sheet	Specific demographic data about client: legal name, identification number, sex, age, birth date, marital status, occupation and employer, health insurance, nearest relative to notify in an emergency, religious preference, name of attending physician, date and time of admission
Physician's order sheet	Record of physician's orders for treatment and medications, with date, time, and physician's signature
Nurse's admission assessment	Summary of nursing history and physical examination
Graphic record and flow sheet	Record of repeated observations and numerical measurements such as vital signs, pain assessment, daily weights, and intake and output
Medical history and examination	Results of initial examination performed by physician, including findings, family history, confirmed diagnoses, and medical plan of care
Nurses' notes	Record of nursing assessment, planning, implementation, and evaluation of care
Medication records	Accurate documentation of all medications administered to client: date, time, dose, route, and nurse's signature
Client education record	Documentation of client's or significant other's response to educational needs and level of understanding of diagnosis and treatment plan
Physician's progress notes	Ongoing record of client's progress and response to medical therapy and review of disease process
Health care discipline's records	Entries made into record by all health-related disciplines (e.g., respiratory therapy, radiology, social work, laboratories)
Discharge summary	Summary of client's condition, progress, prognosis, rehabilitation, and teaching needs at time of dismissal from hospital or health care agency

Source Records

In a **source record** the client's chart is organized so that each discipline (e.g., nursing, medicine, social work, respiratory therapy) has a separate section in which to record data. Unlike the POMR, this format does not organize the information by client problems. The advantage of a source record is that caregivers can easily locate the proper section of the record in which to make entries. Components of a source record are summarized in Table 7-2.

A disadvantage of source records is fragmented data. Information is well organized but not according to the client's problems. Details about a particular problem may be distributed throughout the record. For example, in the case of a wound infection, the nurse describes the appearance of the wound in the nurses' notes. The physician notes in a separate section the progress of the wound's healing and the proposed course of therapy. The results of tests measuring growth of bacteria from the wound can be found in the laboratory test section. Thus any data relevant to a single problem requires careful investigation to locate.

In the source record you chart a narrative description of nursing care delivered. In a hospital, entries are made in the client's record during each shift of duty. If a client is seen in a clinic or at home, you document the care provided during each visit or telephone contact, including a description that summarizes important observations relating to the client's condition, nursing care, and evaluation of response.

Charting by Exception

Charting by exception (CBE) is an innovative approach to reduce the time required to complete documentation. Standards of practice and predetermined criteria for nursing assessments and interventions are defined. You write a nar-

rative note *only* when the standardized statement on the form does not match the client's status (Short, 1997). Therefore when you see any entries in the chart, you know that something out of the ordinary has been observed. This makes it easier to track unexpected changes in a client's condition as they develop. This charting system helps eliminate repetition, decreases subjective data, and decreases documentation time (Cummins, 1999).

Focus Charting

Focus charting allows the documentation of any client situation rather than charting only problems and does not label client concerns as "problems." This allows for greater flexibility in client documentation. Focus charting includes a sign or symptom, a condition, a nursing diagnosis, a behavior, a significant event, or an acute change in a client's condition. Each entry includes **data, actions, and client response (DAR)** for the particular client situation.

Case Management Plan and Critical Pathways

The case management model of delivering care includes a multidisciplinary approach to documenting client care. The standardized plan of care is summarized into **critical pathways** (or care maps) within a **case management plan.** These standardized documents include one- to two-page care plans for the problems, key interventions, and expected outcomes for clients with a specific disease or condition (see Figure 6-5, p. 89). Multidisciplinary health care team members use the critical pathway to monitor the client's progress during client care, using one critical pathway as a monitoring and documentation tool. Critical pathways incorporated into documentation tools can be developed to eliminate other nursing forms and thus reduce duplication and the amount of charting (Lavin and Enright, 1996).

The critical pathways are used to direct and monitor the flow of client care. The critical pathways define client-focused outcomes and specify those interventions provided for each given day of care. Because of the nature of human response, there are **variances** in the client outcomes when the client deviates from the critical path plan. These variances refer to either positive or negative changes, depending on the clinical situation. A positive variance occurs when a client progresses more rapidly than the case management plan expected (e.g., a nasogastric tube may be discontinued a day early). A negative variance occurs when the activities on the clinical pathway are not completed as predicted or the client does not meet the expected outcomes. An example of a negative variance is the addition of oxygen therapy for a postoperative client experiencing breathing problems. Deviations from the case management plan can be classified into operational-, community-, practitioner-, or client-caused variances. Your responsibility is to determine why the problem arose and to implement changes to eliminate the variance or to justify the actions taken to manage the critical path deviation (Iyer and Camp, 1999).

COMMON RECORD-KEEPING FORMS

The client chart includes a variety of forms to make documentation easy, quick, and comprehensive. Duplication within the record should be avoided.

Admission Nursing History Forms

Admission nursing history forms provide baseline data for later comparisons with changes in the client's condition. The form allows the admitting nurse to make a thorough assessment (e.g., biographical data, holistic assessment, and review of health risk factors) and to identify relevant nursing diagnoses or problems for the client's care pathway. Each institution designs nursing history forms based on its standards of practice and philosophy of nursing care. Figure 7-2 is an example of an admission nursing history form.

Flow Sheets and Graphic Records

Flow sheets and **graphic records** allow documentation of certain routine observations or specific measurements made repeatedly, such as the bath, vital signs, pain assessment, and intake and output. Flow sheets provide a quick and easy reference for assessing changes in a client's status. Critical care units commonly use flow sheets for many types of data. The flow sheets are an effective way to record information so that you can observe trends over time. Flow sheets are part of the permanent record. Figure 7-3 is an example of a nursing flow sheet.

When a significant change is noted on a flow sheet, you describe this in the progress notes and describe nursing measures implemented in response to the change. For example, if a client's blood pressure becomes dangerously high, record in the progress note the blood pressure and the medication

administered to lower the pressure. Also include evaluation of the client's subsequent blood pressures and other pertinent interventions.

Client Education Record

Client teaching is an essential part of nursing interventions. Many hospitals have an education record that identifies clients' level of knowledge related to diagnosis, treatment, and medications. The goal of client and family education is to improve health outcomes by promoting healthy behavior and self-care and involving the client and/or family in care decisions. Education supports recovery and a rapid return to function (see Chapter 9). Standards for client education include assessment of needs, abilities, learning preferences, and readiness to learn. Based on this assessment, client education needs to include safe and effective use of medications, nutrition and diet modifications, safety and safe use of medical equipment, pain management, rehabilitation techniques to promote functional independence and self-care activities, and available resources (CAMH, 2000).

Client Care Summary or Kardex

Many hospitals now have computerized systems that provide certain basic information in the form of a client care summary. This is printed for each client during each shift. Data are automatically updated as orders are entered and as nursing decisions are made. In some settings a **Kardex** (flip-over card file) is kept at the nurses' station to make certain information for the daily care of a client readily accessible. It often has two parts: an activity and treatment section and a nursing care plan section. The updated information in the Kardex eliminates the need for you to refer repeatedly to the client's chart. Information commonly found in the Kardex or client care summary includes the following:

1. Basic demographic data (name, age, sex)
2. Primary medical diagnosis
3. Current physician's orders (e.g., diet, activity, vital signs)
4. A nursing care plan
5. Nursing orders or nursing interventions (e.g., intake and output, positioning, comfort measures, teaching)
6. Scheduled tests and procedures
7. Safety precautions used in the client's care
8. Factors related to activities of daily living
9. Nearest relative/guardian or person to contact in an emergency
10. Emergency code status
11. Allergies

Acuity Charting

Acuity charting provides a method of determining the hours of care and staff required for a given group of clients based on the type and number of nursing interventions required for each client. The acuity level determined by the nursing care allows clients to be rated in comparison with one another. For example, an acuity system might rate clients from 1 to 5 (1 requires the most time, 5 requires the least amount of time). A client returning from surgery with many assess-

Ashland Community Hospital

ADMIT FORM

Part I: Admission Routine

Date _____ Time _____ Temp. _____ Pulse _____ Resp. _____

Mode ☐ amb. ☐ gurney ☐ wc ☐ other _____ B/P _____

Via ☐ admitting ☐ ER ☐ other _____ Height _____ Actual Weight _____

Admitting Physician: _____ Family Physician: _____

Admitting Diagnosis: _____

Most Recent Adm. (hosp./date/reason) _____

Patient's Statement (of present complaint) _____

Allergies: _____
Type of Reaction _____

Medications Patient's significant other understands purpose ☐ yes ☐ no   Disposition of meds:

Medication and strength	freq.	time last dose		Medication and strength		
1.				6.		☐ did not bring
2.				7.		☐ patient has
3.				8.		☐ family has
4.				9.		☐ pharmacy
5.				10.		

Valuables List: (jewelry, clothing, etc.) _____

☐ glasses   ☐ contact lenses   ☐ dentures—   ☐ bridge/partial   ☐ other

Oriented to   ☐ room   ☐ bed   ☐ phone   ☐ call light/TV   ☐ visiting hours   ☐ safety/smoking policy
☐ doctor's orders   ☐ armband

Part II: Patient/Family History

Patient History (major illnesses/operations/major injuries) include endocrine history/problems—past pregnancies

1	4	7
2	5	8
3	6	9

Use of tobacco ☐ no ☐ yes   Type _____ Daily amount _____

Use of alcohol ☐ no ☐ yes   Type _____ Daily amount _____

Organ donor ☐ no ☐ yes   Living will ☐ no ☐ yes   If yes, copy at ACH ☐ no ☐ yes

Other pertinent information:

Family History ☐ heart disease ☐ stroke ☐ hypertension ☐ asthma ☐ TB ☐ diabetes ☐ cancer
☐ kidney disease ☐ allergy ☐ epilepsy ☐ blood disorder ☐ mental disorder ☐ other

Socio/Economic   Religion: _____   Marital status: ☐ single ☐ married ☐ divorced ☐ widowed

Family ☐ lives with ☐ lives alone ☐ no family ☐ house ☐ apt. ☐ other
Lives in

Occupation _____   ☐ full time ☐ part time ☐ retired ☐ other

ADL ☐ independent ☐ needs assist with (specify what kind of help is needed and who provides it)

Anticipated Discharge Needs: ☐ self care ☐ community agency ☐ discharge planner ☐ other

Comments/plan: _____

Notify in emergency: _____ relation _____ phone _____

Nearest relative: _____ relation _____ phone _____

Info obtained from ☐ patient ☐ family ☐ other   Admitting Nurse: _____

ACH 144

Part III: System Assessment

Place an "X" in area of abnormality. If unable to assess, indicate reason.

Assess eyes, ears, nose, throat for abnormality.

| E E N T | impaired vision | blind | pain | reddened | drainage | gums | (other) ☐ No problem |
| | hard of hearing | deaf | burning | edema | lesion | teeth | |

Explain: _____

Assess chest configuration, resp. rate, rhythm, depth, pattern, breath sounds, comfort.

R E S P	asymmetric	tachypnea	apnea	rales	cough	absent	(other) ☐ No problem
	barrel-chest	bradypnea	shallow	rhonchi	sputum	diminished	
	dyspnea	orthopnea	labored	wheezing	pain	cyanotic	

Explain: _____

Assess heart sounds, rate rhythm, pulse, blood pressure, circulation, fluid retention, comfort.

C V	arrhythmia	rub	numbness	dimin. pulses	edema	(other) ☐ No problem
	irregular	bradycardia	murmur	tingling	absent pulses		
	pain	S₁ or S₂	fatigue				

Explain: _____

Assess weight, abdomen, bowel habits, swallowing, bowel sounds, comfort.
Home diet/food habits/caffeine amount—

| G I | weight loss | N or V | anorexia | diarrhea | distention | hypoactive BS | mass | (other) ☐ No problem |
| | obese | thirst | dysphagic | constipation | rigidity | hyperactive BS | pain | |

Explain: _____ stool color _____

Assess urine freq., control, color, consistency, odor, comfort/Gyn—bleeding, discharge, pregnancy.
Birth control method _____ last menses _____ last Pap smear _____

| G U and G Y N | pain | hesitancy | oliguria | dysuria | urine color | vaginal bleeding | circumcised | (other) ☐ No problem |
| | frequency | incontinent | nocturia | hematuria | discharge | pregnancy | æ circumcised | |

Explain: _____

Assess motor function, sensation, LOC, strength, grip, gait, coordination, orientation, speech, vision.

N E U R O	weakness	numbness	headache	paralysis	stuporous	pupils	(other) ☐ No problem
	unsteady	tingling	seizures	lethargic	comatose	speech	
	vertigo	pain	tremors	confused	vision	grip	

Explain: _____

Assess mobility, motion, gait, alignment, joint function/Skin color, texture, turgor, integrity.

M S and S K I N	appliance	stiffness	itching	petechiae	hot	drainage	(other) ☐ No problem
	prosthesis	swelling	lesion	poor turgor	cool		
	deformity	wound	rash	skin color	flushed		
	atrophy	pain	ecchymosis	diaphoretic	moist		

Explain: _____

Date: _____ Time: _____ R.N. Signature: _____

FIGURE **7-2**   Admission nursing history form. (Courtesy Ashland Community Hospital, Ashland, Ore.)

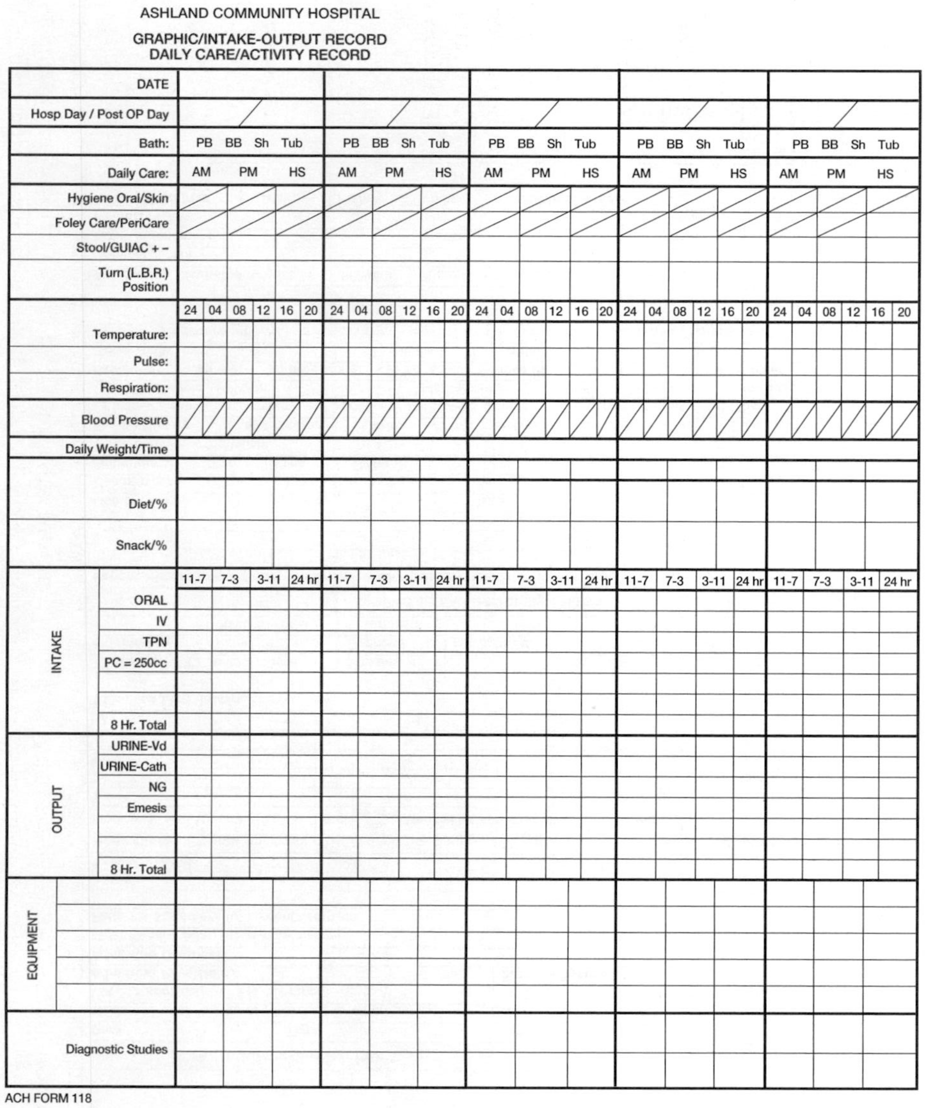

ASHLAND COMMUNITY HOSPITAL
GRAPHIC/INTAKE-OUTPUT RECORD
DAILY CARE/ACTIVITY RECORD

DATE
Hosp Day / Post OP Day
Bath: PB BB Sh Tub
Daily Care: AM PM HS
Hygiene Oral/Skin
Foley Care/PeriCare
Stool/GUIAC + −
Turn (L.B.R.) Position
24 04 08 12 16 20
Temperature:
Pulse:
Respiration:
Blood Pressure
Daily Weight/Time
Diet/%
Snack/%
11-7 7-3 3-11 24 hr
INTAKE: ORAL, IV, TPN, PC = 250cc, 8 Hr. Total
OUTPUT: URINE-Vd, URINE-Cath, NG, Emesis, 8 Hr. Total
EQUIPMENT
Diagnostic Studies
ACH FORM 118

FIGURE 7-3 Nursing assessment flow sheet. (Courtesy Ashland Community Hospital, Ashland, Ore.)

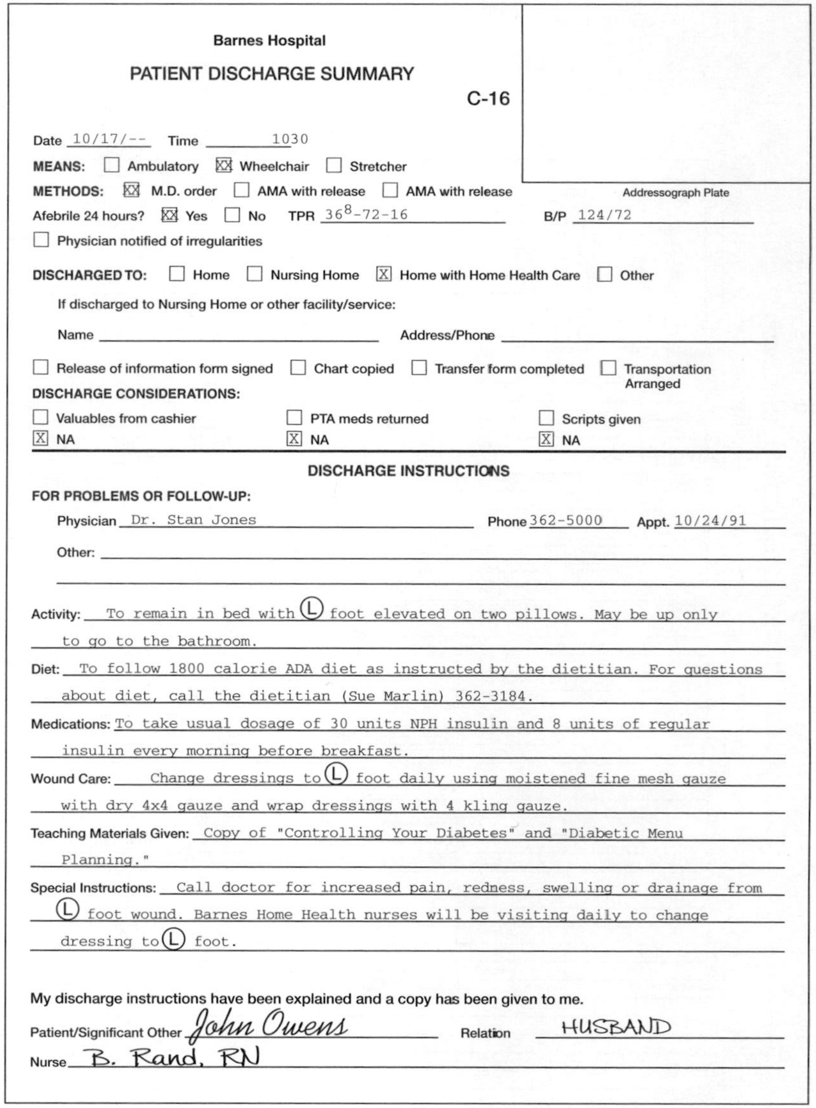

Barnes Hospital
PATIENT DISCHARGE SUMMARY
C-16

Addressograph Plate

Date 10/17/-- Time 1030
MEANS: ☐ Ambulatory ☒ Wheelchair ☐ Stretcher
METHODS: ☒ M.D. order ☐ AMA with release ☐ AMA with release
Afebrile 24 hours? ☒ Yes ☐ No TPR 36⁸-72-16 B/P 124/72
☐ Physician notified of irregularities
DISCHARGED TO: ☐ Home ☐ Nursing Home ☒ Home with Home Health Care ☐ Other
If discharged to Nursing Home or other facility/service:
Name ______ Address/Phone ______
☐ Release of information form signed ☐ Chart copied ☐ Transfer form completed ☐ Transportation Arranged
DISCHARGE CONSIDERATIONS:
☐ Valuables from cashier ☒ NA
☐ PTA meds returned ☒ NA
☐ Scripts given ☒ NA

DISCHARGE INSTRUCTIONS
FOR PROBLEMS OR FOLLOW-UP:
Physician Dr. Stan Jones Phone 362-5000 Appt. 10/24/91
Other:

Activity: To remain in bed with Ⓛ foot elevated on two pillows. May be up only to go to the bathroom.
Diet: To follow 1800 calorie ADA diet as instructed by the dietitian. For questions about diet, call the dietitian (Sue Marlin) 362-3184.
Medications: To take usual dosage of 30 units NPH insulin and 8 units of regular insulin every morning before breakfast.
Wound Care: Change dressings to Ⓛ foot daily using moistened fine mesh gauze with dry 4x4 gauze and wrap dressings with 4 kling gauze.
Teaching Materials Given: Copy of "Controlling Your Diabetes" and "Diabetic Menu Planning."
Special Instructions: Call doctor for increased pain, redness, swelling or drainage from Ⓛ foot wound. Barnes Home Health nurses will be visiting daily to change dressing to Ⓛ foot.

My discharge instructions have been explained and a copy has been given to me.
Patient/Significant Other John Owens Relation HUSBAND
Nurse B. Rand, RN

FIGURE 7-4 Discharge summary form. (Courtesy Barnes-Jewish Hospital, St. Louis.)

ments and interventions is rated as an acuity level 1. On the same continuum, another client awaiting discharge after a very successful recovery from surgery is rated as an acuity level 5. Staffing patterns can then be determined by examining the total acuity points of the clients on a particular nursing unit.

Standardized Care Plans

Some institutions use **standardized care plans** to make documentation more efficient. The plans, based on the institution's standards of nursing practice, are preprinted established guidelines used to care for clients with similar health problems. After you complete a nursing assessment, the appropriate standard care plans are placed in your client's record. It is very important that you make necessary modifications to individualize the nursing plan of care. Most standardized plans also allow the addition of specific desired outcomes and the dates when these outcomes should be achieved (see Chapter 6).

Discharge Summary Forms

Much emphasis is placed on preparing a client for a timely discharge from a health care institution (Ebert and Bethel, 1996). Ideally you begin discharge planning on admission and in some cases even before admission, as is necessary with same-day surgery admissions and childbirth. When doing discharge planning, you need to be responsive to changes in the client's condition and to involve clients and family in the discharge planning process (see Chapter 2).

A discharge summary provides important information pertaining to the client's unresolved problems and continued health care after discharge (Anthony and Hudson-Barr, 1998). You will need to include the reason for hospitalization, significant findings, client's status, and any specific teaching plan that is given to the client and/or family (JCAHO, 1999). Discharge summary forms (Figure 7-4) make the summary concise and instructive. Many forms include copies that you give to the client, family members, or home care nurses. Home care agencies or extended nursing care facilities can also benefit from receiving information on the summary forms (Box 7-2) to enhance continuity of care.

COMPUTERIZED DOCUMENTATION

The technology that exists is virtually unlimited, and the future holds incredible potential for computerization in the health care delivery system. There are many benefits to computerized documentation. Documentation systems that are now available minimize repetitive clerical and monitoring tasks and increase your time available for direct client care. Software programs allow access to specific assessment data quickly, and the information can be automatically transferred to different reports. Computers also help you reduce errors (e.g., better legibility than handwritten notations), standardize nursing care plans, increase your job satisfaction and productivity, and document all facets of client care (Eggland, 1997). Another benefit of computerized documentation is the enhancement of quality improvement activities.

Computerized documentation will potentially change drastically with the increased use of new technology. Therefore in the future, nursing will potentially use either pen-based or voice recognition computers in documentation. A notebook-sized computer with handwriting recognition capabilities would allow documentation with an ease and flexibility not possible in the current systems.

Another form of computerized documentation is a complete **computer-based client record (CCR)**. The CCR is a comprehensive system that utilizes many components of data collection and has a much broader scope than current charting systems. You must know the legal risks of computerized documentation. Confidentiality issues must be addressed because there is an increased risk of access to information by unauthorized individuals. Consequently, the American Nurses Association, the American Medical Record Association, and the Canadian Nurses Association developed guidelines for safe computer charting:

1. The password that is used to enter and sign off computer files should not be shared with another caregiver. A good system requires frequent changes in personal passwords to prevent unauthorized persons from accessing and tampering with records (Eggland, 1997).
2. Avoid leaving the computer terminal unattended after being logged on.
3. Follow the correct protocol for correcting errors according to agency policy.
4. Software systems have a system for backup files. If you inadvertently delete part of the permanent record, follow agency policy. It may be necessary to type an explanation into the computer file with the date, time, and your initials and to submit an explanation in writing to your manager (Smith, 2000).
5. Avoid leaving information about a client displayed on a monitor where others may see it. Keep a log that accounts for every copy of a computerized file that you have generated from the system.
6. Follow the agency's confidentiality procedures for documenting sensitive material, such as a diagnosis of HIV infection.
7. Printouts of computerized records should be protected. Shredding of printouts and the logging of the number of copies generated by each caregiver are ways to minimize duplicate records and protect the confidentiality of client information.

HOME CARE DOCUMENTATION

Home care continues to grow as increasing numbers of older adults use home care services. Medicare has specific guidelines for establishing eligibility for home care reimbursement. Documentation in the home care system has different implications than in other areas of nursing. The documentation is both the quality control and the justification for reimbursement from Medicare, Medicaid, or private insurance companies. You must document all of your services for payment (e.g., direct skilled care, client instructions, skilled observation, and evaluation visits) (JCAHO, 1999).

LONG-TERM CARE DOCUMENTATION

Increasing numbers of older adults and disabled people in the United States are requiring care in long-term health care facilities. Nursing personnel often face challenges much different from those in the acute care setting. Changes in the Medicare program in the form of the prospective payment system (PPS) determine the standards and policies for reimbursement and documentation in long-term health care (Boroughs, 1999).

Each resident in long-term care is assessed by using the Resident Assessment Instrument, an eight-page tool, mandated by the Omnibus Budget Reconciliation Act of 1989 (OBRA). Documentation supports a multidisciplinary approach to the assessment and planning process for clients. Communication among nurses, social workers, recreational therapists, and dietitians is essential in the regulated documentation process. The fiscal support for long-term care residents hinges on the justification of nursing care as demonstrated in sound documentation of the services rendered. The ultimate goal is to provide the highest quality care at the lowest cost per resident (Boroughs, 1999).

REPORTING

Reports provide a summary of activities or observations seen, performed, or heard that are exchanged among health care team members. For example, after completing a work shift, you give a verbal report to nurses on the next shift and the laboratory submits written reports describing the results of diagnostic tests for inclusion in the permanent medical record.

Change-of-Shift Report

The **change-of-shift report** occurs at least twice a day in all types of nursing units. At the end of each shift, information about your assigned clients is given to nurses working on the next shift. The purpose of the report is to provide better continuity and individualized care for clients. For example, if you find that a certain position increases a client's breathing, you relay that information to the next nurse caring for the client.

Change-of-shift reports are given orally in person, by audiotape recordings, or during rounds at the client's bedside. Oral reports are given in person, with staff members from both shifts participating. Audiotaped reports may be done before the end of the shift, which can increase efficiency and minimize social interactions. An opportunity for a last-minute update on events that occur after taping and for clarification when there are questions is essential. Reports given in person or during rounds allow you to obtain immediate feedback when questions are raised about a client's care. When you make rounds, the client and family members also have the opportunity to participate in any decisions.

The change-of-shift report should be given quickly and efficiently. A good report provides a baseline for comparisons and indicates the kind of care to be anticipated for the next shift. An organized and concise approach helps you set goals and anticipate client needs and lessens the chance of important information being overlooked. A sample format is as follows: background information (name, age, medical diagnosis), primary health problem, nursing diagnoses, observations of the client's condition and response to therapies, progress with teaching, interventions, and family involvement. It is especially important to report any recent changes or priority situations concerning the client's condition.

When giving a report, you must maintain a professional manner. Describe interactions in objective terms, avoiding such judgmental labels as "uncooperative," "difficult," or "bad" when describing client behaviors. This kind of language can contribute to prejudicial opinions about the client. Judgmental statements overheard by the client or family could also lead to legal charges.

Telephone Reports and Orders

TELEPHONE ORDERS.   When significant events or changes in a client's condition have occurred, a telephone report needs to include clear, accurate, and concise information. When documenting the phone call, include when the call was made, who made it (if you did not make the call), who was called, to whom information was given, what information was given, and what information was received (Figure 7-5). An example follows: "Laboratory technician J. Ignacio, reported a potassium level of 5.9. Dr. Wade notified at 2030. D. Markle, RN."

TELEPHONE ORDERS (TOS) AND VERBAL ORDERS (VOS).   A telephone order involves a physician's stating a prescribed therapy over the phone to a registered nurse, and verbal orders are stated by the physician and written by the nurse. Telephone and verbal orders are frequently given at night or during an emergency. It is important to verify the order by repeating it clearly. Clarification may be needed. Then the order is written on the physician's order sheet in the client's permanent record and signatures are included. An example follows: "10/16/96: 0815, Tylenol #3 tabs 2 q6 hours for incisional pain. T.O. Dr. Knight/J. Woods, RN." The physician later verifies the telephone or verbal order legally by signing it within a set time (e.g., 24 hours) as stipulated by hospital policy. Telephone and verbal orders should be used only when absolutely necessary and not for the sake of

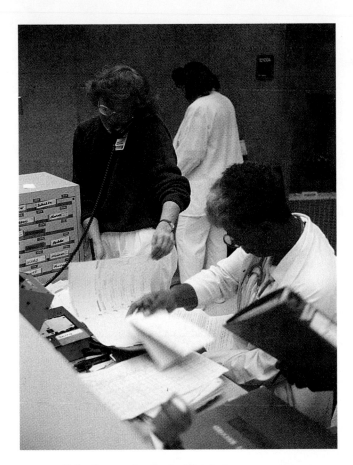

FIGURE **7-5** Persons involved with telephone reports must verify that information is accurate.

be given by phone or in person. When giving a transfer report, the following information is included:

1. Client's name, age, primary physician, and medical diagnosis
2. Summary of medical progress up to the time of transfer
3. Current health status (physical and psychosocial)
4. Allergies
5. Emergency code status
6. Family support
7. Current nursing diagnoses or problems and care plan
8. Any critical assessments or interventions to be completed shortly after transfer (helps receiving nurse to establish priorities of care)
9. Need for any special equipment

At the completion of the transfer report, the receiving nurse may clarify information by asking questions about the client's status.

Incident Reports

An incident is any event not consistent with the routine operation of a health care unit or routine care of a client. Examples include client falls, needle-stick injuries, a visitor becoming ill, and medication errors. An **incident report** is filed when there is an actual or potential injury and is not a part of the patient record. Therefore an objective description of what was observed and follow-up actions taken are documented in the client's medical record without reference to the existence of the incident report (see Chapter 3).

convenience. Box 7-3 provides guidelines that promote accuracy when receiving telephone orders.

Transfer Reports

Clients may be transferred from one unit to another or to another facility to receive different levels of care. For example, clients transfer from intensive care units to general nursing units when the level of care no longer requires intense monitoring. A **transfer report** involves communication of information about clients from the nurse on the sending unit to the nurse on the receiving unit. Transfer reports may

Key Terms

accreditation, *p. 101*
acuity charting, *p. 106*
case management plan, *p. 105*
change-of-shift report, *p. 110*
charting by exception (CBE), *p. 105*
computer-based client record (CCR), *p. 108*
critical pathways, *p. 105*

DAR (data, action, client response), *p. 105*
diagnosis-related groups (DRGs), *p. 101*
documentation, *p. 101*
flow sheets, *p. 106*
focus charting, *p. 105*
graphic records, *p. 106*
incident report, *p. 111*
Kardex, *p. 106*

PIE note, *p. 104*
problem-oriented medical record (POMR), *p. 104*
record, *p. 101*
reports, *p. 101*
SOAP note, *p. 104*
source record, *p. 105*
standardized care plans, *p. 108*
transfer report, *p. 111*
variances, *p. 106*

Key Concepts

- A client's health care record is written legal documentation of the care received.
- All information pertaining to a client's health care management is confidential.
- The medical record is a client's bill or financial record that serves as the basis for reimbursement to health care agencies.
- Your signature on an entry in a record designates accountability for the contents of that entry.
- Accurate record keeping requires an objective interpretation of data with precise measurements, correct spelling, and proper use of abbreviations.
- Document changes in a client's condition to keep a record current.
- Problem-oriented medical records are organized by the client's health care problems.
- Critical pathways are instrumental in the evolving documentation methods that focus on client outcomes.
- There are a variety of record-keeping forms used in client documentation (e.g., admission nursing history forms, flow sheets).
- Medicare guidelines for establishing a client's home care reimbursement are the basis for documentation by home health nurses.
- Long-term care documentation is multidisciplinary and closely linked with fiscal requirements of outside agencies.
- Computerized information systems provide information about clients in an organized and easily accessible fashion.
- The major purpose of the change-of-shift report is to maintain continuity of care.
- When information pertinent to care is communicated by telephone, the information must be verified.
- Incident reports objectively describe any event not consistent with the routine care of a client.

Critical Thinking Activities

1. Observe a change-of-shift report at a health care facility, and using the chapter discussion and the guidelines in Box 7-1, critique the effectiveness of the exchange.
2. Compare and contrast the content of the following formats: charting by exception, narrative documentation, focus charting, and SOAP charting. Identify the advantages of each.
3. Separate information from a client interview into objective and subjective data.
4. Attend a discharge planning conference to find out how each of the following members of the health care team is involved in discharge planning: nurse, social worker, dietitian, physician, and physical therapist.

Review Questions

1. An advantage of charting by exception (CBE) is that:
   1. entries follow the format of the nursing process.
   2. it originated from a nursing model rather than a medical model.
   3. it moves away from charting only problems, allowing greater flexibility.
   4. it is easy to track unexpected changes because detailed descriptions are used only when standard criteria do not match the client status.
2. Critical pathways define client-focused outcomes. Benefits of critical pathways include identification of variances that communicate:
   1. achievement of expected outcomes.
   2. trends for implementing an action plan in response to identified problems.
   3. use of clear, concise descriptions using the client's own language to identify problems.
   4. description of changes that occur when the client does not meet or exceeds expected outcomes.
3. When comparing documentation for acute care in hospitals with documentation for long-term care, major differences are related to:
   1. the goal of the highest quality care at the lowest cost.
   2. using a multidisciplinary approach for assessment and planning.
   3. the prospective payment system determining the standards for reimbursement.
   4. increasing numbers of older adults and disabled people in the United States requiring long-term care.
4. When giving a change-of-shift report, you are expected to:
   1. include community resources that the client can contact.
   2. include a step-by-step description of how to perform procedures.
   3. provide an organized and concise description of client status and anticipated needs.
   4. review signs and symptoms of complications that should be reported to the physician.
5. When you receive telephone orders from a physician, it is common for agencies to require you to:
   1. make a photocopy of the order to avoid errors.
   2. repeat prescribed orders back to the physician to verify accuracy.
   3. delay implementation of telephone orders until they have been verified.
   4. include a description of the reason the telephone order was needed, using concise, objective terms.
6. Incident reports are an important part of quality improvement programs. The intended goal of incident reports is:
   1. to provide information in the medical record.
   2. to reprimand individuals involved in the incident.
   3. to identify changes needed to prevent reoccurrences.
   4. to document actual injury and follow-up actions taken.

7. A nurse makes the following documentation in the client record: "0830 Client appears to be in severe pain and refuses to ambulate. Blood pressure and pulse are elevated. Physician notified and analgesic administered as ordered with adequate relief. J. Doe, RN." The most significant statement about the documentation would be that it is:
   1. inadequate because the pain is not described on a scale of 1 to 10.
   2. good because it shows immediate responsiveness to the problem.
   3. acceptable because it includes assessment, intervention, and evaluation.
   4. unacceptable because it is vague subjective data without supportive data.

8. Documentation of assessment of a client recovering from surgery included the following information: complete bath, level of pain is 6 (scale 0 to 10), turning in bed with assist of one, and dressing clean, dry, and intact. The least appropriate information is:
   1. complete bath.
   2. level of pain is 6 (scale 0 to 10).
   3. turning in bed with assist of one.
   4. dressing clean, dry, and intact.

9. A nurse documents an assessment completed at 1700. In civilian time this is:
   1. 9 PM.
   2. 6 PM.
   3. 5 PM.
   4. 7 PM.

10. A client is nauseated and vomits three times after breakfast. You give medication that the doctor ordered when you called to report the change in status. The medication relieves the nausea. The first data to appear in this documentation should be:
    1. physician orders.
    2. change in status.
    3. time of breakfast.
    4. medication given.

11. The best description of narrative documentation is that it:
    1. organizes data by problem or diagnosis.
    2. describes occurrences in chronological order.
    3. includes subjective data, objective data, assessment, and plan.
    4. originated from the medical model.

12. A nurse's assessment includes the following data. The information that is objective data is:
    1. information about educational and cultural influences.
    2. a description of joint mobility based on the client's report.
    3. assessment of breath sounds, coughing, and respiratory rate.
    4. a description of pain including onset, intensity, and precipitating factors.

References

Anthony MK, Hudson-Barr DC: Successful client discharge: a comprehensive model of facilitators and barriers, *J Nurs Adm* 28(3):48, 1998.

Boroughs DS: Documentation in the long-term care setting, *J Nurs Adm* 29(12):46, 1999.

Cummins KM: Charting by exception, a timely format for you? *Am J Nurs* 99(3):24G, 1999.

Ebert V, Bethel S: Mission accomplished: a system for discharge planning, *Nurs Manage* 27(8):27, 1996.

Eggland ET: Using computers to document, *Nursing* 27(1):17, 1997.

Health insurance portability and accountability act of 1996, 64 *Federal Register* 60053 (1999).

Iyer P, Camp NH: Nursing documentation: a nursing process approach, St. Louis, 1999, Mosby.

Joint Commission on Accreditation of Healthcare Organizations: *Comprehensive accreditation manual for hospitals (CAMH)*, update 3, Chicago, 2000, The Commission.

Joint Commission on Accreditation of Healthcare Organizations, *Standards for the accreditation of health care organizations*, Chicago, 1999, The Commission.

Ladebauche P: Limiting liability to avoid malpractice litigation, *MCN Am J Matern Child Nurs* 20(5):243, 1995.

Lavin J, Enright B: Charting with managed care in mind, *RN* 59(8):47, 1996.

Omnibus Budget Reconciliation Act of 1989, Pub L No. 101-239, 103 Stat 2106.

Phillips DM: JCAHO pain management standards are unveiled, *JAMA* 284(4):428, 2000.

Platt A, Reed B: Meet new pain standard with new technology: documentation takes a leap into the palm of your hand, *Nurs Manage* 32(3):40, 2001.

Short MS: Charting by exception on a clinical pathway, *Nurs Manage* 28(8):45, 1997.

Smith LS: Safe computer charting, *Nursing* 30(9):85, 2000.

8

Communication

Objectives

- Define the key terms listed.
- Identify situations that require careful communication decision making.
- Describe the elements of the communication process.
- Describe the three levels of communication and their uses in nursing.
- Differentiate aspects of verbal and nonverbal communication.
- Identify features and expected outcomes of the nurse-client helping relationship.
- List nursing focus areas within each phase of a therapeutic nurse-client helping relationship.
- Describe behaviors and techniques that affect communication.
- Explain the focus of communication within each phase of the nursing process.
- Discuss effective communication for clients of varying developmental levels.
- Identify client health states or responses that contribute to impaired communication.
- Explain techniques used to assist clients with special communication needs.

*C*ommunication is the process of transmitting messages and interpreting meaning (Wilson and others, 1995). As an important nursing skill, communication competency is acquired through study and application. Caring relationships are the heart of nurses' work. Watson (1985) identified the "carative factors" that demonstrate human-to-human caring. These factors are instilling faith and hope, cultivating sensitivity to self and to others, developing a helping-trust relationship, promoting and accepting the expression of positive and negative feelings, using scientific problem solving for decision making, promoting interpersonal teaching-learning, providing a supportive environment, assisting with gratification of human needs, and allowing for spiritual forces and phenomena. These aspects of caring within interpersonal relationships are intimately connected to your ability to communicate effectively.

You will use nonverbal, verbal, and technological skills to communicate in both personal and impersonal situations. You send and receive information through many different channels, including in person, in writing, over the telephone, through fax and electronic mail, and through the Internet. Communication in all these modes is an ongoing, dynamic, and often complex process.

THE POWER OF COMMUNICATION

Like any therapeutic agent, communication can result in both harm and good. Every nuance of your posture, each small expression and gesture, every word you choose, and every phrase uttered can hurt or heal through the messages they send. Even techniques meant to be therapeutic can have unexpected negative effects, yet nontherapeutic techniques can at times bring comfort and achieve goals. Failure to communicate leads to serious problems, increases liability, and threatens professional credibility. Inappropriate or missing communication can cause "glitches" in the health care system with added cost to the client and agency. Communication must be respected for its potential power and not misused to manipulate, bully, or coerce others. At its best, good communication empowers others and enables people to know themselves and to make their own choices (Beebe and others, 1996). As you grow in self-awareness and learn from situations that did not go as well as you had planned, you can celebrate the joy of being part of helping relationships. Rowe (1999) suggests keeping a journal in which you can learn from reflection. Describe a difficult event and the client's reaction to you. Reflect on and write lessons learned to help in similar situations. The good news is this is a lifelong learning process.

DECISION MAKING AND COMMUNICATION

As a nurse you constantly make decisions about what, when, where, why, and how to convey messages to others. Deciding which techniques best fit each unique nursing scenario is challenging. Notice that examples are provided to guide you.

Challenging Communication Situations   Box 8-1

The *silent, withdrawn* person who does not express any feelings or needs

The *sad, depressed* person who has slow mental and motor responses

The *angry, hostile* person who does not listen to explanations

The *sullen, uncooperative* person who resents being asked to do something

The *talkative, lonely* person who wants someone with him or her all the time

The *demanding* person who wants someone to wait on him or her or meet his or her requests

The *ranting and raving* person who blames nursing staff unfairly

The *sensory impaired* person who cannot hear or see well

The *verbally impaired* person who cannot articulate words

The *gossiping, catty* person who violates confidentiality and stirs up trouble

The *bitter, complaining* person who is negative about everything

The *mentally handicapped* person who is frightened and distrustful

The *confused, disoriented* person who is bewildered and uncooperative

The *anxious, nervous* person who cannot cope with what is happening

The *grieving, crying* person who has had a major loss

The *unresponsive, comatose* person who cannot communicate at all

Situations that challenge your decision-making skills and call for careful use of therapeutic techniques often involve persons such as those described in Box 8-1. Practice helps! Take the initiative to discuss and role play these scenarios before encountering them in the clinical setting.

BASIC ELEMENTS OF THE COMMUNICATION PROCESS

Examine Figure 8-1, the basic elements of the communication process. Although this model oversimplifies, it helps you identify essential components. People in conversation rarely analyze the meaning of every gesture or word. In your professional role you will learn to pay attention to each aspect so that interactions can be purposeful and effective.

The **referent** motivates one person to communicate with another. In a health care environment, sights, sounds, odors, time schedules, messages, objects, emotions, sensations, perceptions, ideas, and other cues initiate communication. Considering the referent during an interaction helps the sender develop and organize the message.

The **sender** is the person who delivers the message. The roles of sender and receiver change back and forth as two persons interact.

The **message** is the verbal and nonverbal information expressed by the sender. The most effective message is clear, organized, and expressed in a manner familiar to the receiver.

The **channel** is the means of conveying and receiving the message through visual, auditory, and tactile senses. The sender's facial expression conveys a visual message, spoken

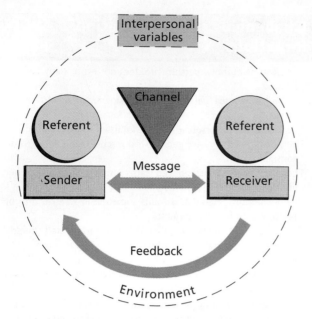

FIGURE **8-1**   Communication as active process between sender and receiver.

words travel through auditory channels, and placing a hand on another person uses the channel of touch. Usually, the more channels the sender uses to convey a message, the more clearly it will be received.

The **receiver** is the person to whom the message is sent. The message then acts as one of the receiver's referents, prompting a response. The more the sender and receiver have in common and the closer the relationship, the more likely the receiver will accurately perceive the sender's meaning and respond appropriately.

The **environment** is the physical and emotional climate in which the interaction takes place. For effective communication, the environment should be comfortable and suited to participants' needs. The more positive an environment the sender and receiver can create, the more successful the exchange.

The **feedback** is the message returned to the original sender by the receiver. Feedback indicates whether the meaning of the sender's message was understood. Your positive intent is not enough to ensure accurate reception of a message. Seek verbal and nonverbal feedback from the receiver to be sure the message has been understood.

Levels of Communication

There are three levels of communication, each with important uses in nursing. **Intrapersonal communication** is a powerful form of communication within an individual. Intrapersonal communication is also called *self-talk, self-verbalization,* and *inner thought* (Balzer Riley, 2000). People "talk to themselves" by forming thoughts internally that strongly influence perceptions, feelings, behavior, and self-concept. Be aware of the nature and content of your thinking and try to replace negative, self-defeating thoughts with positive assertions. Positive self-talk can be used as a tool to

improve health and self-esteem. In forms such as imagery or meditation, it can be used to enhance coping and reduce stress. Self-instruction can provide a mental rehearsal for difficult tasks or situations so individuals can deal with them more effectively. During interactions, participants engage in both intrapersonal and interpersonal or public communication.

Interpersonal communication is interaction that occurs between two people or within a small group. It refers to nonverbal and verbal behavior within a social context and includes symbols and cues used to give and receive meaning. Because messages received may be different from messages intended, meaning must be validated, or mutually negotiated, between participants. Effective interpersonal communication includes idea sharing, problem solving, expression of feelings, decision making, goal accomplishment, team building, and personal growth.

Public communication is the interaction of one individual with large groups of people. You will have opportunities to speak with groups of clients or consumers about health-related topics. Consider special adaptations in eye contact, posture, gestures, voice inflection, and use of media materials to communicate messages effectively.

■ FORMS OF COMMUNICATION

Messages are conveyed verbally and nonverbally, concretely, and symbolically. People express themselves through language, movements, gestures, voice inflection, facial expressions, and use of space. Many forms of communication merge to create meaning in the sender's message.

Verbal Communication

Verbal communication involves the spoken or written word. Verbal **language** is a code that conveys specific meaning as words are combined. The most important aspects of verbal communication are discussed in the following sections.

VOCABULARY.   Communication is unsuccessful if the receiver cannot translate the sender's words and phrases. You work with persons of various cultures who speak different languages. Those who speak your language may use subcultural variations of words (e.g., *dinner* may mean a midday meal or the last meal of the day). Medical jargon may sound like a foreign language. Children may use special words to describe bodily functions or a favorite blanket or toy. Adolescents often use words in unique ways that are unfamiliar to adults.

DENOTATIVE AND CONNOTATIVE MEANING.   A single word can have several meanings. The **denotative meaning** is shared by individuals who use a common language. The word *baseball* has the same meaning for all individuals who speak English, but the word *code* denotes cardiac arrest primarily to health care providers. The **connotative meaning** is the shade or interpretation of a word's meaning influenced by the thoughts, feelings, or ideas people have about the word. Families who are told a loved one is in serious condition may believe that death is near, but to nurses the term *serious* may simply describe the nature of the illness.

PACING.   Talking rapidly, using awkward pauses, or speaking slowly and deliberately can convey an unintended message. Consider the following exchange:

> Client: "Do you know if the doctor found anything wrong?"
> Nurse: "No . . . but I'm sure if he did . . . he would have come to explain things to you. (then very rapidly) Now let's get back to where we were."

Long pauses and rapid shift to another subject may give the impression that you are hiding the truth. Speak slowly enough to enunciate clearly, and use pauses to accentuate or stress a particular point to give the listener time to understand.

INTONATION.   Tone of voice dramatically affects a message's meaning, and emotions directly influence tone of voice. A simple question or statement can express enthusiasm, anger, or concern. Be aware of your intonation to avoid sending unintended messages. If the client interprets your message as uncaring or condescending, further communication may be inhibited. Pay attention to a client's intonation for information about his or her emotional state or energy level.

CLARITY AND BREVITY.   Effective communication is simple, short, and to the point to minimize confusion. Avoid phrases such as "you know" or "OK?" at the end of every sentence. Give examples to clarify messages for the receiver. Use short sentences and words that express an idea simply and directly.

TIMING AND RELEVANCE.   Timing is critical in communication. Even if a message is clear, poor timing can prevent it from being effective. Do not begin routine teaching when a client is in severe pain or emotional distress. The best time for interaction is when a client expresses an interest in communicating. Relevant messages are more effective. When a client is facing emergency surgery, discussing the risks of smoking is less relevant than explaining perioperative procedures.

Nonverbal Communication

Nonverbal communication includes messages sent through the language of the body, without using words. Nonverbal forms of communication include facial expressions; vocal cues; eye contact; gestures; posture; touch; odor; physical appearance; dress; silence; and the use of space, time, and objects (Yerby and others, 1995). Nonverbal communication often accurately reveals true feelings, because one has less control over nonverbal reactions. A client who says he feels fine but grimaces with each movement and holds his body rigidly is probably in pain. Nonverbal cues add meaning to verbal communication and help you judge the reliability of verbal messages.

Because nonverbal messages are usually more subtle than verbal messages, practice to become an astute observer of nonverbal behavior. Try to be sure your nonverbal and verbal messages match. If you say a client is getting better but wear an expression of doubt, you will not relieve the client's anxiety.

Metacommunication is the deeper "message within a message." It conveys the sender's attitude toward self and the message, as well as attitudes, feelings, and intentions toward the receiver. Metacommunication can be an explicit statement or an implicit, nonverbal demonstration of feelings. The client who has had facial reconstructive surgery tells you, "This scar doesn't look as bad as I thought it would," but is teary and appears apprehensive. In this case, you explore further the client's feelings and concerns.

PERSONAL APPEARANCE.   Physical characteristics, manner of dress and grooming, and jewelry are indicators of well-being, personality, social status, occupation, religion, culture, and self-concept. First impressions are largely based on appearance, and your physical appearance influences the client's perception of care. You may wear uniforms, scrubsuits, laboratory coats, business suits, and street clothes as practice roles dictate. Although the traditional white uniform does not reflect your abilities, it may take longer to establish trust if your clothing differs from the client's preconceived image.

POSTURE AND GAIT.   The way people sit, stand, and move is a form of self-expression. Posture and gait reflect emotions, self-concept, and health status. An erect posture and a quick, purposeful gait communicate a sense of well-being and assuredness. A slumped posture and slow, shuffling gait may indicate depression or fatigue. Leaning forward conveys attention. Leaning backward in a more relaxed manner may show less interest or indicate caution.

FACIAL EXPRESSION.   The face, the most expressive part of the body, reveals emotions such as surprise, fear, anger, disgust, happiness, and sadness. The sender's facial expressions often become the basis for important judgments by the receiver, although because of the diversity in facial expressions, meaning may be misunderstood. Facial expressions may reveal, contradict, or suppress true emotions. People may be unaware of the messages their expressions convey. When facial expressions are unclear, verbal feedback should be sought to be sure of the sender's intent. A client who frowns after receiving information may be confused, angry, disapproving, or simply concentrating on a reply. You might say, "I notice you're frowning," and encourage further clarification of the client's response.

Nurses are watched closely by clients. Consider the impact your facial expression might have on a client who asks, "Am I going to die?" The slightest change in the eyes, lips, or face can reveal your true feelings. Understanding this you will learn to avoid showing overt shock, disgust, dismay, or other distressing reactions in the client's presence.

EYE CONTACT.   Eye contact signals a readiness to communicate. By maintaining eye contact during conversa-

Nursing Actions Within the Zones of Personal Space and Touch   Box 8-2

ZONES OF PERSONAL SPACE
Intimate Zone (0 to 18 inches)
Holding a crying infant
Performing physical assessment
Bathing, grooming, dressing, feeding, and toileting a client
Changing a client's dressing

Personal Zone (18 inches to 4 feet)
Sitting at a client's bedside
Taking the client's nursing history
Teaching an individual client
Exchanging information at change-of-shift

Social Zone (4 to 12 feet)
Making rounds with a physician
Sitting at the head of a conference table
Teaching a class for clients with diabetes
Conducting a family support group

Public Zone (12 feet and greater)
Speaking at a community forum

Testifying at a legislative hearing
Lecturing to a class of students

ZONES OF TOUCH
Social Zone (permission not needed)
Hands
Arms
Shoulders
Back

Consent Zone (permission needed)
Mouth
Wrists
Feet

Vulnerable Zone (special care needed)
Face
Neck
Front of body

Intimate Zone (great sensitivity needed)
Genitalia

---

tion, those involved communicate respect for one another and a willingness to listen. Eye contact also allows one to closely observe another. Lack of eye contact may indicate anxiety, defensiveness, discomfort, or lack of confidence in communicating. Some cultures, such as Asian and Indochinese, Native American, and Appalachian, consider eye contact to be intrusive, threatening, or harmful and minimize its use.

Eye movements communicate feelings and emotions. Wide eyes express frankness, terror, and naivete. Downward glances show modesty. Raised upper eyelids reveal displeasure, and a constant stare may be associated with hatred or coldness. Looking down on a person establishes authority, whereas interacting at the same eye level indicates equality in the relationship. You appear less dominant and less threatening when interacting at the client's eye level. Rising to the same eye level of an angry person helps establish your autonomy.

GESTURES.   A salute, a thumbs-up, and a tapping foot are types of gestures. Hands and feet emphasize, punctuate, and clarify the spoken word. Gestures alone carry specific meanings, or they may create messages with other communication cues. A finger pointed toward a person may communicate several meanings, but when accompanied by a frown and a stern tone of voice, the gesture becomes a sign of accusation or threat.

TERRITORIALITY AND SPACE.   Territoriality is the need to gain, maintain, and defend one's exclusive right to space. *Territory* can be separated and made visible to others, such as a fence around a yard, a towel on the beach, or a bed in a hospital room. *Personal space* is invisible, individual, and travels with the person. During interpersonal interaction, people consciously maintain varying distances between themselves, depending on the nature of the relationship and

situation. When personal space becomes threatened, people respond defensively and communicate less effectively. Examples of nursing actions within the four zones of personal space are listed in Box 8-2.

You must frequently move into clients' territory and personal space because of the nature of care giving. Convey confidence, gentleness, and respect for privacy, especially when actions require intimate contact. As the distance between you becomes greater, the client and you may feel less threatened or constrained.

FACTORS INFLUENCING COMMUNICATION

Situations have several contextual aspects that influence the nature of communication and interpersonal relationships (Beebe and others, 1996). These include the participants' physical and emotional status, the nature of their relationship, their environment, the situation prompting communication, and the sociocultural elements present. The many factors influencing communication within these contexts are described in Box 8-3. Awareness of these factors helps the nurse make sound decisions during the communication process.

THE NURSE–CLIENT HELPING RELATIONSHIP

A helping relationship between you and your client does not just happen—it is created with care and skill, and it is built on the client's trust in you as a nurse. Through **therapeutic communication** you develop a relationship with the client to fulfill several purposes. Imogene King (1971) calls the nurse-client relationship "learning experiences whereby two people interact to face an immediate health problem, to share, if possible, in resolving it, and to discover ways to adapt to the situation." Clients are helped to clarify needs

Contextual Factors Influencing Communication

Box 8-3

PSYCHOPHYSIOLOGICAL CONTEXT

The *internal factors* influencing communication:

Physiological status

Emotional status

Growth and development status

Unmet needs

Attitudes, values, and beliefs

Perceptions and personality

Self-concept and self-esteem

RELATIONAL CONTEXT

The *nature of the relationship* between the participants:

Social, helping, or working relationship

Level of trust between participants

Level of self-disclosure between participants

Shared history of participants

Balance of power and control

SITUATIONAL CONTEXT

The *reason for* the communication:

Information exchange

Goal achievement

Problem resolution

Expression of feelings

ENVIRONMENTAL CONTEXT

The *physical surroundings* in which communication takes place:

Degree of privacy

Degree of comfort and safety

Noise level

Presence of distractions

CULTURAL CONTEXT

The *sociocultural elements* that affect the interaction:

Educational level of participants

Language and self-expression patterns

Customs and expectations

Phases of the Helping Relationship

Box 8-4

PREINTERACTION PHASE

Before meeting the client, you:

Review available data, including the medical and nursing history

Talk to other caregivers who may have information about the client

Anticipate health concerns or issues that may arise

Identify a location and setting that will foster comfortable, private interaction

Plan enough time for the initial interaction

ORIENTATION PHASE

When you and the client meet and get to know one another, you:

Set the tone for the relationship by adopting a warm, empathetic, caring manner

Recognize that the initial relationship may be superficial, uncertain, and tentative

Expect the client to test your competence and commitment

Closely observe the client and expect to be closely observed by the client

Begin to make inferences and form judgments about client messages and behavior

Assess the client's health status

Prioritize client problems and identify client goals

Clarify the client's and your roles

Form contracts with the client to specify who will do what

ORIENTATION PHASE—cont'd

Let the client know when to expect the relationship to be terminated

WORKING PHASE

When you and the client work together to solve problems and accomplish goals, you:

Encourage and help the client to express feelings about his or her health

Encourage and help the client with self-exploration

Provide information needed to understand and change behavior

Encourage and help the client to set goals

Take actions to meet the goals set with the client

Use therapeutic communication skills to facilitate successful interactions

Use appropriate self-disclosure and confrontation

TERMINATION PHASE

During the ending of the relationship, you:

Remind the client that termination is near

Evaluate goal achievement with the client

Reminisce about the relationship with the client

Separate from the client by relinquishing responsibility for his or her care

Achieve a smooth transition for the client to other caregivers as needed

and goals, solve problems, cope with situational or maturational crises, clarify and strengthen values, reduce stress and anxiety, and gain insight and self-understanding (Edelman and Mandle, 1998). Creating this therapeutic environment depends on your ability to communicate, provide comfort, and help the client meet his or her needs. Comforting strategies include gentle humor, physical comfort measures, emotionally supportive statements, and comforting and connecting touch. You provide information, support clients' active decision making, and offer opportunities for clients to engage in social exchange. These comforting strategies demonstrate caring and depend on your skill in communi-

cation and relationship building (Bottorff and others, 1995). Use Box 8-4 to guide you through the phases of the helping relationship with clients you care for in a variety of settings.

NURSE–HEALTH TEAM MEMBER RELATIONSHIPS

As a member of the health care community you interact with multiple health team members. Many elements of the nurse-client helping relationship are also applied in these collegial relationships, focused on accomplishing the work and goals of the clinical setting. Communication in such relationships may be geared toward team building, facilitating the group process, collaboration, consultation, delegation, supervision, leadership, and management.

Social, informational, and therapeutic interactions are all needed among the nurse and health team members to build morale, accomplish goals, and strengthen working relationships. Everyone has interpersonal needs for inclusion, such as feeling accepted, wanted, and a part of the group; identity; privacy; power and control; and affection (Stewart and Logan, 1997; Wilson and others, 1995). You will need friendship, support, guidance, and encouragement from other nurses and team members to cope with the many stressors imposed by the nursing role. Extend the same caring communication used with clients to build positive relationships with colleagues and co-workers.

COMMUNICATION WITHIN CARING RELATIONSHIPS

Principles and guidelines for using effective communication techniques can strengthen all caring relationships established within the professional role. Caring and helping relationships are manifested by the qualities and behavior explained in the following sections of the text. Examples of nurses using both effective and ineffective techniques are integrated throughout each section, as are suggestions for improving ineffective responses. Although some of the techniques may seem artificial or unnatural at first, your skill and comfort will increase with practice and experience, and tremendous satisfaction will result as therapeutic relationships and outcomes are achieved.

Professionalism
Verbal and nonverbal behavior greatly influence the helping relationship. The client's acceptance of you as a professional often depends on the manner in which you present a professional and caring image. Professional appearance, demeanor, and behavior are important in establishing trustworthiness and competence. They communicate that you have assumed the professional helping role, are clinically skilled, and are focused on the client rather than yourself. Nothing harms nursing's image like inappropriate appearance and behavior in those who hold a professional role. Consider the level of trust one might feel while being cared for by each of the following nurses.

> Annie Robbins is late for her shift. She left her stethoscope and note pad at home. She is chewing gum, she has a large chunky necklace and long dangling hair, and her underwear is visible beneath her uniform. She is wearing heavy makeup and perfume, has long painted fingernails, and there is smoke on her breath and clothing. She giggles, talks loudly, uses slang, rolls her eyes, sulks, grimaces, writes vital signs on the skin of her hand, and reacts to problems by blaming others and behaving immaturely.
>
> Mary Kline arrives at work on time, and is organized, well prepared, and equipped for the responsibilities of her nursing role. She is clean, neat, well groomed, appropriately

dressed, and scent- and odor-free. Her behavior reflects warmth, friendliness, confidence, and competence. She speaks in a clear well-modulated voice, uses good grammar, listens to others, helps and supports teammates, communicates effectively, and handles problems in a mature manner.

Courtesy
Common courtesy is important to your role. It conveys respect for others and oneself. Courtesy techniques include saying hello and goodbye, knocking on doors before entering, introducing oneself and stating one's purpose, addressing people by name, saying "please" and "thank you" to team members, and apologizing for inadvertently making an error or causing someone distress—all are integral parts of good professional communication. Being discourteous causes you to be perceived as rude, crude, or insensitive. It sets up barriers between you and the client and causes friction among team members.

Self-introduction is especially important. Failure to give your name, indicate your professional status, or acknowledge the client can create uncertainty about the interaction and conveys an impersonal lack of commitment or caring. Make eye contact and smile. Acknowledging others by name shows your respect for human dignity and for the uniqueness of the other person. Because using last names conveys respect in most cultures, begin initial interactions by using the client's last name. Ask others how they would like to be addressed and let them know your personal preference as well. Using first names is appropriate for infants, young children, confused or unconscious clients, and close team members.

AVOID TERMS OF ENDEARMENT. Calling the client "honey," "dear," "Grandpa," or "sweetheart" rather than by a personal name is inappropriate. Most people are offended by such casual familiarity from caregivers.

AVOID REFERRING TO CLIENTS BY DIAGNOSIS, ROOM NUMBER, OR OTHER ATTRIBUTE. Referring to clients by attributes rather than their names is demeaning and sends the message that you do not care enough about the person to know him or her as an individual.

Confidentiality
It is essential that you safeguard the client's right to privacy by carefully protecting information of a confidential nature. This is accomplished by reassuring the person that information will be kept private and then keeping that promise. It is often tempting to share exciting or shocking information or to share information with those who are genuinely interested and concerned, but resist that temptation. In situations in which you are obligated to report information to others, the client should be told in advance if at all possible.

> Client: "What's wrong with my roommate? She seems so sick."
> Nurse: "I know you're concerned about Mrs. Hoover, but I can't share any personal information about a client without his or her permission."

AVOID VIOLATING CONFIDENTIALITY. Sharing personal information or gossiping about others violates both nursing's ethical code and practice standards. It sends the message that you cannot be trusted and damages interpersonal relationships.

Trust

Trust is an essential building block of the helping relationship and must not be allowed to "leak away" (Salvage, 2000) in times when being "too busy" becomes a protective excuse for not being involved (Hills and Hupcey, 1998). You foster trust when you communicate warmth and caring and demonstrate consistency, reliability, honesty, and competence. Trusting another person involves risk and vulnerability, but it also fosters open, therapeutic communication and enhances the expression of feelings, thoughts, and needs.

Being untrustworthy or dishonest seriously undermines relationships and violates legal and ethical standards of practice. Do not withhold key information, lie, or distort the truth. This is not always easy.

> Nurse, lying to a client who asked why his 24-hour urine collection was being repeated: "The lab wants us to repeat the test, because their machine broke down during the analysis and they need a fresh specimen."
>
> A better response would be, "I'm sorry, Mr. Gottleib. One of the staff didn't save some of your urine by mistake. We will make every effort to make sure it is all saved this time."

Availability

Availability means being present for the other person when needed and offering your presence even when the need is not expressed verbally. You can express a willingness to be available, although the other person may not verbalize such a need, you show a caring attitude, demonstrating your willingness to listen, talk, or just be physically present. Be aware of the tendency to avoid clients whose behavior is troublesome. Such avoidance may escalate negative behavior. Being *task oriented*, making the technical procedure the focus of the interaction, may be another way of not being emotionally available and means you miss opportunities to assess the client, explore concerns, allay anxiety, demonstrate empathy, integrate client teaching, and involve the client in care. You may be perceived as cold, uncaring, and unapproachable. As a student, when you first perform technical skills, it is difficult to integrate therapeutic communication because of the need to focus on the procedure. In time, you learn to do both and promote more satisfactory interactions. Consider the quality of care given in each of the following scenarios.

> Nurse A silently enters the client's room: "It's time for your pain shot."
>
> Client, Mr. Stewart, is mildly startled and grimaces. As he starts to ask a question, Nurse A quickly reaches for his arm, gives the injection, then leaves.
>
> Nurse B, calling the client's name as she enters the room: "Mr. Stewart, I have your pain medication. Are you feeling as uncomfortable as you look?"

> Client: "Yes, my back feels like a knife went through it. Will the pain ever go away?"
>
> Nurse B lays syringe down and sits by client: "It's normal to have severe pain the first few days after surgery. This medicine should help. I'll give the shot, then show you how to move in bed so the pain won't get worse. If you have breakthrough pain, I will call the doctor to see about adjusting your medicine."

Empathy

Empathy is the ability to understand and accept another person's reality, to accurately perceive feelings, and to communicate this understanding to the other. Balzer Riley (2000) writes, "When clients or colleagues are hurting, confused, troubled, anxious, doubtful of self-worth, or uncertain as to identity, then understanding is called for." Such empathetic understanding requires sensitivity and imagination, especially if you have not had similar experiences. You cannot be empathetic in all situations, but it is an important goal—a key to unlocking concern and communicating emotional support for others. Alligood and May (2000) increase our understanding of the impact of empathy, proposing that ". . . empathy organizes perceptions; facilitates awareness of self and others; increases sensitivity; promotes shared respect, mutual goals, and social awareness; and cultivates understanding of individuals within a historical and social context."

Empathy statements reflect an understanding of what has been communicated and tell the person that you heard both the feeling and the factual content of the communication. Empathy statements are neutral and nonjudgmental. They can be used to establish trust in very difficult situations.

> Nurse to client who has received bad news: "That must have been a difficult thing to hear."
>
> Nurse to family member: "It sounds like you're really afraid of what might happen to your husband."

Sympathy

Sympathy is the concern, sorrow, or pity you feel for the client, when you personally identify with the client's needs. Sympathy is a subjective look at another person's world that prevents a clear perspective of all sides of the issues confronting that person. Sharing sympathy with another feels good, creates a bond, and minimizes differences. Although sympathy is a compassionate response to another's situation, it is not as therapeutic as empathy because your own emotional issues can prevent effective problem solving and impair good judgment. Stuart and Laraia (2000) explain that sympathy can cause problems in a helping relationship, because helpers who share the client's needs may be unable to help the client select realistic solutions for problems and may assume the client's feelings are similar to their own.

> Nurse to client who is grieving over an amputation: "I'm so sorry about your amputation. I know just how you feel."
>
> A better response would be, "I can only imagine how hard it might be to lose a leg."

Listening and Responding

Active listening means listening attentively with the whole person—mind, body, and spirit. It includes listening for main and supportive ideas; acknowledging and responding; giving appropriate feedback; and paying attention to the other person's total communication, including the content, the intent, and the feelings expressed (Berko and others, 1997). Attentive listening allows you to better understand the message being communicated and is an excellent way to build trust. In many situations, the person just wants someone to listen.

To listen attentively, face the client at a distance of about 3 feet, remove physical barriers, maintain eye contact, assume a relaxed posture, lean forward slightly, and nod in acknowledgment to give feedback and encouragement as the client speaks.

PROVIDE INFORMATION. Giving information, whether factual information or professional advice, helps the other person make decisions. It helps reduce anxiety and meet client needs for safety and security. When offering suggestions, stress that the client has the right to make decisions about options so that client autonomy is maintained. Speak in simple language and translate medical terms.

> Nurse: "Mr. Valdez, this new medicine is called Lanoxin. It acts as a cardiotonic and antidysrhythmic—that means it will help your heart have a stronger and more regular beat."

PARAPHRASE COMMUNICATION. *Paraphrasing* is restating what was said in the receiver's own words to make sure information has been accurately received.

CLARIFY COMMUNICATION. *Clarifying* is used to validate whether the message was interpreted correctly. Try to restate an unclear or ambiguous message or ask the other person to restate it, explain further, or give an example of what was meant.

FOCUS COMMUNICATION. *Focusing* directs conversation to a specific topic or issue when a discussion becomes unclear and limits the area to which the sender can respond. Use it when the sender rambles or introduces many unrelated topics in the same conversation.

SUMMARIZE COMMUNICATION. *Summarizing* provides a concise review of main ideas from a discussion. It can bring a sense of satisfaction and closure to an individual conversation, or it can be used during the termination phase of a nurse-client relationship. By reviewing a conversation, you can focus on key issues and obtain additional relevant information as needed.

> Nurse to client: "We've talked about what to expect when you go home and the self-care you'll need to do, and you feel like you're ready, but you still need to make arrangements for a leave of absence from work."
> Client to nurse: "Yes, and I also have to fill out workers' compensation papers."

USE APPROPRIATE SELF-DISCLOSURE. *Self-disclosure* is used during the working phase of a helping relationship. Self-disclosures are personal statements, intentionally revealed to the other person to model and educate, foster a therapeutic alliance, validate reality, and encourage autonomy (Stuart and Laraia, 2000). Keep self-disclosures relevant, appropriate, made to benefit the client, not you, and used sparingly so that the client remains the focus of the interaction. Tie your comments back to the client focus (Balzer Riley, 2000).

> Nurse to client: "When my mother was dying, I was torn between wanting to stay with her every moment and trying to meet the needs of my small children. Is that how it is for you?"

AVOID INATTENTIVE LISTENING. Fidgeting, breaking eye contact, daydreaming during conversation, and "pseudo listening"—pretending to listen when one really is not—convey the message that what the sender has to say is not important. These behaviors inhibit conversation and undermine trust.

> Nurse looks at watch and taps foot impatiently, gazing out the window as client talks.

AVOID MEDICAL VOCABULARY. Technical words can cause confusion and anxiety and should be avoided or translated.

> Nurse to client: "Sit up while your lungs are auscultated."
> A better response would be, "Let me help you sit up while I listen to your lungs."
> Nurse to young child: "Do you need to urinate?"
> A better response would be, "Do you need to use the potty?"

AVOID GIVING PERSONAL OPINIONS. When you give a personal opinion, it takes decision making away from the client, unlike professional advice, information about options that are available. The problem and its solution belong to the client rather than the nurse.

> Client: "I don't know how much longer I'll be able to take care of my husband. I just don't know what to do."
> Nurse: "If I were you, I'd put my husband in a nursing home."
> A better response would be, "Sounds like that's a difficult decision. Let's talk about what choices are available for someone like your husband who needs a lot of care."

AVOID PRYNG. Asking irrelevant personal questions to satisfy your curiosity is inappropriate and invasive. If clients wish to share private information, they will.

AVOID CHANGING THE SUBJECT. Changing the subject is insensitive and tends to block further communication. If changing the subject is necessary, explain why.

Client: "I really miss my kids. I cry every time I think of them."

Nurse: "Dr. Marcus will be here in a minute to take out your chest tube."

A better response would be, "It must be hard to be apart from your children. Maybe we can talk about it after Dr. Marcus takes out your chest tube."

Acceptance and Respect

Conveying acceptance is an important part of therapeutic communication. It means you are nonjudgmental. As a nurse you are expected to provide high-quality care regardless of social or economic status, personal attributes, or the nature of the illness. Acceptance is a willingness to hear a message or to acknowledge feelings yet does not mean that you agree or approve. Acceptance includes giving positive feedback, making sure verbal and nonverbal cues match, using touch, being empathetic, restating, and avoiding arguments.

ASKING FOR EXPLANATIONS.   Asking "why" may imply an accusation and can result in resentment, insecurity, and mistrust. Try to phrase a question to avoid using "why."

Client: "I don't follow the diabetic diet the doctor talked about."

Nurse: "What problems have you had with the eating plan?"

AVOID APPROVAL OR DISAPPROVAL.   Do not impose your own attitudes, values, beliefs, and moral standards on others while in the professional helping role. People have the right to be themselves and make their own decisions. Avoid using terms such as *should, ought, good, bad, right,* or *wrong.* Agreeing or disagreeing sends the subtle message that you have the right to make value judgments about client decisions. Instead, help the other person anticipate the consequences of decisions.

AVOID ARGUING.   Challenging or arguing with someone's perceptions denies that they are real and may imply that the person is lying, misinformed, or uneducated. Present information or reality in a way that avoids argument.

Client: "My husband does not like it when I complain to the doctor about side effects of my drugs. He says the doctor is too busy."

Nurse: "It is true that the physicians here have many clients and your husband is thoughtful to be concerned, but such information can help the doctor prescribe the best medication for you and save everyone time."

AVOID BEING DEFENSIVE.   Defensiveness in the face of criticism implies the sender has no right to an opinion. The sender's concerns may be ignored when you focus on the need for self-defense, defense of the health care team, or defense of others.

Client: "The other nurse did the bandage differently. Don't you know what you are doing?"

Nurse: "I would appreciate it if you would tell me in what way the dressing is different so we can work together to get it just right for you."

Silence

It takes time and experience to become comfortable with silence. We fill empty spaces with words, but quiet can serve as time for you to observe, to sort out feelings, to think how to say things, and to consider what has been communicated. Interrupting a meaningful silence can be seen as disrespectful. Silence is therapeutic in times of profound sadness, deep thought, or grief when there are no "right" words. Relax your body, pay attention to slowing your breathing, and concentrate on offering your presence rather than words. Silence is a gift you give.

Mrs. Hartz, who is dying of renal failure, has just voiced feelings of deep grief about having to leave her family and friends behind. The nurse sits quietly while they both wipe away tears, think about love and loss, and appreciate the sharing that is taking place between them.

Hope and Encouragement

Hope is essential for healing and communicates a "sense of possibility" to others (Benner, 1984). Encouragement and positive feedback are important in fostering hope and self-confidence and for helping people achieve their potential and reach their goals. You can give hope and encouragement by commenting on the positive aspects of the other person's behavior, performance, or response. Hope can also be strengthened by sharing a vision of the future and reminding others of their resources and strengths. Offer an example of a client who recovered from serious illness and emphasize that people are different and some make exceptional progress (Laubach, 2000).

AVOID FALSE REASSURANCE THAT CAN DO MORE HARM THAN GOOD.   Although false reassurance might be intended kindly and help you avoid distress, you tend to block conversation and discourage further expression of feelings.

Client: "I don't think I'm going to beat this lupus."

Nurse: "Don't worry, I'm sure everything will be all right."

A better response would be, "Tell me more about what you're thinking," or "What's it like to feel that way?"

Socializing

Socializing is an important component of your communication as a nurse. You use it as a tool to get to know one another and to help people relax. At the beginning of an interaction use social conversation that is easy and superficial to make connections and help the client feel comfortable in sharing feelings and concerns. A friendly, informal, and warm communication style helps establish trust.

Nurse: "It certainly is a lovely day, Mrs. Spier."

Client: "Yes, isn't it? If I were home and feeling better, I'd be planting my garden."

Nurse: "You're a gardener? What types of plants do you grow?"

Client: "Oh, a little of everything. I like some tomatoes, lettuce, radishes, and maybe some squash."

AVOID INAPPROPRIATE SOCIALIZING.   Move beyond social conversation to talk about issues or concerns affecting the client's health.

Assertiveness and Autonomy

Assertive communication is based on a philosophy of protecting individual rights and responsibilities. It includes the ability to be self-directive in acting to accomplish goals and advocate for others. Assertive responses promote self-esteem and uphold personal and professional rights. They are characterized by feelings of security, competence, power, and professionalism. Assertive statements convey a message without resorting to sarcasm, whining, anger, blaming, or manipulation. Assertive responses are good tools to deal with criticism, change, negative conditions in personal or professional life, and conflict or stress in relationships.

Assertive responses often contain "I" messages, such as "I want," "I need," "I think," or "I feel." Simple assertive messages are usually stated in three parts, referencing the nurse, the other individual's behavior, and its effect.

Nurse to nurse: "When you are late for work, I have to stay late and am delayed picking up my children from the babysitter."

You can state a more complex assertive message by using the ASSERT formula: Describe the *Action* that prompted the need for the message; express a *Subjective* interpretation of the action; express *Sensations* related to the action; indicate the *Effects* of the action; make a *Request* of the other person; and *Tell* your intentions if the request is not met (Berko and others, 1997).

Nurse to supervisor: "When you say I'm not performing well, that sounds serious. I feel surprised and confused, because I had a sense that I was doing a good job. Please give me some examples of what you mean. If there are none, I'll discuss this evaluation with the director of nursing."

AVOID PASSIVE RESPONSES.   Passive responses avoid issues or conflict and are characterized by feelings of sadness, depression, anxiety, and hopelessness.

Nurse to co-worker, hopelessly: "I guess there's nothing we can do about it."

Nurse to spouse during argument: "Whatever you say."

A better response would be, "What can we do to make things better?"

AVOID AGGRESSIVE RESPONSES.   Aggressive responses provoke confrontation at the other person's expense. They are characterized by feelings of anger, frustration, resentment, and stress.

Nurse to spouse during argument: "You just always have to have the last word, don't you?"

A better response would be, "I want to hear your concerns, too. Let's take one thing at a time. Do you want to start or shall I?"

Humor

Humor is a coping strategy that adds perspective and helps you and the client adjust to stress. The American Association for Therapeutic Humor (2000) defines therapeutic humor as any intervention that promotes health and wellness by stimulating expression or appreciation of the absurdity of life's incongruity. Laughter is a diversion from stress-related tension, provides a sense of well-being, and more of a feeling of control or mastery. Humor can help provide emotional support to clients and can humanize the illness experience. Laughter provides both a psychological and physical release for you and the client, promotes open, relaxed interaction, and illustrates our shared experience in being human.

You can assess whether humor is appropriate by noticing if clients use humor in their conversations. Start with small doses to see if this is helpful. To offer positive humor, share humorous incidents or situations, offer a clown nose to someone who could use a laugh, or share puns or simple jokes that are not offensive. Positive humor is associated with hope and love and joy with the intent to bring people closer. Avoid negative humor, which is inappropriate, such as ethnic, religious, sexist, ageist, or put-down humor, which creates distance. Realize that humor can backfire; not everyone will appreciate a humorous approach because of negative moods, stress, or physical discomfort. Humor may be a signal for closer attention. When a client preparing for surgery quips, "Well, I won't die from it," gently explore concerns of the client.

Health care staff may use dark, negative humor after difficult or traumatic situations to survive intact and defuse tension and stress. This "coping humor" may be seen as callous or uncaring by those not involved in the situation. Avoid using "coping humor" within earshot of clients or their loved ones. Understand that humor is a release but timing, content, and receptivity are important in the use of therapeutic humor (Balzer Riley, 2000).

Touch

Touch is a powerful form of communication. It is an integral part of human behavior; from birth until death, people need to be touched and to touch others (Rousalato, 1996b). You are privileged to experience more of this intimate form of personal contact than almost any other professional. Messages such as affection, emotional support, encouragement, and tenderness are conveyed through touch (Bottorff, 1995). Comfort touch is important for vulnerable clients experiencing severe illness with its accompanying physical and emotional losses (Butts and Janes, 1995). Nurses use non-procedural touch with clients to get their attention, to arouse them from sleep, to begin a nursing intervention, to add emphasis to explanations, to make requests, to comfort, to emphasize or point things out, to tease, to thank, and to reprimand (Rousalato, 1996a). Touch may also convey understanding better than words or gestures. Therapeutic Touch is a special form of alternative touch therapy used by nurses to achieve health assessment, pain reduction, and relaxation by influencing a client's energy fields. Learning Therapeutic touch involves knowing how to meditate, acquiring experimental knowledge of energy fields, and practicing with guidance from specially trained advanced practice nurses (Edelman and Mandle, 1998).

Because much of what you do involves touching, learn to use touch wisely. The zones of touch (Rousalato, 1996a) are described in Box 8-2. Touch delivered in the social or consent zones is less anxiety producing than touch delivered in the vulnerable or intimate zones. Seed (1995) discovered that students may initially find giving intimate care stressful, especially with clients of the opposite sex, and that students learn to cope with intimate contact by changing their perception of the situation. Similarly, the client who is ill and dependent must permit closer physical contact than is normally tolerated and may be uncomfortable with touch. Remain sensitive to your own responses and to clients' feelings. If a client refuses to hold your hand during an episode of pain or pulls away from physical contact, it may mean the client is uncomfortable with being touched. Touch may be perceived negatively when it is given without consent; used within a hostile or nontrusting relationship; and delivered to a vulnerable, intimate, or painful area of the body. Your touch should never be angry, rough, violent, overly stimulating, threatening, overly tentative, sexual, or unnecessarily painful.

Cultural Sensitivity

Persons of different cultures use different types of eye contact, personal space, gestures, loudness of voice, pace of speech, touch, silence, and meaning of language (Davidhizar and Giger, 1994; Grossman, 1994; Nance, 1995). Make a conscious effort not to interpret messages through your own cultural perspective; instead consider the context of the other individual's background (see Chapter 16). Consider the cultural sensitivity demonstrated by the nurse in the following example (Jambunathan and Stewart, 1995).

> Carrie Barton is caring for Huan Mi, a young female refugee from Vietnam's Hmong Delta who has just delivered a small baby boy. Carrie understands that childbirth in different cultures is treated as a traumatic life crisis and a time of vulnerability for the mother and infant. She knows that Ms. Huan's lack of prenatal care was related to the woman's fear of miscarriage if touched by doctors or nurses, and she is careful in her use of touch with Ms. Huan. Carrie has learned that touching the head is considered dangerous. Carrie did not try to argue with Ms. Huan's refusal of an episiotomy because she preferred to tear and heal naturally. She also respected Ms. Huan's decision that having the baby circumcised would be "unnatural." When teaching her about birth

control, Carrie was aware that Ms. Huan might have difficulties practicing the techniques because of male/female role expectations. She was careful in how she sought feedback about Ms. Huan's understanding of the information, recognizing that Asian persons often agree with the speaker to be polite rather than to indicate agreement or understanding.

Cultural insensitivity in communication takes many forms, including making fun of another's culture, ethnicity, language, or dress; telling jokes that make fun of specific cultures; stereotyping; patronizing; and incorrectly interpreting culturally based behavior. It also includes behaving in ways that offend the cultural practices of others. Carrie simply avoided touching Mrs. Huan's head. She did not laugh at her fears.

Gender Sensitivity

Gender influences how we think, act, feel, and communicate. *Gender sensitivity* means recognizing the differences in male and female communication patterns. Males grow up using communication to achieve goals, establish individual status and authority, and compete for attention and power. Females grow up using communication to build connections with others; include others; and cooperate with, respond to, show interest in, and support others. Men typically prefer to talk about topics that do not expose personal feelings, whereas women enjoy discussing feelings and personal issues. Men find closeness in doing, and women find closeness in dialogue (Wood, 1996). Men tend to speak directly when giving criticism or orders. Women speak indirectly, couching criticism and commands in praise or vagueness to avoid causing offense or hurt feelings. A male nurse might say to his colleague, "Help me turn Jeremy." A female nurse might say, "Jeremy needs to be turned," expecting her colleague to understand the implied request for help. Men use more banter, teasing, and playful "put-downs." They sometimes hesitate to ask questions for fear of appearing unknowledgeable, whereas women ask questions to elicit information. Men usually want others to know of their accomplishments; women may tend to downplay their achievements (Beebe and others, 1996). Research has shown that gender differences also influence the way male and female nurses use silence, touch, and humor in their practice (Perry, 1996).

Gender-insensitive communication means a nurse of one gender misinterprets or reacts to messages differently than they were intended by the other gender and includes conversation with sexual innuendoes, gender-denigrating jokes, and male-female stereotyping.

COMMUNICATION WITHIN THE NURSING PROCESS

You use communication skills to gather, analyze, and transmit information and to accomplish the work of each phase of the nursing process. Although the nursing process is a reliable framework for delivering comprehensive client care, it will not

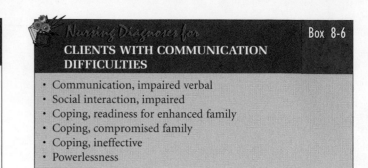

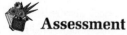

Communication Through the Nursing Process   Box 8-5

ASSESSMENT
Interviewing and history taking
Physical examination (use of visual, auditory, and tactile channels)
Observation of nonverbal behavior
Review of medical records, literature, diagnostic tests

NURSING DIAGNOSIS
Written analysis of assessment findings
Discussion of health care needs and priorities with client and family

PLANNING
Written care plans
Health team planning sessions
Discussions with client and family to determine methods of implementation
Making referrals

IMPLEMENTATION
Discussion with other health professionals
Health teaching
Provision of therapeutic support
Contact with other health resources
Record of client's progress in care plan and nurse's notes

EVALUATION
Acquisition of verbal and nonverbal feedback
Written results of expected outcomes
Update of written care plan
Explanation of revisions to client

Nursing Diagnoses for CLIENTS WITH COMMUNICATION DIFFICULTIES   Box 8-6

- Communication, impaired verbal
- Social interaction, impaired
- Coping, readiness for enhanced family
- Coping, compromised family
- Coping, ineffective
- Powerlessness

work well unless you master the art of effective interpersonal communication. Successful communication occurs with knowledge acquired from books, experiences, and observation of others' communication skills. Communication techniques used within the nursing process are also applied during the problem-solving process with team members to resolve problems or accomplish goals within the clinical setting that are not directly related to client care (Box 8-5). A few techniques deserve special mention because of their importance in the nursing and problem-solving processes.

Assessment

When you assess a client's communication ability, systematically collect data, organize the data collected, and document information that has been obtained from the client, family, and significant others. This is the beginning of a beneficial nurse-client relationship with the rapport needed for good communication.

Information Gathering

Ask relevant questions to gather data about the client or problem. Use *focused questions* to elicit more information about a particular subject. A focused question that is open ended, "What is your usual sleep pattern?" cannot be answered with a yes/no or one-word response. A closed question, "How many hours of sleep do you average each night?" requires a more specific answer.

Overuse of information-seeking as a therapeutic communication technique can be dehumanizing, because informational interactions do not allow you to establish a more meaningful relationship or deal with important emotional issues. It may be a way for you to ignore uncomfortable areas in favor of more comfortable, neutral topics.

> Client, worried: "I don't know what to do about my daughter; her tantrums are driving me crazy. The doctor thinks she might be either hyperactive or mentally retarded."
> Nurse: "What's your daughter's name?" or "How long has she been having tantrums?"
> A better response yielding more assessment data would be, "You sound worried about this. Tell me what happens when your daughter has a tantrum."

Nursing Diagnosis

After collecting assessment data, cluster pertinent defining characteristics for patterns and problems. Success in accurately identifying the client's communication problem will ensure the formulation of an accurate nursing diagnosis (Box 8-6). The related factor should focus on the cause of the communication disorder so that you can select appropriate nursing interventions.

Impaired verbal communication is the nursing diagnostic label to describe the client who has limited or no ability to communicate verbally. This diagnosis is useful for a wide variety of clients with special problems and needs related to communication. It is defined as "decreased, delayed, or absent ability to receive, process, transmit, and use a system of symbols" (NANDA, 2001).

Planning

As you use assessment data to formulate and support nursing diagnoses, you now must direct your focus to appropriate actions to assist in addressing the identified problem or need. In planning, begin to establish goals and expected outcomes of care and determine specific nursing interventions to assist with the client's communication difficulties. Select interventions and communication techniques appropriate for the client's age, cultural beliefs, and practices. When possible, collaborate with the client, family, friends, and other health care team members. Often the family can suggest ways that foster communication with the client. Make the establishment of goals for care a mutual process between you

Communicating With Clients Who Have Special Needs

Box 8-7

CLIENTS WITH DIFFICULTY HEARING

Avoid shouting.

Use simple sentences.

Punctuate speech with facial expression and gestures.

CLIENTS WITH DIFFICULTY SEEING

Communicate verbally before touching the client.

Orient the client to sounds in the environment.

Inform the client when the conversation is over and when you are leaving the room.

CLIENTS WHO ARE MUTE OR CANNOT SPEAK CLEARLY

Place sign by unit call system to answer call light in person.

Listen attentively, be patient, and do not interrupt.

Do not finish client's sentences for them.

Ask simple questions that require "yes" or "no" answers.

Allow time for understanding and responses.

Use visual cues (e.g., words, pictures, objects) when possible.

Allow only one person to speak at time.

Do not shout or speak too loudly.

Encourage the client to converse.

Let the client know if you do not understand.

Use communication aids as needed:

  Pad and felt-tipped pen or magic slate

  Flash cards

  Communication board with words, letters, or pictures denoting basic needs

  Computer toy ("speak and spell" type)

  Call bells or alarms

  Sign language

  Use of eye blinks or movement of fingers for simple responses ("yes" or "no")

CLIENTS WHO ARE COGNITIVELY IMPAIRED

Reduce environmental distractions while conversing.

Get the client's attention before speaking.

Use simple sentences and avoid long explanations.

Avoid shifting from subject to subject.

Ask one question at a time.

Allow time for the client to respond.

Include family and friends to conversations, especially in subjects known to the client.

CLIENTS WHO ARE UNRESPONSIVE

Call the client by name during interactions.

Communicate both verbally and by touch.

Speak to the client as though he or she could hear.

Explain all procedures and sensations.

CLIENTS WHO DO NOT SPEAK ENGLISH

Speak to the client in a normal tone of voice (shouting may be interpreted as anger).

Establish a method for the client to signal the desire to communicate (call light or bell).

Provide an interpreter (translator) as needed:

  Use a person familiar with the client's culture and with biomedicine if possible.

  Allow plenty of time for the interpreter to transmit messages.

  Communicate directly to the client and family rather than the interpreter.

  Ask one question at a time.

  Avoid making comments to the interpreter about the client or family (they may understand some English).

Develop a communication board, pictures, or cards using words translated into English for the client to make basic requests (e.g., pain medication, water, elimination).

Have a dictionary (English/Spanish or appropriate) available if the client can read.

---

and the client. Success in promoting a client's ability to communicate depends not only on the client's participation in goal setting but also on your style of communication and ability to establish a therapeutic relationship. Therapeutic communication skills enable you to perceive, react to, and respect the client's uniqueness.

Collaboration

Remember to include family caregivers during the planning and intervention phases of the nursing process. Davidhizar and Rexroth (1994) write that such collaboration can provide support to the family and client, increase the caregiver's understanding, increase compliance, increase the nurse's understanding, reinforce teaching, decrease manipulative behavior, promote communication among family members, and facilitate positive client-family relationships. Encourage collaboration by asking others for ideas and suggestions about what should be done to reach goals. It gives others the opportunity to express themselves and strengthens problem-solving ability.

When you fail to collaborate with clients, families, and other providers, the nursing interventions have less chance of success. Clients are denied the collective expertise that can make a crucial difference in health outcomes.

 Implementation

Many altered health states and human responses contribute to impaired communication, such as: the infant whose self-expression is limited to crying, body movement, and facial expression; the person who receives messages through fewer channels because of hearing or visual impairment; the person who cannot understand or form words because of a stroke or late-stage Alzheimer's disease; the person with autism or schizophrenia who responds to internal stimuli and misinterprets external stimuli; the person who does not speak or understand English; the client with learning disabilities and limited vocal skills who uses gaze and body orientation to display a readiness to communicate; and the unresponsive or heavily sedated person who cannot send or receive verbal messages.

The client who cannot communicate effectively has difficulty expressing needs and responding appropriately to the environment and requires special thought and sensitivity. Such persons benefit greatly when you adapt communication techniques to their circumstances (Box 8-7). When caring for a client with impaired verbal communication related to cultural difference, you may provide a table of simple words in the client's language to meet the expected outcome that the client will communicate basic needs such as food, water, toileting, rest, sleep, and pain relief. Collaborate with team members to design the best communication strategies. A speech therapist can help the client with aphasia, an interpreter (translator) may be needed for the client who speaks a foreign language, and a psychiatric nurse specialist might help an angry or highly anxious client to communicate.

Good communication will improve the quality of your client's interpersonal relationships and well-being; it is a very important aspect of holistic health. If the client uses ineffective communication techniques that interfere with coping or interpersonal relationships, intervene to help your client send, receive, and interpret messages more effectively. Serve as a communication role model and teacher to help clients express needs, feelings, and concerns; develop social interaction skills; communicate thoughts and feelings clearly; interpret messages sent from others; and increase feelings of autonomy and assertiveness. Methods such as role playing can allow clients to practice situations in which they have difficulty communicating.

Providing Alternative Communication Methods

Clients with physical communication barriers (e.g., those with a laryngectomy or endotracheal tube) may be unable to speak, or the clarity of speech may be so poor that alternative methods of communication are needed (see Box 8-7, p. 127). For these clients, provide simple communication methods to decrease frustration. Remember to be patient as the client tries to communicate. The client must be physically able to use the method you provide (e.g., communication boards, pencil and pad). A client who is unable to speak can be at risk for injury unless personal needs can be quickly communicated.

Communicating With Children

Communication with a child requires special considerations to develop a working relationship with the child and family. Because contact between parent and child is usually close, the information communicated by parents can be assumed to be reliable, although some parents may exaggerate. Offer a child toys or materials so the parent can give full attention to your information gathering. Give periodic attention to infants and younger children as they play to include them. An older child can be actively involved in communication. Consider the influence of development on language and thought processes.

Children, particularly the young, are especially responsive to nonverbal messages. Sudden movements or threatening gestures can be frightening. Remain calm and gentle and, if possible, let the child make the first move. Use a quiet, friendly, confident tone of voice. The child feels helpless in most situations involving health care personnel. When it is necessary to give explanations or directions, use simple, direct language and be honest. To minimize fear and anxiety,

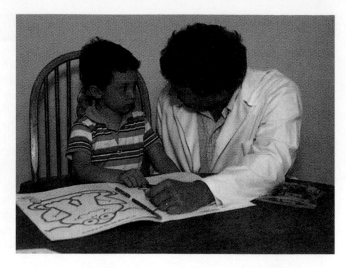

FIGURE **8-2** Drawing helps children communicate.

prepare the child by explaining what to expect. Avoid staring and meet the child at eye level.

Drawing and playing with young children allow the child to communicate nonverbally (making the drawing) and verbally (explaining the picture) (Figure 8-2). Use a child's drawing as a basis for beginning a conversation.

Communicating With Older Adult Clients

Sensory alterations prevent receiving messages clearly. Motor disturbances such as dysarthria interfere with speech clarity. Many older adults adapt to sensory losses and can learn to communicate effectively. When obvious deficits exist, maximize existing motor and sensory function to help the client communicate more effectively (see Box 8-7, p. 127). Ebersole and Hess (1998) indicate that older adults may suffer from other sensory deprivations (elimination of order or meaning and restricting the environment to dull monotony) and sensory overload (Box 8-8). Identify these challenges and work with the client to enhance effective communication. Attend to wisdom these clients have to offer you and think of them as teachers about living.

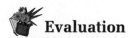 **Evaluation**

Client Care

Evaluating whether communication has been therapeutic is based on the client's progress or lack of progress toward goals and expected outcomes. You evaluate whether nursing interventions met established outcomes to determine if goals were achieved. If so, interventions were effective. For example, the nurse delivering care to the client with *impaired verbal communication related to cerebral dysfunction* may have established the goal of the client being able to communicate basic needs (e.g., water, food, toileting). The outcome would then be that the client uses a communication board to request water, food, and assistance with

Gerontological Nursing Practice   Box 8-8

In dealing with impaired communications with older adults, the primary goal is to establish a reliable communication system that is easily understood by all health care team members because nursing care of the older adult is ideally delivered by an interdisciplinary model. Communication with older adults requires special attention. The nurse must be aware of the physical, psychological, and social changes of aging.

The nurse can use the following interventions to assist with impaired communication with older adults:

- During conversation, maintain a quiet environment that is free from background noise.
- Avoid shifting from subject to subject; allow time for conversation.
- Be an attentive listener. Use explorative questions to facilitate conversation (e.g., "How do you feel?").
- Avoid long sentences to explain the subject. Try to keep it short, simple, and to the point.
- Allow the older adult the opportunity to reminisce. Reminiscing has therapeutic properties that increase the sense of well-being.
- If you are experiencing problems understanding the client (e.g., dysarthria), let the client know and facilitate methods that help the client speak more clearly. The nurse may need to consult with a speech therapist.
- Include the client's family and friends in conversations, particularly in known subjects to the client.
- Be aware of cultural differences among clients.

toileting. While caring for the client, the nurse observes whether the client uses the communication board easily and effectively. Was the client able to communicate basic needs with the staff, and thus were the needs met? The nurse might question the client about whether needs were adequately met. If the goal was met, interventions were appropriate for the client. If not, the plan of care should be modified to achieve the goal and outcome. This modification process is ongoing and continues until the time of discharge.

For clients with actual communication alterations, a variety of approaches can be used to evaluate the success of the plan of care. Goals, outcomes, and corresponding evaluative measures for the problem of impaired communication should include client's expectations.

Client Expectations

Reviewing the client's expectations of care and determining if these expectations were achieved is also an important part of the evaluation process. This aspect of evaluation can be encouraged by asking clients and their families for input about goal achievement, factors that affected outcomes, and suggestions for changes that might be made in the plan of care.

> Nurse to client: "You wanted to increase your weight. Let's look at what you've accomplished so far with your goal of increasing your calorie intake."
>
> Nurse to client: "Because your calorie intake hasn't increased as much as we would like, let's figure out what's preventing that from happening."
>
> Nurse to client: "John, did it help your appetite to brush your teeth and get up in a chair before eating?"

Avoiding client input into evaluation and its resultant care plan modification leads to a task-oriented rather than a critical thinking, client-centered approach to nursing. It denies the client's right to see the total picture of care and to be involved in all phases of the nursing process.

Key Terms

active listening, *p. 122*
assertive communication, *p. 124*
channel, *p. 115*
communication, *p. 115*
connotative meaning, *p. 116*
denotative meaning, *p. 116*
empathy, *p. 121*

environment, *p. 116*
feedback, *p. 116*
humor, *p. 124*
interpersonal communication, *p. 116*
intrapersonal communication, *p. 116*
language, *p. 116*
message, *p. 115*
metacommunication, *p. 117*
nonverbal communication, *p. 117*

public communication, *p. 116*
receiver, *p. 116*
referent, *p. 115*
sender, *p. 115*
sympathy, *p. 121*
therapeutic communication, *p. 118*
verbal communication, *p. 116*

Key Concepts

- Communication is a powerful therapeutic tool and an essential nursing skill used to influence others and achieve positive health outcomes.
- Nurses consider many contexts and factors influencing communication when making decisions about what, when, where, how, why, and with whom to communicate.

- Communication is most effective when the receiver and sender accurately perceive the meaning of one another's messages.
- The sender's and receiver's physical and developmental status, perceptions, values, emotions, knowledge, sociocultural background, roles, and environment influence message transmission.

Continued

Key Concepts—cont'd

- Effective verbal communication requires appropriate intonation, clear and concise phrasing, proper pacing of statements, and proper timing and relevance of a message.
- Effective nonverbal communication complements and strengthens the message conveyed by verbal communication.
- Nurses use intrapersonal, interpersonal, and public interaction to achieve positive change and health goals.
- Helping relationships are strengthened when the nurse demonstrates caring by establishing trust, empathy, autonomy, confidentiality, and professional competence.
- Effective communication techniques are facilitative and tend to encourage the other person to openly express ideas, feelings, or concerns.
- Ineffective communication techniques are inhibiting and tend to block the other person's willingness to openly express ideas, feelings, or concerns.
- The nurse must blend social and informational interactions with therapeutic communication techniques so that others can explore feelings and manage health issues.
- When using therapeutic humor, consider timing, receptivity, and content of the humorous intervention.
- Methods that facilitate communication with children include sitting at eye level; interacting with parents; using simple, direct language; and incorporating play activities.
- Older adult clients with sensory, motor, or cognitive impairments require the adaptation of communication techniques to compensate for their loss of function and special needs.
- Clients with impaired verbal communication require special consideration and alterations in communication techniques to facilitate the sending, receiving, and interpreting of messages.
- Desired outcomes for clients with impaired verbal communication include increased satisfaction with interpersonal interactions, the ability to send and receive clear messages, and attendance to and accurate interpretation of verbal and nonverbal cues.

Critical Thinking Activities

1. Walter Jordan is a 34-year-old man brought to the emergency department with crushing chest pain, shortness of breath, and exercise intolerance. His wife is at his side, in tears, moaning, "He's dying." What factors influencing communication are present in this scenario, and how would they affect your communication?
2. You take Mrs. Jordan's arm to escort her to the waiting room. She reacts angrily, wrenching her arm out of your grasp. What should you do now?
3. The couple's son, a 4-year-old boy, is in the emergency department. His eyes are wide open, his skin is pale, and his eyes are tearing. How would you explain to him what is happening with his father?
4. The Jordans' 16-year-old daughter is pacing and picking at her nails. Construct a way to establish a helping-trust relationship with her.
5. You notice Emily, a team member, going into the bathroom in tears. How can you offer help without invading privacy?

Review Questions

1. "Communication is not the message that was intended but rather the message that was received." The statement that best helps explain this is:
   1. clear communication can ensure the client will receive the message intended.
   2. sincerity in communication is the responsibility of the sender and the receiver.
   3. attention to personal space can minimize misinterpretation of communication.
   4. contextual factors such as attitudes, values, beliefs, and self-concept influence communication.
2. You demonstrate active listening by:
   1. agreeing with the client.
   2. repeating everything the client says to clarify.
   3. assuming a relaxed posture and leaning toward the client.
   4. smiling and nodding continuously throughout the interview.
3. As a nurse you build helping, caring relationships by:
   1. using touch for calming and comfort.
   2. not asking the client to do anything painful.
   3. establishing trust and demonstrating empathy.
   4. being sympathetic and protective of the client.
4. Gender influences how we think, act, feel, and communicate. In Western culture it is important to remember when you are trying to be sensitive to gender in communication that:
   1. males use indirect communication to meet their needs, whereas females communicate directly.
   2. males grow up using aggressive communication, whereas females use passive communication.
   3. males and females should be treated equally, therefore it serves no purpose to distinguish between genders in communication.
   4. males grow up using communication to achieve goals, whereas females use communication to build connections with others.
5. A nursing assistant comes to you to complain about a nurse on the unit where you work. The most effective response would be:
   1. to call the supervisor to ask for advice.
   2. to tell him it is none of your business.
   3. to listen sympathetically to help build team spirit.
   4. to suggest he talk with the nurse to resolve the issue.
6. The statement that best explains the role of collaboration with others for the client's plan of care is:
   1. the professional nurse consults the physician for direction in establishing goals for clients.

2. the professional nurse depends on the latest literature to complete an excellent plan of care for clients.

3. the professional nurse works independently to plan and deliver care and does not depend on other staff for assistance.

4. the professional nurse collaborates with colleagues and the client's family to provide combined expertise in planning care.

7. When working with an older adult, you should remember to:
   1. avoid touching the client.
   2. avoid shifting from subject to subject.
   3. avoid allowing the client to reminisce.
   4. avoid asking the client how he or she feels.

8. When giving nursing care to a client who is unresponsive, remember to:
   1. speak loudly.
   2. use touch sparingly to avoid startling the client.
   3. use the client's name and explain procedures as if the client can hear.
   4. spend as little time as possible with the client to minimize stimulation.

References

Alligood M, May BA: A nursing theory of personal system empathy: interpreting a conceptualization of empathy in King's interaction systems, *Nurs Sci Q* 13(3):243, 2000.

American Association for Therapeutic Humor, www.AATH.org , 2000.

Balzer Riley J: *Communication in nursing,* ed 4, St. Louis, 2000, Mosby.

Beebe SA and others: *Interpersonal communication: relating to others,* Boston, 1996, Allyn & Bacon.

Benner P: *From novice to expert: excellence and power in clinical nursing practice,* Englewood Cliffs, NJ, 1984, Prentice Hall.

Berko MR and others: *Connecting: a culture-sensitive approach to interpersonal communication competency,* ed 2, Philadelphia, 1997, Harcourt Brace.

Bottorff JL and others: Comforting: exploring the work of cancer nurses, *J Adv Nurs* 22(6):1077, 1995.

Butts JB, Janes S: Transcending the latex barrier: the therapeutics of comfort touch in patients with acquired immunodeficiency syndrome, *Holistic Nurs Pract* 10(1):61, 1995.

Davidhizar R, Giger JN: When your patient is silent, *J Adv Nurs* 20(4):703, 1994.

Davidhizar R, Rexroth R: The benefits of triad communication in home health care, *Rehabil Nurs* 19(6):352, 1994.

Ebersole P, Hess P: *Toward a healthy aging,* ed 5, St. Louis, 1998, Mosby.

Edelman CL, Mandle CL: *Health promotion throughout the lifespan,* ed 4, St. Louis, 1998, Mosby.

Grossman D: Enhancing your "cultural competence," *Am J Nurs* 94(7):58, 1994.

Hills B, Hupcey J: Establishing the nurse-family relationship in the intensive care unit, *West J Nurs Res* 20(2):180, 1998.

Jambunathan J, Stewart S: Among women in Wisconsin: what are their concerns in pregnancy and childbirth? *Birth* 22(4):204, 1995.

King I: *Toward a theory for nursing,* New York, 1971, John Wiley & Sons.

Laubach EW: How to communicate with seriously ill patients, *Nurs Manage* 31(4):24H, 2000.

Nance TA: Intercultural communication: finding common ground, *J Obstet Gynecol Neonatal Nurs* 24(3):249, 1995.

North American Nursing Diagnosis Association (NANDA): *Nursing diagnoses: definitions and classifications, 2001-2002,* Philadelphia, 2001, The Association.

Perry B: Influence of nurse gender on the use of silence, touch, and humor, *Int J Palliative Nurs* 2(1):7, 1996.

Rousalato P: Non-necessary touch in the nursing care of elderly people, *J Adv Nurs* 23(5):904, 1996a.

Rousalato P: The right to touch and be touched, *Nurs Ethics* 3(2):165, 1996b.

Rowe J: Self-awareness: improving nurse-client interactions, *Nurs Stand* 4(8):37, 1999.

Salvage J: Time to clean up our act, *Nurs Times* 96(7):23, 2000.

Seed A: Crossing the boundaries: experiences of neophyte nurses, *J Adv Nurs* 21(6):1136, 1995.

Stewart J, Logan C: *Together: communicating interpersonally,* ed 5, New York, 1997, McGraw Hill.

Stuart GW, Laraia MT: *Principles and practice of psychiatric nursing,* ed 7, St. Louis, 2000, Mosby.

Watson J: *Nursing: human science and health care,* Norwalk, Conn, 1985, Appleton-Century-Crofts.

Wilson GL and others: *Interpersonal communication,* ed 4, Madison, Wis, 1995, Brown & Benchmark.

Wood JT: *Gendered relationships,* Mountain View, Calif, 1996, Mayfield.

Yerby J and others: *Understanding family communication,* ed 2, Scottsdale, Ariz, 1995, Gorsuch Scarisbrick.

9

Client Education

Objectives

- Define key terms.
- Identify appropriate topics for a client's health education needs.
- Describe the similarities and differences between teaching and learning.
- Identify the purposes of client education.
- Compare the communication and teaching processes.
- Describe the domains of learning.
- Differentiate factors that determine readiness to learn from those that determine ability to learn.
- Compare the nursing and teaching processes.
- Write learning objectives for a teaching plan.
- Describe the characteristics of a good learning environment.
- Identify the principles of effective teaching.
- Describe ways to adapt teaching for clients with different learning needs.
- Describe ways to incorporate teaching with routine nursing care.
- Identify the methods for evaluating learning.

Client education will be one of your most important roles in nursing, regardless of the health care setting. Factors such as shorter hospital stays and the increased demand on nurses' time can complicate your ability to provide client education. As nurses try to find the most effective way to educate clients, health care consumers have become more assertive in seeking knowledge and understanding of their health and the resources available within the health care system. Providing your clients with needed information for self-care is necessary to ensure continuity of care from the hospital to the home (Chachkes and Christ, 1996). Client education is important because the client has a right to know and to be informed about diagnosis, prognosis, treatments, and risks. Creating a well-designed, comprehensive teaching plan that fits your client's learning needs can reduce health care costs, improve the quality of care, provide informed consent for treatments, and help clients to gain optimum wellness and increased independence.

STANDARDS FOR CLIENT EDUCATION

Accrediting agencies set guidelines for providing client education in health care institutions. These guidelines ensure that clients and their families receive information necessary to maintain the client's optimal level of health. In the United States, the Joint Commission on Accreditation of Healthcare Organizations (JCAHO) (2001) sets standards for client and family education (Box 9-1). All health care professionals must participate in client education to meet these standards. It is important to document evidence of successful client education in your client's medical record.

PURPOSES OF CLIENT EDUCATION

The goal of client education is to assist individuals, families, or communities in achieving optimal levels of health (Edelman and Mandle, 1998). In today's health care arena, clients know more about health and want to be involved in health maintenance. To meet this need, you need to provide education to clients in convenient and familiar places (e.g., in their homes, churches, or schools). Comprehensive client education includes three important purposes, each involving a separate phase of health care, which are detailed in the following sections.

Maintenance and Promotion of Health and Illness Prevention

Health care consumers have become more health conscious. Participation in regular exercise activities and in health-screening programs are examples of how people maintain their health. In the school, home, clinic, or workplace, information and skills are provided to clients to help them assume healthier behaviors (Box 9-2). For example, in childbearing classes, expectant parents learn about physical and psychological changes in the woman and about fetal development. After learning about normal childbearing, the mother is more likely to engage in physical exercise, and

---

JCAHO Patient and Family Education and Responsibilities   Box 9-1

PF.1   The hospital plans for and supports the provision and coordination of patient education activities.

PF.1.1   The hospital identifies and provides the resources necessary for achieving educational objectives.

PF.2   The patient education process is coordinated among appropriate staff or disciplines who are providing care or services.

PF.3   The patient receives education and training specific to the patient's assessed needs, abilities, learning preferences, and readiness to learn as appropriate to the care and services provided by the hospital.

PF.3.1   Based on assessed needs, the patient is educated about how to safely and effectively use medications, according to law and regulation, and the hospital's scope of services, as appropriate.

PF.3.2   The patient is educated about nutrition interventions, modified diets, or oral health, when applicable.

PF.3.3   The hospital assures that the patient is educated about how to safely and effectively use medical equipment or supplies, as appropriate.

PF.3.4   Patients are educated about pain and managing pain as part of treatment, as appropriate.*

PF.3.5   Patients are educated about habilitation or rehabilitation techniques to help them be more functionally independent, as appropriate.

PF.3.6   The patient is educated about other available resources, and when necessary, how to obtain further care, services, or treatment to meet his or her identified needs.

PF.3.7   Education includes information about patient responsibilities in the patient's care.

PF.3.8   Education includes self-care activities, as appropriate.

PF.3.9   Discharge instructions are given to the patient and those responsible for providing continuing care.

PF.3.10   Academic education is provided to children and adolescents either directly by the hospital or through other arrangements, when appropriate.

From Joint Commission on Accreditation of Healthcare Organizations: *Accreditation manual of hospitals,* Oakbrook Terrace, Ill, 2001, The Commission.
*Effective January 1, 2001.

---

the father is more likely to support the mother during her pregnancy.

The Internet has had a tremendous impact on the importance of client education. Today your clients have more access to information about their health. Regardless of the source of information, promoting healthful behavior through education increases self-esteem by encouraging your clients to assume more responsibility for health. When clients become more health conscious, they are more likely to seek early diagnosis of health problems (Redman, 2001).

Restoration of Health

Injured or ill clients need information or skills that will help them regain improved levels of health (see Box 9-2, p. 134). Clients recovering from illness or injury and adapting to resulting changes seek information about their health. However, clients who find it difficult to adapt to illness may become passive and uninterested in learn-

Topics for Health Education

Box 9-2

HEALTH MAINTENANCE AND PROMOTION AND ILLNESS PREVENTION
First aid
Avoidance of risk factors (e.g., smoking, alcohol)
Growth and development
Hygiene
Immunizations
Prenatal care and normal childbearing
Nutrition
Exercise
Safety (e.g., in home, car, workplace, hospital)
Screening (e.g., blood pressure, vision, cholesterol level)

RESTORATION OF HEALTH
Client's disease or condition
  Anatomy and physiology of body system affected
  Cause of disease
  Origin of symptoms
  Expected effects on other body systems
  Prognosis
  Limitations on function
  Rationale for treatment
  Medications
  Tests and therapies

RESTORATION OF HEALTH—cont'd
  Nursing measures
  Surgical intervention
  Expected duration of care
  Hospital or clinic environment
  Hospital or clinic staff
  Long-term care
  Methods for client participation in care

COPING WITH IMPAIRED FUNCTION
Home care
  Medications
  Diet
  Activity
  Self-help devices
Rehabilitation of remaining function
  Physical therapy
  Occupational therapy
  Speech therapy
Prevention of complications
  Knowledge of risk factors
  Implications of noncompliance with therapy
  Environmental alterations

---

ing. Identify the client's willingness to learn, and motivate the client to learn.

Family or friends are often a vital part of your client's return to health and may need to know as much as the client. When these individuals are excluded from a client's teaching plan, conflicts may arise. For example, if the family does not understand a client's need to regain independent function, their efforts may cause the client to become unnecessarily dependent and slow the client's recovery. However, for education to be successful, do not assume the family should be involved. Assess the client-family relationship before education begins.

Coping With Impaired Functioning

Not all clients fully recover from illness or injury. Many must learn to cope with permanent health changes. New knowledge and skills are often needed for clients to continue activities of daily living (see Box 9-2). For example, the client whose ability to speak is lost after surgery of the larynx learns new ways of communicating, and the client with severe heart disease learns about diet, medication, and exercise to reduce further heart damage.

In the case of serious disability, the client's role in the family or community may change. In these cases, family members and friends need to be supportive and accepting. The ability to provide support results from education, which begins as soon as the client's needs are identified and a willingness of family and friends to help is identified. Your client education may focus on assisting clients with health care management. This includes, for example, giving medications and baths and applying dressings. Adaptation to the additional emotional effects of these chronic conditions must

also be taught. If the client has no family or friends, or if no one is willing to help the client, you will need to make other arrangements for the client's continuing care based on the client's needs, such as referring the client to a long-term care facility or setting up multidisciplinary home care.

TEACHING AND LEARNING

It is impossible to separate **teaching** from **learning.** Teaching is an interactive process that promotes learning. It consists of a conscious and deliberate set of actions that helps individuals gain new knowledge or perform new skills (Redman, 2001). A teacher provides information that prompts the learner to engage in activities that lead to a desired change or health behavior.

Learning is the acquisition of new knowledge or skills through reinforced practice and experience. Generally teaching and learning begin when a person identifies a need for knowing or acquiring an ability to do something. Teaching is most effective when it responds to a learner's needs. The teacher identifies these needs by asking questions and determining the learner's interests. Interpersonal communication is essential for successful teaching.

Role of the Nurse in Teaching and Learning

You have many roles in the teaching and learning process. These roles include:

- Answering your client's questions
- Providing information based on your client's health needs or treatment plans
- Clarifying information from a variety of sources (e.g., physicians, newspapers, television, and the Internet)

Comparison of Terms Used in Teaching and Communication — Table 9-1

Communication	Teaching
Referent Idea that initiates reason for communication	Perceived need to provide person with information, establishment of relevant learning objectives by teacher
Sender Person who conveys message to another	Teacher who performs activities aimed at assisting other person to learn
Intrapersonal Variables (Sender) Knowledge, values, emotions, and sociocultural influences that affect senders' thoughts	Teacher's philosophy of education (based on learning theory), knowledge of teaching content, teaching approach, experiences in teaching, emotions, and values
Message Information expressed or transmitted by sender	Content or information taught
Channels Methods used to transmit message (visual, auditory, touch)	Methods used to present content (visual and auditory materials, touch, taste, smell)
Receiver Person to whom message is transmitted	Learner
Intrapersonal Variables (Receiver) Knowledge, values, emotions, and sociocultural influences that affect receiver's thoughts	Willingness and ability to learn (physical and emotional health, education, experience, developmental level)
Feedback Information revealing that true meaning of message was received	Determination of whether learning objectives were achieved

To be an effective educator, you must engage the client as a partner in learning and not merely pass on facts (Hinchliff, 1999). Carefully determine what your clients need to know and find the time when they are ready to learn. When client education is valued and implemented, clients can become better prepared to assume health care responsibilities. The relationship between client education and favorable client outcomes is important in nursing. For example, children with asthma must learn to use inhalers correctly to prevent respiratory distress. By including the child and by tailoring your educational approach based on the child's developmental level and previous experience with inhalers, you can help the child control the disease, have improved self-esteem, and remain out of the acute care setting.

TEACHING AS COMMUNICATION

The teaching process closely parallels the communication process (see Chapter 8). Effective teaching depends in part on the effectiveness of your communication skills. A teacher applies each element of the communication process while giving information to learners. Thus the teacher and learner become involved in a teaching process that increases the learner's knowledge and skills.

The steps of the teaching process can be compared with those of the communication process (Table 9-1). In teaching, you need to provide the client with information. Either you or the client may identify the educational need. Then, specific learning objectives are identified. A **learning objective** describes what the client will be able to do after successful instruction.

You are the sender who wants to convey a message to the client. Learning is promoted by communicating in a language recognized by the client. Many interpersonal variables influence your style and approach. Attitudes, values, cultural preferences, emotions, and knowledge influence the way you send messages (Hinchliff, 1999). Evaluating past experiences with teaching will help you choose the best way to present information.

Deliver the content clearly and precisely. Organize your information in a logical sequence so that your client will easily understand the skills or ideas. Each lesson progresses from the simple to the more complex skills or ideas (Houston and Haire-Joshu, 1996).

You can teach your client in a variety of ways. All the senses are channels for presenting information. The auditory channel is the simplest, as in a lecture or discussion. The learning process becomes more active and stimulating when you use visual and psychomotor channels as well.

The receiver in the teaching-learning process is the learner. Interpersonal variables affect your client's willingness and ability to learn. Language, attitudes, anxiety, cultural preferences, and values influence the ability to understand a message. The ability to learn depends on emotional and physical health, stage of development, and previous knowledge.

To be an effective teacher, you must also have a method to evaluate the success of a teaching plan. **Return demonstration** is a good form of feedback. The learner restates the received information or demonstrates learned skills, which allows you to assess the success of learning.

DOMAINS OF LEARNING

Learning occurs in the cognitive (understanding), affective (values), and psychomotor (motor skills) domains. Any topic to be learned may involve all domains or only one. You will work with clients who need to learn in each domain.

Cognitive learning includes all intellectual behaviors such as the acquisition of knowledge, comprehension (ability to understand), application (using abstract ideas in concrete situations), analysis (relating ideas in an organized way), synthesis (recognizing parts of information as a whole), and evaluation (judging the worth of a body of information).

Affective learning deals with the expression of feelings related to attitudes, opinions, or values. The learner receives the information, responds to the information and the teacher, values the worth of the teacher and the information, organizes values, and responds with a consistent value system.

Psychomotor learning involves acquiring skills that require the integration of mental and motor activity such as the ability to walk, to use an eating utensil, or to give an insulin injection. Guide the learner's response, leading to the confidence to perform the desired behavior in gradually more complex ways. Adaptation occurs when your client can change a response when unexpected problems arise. This results in originating, which involves creating new patterns of behavior.

Teaching your client a specific behavior often involves incorporating behaviors from all three learning domains. A client being taught the proper method of giving an injection must first understand the reasons injections are needed and then must know the proper location for administering the injection and the importance of using sterile technique (cognitive). The techniques of locating an acceptable area on the skin and introducing the needle use the senses of touch and vision (psychomotor). In addition, the client must be willing to accept the need for injections and must overcome any fear of or distaste for injections (affective).

BASIC LEARNING PRINCIPLES

To teach effectively and efficiently, you must first understand how people learn. Learning depends on the motivation to learn, the ability to learn, and the learning environment. The ability to learn depends on physical and cognitive attributes, one's developmental level, physical wellness, and intellectual thought processes. The environment also affects the ability to learn. You must manipulate environmental conditions to facilitate client learning.

Motivation to Learn

Motivation is an internal impulse (e.g., an idea, an emotion, or a physical need) that causes a person to take action and addresses a person's desire to learn (Redman, 2001). Previous knowledge, attitudes, and sociocultural factors influence motivation. If a person does not want to learn, it is unlikely that learning will occur. Often client motives are physical. A client with a physical change in function may be motivated to learn strategies to help adapt to the functional change. For example, a client with a lower limb amputation may be motivated to learn to ambulate with a prosthesis.

An **attentional set** is the mental state that allows the learner to focus on and comprehend the material. People often use mental pictures to visualize ideas. Before learning anything, clients must give attention to, or concentrate on, the information to be learned. Physical discomfort, anxiety, and environmental distractions can influence the ability to attend. Any physical condition that impairs your client's ability to concentrate (e.g., pain, fatigue, or hunger) interferes with learning. Assess your client for factors that diminish attention before beginning a teaching plan. Verbal and nonverbal cues can reveal that your client is not ready to learn.

Anxiety may increase or decrease the ability of a person to pay attention. Anxiety is uneasiness or uncertainty resulting from anticipating a threat or danger. When faced with change or the need to act differently, your client may feel anxious. Learning requires a change in behavior and thus produces anxiety. A mild level of anxiety may motivate learning. However, a high level of anxiety prevents learning from taking place. It incapacitates a person, creating an inability to attend to anything other than relieving the anxiety.

Your client's **health beliefs** are powerful motivators and are influenced by a number of variables (see Chapter 1). Know your client's health beliefs to determine the factors that will motivate learning. Your client's view of health may not be congruent with your view of health.

In addition, health teaching often involves changing attitudes and values that cannot be altered by simply teaching facts. Therefore assess your client's view of health, motivation to learn, and what knowledge is needed to adhere to the prescribed therapy. You must also include beliefs that motivate your client to learn in the teaching plan. For example, if your client is a busy executive with high blood pressure, you could use the client's desire to succeed and the concern that illness will impair work to motivate behavioral change. To facilitate successful teaching, the motivating factor should be stressed and encouraged for several months after the initial teaching intervention.

Learning is also enhanced when clients are actively involved in the educational session (Edelman and Mandle, 1998). A client's involvement in learning implies an eagerness to acquire knowledge or skills and allows the client to make decisions during teaching sessions. For example, a client with diabetes learns to monitor blood glucose levels to gain control of the disease. Assist the client in choosing a blood glucose meter and adapting a monitoring system and schedule to personal lifestyle patterns (Figure 9-1).

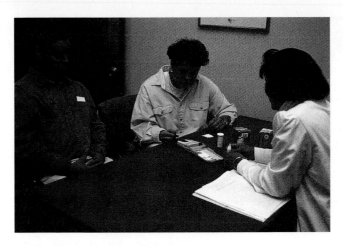

FIGURE **9-1**   Nurse instructing a client with a glucose meter. (Courtesy Steve Frazier, Barnes-Jewish Hospital, St. Louis.)

READINESS TO LEARN.   Readiness to learn is significant. Your clients cannot learn when they are unwilling or unable to accept the reality of illness. A temporary or permanent loss of health is difficult for clients to accept. The stages of grieving (see Chapter 22) encompass a series of responses clients experience during illness. People experience these stages at different rates. It is important for you to properly time client teaching to facilitate your client's adjustment to illness or disability (Table 9-2). Introduce the teaching plan when your client enters the stage of acceptance, which is most compatible with learning.

Ability to Learn

The ability to learn is influenced by your client's developmental level and physical capabilities. You must consider these important factors in developing an effective teaching plan.

DEVELOPMENTAL CAPABILITY.   Cognitive development influences your client's ability to learn. Learning occurs more readily when new information complements existing knowledge. Therefore your client's stage of development and intellectual abilities must be considered for teaching to be successful. For example, if teaching booklets and brochures are shared with a client who cannot read, the information provided is not helpful to the client. Learning, like developmental growth, is an evolving process. Assess the client's level of knowledge and intellectual skills before beginning a teaching plan. For example, reading a medication label or instructions in a teaching booklet requires reading and comprehension skills.

AGE-GROUP.   Age reflects the developmental capability for learning and learning behaviors that can be acquired. Without proper biological, motor, language, and personal-social development, many types of learning cannot take place (see Chapter 18). Learning occurs when behavior changes as a result of experience or growth (Wong and others, 1999). Box 9-3 summarizes teaching methods to adapt based on a client's developmental level.

PHYSICAL CAPABILITY.   The ability to learn often depends on a person's level of physical development and overall physical health. To learn psychomotor skills, your client must have the necessary level of strength, coordination, and sensory acuity. For example, it would be useless for you to teach your client to transfer from a bed to a wheelchair if there is insufficient upper body strength. Therefore you should not overestimate the client's physical abilities. The following physical attributes are required to learn psychomotor skills:

1. Size (height and weight that match the task to be performed or the equipment to be used [e.g., crutch walking])
2. Strength (ability of the client to follow strenuous exercise program)
3. Coordination (dexterity needed for complicated motor skills such as using utensils or changing a bandage)
4. Sensory acuity (visual, auditory, tactile, gustatory, and olfactory: sensory resources needed to receive and respond to messages taught)

Any condition (e.g., pain) that depletes a person's energy will also impair the ability to learn. For example, when an illness becomes aggravated by complications such as a high fever or respiratory difficulty, teaching should be postponed. After working with your client, assess the client's energy level by noting the client's willingness to communicate, amount of activity initiated, and responsiveness toward questions. You may stop teaching temporarily when your client needs rest. You should resume teaching when your client is rested and free of pain.

Learning Environment

Factors in the physical environment where teaching takes place can make learning a pleasant or difficult experience. Choose a setting that helps your client focus attention on the learning task. The number of persons being taught, need for privacy, room temperature, room lighting, noise, room ventilation, and room furniture are important considerations when choosing the setting.

The ideal environment for promoting learning is a room that has good lighting and ventilation, appropriate furniture, and a comfortable temperature (Figure 9-2). A darkened room interferes with the client's ability to see the demonstration of a skill or visual aids such as posters or pamphlets. A room that is too cold, hot, or stuffy will make the client too uncomfortable to pay attention to you. Comfortable furniture helps to eliminate distractions such as the need to change position or shift body weight.

It is also important for you to choose a quiet setting that offers privacy and where interruptions are infrequent. If your client desires, family members might share in discussions. However, the client may be reluctant to discuss the nature of the illness when other persons, even family members, are in the room.

Teaching a group of clients requires a room that allows all persons to be seated comfortably and within hearing distance of the teacher. The size of the room should not over-

Relationship Between Psychosocial Adaptation to Illness and Learning   Table 9-2

Stage	Client's Behavior	Learning Implications	Rationale
Denial or disbelief	Client avoids discussion of illness ("There's nothing wrong with me") and disregards physical restrictions. Client suppresses and distorts information that has not been presented clearly.	Provide support, empathy, and careful explanations of all procedures while they are being done. Let client know you are available for discussion. Explain situation to family. Teach in present tense (explain current therapy).	Client is not prepared to deal with problem. Any attempt to convince or tell client about illness will result in further anger or withdrawal. Provide only information client pursues or absolutely requires.
Anger	Client blames and complains and often directs anger at nurse.	Do not argue with client, but listen to concerns. Teach in present tense. Reassure family of client's normality.	Client needs opportunity to express feelings and anger. Client is still not prepared to face future.
Bargaining	Client offers to live better life in exchange for promise of better health ("If God lets me live, I promise to be more careful").	Continue to introduce only reality. Teach only in present tense.	Client is still unwilling to accept limitations.
Resolution	Client begins to express emotions openly, realizes that illness has created changes, and begins to ask questions.	Encourage expression of feelings. Begin to share information needed for future, and set aside formal times for discussion.	Client begins to perceive need for assistance and is ready to accept responsibility for learning.
Acceptance	Client recognizes reality of condition, actively pursues information, and strives for independence.	Focus teaching on future skills and knowledge required. Continue to teach about present occurrences. Involve family in teaching information for discharge.	Client is more easily motivated to learn. Acceptance of illness reflects willingness to deal with its implications.

Teaching Methods Based on Client's Developmental Capacity   Box 9-3

INFANT
Keep routines (e.g., feeding, bathing) consistent.

Hold infant firmly while smiling and speaking softly to convey sense of trust.

Have infant touch different textures (e.g., soft fabric, hard plastic).

TODDLER
Use play to teach procedure or activity (e.g., handling examination equipment, applying bandage to doll).

Offer picture books that describe story of children in hospital or clinic.

Use simple words such as *cut* instead of *laceration* to promote understanding.

PRESCHOOLER
Use role playing, imitation, and play to make it fun for preschoolers to learn.

Encourage questions and offer explanations. Use simple explanations and demonstrations.

Encourage children to learn together through pictures and short stories about how to perform hygiene.

SCHOOL-AGE CHILD
Teach psychomotor skills needed to maintain health. (Complicated skills, such as learning to use a syringe, may take considerable practice.)

SCHOOL-AGE CHILD—cont'd
Offer opportunities to discuss health problems and answer questions.

ADOLESCENT
Help adolescent learn about feelings and need for self-expression.

Use teaching as collaborative activity.

Allow adolescents to make decisions about health and health promotion (safety, sex education, substance abuse).

Use problem solving to help adolescents make choices.

YOUNG OR MIDDLE ADULT
Encourage participation in teaching plan by setting mutual goals.

Encourage independent learning.

Offer information so that adult can understand effects of health problem.

OLDER ADULT
Teach when client is alert and rested.

Involve adult in discussion or activity.

Focus on wellness and the person's strength.

Use approaches that enhance sensorially impaired client's reception of stimuli (see Chapter 35).

Keep teaching sessions short.

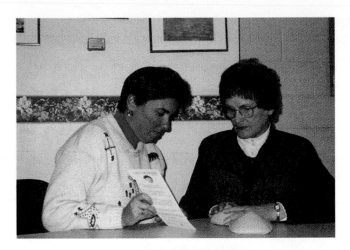

FIGURE 9-2 Choosing comfortable, pleasant environments enhances the learning experience. The nurse is explaining the breast self-examination procedure to the client.

whelm the group, tempting participants to sit outside the group along the perimeter. Arranging the group to allow participants to observe one another further enhances learning. More effective communication occurs as learners observe others' verbal and nonverbal interactions.

INTEGRATING THE NURSING AND TEACHING PROCESSES

There are distinct comparisons between the nursing process and the teaching process. During the nursing process, assessment reveals your client's health care needs. The nursing diagnoses identified are unique to your client's situation. You develop an individualized plan of care with appropriate interventions that are implemented. Evaluation determines the level of success in meeting goals of care.

While assessing and diagnosing your client's health care problems, you may identify the need for education. When education becomes a part of the care plan, the teaching process begins. Like the nursing process, the teaching process requires assessment; in this case it requires you to analyze the client's need, motivation, and ability to learn (Table 9-3). A diagnostic statement specifies the information or skills your client requires. Specific learning objectives are set, and the teaching plan is implemented, using teaching and learning principles to ensure that your client acquires knowledge and skills. Finally, the teaching process requires an evaluation of learning based on learning objectives.

The nursing and teaching processes are not the same. The nursing process requires assessment of all sources of data to determine a client's total health care needs, whereas the teaching process focuses on the client's learning needs, resources, and willingness and ability to learn.

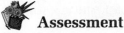 **Assessment**

Assessment brings the scope of a teaching plan into focus. Successful client teaching requires that you assess the client's learning needs to determine teaching content (Redman, 2001). Other factors that influence relevant content include learning resources and the client's ability and willingness to learn. A thorough assessment will help you choose the best teaching methods and ensures a more individualized approach toward client education.

LEARNING NEEDS.   Together, you and your client identify information critical for the client to learn. Questions such as "What do you believe is important for you to know to care for yourself?" allow the client to be an active participant in planning self-care. Learning needs may change depending on where your client is in the recovery process. Assessment of learning needs is an ongoing activity. Some examples of key areas of assessment are (1) questions raised by the client or family about health issues; (2) the client's level of understanding of current health status, implications of illness, types of therapy, and prognosis; (3) information or skills needed to perform self-care; (4) experiences that influence the client's need to learn; and (5) information necessary for family members to support the client's needs.

MOTIVATION TO LEARN.   Ask questions that identify your client's motivation to learn. These questions help determine whether the client is prepared and willing to learn. Ask questions that relate to the client's learning behaviors, health beliefs, attitudes about health care providers, knowledge of information to be learned, physical symptoms that interfere with learning (e.g., fatigue, pain, or dizziness), sociocultural background, and learning-style preference.

ABILITY TO LEARN.   Determine the client's physical and cognitive levels. Many factors can impair the ability to learn. You need to assess the client's physical strength and coordination, any sensory deficits, the client's reading and developmental level (see Box 9-3), and the client's level of cognitive functioning (Chapter 18).

TEACHING ENVIRONMENT.   Create an environment for a teaching session that is conducive to learning. Assess for distractions, noise, the client's comfort level, and the availability of rooms and equipment. In the home setting, lighting, space, and equipment availability are especially important to assess.

RESOURCES FOR LEARNING.   Identify resources for learning, which may include the support of family members or significant others. In these cases, you must assess the readiness of family and friends to learn any information necessary to help care for the client. Family perceptions of the client's illness, the client's willingness to involve family members in care, the family's willingness to help provide care, resources available in the home, and needed teaching tools must also be determined. Ensure that available teaching resources such as brochures, audiovisual materials, and posters are available when needed and that the most appropriate teaching tool for the client's needs and ability to learn

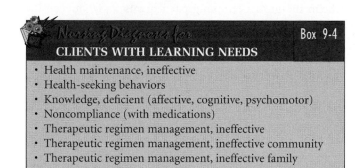

Comparison of the Nursing and Teaching Processes		Table 9-3
Basic Steps	Nursing Process	Teaching Process
Assessment	Collect data about client's physical, psychological, social, cultural, developmental, and spiritual needs from client, family, diagnostic tests, medical record, nursing history, and literature.	Gather data about client's learning needs, motivation, ability to learn, and teaching resources from client, family, learning environment, medical record, nursing history, and literature.
Nursing diagnosis	Identify appropriate nursing diagnoses.	Identify client's learning needs on basis of three domains of learning.
Planning	Develop individualized care plan. Set diagnosis priorities based on client's immediate needs. Collaborate with client on care plan.	Establish learning objectives, stated in behavioral terms. Identify priorities regarding learning needs. Collaborate with client on teaching plan. Identify type of teaching method to use.
Implementation	Perform nursing care therapies. Include client as active participant in care. Involve family in care as appropriate.	Implement teaching methods. Actively involve client in learning activities. Include family participation as appropriate.
Evaluation	Identify success in meeting desired outcomes and goals of nursing care.	Determine outcomes of teaching-learning process. Measure client's ability to achieve learning objectives. Reteach as needed.

is selected. Written materials should be assessed for reading level. There are computer programs designed to facilitate this task. Also, organizations such as a literacy council can be of great assistance.

CULTURAL CONSIDERATIONS. Assess the language the client most commonly uses. Brochures should be written in your client's native language. The client's role in the family and how illness is perceived culturally must be determined. You must also explore the significance of prescribed medications and therapies in the client's culture and explore alternative therapies the client uses. Teaching that does not include cultural considerations is ineffective.

Nursing Diagnosis

After assessing information related to your client's ability and need to learn, interpret the data to form diagnoses that reflect the client's specific learning needs (Box 9-4). This ensures that teaching will be goal directed and individualized. If a client has several learning needs, nursing diagnoses allow for priority setting.

Several nursing diagnoses apply to learning needs. Each diagnostic statement describes the specific type of learning need and its cause. Classifying diagnoses by the three learning domains helps you focus specifically on the subject matter and teaching methods.

Some health care problems can be managed or eliminated through education. In these situations, the related factor of the diagnostic statement is *knowledge, deficient.* For example, your client may not be taking a medication at the appropriate time because of a lack of understanding about how the medication works.

Some nursing diagnoses may indicate that barriers to learning exist (e.g., *pain* and *activity intolerance*). In these cases, teaching is delayed until the nursing diagnosis is resolved or the health problem is controlled.

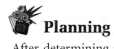

Nursing Diagnoses for	Box 9-4
CLIENTS WITH LEARNING NEEDS	

- Health maintenance, ineffective
- Health-seeking behaviors
- Knowledge, deficient (affective, cognitive, psychomotor)
- Noncompliance (with medications)
- Therapeutic regimen management, ineffective
- Therapeutic regimen management, ineffective community
- Therapeutic regimen management, ineffective family

Planning

After determining nursing diagnoses that identify a client's learning needs, develop a teaching plan. The plan includes topics for instruction, teaching resources (e.g., equipment or booklets), recommendations for involving family, and objectives. The setting may influence the complexity of the plan. No matter what the length, the teaching plan should provide continuity of instruction, especially when several nurses or disciplines are collaborating in educating the client.

It is very important that you establish clear goals and measurable outcomes so that client education is effectively evaluated and modified as needed. Expected outcomes guide the choice of teaching strategies and who is involved in the plan. Client participation ensures a more relevant and meaningful plan (see care plan). In many situations, the client's family should be included in the teaching plan. For example, a client with a spinal cord injury who needs to know how to perform self–urinary catheterization may need assistance with this procedure at home. In this case, it would be appropriate to include family members and other possible caregivers in the educational plan.

Clients receive education in multiple health care settings. Your responsibility is to identify the client's learning needs and to refer the client to appropriate multidisciplinary health care providers. For example, you should refer a client

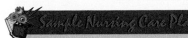

Sample Nursing Care Plan

ASSESSMENT

Mrs. Fairchild is being prepared for her abdominal hysterectomy scheduled for today. You assess Mrs. Fairchild's knowledge of the surgery and what she can expect postoperatively. Mrs. Fairchild's medical record reflects that she attended the prehysterectomy course offered at the medical center. Although she has a good understanding of why she must have the surgery, Mrs. Fairchild states **she cannot remember all the details about what is expected of her after surgery.** She is **moderately anxious and is verbalizing questions about her activity level postoperatively.** In addition, she is **unable to verbalize** how to cough and deep breathe.

*Defining characteristics are shown in bold type.

NURSING DIAGNOSIS

Knowledge, deficient (cognitive) regarding postoperative care related to lack of recall of information.

PLANNING

GOAL

Mrs. Fairchild will describe routine postoperative care before her surgery.

Mrs. Fairchild will participate in postoperative surgical care during her hospitalization.

EXPECTED OUTCOMES

Mrs. Fairchild will verbalize what to expect during the postoperative period, including pain management, monitoring of vaginal discharge, progression of diet, and activity level with related rationale before her surgery.

Mrs. Fairchild will explain the importance of and will demonstrate how to cough and deep breathe before her surgery.

Mrs. Fairchild will cough and deep breathe and increase her activity level appropriately after her surgery.

IMPLEMENTATION

STEPS

1. Determine readiness to learn and learning needs.

2. Describe anticipated routine postoperative care with rationale, including pain management, progression of diet, monitoring vaginal discharge and expected activity level. Allow client to see and touch patient-controlled analgesia pump.

3. Explain, demonstrate, and have client perform return demonstration of coughing and deep breathing.

4. Make follow-up phone call 48 hours after discharge to answer questions and reinforce instructions.

RATIONALE

Client must demonstrate readiness to learn, and information must be perceived as important for the adult to learn effectively (Fox, 1998).

Providing structured information about postoperative procedures and allowing clients to see and touch equipment before surgery enhances learning and decreases anxiety. Understanding the importance of care enhances compliance with postoperative routine (Redman, 2001).

Using role modeling and having the client perform behaviors enhances healthy behaviors (Bandura, 1997).

Repetition and learning information over time will enhance the client's understanding (Redman, 2001).

EVALUATION

- Have client describe routine postoperative care.
- Observe client as she demonstrates coughing and deep breathing.
- Assess level of pain, anxiety, and progression of activity level and diet postoperatively.
- Observe client's verbal and nonverbal behavior before and after surgery.

---

with a new diagnosis of chronic renal failure to a dietitian for dietary considerations. Clients in acute care settings often require assistance from discharge planners, case managers, and community agencies to be successfully discharged. It is your responsibility to collaborate with and include these multidisciplinary health care team members in the teaching plan.

Clients are also members of communities. Teaching plans often include information necessary to assist clients in returning to their communities as functioning members. Therefore, you must also consider the client's community when planning an educational session. For example, when teaching transfer techniques to the client with the spinal cord injury, you may need to include how the client will transfer onto and off of public transportation that is available in the client's community.

SETTING PRIORITIES. Learning objectives identify the expected outcomes of a planned learning experience, which help establish priorities for learning. Learning needs must be prioritized based on your client's nursing diagnoses, needs, and previous knowledge. In most situations it is inappropriate to delegate educational interventions to assistive personnel. You are ultimately responsible for ensuring that all teaching needs have been met. Therefore you will need to determine and prioritize what the client needs to know. Usually, teaching needs focused on client safety issues are the most important. For example, a client with newly diagnosed hypertension and angina needs to learn about newly prescribed medications, which include nitroglycerine spray for angina and a calcium channel blocker. In this situation, knowledge regarding the early identification of chest pain and appropriate use of the nitroglycerine spray is the learning priority.

Learning objectives are either short term (relating to immediate learning needs) or long term (relating to permanent adaptation to a health problem). You and the client should develop learning objectives together. Each objective is a statement of a single behavior that identifies the client's ability to do something after a learning experience. The objective contains an active verb describing what the learner will do after the objective is met, such as perform a crutch gait, administer an injection, or identify drug doses. The verb should have few interpretations and be stated in terms of how the client is to demonstrate learning (Redman, 2001).

Behavioral objectives are measurable and observable, indicating how learning is evidenced (e.g., to perform the three-point crutch gait) and describing the conditions or timing under which the behavior occurs. Conditions or time frames should be realistic and designed for the learner's needs. It helps to consider the conditions under which the client or family will typically perform the learned behavior (e.g., to walk from bedroom to bath using crutches).

Criteria for acceptable performance set a standard by which achievement is measured. Set criteria on the basis of a desired level of accuracy, success, or satisfaction. For example, a client undergoing therapy for a fractured leg will walk on crutches to the end of the hall within 3 days. You and the client use these criteria for self-evaluation, which is a powerful motivator of behavior.

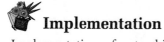

Implementation

Implementation of a teaching plan involves applying all teaching and learning principles. Implementation involves believing that each interaction with a client is an opportunity to teach. Maximize opportunities for effective learning, and create an active learning environment. Because learning situations vary, there is no single correct way to teach. The principles of teaching are, in effect, techniques that incorporate the principles of learning.

TIMING.   When is the right time to teach? When a client first enters a clinic or hospital? At discharge? At home? Each may be appropriate because clients continue to have learning needs and opportunities as long as they stay in the health care system. Plan to teach when the client is most attentive, receptive, and alert. The frequency of sessions depends on the learner's abilities and the complexity of the material.

The length of teaching sessions also affects learning. Prolonged sessions cause clients to lose concentration and attentiveness, especially older adult clients. Frequent sessions lasting 20 to 30 minutes are more easily tolerated and retain the client's interest in the material. Nonverbal cues, such as

poor eye contact or slumped posture, indicate a client's loss of concentration. After loss of concentration is noted, the session should be stopped.

ORGANIZING TEACHING MATERIAL.   Give careful consideration to the order of information presented. An outline of content helps to organize information into a logical sequence. Material should progress from simple to complex ideas because a person must learn simple facts and concepts before learning how to make associations or complex interpretations of ideas. For example, to teach a woman how to feed her husband who has a gastric tube, first teach the wife how to measure the tube feeding and how to manipulate the equipment. Once this is accomplished, teach her how to administer the feeding.

Because clients are more likely to remember information taught in the beginning of a teaching session, present essential information first. Informative but less critical content should follow the essential information. Other interventions that reinforce learning include using repetition and summarizing key points (Murphy and Davis, 1997).

TEACHING APPROACHES.   To be a successful teacher, choose a teaching approach that matches your client's needs. A client's learning needs may change over time. Therefore, teaching approaches may need to be modified as you care for the client over time.

TELLING.   The telling approach is useful when limited information must be taught (e.g., when preparing the client for an emergent diagnostic procedure). When this approach is used, the task to be done by the client is outlined and explicit instructions are given. There is no time for feedback with this method.

SELLING.   The selling approach uses two-way communication. Instruction is based on the client's response. Specific feedback is given to the client who shows success at learning. For example, the client learns a step-by-step procedure for changing a dressing. Information from the client is used to adapt the teaching approach.

PARTICIPATING.   The participating approach involves you and the client in setting objectives and participating in the learning process together. The client helps decide content, and you guide and counsel the client. For example, a parent with a child diagnosed with sickle cell disease works with you to manage the child's pain. In this method there is opportunity for discussion, feedback, and revision of the teaching plan.

ENTRUSTING.   The entrusting approach provides the client the opportunity to manage self-care. The client accepts responsibilities and performs the tasks well, while you observe the client's progress and remain available for assistance. For example, a client who is receiving continuous intravenous pain medication at home for end-stage cancer requires a higher dose of pain medication. The client understands the dosage of the medication and how the medication pump works. You help the client determine an appropriate new pain medication dosage and allow the client to adjust the settings on the medication pump.

REINFORCING. The principle of **reinforcement** applies to the process of learning. The teacher is often the source of reinforcement. Reinforcement is using a stimulus that increases the probability of a response. A learner who receives reinforcement before or after a desired learning behavior will likely repeat the behavior. Feedback is a common form of reinforcement.

Reinforcers are positive or negative. Positive reinforcement such as a smile or praise and approval produces the desired responses. Although negative reinforcement (e.g., frowning) may work, people usually respond better to positive reinforcement.

Three types of reinforcers are social, material, and activity. Most reinforcers are social (e.g., smiles, compliments, words of encouragement, or physical contact), which are used to acknowledge a learned behavior. Examples of material reinforcers are food, toys, and music. These work best with young children. Activity reinforcers rely on the principle that a person is motivated to engage in an activity if promised that, after its completion, the opportunity to engage in more desirable activity will be available. For example, a client will more likely perform painful physical therapy exercises if given the chance to rest afterward.

Choosing an appropriate reinforcer involves careful thought and attention to individual preferences. Reinforcers should never be used as threats. Reinforcement is not always effective with every client.

INCORPORATING TEACHING WITH NURSING CARE. You can teach effectively while delivering nursing care. For example, you might choose to educate your client on the actions of medications while you are administering them. When you follow a teaching plan informally, your client feels less pressure to perform and learning becomes more of a shared activity. Teaching during routine care is efficient and cost-effective.

TEACHING METHODS. Active participation is a key to learning. By actively experiencing a learning event, the person is more likely to retain knowledge. A teaching method is the way you deliver information and is based on the client's learning needs (Box 9-5). The instructional method you choose depends on the time available for teaching, the setting, the resources available, and your comfort level with teaching. Skilled teachers are flexible and combine more than one method into a teaching plan.

ONE-ON-ONE DISCUSSION. When teaching a client at the bedside, in a physician's office, or in the home, information is shared through one-on-one discussion. Information is provided informally, allowing the client to ask questions or share concerns. Various teaching aids can be used during the discussion, depending on the client's learning needs.

Teaching Methods Based on Client's Learning Needs   Box 9-5

COGNITIVE
Discussion (One-on-One or Group)
May involve nurse and client or nurse with several clients
Promotes active participation and focuses on topics of interest to client
Allows peer support
Enhances application and analysis of new information

Lecture
Is more formal method of instruction because it is controlled by teacher
Helps learner acquire new knowledge and gain comprehension

Question-and-Answer Session
Is designed specifically to address client's concerns
Assists client in applying knowledge

Role Play, Discovery
Allows client to actively apply knowledge in controlled situation
Promotes synthesis of information and problem solving

Independent Project (Computer-Assisted Instruction), Field Experience
Allows client to assume responsibility for completing learning activities at own pace
Promotes analysis, synthesis, and evaluation of new information and skills

AFFECTIVE
Role Play
Allows expression of values, feelings, and attitudes

AFFECTIVE—cont'd
Discussion (Group)
Allows client to acquire support from others in group
Permits client to learn from others' experiences
Promotes responding, valuing, and organization

Discussion (One-on-One)
Allows discussion of personal, sensitive topics of interest or concern

PSYCHOMOTOR
Demonstration
Provides presentation of procedures or skills by nurse
Permits client to incorporate modeling of nurse's behavior
Allows nurse to control questioning during demonstration

Practice
Gives client opportunity to perform skills using equipment
Provides repetition

Return Demonstration
Permits client to perform skills as nurse observes
Is excellent source of feedback and reinforcement

Independent Project, Game
Requires teaching method that promotes adaptation and origination of psychomotor learning
Permits learner to use new skills

GROUP INSTRUCTION.   Group instruction is used because groups offer an economical way to teach a number of clients at one time, and often the experience of being part of a group may provide the support necessary for clients to meet learning objectives (Redman, 2001). Group instruction may involve both lecture and discussion. Lectures are efficient in helping groups of clients learn standard content about a subject. After hearing information from a lecture, learners need the opportunity to share ideas and seek clarification. Group discussions allow clients and families to learn from each other as they review common experiences (Redman, 2001).

PREPARATORY INSTRUCTION.   Clients frequently face unfamiliar tests or procedures that create anxiety. Providing information about procedures helps clients form realistic images of what to anticipate. The following are guidelines for giving preparatory explanations:

1. Physical sensations during the procedure are described but not evaluated. When drawing a blood specimen, explain that the client will feel a sticking sensation as the needle punctures the skin.
2. The cause of the sensation is described, preventing misinterpretation of the experience. Explain that a needle insertion burns because alcohol used to cleanse the skin enters the puncture site.
3. Clients are prepared only for aspects of the experience that have commonly been noticed by other clients. Explain that it is normal for a tight tourniquet to cause a person's hand to tingle and feel numb.

The client finds comfort in knowing what to expect. When preparatory instructions accurately portray the actual experience, the client is able to cope more effectively with the stress from procedures and therapies (Redman, 2001).

DEMONSTRATIONS.   Demonstrations are useful methods for teaching psychomotor skills. An effective demonstration requires advance planning, including the following:

1. Assemble and organize equipment.
2. Perform each step in sequence while analyzing the knowledge and skills involved.
3. Determine when explanations need to be given, considering the client's learning needs.
4. Judge the proper speed and timing of the demonstration, based on the client's cognitive abilities and anxiety level.

Demonstrate the procedure or skill in the same order in which the client will perform it. Encourage the client to ask questions so that each step is clearly understood. To enable the client to easily observe each step of the procedure, demonstrations should be performed slowly, avoiding a hurried approach. Give the client the opportunity to practice the procedure under supervision. Ultimately the client demonstrates the procedure independently to ensure acquisition of the skill. This demonstration should occur under the same conditions that the client will experience at home.

ANALOGIES.   Learning occurs when a teacher translates complex language or ideas into words or concepts that the client understands. **Analogies** supplement verbal instruction with familiar images that make complex information more real and understandable (Redman, 2001). For example, comparing arterial blood pressure to the flow of water through a hose is an analogy that might be useful when explaining hypertension to a client. When using analogies, you must be familiar with the concept; be aware of the client's background, experience, and culture; and keep the analogy simple and clear.

ROLE PLAYING.   Role play is used to teach ideas and attitudes. An example might include teaching family caregivers better ways of communicating with older adult parents. The technique involves rehearsing a desired behavior, and as a result, clients are taught required skills and feel more confident in performing them independently.

DISCOVERY.   Discovery is a useful technique for teaching problem solving, application, and independent thinking. During individual or group discussion a problem or situation pertaining to the clients' learning needs is presented for clients to solve. For example, clients with heart disease may be asked to plan a meal low in cholesterol.

MAINTAINING ATTENTION AND PARTICIPATION.   Your actions can also increase learner attention and participation. When conducting a discussion with a client, change the tone and intensity of your voice, make eye contact, and use gestures that accentuate key points of discussion. A learner remains interested in a teacher who is actively enthusiastic about the subject under discussion (Hinchliff, 1999).

THE PROBLEM OF ILLITERACY.   The National Adult Literacy Survey, conducted in the United States, found that 40 to 44 million Americans could not read or write and another 50 million Americans had only marginal reading skills. Although illiteracy existed among all races, African-American, American Indian/Alaska Native, Hispanic, and Asian/Pacific Islander adults were more likely to be illiterate than white adults (National Center for Education Statistics, 1996). Low literacy may decrease compliance with health instructions, interfere with the ability to provide informed consent, increase the frequency of hospitalizations, and have an overall negative impact on the client's health status (American Medical Association, 1999). A significant problem for health care providers is **functional illiteracy.** Clients who are functionally illiterate are able to find ways to hide their inability to read (Brooks, 1998). Therefore you must carefully assess your client's ability to read before providing client education.

To compound the problem of illiteracy, the readability of health education material has been found to range from elementary school level to college level (Wilson, 1996; Duffy and Snyder, 1999). Thus it appears that written health information available to a client often exceeds the client's reading ability. Box 9-6 provides interventions you may use when teaching the illiterate client.

CULTURAL VARIABLES.   Health education materials often fail to recognize cultural beliefs, values, language, per-

Client Teaching Strategies for the Illiterate Client   Box 9-6

- Use simple words the client can understand.
- Use the active voice when providing instructions (e.g., tell client to "take medication before bedtime" instead of "medication should be taken at bedtime").
- Use examples to keep the client an active participant in learning.
- Present the most important information first, and summarize it at the end of the session.
- Teaching materials should reflect the reading level of the client, and information should be spaced out to decrease intimidation.
- Use pictures or illustrations when possible.
- Ask specific questions and address what you have taught (e.g., "When will you take this medication?"). Just asking if the client has any questions is not helpful because the illiterate client often does not have the ability to process information.
- Observe the client's ability to perform desired behaviors.

Data from Brooks DA: Techniques for teaching ED patients with low literacy skills, *J Emerg Nurs* 24(6):601, 1998.

Gerontological Nursing Practice   Box 9-7

- Present information slowly.
- Give information in short frequent sessions.
- Repeat information frequently.
- Reinforce teaching with audiovisual material, written exercises, and practice.
- Use examples.
- Allow more time for learners to express themselves, demonstrate learning, and ask questions.
- Establish reachable short-term goals.
- Apply teaching to present situations.
- Base new information on clients' previous level of learning.

Data from Barry CB: Teaching the older patient in the home assessment and adaptation, *Home Health Nurse* 18(6):374, 2000; Edelman CL, Mandle CL: *Health promotion throughout the lifespan,* ed 4, St. Louis, 1998, Mosby; Tiivel J: Increasing the effectiveness of your teaching program for the elderly: assessing the client's readiness to learn, *Perspectives* 21(3):7, 1997.

ceptions, and attitudes held by clients and families (Wilson, 1996). You must be aware of the client's cultural background, beliefs, and ability to understand instructions developed outside of the native language. Cultural diversity is widespread and poses a great challenge to provide culturally sensitive health care and client education. When educating clients of different ethnic groups, do the following:

1. Become aware of each culture's distinctive aspects.
2. Collaborate with other nurses and educators to assist in dealing with cultural diversity.
3. Enlist the help of people in the cultural group to share values and beliefs.
4. Use input and experiences of ethnic nurses in providing care to members of their community (Edelman and Mandle, 1998).

SPECIAL NEEDS OF CHILDREN AND OLDER ADULTS.

The choice of instructional methods and application of teaching-learning principles is based on a client's age. Children, adults, and older adults learn differently. Adapt teaching strategies to each learner's abilities and developmental stage.

Children pass through several developmental stages (see Chapter 18). In each stage, children acquire new cognitive and psychomotor abilities that respond to different types of learning. Parental input and participation are needed in implementing health education for children.

Older adults experience numerous physical and psychological changes as they age. These changes can create barriers to learning. Sensory changes require teaching methods that enhance the client's functioning. Research shows that older adults learn and remember effectively if the learning is paced properly and the material is relevant to the learner's needs and abilities (Rankin and Stallings, 1996; Tiivel, 1997). Educational strategies for gerontological nursing practice are highlighted in Box 9-7.

 Evaluation

CLIENT CARE.   Client education is not complete until you evaluate the outcomes of the teaching-learning process. Success depends on the client's ability to meet the established performance criteria.

Return demonstrations, use of questions, observation of client behaviors, role playing, and discussions can be used to evaluate your client's learning. For example, the client who will use a three-point crutch gait while walking to the end of the hall must demonstrate the actual crutch-walking technique.

If evaluation indicates a knowledge or skill deficit still exists, modify the teaching plan. Alternative teaching methods often help to clarify information or strengthen skills that the client was unable to comprehend or perform originally. Evaluation may also reveal new learning needs or new factors that may interfere with the client's ability to learn. Use this information to update the teaching plan and make it relevant to client needs. Like the nursing process, the teaching process is continuous and ever changing.

CLIENT EXPECTATIONS.   After you educate clients to manage their health promotion activities, disease process, and their physical and functional limitations, you send them back to their home and community. It is important to have a method for evaluating your client's expectations regarding client education. Did your client and family receive the education they expected? Were the expectations regarding self-care met? Are there some education expectations remaining? Did the educational program increase your clients' comfort in managing their health status in their home? If your clients' expectations are not met, then you increase the risk that your clients will not adhere to the prescribed treatment plan, will be less independent, and perhaps will ignore signs and/or symptoms indicating a need to make an appointment with their health care provider.

DOCUMENTATION OF CLIENT TEACHING

Because client teaching often occurs informally (e.g., during medication administration or physical examination), it is difficult to document client education consistently. However, because you are legally responsible for providing accurate and timely information to clients, quality documentation is essential. Smalley (1997) suggests the following for documenting client education:

1. *Specific content:* Specifically describe subject matter so that other nurses can follow up and reinforce teaching (e.g., "verbalized side effects of digoxin").

2. *Evaluation of learning:* Document evidence of learning (e.g., a return demonstration of coughing and deep breathing). This informs staff about the client's progress and determines material that still needs to be taught.

3. *Method of teaching:* Describe teaching methods used. Knowing methods used in instruction (e.g., demonstrations, discussion) helps staff to follow up more efficiently or offer alternative teaching methods if learning does not occur. Resources used, such as pamphlets or audiovisual materials, are included in the client's record. Many institutions have special forms or teaching flow sheets that document the plan, implementation, and evaluation of client teaching (Snyder, 1996).

Key Terms

affective learning, *p. 136*

analogies, *p. 144*

attentional set, *p. 136*

cognitive learning, *p. 136*

functional illiteracy, *p. 144*

health beliefs, *p. 136*

learning, *p. 134*

learning objective, *p. 135*

motivation, *p. 136*

psychomotor learning, *p. 136*

reinforcement, *p. 143*

return demonstration, *p. 136*

teaching, *p. 134*

Key Concepts

- In the present health care system, there is greater emphasis on providing quality health education.
- You must ensure that clients, families, and communities receive information needed to maintain optimal health.
- Health education is aimed at the promotion, restoration, and maintenance of health.
- Teaching is most effective when it is responsive to the learner's needs.
- Teaching is a form of interpersonal communication, with teacher and student actively involved in a process that increases the student's knowledge and skills.
- Teaching a client a specific behavior can involve incorporation of behaviors from all three learning domains.
- The client's ability to attend to the learning process depends on physical comfort and anxiety level and the presence of environmental distraction.

- A person's health beliefs influence the willingness to gain the knowledge and skills necessary to maintain health.
- Clients of different age-groups require different teaching strategies as a result of developmental capabilities.
- Presentation of teaching content should progress from simple to more complex ideas.
- The client should be an active participant in a teaching plan, agreeing to the plan, helping to choose instructional methods, and recommending times for instruction.
- A combination of teaching methods improves the learner's attentiveness and involvement.
- Teaching methodologies should match the client's learning need.
- Learning objectives describe what a person is to learn in behavioral terms.
- You evaluate a client's learning by observing the performance of expected learning behaviors under desired conditions.

Critical Thinking Activities

1. A group of day care teachers has asked you to present information on common childhood illnesses. Describe the steps you would take and the factors you would consider in developing, presenting, and evaluating your presentation.

2. Mr. Green has been newly diagnosed with type 2 diabetes. As you are teaching him, you suspect that he is unable to read and comprehend the information in the brochures you have given him. Describe the interventions you would employ in developing a teaching plan for this client.

3. Mrs. Trap, a 38-year-old woman, has just had abdominal surgery for ovarian cancer. She is avoiding discussing her change in health status and has misinterpreted what her physician has told her. Which stage of grieving is she in? Describe your teaching priorities for this client.

4. Isaac Garrett is a 16-year-old who is having surgery for appendicitis. He and his parents need preoperative teaching. Describe teaching methods that are effective with an adolescent.

Review Questions

1. A client must learn to use a walker. Acquisition of this skill will require learning in the:
   1. cognitive domain.
   2. affective domain.
   3. psychomotor domain.
   4. attentional domain.
2. You should plan to teach a client about the importance of exercise:
   1. when there are visitors in the room.
   2. when the client's pain medications are working.
   3. just before lunch, when the client is most awake and alert.
   4. when the client is talking about current stressors in his or her life.
3. A client newly diagnosed with cervical cancer is going home. The client is avoiding discussion of her illness and postoperative orders. In teaching the client about discharge instructions, you should:
   1. teach the client's spouse.
   2. focus on knowledge the client will need in a few weeks.
   3. provide only the information the client needs to go home.
   4. convince the client that learning about her health is necessary.
4. The school nurse is about to teach a freshman-level health class about nutrition. To achieve the best learning outcomes, the nurse should:
   1. provide information using a lecture.
   2. use simple words to promote understanding.
   3. develop topics for discussion that require problem solving.
   4. complete an extensive literature search focusing on eating disorders.
5. A nurse is going to teach a client how to perform a breast self-examination. The behavioral objective that would best measure the client's ability to perform the examination is:
   1. the client will verbalize the steps involved in breast self-examination within 1 week.
   2. the nurse will explain the importance of performing breast self-examination once a month.
   3. the client will perform breast self-examination correctly on herself before the end of the teaching session.
   4. the nurse will demonstrate breast self-examination on a breast model provided by the American Cancer Association.
6. A client who is having chest pain is going for an emergency cardiac catheterization. The most appropriate teaching approach in this situation is the:
   1. telling approach.
   2. selling approach.
   3. entrusting approach.
   4. participating approach.
7. You are teaching a parenting class to a group of pregnant adolescents and have given the adolescents baby dolls to bathe and talk to. This is an example of:
   1. discovery.
   2. an analogy.
   3. role playing.
   4. a demonstration.
8. An older adult is being started on a new antihypertensive medication. In teaching the client about the medication, you should:
   1. speak loudly.
   2. present the information once.
   3. expect the client to understand the information quickly.
   4. allow the client time to express himself or herself and ask questions.
9. A client must learn how to administer a subcutaneous injection. You know the client is ready to learn when the client:
   1. has walked 400 feet.
   2. expresses the importance of learning the skill.
   3. can see and understand the markings on the syringe.
   4. has the dexterity needed to prepare and inject the medication.
10. A client who is hospitalized has just been diagnosed with chronic renal failure. The best time to start teaching the client about the management of renal failure is:
   1. the day of discharge.
   2. when the client's family is available to support the client.
   3. as soon as the doctors have told the client about his or her illness.
   4. as soon as the client demonstrates a willingness to learn.

References

American Medical Association: Health literacy: report on the council of scientific affairs, *JAMA* 281(6):552, 1999.

Bandura A: *Self-efficacy: the exercise of control,* New York, 1997, WH Freeman.

Barry CB: Teaching the older patient in the home assessment and adaptation, *Home Healthc Nurse* 18(6):374, 2000.

Brooks DA: Techniques for teaching ED patients with low literacy skills, *J Emerg Nurs* 24(6):601, 1998.

Chachkes E, Christ G: Cross cultural issues in patient education, *Patient Educ Couns* 27:13, 1996.

Duffy MM, Snyder K: Can ED patients read your patient education materials? *J Emerg Nurs* 25(4):294, 1999.

Edelman CL, Mandle CL: *Health promotion throughout the lifespan,* ed 4, St. Louis, 1998, Mosby.

Fox VJ: Postoperative education that works, *AORN J* 67(5):1010, 1998.

Hinchliff S: *The practitioner as teacher,* Edinburgh, 1999, Bailliere Tindall.

Houston C, Haire-Joshu D: Application of health behavior models to promote behavior change. In Haire-Joshu D, editor: *Management of diabetes mellitus: perspective of care across the life span,* ed 2, St. Louis, 1996, Mosby.

Joint Commission on Accreditation of Healthcare Organizations: *Accreditation manual of hospitals,* Chicago, 2001, The Commission.

Murphy PW, Davis TC: When low literacy blocks compliance, *RN* 60(10):58, 1997.

National Center for Education Statistics: *1992 National adult literacy survey,* 1996, http://nces.ed.gov/nadlits/.

Rankin SH, Stallings KD: *Patient education: issues, principles, practices,* ed 3, Philadelphia, 1996, JB Lippincott.

Redman B: *The practice of patient education,* ed 9, St. Louis, 2001, Mosby.

Smalley R: Taking charge: patient education—we have a better system now, *RN* 60(6):19, 24, 1997.

Snyder B: An easy way to document patient ed, *RN* 59(3):43, 1996.

Tiivel J: Increasing the effectiveness of your teaching program for the elderly: assessing the client's readiness to learn, *Perspectives* 21(3):7, 1997.

Wilson F: Patient education materials nurses use in community health, *West J Nurs Res* 18(2):195, 1996.

Wong D and others: *Whaley and Wong's nursing care of infants and children,* ed 6, St. Louis, 1999, Mosby.

10

Infection Control

Objectives

- Define key terms.
- Identify the body's normal defenses against infection.
- Discuss the events in the inflammatory response.
- Describe the signs and symptoms of a localized or systemic infection.
- Describe characteristics of each link of the infection chain.
- Assess clients at risk for acquiring an infection.
- Explain conditions that could promote development of nosocomial infections.
- Describe strategies for standard precautions.
- Identify principles of surgical asepsis.
- Describe nursing interventions designed to break each link in the infection chain.
- Correctly perform barrier isolation techniques.
- Perform proper procedures for hand washing.
- Properly apply a surgical mask and gloves.
- Describe infection-control interventions unique to health promotion versus acute care versus restorative care settings.

*C*urrent trends and rising costs in health care delivery have increased interest in infection prevention and control practices. Increases in drug-resistant microorganisms and concern about occupational exposure to tuberculosis, human immunodeficiency virus (HIV), and hepatitis have increased concern about transmission of infections. As a nurse, you have an opportunity to participate in cost-effective quality health care by focusing on strategies that prevent and control infections.

Infection prevention and control and prevention are some of the most important functions you can perform. Knowledge of the infectious process and the critical thinking skills involved in aseptic technique and barrier protection cannot be overemphasized. This chapter emphasizes techniques for prevention and control of infections and the critical thinking skills necessary to achieve these goals.

SCIENTIFIC KNOWLEDGE BASE
Nature of Infection

An **infection** is the invasion of a susceptible host by pathogens or **microorganisms,** resulting in disease. The principal infecting agents are bacteria, viruses, fungi, and protozoa (Table 10-1). It is important to know the difference between an infection and colonization. If a microorganism is present or invades a host, grows, and/or multiplies but does not cause disease or infection, this is referred to as **colonization.** Disease or infections result only if the **pathogens** multiply and alter normal tissue function. If the infectious disease can be transmitted directly from one person to another, it is considered a contagious or **communicable disease** (Jackson and Tweeten, 2000).

Chain of Infection

The presence of a pathogen does not mean that an infection will begin. Development of an infection occurs in a cyclical process that depends on the presence of the following elements: the infectious agent or pathogen, reservoir for pathogen growth, portal of exit from the reservoir, mode of transmission or vehicle, portal of entry, and a susceptible host (Figure 10-1). Infection develops if this chain stays intact. Your efforts to control and prevent infections are directed at breaking this chain.

INFECTIOUS AGENT.   The development of an infectious disease depends on the number of organisms present; their **virulence,** or ability to produce disease; their ability to enter and survive in the host; and the susceptibility of the host.

RESERVOIR.   Places where microorganisms can survive, multiply, and await transfer to a susceptible host are called

Common Pathogens and Some Infections or Diseases They Produce		Table 10-1
Organism	Major Reservoir(s)	Major Diseases/Infections
Bacteria		
Staphylococcus aureus	Skin, hair, upper respiratory	Wound infection, abscess, cellulitis, osteomyelitis, pneumonia, food poisoning
Staphylococcus epidermidis	Skin	IV line infection, bacteremia, endocarditis
Streptococcus pyogenes	Skin, upper respiratory, perianal	Wound infection, impetigo, strep throat, puerperal sepsis (postpartum sepsis)
Escherichia coli	Colon	Gastroenteritis, urinary tract infection
Pseudomonas aeruginosa	Water, soil	Wound or burn infections, urinary tract infection, pneumonia
Neisseria gonorrhoeae	Genitourinary tract, rectum, mouth	Sexually transmitted disease (gonorrhea), pelvic inflammatory disease, septic arthritis
Chlamydia trachomatis	Genitourinary tract, rectum	Sexually transmitted disease (chlamydia), pelvic inflammatory disease, neonatal eye and lung infections
Mycobacterium tuberculosis	Droplet nuclei from lungs	Tuberculosis
Viruses		
Hepatitis A virus	Feces	Hepatitis A
Hepatitis B virus	Blood and some body fluids	Hepatitis B
Hepatitis C virus	Blood	Hepatitis C
Herpes simplex virus (Types I and II)	Lesions of mouth, skin, genitals	Cold sores, herpetic whitlow, sexually transmitted disease
Varicella-zoster virus	Vesicle fluid, respiratory tract infection	Varicella (chickenpox) primary infection, herpes zoster (shingles) reactivation
Fungi		
Candida albicans	Skin, mouth, genital tract	Bacteremia, pneumonia, wound infection
Protozoa		
Plasmodium falciparum	Blood, infected female Anopheles mosquito	Malaria

From Rosen-Kotilainen H: Laboratory diagnostics. In Pfeiffer J, editor: *APIC text of infection control and epidemiology,* Washington, DC, 2000, Association for Professionals in Infection Control and Epidemiology, Inc.

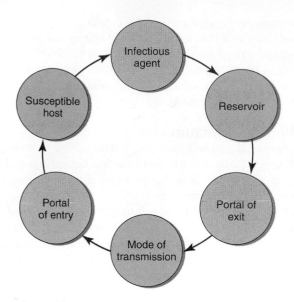

FIGURE **10-1** Chain of infection.

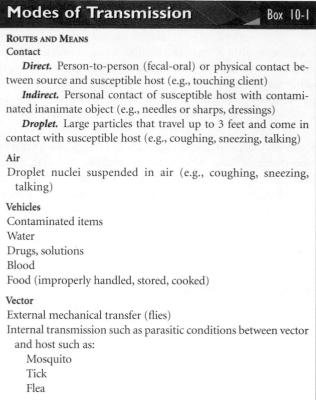

reservoirs. Common reservoirs are humans and animals (hosts), insects, food, water, and organic matter on inanimate surfaces (fomites). Frequent reservoirs for nosocomial infections include health care workers, clients, equipment, and the environment. Human reservoirs are divided into two types: those with acute or symptomatic disease and those who show no signs of disease but are **carriers** of the disease. Microorganisms or disease can be transmitted in either case.

PORTAL OF EXIT. After microorganisms find a site in which to grow and multiply, they must find a portal of exit if they are to enter another host and cause disease. Microorganisms can exit through a variety of sites such as skin and mucous membranes, respiratory tract, gastrointestinal tract, reproductive tract, and blood.

MODE OF TRANSMISSION. Many times there is little that you can do about the infectious agent or the susceptible host, but by practicing infection prevention and control techniques, such as hand washing, you can interrupt the mode of transmission (Box 10-1). The same microorganism may be transmitted by more than one route. For example, the virus that causes chickenpox may be spread by airborne route in droplet nuclei and also by direct contact with vesicle fluid.

PORTAL OF ENTRY. Organisms can enter the body through the same routes they use for exiting. Common portals of entry include nonintact skin, mucous membranes, genitourinary (GU) tract, gastrointestinal (GI) tract, and respiratory tract. For example, obstruction to the flow of urine from a urinary catheter allows organisms to ascend the urethra.

SUSCEPTIBLE HOST. Susceptibility to an infectious agent depends on the individual's degree of resistance to pathogens. Although everyone is constantly in contact with large numbers of organisms, an infection does not develop until an in-

dividual becomes susceptible to the strength and numbers of those microorganisms. A person's natural defenses against infection and certain risk factors (see Assessment section) affect susceptibility.

A host is no longer considered susceptible if it has acquired **immunity** from either a natural or artificially induced event. Natural active immunity results from having a certain disease, such as measles, and mounting an immune response that usually lasts a lifetime. Natural passive immunity is the acquisition of an **antibody** by one person from another, such as the baby that is born with its mother's antibodies. These antibodies are acquired through the placenta during the last months of pregnancy. This type of immunity is of short duration, usually lasting only a few weeks to months.

Course of Infection

Infections follow a progressive course (Figure 10-2). The severity depends on the extent of the infection, the **pathogenicity** and virulence of the causative microorganisms, and the host's susceptibility. If infection is localized, such as in a wound, antibiotic therapy and proper wound care may control the infection's spread and minimize the illness. The client will experience only localized symptoms such as pain, tenderness, and swelling at the wound site. An infection that affects the entire body instead of just a single organ or part is systemic and can be fatal.

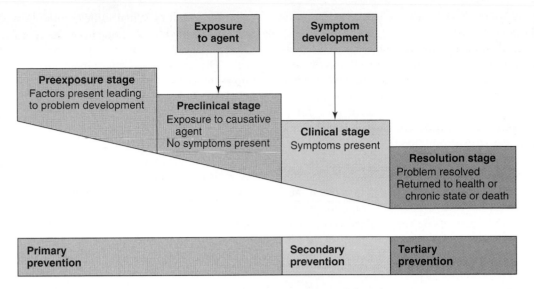

FIGURE **10-2**   Stages of the natural history of a condition and their relationship to primary, secondary, and tertiary levels of prevention. (From Jackson M, Tweeten S: General principles of epidemiology. In Pfeiffer J, editor: *APIC text of infection control and epidemiology,* Washington, DC, 2000, Association for Professionals in Infection Control and Epidemiology, Inc.; redrawn from Clark MJ: *Nursing in the community,* Norwalk, Conn, Appleton & Lange, 1992. Modified by permission of Pearson Education, Inc, Upper Saddle River, NJ.)

Defenses Against Infection

The body has normal defenses against infection. Normal flora, body system defenses, and inflammation are nonspecific defenses that protect against microorganisms, regardless of prior exposure. The immune system is composed of separate cells and molecules, some of which fight specific pathogens.

NORMAL FLORA.   The body usually contains normal **flora** or large numbers of microorganisms that reside on the surface and deep layers of the skin, in the saliva and oral mucosa, and in the intestinal walls. Normal flora do not cause disease but instead help to maintain health. For example, the skin's flora inhibit multiplication of organisms landing on the skin. The number of flora maintains a sensitive balance with other microorganisms to prevent infection. Any factor that disrupts this balance places a person at serious risk for infection. For example, the use of broad-spectrum antibiotics for the treatment of infection can eliminate or change normal bacterial flora, leading to **suprainfection.** Microorganisms resistant to antibiotics can then cause serious infection (Williams and Peterson, 2000).

BODY SYSTEM DEFENSES.   Microorganisms can easily enter the skin, respiratory tract, and gastrointestinal tract. However, these body systems also have unique defenses against infection, physiologically suited to their structure and function (Table 10-2). Any condition that impairs an organ's specialized defenses increases susceptibility to infection. When a person ages, there are normal physiological changes that influence susceptibility to infection (Box 10-2, p. 153).

INFLAMMATION.   The body's cellular response to injury or infection is **inflammation.** Inflammation is a protective vascular reaction that delivers fluid, blood products, and nutrients to interstitial tissues in an area of injury. This process neutralizes and eliminates pathogens or **necrotic** tissues and establishes a means of repairing body cells and tissues (Table 10-3). Signs of inflammation include swelling, redness, heat, pain or tenderness, and loss of function in the affected body part. When inflammation becomes systemic, signs and symptoms may include fever, leukocytosis (increased number of white blood cells), malaise, anorexia, nausea, vomiting, and lymph node enlargement. The inflammatory response may be triggered by many physical agents (e.g., temperature extremes and radiation), chemical agents (e.g., gastric acid or poisons), and microorganisms.

IMMUNE RESPONSE.   When a foreign material (**antigen**) enters the body, a series of responses changes the body's biological makeup. The next time that antigen enters the body, the antigen is either neutralized, destroyed, or eliminated.

Nosocomial Infection

Clients in health care settings, especially acute care hospitals and long-term care facilities, are at a higher risk for infection than those clients seen in the home setting. Clients in health care settings often have multiple illnesses and are older adults and poorly nourished, thus more susceptible to infections. In addition, many clients have a lowered resistance to microorganisms because of underlying medical conditions (e.g., HIV, diabetes mellitus, or malignancies) that impair the body's immune response. Invasive treatment devices such as intravenous (IV) catheters or urinary catheters impair the body's natural defenses against microorganisms. Several invasive diagnostic examinations such as bronchoscopy or gastroscopy and treatment with broad-spectrum antibiotics have also been shown to increase the risk for certain infections (Schaffer and others, 1996).

When a client who develops an infection that was not present or incubating at the time of admission to a health care setting it is called a **nosocomial infection.** A community-acquired infection is one that was present in a client when admitted to a health care facility. The incidence of nosocomial infections may be lowered if nurses conscientiously practice hand washing and aseptic techniques.

Nosocomial infections are exogenous or endogenous. An **exogenous infection** arises from microorganisms outside the individual, such as *Salmonella, Clostridium tetani,* and *Aspergillus,* which do not exist as normal flora. **Endogenous infection** occurs when part of the client's flora becomes altered and an overgrowth results (e.g., infections caused by enterococci, yeasts, and streptococci). This often happens when the client receives broad-spectrum antibiotics that can alter normal flora. When sufficient numbers of microorganisms normally found in one body cavity or lining are transferred to another body site, an endogenous infection develops. The number of microorganisms needed to cause a nosocomial infection depends on the virulence of the organism, the host's susceptibility, and the body site affected (Box 10-3).

ASEPSIS. Efforts to minimize the onset and spread of infection are based on the principles of aseptic technique. **Aseptic technique** is an effort to keep the client as free from exposure to infection-causing pathogens as possible. The term **asepsis** means the absence of disease-producing microorganisms. The two types of aseptic technique are medical asepsis and surgical asepsis.

Medical asepsis (clean techniques) includes procedures used to reduce the number of microorganisms and prevent

Normal Body System Defense Mechanisms Against Infection

Table 10-2

Defense Mechanisms	Action	Factors That May Alter Defense
Skin		
Intact multilayered surface, body's first line of defense against infection	Provides mechanical barrier to microorganisms	Cuts, abrasions, puncture wounds, areas of maceration
Shedding of outer layer of skin cells	Removes organisms that adhere to skin's outer layers	Failure to bathe regularly
Sebum	Contains fatty acid that kills some bacteria	Excessive bathing
Mouth		
Intact multilayered mucosa	Provides mechanical barrier to microorganisms	Lacerations, trauma, extracted teeth
Saliva	Washes away particles containing microorganisms	Poor oral hygiene, dehydration
	Contains microbial inhibitors (e.g., lysozyme)	
Respiratory Tract		
Cilia lining upper airways, coated by sticky mucous blanket	Trap inhaled microbes and sweep them outward in mucus to be expectorated or swallowed	Smoking, high concentration of oxygen and carbon dioxide, decreased humidity, cold air
Macrophages	Engulf and destroy microorganisms that reach lung's alveoli	Smoking
Urinary Tract		
Flushing action of urine flow	Washes away microorganisms on lining of bladder and urethra	Obstruction to normal flow by urinary catheter placement, obstruction from growth or tumor, or delayed micturition
Intact multilayered epithelium	Provides barrier to microorganisms	Introduction of urinary catheter, continual movement of catheter in urethra
Gastrointestinal Tract		
Acidity of gastric secretions	Chemically destroys microorganisms incapable of surviving low pH	Administration of antacids
Rapid peristalsis in small intestine	Prevents retention of bacterial contents	Delayed motility from impaction of fecal contents in large bowel or mechanical obstruction by masses
Vagina		
At puberty, normal flora cause vaginal secretions to achieve low pH	Acidic secretions inhibit growth of many microorganisms	Antibiotics and birth control pills that disrupt normal flora

Gerontological Nursing Practice   Box 10-2

The older adult experiences a number of age-associated physiological changes that influence susceptibility to infection. These changes include the following:

- There are decreased tears to flush and remove debris from the eye and a decrease in lysozymes that affect certain microorganisms. A decreased blink reflex can lead to corneal dryness. Caution clients and families to observe for eye infections and use artificial tears when necessary.
- Drying of the oral mucosa and recession and weakening of gingival tissues require frequent oral hygiene and regular dental care.
- An increased chest diameter and rigidity, weakened cough, decreased ability to swallow, and decreased elastic tissue surrounding alveoli predispose older adults to ventilatory problems. Aspiration and postoperative pneumonia are common complications. When caring for older adult clients, elevate the head of the bed and encourage the client to ambulate as soon as possible (unless contraindicated). Instruct and assist client in deep breathing and coughing techniques.
- A decrease in production of digestive juices and a reduction in intestinal motility affect removal of potential pathogens in the bowel. Clients and families should learn about safe food preparation and eat foods that are nutritionally good and easy to digest.
- A thinning of the dermal and epidermal skin layers, along with a decrease in skin elasticity predisposes older adults to skin tearing. Rigorous nursing care is necessary to prevent pressure ulcers in bedridden clients (see Chapter 38).
- With aging there is a decreased production of T-lymphocytes and B-lymphocytes. With reduced immunity it is important for older adults to receive regular immunizations and medical checkups.

Modified from Gantz NM and others: Geriatric infections. In Pfeiffer J, editor: *APIC text of infection control and epidemiology*, Washington, DC, 2000, Association for Professionals in Infection Control and Epidemiology, Inc.

their spread. Hand washing, barrier techniques, and routine environmental cleaning are examples of medical asepsis.

Surgical asepsis (sterile techniques) are used during client care, including surgery, to prevent microbial contamination of an open wound or a sterile item. These techniques can be practiced by nurses in the operating room or at the bedside. Surgical asepsis demands the highest level of aseptic technique and requires that all areas be kept free of infectious microorganisms. In medical asepsis, an area or object is considered contaminated only if it is suspected of containing pathogens (e.g., a used bedpan or wet piece of gauze). In surgical asepsis, an area or object may be considered contaminated if touched by an object that is not sterile (e.g., a tear in a surgical glove during a procedure or a sterile instrument placed on an unsterile surface).

You are responsible for providing a safe environment for the client. It is easy to forget key procedural steps or to take shortcuts that break aseptic procedures when hurried. Failure to use good technique places clients at risk for an infection that can seriously impair their recovery.

NURSING KNOWLEDGE BASE

The experience of having a serious infection creates feelings of anxiety, frustration, and anger in clients or their families. These feelings can worsen when clients are isolated to prevent transmission of a microorganism to other clients or health care staff. The solitude of isolation limits normal social interactions. Emotional reactions are likely to occur. Family members may fear the possibility of developing the infection themselves and may avoid contact with the client. Even the simple procedures of proper hand washing or gloving may communicate feelings of rejection. You can help clients and families reduce some of these feelings by discussing the disease process, explaining isolation procedures, and maintaining a friendly, understanding manner.

Inflammation	Table 10-3
Physiological Response	**Signs and Symptoms**
Vascular and Cellular Response	
Arterioles supplying infected or injured area dilate, delivering blood and leukocytes.	Redness Warmth
Tissue necrosis causes release of histamine, bradykinin, prostaglandin, and serotonin, which increase blood vessel permeability.	Edema
Fluid, protein, and cells enter interstitial spaces to cause swelling.	Pain
White blood cells (WBCs) enter tissues and phagocytose microorganisms. More WBCs are released into bloodstream.	WBC count normally 5000 to 10,000/mm^3; 15,000 to 20,000/mm^3 common with inflammation
Phagocytic release of pyrogens from bacteria occurs.	Fever
Inflammatory Exudate	
Fluid, dead cells, and WBCs form **exudate** at inflammatory site that later clears with lymphatic drainage.	Serous or sanguineous exudate
Tissue Repair	
Damaged cells are replaced with healthy new cells. Cells mature to take on structural characteristics and appearance of injured cells.	Tissue defects heal and close

Examples of Sites and Potential Causes for Nosocomial Infections*   Box 10-3

SURGICAL OR TRAUMATIC WOUND INFECTIONS
Improper surgical technique
Improper skin preparation before surgery (shaving or incorrect antiseptic scrub)
Improper aseptic technique during dressing change
Client risk factors such as malnutrition

PRIMARY BLOODSTREAM INFECTION/SEPSIS
Improper skin prep before insertion of intravascular access device
Failure to change intravenous site when inflammation first appears
Contamination of intravenous fluids, needles, or catheters
Improper technique during the insertion of drug additive into intravenous fluids
Improper care of peritoneal or hemodialysis shunts
Improper technique when adding stopcocks or connecting tubes to intravenous fluids
Use of multiple lumen central venous catheters

PNEUMONIA
Improper aseptic technique during suctioning
Displacement of nasogastric tube
Use of H_2 blocker/antacids
Client risk factors such as immobility or decreased gag reflex

URINARY TRACT INFECTION
Improper insertion of urinary catheter
Open or disconnected drainage system

Improper specimen collection technique
Obstruction of drainage
Reflux of urine into bladder
Contaminated catheter or equipment
Improper hand-washing technique

BONE AND JOINT INFECTION
Improper aseptic technique during pin care or dressing care

CARDIOVASCULAR SYSTEM INFECTION
Improper aseptic technique during dressing change or following cardiac surgery

CENTRAL NERVOUS SYSTEM INFECTION
Improper aseptic techniques during dressing changes or during monitoring of intracranial monitoring device

GASTROINTESTINAL SYSTEM INFECTION
Contaminated food or water
Overuse of antibiotics

SKIN AND SOFT TISSUE
Improper skin care
Client risk factors such as poor nutrition and hydration

*All forms of nosocomial infection can result from improper hand washing or use of contaminated equipment.

Cultural, religious, or social beliefs not only can influence how a client reacts to an infectious disease but can also influence infection prevention. For example, social support for clients may promote their adherence to treatment for infectious diseases. Rubel and Garro (1992) report that during an outbreak of pulmonary tuberculosis (TB) on a Navajo Indian reservation, traditional healers received specific education about TB control practices. These healers then successfully incorporated recommended interventions into the traditional health beliefs of the community.

Why a client may react to an infection or infectious disease is important for you to know in establishing a plan of care. The challenge is to identify and support those behaviors that maintain human health or prevent infection.

NURSING PROCESS

 Assessment

You must assess the client's susceptibility to and risk factors for infection (Box 10-4). A review of the medical history with the client and family may reveal a recent exposure to a communicable disease. By assessing existing signs and symptoms, you can determine whether a client's clinical condition indicates the onset or extension of an infection. During the interview process, you also have an opportunity to assess the client's and family's knowledge of a known infection or disease.

Because a client's nutritional health can directly influence susceptibility to infection, a thorough diet history is necessary. Determine a client's normal daily nutrient intake and whether preexisting problems such as impaired swallowing or oral pain alter food intake.

Assess laboratory data as soon as they are available (Table 10-4). Laboratory values such as increased white blood cells (WBCs) and/or a positive blood culture may indicate infection. When assessing laboratory data, consider the age of the client. For example, in the older adult, bacterial growth in urine without clinical symptoms may not indicate the presence of a urinary tract infection (Gantz and others, 2000).

Sometimes abnormal laboratory results may indicate the client's risk for infection and the need for the use of barrier precautions or protective isolation. Consult with the infection-control professional or refer to the facility's policy for assistance. The early recognition of infection will assist you in making the correct nursing diagnosis and establishing a treatment plan. In addition, you can alert other members of the health care team to the need for further investigation of the client's condition, facilitating initiation of prompt therapy and barrier protection.

Also assess the ways in which an infection affects the client and family. Clients with chronic or serious infection such as tuberculosis or acquired immunodeficiency syndrome (AIDS) may experience psychological and social problems from self-imposed isolation or rejection by friends and family. Ask the client how the infection is af-

Factors Affecting Susceptibility to Infection

Box 10-4

AGE

Infants have immature immune systems.

Children acquire more immunity but are susceptible to infectious diseases such as mumps and measles.

Young and middle-age adults have refined body system defenses and immunity.

Older adults' immune responses decline, and the structure and function of major organs change.

HEREDITY

Certain congenital and genetic chromosomal disorders can have an effect on humoral or cellular immunity.

Clients with diabetes, some types of which are hereditary, can be more at risk for infections and delayed wound healing.

CULTURAL PRACTICES

Various cultural or religious beliefs or practices can influence clients' decisions to seek treatment for an infection or to use methods to prevent infections (e.g., a Native American or Latino client may seek treatment from a "healer" rather than a physician, or the decision on whether to use a condom may be determined by the client's religious belief).

NUTRITIONAL STATUS

A reduction in protein, carbohydrates, and fats as a result of illness, inadequate diet, or debility increases a client's susceptibility to infection and delays wound repair.

STRESS

Increased stress elevates cortisone levels, causing decreased resistance to infection.

Continuous stress exhausts energy stores.

REST AND EXERCISE

Inadequate rest and exercise can increase stress and decrease body functions such as elimination and circulation.

INADEQUATE DEFENSES

Primary and secondary defenses may be altered (e.g., broken skin or mucosa, traumatized tissue, suppressed immune response).

PERSONAL HABITS

Smoking inhibits respiratory ciliary action and decreases resistance to respiratory infections.

Alcohol ingestion can impair the effect of antibiotics.

Risky sexual behavior, such as multiple sex partners, increases the chance for exposure to HIV and other sexually transmitted diseases.

ENVIRONMENTAL FACTORS

Crowded living conditions and adequacy and safety of water supply can influence the client's susceptibility to infections.

Inadequate refrigeration and cooking facilities can increase a client's exposure to food-borne illness such as *Shigella* or *Escherichia coli.*

IMMUNIZATION/DISEASE HISTORY

Clients who have not received recommended immunizations are at risk for vaccine-preventable diseases such as measles, mumps, and rubella.

Older adults with underlying medical conditions can decrease their susceptibility to influenza and pneumococcal pneumonia through immunizations.

Recent exposure to a communicable disease may increase the client's susceptibility.

MEDICAL THERAPIES

Certain drugs, such as cortisone, and certain invasive therapies, such as intravenous catheters or surgeries, can increase the risk for infection.

CLINICAL APPEARANCE/DATA

Localized infections usually present with redness, swelling, and pain or tenderness. There may be a purulent drainage from wounds or lesions.

Systemic infections may present with fever, chills, nausea and vomiting, loss of appetite, or lymph node enlargement.

Clinical data may show an increase in white blood cells (WBCs), positive culture, or an abnormal x-ray examination.

---

fecting the ability to maintain relationships. Determine whether chronic infection has drained the client's financial resources.

CLIENT EXPECTATIONS.   Assess clients' expectations about their care and involve them in all aspects of care planning. Some clients and their families may wish to know more about the disease process, whereas others may only want to know the interventions necessary to treat the infection. Encourage clients to verbalize their expectations so that you can establish interventions to meet clients' priorities.

 Nursing Diagnosis

Following assessment, review all of your findings and analyze data to identify relevant nursing diagnoses. For the nursing diagnosis *risk for infection,* defining characteristics include risk factors such as inadequate primary defenses (e.g., broken skin or stasis of body fluids), inadequate sec-

ondary defenses (e.g., decreased hemoglobin and white blood cells), or chronic disease.

Clusters of defining characteristics lead to the selection of a nursing diagnosis. The related factors, revealed in the assessment, ensure individualization of the diagnosis. For example, *risk for infection related to intravenous catheter placement* may be diagnosed in a client with a decreased WBC count, multiple intravenous catheters, and inflammation around a single catheter site. The related factor, *intravenous catheter placement,* will direct you to change the catheter regularly and take measures to minimize microorganism transfer through the intravenous system. An accurate related factor ensures a more appropriate care plan.

Infection or its associated treatment may be the related factor for a number of nursing diagnoses (Box 10-5). In the case of the diagnosis *social isolation,* the related factor may be the isolation precautions used for the client. Nursing interventions would then be directed at minimizing the effect isolation has on the client's ability to socialize.

Laboratory Tests to Screen for Infection		Table 10-4
Laboratory Value	Normal (Adult) Values	Indication of Infection
WBC count	5000-10,000/mm³	Increased in acute infection, decreased in certain viral or overwhelming infections
Erythrocyte sedimentation rate	Up to 15 mm/hr for men and 20 mm/hr for women	Elevated in presence of inflammatory process
Iron level	60-90 µg/100 ml	Decreased in chronic infection
Cultures of blood	Normally sterile, without microorganism growth	Presence of infectious microorganism growth
Cultures of wound, sputum, and throat	Possible normal flora	Presence of infectious microorganism growth
Urinalysis	Nitrite and leukocyte negative, WBC 0-10/mm³ esterases	Nitrite positive, leukocyte positive, WBC greater than 20/mm³
Differential Count (Percentage of Each Type of WBC)		
Neutrophils	55%-70%	Increased in acute suppurative infection, decreased in overwhelming bacterial infection (older adult)
Lymphocytes	20%-40%	Increased in chronic bacterial and viral infection, decreased in sepsis
Monocytes	2%-8%	Increased in protozoal, rickettsial, and tuberculosis infections
Eosinophils	1%-4%	Increased in parasitic infection
Basophils	0.5%-1%	Normal during infection

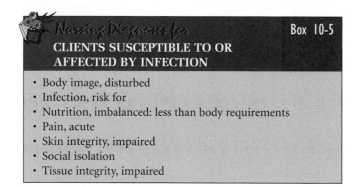

Box 10-5

CLIENTS SUSCEPTIBLE TO OR AFFECTED BY INFECTION

- Body image, disturbed
- Infection, risk for
- Nutrition, imbalanced: less than body requirements
- Pain, acute
- Skin integrity, impaired
- Social isolation
- Tissue integrity, impaired

The presence of an actual infection poses a collaborative problem requiring your intervention. An actual infection might be indicated by objective data such as an elevated temperature, open draining wound, inflammation of a wound site, and laboratory values revealing an increased WBC count. Subjective findings might include client complaint of chills, malaise, or tenderness at the wound site. Work with physicians, dietitians, and other team members in monitoring the infection, providing therapies such as antibiotic administration and wound care, and implementing appropriate infection control measures.

Planning

Develop the client's care plan based on each nursing diagnosis. For each diagnosis it is important to identify specific goals and outcomes, set priorities, and plan for continuing care after discharge.

GOALS AND OUTCOMES. Select achievable goals in collaboration with the client, family, and other health care team members. For example, in an acute care setting, the goal for the diagnosis *risk for infection* might be "to control or decrease the progression of infection" and the outcome might be "Client's wound drainage decreases in 3 days." In this plan other members of the health care team such as the infection-control nurse or the enterostomy therapist might be involved.

SETTING PRIORITIES. Set the priorities for care based on the client's nursing diagnoses. Give special attention to any urgent needs created by the infection. For example, if the client's infection becomes systemic, you will need to attend to managing fever and preventing dehydration. Once the infection begins to resolve, priorities may focus on client education and emotional support.

CONTINUITY OF CARE. It is important that the client's required level of care continue after discharge from the health care setting. Assess the client, family, and other caregivers for their ability to provide continuity of care. For example, assess whether the client or family can perform necessary dressing changes. Other members of the health care team such as the discharge planner or social services might be involved. Community resources may be available to assist in providing care after discharge from the acute care setting.

Implementation

Your care plan includes nursing interventions designed to control and prevent infection.

HEALTH PROMOTION. Good infection control begins with prevention. Review with clients and their families preventive measures that strengthen the host's defenses, such as nutrition, recommended immunizations, personal hygiene, and regular rest and exercise. In addition, explain infection-control principles, such as hand washing, designed to prevent infections from occurring.

NUTRITION.   Nutrition has a major influence on resistance to infection. Some increased risks for infection usually associated with aging may in fact be related to nutrition due to loss of appetite (Thompson, 2000). A proper diet is one that promotes optimal immune functioning and consists of a variety of foods from all food groups (see Chapter 30).

In collaboration with dietitians or alone, design education programs specific to clients' needs. After assessment and input from the client, teach the client the importance a proper diet plays in maintaining immunity and preventing infection. Incorporate the client's food preferences when possible.

HYGIENE.   One infection-control goal of personal hygiene for the client is to reduce the microbial load of the skin and maintain the well-being of mucous membranes such as the mouth and vagina (Fauerbach, 2000). For example, teach the client to wash from clean to dirty, from the urethra down toward the rectum, using a clean wash cloth (Chapter 26). Also encourage the client to maintain good oral hygiene.

IMMUNIZATION.   Immunization programs for infants and children have decreased the occurrence of many childhood, vaccine-preventable diseases such as diphtheria, whooping cough, and measles. New vaccines for hepatitis A and chickenpox (varicella) have provided immunity to both adults and children for highly communicable diseases. In addition, specific vaccines such as influenza and pneumococcal pneumonia have decreased the mortality and morbidity previously seen in older adults or clients with underlying medical problems such as chronic obstructive pulmonary disease (COPD). Advise clients about the advantages of immunizations, but also make them aware of the contraindications for particular vaccines, especially for pregnant or lactating women.

ADEQUATE REST AND REGULAR EXERCISE.   Adequate rest and regular exercise help prevent infection. Physical exercise increases lung capacity, circulation, energy, and endurance. It also decreases stress and improves appetite, sleeping, and elimination. Balancing the need for regular exercise is the need for rest and sleep. Some clients may need education stressing the importance of sleep and rest for infection prevention.

ACUTE CARE.   A client with an infection has many needs. By monitoring the course of the infection carefully, you can choose the most appropriate measures to maintain or restore the client's health. Disinfection and sterilization of supplies and good hand washing are examples of aseptic methods used to control the spread of microorganisms.

When a client develops an infection, continue preventive care so that health care personnel and other clients do not acquire the infection. Good hand washing and use of barrier precautions, such as gloves or masks, minimize exposure of staff and clients to infection. Clients with communicable diseases and infections that are easily transmissible to others

require special precautions. Isolation precautions involve control of a client's environment by forming barriers against bacterial spread.

Treatment of an infection includes identification and elimination of the organism and support of the client's defenses. Specimens of body fluids or drainage from infected body sites may be collected for cultures. When the disease process or causative organism has been identified, the physician may prescribe an antibiotic. Administer antibiotics carefully, watching for allergic reactions and assessing the progress of the client's infection.

Systemic infections, those that affect the body as a whole, require measures to prevent the complications of fever (see Chapter 11). Maintaining intake of fluids prevents dehydration resulting from diaphoresis. Increased metabolism requires an adequate nutritional intake. Rest preserves energy for the healing process.

Localized infections often require measures to facilitate removal of infectious organisms. Apply wet-to-dry dressings (see Chapter 34) to remove infected drainage from wound sites. Application of heat compresses promotes blood flow to an infected site and thus the delivery of blood components needed to fight an infection. Drainage tubes may be inserted to remove infected drainage from body cavities. Use medical and surgical aseptic techniques to manage wounds and ensure the correct handling of infected drainage or body fluids.

During any infection the client's body defense mechanisms must be supported. For example, if a client is known to have diarrhea, you must cleanse the skin promptly and dry thoroughly to prevent breakdown and entrance of microorganisms.

MEDICAL SEPSIS.   Basic medical aseptic techniques break the infection chain. Precautions are used for all clients, even when an infection has not been diagnosed. Aggressive preventive measures can be highly effective in reducing nosocomial infections.

Control or Elimination of Infectious Agents.   With the increased use of disposable equipment, nurses may be less aware of disinfection and sterilization procedures. The proper cleaning, disinfection, and sterilization of contaminated objects significantly reduce and often eliminate microorganisms.

Cleaning.   Cleaning involves the removal of foreign materials (e.g., organic material such as blood or inorganic material such as soil) from objects. Generally this involves the use of water, a detergent, and proper mechanical scrubbing action. Cleaning must occur before disinfection and sterilization procedures (Rutala 1996). Check the policy of the health care facility before cleaning. In most institutions technicians will clean equipment. When cleaning objects soiled by blood or body fluids, apply personal protection equipment (PPE) such as gloves, goggles, and mask to protect from splashing fluids.

Disinfection and Sterilization.   Physical and chemical processes are used for disinfection and sterilization. Both processes disrupt the internal functioning of microorganisms

Categories for Sterilization, Disinfection, and Cleaning   Box 10-6

CRITICAL ITEMS—STERILIZATION

Items that enter sterile tissue or the vascular system present a high risk of infection if the items are contaminated with any microorganisms and spores. Items must be sterile. These items include surgical instruments, cardiac and urinary catheters, needles, and implants.

SEMICRITICAL ITEMS—DISINFECTION

Items that come in contact with skin that is not intact or with mucous membranes also present risks. These objects must be free of all microorganisms (except bacterial spores). These items include respiratory therapy equipment, endotracheal tubes, gastrointestinal endoscopes, and reusable mercury thermometers.

NONCRITICAL ITEMS—CLEANING

Items that come in contact with intact skin but not with mucous membranes must be clean. These items include bedpans, blood pressure cuffs, crutches, linens, and food utensils.

Control and Prevention to Reduce Reservoirs of Infection   Box 10-7

Hand washing. Use appropriate soap and warm water to wash hands before and after client care.

Bathing. Use soap and water to remove drainage, dried secretions, excess perspiration, or sediment from antiseptics.

Dressing changes. Change dressings that become wet or soiled (see Chapter 34).

Contaminated articles. Place tissues, soiled dressings, or soiled linen in moisture-resistant bags for proper disposal.

Contaminated needles. Place syringes, hypodermic needles, and intravenous needles in puncture-proof containers. (Do not recap needles or attempt to break them.)

Bedside unit. Keep table surfaces clean and dry.

Bottled solutions. Keep solutions tightly capped. Date solutions once opened.

Surgical wounds. Keep drainage tubes and collection bags patent to prevent accumulation of fluid under the skin's surface.

Drainage bottles and bags. Dispose of suction bottles according to agency policy. Empty all drainage systems on each shift unless otherwise ordered by a physician.

by destroying cell proteins. **Disinfection** is a process that eliminates almost all pathogenic organisms on objects, with the exception of bacterial spores. **Sterilization** is a process that eliminates or destroys all forms of microbial life (Rutala, 1996). Examples of sterilization are processing items using steam, dry heat, hydrogen peroxide plasma, or ethylene oxide (ETO). The level of disinfection and sterilization required depends on the type and use of the contaminated item (Box 10-6). You have the responsibility of checking for package integrity and/or expiration dates before using an object designated as sterile. Items not meeting the criteria for being sterile should be disposed of or sent to the sterilization-processing department (check agency policy).

CONTROL OR ELIMINATION OF RESERVOIRS. To control or eliminate infection in reservoir sites, eliminate sources of body fluids, drainage, or solutions that might harbor microorganisms. In addition, carefully discard disposable articles that become contaminated with infectious material (Box 10-7).

CONTROL OF PORTALS OF EXIT. To control organisms exiting through the respiratory tract, avoid talking, sneezing, or coughing directly over a surgical wound or sterile dressing field. Also teach clients to protect others when they sneeze or cough, and give clients disposable wipes or tissues to control spread of microorganisms. Refrain from working with clients who are highly susceptible to infection if you have a cold or other communicable infection.

Another way of controlling the exit of microorganisms is the careful handling of body fluids such as urine, feces, and wound drainage. Wear disposable gloves if there is a chance of contact with any blood or body fluids and wash hands after providing care. Be sure to bag contaminated items appropriately.

CONTROL OF TRANSMISSION. Effective infection control requires that you know the modes of transmission of microor-

ganisms and the methods of control. In any health care setting a client should have a personal set of care items. Sharing graduated containers for measuring urine, bath basins, and eating utensils can easily lead to transmission of infection. When using a stethoscope, always wash off the bell or diaphragm with a disinfectant before proceeding to the next client.

Because certain microorganisms travel easily through the air, do not shake linens or bedclothes. Dust with a treated or dampened cloth to prevent dust particles from entering the air.

To prevent transmission of microorganisms through indirect contact, do not allow soiled items and equipment to touch your clothing. A common error is to carry dirty linen in the arms against the uniform. Use special linen bags, or carry soiled linen with the hands held out from the body. Clean or soiled linen should never be put on the floor.

Hand Washing. The most important and most basic technique in preventing and controlling transmission of pathogens is hand washing. Hand washing is a vigorous, brief rubbing together of all surfaces of lathered hands, followed by rinsing under a stream of water (Larson, 2000). The need for hand washing depends on the following: the intensity of contact with the client or contaminated object, the degree or amount of contamination that could occur with that contact, the susceptibility of the client or health care worker to infection, and the procedure or activity to be performed (Larson, 2000). For example, if you simply touch an object that is not visibly soiled, hand washing is not required. In contrast, contact with any client, especially one with wound drainage, requires thorough hand washing. Larson (2000) recommends that hands be washed in the following situations:

1. When visibly soiled

2. Before and after client contact
3. Before performing invasive procedures such as urinary catheterization or placement of an intravascular catheter (antimicrobial soap is recommended)
4. After contact with a source of microorganisms (blood or body fluid, mucous membranes, nonintact skin, or inanimate objects that might be contaminated)
5. After removing gloves (wearing gloves does not remove the need to wash hands)

The Centers for Disease Control and Prevention (CDC) note that washing hands for at least 10 to 15 seconds is necessary to remove transient microorganisms from the skin. Hands that are more heavily soiled may require a longer time for washing (Garner, 1996a). The frequency of washing also affects the type and number of microorganisms on the hands. Skill 10-1 lists the correct steps for hand washing.

Use of antimicrobial soap (antiseptic) is encouraged when nurses work in special care units, perform invasive procedures, or care for clients who are **immunocompromised,** have damage to their integumentary system (wounds), or are infected or colonized with epidemiologically significant organisms (e.g., methicillin-resistant *Staphylococcus aureus* [MRSA] or vancomycin-resistant enterococcus [VRE]). There are several effective antimicrobials, including solutions containing chlorhexidine gluconate, alcohol, or an iodophor. Certain antimicrobial soaps can irritate the skin, and the need for antimicrobial soap must be evaluated against potential skin irritations.

Isolation and Barrier Protection. When a client has a known infection, nurses follow specific infection control practices, but not all sources of infection are obvious. The majority of microorganisms that cause infections or disease are found in colonized body substances of clients, regardless of whether a culture has confirmed an infection and a diagnosis has been made. Because of increased attention to the prevention of blood-borne pathogens and tuberculosis, the CDC and the Occupational Safety and Health Administration (OSHA) have stressed the importance of barrier protection (CDC, 1988; OSHA, 1991).

Isolation or barrier protection includes the appropriate use of personal protection equipment such as gloves, masks or respirators, eyewear, and gowns. Assess the need for barrier precautions based on potential transmission of infection, regardless of the client's diagnosis. For example, because TB is transmitted by droplet nuclei, only a mask or respirator is needed as a barrier protection. When suctioning a client with a tracheostomy, wearing eyewear and a mask is appropriate protection.

In 1996 the CDC published revised guidelines for isolation precautions. These guidelines can be modified in facilities, according to need and as dictated by state or local regulations (Hospital Infection Control Practices Advisory Committee [HICPAC] 1996; Garner, 1996a). The CDC recommendations contain two tiers of precautions (Table 10-5). The first and most important tier is called **standard precautions** and is designed to be used for care of all clients, in all settings, regardless of diagnosis. Standard precautions apply to contact with blood, body fluid, nonintact skin, and mucous membranes from all clients. These precautions protect the client and provide protection for the health care worker as directed by OSHA.

The second tier of precautions is designed for care of clients with specific types of infection. The precautions are used for clients known or suspected to be infected or colonized with microorganisms transmitted by droplets, by airborne route, or by contact with contaminated surfaces or dry skin. There are three types of transmission-based precautions: **airborne, droplet,** and **contact.** They may be used singly or in combination for diseases (e.g., chickenpox) that have multiple routes of transmission. Use them in addition to standard precautions.

Because of the resurgence of TB, the CDC (1994) has produced guidelines for the prevention of transmission of TB in the health care worker and stresses the importance of isolation for the known or suspected TB client in a special negative-pressure room. Close the doors to the client's room to control direction of airflow. A special high-filtration particulate respirator is worn when entering a respiratory isolation room. Respirators must be able to fit health care workers with different facial sizes and characteristics. When worn correctly, particulate respirators and masks (Figures 10-3 and 10-4) have a tighter face seal and filter at a higher level than routine surgical masks (OSHA, 1995).

Additional guidelines for prevention of transmission of certain drug-resistant organisms have been published by the CDC (HICPAC, 1995). These guidelines, primarily for microorganisms such as VRE, are more stringent than other published recommendations.

Regardless of the type of isolation or barrier protection used, certain basic principles must be followed when delivering care in a client's room (Box 10-8). You should understand how certain diseases are transmitted and what barriers are needed to prevent transmission. For example, you do not routinely need to wear a gown or gloves when giving oral medications but may need these barriers when changing a dressing from a draining wound. However, gloves are appropriate when assisting a client with an oral medication if the client has a visible draining oral herpes simplex lesion.

Care should be taken to avoid exposing an article brought into a client's room to any infectious material. Bag any contaminated article (e.g., blood pressure cuff) according to agency policy and send it for decontamination. Do not use a contaminated article or bring the article into the room of another client.

Before you institute isolation measures, explain to the client and family the nature of the client's condition, the purpose of the isolation barriers, and ways to carry out specific precautions. Teach the client and family the proper way to wash hands and apply gloves, masks, or gowns. Demonstrate each procedure, and give the client and family an opportunity to practice. Explain methods of transmission of infectious organisms so that the client un-

Skill 10-1
HAND WASHING

DELEGATION CONSIDERATIONS

Hand washing is a basic procedure that should be performed correctly by all caregivers. If you observe assistive personnel, physicians or therapists, and family caregivers incorrectly perform hand washing, reinforce the importance of the technique and the correct procedural steps.

EQUIPMENT

- Easy-to-reach sink with warm running water
- Antimicrobial or regular soap
- Paper towels or air dryer
- Clean orangewood stick (optional)

STEPS	RATIONALE
1. Inspect surface of hands for breaks or cuts in skin or cuticles. Note condition of nails. Artificial nails and long or unkept nails should be avoided. Report and cover any skin lesions before providing client care.	Open cuts or wounds can harbor high concentrations of microorganisms. Long nails and chipped or old polish increase number of bacteria residing on nails, requiring more vigorous hand washing. Artificial nails may increase the microbial load on hands (Larson, 1995). Agency policy may prevent nurse from caring for high-risk clients if open lesions are present on hands.
2. Inspect hands for heavy soiling.	Requires lengthier hand washing.
3. Assess client's risk for or extent of infection, for example, white blood cell count, extent of open wounds, or known medical diagnosis.	Use of antimicrobial soaps is encouraged for clients who are immunosuppressed (Larson, 1995).
4. Push wristwatch and long uniform sleeves above wrists. Avoid wearing rings. If worn, remove during washing.	Provides complete access to fingers, hands, wrists. Wearing of rings increases number of microorganisms on hands (Garner, 1995).
5. Be sure fingernails are short, filed, and smooth.	Many microorganisms on hands come from the subungual region (beneath the fingernails).
6. Stand in front of sink, keeping hands and uniform away from sink surface. (If hands touch sink during hand washing, repeat.)	Inside of sink is a contaminated area. Reaching over sink increases risk of touching edge, which is contaminated.
7. Turn on water. Turn faucet on (see illustration) or push knee pedals laterally or press pedals with foot to regulate flow and temperature.	
8. Avoid splashing water against uniform.	Microorganisms travel and grow in moisture.
9. Regulate flow of water so that temperature is warm.	Warm water removes less of the protective oils than hot water.
10. Wet hands and wrists thoroughly under running water. Keep hands and forearms lower than elbows during washing.	Hands are the most contaminated parts to be washed. Water flows from least to most contaminated area, rinsing microorganisms into sink.
11. Apply a small amount of soap or antiseptic, lathering thoroughly (see illustration). Soap granules and leaflet preparations may be used.	The use of antiseptic exclusively can be drying to the hands and cause skin irritations.

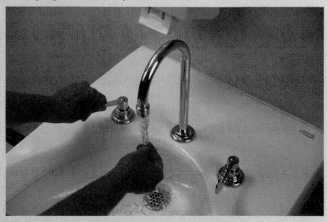

STEP 7   Turning on water.

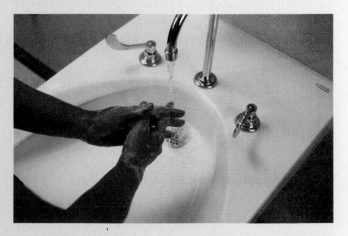

STEP 11   Lathering hands thoroughly.

- *Critical Decision Point*
  The decision whether to use an antiseptic or not should be dependent on the procedure to be performed and the client's immune status.

12. Wash hands using plenty of lather and friction for at least 10 to 15 seconds. Interlace fingers and rub palms and back of hands with circular motion at least 5 times each. Keep fingertips down to facilitate removal of microorganisms.	Soap cleanses by emulsifying fat and oil and lowering surface tension. Friction and rubbing mechanically loosen and remove dirt and transient bacteria. Interlacing fingers and thumbs ensures that all surfaces are cleansed.
13. Areas underlying fingernails are often soiled. Clean them with fingernails of other hand and additional soap or clean orangewood stick.	Area under nails can be highly contaminated, which will increase the risk for infections for you or the client.

- *Critical Decision Point*
  Do not tear or cut skin under or around nail.

14. Rinse hands and wrists thoroughly, keeping hands down and elbows up (see illustration).	Rinsing mechanically washes away dirt and microorganisms.
15. Dry hands thoroughly from fingers to wrists and forearms with paper towel, single-use cloth, or warm air dryer.	Drying from cleanest (fingertips) to least clean (forearms) area avoids contamination. Drying hands prevents chapping and roughened skin.
16. If used, discard paper towel in proper receptacle.	Prevents transfer of microorganisms.
17. To turn off hand faucet, use clean, dry paper towel, avoiding touching handles with hands (see illustration). Turn off water with foot or knee pedals (if applicable).	Wet towel and hands allow transfer of pathogens by capillary action.
18. Inspect surface of hands for obvious signs of dirt or other contaminants.	Determines if hand washing is adequate.

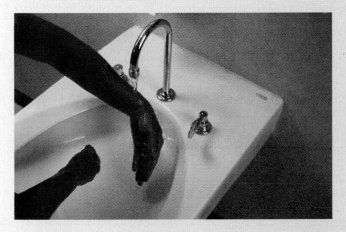

STEP 14   Rinsing hands.

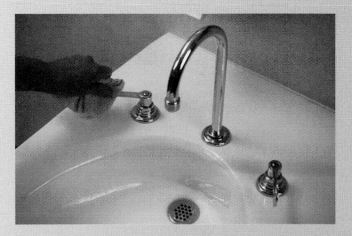

STEP 17   Turning off faucet.

UNEXPECTED OUTCOMES AND RELATED INTERVENTIONS
- Hands or areas under fingernails remain soiled.
  - You must repeat hand washing.
  - Wear gloves. (This should be on a temporary basis because glove wearing can increase bacterial growth and may increase latex allergies among clients and health care workers.)
- Repeated use of soaps or antiseptic may cause dermatitis or cracked skin.
  - Requires methods to alleviate complications of hand washing: Rinse and dry hands thoroughly, avoid excessive amounts of soap or antiseptic, try various products, use hand lotions or barrier creams (small individual-use containers are preferred because large containers have been associated with nosocomial infections).

RECORDING AND REPORTING
- It is not necessary to record or report this procedure.
- Report any dermatitis to employee health and/or infection control per your agency's policy.

CDC Isolation Guidelines

Table 10-5

Standard Precautions (Tier One)

Standard precautions apply to blood, all body fluids, secretions, excretions (except sweat), nonintact skin, and mucous membranes.

Hands are washed between client contacts; after contact with blood, body fluids, secretions, and excretions and after contact with equipment or articles contaminated by them; and immediately after gloves are removed.

Gloves are worn when touching blood, body fluids, secretions, excretions, nonintact skin, mucous membranes, or contaminated items. Gloves should be removed and hands washed between client care.

Masks, eye protection, or face shields are worn if client care activities may generate splashes or sprays of blood or body fluid.

Gowns are worn if soiling of clothing is likely from blood or body fluid. Wash hands after removing gown.

Client care equipment is properly cleaned and reprocessed and single-use items are discarded.

Contaminated linen is placed in a leakproof bag and handled to prevent skin and mucous membrane exposure.

All sharp instruments and needles are discarded in a puncture-resistant container. CDC recommends that needles be disposed of uncapped or that a mechanical device be used for recapping.

A private room is unnecessary unless the client's hygiene is unacceptable. Check with an infection control professional.

Transmission Categories (Tier Two)

Category	Disease	Barrier Protection
Airborne precautions	Droplet nuclei smaller than 5 microns; measles; chickenpox (varicella); disseminated varicella zoster; pulmonary or laryngeal TB	Private room, negative airflow of at least six exchanges per hour, mask or respiratory protection device (see CDC TB guidelines)
Droplet precautions	Droplets larger than 5 microns; diphtheria (pharyngeal); rubella; streptococcal pharyngitis, pneumonia, or scarlet fever in infants and young children; pertussis; mumps; mycoplasma pneumonia; meningococcal pneumonia or sepsis; pneumonic plague	Private room or cohort clients; mask
Contact precautions	Direct client or environmental contact; colonization or infection with multidrug-resistant organism; respiratory syncytial virus; shigella and other enteric pathogens; major wound infections; herpes simplex; scabies, varicella zoster (disseminated)	Private room or cohort clients; gloves, gowns

Modified from Garner JS: Guidelines for isolation precautions for hospitals, *Infect Control Hosp Epidemiol* 17(1):54, 1996.

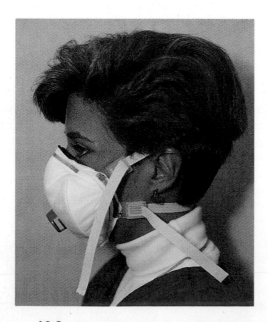

FIGURE **10-3** Disposable HEPA air-purifying respirator.

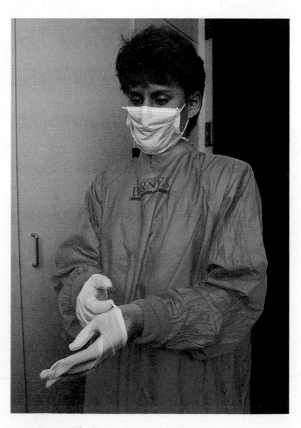

FIGURE **10-4** Nurse wearing an N-95 respirator.

derstands the difference between contaminated and clean objects.

Provide for the client's sensory stimulation during isolation. Reading materials, a radio or television set, a clock, and hobby materials should be available. Take the opportunity to listen to the client's concerns or interests. If care is rushed or you show a lack of interest in the client's needs, the client will feel rejected and even more isolated. Explain the client's potential risk of depression or loneliness to family members. Encourage visitors to avoid negative expressions or actions concerning isolation. Advise family members on ways to provide meaningful stimulation.

Protective Environment. Special rooms for highly susceptible clients such as transplant recipients may be used. When a private room is recommended, post a card on the client's room door, listing the precautions for the isolation category (check agency policy). The card is a handy reference for health care workers and visitors and alerts all who enter the room of any special precautions.

The isolation room or an adjoining anteroom should contain hand washing, bathing, and toilet facilities. Soap and antiseptic solutions should also be available. Personnel and visitors wash their hands before coming to the client's bedside and again before leaving the room. If toilet facilities are unavailable, there are special procedures for handling portable commodes, bedpans, or urinals (check agency policy). Personal protective equipment (PPE) should be stored in an anteroom between the room and hallway or in a convenient location close to the point of use. Resupply PPE as needed.

Each client care room, including those used for isolation, contains a special impervious bag for soiled or contaminated linen and a trash container with plastic liners. These receptacles prevent transmission of microorganisms by preventing seepage to and soiling of the outside surface. A dispos-

---

Procedural Guidelines for   **Box 10-8**
Caring for a Client in Isolation Precautions

1. Assess isolation indications (e.g., current laboratory tests or client's history of exposure).
2. Review agency policies and precautions necessary for the specific isolation system and consider care measures to be performed while in client's room.
3. Review nurses' notes or confer with colleagues regarding client's emotional state and adjustment to isolation.
4. Wash hands and prepare all equipment to be taken into client's room.
5. Prepare for entrance into isolation room:
   a. Apply either surgical mask or respirator around mouth and nose. (Type will depend on type of isolation and facility policy.)
   b. Apply eyewear or goggles snugly around face and eyes (when needed).
   c. Apply gown, being sure it covers all outer garments. Pull sleeves down to wrist. Tie securely at neck and waist (see illustration).
   d. Apply disposable gloves (NOTE: Unpowdered, latex-free gloves should be worn if the client or the health care worker has a latex allergy). If gloves are worn with gown, bring glove cuffs over edge of gown sleeves.
6. Enter client's room. Arrange supplies and equipment. (If equipment will be removed from room for reuse, place on clean paper towel.)
7. Explain purpose of isolation and necessary precautions to client and family. Offer opportunity to ask questions. Assess for evidence of emotional problems that may be caused by being in isolation.
8. Assess vital signs.
   a. If client is infected or colonized with a resistant organism (e.g., VRE, MRSA), equipment remains in room. Proceed to assess vital signs by routine procedures. Avoid contact of stethoscope or blood pressure cuff with infective material.
   b. If stethoscope is to be reused, clean diaphragm or bell with alcohol. Set aside on clean surface.
   c. Individual or disposable thermometers should be used.

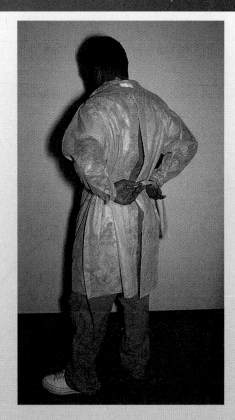

STEP 5C

9. Administer medications (see Chapter 13):
   a. Give oral medication in wrapper or cup.
   b. Dispose of wrapper or cup in plastic-lined receptacle.
   c. Administer injection, being sure gloves are worn.
   d. Discard syringe and uncapped needle or sheathed needle into special container.
   e. If gloves are not worn and hands contact contaminated article or body fluids, wash hands immediately.

Continued

10. Administer hygiene, encouraging the client to discuss questions or concerns about isolation. Informal teaching can be used at this time.
    a. Avoid allowing gown to become wet.
    b. Remove linen from bed; if excessively soiled, avoid contact with gown. Place in impervious linen bag.
    c. Change gloves and wash hands if they become excessively soiled and further care is necessary.
11. Collect specimens:
    a. Place specimen containers on clean paper towel in client's bathroom.
    b. Follow procedure for collecting specimen of body fluids.
    c. Transfer specimen to container without soiling outside of container. Place container in plastic bag and place label on outside of bag or as per facility policy.
12. Dispose of linen and trash bags as they become full:
    a. Use sturdy, moisture-impervious single bags to contain soiled articles.
    b. Tie bags securely at top in knot (see illustration).
13. Resupply room as needed.
14. Leave isolation room.
    a. Remove gloves. Remove one glove by grasping cuff and pulling glove inside out over hand. Discard glove. With ungloved hand, tuck finger inside cuff of remaining glove and pull it off, inside out.
    b. Untie *top* mask string and then bottom strings, pull mask away from face and drop into trash receptacle. (Do not touch outer surface of mask.)
    c. Untie waist and neck strings of gown. Allow gown to fall from shoulders. Remove hands from sleeves without touching outside of gown. Hold gown inside at shoulder seams and fold inside out; discard in laundry bag.
    d. Remove eyewear or goggles.
    e. Wash hands minimum of 10 seconds.
    f. Explain to client when you plan to return to room. Ask whether client requires any personal care items, books, or magazines.

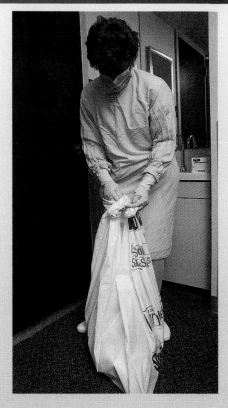

STEP 12B

    g. Leave room and close door, if necessary. (Door should be closed if client is on airborne precautions.)
    h. All contaminated supplies and equipment should be disposed of in a manner that prevents spread of microorganisms to other persons (see agency policy).

able, rigid container should be available in the room to discard used needles, sharps, and syringes.

Depending on the microorganisms and mode of transmission, you must critically evaluate what articles or equipment can be taken into an isolation room. For example, the Hospital Infection Control Practices Advisory Committee (HICPAC) of CDC recommends only dedicated articles be taken into an isolation room of a client infected or colonized with vancomycin-resistant enterococci (HICPAC, 1995).

Personal Protective Equipment (PPE). Gowns or cover-ups protect health care workers from coming in contact with infected blood and body fluids or materials. Gowns used for barrier protection are made of a fluid-resistant material and should be changed immediately if damaged or heavily contaminated.

Isolation gowns usually open at the back and have ties or snaps at the neck and waist to keep the gown closed and se-

cure. A gown should be long enough to cover all outer garments. Long sleeves with tight-fitting cuffs provide added protection. No special technique is required for applying a gown as long as it is fastened securely. Occasionally you may reuse an isolation gown but only for the same client. Evaluate the cost of the gown and cover-up, and reuse the isolation gown for the same client if the gown is not visibly soiled.

Wear a mask or respirator when splashing or spraying of blood or body fluids is anticipated. The mask also protects you from inhaling microorganisms from a client's respiratory tract and prevents the transmission of pathogens from your respiratory tract. Occasionally a client who is susceptible to infection may wear a mask to prevent inhalation of pathogens. Clients requiring respiratory precautions should wear masks when ambulating or being transported outside of their room to protect other clients and personnel.

Masks may prevent the transmission of infections caused by direct contact with mucous membranes. A mask discour-

Procedural Guidelines for
Donning a Surgical Type of Mask   Box 10-9

1. Find top edge of mask (usually has thin metal strip along edge). Pliable metal fits snugly against bridge of nose
2. Hold mask by top two strings or loops. Tie two top ties at top of back of head (see illustration), with ties above ears. (Alternative: slip loops over each ear.)

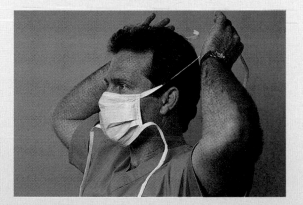

STEP 2

3. Tie two lower ties snugly around neck with mask well under chin (see illustration).

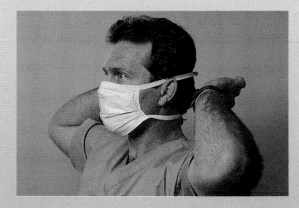

STEP 3

4. Gently pinch upper metal band around bridge of nose.
NOTE: Mask should be changed if wet, moist, or contaminated.

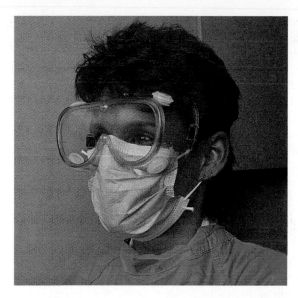

FIGURE **10-5**   Nurse wearing protective goggles and mask.

ages the wearer from touching the nose or mouth. A properly applied mask fits snugly over the mouth and nose so that the pathogens and body fluids cannot enter or escape through the sides (Box 10-9). If a person wears glasses, the top edge of the mask fits below the glasses so they will not cloud over as the person exhales. Keep talking to a minimum while wearing a mask. A mask that has become moist is ineffective and should be discarded. Warn clients and family members that a mask can cause a sensation of smothering. If family members become uncomfortable, they should leave the room and discard the mask.

Apply gloves when there is a risk of exposing the hands to blood, body fluids, or potentially infectious material. In addition, gloves are recommended when you have scratches or breaks in the skin and when performing venipuncture or finger or heel sticks. In most cases disposable, single-use gloves are worn. Gloves may be worn alone or in combination with other PPE. When other PPE is necessary, first don a mask and eyewear (if required), apply a gown (if required), and then apply gloves. Pull the glove cuffs up over the wrists or cuffs of a gown.

After contacting infectious material, change gloves and wash your hands if care is not completed. If your actions do not involve more client contact, it is unnecessary to reapply gloves. Clients and their families can be taught the reasons for wearing gloves and the correct method for applying gloves.

Many gloves used for barrier protection or surgical asepsis are made of latex. Before applying latex gloves, assess the potential for latex allergies. The symptoms range from mild dermatitis to severe anaphylactic shock. Clients and health care workers can become sensitized to latex by repeated contact or by inhaling aerosolized latex allergens contained in the glove powder.

The American Nurses Association (ANA) (1996) provides the following suggestions for nurses to avoid becoming latex allergic:

1. Whenever possible, wear powder-free gloves (they are lower in protein allergens).
2. Wear gloves that are appropriate for the task (e.g., avoid use for cleaning).
3. Wash with a pH-balanced soap immediately after removing gloves.
4. Apply only non–oil-based hand care products (oil-based products break down latex allergens).
5. If a reaction or dermatitis occurs, report to employee health and/or seek medical treatment immediately.

Wear eyewear and face shields, properly fitted, during procedures in which the eyes or face could be splattered by blood or other infectious material (Figure 10-5). In many instances caregivers purchase their own eyewear with prescription lenses. Regular glasses are insufficient. Glasses must have side shields to prevent material from entering the eye between the glasses and face.

Specimen Collection.   A client with a suspected or actual infectious disease may undergo many laboratory studies. Body fluids and materials suspected of containing infectious organisms are collected for culture and sensitivity tests. The specimen is placed in a special medium that promotes the growth of organisms. A laboratory technologist then identifies the type of microorganisms growing in the culture. Additional sensitivity test results indicate the antibiotics to which the organisms are resistant or sensitive so that the proper medications will be used in the client's treatment.

Obtain all culture specimens with sterile equipment. Collecting fresh material from the site of infection, as in the case of wound drainage, ensures that the specimen will not be contaminated by resident flora. Seal all specimen containers tightly to prevent spillage and contamination of the outside of the container (Box 10-10). After the specimens are transferred to containers, label each specimen properly with the client's name, client identifier, date and time, and type of specimen. Place the specimen containers in labeled impervious bags before transporting them to the laboratory if required by facility policy.

Bagging.   Bagging articles generally is the same for all client's rooms regardless of whether the room is an isolation room. Bagging articles prevents accidental exposure of personnel to contaminated articles and prevents contamination of the surrounding environment. Garner (1996b) recommends that a single bag is adequate for discarding or wrapping items if the bag is impervious and sturdy and if the article can be placed in the bag without contaminating the outside of the bag. Typically you would place reusable equipment such as stethoscopes, forceps, or suction bottles in single bags according to agency policy.

Place all soiled linen in a designated waterproof impervious bag in the client's room. Do not overfill the bag. Linen that is visibly soiled with blood or body fluids should be handled, transported, and processed in a manner that will prevent exposure of skin or mucous membrane and/or contamination of the health care worker's clothing. Double bagging still may be required in some hospitals. A standard-sized linen bag, not overfilled, tied securely and intact is adequate to prevent infection transmission. Consult agency policy and any applicable regulations for the proper procedure.

Biohazardous waste includes both infectious and medical waste that must be disposed of in special red bags. Red-bagged or infectious trash must be disposed of by incineration and special handling. These special procedures are a high expense for health care facilities. The following waste materials should be considered infectious or medical waste (Luebbert, 2000):

1. Cultures, including discarded cultures of infectious organisms

---

Specimen Collection Techniques*   Box 10-10

WOUND SPECIMEN

Clean site with sterile water or saline before wound specimen collection. Wear gloves and use cotton-tipped swab or syringe to collect as much drainage as possible. Have clean test tube or culture tube on clean paper towel. After swabbing center of wound site, grasp collection tube by holding it with paper towel. Carefully insert swab without touching outside of tube. After securing tube's top, transfer tube into bag for transport and then wash hands.

BLOOD SPECIMEN

Wearing gloves, use syringe and culture media bottles to collect up to 10 ml of blood per culture bottle (check agency policy). After prepping, perform venipuncture at two different sites to decrease likelihood of both specimens being contaminated with skin flora. Place blood culture bottles on bedside table or other surface; swab off bottle tops with alcohol. Inject appropriate amount of blood into each bottle. Remove gloves and transfer specimen into clean, labeled bag for transport. Wash hands.

STOOL SPECIMEN

Wearing gloves, use clean cup with seal top (need not be sterile) and tongue blade to collect small amount of stool, approximately the size of a walnut. Place cup on clean paper towel in client's bathroom. Using tongue blade, collect needed amount of feces from client's bedpan. Transfer feces to cup without touching cup's outside surface. Dispose of tongue blade, and place seal on cup. Transfer specimen into clean bag for transport. Remove gloves and wash hands.

URINE SPECIMEN

Wearing gloves, use syringe and sterile cup to collect 1 to 5 ml of urine. Place cup or tube on clean towel in client's bathroom. If client has a urinary catheter, use syringe to collect specimen. Have client follow procedure to obtain a clean-voided specimen (see Chapter 31) if not catheterized. Transfer urine into sterile container by injecting urine from syringe or pouring it from used collection cup. Secure top of container and transfer specimen into clean, labeled bag for transport. Remove gloves and wash hands.

Data from Rosen-Kotilainen H: Laboratory diagnostics. In Pfeiffer J, editor: *APIC text of infection control and epidemiology,* Washington, DC, 2000, Association for Professionals in Infection Control and Epidemiology, Inc.
*Agency policies may differ on type of containers and amount of specimen material required.

---

2. Pathological waste, such as discarded human tissue, organs, and body parts
3. Blood and blood products, including discarded serum or plasma and materials containing free-flowing blood
4. Sharps, including discarded needles, syringes, scalpels, blood vials, broken or unbroken glass, and pipettes
5. Selected isolation material, discarded waste material from clients with highly communicable diseases

Removal of Protective Equipment.   The method of removing protective clothing, gloves, mask, eyewear, and gown before leaving an isolation room depends on the protective equipment worn at the time. In the example in which all

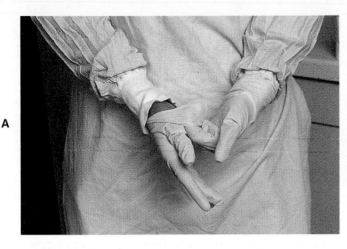
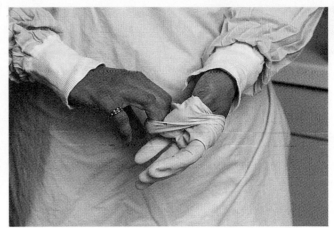

A   B

FIGURE **10-6**   Removing disposable gloves. **A,** Nurse places gloved finger inside cuff to pull first glove off hand. **B,** Second glove is removed as nurse slides fingers inside glove cuff and pulls.

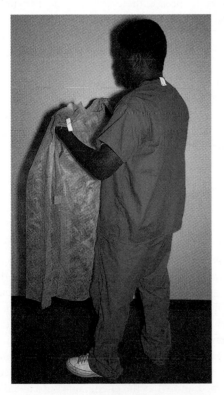

FIGURE **10-7**   Nurse removing isolation gown.

four protective items are worn, first remove the gloves because they are most likely to be contaminated. If you untie a gown with gloves still on, there is a chance of contaminating your hair or a portion of the uniform. When pulling gloves off, grasp the cuff with the other gloved hand and pull it off, turning the glove inside out. Tuck the fingers of the ungloved hand inside the cuff of the remaining glove and pull it off, turning the glove inside out (Figure 10-6). Discard the gloves in a plastic-lined receptacle.

Isolation masks are disposable and made of a specially prepared paper or natural fiber. Untie the top string first, then the bottom, and pull the mask away from the face while holding the strings. Do not touch the outside surface of the mask. Discard the mask in a plastic-lined receptacle. Check agency policy for frequency of disposal of high efficiency particulate arresting (HEPA) and other types of respirators.

To remove a gown, first untie the waist and neck ties. Allow the gown to fall gently from the shoulders. Take care to remove the hands from the sleeves without touching the outside of the gown (Figure 10-7). Do not allow the sleeves to turn inside out. Hold the gown at the shoulder seams, and fold it in half with the outside surfaces touching to reduce contact with the soiled gown. Then discard the gown in an appropriate receptacle.

The last step is to remove eyewear. Some goggles and glasses are reusable. Refer to agency policy for cleaning procedures. Once eyewear is removed, complete thorough hand washing.

Transporting Clients.   Clients infected with highly communicable organisms, such as TB, should leave their rooms only for essential purposes such as diagnostic procedures or surgery. Before transferring the client to a wheelchair or stretcher, give the client the appropriate barrier protection. For example, a client who is infected by an organism transmitted by the respiratory tract must wear a mask. Personnel transporting the client should practice the appropriate precautions while in the client's room. Personnel in diagnostic areas or the operating room should be notified that the client is on isolation. Record the type of isolation on the client's chart, and explain ways to avoid transmitting infection during transport.

CONTROL OF PORTALS OF ENTRY.   Many measures that control the exit of microorganisms also control the entrance of pathogens. Evaluate the client, and provide interventions to control and prevent organisms from gaining a portal of entry (Box 10-11).

PROTECTION OF THE SUSCEPTIBLE HOST.   A client's resistance to infection improves by initiating measures that

Infection Control of Portals of Entry Box 10-11

INTACT SKIN AND MUCOSA

Keep skin clean and well lubricated.

Avoid positioning clients on tubes or objects that might cause breaks in skin.

Use dry, wrinkle-free linen.

Offer frequent oral hygiene (see Chapter 26).

Provide frequent position changes for clients with impaired mobility.

URINARY TRACT

Teach women to clean rectum and perineum by wiping from area of least contamination (urinary meatus) toward area of most contamination (rectum).

Do not allow urine in drainage bags and tubes to flow back into the bladder. Never raise a drainage system above the level of the bladder.

Keep points of connection between catheter or drain and tubing closed.

INVASIVE TUBES AND LINES

When obtaining specimens from drainage tubes or inserting needles into intravenous lines, disinfect tubes and ports by wiping them liberally with a disinfectant solution before entering the system.

WOUND CARE

Keep draining wounds covered so that drainage is contained.

Clean outward from a wound site using a clean swab for each application.

---

protect normal body defense mechanisms. In the acute care setting, many of the interventions either promote existing body defense mechanisms or control exposure to microorganisms. Regular bathing removes transient microorganisms from the skin. Lubrication helps to keep the skin hydrated and intact. Regular oral hygiene removes proteins in the saliva that attract microorganisms. Flossing removes tartar and plaque that can cause infection. An adequate fluid intake promotes normal urine formation and a resultant outflow of urine to flush the bladder and urethra of microorganisms. For immobilized or dependent clients, regular coughing and deep breathing exercises remove mucus from lower airways.

ROLE OF THE INFECTION PREVENTION AND CONTROL DEPARTMENT.

Most health care facilities employ health professionals who are specially trained in the area of infection control. Their roles and responsibilities include providing consultations, educational offerings, and program development in infection control and prevention.

HEALTH PROMOTION IN HEALTH CARE WORKERS AND CLIENTS.

A health care worker who becomes ill can expose susceptible clients to infectious diseases. An institution's employee health service provides programs to assist in infection control, such as immunization programs, recommendations for work restrictions and protocols for management of job-related exposures to infectious diseases.

SURGICAL ASEPSIS. Surgical asepsis or aseptic technique is designed to eliminate all microorganisms, including spores and pathogens, from an object and to protect an area from these microorganisms. Surgical asepsis requires more precautions than medical asepsis. Breaks in technique could result in contamination, thus increasing the client's risk for infection (DeCastro, 2000).

Although surgical asepsis is commonly practiced in the operating room, labor and delivery area, and major diagnostic or procedural areas, surgical aseptic techniques may also be used at the client's bedside (e.g., when inserting intravenous catheters). Surgical asepsis is indicated during procedures that require intentional perforation of the client's skin (e.g., surgical incision), when the skin's integrity is broken related to trauma or burns, and during procedures that involve insertion of a catheter or surgical instruments into sterile body cavities (DeCastro, 2000).

A series of steps involving sterile technique are used in the operating room, such as applying a mask, protective eyewear, and a cap; performing a surgical scrub; and applying a sterile gown and gloves. In contrast, performing a sterile dressing change at a client's bedside may only require hand washing and donning sterile gloves (Box 10-12). Regardless of the procedures followed in different settings, the use of surgical asepsis depends on developing an aseptic conscience. Always recognize the importance of strict adherence to aseptic principles. You can also be an excellent role model and client advocate, reinforcing proper practice for other caregivers.

PREPARATION FOR STERILE PROCEDURES. In the operating room, control of aseptic technique is more easily enforced. In treatment rooms and at the bedside it is important to have a client's full cooperation. Therefore assess the client's understanding of sterile procedure and the reasons for not moving or interfering with the procedure. Special precautions, such as masking the client or changing the client's position, may be necessary to prevent contamination during procedures. Determine whether a client has undergone a sterile procedure in the past. Explain how the procedure will be performed and what the client can do to avoid contaminating sterile objects:

1. Avoid sudden movements of body parts covered by sterile drapes.
2. Refrain from touching sterile supplies, drapes, or your sterile gloves and gown.
3. Avoid coughing, sneezing, or talking over a sterile area.

Certain sterile procedures may last for an extended time. Assess the client's needs (e.g., pain control or elimination) in advance and anticipate factors that may disrupt a procedure. If a client is in pain, try to administer analgesics no more than 30 minutes before a sterile procedure begins. Clients often assume relatively uncomfortable positions during sterile procedures. Help the client to assume the most comfortable

Procedural Guidelines for
OPEN GLOVING

Box 10-12

1. Consider the procedure to be performed, and consult agency policy on use of gloves.
2. Inspect hands for cuts, open lesions, or abrasions.
3. Assess if the client or health care worker has a known allergy to latex.
4. Examine glove package to ensure package is not wet, torn, or discolored.
5. Perform thorough hand washing, and determine correct glove size and type of glove material to be used.
6. Remove outer glove package wrapper by carefully separating and peeling apart sides.
7. Grasp inner package and lay it on clean, flat surface just above waist level. Open package, keeping gloves on wrapper's inside surface.
8. Identify right and left glove. Each glove has cuff approximately 5 cm (2 inches) wide. Glove dominant hand first.
9. With thumb and first two fingers of nondominant hand, grasp edge of cuff of the glove for the dominant hand. Touch only glove's inside surface.
10. Carefully pull glove over dominant hand (see illustration) leaving a cuff and being sure the cuff does not roll up wrist. Be sure thumb and fingers are in proper spaces (see illustration).
11. With gloved dominant hand, slip fingers underneath second glove's cuff (see illustration).
12. Carefully pull second glove over nondominant hand (see illustration). Do not allow fingers and thumb of gloved dominant hand to touch any part of exposed nondominant hand. Keep thumb of dominant hand abducted.
13. After second glove is on, interlock hands (see illustration). Cuffs usually fall down after application. Be sure to touch only sterile sides.

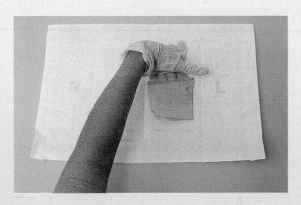

STEP 11

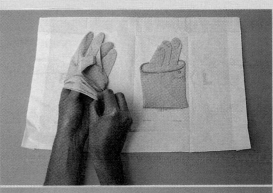

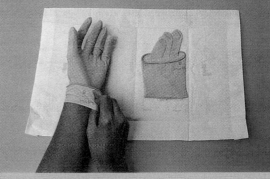

STEP 10

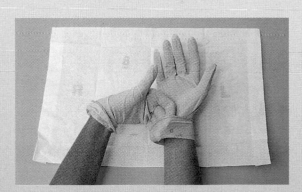

STEP 12

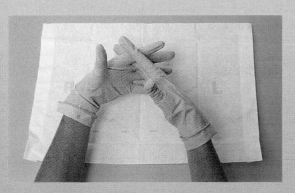

STEP 13

position possible. Finally, the client's condition may result in events that contaminate a sterile field (e.g., the client with a respiratory infection who transmits organisms by coughing or breathing). Anticipate such a problem (e.g., offering a mask to the client before the procedure begins).

PRINCIPLES OF SURGICAL ASEPSIS.   When beginning a surgically aseptic procedure, explain principles to ensure maintenance of asepsis must be followed. Failure to follow each principle conscientiously endangers clients, placing them at risk for an infection. Principles of surgical asepsis include the following:

1. *A sterile object remains sterile only when touched by another sterile object.* The following principles guide you in placement and handling of sterile objects:
   - Sterile touching sterile remains sterile; for example, sterile gloves are worn to handle objects on a sterile field.
   - Sterile touching clean becomes contaminated; for example, if the tip of a syringe touches the surface of a clean disposable glove, the syringe is contaminated.
   - Sterile touching contaminated becomes contaminated; for example, when you touch a sterile object with an ungloved hand, the object is contaminated.
   - Sterile touching questionable is contaminated; for example, when a tear or break in the covering of a sterile object is found, it is discarded or reprocessed regardless of whether the object appears untouched.
2. *Only sterile objects may be placed on a sterile field.* All items are properly sterilized before use. The package or container holding a sterile object must be intact and dry. A package that is torn, punctured, wet, or open is unsterile (Figures 10-8 and 10-9).
3. *A sterile object or field out of the range of vision or an object held below a person's waist is contaminated.* Never turn your back on a sterile tray or leave it unattended. Any object held below waist level is considered contaminated because it cannot be viewed at all times. Sterile objects should be kept either on or out over the sterile field.
4. *A sterile object or field becomes contaminated by prolonged exposure to the air.* Avoid activities that may create air currents, such as excessive movements or rearranging linen after a sterile object or field becomes exposed. When opening sterile packages, minimize the number of people walking into the area. Microorganisms also travel by droplet through the air. No one should talk, laugh, sneeze, or cough over a sterile field or when gathering and using sterile equipment. When opening a tray and adding sterile equipment, wear a mask. Microorganisms traveling through the air can fall on sterile items or fields if you reach over the work area (Box 10-13).
5. *A sterile object or field becomes contaminated by capillary action when a sterile surface comes in contact with a wet contaminated surface.* Moisture seeps through a sterile package's protective covering, allowing microorganisms to travel to the sterile object. When stored sterile packages become wet, discard the objects immediately or send the equipment for resterilization. Spilling solution over a sterile drape contaminates the field unless the drape cannot be penetrated by moisture.
6. *Because fluid flows in the direction of gravity, a sterile object becomes contaminated if gravity causes a contaminated liquid to flow over the object's surface.* To avoid contamination during a surgical hand scrub, hold your hands above the elbows. This allows water to flow downward without contaminating your hands and fingers. The principle of water flow by gravity is also the reason for drying from fingers to elbows with the hands held up, after the scrub.
7. *The edges of a sterile field or container are contaminated.* A 2.5-cm (1-inch) border around a sterile towel or drape is considered contaminated (Box 10-14). The edges of sterile containers become exposed to air after they are open and are thus contaminated. After a sterile needle is removed from its protective cap or after forceps are removed from a container, the objects must not touch the container's edge. The lip of an opened bottle of solution also becomes contaminated after it is exposed to air. When pouring a sterile liquid, first pour a small amount of solution and discard it. The solution washes away any microorganisms on the bottle lip. Then

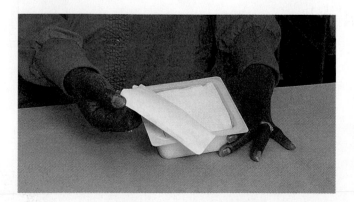

FIGURE **10-8**   Opening a commercially packaged sterile item.

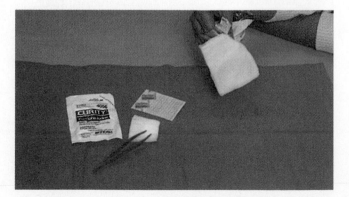

FIGURE **10-9**   Adding item to a sterile field, being sure not to hold arm over sterile field.

pour the liquid a second time to fill a sterile container with the desired amount of solution.

RESTORATIVE CARE.   The need for infection control is also present when clients are in the restorative phase of their care. Nurses in long-term care settings can contribute to quality health care by practicing skills and techniques necessary to prevent infections.

LONG-TERM CARE.   Some of the same risks for infections that are present in acute care can apply in long-term care facilities, such as skilled nursing homes (Gantz and others, 2000). Certain risks of nosocomial infections are increased because of the usual age of clients seen in long-term care facilities. For example, in older adults several age-associated physical changes can alter the natural barriers to infections (see Box 10-2, p. 153).

Some of the major infections common to clients in long-term care are urinary tract infections, pressure ulcer infections, and pneumonia, which are the three most common infections in long-term care facilities. You can play an important role in the control of these infections by using critical thinking skills and knowledge of how these infections can be prevented. See Chapters 27, 31, and 34 for additional information on these infections.

 Evaluation

CLIENT CARE.   As you deliver care to the client, it is important to evaluate the result of interventions so that you can continue or revise nursing care therapies or determine that a problem has been resolved. Evaluation of nursing care is based on the goals and outcomes established during the planning phase of the nursing process. Because a client's condition can change at any time, evaluation is ongoing. You should use assessment skills to determine the client's progress over time. For example, evaluate if inflammation is increasing, if the WBC count is decreasing, or if the client's sputum is clearing.

Procedural Guidelines for   **Box 10-13**

OPENING WRAPPED STERILE ITEMS

1. Place sterile kit or package containing sterile items on clean, dry, flat work surface above waist level.
2. Open outside cover, and remove kit from dust cover. Place on work surface.
3. Grasp outer surface of tip of outermost flap.
4. Open outermost flap away from body, keeping arm outstretched and away from sterile field (see illustration).
5. Grasp outside surface of edge of first side flap.
6. Open side flap, pulling to side, allowing it to lie flat on table surface. Keep your arm to side and not over sterile surface (see illustration). Do not allow flaps to spring back over sterile contents.
7. Repeat steps for second side flap.
8. Grasp outside border of last and innermost flap.
9. Stand away from sterile package, and pull flap back, allowing it to fall flat on table (see illustration).
10. Use the inner surface of the package (except for the 1-inch border around the edges) as a field to add additional items because it is sterile. Grasp the 1-inch border to move the field over the work surface.

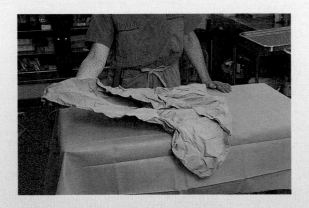

STEP 6

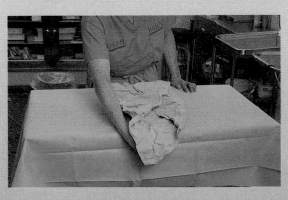

STEP 4

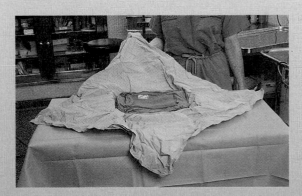

STEP 9

Procedural Guidelines for
PREPARATION OF A STERILE FIELD

Box 10-14

1. Wash hands.
2. Place pack containing sterile drape on work surface, and open as described under "Opening Wrapped Sterile Item."
3. Apply sterile gloves (optional, see agency policy).
4. With fingertips of one hand, pick up the folded top edge of the sterile drape.
5. Gently lift the drape up from its outer cover and let it unfold by itself without touching any object. Keep it above the waist. Discard the outer cover with the other hand.

6. With the other hand, grasp an adjacent corner of the drape and hold it straight up and away from the body (see illustration).
7. Holding the drape, first position and lay the bottom half over the intended work surface (see illustration).
8. Allow the top half of the drape to be placed over the work surface last (see illustration).
9. Grasp the 1-inch border around the edge to position as needed.

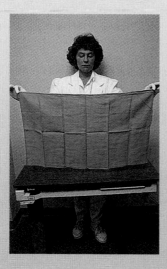

STEP 6

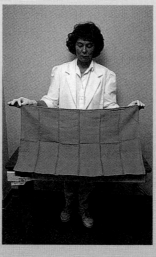

STEP 7

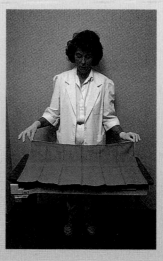

STEP 8

Evaluative measures are used for each of the established expected outcomes. The information gathered determines the status of each client goal. For example, if the goal is "Wound heals within 2 weeks" and the outcome is "Client's wound drainage decreases in 3 days," the evaluative measure involves inspecting the amount of drainage on a dressing or measuring the amount of drainage collected in a drainage device. Your evaluation will determine if interventions should continue, if revisions are needed in therapies, if new therapies are required, or if the client has developed new nursing diagnoses.

CLIENT EXPECTATIONS.   Always remember to ask the client if expectations of care have been met. Has the client gained the information he or she desires to understand therapies and to manage treatment of an infection at home? Does the client believe that you performed knowledgeably and competently? Was the client on isolation treated with respect and dignity? You must not assume you know the client's expectations. Your evaluation reviews expectations gathered during assessment and then reassesses the client's perceptions and opinions about care.

Key Terms

airborne precautions, *p. 159*
antibody, *p. 150*
antigen, *p. 151*
asepsis, *p. 152*
aseptic technique, *p. 152*
carriers, *p. 150*
colonization, *p. 149*
communicable disease, *p. 149*
contact precautions, *p. 159*

disinfection, *p. 158*
droplet precautions, *p. 159*
endogenous infection, *p. 152*
exogenous infection, *p. 152*
exudate, *p. 153*
flora, *p. 151*
immunity, *p. 150*
immunocompromised, *p. 159*
infection, *p. 149*
inflammation, *p. 151*
isolation, *p. 159*

medical asepsis, *p. 152*
microorganisms, *p. 149*
necrotic, *p. 151*
nosocomial infection, *p. 152*
pathogenicity, *p. 150*
pathogens, *p. 149*
standard precautions, *p. 159*
sterilization, *p. 158*
suprainfection, *p. 151*
surgical asepsis, *p. 153*
virulence, *p. 149*

Key Concepts

- Normal body flora resist infection by inhibiting multiplication of pathogenic microorganisms.
- Immunity to infection is measured by the capacity to produce antibodies in response to exposure to an antigen.
- An infection can develop as long as the six elements constituting the infection chain are uninterrupted.
- A microorganism's virulence depends on its ability to resist attack by the body's normal defenses.
- Microorganisms are transmitted by direct and indirect contact, by airborne spread, and by vectors and contaminated vehicles.
- Increasing age, poor nutrition, stress, inherited conditions, chronic disease, and treatments or conditions that compromise the immune response increase susceptibility to infection.
- Gloves, gowns, and masks in combination with eye protection devices such as goggles or glasses with solid side shields should be worn when in contact with blood or potentially infectious material or whenever splashes or spray of blood or potentially infectious material may be generated.
- Invasive procedures, medical therapies, long hospitalization, and contact with health care personnel increase a hospitalized client's risk for acquiring a nosocomial infection.
- Surgical asepsis requires more stringent techniques than medical asepsis and is directed toward eliminating microorganisms.
- The CDC recommends that all clients be considered as potentially infected with HIV and other blood-borne pathogens; therefore health care workers should reduce the risk of exposure to blood and body fluids.
- Standard precautions involve using barrier protection with all clients regardless of presence of infection.
- Following aseptic principles is the key to your success in preventing clients from acquiring infections.
- A client receiving isolation precautions is subject to sensory deprivation because of the restricted environment.
- Lack of hand washing is the main cause of nosocomial infections.
- An infection-control health professional provides educational and consultative services to maintain aseptic practices.
- If the skin is broken or if you perform an invasive procedure into a body cavity normally free of microorganisms, surgical aseptic practices are enforced.
- A sterile object becomes contaminated by direct contact with a clean or contaminated object, by exposure to airborne microorganisms, or by contact with a wet surface containing microorganisms.

Critical Thinking Activities

1. During a home care visit, it is reported that several members of a family have had diarrhea and vomiting after eating a dinner of turkey and stuffing. After further investigation, it is determined that the turkey was thawed at room temperature instead of following the recommendation to thaw in the refrigerator and that the stuffing was placed in the turkey's cavity before the turkey was completely thawed. The nurse reports this immediately to the physician, and stool cultures are ordered. Three members of the family are diagnosed as having *Salmonella* food-borne illness. Describe in this case (using the chain of infection) how the infection occurred and how you can assist the clients in preventing further food-borne illness.
2. In the following client care situations, select the appropriate PPE and give the rationale: (a) starting an IV catheter, (b) blood pressure checks on a client with hepatitis B, (c) changing the bed linen for an incontinent client, (d) entering the room of a client with meningococcal meningitis, (e) entering the room of a client with *Mycobacterium avium*, (f) emptying a suction bottle containing bloody fluid, and (g) changing an infected wound dressing on a client in a home situation.
3. Mrs. Smith is admitted for a major surgical procedure. During the admission procedure, you notice that Mrs. Smith has a productive cough that she says she has had for about 6 weeks. She further states that she has occasionally seen blood in her sputum and has lost weight over the past 4 weeks. Mrs. Smith also tells you that one of the members of her immediate household has been recently diagnosed with tuberculosis. With this additional history, what should you do?

Review Questions

1. The *most* effective way to break the chain of infection is by:
   1. hand washing.
   2. wearing gloves.
   3. placing clients in isolation.
   4. providing private rooms for all clients.
2. A client's surgical wound has become swollen, red, and tender. You note that the client has a new fever and leukocytosis. Your best immediate intervention would be to:
   1. use surgical technique to change the dressing.
   2. reassure the client and recheck the wound later.
   3. notify the physician and support the client's fluid and nutritional needs.
   4. alert the client and caregivers to the presence of an infection to ensure care after discharge.
3. A client is isolated for pulmonary tuberculosis. You note the client seems to be angry, but you know this is a normal response to isolation. The best intervention would be to:
   1. provide a dark, quiet room to calm the client.
   2. explain isolation procedures and provide meaningful stimulation.
   3. reduce the level of precautions to keep the client from becoming angry.

Continued

Review Questions—cont'd

4. limit family and other caregiver visits to reduce the risk of spreading the infection.

4. A client has an indwelling urinary catheter. You recognize that the catheter represents a risk for urinary tract infection because:
   1. it keeps an incontinent client's skin dry.
   2. it can get caught in the linens or equipment.
   3. it obstructs the normal flushing action of urine flow.
   4. it allows the client to remain hydrated without having to urinate.

5. You have redressed a client's wound and now plan to administer a medication to the client. It is important to:
   1. remove gloves and wash hands before leaving the room.
   2. remove gloves and wash hands before administering the medication.
   3. leave the gloves on to administer the medication.
   4. leave the medication on the bedside table to avoid having to remove gloves.

6. A gown should be worn when working with a client:
   1. if the client's hygiene is poor.
   2. if the client has AIDS or hepatitis.
   3. if you are assisting with medication administration.
   4. if blood or body fluids may get on your clothing from a task you plan to perform.

7. Gloves should be removed and hands washed:
   1. only after wound care.
   2. when leaving the room.
   3. when you have completed all tasks for the client.
   4. when the specific task you put them on for is completed.

8. A complication for postoperative clients is pneumonia. To prevent pneumonia, your best intervention is to:
   1. ensure rest, avoiding disturbing the client.
   2. discourage ambulation because this could disrupt the wound.
   3. provide adequate fluid and nutrition support postoperatively.
   4. provide adequate pain control and encourage the client to breathe deeply and cough regularly.

References

Advisory Committee on Immunization Practices, Centers for Disease Control and Prevention: *MMWR Morb Mortal Wkly Rep* 5/17/98, 1/12/01.

American Nurses Association: *Latex allergy, WP-70M,* 1996, Washington, DC, 1996, The Association.

Centers for Disease Control and Prevention: Update: universal precautions for prevention of transmission of human immunodeficiency virus, hepatitis B, and other bloodborne pathogens in health care setting, *MMWR Morb Mortal Wkly Rep* 37(24):377, 1988.

Centers for Disease Control and Prevention: Guidelines for preventing the transmission of tuberculosis in health care facilities, *MMWR Morb Mortal Wkly Rep* 43(RR-13):1, 1994.

DeCastro H: Laboratory diagnostics. In Pfeiffer J, editor: *APIC text of infection control and epidemiology,* Washington, DC, 2000, Association for Professionals in Infection Control and Epidemiology, Inc.

Fauerbach L: Risk factors for infection transmission. In Pfeiffer J, editor: *APIC text of infection control and epidemiology,* Washington, DC, 2000, Association for Professionals in Infection Control and Epidemiology, Inc.

Gantz NM and others: Geriatric infections. In Pfeiffer J editor: *APIC text of infection control and epidemiology,* Washington, DC, 2000, Association for Professionals in Infection Control and Epidemiology, Inc.

Garner B: Infection control. In Meeker MH, Rothrock JC, editors: *Alexander's care of the patient in surgery,* ed 11, St. Louis, 1999, Mosby.

Garner J: Isolation systems. In Olmsted R, editor: *APIC infection control and applied epidemiology,* St. Louis, 1996b, Mosby.

Garner JS: Guidelines for isolation precautions for hospitals, *Infect Control Hosp Epidemiol* 17(1):54, 1996a.

Hospital Infection Control Practices Advisory Committee: Recommendations for preventing the spread of vancomycin-resistant organisms, *Am J Infect Control* 23:87, 1995.

Hospital Infection Control Practices Advisory Committee: Guidelines for isolation precautions in hospitals, *Am J Infect Control* 24:24, 1996.

Jackson M, Tweeten S: General principles of epidemiology. In Pfeiffer J, editor: *APIC text of infection control and epidemiology,* Washington, DC, 2000, Association for Professionals in Infection Control and Epidemiology, Inc.

Larson E: APIL guidelines for hand washing and hand antisepsis in health care settings, *Am J Infect Control* 23(4):251, 1995.

Larson E: APIC guidelines for hand washing and hand antisepsis in health care settings. In Pfeiffer J, editor: *APIC text of infection control and epidemiology,* Washington, DC, 2000, Association for Professionals in Infection Control and Epidemiology, Inc.

Luebbert P: Infection control in clinical laboratories. In Pfeiffer J, editor: *APIC text of infection control and epidemiology,* Washington, DC, 2000, Association for Professionals in Infection Control and Epidemiology, Inc.

Occupational Safety and Health Administration: Occupational exposure to blood borne pathogens: final rule, 29 CFR 1919:1030, *Federal Register* 56:64175, 1991.

Occupational Safety and Health Administration: Respiratory protective devices: final rules and notice, *Federal Register* 60:30336, 1995.

Rosen-Kotilainen H: Laboratory diagnostics. In Pfeiffer J, editor: *APIC text of infection control and epidemiology,* Washington, DC, 2000, Association for Professionals in Infection Control and Epidemiology, Inc.

Rubel A, Garro I: Social and cultural factors in successful control of tuberculosis, *Public Health Rep* 107(6):626, 1992.

Rutala W: Disinfection and sterilization of patient-care items, *Infect Control Hosp Epidemiol* 17(6):377, 1996.

Schaffer S and others: *Infection prevention and safe practice,* St. Louis, 1996, Mosby.

Thompson C: Nutrition and immune function. In Pfeiffer J, editor: *APIC text of infection control and epidemiology,* Washington, DC, 2000, Association for Professionals in Infection Control and Epidemiology, Inc.

Williams D, Peterson P: Antimicrobial use and development of resistance. In Pfeiffer J, editor: *APIC text of infection control and epidemiology,* Washington, DC, 2000, Association for Professionals in Infection Control and Epidemiology, Inc.

Vital Signs

Objectives

- Define the key terms listed.
- Explain the principles and mechanisms of thermoregulation.
- Describe nursing measures that promote heat loss and heat conservation.
- Discuss physiological changes associated with fever.
- Accurately assess body temperature.
- Accurately assess pulse, respiration, oxygen saturation, and blood pressure.
- Describe factors that cause variations in vital signs.
- Identify ranges of acceptable vital sign values for an adult, child, and infant.
- Explain variations in technique used to assess an infant's, child's, and adult's vital signs.
- Appropriately delegate vital sign measurement to assistive personnel.

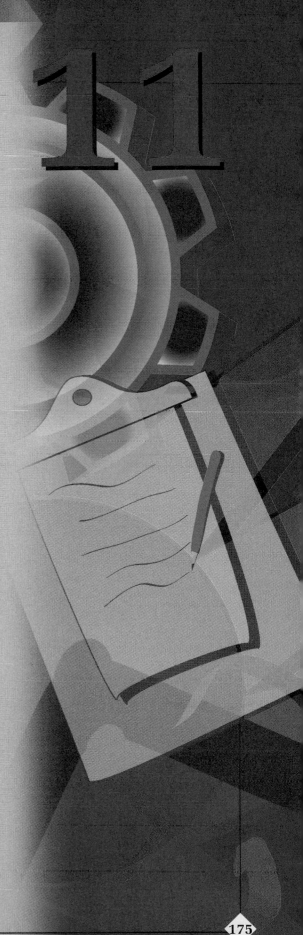

The cardinal **vital signs** are temperature, pulse, respiration, blood pressure (BP), and oxygen saturation. A sixth vital sign, assessment of pain, is a standard of care in health care settings. Frequently pain and discomfort may be the signs that lead a client to seek health care. For this reason, assessment of your client's pain is key to understanding the client's clinical status and progress. Many factors such as the temperature of the environment, physical exertion, and the effects of illness cause vital signs to change, sometimes outside the acceptable range. Measurement of vital signs and the assessment of pain (see Chapter 29) provide data to determine a client's usual state of health (baseline data) and response to physical and psychological stress and medical and nursing therapy. A change in vital signs can indicate a change in physiological functioning or a change in comfort. An alteration in vital signs may signal the need for medical or nursing intervention.

Measurement of vital signs is a quick and efficient way of monitoring a client's condition or identifying problems and evaluating the client's response to intervention. The basic skills required to measure vital signs are simple but should not be taken for granted. Vital signs and other physiological measurements are the basis for clinical problem solving.

GUIDELINES FOR MEASURING VITAL SIGNS

Vital signs are assessed whenever a client enters a health care agency. Vital signs are included in a complete physical assessment (see Chapter 12) or obtained individually to assess a client's condition. The client's needs and condition determine when, where, how, and by whom vital signs are measured. You must be able to measure vital signs correctly, understand and interpret the values, communicate findings appropriately, and begin interventions as needed. The following guidelines will help you incorporate vital sign measurement into nursing practice:

1. When caring for the client, you are responsible for vital sign measurement. You can delegate the measurement of selected vital signs to assistive personnel. However, you must review vital sign measurements, interpret their significance, and make decisions about interventions.
2. Equipment should be functional and appropriate to ensure accurate findings.
3. Equipment should be selected based on the client's condition and characteristics (e.g., an adult-size blood pressure cuff is not used for a child).
4. Know the client's usual range of vital signs. A client's usual values may differ from the standard range for that age or physical state. You will be using the client's usual values as a baseline for comparison with findings taken later.
5. Know the client's medical history, therapies, and prescribed medications. Some illnesses or treatments cause predictable vital sign changes.
6. Control or minimize environmental factors that may affect vital signs. Measuring the pulse after the client

When to Measure Vital Signs   Box 11-1

When the client is admitted to a health care facility
In a hospital on a routine schedule according to a physician's order or hospital standards of practice
Before and after a surgical procedure
Before and after an invasive diagnostic procedure
Before, during, and after a transfusion of blood products
Before, during, and after the administration of medications that affect cardiovascular, respiratory, and temperature-control function
When the client's general physical condition changes (as with loss of consciousness or increased intensity of pain)
Before and after nursing interventions that influence a vital sign (e.g., before and after a client currently on bed rest ambulates, before and after a client performs range-of-motion exercises)
When the client reports nonspecific symptoms of physical distress (e.g., feeling "funny" or "different")

exercises may yield a value that is not a true indicator of the client's condition.
7. Use an organized, systematic approach when measuring vital signs.
8. Based on the client's condition, collaborate with the physician to decide the frequency of vital sign assessment. In the hospital the physician orders a minimum frequency of vital sign measurements for each client. After surgery or treatment intervention, vital signs are measured frequently to detect complications. As a client's physical condition worsens, it may be necessary to monitor vital signs as often as every 5 to 10 minutes. You will use vital sign assessment during medication administration. The physician may order certain cardiac drugs to be given only within a range of pulse or blood pressure values. Outside of the hospital, vital sign assessment occurs whenever the client seeks care from a health care provider. In either environment you are responsible for judging whether more frequent assessments are needed (Box 11-1).
9. Analyze the results of vital sign measurement. Vital signs are not interpreted in isolation. Know other physical signs or symptoms and be aware of your client's ongoing health status.
10. Verify and communicate significant changes in vital signs. Baseline measurements will allow you to identify changes in vital signs. When vital signs appear abnormal, it may help to have another nurse or a physician repeat the measurement. Inform the physician of abnormal vital signs and document and report vital sign changes to nurses working the next shift.

BODY TEMPERATURE

The body temperature is the difference between the amount of heat produced by body processes and the amount of heat lost to the external environment.

   Heat produced − Heat lost = Body temperature

Despite environmental temperature extremes and physical activity, temperature-control mechanisms of human beings keep the body's core temperature or temperature of deep tissues relatively constant within a range as low as 35° C (95° F) during sleep and cold exposure to 40° C (104° F) during strenuous exercise. However, surface temperature fluctuates, depending on blood flow to the skin and the amount of heat lost to the external environment. Because of these surface temperature fluctuations, the acceptable temperature of human beings ranges from 36° to 38° C (96.8° to 100.4° F). The body's tissues and cells function best within this relatively narrow temperature range. For healthy young adults the average oral temperature is 37° C (98.6° F). No single temperature is normal for all people. The measurement of body temperature is aimed at obtaining a representative average temperature of core body tissues.

Average normal temperatures vary depending on the measurement site. Sites reflecting **core temperature**, such as the pulmonary artery, are more reliable indicators of body temperature than sites reflecting surface temperature. The pulmonary artery offers accurate readings because of the blood mix from all regions of the body, and is the standard against which all other sites are judged for accuracy.

Body Temperature Regulation

Body temperature is precisely regulated by physiological and behavioral mechanisms. For the body temperature to stay constant and within an acceptable range, the relationship between heat production and heat loss must be maintained.

NEURAL AND VASCULAR CONTROL.   The hypothalamus, located between the cerebral hemispheres of the brain, controls body temperature. The hypothalamus attempts to maintain a comfortable temperature or "set point." When the hypothalamus senses an increase in body temperature, impulses are sent out to reduce body temperature by sweating and **vasodilation** (widening of blood vessels). If the hypothalamus senses the body's temperature lower than set point, signals are sent out to increase heat production by muscle shivering or heat conservation by **vasoconstriction** (narrowing of surface blood vessels). Disease or trauma to the hypothalamus or spinal cord, which carries hypothalamic messages, decreases the body's ability to control body temperature.

HEAT PRODUCTION.   **Thermoregulation** requires normal heat production processes. Heat is produced as a by-product of metabolism. As metabolism increases, additional heat is produced. When metabolism decreases, less heat is produced. Heat production occurs during rest, voluntary movements, involuntary shivering, and **nonshivering thermogenesis.**

1. Basal metabolism accounts for the heat produced by the body at absolute rest. The average **basal metabolic rate (BMR)** depends on the body surface area.
2. Voluntary movements such as muscular activity during exercise require additional energy. The metabolic rate increases during activity and heat production can increase up to 50 times normal.
3. Shivering is an involuntary response to temperature differences in the body. The skeletal muscle movement during shivering requires significant energy. Shivering can increase heat production to four to five times normal.
4. Nonshivering thermogenesis occurs primarily in neonates. Because neonates cannot shiver, a limited amount of vascular brown adipose tissue present at birth can be metabolized for heat production.

HEAT LOSS.   Heat loss and heat production occur simultaneously. The skin's structure and exposure to the environment result in constant, normal heat loss through radiation, conduction, convection, and evaporation.

Radiation is the transfer of heat between two objects without physical contact. Heat radiates from the skin to any surrounding cooler object. Up to 85% of the human body's surface area radiates heat to the environment.

Conduction is the transfer of heat from one object to another with direct contact. When the warm skin touches a cooler object, heat is lost until their temperatures are similar. Heat conducts through solids, gases, and liquids. Conduction normally accounts for a small amount of heat loss. You can increase a client's conductive heat loss by applying an ice pack or bathing a client with cool water. Applying several layers of clothing reduces conductive loss. The body gains heat by conduction when contact is made with materials warmer than skin temperature.

Convection is the transfer of heat away by air movement. An electric fan promotes heat loss through convection. Convective heat loss increases when moistened skin comes into contact with slightly moving air.

Evaporation is the transfer of heat energy when a liquid is changed to a gas. The body continuously loses heat by evaporation. About 600 to 900 ml of water a day evaporates from the skin and lungs, resulting in water and heat loss. By regulating perspiration or sweating, the body promotes additional evaporative heat loss. **Diaphoresis** is visual perspiration of the forehead and upper thorax. When diaphoresis occurs, the body temperature is reduced.

BEHAVIORAL CONTROL.   When the environmental temperature falls, a person can add clothing, move to a warmer place, raise the thermostat setting on a furnace, increase muscular activity by running in place, or sit with arms and legs tightly wrapped together. In contrast, when the temperature becomes hot, a person can remove clothing, stop activity, lower the thermostat setting on an air conditioner, seek a cooler place, or take a cool shower.

Temperature Alterations

Changes in body temperature can be related to excess heat production, heat loss, minimal heat production, or any combination of these alterations. The nature of the change affects the type of clinical problems a client experiences.

Patterns of Fever Box 11-2

Sustained	A constant body temperature continuously above 38° C (100.4° F) that demonstrates little fluctuation
Intermittent	Fever spikes interspersed with usual temperature levels; temperature returns to acceptable value at least once in 24 hours
Remittent	Fever spikes and falls without a return to normal temperature levels
Relapsing	Periods of febrile episodes interspersed with acceptable temperature values; febrile episodes and periods of normothermia may be longer than 24 hours

Classification of Hypothermia Table 11-1

	C	F
Mild	34°-36°	93.2°-96.8°
Moderate	30°-33°	86.0°-93.2°
Severe	<30°	<86.0°

Hypothermia ↓ 36°

FEVER. Pyrexia, or **fever,** occurs because heat loss mechanisms are unable to keep pace with excess heat production, resulting in an abnormal rise in body temperature. A fever is usually not harmful if it stays below 39° C (102° F) and a single temperature reading may not indicate a fever. In addition to physical signs and symptoms of infection, a fever determination is based on several temperature readings at different times of the day compared with the usual value for that person at that time.

A true fever results from an alteration in the hypothalamic set point. Substances that trigger the immune system, or **pyrogens,** stimulate the release of hormones in an effort to promote the body's defense against infection. These hormones also trigger the hypothalamus to raise the set point, inducing a **febrile** episode. To meet the new set point, the body produces and conserves heat. The person can experience chills, shivers, and can feel cold, even though the body temperature is rising. If the set point has been "overshot" or the pyrogens are removed, the skin becomes warm and flushed because of vasodilation. Diaphoresis assists in evaporative heat loss. When the fever "breaks," the temperature returns to an acceptable range and the client becomes **afebrile.**

Fever, or **pyrexia,** is an important defense mechanism. Mild temperature elevations up to 39° C (102° F) enhance the body's immune system by stimulating white blood cell production. Increased temperature reduces the concentration of iron in the blood plasma, suppressing the growth of bacteria. Fever also fights viral infections by stimulating interferon, the body's natural virus-fighting substance.

Fevers also serve a diagnostic purpose. Fever patterns can differ depending on the causative pyrogen (Box 11-2). The duration and degree of fever depend on the pyrogen's strength and the ability of the individual to respond. The term *fever of unknown origin* (FUO) refers to a fever whose etiology (cause) cannot be determined.

HYPERTHEMIA. An elevated body temperature related to the body's inability to promote heat loss or reduce heat production is **hyperthermia.** Any disease or trauma to the hypothalamus can impair heat loss mechanisms. **Malignant** hyperthermia is a hereditary condition of uncontrolled heat production. Malignant hyperthermia occurs when susceptible persons receive certain anesthetic drugs.

Prolonged exposure to the sun or high environmental temperatures can overwhelm the body's heat loss mechanisms. Heat also depresses hypothalamic function. These conditions cause **heat stroke,** a dangerous heat emergency. Signs and symptoms of heat stroke include giddiness, confusion, delirium, excess thirst, nausea, muscle cramps, visual disturbances, and even incontinence. The most important sign of heat stroke is hot, dry skin.

HYPOTHERMIA. Heat loss during prolonged exposure to cold overwhelms the body's ability to produce heat, causing **hypothermia.** Hypothermia is classified by core temperature measurements (Table 11-1). It can be accidental or intentional.

Accidental hypothermia develops gradually and may go unnoticed for several hours. The hypothermic client suffers uncontrolled shivering, loss of memory, depression, and poor judgment. As the body temperature falls below 34° C (93.2° F), heart and respiratory rates and blood pressure fall.

NURSING PROCESS

Knowledge of body temperature physiology assists you when assessing your client's response to temperature alterations and helps you intervene safely.

Assessment

Assessment of thermoregulation requires you to make judgments about the site for temperature measurement, type of thermometer, and frequency of measurement. Table 11-2 presents an example of a focused client assessment for temperature measurement.

SITES. There are several sites for measuring core and surface body temperature. The core temperatures of the pulmonary artery, esophagus, and urinary bladder are often used in intensive care settings and require continuous invasive monitoring devices placed in body cavities or organs.

Intermittent temperature measurements are obtained from the routinely used invasive sites of the tympanic membrane, mouth, rectum, and axilla. Noninvasive special chemically prepared thermometer patches can also be applied to the skin.

Factors to Assess	Questions and Approaches	Physical Assessment Strategies
Temperature measurement site	Ask client preferred route Ask client if hearing aids in use Ask if client has recently ingested liquid or smoked Inquire about client's recent physical activity	Assess client's ability to position self Identify any signs of trauma to oral mucosa, aural drainage, diaphoresis Assess client's level of consciousness Assess for dyspnea
Frequency of temperature measurement	Note physician order for temperature monitoring in chart Note previous temperature, onset and duration of febrile episode Assess client comfort and well-being Assess environmental comfort	Assess for flushed, warm, dry skin Note shivering or diaphoresis

Table 11-2 *Example of a Focused Client Assessment*

To ensure accurate temperature readings, each site must be measured correctly (Skill 11-1). The temperature obtained varies depending on the site used but should be between 36.0° C (96.8° F) and 38.0° C (100.4° F). Rectal temperatures are usually 0.5° C (0.9° F) higher than oral temperatures. Axillary temperatures are usually 0.5° C (0.9° F) lower than oral temperatures. Each of the common temperature measurement sites has advantages and disadvantages (Box 11-3). You must select the safest and most accurate site for the client. The same site should be used if possible when repeated measurements are necessary.

THERMOMETERS.   Two types of thermometers are commonly available for measuring body temperature: electronic and disposable. A third type, the mercury-in-glass thermometer, was once the standard device found in the clinical setting. However, many municipalities have prohibited the sale or use of mercury-containing medical devices because of the potential hazards.

Each device measures temperature in either the **centigrade** or **Fahrenheit** scale. Electronic thermometers allow you to convert scales by activating a switch. When it is necessary to manually convert temperature readings, the following formulas can be used:

1. To convert Fahrenheit to centigrade, subtract 32 from the Fahrenheit reading and multiply the result by 5/9.

    Example: (104° F − 32° F) × 5/9 = 40° C

2. To convert centigrade to Fahrenheit, multiply the centigrade reading by 9/5 and add 32 to the product.

    Example: (9/5 × 40° C) + 32 = 104° F

ELECTRONIC THERMOMETERS.   The electronic thermometer consists of a rechargeable battery-powered display unit, a thin wire cord, and a temperature-processing probe covered by a disposable plastic sheath (Figure 11-1). One form of electronic thermometer uses a pencil-like probe. Separate unbreakable probes are available for oral and rectal use. The oral probe can also be used for axillary temperature measurement. Within 20 to 50 seconds of insertion, a reading appears on the display unit. A sound signals when the peak temperature reading has been measured.

Another form of electronic thermometer is used exclusively for tympanic temperature measurement. An otoscope-like speculum with an infrared sensor tip detects heat radiated from the tympanic membrane. Within 2 to 5 seconds of placement in the auditory canal, a reading appears on the display unit. A sound signals when the peak temperature reading has been measured.

DISPOSABLE THERMOMETERS.   Disposable, single-use thermometers are thin strips of plastic with chemically impregnated paper. They are used for measurement of oral or axillary temperatures, particularly in children (Figure 11-2). They are useful when caring for clients on protective isolation (see Chapter 10). They are inserted the same way as an oral or axillary thermometer and used only once. Chemical dots on the thermometer change color to reflect the temperature reading. Sixty seconds are needed to measure a temperature, and then an additional 10 seconds are needed to ensure the temperature reading has stabilized (Erickson and others, 1996).

Another form of disposable thermometer is a temperature-sensitive patch or tape. Applied to the forehead or abdomen, the patch changes color at different temperatures.

GLASS THERMOMETERS.   The mercury-in-glass thermometer is a glass tube sealed at one end, with a mercury-filled bulb at the other. Exposure of the bulb to heat causes the mercury to expand and rise in the enclosed tube. The length of the thermometer is marked with Fahrenheit or centigrade calibrations.

Obtaining a temperature with a mercury-in-glass thermometer requires careful preparation of the device (Box 11-4). In addition to proper positioning of the thermometer using the oral, rectal, or axillary site, you must maintain this position for at least 3 minutes to obtain an accurate reading. In addition to the time delay, the mercury-in-glass device is easily breakable, and when broken, releases hazardous mercury. Many agencies no longer use glass thermometers. However, many clients may have mercury-in-glass

Text continued on p. 184

Skill 11-1
MEASURING BODY TEMPERATURE

DELEGATION CONSIDERATIONS

You may delegate the skill of temperature measurement to assistive personnel.

- Inform caregiver of appropriate route and device to measure temperature.
- Inform caregiver of proper position for client receiving rectal temperature measurement.
- Inform caregiver of specific factors related to client that can falsely raise or lower temperature.
- Inform caregiver of the frequency of temperature measurement.
- Determine that caregiver is aware of the usual temperature values for the client.
- Inform caregiver of the need to report any abnormal temperatures that you will need to confirm.

EQUIPMENT

- Appropriate thermometer
- Tissue or soft wipe
- Lubricant (for rectal measurements only)
- Pen, pencil, vital sign flow sheet or record form
- Disposable gloves, plastic thermometer sleeve or disposable probe cover

STEPS	RATIONALE
1. Assess for signs and symptoms of temperature alterations and for factors that influence body temperature.	Physical signs and symptoms may indicate abnormal temperature. You can accurately assess nature of variations.
2. Determine any previous activity that would interfere with accuracy of temperature measurement. When taking oral temperature, wait 20 to 30 minutes before measuring temperature if client has smoked or ingested hot or cold liquid or food.	Smoking and hot or cold substances can cause false temperature readings in oral cavity.
3. Determine appropriate site and measurement device to be used.	Chosen on basis of preferred site for temperature measurement and any client contraindications (see Box 11-3, p. 185).
4. Explain route by which temperature will be taken and importance of maintaining proper position until reading is complete.	Clients are often curious about such measurements and should be cautioned against prematurely removing thermometer to read results.
5. Wash hands.	Reduces transmission of microorganisms.
6. Assist client in assuming comfortable position that provides easy access to route through which temperature is to be measured.	Ensures comfort and accuracy of temperature reading.
7. Obtain temperature reading.	
A. Oral Temperature Measurement With Electronic Thermometer:	
(1) Apply disposable gloves (optional).	Use of oral probe cover, which can be removed without physical contact, minimizes need to wear gloves.
(2) Remove thermometer pack from charging unit. Attach oral probe (blue tip) to thermometer unit. Grasp top of probe stem, being careful not to apply pressure on the ejection button.	Charging provides battery power. Ejection button releases plastic cover from probe.
(3) Slide disposable plastic probe cover over thermometer probe until cover locks in place (see illustration).	Soft plastic cover will not break in client's mouth and prevents transmission of microorganisms between clients.
(4) Ask client to open mouth; then gently place thermometer probe under tongue in posterior sublingual pocket lateral to center of lower jaw.	Heat from superficial blood vessels in sublingual pocket produces temperature reading. With electronic thermometer, temperatures in right and left posterior sublingual pocket are significantly higher than in area under front of tongue.
(5) Ask client to hold thermometer probe with lips closed.	Maintains proper position of thermometer during recording.
(6) Leave thermometer probe in place until audible signal occurs and client's temperature appears on digital display; remove thermometer probe from under client's tongue.	Probe must stay in place until signal occurs to ensure accurate reading.

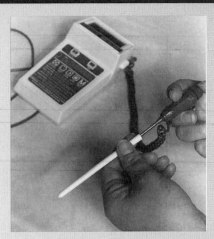

STEP 7A(3)   Disposable plastic cover is placed over the probe.

(7) Push ejection button on thermometer stem to discard plastic probe cover into appropriate receptacle.

Reduces transmission of microorganisms.

(8) Return thermometer stem to storage well of recording unit.

Protects probe from damage. Returning probe automatically causes digital reading to disappear.

(9) If gloves worn, remove and dispose in appropriate receptacle. Wash hands.

Reduces transmission of microorganisms.

(10) Return thermometer to charger.

Maintains battery charge.

B. Rectal Temperature Measurement With Electronic Thermometer:

(1) Draw curtain around bed and/or close room door. Assist client to Sims' position with upper leg flexed. Move aside bed linen to expose only anal area. Keep client's upper body and lower extremities covered with sheet or blanket.

Maintains client's privacy, minimizes embarrassment, and promotes comfort. Exposes anal area for correct thermometer placement.

(2) Apply disposable gloves.

Maintains standard precautions when exposed to items soiled with body fluids (e.g., feces).

(3) Remove thermometer pack from charging unit. Attach rectal probe (red tip) to thermometer unit. Grasp top of probe stem, being careful not to apply pressure on the ejection button.

Charging provides battery power. Ejection button releases plastic cover from probe.

(4) Slide disposable plastic probe cover over thermometer probe until it locks in place.

Probe cover prevents transmission of microorganisms between clients.

(5) Squeeze liberal portion of lubricant onto tissue. Dip probe cover's end into lubricant, covering 2.5 to 3.5 cm (1 to 1½ inches) for adult.

Lubrication minimizes trauma to rectal mucosa during insertion. Tissue avoids contamination of remaining lubricant in container.

(6) With nondominant hand, separate client's buttocks to expose anus. Ask client to breathe slowly and relax.

Fully exposes anus for thermometer insertion. Relaxes anal sphincter for easier thermometer insertion.

(7) Gently insert thermometer probe into anus in direction of umbilicus 3.5 cm (1½ inches) for adult. Do not force thermometer.

Ensures adequate exposure against blood vessels in rectal wall.

Critical Decision Point
If thermometer cannot be adequately inserted into rectum, remove thermometer and consider alternative method for obtaining temperature.

STEPS	RATIONALE
(8) Leave thermometer probe in place until audible signal occurs and client's temperature appears on digital display; remove thermometer probe from anus (see illustration).	Probe must stay in place until signal occurs to ensure accurate reading.

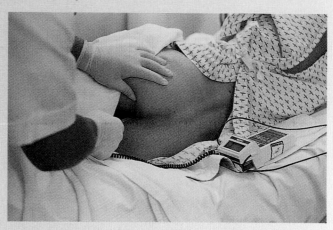

STEP 7B(8) Probe removed smoothly from anus.

STEPS	RATIONALE
(9) Push ejection button on thermometer stem to discard plastic probe cover into appropriate receptacle.	Reduces transmission of microorganisms.
(10) Return thermometer stem to storage well of recording unit.	Protects probe from damage. Returning probe automatically causes digital reading to disappear.
(11) Wipe client's anal area with tissue or soft wipe to remove lubricant or feces and discard tissue. Assist client in assuming a comfortable position.	Provides for comfort and hygiene.
(12) Remove and dispose of gloves in appropriate receptacle. Wash hands.	Reduces transmission of microorganisms.
(13) Return thermometer to charger.	Maintains battery charge.

C. Axillary Temperature Measurement With Electronic Thermometer:

STEPS	RATIONALE
(1) Wash hands.	Reduces transmission of microorganisms.
(2) Draw curtain around bed and/or close room door. Assist client to supine or sitting position. Move clothing or gown away from shoulder and arm.	Maintains client's privacy, minimizes embarrassment, and promotes comfort. Exposes axilla for correct thermometer placement.
(3) Remove thermometer pack from charging unit. Be sure oral probe (blue tip) is attached to thermometer unit. Grasp top of probe stem, being careful not to apply pressure on ejection button.	Ejection button releases plastic cover from probe.
(4) Slide disposable plastic probe cover over thermometer probe until it locks in place.	Soft plastic cover prevents transmission of microorganisms between clients.
(5) Raise client's arm away from torso, inspect for skin lesions and excessive perspiration. Insert probe into center of axilla, lower arm over probe, and place arm across chest.	Maintains proper position of probe against blood vessels in axilla.

Critical Decision Point

Do not use axilla if skin lesions present because local temperature may be altered and area may be painful to touch.

STEPS	RATIONALE
(6) Hold probe in place until audible signal occurs and temperature appears on digital display.	Probe must stay in place until signal occurs to ensure accurate reading.
(7) Push ejection button on thermometer stem to discard plastic probe cover into appropriate receptacle.	Reduces transmission of microorganisms.

STEPS	RATIONALE
(8) Return thermometer stem to storage well of recording unit.	Protects probe from damage. Returning probe automatically causes digital reading to disappear.
(9) Assist client in assuming a comfortable position, replacing linen or gown.	Restores comfort and sense of well-being.
(10) Wash hands.	Reduces transmission of microorganisms.
(11) Return thermometer to charger.	Maintains battery charge.

D. Tympanic Membrane Temperature With Electronic Tympanic Thermometer:

STEPS	RATIONALE
(1) Assist client in assuming comfortable position with head turned toward side, away from you. Right-handed persons should obtain temperature from client's right ear. Left-handed persons should obtain temperature from client's left ear.	Ensures comfort and exposes auditory canal for accurate temperature measurement. The less acute angle of approach, the better the probe seal with the auditory canal.
(2) Note if there is obvious earwax in the client's ear canal.	Lens cover of speculum must not be impeded by earwax, to ensure clear optical pathway. Switch to other ear or select alternative measurement site.
(3) Remove thermometer handheld unit from charging base, being careful not to apply pressure on the ejection button.	Base provides battery power. Removal of handheld unit from base prepares it to measure temperature. Ejection button releases plastic probe cover from thermometer tip.
(4) Slide disposable speculum cover over otoscope-like tip until it locks into place. Be careful not to touch lens cover.	Soft plastic probe cover prevents transmission of microorganisms between clients. Lens cover must be unimpeded by dust, fingerprints, or earwax to ensure clear optical pathway.
(5) Insert speculum into ear canal following manufacturer's instructions for tympanic probe positioning (see illustration):	

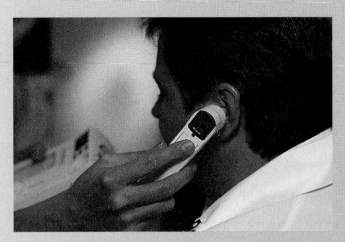

STEP 7D(5)   Tympanic membrane thermometer with probe cover placed in client's ear.

STEPS	RATIONALE
(a) Pull ear pinna backward, up and out for an adult.	Correct positioning of the probe with respect to ear canal ensures accurate readings. The ear tug straightens the external auditory canal, allowing maximum exposure of the tympanic membrane.
(b) Move thermometer in a figure-eight pattern.	Some manufacturers recommend movement of the speculum tip in a figure-eight pattern that allows the sensor to detect maximum tympanic membrane heat radiation.
(c) Fit otoscope probe snugly into canal and do not move.	Gentle pressure seals ear canal from ambient air temperature, which can alter readings as much as 2.8° C (5° F) (Braun and others, 1998). Operator error can lead to false low temperatures (Weiss and others, 1998).

STEPS	RATIONALE
(d) Point speculum tip toward nose.	
(6) As soon as probe is in place, depress scan button on handheld unit. Leave thermometer probe in place until audible signal occurs and client's temperature appears on digital display.	Depression of scan button causes infrared energy to be detected. Otoscope tip must stay in place until signal occurs to ensure accurate reading.
(7) Carefully remove speculum from auditory meatus.	Prevents rubbing of sensitive outer ear lining.
(8) Push ejection button on handheld unit to discard plastic probe cover into appropriate receptacle. If a second reading is necessary replace probe lens cover and wait 2 minutes before inserting the probe tip.	Reduces transmission of microorganisms. Automatically causes digital reading to disappear. Time allows ear canal to regain usual temperature (Giuliano and others, 2000).
(9) Return handheld unit to charging base.	Protects sensory tip from damage.
(10) Assist client in assuming a comfortable position.	Restores comfort and sense of well-being.
(11) Wash hands.	Reduces transmission of microorganisms.
8. Discuss findings with client as needed.	Promotes participation in care and understanding of health status.
9. If temperature is assessed for the first time, establish temperature as baseline if it is within normal range.	Used to compare future temperature measurements.
10. Compare temperature reading with client's previous temperature and normal temperature range for client's age-group.	Normal body temperature fluctuates within narrow range; comparison reveals presence of abnormality. Improper placement or movement of thermometer can cause inaccuracies. Second measurement confirms initial findings of abnormal body temperature.

UNEXPECTED OUTCOMES AND RELATED INTERVENTIONS

- Temperature 1° C above usual range.
  - Assess possible sites for localized infection and for related data suggesting systemic infection.
  - Follow interventions listed in Box 11-7.
- If fever persists or reaches unacceptable level as defined by physician, administer antipyretics and antibiotics as ordered.
- Temperature 1° C below usual range.
  - Remove any wet clothing or linen and cover client with warm blankets.
  - Close room doors or windows to eliminate drafts.

- Encourage warm liquids.
- Monitor apical pulse rate and rhythm (see Skill 11-2, p. 190) because hypothermia may cause bradycardia and dysrhythmias.

RECORDING AND REPORTING

- Record temperature in nurses' notes or vital sign flow sheet. Measurement of temperature after administration of specific therapies should be documented in narrative form in nurses' notes.
- Report abnormal findings to nurse in charge or physician.

---

thermometers in their homes. If you break a thermometer or suspect a mercury spill you are required to take immediate action (Box 11-5). It is also important that you teach your clients and their families what to do in the event of breakage of a mercury-in-glass thermometer.

Nursing Diagnosis

After assessment, you will review all of the available data and look for patterns and trends that are suggestive of a health problem relating to temperature imbalance (Box 11-6). For example, an increase in body temperature, flushed skin, skin that is warm to touch, and tachycardia are defining characteristics for the diagnosis of *hyperthermia*. You will validate findings to ensure the accuracy of the diagnosis.

Once a diagnosis is determined, you must determine the factor that likely caused the client's health problem. The related factor allows the nurse to select appropriate nursing interventions. In the example of *hyperthermia*, the related factor of vigorous activity will result in much different interventions than the related factor of infectious process.

Planning

The plan of care (see care plan) depends on your assessment of the client's perception and acceptance of the body temperature alteration. It also depends on the extent to which the client's internal compensatory mechanisms and behavior have adjusted to the temperature alteration. The client should actively participate in choosing therapies for the care plan when able.

Advantages and Disadvantages of Select Temperature Measurement Sites   Box 11-3

TYMPANIC MEMBRANE

Advantages

Easily accessible site

Minimal client repositioning required

Provides accurate core reading

Very rapid measurement (2 to 5 seconds)

Can be obtained without disturbing or waking client

Eardrum close to hypothalamus; sensitive to core temperature changes

Unaffected by oral intake of food, fluid, smoking

Can be used for tachypneic clients

Disadvantages

Variability of measurement exceeds that of other core temperature devices (Leicke-Rude and Bloom, 1998)

Reduced sensitivity to detect fever compared to oral sensor

Cerumen impaction can lower readings (Giuliano and others, 2000)

Hearing aids must be removed before measurement

Should not be used with clients who have had surgery of the ear or tympanic membrane

Requires disposable probe cover

Does not accurately measure core temperature changes during and after exercise (Yeo and Scarborough, 1996)

Measurement accuracy in newborns has been questioned (Cusson and others, 1997)

Affected by ambient temperature devices such as incubators, radiant warmers, and facial fans (Giuliano and others, 2000)

Cannot obtain continuous measurement

Expensive

RECTAL

Advantages

Reflects core temperature

Disadvantages

May lag behind core temperature during rapid temperature changes (Giuliano and others, 2000)

Should not be used for children with diarrhea, clients who have had rectal surgery, a rectal disorder, or decreased platelets (Haddock and others, 1996)

Should not be used for routine vital signs in newborns (Cusson and others, 1997)

Requires positioning and may be source of client embarrassment and anxiety

Risk of body fluid exposure

Requires lubrication

ORAL

Advantages

Accessible—requires no position change

Comfortable for client

Provides accurate surface temperature reading

Reflects rapid change in core temperature

Acceptable route for clients with endotracheal tube in place (Fallis, 2000).

Disadvantages

Affected by ingestion of fluid or food, smoking

Should not be used with clients who have had oral surgery, trauma, history of epilepsy, or shaking chills

Should not be used with infants, small children, or confused, unconscious, or uncooperative clients

Risk of body fluid exposure

AXILLA

Advantages

Safe and noninvasive

Can be used with newborns and uncooperative clients

Disadvantages

Long measurement time

Requires continuous positioning by nurse

Measurement lags behind core temperature during rapid temperature changes

Requires exposure of thorax

Not recommended for detection of fever in infants and young children (Haddock and others, 1996)

SKIN

Advantages

Inexpensive

Provides continuous reading

Safe and noninvasive

Does not require disturbing client

Can be used for neonates

Easy to read

Disadvantages

Lags behind other sites during temperature changes, especially during hyperthermia

Diaphoresis or sweat can impair adhesion

Measurement can vary at different body sites

Can be affected by environmental temperature

Unreliable during chill phase of fever (Holtzclaw, 1998)

Priorities of care must be set with regard to the extent the temperature alteration affects a client. Safety is a top priority.

 Implementation

HEALTH PROMOTION.   Health promotion for clients at risk for altered body temperature is directed toward promoting balance between heat production and heat loss. Client activity, temperature of the environment, and clothing are all considered. Teach clients to avoid strenuous exercise in hot, humid weather; to drink fluids such as water and clear fruit juices before, during, and after exercise; to wear light, loose-fitting, light-colored clothing; to avoid exercising in areas with poor ventilation; to wear a protective covering over the head when outdoors; and to expose themselves to hot climates gradually.

Prevention is the key for clients at risk for hypothermia. Prevention involves educating clients, family members, and friends. Clients most at risk include the very young and the very old and persons debilitated by trauma, stroke, diabetes, drug or alcohol intoxication, sepsis, and Raynaud's disease. Mentally ill or handicapped clients may fall victim to hypothermia because they are unaware of the dangers of cold conditions. Persons without adequate home heating, shelter, diet, or clothing are also at risk.

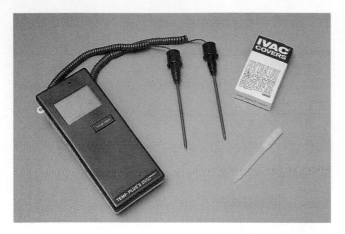

FIGURE 11-1 Electronic thermometer used for oral, rectal, or axillary measurements.

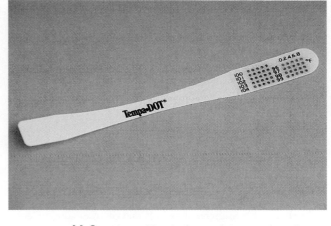

FIGURE 11-2 Disposable, single-use thermometer strip.

Procedural Guidelines for Box 11-4
PREPARATION OF MERCURY-IN-GLASS THERMOMETER

Equipment
- Mercury in glass thermometer (rectal or oral)
- Plastic sleeve
- Lubricating jelly (rectal only)
- Disposable gloves

1. Apply disposable gloves to avoid contact with body fluids (e.g., saliva, stool).
2. Hold end (if color-coded, tip will be blue or red) of glass thermometer with fingertips to reduce contamination of bulb.
3. Read mercury level while gently rotating thermometer at eye level. If mercury is above desired level, grasp tip of thermometer securely, stand away from solid objects, and sharply flick wrist downward. Brisk shaking lowers mercury level in glass tube. Continue shaking until reading is below 35.5° C (96° F). Thermometer reading must be below client's actual temperature before use.
4. Insert thermometer into plastic sleeve cover to protect from body secretions (e.g., saliva, stool). Apply lubricant to cover 2.5 to 3.5 cm (1 to 1.5 inch) on rectal thermometer.
5. Place thermometer using technique appropriate to oral, rectal, or axillary site.
6. Leave thermometer in place 3 minutes for rectal temperature, 2 minutes for axillary temperature, or according to agency policy.
7. Remove the thermometer. Carefully discard the plastic sleeve. Wipe off secretions with clean tissue, moving toward the bulb.
8. Read thermometer at eye level, read findings, store thermometer in storage container. Remove gloves and wash hands.

Steps to Take in the Event of a Mercury Spill Box 11-5

1. Do NOT touch spilled mercury droplets. If skin contact occurs, immediately flush area with water for 15 minutes.
2. If possible, remove client from immediate contaminated environment.
3. Change any clothing or linen that has been contaminated with mercury. Wash hands thoroughly after changing.
4. Notify agency's environmental services department or obtain a mercury spill kit if available.
5. Follow procedures for mercury removal as directed by Material Safety Data Sheet (MSDS). Spills are removed using special absorbent materials, filtered vacuum equipment, and protective clothing.
6. Promote exhaust ventilation to reduce concentration of mercury vapors.
7. Follow agency guidelines for laundering clothing.
8. Complete occurrence report as directed by institution procedure.

Nursing Diagnoses for Box 11-6
CLIENTS WITH BODY TEMPERATURE ALTERATIONS

- Body temperature, risk for imbalanced
- Hyperthermia
- Hypothermia
- Thermoregulation, ineffective

ACUTE CARE

HYPERTHERMIA. Treatment for an elevated temperature depends on the fever's cause, any adverse effects, and the strength, intensity, and duration of the fever. You play a key role in assessing fever and implementing temperature-reducing strategies (Box 11-7). The physician may try to determine the cause of the fever by isolating the causative pyrogen. You may be requested to obtain necessary culture specimens for laboratory analysis, such as urine, blood, sputum, and from wound sites. The physician will order antibiotics to be given after the cultures have been obtained. Antibiotics destroy pyrogenic bacteria and eliminate the body's stimulus for fever.

The objective of fever therapy is to increase heat loss, reduce heat production, and prevent complications. Nonpharmacological therapy for fever uses methods that increase heat loss by evaporation, conduction, convection, or radiation.

Sample Nursing Care Plan **HYPERTHERMIA**

ASSESSMENT
Mr. Coburn is a 45-year-old school teacher who arrives at the outpatient clinic with the complaint of malaise. His skin is **warm and dry to touch.** His face is **flushed** and he appears to have **labored breathing.** He admits to smoking one pack of cigarettes per day and recently began expectorating yellow-green sputum. Vital signs obtained are: BP RA 116/62, LA 114/64; right radial **pulse 128,** regular and bounding; **RR 26;** SpO$_2$ 98% on room air; tympanic **temperature 39.2° C (102.6° F).**

*Defining characteristics are shown in bold type.

NURSING DIAGNOSIS
Hyperthermia related to infectious process

PLANNING

GOALS	EXPECTED OUTCOMES
Client will regain normal range of body temperature within next 24 hours.	Body temperature will decline at least 1° C (1.8° F) within next 8 hours.
Client will attain sense of comfort and rest within next 48 hours.	Client will verbalize increased satisfaction with rest and sleep pattern.
	Client will report increase in energy level within next 3 days.
Fluid and electrolyte balance will be maintained during next 3 days.	Intake will equal output within next 24 hours.
	Postural hypotension will not be evident during ambulation.

IMPLEMENTATION

STEPS	RATIONALE
1. Instruct client to reduce external coverings and keep clothing and bed linen dry.	Promotes heat loss through conduction and convection.
2. Instruct client to monitor temperature at home and administer acetaminophen every 4 hours as ordered for temperature over 39° C (102° F).	Antipyretics reduce set point (Holtzclaw, 1998) and promote comfort.
3. Instruct client to limit physical activity and increase frequency of rest periods over next 2 days.	Activity and stress increase metabolic rate, contributing to heat production.
4. Instruct client to increase oral fluids of choice.	Fluids lost through insensible water loss require replacement.
5. Instruct client to take oral antibiotics as prescribed.	Antibiotics must be taken for the prescribed period for maximum effectiveness.

EVALUATION
• During ambulatory center follow-up phone call, ask client to identify temperature and describe energy level.

Nursing Measures for Clients With a Fever   Box II-7

ASSESSMENT
Obtain frequent core temperature readings (i.e., tympanic, rectal) during the febrile episode.

Assess for contributing factors such as dehydration, infection, or environmental temperature.

Identify physiological response to fever.

Obtain all vital signs.

Assess skin color and temperature, presence of thirst, malaise; observe for shivering and diaphoresis.

Assess client comfort and well-being.

INTERVENTIONS (UNLESS CONTRAINDICATED)
Obtain blood cultures when ordered (see Chapter 10). Blood specimens are obtained to coincide with temperature spikes when the antigen-producing organism is most prevalent.

Minimize heat production: reduce the frequency of activities that increase oxygen demand such as excessive turning and ambulation; allow rest periods; limit physical activity.

Maximize heat loss: reduce external covering on client's body without causing shivering; keep clothing and bed linen dry.

Satisfy requirements for increased metabolic rate: provide supplemental oxygen therapy as ordered to improve oxygen delivery to body cells; provide measures to stimulate appetite, and offer well-balanced meals; provide fluids (at least 3 L/day for a client with normal cardiac and renal function) to replace fluids lost through insensible water loss and sweating.

Promote client comfort: encourage oral hygiene because oral mucous membranes dry easily from dehydration; control temperature of the environment without inducing shivering; apply damp cloth to client forehead.

Identify onset and duration of febrile episode phases: examine previous temperature measurements for trends.

Initiate health teaching as indicated.

Control environmental temperature to 21° to 27° C (70° to 80° F).

Outcome Evaluation for MR. COBURN   Box 11-8

Nursing Action	Client Response/Finding	Achievement of Outcome
Ask Mr. Coburn to keep a diary of temperature and acetaminophen use for next 24 hours.	Diary completed.	Temperature between 98° F and 100.8° F; four doses of acetaminophen used appropriately
Ask Mr. Coburn to implement rest periods over next 48 hours.	Mr. Coburn remained home from work, reports less malaise.	Energy level returning to baseline
Ask Mr. Coburn to describe fluid intake for past 24 hours.	Fluids increased to 8 ounces water or fruit juice every 4 hours while awake.	Adequate fluid intake

Nursing measures to enhance body cooling must avoid stimulating shivering. Shivering is counterproductive because of the heat produced by muscle activity.

Antipyretics are drugs that reduce fever. Nonsteroidal drugs such as acetaminophen, salicylates, indomethacin, ibuprofen, and ketorolac reduce fever by increasing heat loss. Corticosteroids reduce heat production by interfering with the hypothalamic response. These drugs mask signs of infection by suppressing the immune system. Corticosteroids are not used to treat a fever. However, you must be aware of their effect on suppressing the ability of the client to develop a fever in response to a pyrogen.

HEAT STROKE.   First aid treatment for victims of heat stroke includes moving the client to a cooler environment, reducing clothing covering the body, placing wet towels over the skin, and using oscillating fans to increase convective heat loss. Emergency medical treatment may include hypothermia blankets, intravenous fluids, and irrigating the stomach and lower bowel with cool solutions.

HYPOTHERMIA.   The priority treatment for hypothermia is to prevent a further decrease in body temperature. Removing wet clothes, replacing them with dry ones, and wrapping the client in blankets is a key nursing intervention. In emergencies away from a health care setting, the client lies under blankets next to a warm person. A conscious client benefits from drinking hot liquids such as soup, while avoiding alcohol and caffeinated fluids. Keeping the head covered, placing the client near a fire or in a warm room, or placing heating pads next to areas of the body (head and neck) that lose heat the quickest helps.

RESTORATIVE AND CONTINUING CARE.   Educate clients about the importance of taking and continuing any antibiotics as directed until the course of treatment is completed.

Children and older adults are especially at risk for deficient fluid volume because they can quickly lose large amounts of fluids in proportion to their body weight. Identifying preferred fluids and encouraging oral fluid intake is an important nursing intervention.

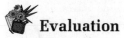

Evaluation

All nursing interventions are evaluated by comparing the client's actual response with the outcomes of the care plan (Box 11-8). This reveals whether goals of care have been met. After any intervention you should measure the client's temperature to evaluate for change. In addition, you may use other evaluative measures such as palpation of the skin and assessment of pulse and respiration. If therapies are effective, body temperature will return to an acceptable range, other vital signs will stabilize, and the client will report a sense of comfort.

PULSE

The pulse is the palpable bounding of the blood flow in a peripheral artery. Blood flows through the body in a continuous circuit. Electrical impulses from the sinoatrial (SA) node travel through heart muscle to stimulate cardiac contraction. Approximately 60 to 70 ml of blood enters the aorta with each contraction (**stroke volume [SV]**). The pulse is felt as a tap when palpating an artery lightly against underlying bone or muscle. The number of pulsing sensations occurring in 1 minute is the pulse rate.

The volume of blood pumped by the heart during 1 minute is the **cardiac output (CO)**, the product of heart rate and the ventricle's stroke volume (SV) (see Chapter 24). The cause of an abnormally slow, rapid, or irregular pulse may ultimately alter cardiac output. Although cardiac output depends on heart rate, a change in heart rate alone does not alter cardiac output.

Locating the Peripheral Pulse

Any accessible artery can be assessed for pulse rate, but the radial and carotid arteries are commonly used because they are easily palpated. When a client's condition suddenly deteriorates, the carotid site is recommended for finding a pulse quickly.

The radial and apical locations are the most common sites for pulse rate assessment. They are often used by persons learning to monitor their own heart rates (e.g., athletes, clients using heart medications). If the radial pulse is abnormal, difficult to palpate, or inaccessible because of a dressing or cast, the apical pulse is assessed. When a client takes a medication that affects the heart rate, the apical pulse provides a more accurate assessment of heart rate. Table 11-3 summarizes pulse sites and criteria for measurement. Skill 11-2 outlines radial and apical pulse rate assessment.

Stethoscope

You will need a stethoscope to assess the apical rate (Figure 11-3). The five major parts of the stethoscope are the ear-

Pulse Sites

Table 11-3

Site	Location	Assessment Criteria
Temporal	Over temporal bone of head, above and lateral to eye	Easily accessible site used to assess pulse in children
Carotid	Along medial edge of sternocleidomastoid muscle in neck	Easily accessible site used during physiological shock or cardiac arrest when other sites are not palpable
Apical	Fourth to fifth intercostal space at left midclavicular line	Site used to auscultate for heart sounds; site used for infants and young children
Brachial	Groove between biceps and triceps muscles at antecubital fossa	Site used to assess pulse rate; site used to auscultate blood pressure
Radial	Radial or thumb side of forearm at wrist	Common site used to assess character of pulse peripherally and assess status of circulation to hand
Ulnar	Ulnar side of forearm at wrist	Site used to assess status of circulation to hand
Femoral	Below inguinal ligament, midway between symphysis pubis and anterior superior iliac spine	Site used to assess character of pulse during physiological shock or cardiac arrest when other pulses are not palpable
Popliteal	Behind knee in popliteal fossa	Site used to auscultate lower extremity blood pressure
Posterior tibial	Inner side of ankle, below medial malleolus	Site used to assess status of circulation to foot
Dorsalis pedis	Along top of foot, between extension tendons of great and first toe	Site used to assess status of circulation to foot

pieces, binaurals, tubing, bell chestpiece, and diaphragm chestpiece.

The plastic or rubber earpieces should fit snugly and comfortably in your ears. The binaurals should be angled and strong enough that the earpieces stay firmly in your ears without causing discomfort. To ensure the best reception of sound, the earpieces follow the contour of your ear canal, pointing toward your face when the stethoscope is in place.

The polyvinyl tubing should be flexible and 30 to 40 cm (12 to 18 inches) long. Longer tubing decreases the transmission of sound waves. The tubing should be thick walled and moderately rigid to eliminate transmission of environmental noise and prevent the tubing from kinking, which distorts sound wave transmission. Stethoscopes can have single or dual tubes.

The chestpiece consists of a bell and a diaphragm that are rotated into position. The diaphragm or bell must be in proper position during use to hear sounds through the stethoscope. To test the position of the chestpiece, tap lightly on the diaphragm to determine which side is functioning. The diaphragm is the circular, flat-surfaced portion of the chestpiece covered with a thin plastic disk. It transmits high-pitched sounds created by the high velocity movement of air and blood. Bowel, lung, and heart sounds are auscultated using the diaphragm. Always place the stethoscope directly on the skin, because clothing can obscure the sound. Position the diaphragm to make a tight seal against the client's skin (Figure 11-4). Exert enough pressure on the diaphragm to leave a temporary red ring on the client's skin when the diaphragm is removed.

The bell is the bowl-shaped chestpiece usually surrounded by a rubber ring. The ring avoids chilling the client with cold metal when you place the bell on the skin. The bell transmits low-pitched sounds created by the low-velocity movement of blood. Heart and vascular sounds are auscul-

tated using the bell. Apply the bell lightly, resting the chestpiece on the skin (Figure 11-5). Compressing the bell against the skin reduces low-pitched sound amplification and creates a "diaphragm of skin."

The size of the stethoscope chestpiece varies from small, used for infants and young children, to large. By assessing the surface area to be auscultated you can determine the appropriate size chestpiece.

The stethoscope is a delicate instrument and requires proper care for optimal function. The earpieces should be removed regularly and cleaned of cerumen (earwax). You should inspect the bell and diaphragm for dust, lint, and body oils, and clean it with mild soap and water.

Assessment of Pulse

PULSE RATE. Before measuring a pulse, review your client's record to obtain a baseline rate for comparison (Table 11-4). When assessing the pulse, consider the variety of factors influencing pulse rate (Table 11-5). A combination of these factors may cause significant changes. If you detect an abnormal rate while palpating a peripheral pulse, the next step is to assess the apical rate. The apical rate requires auscultation of the heart sounds, which provides a more accurate assessment of cardiac contraction.

The **apical pulse** is assessed by listening for heart sounds (see Chapter 12). After properly positioning the bell or the diaphragm of the stethoscope on the chest, try to identify the first and second heart sounds (S_1 and S_2). At normal slow rates, S_1 is low pitched and dull, sounding like a "lub." S_2 is a higher pitched and shorter sound and creates the sound "dub." Each set of "lub-dub" is counted as one heartbeat. Count the number of "lub-dubs" occurring in 1 minute.

Pulse rate assessment may reveal variations in heart rate. Two common abnormalities in pulse rate are **tachycardia** and **bradycardia.** Tachycardia is an abnormally elevated heart rate,

Text continued on p. 194

Skill 11-2

ASSESSING THE RADIAL AND APICAL PULSES

DELEGATION CONSIDERATIONS

The skill of pulse measurement can be delegated to assistive personnel if client is stable and not at high risk for cardiac irregularity.

- Inform caregiver of appropriate client position when obtaining apical pulse measurement.
- Inform caregiver of client history or risk for irregular pulse.
- Inform caregiver of frequency of pulse measurements.

- Determine that caregiver is aware of the usual values for the client.
- Inform caregiver of the need to report any abnormalities that you should confirm.

EQUIPMENT

- Stethoscope (apical pulse only)
- Wristwatch with second hand or digital display
- Pen, pencil, vital sign flow sheet or record form
- Alcohol swab

STEPS	RATIONALE
1. Determine need to assess radial and/or apical pulse: a. Note risk factors for alterations in pulse.	Certain conditions place clients at risk for pulse alterations: a history of heart disease, cardiac dysrhythmia, onset of sudden chest pain or acute pain from any site, invasive cardiovascular diagnostic tests, surgery, sudden infusion of large volume of intravenous (IV) fluid, internal or external hemorrhage, or administration of medications that alter cardiac function. A history of peripheral vascular disease can alter pulse rate and quality.
b. Note signs and symptoms of altered SV and CO, such as dyspnea, fatigue, chest pain, orthopnea, syncope, palpitations (person's unpleasant awareness of heartbeat), jugular venous distention, edema of dependent body parts, cyanosis or pallor of skin.	Physical signs and symptoms may indicate alteration in cardiac function, which affects pulse rate and rhythm.
c. Client has signs and symptoms of peripheral vascular disease such as pale, cool extremities; thin, shiny skin with decreased hair growth; thickened nails.	Physical signs and symptoms may indicate alteration in local arterial blood flow.
2. Assess for factors that influence pulse rate and rhythm: age, exercise, position changes, fluid balance, medications, temperature, sympathetic stimulation.	Allows you to accurately assess presence and significance of pulse alterations. Acceptable range of pulse rate changes with age (see Table 11-4, p. 195).
3. Determine client's previous baseline pulse rate (if available) from client's record.	Allows you to assess for change in condition. Provides comparison with future pulse measurements.
4. Explain that pulse or heart rate is to be assessed. Encourage client to relax and not speak.	Activity and anxiety can elevate heart rate. Client's voice interferes with your ability to hear sound when apical pulse is measured.
5. Wash hands.	Reduces transmission of microorganisms.
6. If necessary, draw curtain around bed and/or close door.	Maintains privacy.

7. Obtain pulse measurement.
  A. **Radial Pulse:**
    (1) Assist client to assume a supine or sitting position.
	Provides easy access to pulse sites.

(2) If supine, place client's forearm straight alongside or across lower chest or upper abdomen with wrist extended straight (see illustration). If sitting, bend client's elbow 90 degrees and support lower arm on chair or on your arm. Slightly flex the wrist with palm down.	Relaxed position of lower arm and flexion of wrist permit full exposure of artery to palpation.
(3) Place tips of first two fingers of your hand over groove along radial or thumbside of client's inner wrist (see illustration).	Fingertips are most sensitive parts of hand to palpate arterial pulsation. The thumb has pulsation that may interfere with accuracy.

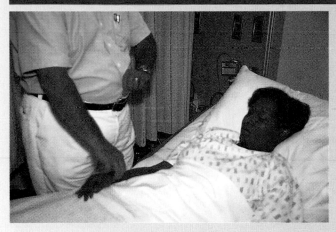

STEP 7A(2)   Pulse check with client's forearm at side with wrist extended.

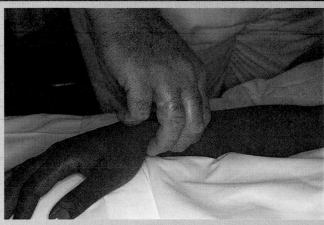

STEP 7A(3)   Hand placement for pulse checks.

(4) Lightly compress against radius, obliterate pulse initially, and then relax pressure so pulse becomes easily palpable.	Pulse is more accurately assessed with moderate pressure. Too much pressure occludes pulse and impairs blood flow.
(5) Determine strength of pulse. Note whether thrust of vessel against fingertips is bounding, strong, weak, or thready.	Strength reflects volume of blood ejected against arterial wall with each heart contraction.
(6) After pulse can be felt regularly, look at watch's second hand and begin to count rate: when sweep hand hits number on dial, start counting with zero, then one, two, and so on.	Rate is determined accurately only after you are assured pulse can be palpated. Timing begins with zero. Count of one is first beat palpated after timing begins.
(7) If pulse is regular, count rate for 30 seconds and multiply total by 2.	A 30-second count is accurate for rapid, slow, or regular pulse rates.
(8) If pulse is irregular, count rate for 60 seconds. Assess frequency and pattern of irregularity.	Inefficient contraction of heart fails to transmit pulse wave, interfering with CO, resulting in irregular pulse. Longer time ensures accurate count.
(9) When pulse is irregular, compare radial pulses bilaterally.	A marked inequality may indicate arterial flow is compromised to one extremity and action should be taken.

- *Critical Decision Point*

If pulse is irregular, assess for pulse deficit. Count apical pulse (Step 7b) while a colleague counts radial pulse. Begin pulse count by calling out loud simultaneously when to begin measuring pulses. If pulse count differs by more than 2, a pulse deficit exists, which may indicate alterations in CO.

B. **Apical Pulse:**

(1) Wash hands.	Reduces transmission of microorganisms.
(2) Draw curtain around bed and/or close door.	Maintains privacy and minimizes embarrassment.
(3) Assist client to supine or sitting position. Move aside bed linen and gown to expose sternum and left side of chest.	Exposes portion of chest wall for selection of auscultatory site.

STEPS	RATIONALE
(4) Locate anatomical landmarks to identify the point of maximal impulse (PMI), also called the apical impulse (see illustration for step 7B[4]A to D). Heart is located behind and to left of sternum with base at top and apex at bottom. Find angle of Louis just below suprasternal notch between sternal body and manubrium; can be felt as a bony prominence. Slip fingers down each side of angle to find second intercostal space (ICS). Carefully move fingers down left side of sternum to fifth ICS and laterally to the left midclavicular line (MCL). A light tap felt within an area 1 to 2 cm (½ to 1 inch) of the PMI is reflected from the apex of the heart.	Use of anatomical landmarks allows correct placement of stethoscope over apex of heart. This position enhances ability to hear heart sounds clearly. If unable to palpate the PMI, reposition client on left side. In the presence of serious heart disease, the PMI may be located to the left of the MCL or at the sixth ICS.
(5) Place diaphragm of stethoscope in palm of hand for 5 to 10 seconds.	Warming of metal or plastic diaphragm prevents client from being startled and promotes comfort.
(6) Place diaphragm of stethoscope over PMI at the fifth ICS, at left MCL, and auscultate for normal S_1 and S_2 heart sounds (heard as "lub dub") (see illustrations).	Allow stethoscope tubing to extend straight without kinks, which distort sound transmission. Normal sounds S_1 and S_2 are high pitched and best heard with the diaphragm.

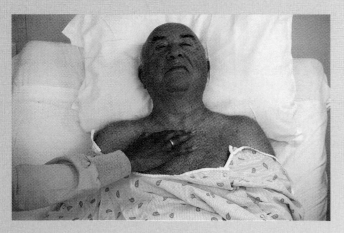

STEP 7B(4A)

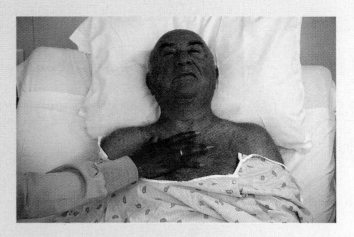

STEP 7B(4B)

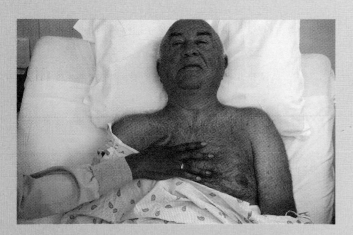

STEP 7B(4C)

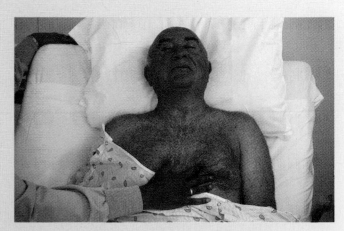

STEP 7B(4D)

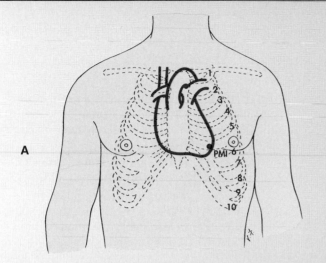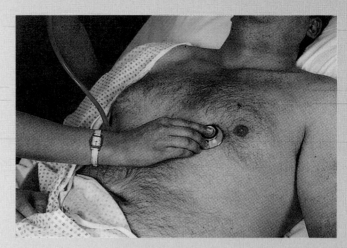

STEP 7B(6)   **A,** Location of PMI in adult. **B,** Stethoscope over PMI.

(7) When S_1 and S_2 are heard with regularity, use watch's second hand and begin to count rate: when sweep hand hits number on dial, start counting with zero, then one, two, and so on.	Apical rate is determined accurately only after you are able to auscultate sounds clearly. Timing begins with zero. Count of one is first sound auscultated after timing begins.
(8) If apical rate is regular, count for 30 seconds and multiply by 2.	Regular apical rate can be assessed within 30 seconds.
(9) If heart rate is irregular or client is receiving cardiovascular medication, count for 1 minute (60 seconds).	Irregular rate is more accurately assessed when measured over longer interval.
(10) Note regularity of any dysrhythmia (S_1 and S_2 occurring early or later after previous sequence of sounds; for example, every third or every fourth beat is skipped).	Regular occurrence of dysrhythmia within 1 minute may indicate inefficient contraction of heart and alteration in CO.
(11) Replace client's gown and bed linen; assist client in returning to comfortable position.	Restores comfort and promotes sense of well-being.
(12) Discuss findings with client as needed.	Promotes participation in care and understanding of health status.
(13) Wash hands.	Reduces transmission of microorganisms.
(14) Clean earpieces and diaphragm of stethoscope with alcohol swab routinely after each use.	Stethoscopes are frequently contaminated with microorganisms. Regular disinfection can control nosocomial infections.
8. Discuss findings with client as needed.	Promotes participation in care and understanding of health status.
9. Wash hands.	Reduces transmission of microorganisms.
10. Compare readings with previous baseline and/or acceptable range of heart rate for client's age (see Table 11-4, p. 195).	Evaluates for change in condition and alterations.
11. Compare peripheral pulse rate with apical rate and note discrepancy.	Differences between measurements indicate pulse deficit and may warn of cardiovascular compromise. Abnormalities may require therapy.
12. Compare radial pulse equality and note discrepancy.	Differences between radial arteries indicate compromised peripheral vascular system.

STEPS	RATIONALE
13. Correlate pulse rate with data obtained from blood pressure and related signs and symptoms (palpitations, dizziness).	Pulse rate and blood pressure are interrelated.

UNEXPECTED OUTCOMES AND RELATED INTERVENTIONS
- Radial pulse is weak, thready, or difficult to palpate.
  - Assess both radial pulses and compare findings. Local obstruction to one extremity (e.g., clot, edema) may decrease peripheral blood flow.
  - Perform complete assessment of all peripheral pulses (see Chapter 12).
  - Observe for symptoms associated with altered tissue perfusion including pallor and cool skin temperature of tissue distal to the weak pulse.
  - Auscultate apical pulse to determine pulse rate and identify pulse deficit.
- Apical pulse is greater than 100 beats/min (tachycardia).
  - Identify related data including pain, fear, anxiety, recent exercise, hypotension, blood loss, fever, or inadequate oxygenation.
  - Observe for signs and symptoms of inadequate CO including fatigue, chest pain, orthopnea, cyanosis.

- Apical pulse is less than 60 beats/min (bradycardia).
  - Observe for factors that may alter heart rate such as digoxin and antidysrhythmics; it may be necessary to withhold prescribed medications until the physician can evaluate the need to adjust the dosage.
  - Observe for signs and symptoms of inadequate CO including fatigue, chest pain, orthopnea, cyanosis.

RECORDING AND REPORTING
- Record pulse rate with assessment site in nurses' notes or vital signs flow sheet.
- Measurement of pulse rate after administration of specific therapies should be documented in narrative form in nurses' notes.
- Report abnormal findings to nurse in charge or physician.

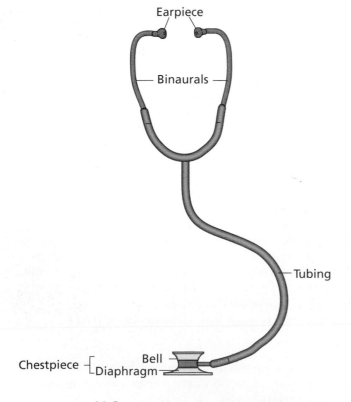

FIGURE 11-3 Parts of a single tubing stethoscope.

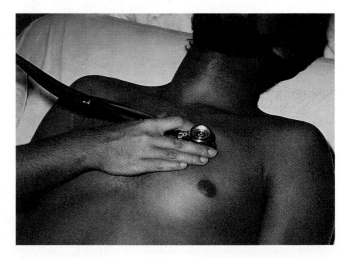

FIGURE 11-4 Positioning the diaphragm of the stethoscope.

more than 100 beats per minute in adults. Bradycardia is a slow rate, less than 60 beats per minute in adults.

PULSE RHYTHM. Normally a regular interval of time occurs between each pulse or heartbeat. An interval interrupted by an early or late beat or a missed beat indicates an abnormal rhythm or **dysrhythmia.** A dysrhythmia may alter cardiac output, particularly if it occurs repetitively. If a dysrhythmia is present, the regularity of its occurrence should be assessed. Dysrhythmias may be described as regularly irregular or irregularly irregular. The physician may order additional tests to evaluate the occurrence of dysrhythmias (see Chapter 24).

An inefficient contraction of the heart that fails to transmit a pulse wave to the peripheral pulse site creates a **pulse deficit.** To assess a pulse deficit ask a colleague to assess the radial pulse rate while you assess the apical rate. When you compare rates and find a difference between the apical and radial pulse rates, a pulse deficit exists. Pulse deficits are frequently associated with dysrhythmias.

STRENGTH AND EQUALITY.   The strength or amplitude of a pulse reflects the volume and pressure of the blood ejected against the arterial wall with each heart contraction

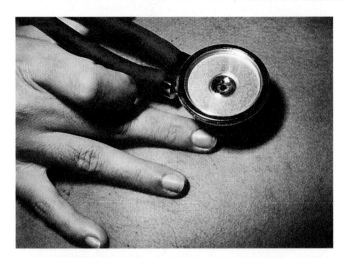

FIGURE 11-5   Positioning the bell of the stethoscope.

Acceptable Ranges of Heart Rate for Age	Table 11-4

Age	Heart Rate (beats/min)
Infants	120-160
Toddlers	90-140
Preschoolers	80-110
School-agers	75-100
Adolescent	60-90
Adult	60-100

Kinney MR and others: *AACN's clinical reference for critical care nursing,* ed 4, St. Louis, 1998, Mosby.

and the condition of the arterial vascular system leading to the pulse site. Normally the pulse strength remains the same with each heartbeat. Assess both radial pulses to compare the characteristics of each. A pulse in one arm may be unequal in strength or absent in many disease states. Pulse strength may be graded or described as bounding, strong, weak, or thready. Evaluating pulse strength and equality is included during assessment of the vascular system (see Chapter 12).

BLOOD PRESSURE

Blood pressure is the force exerted on the walls of an artery created by the pulsing blood under pressure from the heart. Blood flows throughout the circulatory system because of pressure changes, moving from an area of high pressure to an area of low pressure. The heart's contraction ejects blood under high pressure into the aorta. The peak of maximum pressure when ejection occurs is the **systolic** blood pressure. When the heart relaxes, the blood remaining in the arteries exerts a minimum or **diastolic** pressure. Diastolic pressure is the lowest pressure exerted against the arterial walls at all times.

The standard unit for measuring blood pressure is millimeters of mercury (mm Hg). The measurement indicates the height to which the blood pressure can raise a column of mercury. Blood pressure is recorded as a ratio with the systolic reading before the diastolic (e.g., 120/80). The difference between systolic and diastolic pressure is the **pulse pressure.** For a blood pressure of 120/80, the pulse pressure is 40.

Physiology of Arterial Blood Pressure

Blood pressure reflects the interrelationships of cardiac output, peripheral vascular resistance, blood volume, blood viscosity, and artery elasticity. An increase in cardiac output can be the result of greater heart muscle contractility, an increase in heart rate, or an increase in blood volume. When peripheral arteries constrict, such as during periods of stress, peripheral vascular resistance increases, which results in an increase in blood pressure. As vessels dilate and resistance falls, blood pressure drops. When blood is forced through the rigid arteries the blood pressure rises.

Factors Influencing Pulse Rates			Table 11-5
Factor	Increase Pulse Rate	Decrease Pulse Rate	
Exercise	Short-term exercise	Long-term exercise conditions the heart, resulting in lower rate at rest and quicker return to resting level after exercise	
Temperature	Fever and heat	Hypothermia	
Emotions	Acute pain and anxiety increase sympathetic stimulation, affecting heart rate	Unrelieved severe pain increases parasympathetic stimulation, affecting heart rate; relaxation	
Drugs	Positive chronotropic drugs such as epinephrine	Negative chronotropic drugs such as digitalis, beta blockers	
Hemorrhage	Loss of blood increases sympathetic stimulation		
Postural changes	Standing or sitting	Lying down	
Pulmonary conditions	Diseases causing poor oxygenation, such as asthma, COPD		

Factors Influencing Blood Pressure
Box 11-9

AGE
Blood pressure tends to rise with advancing age:

Age	Arterial Pressure (mm Hg)
Newborn (3000 g [6.6 lb])	40 (mean)
1 month	85/54
1 year	95/65
6 years	105/65
10-13 years	110/65
14-17 years	120/75
Middle-age adult	120/80
Older adult	140-160/80-90

Level of a child's or adolescent's blood pressure is assessed with respect to body size and age. Larger children have higher blood pressures than smaller children of the same age. Older adults have a rise in systolic pressure related to decreased elasticity.

STRESS
Anxiety, fear, and pain can initially increase blood pressure because of increased heart rate, increased cardiac output, and increased peripheral vascular resistance.

GENDER
There is no clinically significant difference in blood pressure levels between boys and girls.
After puberty, males have higher readings.
With menopause, women tend to have higher levels of blood pressure than men of the same age.

RACE
The incidence of hypertension is greater in urban African Americans than European Americans.
African Americans tend to develop more severe hypertension at an earlier age and have twice the risk for complications of hypertension such as stroke and heart attack.

DAILY VARIATION
Variations may include a lower blood pressure during sleep, highest blood pressure in the afternoon, a decrease in the evening, and an increase beginning at 4 to 6 AM.

MEDICATIONS
Some medications directly or indirectly affect blood pressure. Antihypertensive medications lower blood pressure. Narcotic analgesics can lower blood pressure. Vasoconstrictors and intravenous fluids such as normal saline can increase blood pressure.

ACTIVITY
Older adults often experience a 5- to 10-mm Hg fall in blood pressure about 1 hour after eating.
Blood pressure can be reduced for several hours after a period of vigorous exercise.

Modified from Thomas SA, DeKeyser F: *Annu Rev Nurs Res* 14:3, 1996; Joint National Committee on Detection, Evaluation, and Treatment of High Blood Pressure: *Arch Intern Med* 157:2413, 1997; Brashers VL: *Clinical application of pathophysiology*, St. Louis, 1998, Mosby; Whaley LF, Wong DL: *Nursing care of infants and children*, ed 6, St. Louis, 1999, Mosby.

If the blood volume decreases, such as during dehydration or hemorrhage, there is less pressure exerted against arterial walls and blood pressure falls. When the hematocrit rises the percentage of red blood cells in the blood increases, causing an increase in blood viscosity. The heart must contract more forcefully to move the viscous blood through the circulatory system, resulting in an increased blood pressure.

Blood Pressure Variations

Blood pressure is continually influenced by many factors during the day. A single blood pressure measurement cannot adequately reflect a client's blood pressure. Blood pressure trends, not individual measurements, guide nursing interventions. Your understanding of the factors that influence blood pressure results in a more accurate interpretation of blood pressure readings. Box 11-9 summarizes factors affecting blood pressure.

HYPERTENSION.   The most common alteration in blood pressure is **hypertension,** an often asymptomatic disorder characterized by persistently elevated blood pressure. The diagnosis of hypertension in adults is made when an average of two or more diastolic readings on at least two subsequent visits is 90 mm Hg or higher or when the average of two or more systolic readings on at least two subsequent visits is consistently higher than 140 mm Hg (Joint National Committee on

Classification of Blood Pressure for Adults
Table 11-6

Category	Systolic (mm Hg)	Diastolic (mm Hg)
Optimal	<120	<80
Normal	<130	<85
High normal	130-139	85-89
Hypertension		
Stage 1 (Mild)	140-159	90-99
Stage 2 (Moderate)	160-179	100-109
Stage 3 (Severe)	180-209	110-119
Stage 4 (Very Severe)	>210	>120

Modified from Joint National Committee on Detection, Evaluation, and Treatment of High Blood Pressure: The sixth report of the Joint National Committee on Detection, Evaluation, and Treatment of High Blood Pressure, *Arch Intern Med* 157:2413, 1997; Brashers VL: *Clinical application of pathophysiology*, St. Louis, 1998, Mosby.

Detection, Evaluation, and Treatment of High Blood Pressure, 1997). Categories of hypertension have been developed and determine medical intervention (Table 11-6).

One elevated blood pressure measurement does not qualify as a diagnosis of hypertension. However, if you assess a high reading during the first blood pressure measurement (e.g., 150/90 mm Hg), instruct your client to return for another checkup at least within 2 months.

Procedural Guidelines for   Box 11-10

Equipment
- Sphygmomanometer
- Stethoscope

1. Obtaining orthostatic blood pressure measurements requires critical thinking and ongoing nursing judgment and is not delegated to assistive personnel.
2. Obtain supine client's blood pressure in each arm. Select arm with highest systolic reading for subsequent measurements.
3. Leaving blood pressure cuff in place, assist client to sitting position. After 1 to 3 minutes with client in sitting position, obtain blood pressure. If orthostatic symptoms occur such as dizziness, weakness, lightheadedness, feeling faint, or sudden pallor, terminate blood pressure measurement and assist client to a supine position.
4. Leaving blood pressure cuff in place, assist client to standing position. After 1 to 3 minutes with client in standing position, obtain blood pressure. If orthostatic symptoms occur (see above), terminate blood pressure measurement and assist client to a supine position. In most cases you will detect orthostatic hypotension within 1 minute of standing (Roper, 1996).
5. Record client's blood pressure in each position; for example: "140/80 supine, 132/72 sitting, 108/60 standing." Note any additional symptoms or complaints.
6. Report findings of orthostatic hypotension or orthostatic symptoms to physician or nurse in charge. Instruct client to obtain assistance when getting out of bed if orthostatic hypotension is present or orthostatic symptoms occur.

Persons with a family history of hypertension are at significant risk. Obesity, cigarette smoking, heavy alcohol consumption, high blood cholesterol levels, and continued exposure to stress are also linked to hypertension.

HYPOTENSION.   **Hypotension** is considered present when the systolic blood pressure falls to 90 mm Hg or below. Although some adults have low blood pressure normally, hypotension is an abnormal finding. Hypotension occurs when arteries dilate, the peripheral vascular resistance decreases, the circulating blood volume decreases, or the heart fails to provide adequate cardiac output. Signs and symptoms associated with hypotension include pallor, skin mottling, clamminess, confusion, dizziness, chest pain, increased heart rate, and decreased urine output. Hypotension is life threatening and is reported to the physician immediately.

Orthostatic hypotension, also referred to as **postural hypotension,** occurs when a client with a normal blood pressure develops symptoms and low blood pressure when rising to an upright position. When a healthy person changes from a lying, to sitting, to standing position the peripheral blood vessels in the legs constrict, preventing the pooling of blood in the legs caused by gravity. Orthostatic hypotension occurs when the peripheral blood vessels in the legs are already constricted or are unable to constrict in response to a change in position. Clients with a decreased blood volume, anemia, dehydration, experiencing prolonged bed rest, with recent blood loss, or taking antihypertensive medications are at risk for orthostatic hypotension. Assess for orthostatic hypotension by obtaining pulse and blood pressure readings with the client supine, sitting, and standing (Box 11-10).

Assessment of Blood Pressure

Arterial blood pressure may be measured either directly (invasively) or indirectly (noninvasively). The direct method requires the insertion of a thin catheter into an artery. The more common noninvasive method requires use of the **sphygmomanometer** and stethoscope. You can measure blood pressure indirectly by auscultation or palpation. Auscultation is the most widely used technique (Skill 11-3).

BLOOD PRESSURE EQUIPMENT.   Before assessing blood pressure you must be comfortable in using a sphygmomanometer and stethoscope. A sphygmomanometer includes a pressure manometer, an occlusive cloth or vinyl cuff that encloses an inflatable rubber bladder, and a pressure bulb with a release valve that inflates the bladder. The two types of sphygmomanometers are the aneroid and the mercury (Figure 11-6). Aneroid manometers have the advantages of being safe, lightweight, portable, and compact. The aneroid manometer has a glass-enclosed circular gauge containing a needle that registers millimeter calibrations. Before using the aneroid model, you must be sure that the needle points to zero and that the manometer is correctly calibrated. Aneroid sphygmomanometers require biomedical calibration at routine intervals to verify their accuracy.

Mercury manometers, once the gold standard, are less common because they contain mercury, a hazardous substance. However, some agencies or specific units, for example, operating rooms or intensive care units, may use the mercury manometer. Pressure created by the inflation of the compression cuff moves the column of mercury upward against the force of gravity. Millimeter calibrations mark the height of the mercury column. To ensure accurate readings, the mercury column should fall freely as pressure is released and should always be at zero when the cuff is deflated. Accurate readings are obtained by looking at the meniscus of the mercury at eye level. Looking up or down at the mercury results in distorted readings. Because many municipalities have prohibited the sale or use of mercury-containing medical devices because of the potential hazards, few mercury manometers are available.

Cloth or disposable vinyl compression cuffs used with the sphygmomanometer come in several sizes. The size selected is proportional to the circumference of the limb being assessed. Ideally, the width of the cuff should be 40% of the circumference (or 20% wider than the diameter) of the midpoint of the limb on which the cuff is to be used. The bladder, enclosed by the cuff, should encircle at least 80% of the arm of an adult and the entire arm of a child (Joint National Committee on Detection, Evaluation, and Treatment of High Blood Pressure, 1997). The lower edge of the cuff should be above the antecubital fossa, allowing room for placement of the stethoscope. An improperly fitting cuff causes inaccurate blood pressure measurement.

Text continued on p. 202

Skill 11-3

MEASURING BLOOD PRESSURE

DELEGATION CONSIDERATIONS
The skill of blood pressure measurement can be delegated to assistive personnel.
- Inform caregiver if client has alterations affecting the appropriate limb for blood pressure measurement.
- Inform caregiver of appropriate size blood pressure cuff for designated extremity.
- Inform caregiver if client is at risk for orthostatic hypotension.
- Inform caregiver of frequency of blood pressure measurements.

- Determine that caregiver is aware of the usual values for the client.
- Inform caregiver of the need to report any abnormalities that you should confirm.

EQUIPMENT
- Aneroid or mercury sphygmomanometer
- Cloth or disposable vinyl pressure cuff of appropriate size for client's extremity
- Stethoscope
- Alcohol swab
- Pen, pencil, vital sign flow sheet or record form

STEPS	RATIONALE
1. Determine need to assess client's BP: a. Note risk factors for alterations in BP.	Certain conditions place clients at risk for BP alterations: history of cardiovascular disease, renal disease, diabetes, circulatory shock (hypovolemic, septic, cardiogenic, or neurogenic), acute or chronic pain, rapid IV infusion of fluids or blood products, increased intracranial pressure, postoperative conditions, toxemia of pregnancy.

b. Observe for signs and symptoms of BP alterations:
    (1) High BP (hypertension) is often asymptomatic until pressure is very high. Assess for headache (usually occipital), flushing of face, nosebleed, and fatigue in older adults.
    (2) Low BP (hypotension) is associated with dizziness; confusion; restlessness; pale, dusky, or cyanotic skin and mucous membranes; cool, mottled skin over extremities.
	Physical signs and symptoms may indicate alterations in BP.

2. Determine best site for BP assessment. Avoid applying cuff to extremity when: intravenous fluids infusing; an arteriovenous shunt or fistula is present; breast or axillary surgery has been performed on that side; extremity has been traumatized, diseased, or requires a cast or bulky bandage. The lower extremities may be used when the brachial arteries are inaccessible.	Inappropriate site selection may result in poor amplification of sounds, causing inaccurate readings. Application of pressure from inflated bladder temporarily impairs blood flow and can further compromise circulation in extremity that already has impaired blood flow.
3. Select appropriate cuff size.	Improper cuff size results in inaccurate readings (see Table 11-7, p. 203). If cuff is too small, it tends to come loose as inflated or results in false-high readings. If the cuff is too large, false-low readings may be recorded.
4. Determine previous baseline BP (if available) from client's record.	Allows you to assess for change in condition. Provides comparison with future BP measurements.
5. Encourage client to avoid exercise and smoking for 30 minutes before assessment of BP.	Exercise and smoking can cause false elevations in BP.
6. Have client assume sitting or lying position. Be sure room is warm, quiet, and relaxing.	Maintains client's comfort during measurement. The client's perceptions that the physical or interpersonal environment is stressful affect the BP measurement (Thomas and DeKeyser, 1996).

STEPS	RATIONALE
7. Explain to client that BP is to be assessed and have client rest at least 5 minutes before measurement. Ask client not to speak when BP is being measured.	Reduces anxiety that can falsely elevate readings. Blood pressure readings taken at different times can be more objectively compared when assessed with client at rest. Talking to a client when the BP is being assessed increases readings 10% to 40% (Thomas and DeKeyser, 1996).
8. Wash hands. With client sitting or lying, position client's forearm or thigh, supported if needed. For arm, turn palm up (see illustration); for thigh, position with knee slightly flexed.	Reduces transmission of microorganisms. If extremity is unsupported, client may perform isometric exercise that can increase diastolic pressure. Placement of arm above the level of the heart causes false-low reading.
9. Expose extremity (arm or leg) fully by removing constricting clothing.	Ensures proper cuff application.
10. Palpate brachial artery (arm) or popliteal artery (leg) (see illustration). Position cuff 2.5 cm (1 inch) above site of pulsation (antecubital or popliteal space).	Inflating bladder directly over artery ensures proper pressure is applied during inflation.
11. Apply bladder of cuff above artery by centering arrows marked on cuff over artery. If no center arrows on cuff, estimate the center of the bladder and place this center over artery (see illustrations). With cuff fully deflated, wrap cuff evenly and snugly around extremity.	Loose-fitting cuff causes false-high readings.
12. If possible position manometer vertically at eye level. Observer should be no farther than 1 m (approximately 1 yard) away.	Accurate readings are obtained by looking at the aneroid needle or meniscus of the mercury at eye level. The meniscus is the point where the crescent-shaped top of the mercury column aligns with the manometer scale. Looking up or down results in distorted readings.

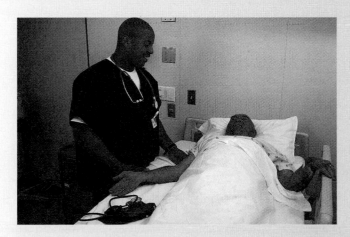

STEP 8   Client's forearm supported in bed.

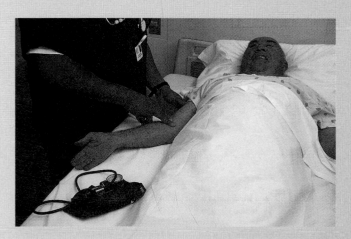

STEP 10   Nurse palpating client's brachial artery.

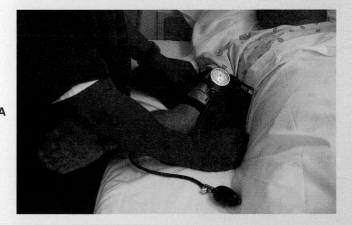

A

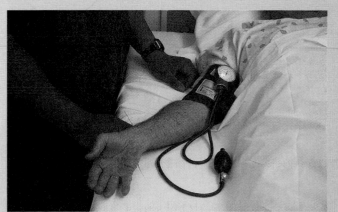

B

STEP 11   **A,** Center bladder of cuff above artery. **B,** Blood pressure cuff wrapped around upper arm.

STEPS	RATIONALE
13. Measure blood pressure.	
A. Two-Step Method:	
(1) Relocate brachial pulse. Palpate artery distal to the cuff with fingertips of nondominant hand while inflating cuff. Note point at which pulse disappears and continue to inflate cuff to a pressure 30 mm Hg above that point. Note the pressure reading. Slowly deflate cuff and note point when pulse reappears. Deflate cuff fully and wait 30 seconds.	Estimating systolic pressure prevents false-low readings, which may result in the presence of an auscultatory gap. Maximal inflation point for accurate reading can be determined by palpation. If unable to palpate artery because of weakened pulse, an ultrasonic stethoscope can be used (see Chapter 12). Completely deflating cuff prevents venous congestion and false-high readings.
(2) Place stethoscope earpieces in ears and be sure sounds are clear, not muffled.	Each earpiece should follow angle of ear canal to facilitate hearing.
(3) Relocate brachial artery and place diaphragm of stethoscope over it. Do not allow chestpiece to touch cuff or clothing (see illustration).	Proper stethoscope placement ensures optimal sound reception. Stethoscope improperly positioned causes muffled sounds that often result in false-low systolic and false-high diastolic readings.
(4) Close valve of pressure bulb clockwise until tight.	Tightening of valve prevents air leak during inflation.
(5) Quickly inflate cuff to 30 mm Hg above client's estimated systolic pressure (see illustration).	Rapid inflation ensures accurate measurement of systolic pressure.
(6) Slowly release pressure bulb valve and allow mercury or needle of aneroid manometer gauge to fall at rate of 2 to 3 mm Hg/sec.	Too rapid or slow a decline in aneroid pressure or mercury level can cause inaccurate readings.
(7) Note point on manometer when first clear sound is heard. The sound will slowly increase in intensity.	First Korotkoff sound indicates systolic pressure.
(8) Continue to deflate cuff gradually, noting point at which sound disappears in adults. Note pressure to nearest 2 mm Hg. Listen for 20 to 30 mm Hg after the last sound and then allow remaining air to escape quickly.	Beginning of the fifth Korotkoff sound is recommended by American Heart Association as indication of diastolic pressure in adults. Fourth Korotkoff sound involves distinct muffling of sounds and is recommended by American Heart Association as indication of diastolic pressure in children.
B. One-Step Method:	
(1) Place stethoscope earpieces in ears and be sure sounds are clear, not muffled.	Earpieces should follow angle of ear canal to facilitate hearing.
(2) Relocate brachial artery and place diaphragm of stethoscope over it. Do not allow chestpiece to touch cuff or clothing.	Proper stethoscope placement ensures optimal sound reception.
(3) Close valve of pressure bulb clockwise until tight.	Tightening of valve prevents air leak during inflation.

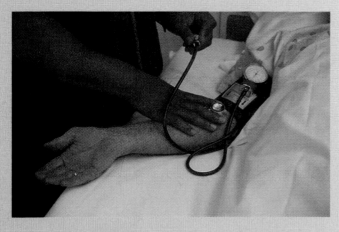

STEP 13A(3)   Stethoscope over brachial artery to measure BP.

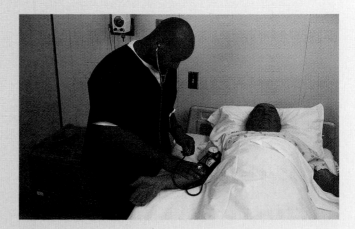

STEP 13A(5)   Inflating BP cuff.

STEPS	RATIONALE
(4) Quickly inflate cuff to 30 mm Hg above client's usual systolic pressure.	Inflation above systolic level ensures accurate measurement of systolic pressure.
(5) Slowly release pressure bulb valve and allow mercury or needle of aneroid manometer gauge to fall at rate of 2 to 3 mm Hg/sec.	Too rapid or slow a decline in aneroid pressure or mercury level can cause inaccurate readings.
(6) Note point on manometer when first clear sound is heard. The sound will slowly increase in intensity.	Record as systolic pressure.
(7) Continue to deflate cuff gradually, noting point at which sound disappears in adults. Note pressure to nearest 2 mm Hg. Listen for 20 to 30 mm Hg after the last sound and then allow remaining air to escape quickly.	Beginning of the fifth Korotkoff sound is recommended by American Heart Association as indication of diastolic pressure in adults. Fourth Korotkoff sound involves distinct muffling of sounds and is recommended by American Heart Association as indication of diastolic pressure in children.
14. Remove cuff from extremity unless measurement must be repeated. If this is the first assessment of client, repeat procedure on the other extremity.	Comparison of BP in both arms detects circulatory problems. (Normal difference of 5 to 10 mm Hg exists between extremities).
15. Assist client in returning to comfortable position and cover upper arm if previously clothed.	Restores comfort and promotes sense of well-being.
16. Discuss findings with client as needed.	Promotes participation in care and understanding of health status.
17. Wash hands.	Reduces transmission of microorganisms.
18. Compare reading with previous baseline and/or acceptable value of blood pressure for client's age.	Evaluates for change in condition and alterations.
19. Compare blood pressure in both arms or both legs.	If using upper extremities, the arm with higher pressure should be used for subsequent assessments unless contraindicated.
20. Correlate blood pressure with data obtained from pulse assessment and related cardiovascular signs and symptoms.	Blood pressure and heart rate are interrelated.

UNEXPECTED OUTCOMES AND RELATED INTERVENTIONS

- Unable to obtain blood pressure reading.
  - Assess for signs and symptoms of decreased CO; if present notify nurse in charge or physician immediately.
  - Palpate radial artery. If radial artery bounding, strong, or weak, reposition blood pressure cuff and repeat measurement. If unable to obtain blood pressure measurement with automatic device or auscultation, use palpation to determine systolic pressure.
  - Reduce environmental noise. Consider electronic blood pressure cuff for home if client has hearing difficulties and if client has sufficient financial resources.
- Blood pressure is less than 90 mm Hg systolic.
  - Assess for signs and symptoms of decreased CO; if present notify nurse in charge or physician immediately.
  - Repeat blood pressure measurement with sphygmomanometer. Electronic blood pressure measurements are less accurate in low blood flow conditions.
  - Position client in supine position to enhance circulation and restrict activity that may be decreasing blood pressure.
  - Administer vasoconstrictor medications and IV solutions as ordered.

- Blood pressure is elevated above client's usual value.
  - Repeat blood pressure measurement in other arm and compare findings. Verify correct selection and placement of cuff.
  - Observe for related symptoms, though symptoms may not be apparent until blood pressure is extremely elevated.
  - Administer antihypertensive medications as ordered.
  - Report elevated blood pressure to nurse in charge or physician to initiate appropriate evaluation and treatment.

RECORDING AND REPORTING

- Inform client of value and need for periodic reassessment.
- Record blood pressure in nurses' notes or vital sign flow sheet.
- Measurement of blood pressure after administration of specific therapies should be documented in narrative form in nurses' notes.
- Report abnormal findings to nurse in charge or physician.

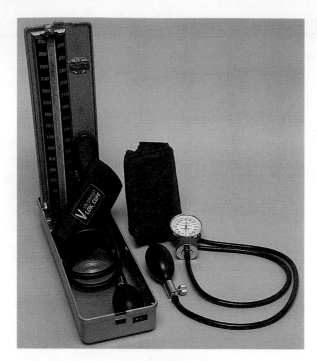

FIGURE **11-6** Sphygmomanometers.

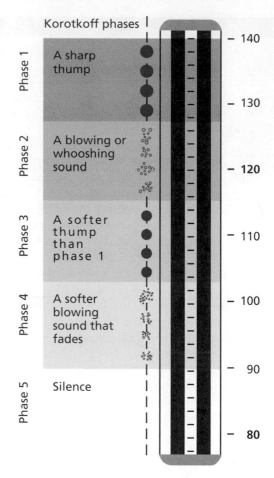

FIGURE **11-7** The sounds auscultated during blood pressure measurement can be differentiated into five Korotkoff phases. In this example, the blood pressure is 140/90.

AUSCULTATION. The best method for blood pressure measurement by auscultation is in a quiet room at a comfortable temperature. Although the client may lie or stand, sitting is the preferred position. The client's position should be the same during each blood pressure measurement to permit a meaningful comparison of values. Before assessment you should attempt to control factors responsible for artificially high readings such as pain, anxiety, or exertion. The client's perception that the physical or interpersonal environment is stressful will affect the blood pressure. Measurements taken at home may be different than those taken at the client's place of employment or in a physician's office.

During the initial assessment obtain and record the blood pressure in both arms. Normally there is a difference of 5 to 10 mm Hg between the right and left arms. In subsequent assessments the blood pressure should be measured in the arm with the higher pressure. Pressure differences greater than 10 mm Hg may indicate vascular problems and should be reported to the physician.

Indirect measurement of arterial blood pressure works on a basic principle of pressure. Blood flows freely through an artery until an inflated cuff applies pressure to tissues and causes the artery to collapse. After the cuff pressure is released, the point at which blood flow returns and sound appears through auscultation is the systolic pressure.

In 1905, Korotkoff, a Russian surgeon, first described the sounds heard over an artery during cuff deflation. The first **Korotkoff sound** is a clear, rhythmic tapping that corresponds to the pulse rate and gradually increases in intensity. Onset of the sound corresponds to the systolic pressure. A murmur or swishing sound appears as the cuff continues to deflate, the second Korotkoff sound. As the artery distends, there is a tur-

bulence in blood flow. The third Korotkoff sound is a crisper and more intense tapping. The fourth Korotkoff sound becomes muffled and low pitched as the cuff is further deflated. Cuff pressure falls below the pressure within the vessel walls. The onset of the fourth Korotkoff sound is recorded as the diastolic pressure in infants and children, pregnant women, and clients with elevated cardiac output or peripheral vasodilation. The fifth Korotkoff sound is the disappearance of sound; in adolescents and most adults, this sound corresponds with the diastolic pressure (Figure 11-7). In some clients the sounds are clear and distinct. In other clients only the beginning and the ending sounds are heard.

The American Heart Association (Joint National Committee on Detection, Evaluation, and Treatment of High Blood Pressure, 1997) recommends recording two numbers for a blood pressure measurement: the point on the manometer when the first sound is heard for systolic and the point on the manometer when the fifth sound is heard for diastolic. Some institutions recommend recording the point when the fourth sound is heard as well, especially for clients with hypertension. The numbers are divided by slashed lines (e.g., 120/80, 120/100/80), and the arm used to measure the blood pressure is noted (e.g., RA 130/70).

Common Mistakes in Blood Pressure Assessment   Table 11-7

Error	Effect
Bladder or cuff too wide	False-low reading
Bladder or cuff too narrow	False-high reading
Cuff wrapped too loosely or unevenly	False-high reading
Deflating cuff too slowly	False-high diastolic reading
Deflating cuff too quickly	False-low systolic and false-high diastolic reading
Arm below heart level	False-high reading
Arm above heart level	False-low reading
Arm not supported	False-high reading
Stethoscope that fits poorly or impairment of the examiner's hearing, causing sounds to be muffled	False-low systolic and false-high diastolic reading
Stethoscope applied too firmly against antecubital fossa	False-low diastolic reading
Inflating too slowly	False-high diastolic reading
Repeating assessments too quickly	False-low systolic reading
Inaccurate inflation level	Inaccurate interpretation of systolic and diastolic readings
Multiple examiners using different Korotkoff sounds for diastolic readings	False-high systolic and low diastolic reading

Many of your decisions and nursing interventions about a client's health care are made on the basis of blood pressure findings in conjunction with other findings. The importance of obtaining an accurate blood pressure cannot be overemphasized. There are several possibilities for error if the auscultation procedure is not followed correctly (Table 11-7). If you are unsure of a reading, ask a colleague to reassess the blood pressure.

ULTRASONIC STETHOSCOPE.   If you are unable to auscultate sounds because of a weakened arterial pulse, an ultrasonic stethoscope can be used (see Chapter 12). This stethoscope allows the nurse to hear low-frequency systolic sounds and is commonly used when measuring the blood pressure of infants and children, and low blood pressure in adults.

PALPATATION.   Indirect measurement of blood pressure by palpation is useful for clients whose arterial pulsations are too weak to create Korotkoff sounds. Severe blood loss and weakened heart contractility are examples of conditions that result in blood pressures too low to auscultate accurately. Only the systolic blood pressure can be assessed by palpation (Box 11-11). The diastolic pressure is difficult to determine by palpation. A subtle change in sensation, usually in the form of a thin, snapping vibration, marks the diastolic level. When the palpation technique is used, the systolic value and the manner in which it was measured are recorded (e.g., RA 78/-, palpated).

The palpation technique is used along with auscultation in some instances. In some hypertensive clients, the sounds usually heard over the brachial artery when the cuff pressure is high disappear as pressure is reduced and then reappear at a lower level. This temporary disappearance of sound is the **auscultatory gap.** It typically occurs between the first and second Korotkoff sounds. The gap in sound may cover a range of 40 mm Hg and thus may cause an underestimation

Procedural Guidelines for   Box 11-11

PALPATING THE SYSTOLIC BLOOD PRESSURE

Equipment
• Sphygmomanometer
1. Apply blood pressure cuff to the upper arm in the same manner used for the auscultation method.
2. Continually palpate the radial artery.
3. Inflate blood pressure cuff 30 mm Hg above the point at which the radial pulse can no longer be palpated.
4. Release valve and allow manometer dial to fall 2 mm Hg per second.
5. As soon as the radial pulse is palpable, note the manometer reading, the systolic blood pressure.

of systolic pressure or overestimation of diastolic pressure. The cuff must be inflated high enough to hear the true systolic pressure before the auscultatory gap. Palpation of the radial artery helps to determine how high to inflate the cuff. You can inflate the cuff 30 mm Hg above the pressure at which the radial pulse was palpated. The range of pressures in which the auscultatory gap occurs is recorded (e.g., "BP RA 180/94 with an auscultatory gap from 180 to 160").

BLOOD PRESSURE ASSESSMENT IN LOWER EXTREMITIES.
Dressings, casts, intravenous catheters, or arteriovenous fistulas or shunts can make the upper extremities inaccessible. Blood pressure must then be measured in the lower extremities. Comparing upper extremity blood pressure with that in the legs is also necessary for clients with certain cardiac and blood pressure abnormalities. The popliteal artery, palpable behind the knee in the popliteal space, is the site for auscultation. Position the cuff with the bladder over the posterior aspect of the midthigh. The cuff must be wide and long enough to allow for the larger girth of the thigh. For most measurements, place the client in a prone position. If such a position is impossible, flex the knee slightly for easier access to the

artery (Figure 11-8). The procedure is identical to brachial artery auscultation. Systolic pressure in the legs is usually higher by 10 to 40 mm Hg than in the brachial artery, but the diastolic pressure is the same.

ASSESSMENT OF BLOOD PRESSURE IN CHILDREN.

All children 3 years of age through adolescence should have blood pressure checked at least yearly. Blood pressure in children changes with growth and development. You can help parents understand the importance of this routine screening to detect children who may be at risk for hypertension. The measurement of blood pressure in infants and children is difficult for several reasons.

1. Different arm size requires careful and appropriate cuff size selection.
2. Readings are difficult to obtain in restless or anxious infants and children.

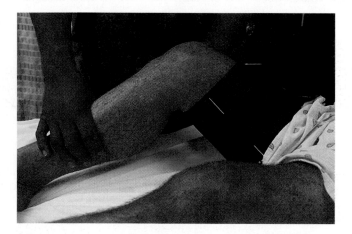

FIGURE **11-8** Lower extremity blood pressure cuff positioned above popliteal artery at midthigh with knee flexed.

3. Placing stethoscope too firmly on the antecubital fossa can cause errors in auscultation sounds.
4. Korotkoff sounds are difficult to hear in children because of low frequency and amplitude.

The same auscultation method used with adults is appropriate for children. An infant or child younger than 5 years of age should lie supine with the arms supported at heart level. Older children may sit. It is important to have the child relaxed and calm. A delay of at least 15 minutes before taking a reading is recommended to allow the child to recover from recent activity or apprehension. Those 15 minutes can be used for other quiet nursing activities. It may help to have a parent nearby. You can prepare the child for the blood pressure cuff's unusual sensation during inflation. Most children understand the analogy of a "tight hug on your arm" and will be more cooperative.

RESPIRATION

Respiration is the mechanism the body uses to exchange gases between the atmosphere and the blood and the cells. Respiration involves three processes: **ventilation** (the mechanical movement of gases into and out of the lungs), **diffusion** (the movement of oxygen [O_2] and carbon dioxide [CO_2] between the alveoli and the red blood cells), and **perfusion** (the distribution of red blood cells to and from the pulmonary capillaries). Analyzing respiratory efficiency requires integrating assessment data from all three processes. Ventilation is assessed by determining respiratory rate, respiratory depth, and respiratory rhythm. Diffusion and perfusion can be assessed by determining oxygen saturation.

Assessment of Ventilation

Adults normally breathe in a smooth, uninterrupted pattern of 12 to 20 breaths per minute. Ventilation is normally regu-

---

Factors Influencing Character of Respirations   Box 11-12

EXERCISE

Exercise increases respiration rate and depth to meet the body's need for additional oxygen and to rid the body of CO_2.

ACUTE PAIN

Pain alters rate and rhythm of respirations, breathing becomes shallow.

Client may inhibit or splint chest wall movement when pain is in area of chest or abdomen.

ANXIETY

Anxiety increases respiration rate and depth as a result of sympathetic stimulation.

SMOKING

Chronic smoking changes the lung's airways, resulting in increased rate of respiration at rest when not smoking.

BODY POSITION

A straight, erect posture promotes full chest expansion.
A stooped or slumped position impairs ventilatory movement.
Lying flat prevents full chest expansion.

MEDICATIONS

Narcotic analgesics, general anesthetics, and sedative hypnotics depress respiration rate and depth.

Amphetamines and cocaine may increase rate and depth.

Bronchodilators slow rate by causing airway dilation.

NEUROLOGICAL INJURY

Injury to the brainstem impairs the respiratory center and inhibits respiratory rate and rhythm.

HEMOGLOBIN FUNCTION

Decreased hemoglobin levels (anemia) reduce oxygen-carrying capacity of the blood, which increases respiratory rate.

Increased altitude lowers the amount of saturated hemoglobin, which increases respiratory rate and depth.

Abnormal blood cell function (e.g., sickle cell disease) reduces ability of hemoglobin to carry oxygen, which increases respiratory rate and depth.

lated by levels of CO_2 in the arterial blood. The normal rate and depth of ventilation, **eupnea,** is interrupted by sighing. The sigh, a prolonged deeper breath, is a protective physiological mechanism for expanding small airways and alveoli not ventilated during a normal breath.

You must first learn to recognize normal thoracic and abdominal movements to assess ventilation. During quiet breathing the chest wall gently rises and falls. When breathing requires greater effort, the intercostal and accessory muscles work actively to move air in and out. The shoulders may rise and fall, and the accessory muscles of ventilation in the neck visibly contract. Diaphragmatic movement becomes less noticeable as costal breathing increases.

Measurement of Respiration

Accurate measurement of respiration requires observation and palpation of chest wall movement. A sudden change in the character of respirations may be important. For example, a reduction in respirations occurring in a client after head trauma may signify injury to the brainstem.

When assessing respiration, you should keep in mind the client's usual ventilatory rate and pattern, the influence any disease or illness has on respiratory function, the relationship between respiratory and cardiovascular function, and the influence of therapies on respiration. Box 11-12 summarizes factors influencing respiration. The objective measurement of respiration includes the rate and depth of breathing and the rhythm of ventilatory movements (Skill 11-4).

RESPIRATORY RATE.   Observe a full inspiration and expiration when counting ventilations or respiratory rate. The respiratory rate varies with age (Table 11-8). A respiratory rate less than 12 per minute or lower than acceptable limits is **bradypnea,** whereas a rate over 20 or greater than the acceptable limits is **tachypnea. Apnea** is the lack of respiratory movements. A respiratory monitoring device that can aid your assessment of respiratory rate is the apnea monitor. This noninvasive device uses leads attached to the client's chest wall to sense movement. An absence of chest wall movement triggers the apnea alarm. Apnea monitoring is

---

Skill 11-4
ASSESSING RESPIRATION

DELEGATION CONSIDERATIONS

The skill of respiration measurement can be delegated to assistive personnel.

- Inform caregiver of client history or risk for increased or decreased respiratory rate or irregular respiration.
- Inform caregiver of frequency of respiration measurement.
- Determine that caregiver is aware of the usual values for the client.
- Inform caregiver of the need to report any abnormalities that you should confirm.

EQUIPMENT

- Wristwatch with second hand or digital display
- Pen, pencil, vital sign flow sheet or record form

STEPS	RATIONALE
1. Determine need to assess client's respiration: a. Note risk factors for respiratory alterations.	Conditions that place client at risk for ventilatory alterations detected by changes in respiratory rate, depth, and rhythm include: fever, pain, anxiety, diseases of chest wall or muscles, constrictive chest or abdominal dressings, presence of abdominal incisions, gastric distention, chronic pulmonary disease (emphysema, bronchitis, asthma), traumatic injury to chest wall, presence of a chest tube, respiratory infection (pneumonia, acute bronchitis), pulmonary edema and emboli, head injury with damage to brainstem, and anemia.
b. Assess for signs and symptoms of respiratory alterations, such as bluish or cyanotic appearance of nail beds, lips, mucous membranes, and skin; restlessness, irritability, confusion, reduced level of consciousness; pain during inspiration; labored or difficult breathing; orthopnea; use of accessory muscles; adventitious breath sounds (see Chapter 12), inability to breathe spontaneously; thick, frothy, blood-tinged, or copious sputum produced on coughing.	Physical signs and symptoms may indicate alterations in respiratory status related to ventilation.

STEPS	RATIONALE

2. Assess pertinent laboratory values:
  a. Arterial blood gases (ABGs) (values may vary slightly within institutions):
    pH 7.35 to 7.45
    $PaCO_2$ 35 to 45 mm Hg
    PaO_2 80 to 100 mm Hg
    SaO_2 94% to 98%
	Arterial blood gases measure arterial blood pH, partial pressure of O_2 and CO_2, and arterial O_2 saturation, which reflect client's oxygenation status.

b. Pulse oximetry (SpO_2): normal SpO_2 90% to 100%; 85% to 89% may be acceptable for certain chronic disease conditions; less than 85% is abnormal.	SpO_2 less than 85% is often accompanied by changes in respiratory rate, depth, and rhythm.
c. Complete blood count (CBC): normal CBC for adults (values may vary within institutions): hemoglobin: 14 to 18 g/100 ml, males; 12 to 16 g/100 ml, females; hematocrit: 40% to 54%, males; 38% to 47%, females; red blood cell count: 4.6 to 6.2 million/mm³, males; 4.2 to 5.4 million/mm³, females.	Complete blood count measures red blood cell count, volume of red blood cells, and concentration of hemoglobin, which reflect client's blood capacity to carry O_2.
3. Determine previous baseline respiratory rate (if available) from client's record.	Allows you to assess for change in condition. Provides comparison with future respiratory measurements.
4. Be sure client is in comfortable position, preferably sitting or lying with the head of the bed elevated 45 to 60 degrees.	Sitting erect promotes full ventilatory movement. Position of discomfort may cause client to breathe more rapidly.

Critical Decision Point

Clients with difficulty breathing (dyspnea) such as those with congestive heart failure or abdominal ascites or in late stages of pregnancy should be assessed in the position of greatest comfort. Repositioning may increase the work of breathing, which will increase respiratory rate.

STEPS	RATIONALE
5. Draw curtain around bed and/or close door. Wash hands.	Maintains privacy. Prevents transmission of microorganisms.
6. Be sure client's chest is visible. If necessary, move bed linen or gown.	Ensures clear view of chest wall and abdominal movements.
7. Place client's arm in relaxed position across the abdomen or lower chest, or place your hand directly over client's upper abdomen (see illustration).	A similar position used during pulse assessment allows respiratory rate assessment to be inconspicuous. Client's hand or your hand rises and falls during respiratory cycle.

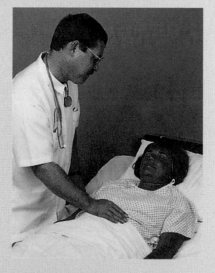

STEP 7   Nurse's hand over client's abdomen to check respiration.

STEPS	RATIONALE
8. Observe complete respiratory cycle (one inspiration and one expiration).	Rate is accurately determined only after you have viewed the entire respiratory cycle.

STEPS	RATIONALE
9. After cycle is observed, look at watch's second hand and begin to count rate: when sweep hand hits number on dial, begin time frame, counting one with first full respiratory cycle.	Timing begins with count of one. Respirations occur more slowly than pulse; thus timing does not begin with zero.
10. If rhythm is regular, count number of respirations in 30 seconds and multiply by 2. If rhythm is irregular, less than 12, or greater than 20, count for 1 full minute. Respiratory rate less than 12 or greater than 20 requires further assessment and may require immediate intervention.	Respiratory rate is equivalent to number of respirations per minute. Suspected irregularities require assessment for at least 1 minute.
11. Note depth of respirations, subjectively assessed by observing degree of chest wall movement while counting rate. You can also objectively assess depth by palpating chest wall excursion or auscultating the posterior thorax (see Chapter 12) after rate has been counted. Depth is shallow, normal, or deep.	Character of ventilatory movement may reveal specific disease state restricting volume of air from moving into and out of the lungs.
12. Note rhythm of ventilatory cycle. Normal breathing is regular and uninterrupted. Sighing should not be confused with abnormal rhythm. Periodically people unconsciously take single deep breaths or sighs to expand small airways prone to collapse.	Character of ventilations can reveal specific types of alterations.

 • **Critical Decision Point**
An irregular respiratory pattern or periods of apnea (the cessation of respiration for several seconds) are a symptom of underlying disease in the adult and must be reported to the physician or nurse in charge. Further assessment may be required (see Chapter 27) and immediate intervention may be needed. An irregular respiratory rate and short apneic spells are normal for newborns.

STEPS	RATIONALE
13. Replace bed linen and client's gown.	Restores comfort and promotes sense of well-being.
14. Wash hands.	Reduces transmission of microorganisms.
15. Discuss findings with client as needed.	Promotes participation in care and understanding of health status.
16. If respiration is assessed for the first time, establish rate, rhythm, and depth as baseline if within normal range.	Used to compare future respiratory assessment.
17. Compare respiration with client's previous baseline and normal rate, rhythm, and depth.	Allows you to assess for changes in client's condition and for presence of respiratory alterations.

UNEXPECTED OUTCOMES AND RELATED INTERVENTIONS

- Client has abnormal respiratory rate, depth, or complains of feeling short of breath.
  - Observe for related factors, including obstructed airway, noisy respirations, cyanosis, restlessness, irritability, confusion, productive cough, and abnormal breath sounds.
  - Assist client to supported sitting position (semi- or high-Fowler's) unless contraindicated, which improves ventilation.
  - Provide oxygen as ordered.
  - Assess for environmental factors that may influence client's respiratory rate such as secondhand smoke, poor ventilation, or gas fumes.

RECORDING AND REPORTING

- Record respiratory rate and character in nurses' notes or vital sign flow sheet.
- Indicate type and amount of oxygen therapy if used by client during assessment.
- Measurement of respiratory rate after administration of specific therapies should be documented in narrative form in nurses' notes.
- Report abnormal findings to nurse in charge or physician.

Acceptable Range of Respiratory Rates for Age	Table 11-8
Age	Rate (breaths/min)
Newborn	35-40
Infant (6 months)	30-50
Toddler (2 years)	25-32
Child	20-30
Adolescent	16-19
Adult	12-16

used frequently with infants in the hospital and at home to observe for prolonged apneic events.

VENTILATORY DEPTH.   The depth of respirations is assessed by observing the degree of excursion or movement in the chest wall. You can subjectively describe ventilatory movements as deep, normal, or shallow. A deep respiration involves a full expansion of the lungs with full exhalation. Respirations are shallow when only a small quantity of air passes through the lungs and ventilatory movement is difficult to see. More objective techniques are required if you observe that chest excursion is unusually shallow (see Chapter 12).

VENTILATORY RHYTHM.   Respiratory rhythm is described as regular or irregular. While assessing respiration, observe the interval between each respiratory cycle. With normal breathing a regular interval occurs between each respiratory cycle. If you observe an irregular ventilatory rhythm, such as periods of apnea with shallow or deep breathing, a more detailed physical assessment is indicated (see Chapter 27). Infants tend to breathe less regularly. The young child may breathe slowly for a few seconds and then suddenly breathe more rapidly.

Measurement of Arterial Oxygen Saturation

A pulse oximeter permits the indirect measurement of **oxygen saturation** for the client's vital sign database (Skill 11-5). The pulse oximeter is a probe with a light-emitting diode (LED) and photosensor connected by cable to an oximeter (Figure 11-9). The LED emits light, which oxygenated and

Skill 11-5
MEASURING OXYGEN SATURATION (PULSE OXIMETRY)

DELEGATION CONSIDERATIONS
The skill of oxygen saturation measurement can be delegated to assistive personnel.
- Inform caregiver of the need to notify you immediately of any reading lower than an SpO_2 of 90%.
- Inform caregiver of appropriate sensor site, probe, and client position for measurement of oxygen saturation.
- Inform caregiver of frequency of oxygen saturation measurements.

- Determine that caregiver is aware of factors that can falsely alter SpO_2 readings (see Box 11-13, p. 211).

EQUIPMENT
- Oximeter
- Oximeter probe appropriate for client and recommended by manufacturer
- Acetone or nail polish remover
- Pen, pencil, vital sign flow sheet or record form

STEPS	RATIONALE
1. Determine need to measure client's oxygen saturation: a. Note risk factors for alteration of oxygen saturation.	Certain conditions place clients at risk for decreased oxygen saturation: acute or chronic compromised respiratory function, recovery from general anesthesia or conscious sedation, traumatic injury to chest wall with or without collapse of underlying lung tissue, ventilator dependence, changes in supplemental oxygen therapy.
b. Assess for signs and symptoms of alterations in oxygen saturation such as altered respiratory rate, depth, or rhythm; adventitious breath sounds (see Chapter 12); cyanotic appearance of nail beds, lips, mucous membranes, skin; restlessness, irritability, confusion; reduced level of consciousness; labored or difficult breathing.	Physical signs and symptoms may indicate abnormal oxygen saturation.
2. Assess for factors that normally influence measurement of SpO_2 such as oxygen therapy, hemoglobin level, and body temperature.	Allows you to accurately assess oxygen saturation variations.
3. Review client's medical record for physician's order or consult agency policy or procedure manual for standard of care.	Medical order may be required to assess oxygen saturation.

STEPS	RATIONALE
4. Determine previous baseline SpO$_2$ (if available) from client's record.	Baseline information provides basis for comparison and assists in assessment of current status and evaluation of interventions.
5. Explain purpose of procedure to client and the way in which oxygen saturation will be measured. Instruct client to breathe normally.	Promotes client cooperation and increases compliance. Prevents large fluctuations in minute ventilation and possible error in SpO$_2$ readings.
6. Assess site most appropriate for sensor probe placement (e.g., digit, earlobe). Site must have adequate local circulation and be free of moisture.	Peripheral vasoconstriction can interfere with SpO$_2$ determination. Moisture impedes ability of sensor to detect SpO$_2$ levels. Finger probes rather than ear, nose, or forehead probes are recommended for clients with poor peripheral perfusion (Jensen and others, 1998).
7. Wash hands.	Reduces transmission of microorganisms.
8. Position client comfortably. If finger is chosen as monitoring site, support lower arm.	Ensures probe positioning and decreases motion artifact that interferes with SpO$_2$ determination.
9. If finger is to be used, remove any fingernail polish with acetone from digit to be assessed. Acrylic nails without polish do not interfere with SpO$_2$ determination.	Ensures accurate readings. Dark nail polish impedes sensor detection of emitted light and produces falsely elevated SpO$_2$ readings (Tittle and Flynn, 1997).
10. Attach sensor probe to monitoring site (see illustration). Instruct client that clip-on probe feels like a clothespin on the finger and will not hurt.	Pressure of sensor probe's spring tension on a peripheral digit or earlobe may be unexpected. Select sensor site based on peripheral circulation and extremity temperature. Peripheral vasoconstriction can alter SpO$_2$.

• *Critical Decision Point*

Do not attach probe to finger, ear, or bridge of nose if area is edematous or skin integrity is compromised. Do not attach probe to fingers that are hypothermic. Earlobe and bridge of nose sensors are not used for infants and toddlers because of skin fragility. Disposable adhesive probes contain latex and should not be used if client has latex allergy.

STEPS	RATIONALE
11. Turn on oximeter by activating power. Observe pulse waveform/intensity display and audible beep. Correlate oximeter pulse rate with client's radial pulse. Differences require reevaluation of oximeter probe placement and may require reassessment of pulse rates.	Pulse waveform/intensity display enables detection of valid pulse or presence of interfering signal. Pitch of audible beep is proportional to SpO$_2$ value. Double-checking pulse rate ensures oximeter accuracy. Oximeter pulse rate, client's radial pulse, and apical pulse rate should be the same. Any difference requires reevaluation of oximeter sensor probe placement and reassessment of pulse rates.
12. Leave probe in place until oximeter readout reaches constant value and pulse display reaches full strength during each cardiac cycle. Inform client that oximeter will alarm if the probe falls off or if the probe is moved. Read SpO$_2$ on digital display.	Reading may take 10 to 30 seconds depending on site selected.
13. If continuous SpO$_2$ monitoring is planned, verify SpO$_2$ alarm limits and alarm volume, which are preset by the manufacturer at a low of 85% and a high of 100%. You must determine the limits for SpO$_2$ and pulse rate alarms based on each client's condition. Verify that alarms are on. Assess skin integrity under sensor probe and relocate sensor probe at least every 2 hours.	Alarms must be set at appropriate limits and volumes to avoid frightening clients and visitors. Spring tension of sensor probe or sensitivity to disposable sensor probe adhesive can cause skin irritation and lead to disruption of skin integrity.
14. Discuss findings with client as needed.	Promotes participation in care and understanding of health status.
15. If intermittent or spot-checking SpO$_2$ measurements are planned, remove probe and turn oximeter power off. Store probe in appropriate location.	Batteries can be depleted if oximeter is left on. Sensor probes are expensive and vulnerable to damage.
16. Assist client in returning to comfortable position.	Restores comfort and promotes sense of well-being.
17. Wash hands.	Reduces transmission of microorganisms.
18. Compare SpO$_2$ readings with client baseline and ac-	Comparison reveals presence of abnormality.

STEPS	RATIONALE
ceptable values.	
19. Correlate SpO₂ with SaO₂ obtained from arterial blood gas (ABG) measurements (see Chapter 27) if available.	Documents reliability of noninvasive assessment. Pulse oximetry can only warn of dangerous low levels of oxygen saturation. Values are not accurate under 80%.
20. Correlate SpO₂ reading with data obtained from respiratory rate, depth, and rhythm assessment (see Skill 11-4, p. 205).	Measurements assessing ventilation, perfusion, and diffusion are interrelated.

UNEXPECTED OUTCOMES AND RELATED INTERVENTIONS

- SpO₂ is less than 90%.
  - Verify that oximeter probe is intact and not influenced by outside light transmission.
  - Observe for signs and symptoms of decreased oxygenation: cyanosis, restlessness, tachycardia.
  - Compare SpO₂ with SaO₂ from ABG to confirm low saturation.
  - Observe for and minimize factors that decrease SpO₂ such as lung secretions, increased activity, hyperthermia.
  - Assist client to a position that maximizes ventilatory effort; for example, place an obese client in a high-Fowler's position.
  - Verify that oxygen delivery system and liter flow are being administered as ordered.
- Pulse rate indicated on oximeter is less than radial or apical pulse rate.
  - Reposition sensor probe to alternative site with increased blood flow.
  - Assess signs and symptoms of cardiac function that would contribute to decreased peripheral blood flow.

- Pulse rate intensity display indicated on oximeter is dampened or irregular.
- Request that client not move extremity or sensor probe site. Motion artifact is a common cause of irregular readings.
- Reposition sensor probe for better contact with underlying skin.
- Protect sensor from room light by covering sensor probe site with opaque covering or washcloth.

RECORDING AND REPORTING

- Record SpO₂ value on nurses' notes or vital sign flow sheet indicating type and amount of oxygen therapy used by client during assessment. Also record any signs and symptoms of reduced oxygen saturation in narrative form in nurses' notes.
- Measurement of SpO₂ after administration of specific therapies is documented in narrative form in nurses' notes.
- Report abnormal findings to nurse in charge or physician.
- Record in nurses' notes client's use of continuous or intermittent pulse oximetry. Documents use of equipment for third-party payers.

---

deoxygenated hemoglobin molecules absorb differently. The photosensor detects the light-absorbing differences between each type of hemoglobin and the oximeter calculates pulse saturation (SpO₂). SpO₂ is a reliable estimate of SaO₂.

The measurement of SpO₂ is affected by factors that affect light transmission or peripheral arterial pulsations. An awareness of these factors will allow you to interpret abnormal SpO₂ measurements accurately (Box 11-13). SpO₂ can be measured intermittently or continuously. Continuous SpO₂ monitoring is used to assess ongoing therapies. Alarm limits can be programmed to alert you if the client's SpO₂ drops to an unacceptable level.

CLIENT TEACHING AND VITAL SIGN MEASUREMENT

The emphasis on health promotion and health maintenance, as well as early discharge from hospital settings, has resulted in an increase in the need for clients and their families to monitor vital signs in the home. Teaching considerations affect all vital sign measurements and should be incorporated into the client's plan of care (Box 11-14). When considering how to

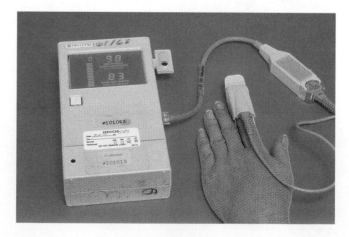

FIGURE 11-9 Pulse oximeter.

teach clients and their families about vital sign measurement, the client's age is an important factor. With the increasing older adult population, there is an increased need for caregivers to be aware of changes from normal vital sign values that are unique to older adults. Box 11-15 identifies some of these variations.

RECORDING VITAL SIGNS

Specific graphic flow sheets exist for recording vital signs (see Chapter 7). Identify and use the agency's policy for recording vital signs. In a community-based setting, vital signs may be recorded on the progress notes for that partic- ular clinic or home visit. In acute care and some restorative care settings a graphic flow sheet is used.

Clients whose care is facilitated through a critical path may have their vital signs listed as outcomes. When a vital sign is above or below the expected value, a note is written regarding the finding and related interventions.

Factors Affecting Determination of Pulse Oxygen Saturation (SpO$_2$) — Box 11-13

INTERFERENCE WITH LIGHT TRANSMISSION

Outside light sources can interfere with the oximeter's ability to process reflected light.

Carbon monoxide (caused by smoke inhalation or poisoning) artificially elevates SpO$_2$ by absorbing light similar to oxygen.

Client motion can interfere with the oximeter's ability to process reflected light.

Jaundice may interfere with the oximeter's ability to process reflected light.

Intravascular dyes (methylene blue) absorb light similar to de-oxyhemoglobin and artificially lower saturation reading.

Dark skin pigment can result in signal loss or overestimation of saturation (Jensen and others, 1998).

INTERFERENCE WITH ARTERIAL PULSATIONS

Peripheral vascular disease (e.g., atherosclerosis) can reduce pulse volume.

Hypothermia at assessment site decreases peripheral blood flow.

Pharmacological vasoconstrictors (e.g., epinephrine) decrease peripheral pulse volume.

Low cardiac output and hypotension decrease blood flow to peripheral arteries.

Peripheral edema can obscure arterial pulsation.

Tight probe will record venous pulsations in the finger that compete with arterial pulsations.

Client Teaching — Box 11-14

VITAL SIGN ASSESSMENT

TEMPERATURE

- Identify client's ability to initiate preventive health measures and recognize alteration in body temperature. Educate clients and family members about measures to prevent body temperature alterations.
- Teach clients risk factors for hypothermia and frostbite: fatigue; malnutrition; cold, wet clothing; alcohol intoxication.
- Teach clients risk factors for heat stroke: strenuous exercise in hot, humid weather; tight-fitting clothing in hot environments; exercising in poorly ventilated areas; sudden exposures to hot climates; poor fluid intake before, during, and after exercise.
- Teach clients the importance of taking and continuing antibiotics as directed until course of treatment is completed.

PULSE RATE

- Clients taking certain prescribed cardiac medications should learn to assess their own pulse rates to detect side effects of medications. Clients undergoing cardiac rehabilitation should learn to assess their own pulse rates to determine their response to exercise.

BLOOD PRESSURE

- Teach client risk factors for hypertension. Persons with family history of hypertension are at significant risk. Obesity, cigarette smoking, heavy alcohol consumption, high blood cholesterol and triglyceride levels, and continued exposure to stress are factors linked to hypertension (Joint National Committee on Detection, Evaluation, and Treatment of High Blood Pressure, 1997).
- Clients with hypertension should learn about their blood pressure values, long-term follow-up care and therapy, the usual lack of symptoms, therapy's ability to control but not cure, and benefits of a consistently followed treatment plan.
- Instruct clients on the importance of appropriate size blood pressure cuff for home use.
- Instruct primary caregiver to take blood pressure reading at same time each day and after client has had a brief rest. Take measurement sitting or lying down, use same position and arm each time pressure is taken.
- Instruct primary caregiver that if it is difficult to hear the pressure, it may be that the cuff is too loose, not big enough, or too narrow; the stethoscope is not over arterial pulse; cuff was deflated too quickly or too slowly; or cuff was not pumped high enough for systolic readings.

RESPIRATION

- Clients who demonstrate decreased ventilation may benefit from being taught deep breathing and coughing exercises (see Chapter 27).
- Instruct family member to contact home care nurse or physician if unusual fluctuations in respiratory rate or rhythm occur.
- Teach client signs and symptoms of hypoxemia: headache, somnolence, confusion, dusky color, shortness of breath, dyspnea.
- Teach client effect of high-risk behaviors such as cigarette smoking on oxygen saturation.

Gerontological Nursing Practice

Box 11-15

TEMPERATURE

- The temperature of older adults is at the lower end of the normal temperature range, 36° C (96.8° F), and therefore temperatures considered within normal range may reflect a fever in an older adult.
- Older adults are very sensitive to slight changes in environment temperature because their thermoregulatory systems are not as efficient (Lueckenotte, 2000).
- A decrease in sweat gland reactivity in the older adult results in a higher threshold for sweating at high temperature, which can lead to hyperthermia and heatstroke (Burke and Walsh, 1997).
- With aging, loss of subcutaneous fat reduces the insulating capacity of the skin; older men are at especially high risk for hypothermia (Burke and Walsh, 1997).

PULSE RATE

- It is often difficult to palpate the pulse of an older adult. A Doppler device will provide a more accurate reading.
- The older adult has a decreased heart rate at rest (Ebersole and Hess, 2001).
- Once elevated, the pulse rate of an older adult takes longer to return to normal resting rate (Ebersole and Hess, 2001).
- When assessing the apical rate of an older woman, the breast tissue is gently lifted and the stethoscope placed at the fifth intercostal space (ICS) or the lower edge of the breast.
- Heart sounds may be muffled or difficult to hear in older adults because of an increase in air space in the lungs.

BLOOD PRESSURE

- Older adults may have decreased upper arm mass, which requires special attention to selection of blood pressure cuff size.
- Older adults may have an increase in systolic pressure related to decreased vessel elasticity while the diastolic pressure remains the same, resulting in a wider pulse pressure (Lueckenotte, 2000).
- Older adults are instructed to change position slowly and wait after each change to avoid postural hypotension and prevent injuries.

RESPIRATION

- Aging causes ossification of costal cartilage and downward slant of ribs, resulting in a more rigid rib cage, which reduces chest wall expansion. Kyphosis and scoliosis that can occur in older adults may also restrict chest expansion and decrease tidal volume (Ebersole and Hess, 2001).
- Older adults may depend more on accessory abdominal muscles during respiration than on weaker thoracic muscles (Burke and Walsh, 1997).
- Responses to hypercapnia and hypoxia are reduced 50% in older adults as compared to young adults (Ebersole and Hess, 2001), limiting the ability of older adults to respond to hypoxia with respiratory changes.
- Identifying an acceptable pulse oximeter probe site may be difficult with older adults because of the likelihood of peripheral vascular disease, decreased cardiac output, cold-induced vasoconstriction, and anemia.

Key Terms

afebrile, p. 178
antipyretic, p. 188
apical pulse, p. 189
apnea, p. 205
auscultatory gap, p. 203
basal metabolic rate (BMR), p. 177
bradycardia, p. 189
bradypnea, p. 205
cardiac output (CO), p. 188
centigrade, p. 179
core temperature, p. 177
diaphoresis, p. 177
diastolic, p. 195
diffusion, p. 204

dysrhythmia, p. 194
eupnea, p. 205
Fahrenheit, p. 179
febrile, p. 178
fever, p. 178
heat stroke, p. 178
hypertension, p. 195
hyperthermia, p. 178
hypotension, p. 197
hypothermia, p. 178
Korotkoff sound, p. 202
malignant hyperthermia, p. 178
nonshivering thermogenesis, p. 197
orthostatic hypotension, p. 208
oxygen saturation, p. 208
perfusion, p. 204

postural hypotension, p. 197
pulse deficit, p. 195
pulse pressure, p. 195
pyrexia, p. 178
pyrogens, p. 178
sphygmomanometer, p. 197
stroke volume (SV), p. 188
systolic, p. 195
tachycardia, p. 189
tachypnea, p. 205
thermoregulation, p. 177
vasoconstriction, p. 177
vasodilation, p. 177
ventilation, p. 204
vital signs, p. 176

Key Concepts

- Vital sign measurement includes the physiological measurement of temperature, pulse, blood pressure, respiration, and oxygen saturation.
- Vital signs are measured as part of a complete physical examination or in a review of a client's condition.

- Vital sign changes are evaluated with other physical assessment findings using clinical judgment to determine measurement frequency.
- Knowledge of the factors influencing vital signs assists in determining and evaluating abnormal values.
- Vital signs provide a basis for evaluating response to nursing interventions.

- Vital signs are best measured when the client is inactive and the environment is controlled for comfort.
- Assist the client in maintaining body temperature by initiating interventions that promote heat loss, production, or conservation.
- A fever is one of the body's normal defense mechanisms.
- The tympanic route is the most accessible site for core temperature measurement.
- To assess cardiac function, pulse rate and rhythm are most easily measured using the radial or apical pulses.
- Respiratory assessment includes determining the effectiveness of ventilation, perfusion, and diffusion.
- Assessment of respiration involves observing ventilatory movements throughout the respiratory cycle.

- Oxygen saturation is influenced by variables affecting ventilation, perfusion, and diffusion.
- Several hemodynamic variables contribute to blood pressure determination.
- Hypertension is diagnosed only after an average of readings made during two or more subsequent visits reveals an elevated blood pressure.
- Selecting and applying the blood pressure measurement cuff improperly can result in errors in blood pressure measurement.
- Changes in one vital sign can influence characteristics of the other vital signs.

Critical Thinking Activities

1. A 68-year-old woman whose husband died last year walks into the wellness clinic of the assisted living facility. She reports that she feels depressed and tired all the time. She provides you with a list of medications, one of which the physician altered in the last 3 weeks, atenolol, a beta-adrenergic blocker. What initial vital signs can you delegate to the assistive personnel at the clinic? What vital sign(s) is (are) the highest priority in this client? State one patient teaching objective you might implement for this client.

2. During a home care visit to a mother and newborn in their two-bedroom mobile home you complete an assessment of the physical environment. The temperature on the wall next to the furnace reads 67.5° F. Cold drafts can be felt around the large windows in the bedrooms and through the cracks in the floorboards. During your infant assessment you note the infant's vital signs are: axillary temperature 34.2° C, heart rate 118 beats per minute, respiration 32. What is your priority nursing diagnosis for this family? Why isn't the infant shivering? What immediate interventions should you initiate? What long-term interventions should you initiate?

3. A 35-year-old obese female client has just returned from the postanesthesia care unit following a laparoscopic cholecystectomy. Her admission database indicates that she is a one pack per day smoker and has a history of

chronic bronchitis with asthma. The postoperative orders are the following: O_2 via nasal catheter to keep SpO_2 over 90, head of bed at 45 degrees, out of bed in evening, clear liquids and medications for pain. List the vital signs to be delegated to assistive personnel. What instructions should be given to assistive personnel about this client?

4. Six hours after your initial assessment, assistive personnel report the last set of frequent vital signs on the postoperative female client in Activity 3 as follows: SpO_2 89, respiration 12, heart rate 98 beats per minute, blood pressure 198/92, tympanic temperature 38.2° C. The client is rousable, but mumbles that she has no pain. The meperidine 75 mg you administered intramuscularly 2 hours ago appears to be effective. Should you reassess any vital signs before notifying the nurse in charge? What nursing diagnoses are evident from these data? State two immediate interventions you should take.

5. As the case manager in the long-term care facility you oversee the assistive personnel. Nurse Wagner reports to you that Ms. Mullen repeatedly charts blood pressure and heart rate readings that are inaccurate during the weekly assessment of the residents. Nurse Wagner notes that many of the blood pressure readings are low, and many of the heart rate readings are also low. What could be the cause of Ms. Mullen's errors? How could you confirm the difficulty Ms. Mullen is having? How would you approach Ms. Mullen?

Review Questions

1. An adult client is assessed to have shallow respirations at a rate of 8 per minute. His heart rate is 46 beats per minute. His vital signs would be described as:
   1. bradycardia and apnea.
   2. tachycardia and apnea.
   3. bradycardia and bradypnea.
   4. tachycardia and bradypnea.

2. Identification of a "pulse deficit" provides information about the heart's ability to perfuse the body adequately. A pulse deficit is:
   1. the difference between the radial and apical pulse rates.
   2. the digital pressure felt when taking radial and ulnar pulses.
   3. the amount of pressure felt when taking radial and ulnar pulses.
   4. the difference between the systolic and diastolic blood pressure readings.

3. The nurse assistant reports to you that Mrs. Rhodes is "feeling funny." Your first action would be to:
   1. notify the physician.
   2. obtain Mrs. Rhodes's vital signs yourself.
   3. delegate the assistant to retake the vital signs.
   4. tell the assistant to keep assessing Mrs. Rhodes and report any further complaints.

4. If a blood pressure cuff is too narrow or wrapped too loosely, the blood pressure measurement will be:
   1. falsely low.

Continued

Review Questions—cont'd

2. falsely high.

3. dependent upon the examiner's hearing acuity.

4. difficult to hear because sounds will be muffled.

5. Patients with apnea experience:
   1. difficult respirations that require effort.
   2. slowness of breathing, followed by rapid breathing.
   3. cessation of breathing, usually temporary.
   4. lack or deficiency of oxygen in body organs and tissues.

6. Poor oxygenation of the blood ordinarily will affect the pulse rate and cause it to become:
   1. bounding.
   2. irregular.
   3. faster than normal.
   4. slower than normal.

7. You obtain a client's supine blood pressure reading of 130/64. One hour later, you obtain a supine blood pressure reading of 134/62, then you obtain a sitting blood pressure reading of 98/58. Your immediate action would be to:
   1. assist client to a supine position.
   2. assess blood pressure in the other arm.
   3. report findings to the nurse in charge.
   4. question the client about lightheadedness.

8. You are taking vital sign measurements and note that the client has a strong radial pulse that diminishes in intensity and that there are interruptions in rhythm about every four to six beats. Your immediate action is to:
   1. report the findings to a physician.
   2. measure a 60-second apical pulse.
   3. connect the client to a cardiac monitor.
   4. obtain a 60-second apical-radial pulse.

9. Nursing interventions such as removing excess blankets from the client and applying cool cloths to the axilla act to decrease body temperature through:
   1. conduction.
   2. convection.
   3. evaporation.
   4. radiation.

References

Brashers VL: *Clinical application of pathophysiology,* St. Louis, 1998, Mosby.

Braun SK and others: Getting a better read on thermometry, *RN* 61(3):57, 1998.

Burke MM, Walsh MB: *Gerontologic nursing,* St. Louis, 1997, Mosby.

Cusson RA and others: The effect of environment on body site temperatures in full-term neonates, *Nurs Res* 46(4):202, 1997.

Ebersole P, Hess P: *Geriatric nursing and healthy aging,* St. Louis, 2001, Mosby.

Erickson RS and others: Accuracy of chemical dot thermometers in critically ill adults and young children, *IMAGE J Nurs Scholarship* 28:23, 1996.

Fallis WM: Oral measurement of temperature in orally intubated critical care patients: state-of-the-science review, *Am J Crit Care* 9:334, 2000.

Giuliano KK and others: Temperature measurement in critically ill adults: a comparison of tympanic and oral methods, *Am J Crit Care* 9(4):254, 2000.

Haddock BJ and others: The falling grace of axillary temperatures, *Pediatr Nurs* 22(2):121, 1996.

Holtzclaw B: Thermal balance. In Kinney and others, editors: *AACN clinical reference for critical care nursing,* ed 4, St. Louis, 1998, Mosby.

Jensen LA and others: Meta-analysis of arterial oxygen saturation monitoring by pulse oximetry in adults, *Heart Lung* 27(9): 387, 1998.

Joint National Committee on Detection, Evaluation, and Treatment of High Blood Pressure: The sixth report of the Joint National Committee on Detection, Evaluation, and Treatment of High Blood Pressure, *Arch Intern Med* 157:2413, 1997.

Jones D and others: A comparison of two noninvasive methods of blood pressure measurement in the triage area, *J Emerg Nurs* 22:111, 1996.

Kinney MR and others: *AACN's clinical reference for critical care nursing,* ed 4, St. Louis, 1998, Mosby.

Leicke-Rude M, Bloom LF: A comparison of temperature taking methods in neonates, *Neonatal Netw* 17(5):21, 1998.

Lueckenotte AG: *Gerontologic nursing,* ed 2, St. Louis, 2000, Mosby.

Roper M: Assessing orthostatic vital signs, *Am J Nurs* 96(8):43, 1996.

Thibodeau GA, Patton KT: *Anatomy and physiology,* ed 4, St. Louis, 1999, Mosby.

Thomas SA, DeKeyser F: Blood pressure, *Annu Rev Nurs Res* 14:3, 1996.

Tittle M, Flynn MB: Correlation of pulse oximetry and co-oximetry, *Dimen Crit Care Nurs* 16(2):88, 1997.

Weiss ME and others: A comparison of temperature measurements using three ear thermometers, *Appl Nurs Res* 11(4):158, 1998.

Whaley LF, Wong DL: *Nursing care of infants and children,* ed 6, St. Louis, 1999, Mosby.

Yeo S, Scarbough M: Exercise-induced hyperthermia may prevent accurate core temperature measurement by tympanic membrane thermometer, *J Nurs Meas* 4(2):143, 1996.

Health Assessment and Physical Examination

12

Objectives

- Define key terms.
- Discuss the purposes of physical examination.
- Describe the techniques used with each physical assessment skill.
- Discuss how cultural diversity can influence health assessment.
- Describe proper client positions for a physical examination.
- List techniques used to prepare a client physically and psychologically before and during an examination.
- Describe interview techniques used to enhance communication during history taking.
- Make environmental preparations before an examination.
- Identify data to collect from the nursing history before an examination.
- Discuss normal physical findings in a young and middle-age adult compared with an older adult.
- Discuss ways to incorporate health teaching into the examination.
- Use physical assessment skills during routine nursing care.
- Describe physical measurements made in assessing each body system.
- Identify self-screening examinations commonly performed by clients.

As a nurse, you will work in many settings, seeking information about clients' health status. You may conduct health assessments at health fairs, clinics, in physicians' offices, in a client's home, or in hospitals. Health screenings focus on a specific physical problem. For example, blood pressure screenings detect the risk for high blood pressure. If a screening determines that a client has a risk for a disease, the client is referred for a more complete physical examination. A complete health assessment involves a health history and behavioral and physical examination. The health history involves a lengthy client interview to gather subjective data about the client's condition. A physical examination is a head-to-toe review of body systems that offers objective information about the client.

You will use physical assessment skills during an examination to make clinical judgments. The client's condition and response affect the extent of your examination. The accuracy of your assessment will influence the choice of therapies a client receives and the evaluation of response to those therapies. Continuity of health care improves when you make ongoing objective and comprehensive assessments.

PURPOSES OF PHYSICAL EXAMINATION

An examination should be designed for the client's needs. If a client is acutely ill, you may assess only the involved body systems. Conduct a more comprehensive examination when the client feels more at ease, so that you then can learn about the client's total health status. A complete physical examination is performed for routine screening to promote wellness behaviors and preventive health care measures; to determine eligibility for health insurance, military service, or a new job; and to admit a client to a hospital setting or long-term care facility.

Physical examination is used to do the following:
1. Gather baseline data about the client's health status
2. Supplement, confirm, or refute data obtained in the history
3. Confirm and identify nursing diagnoses
4. Make clinical judgments about a client's changing health status and management
5. Evaluate the physiological outcomes of care

Gathering a Database

You initially gather information about the client's health status from the health history. A subsequent physical examination may reveal information that refutes, confirms, or supplements the history. You need a complete and thorough assessment to make a nursing diagnosis. Group significant findings into patterns of data that reveal actual or at-risk nursing diagnoses. Gather additional information about any abnormal findings. All of the information obtained during the initial physical examination provides a baseline of the client's condition. The baseline is not the normal range of findings for the average person. It is, rather, the pattern of findings you identified when you first assessed the client. You will use this baseline as a comparison for future findings.

CULTURAL SENSITIVITY

Respect the cultural differences of your clients when completing an examination. It is important for you to remember that cultural differences influence a client's behavior. A client's health beliefs, use of alternative therapies, nutritional habits, relationships with family, and comfort with your physical closeness must be considered during examination and history taking.

You must be culturally aware and avoid stereotyping on the basis of gender or race. There is a difference between cultural and physical characteristics. It is important for you to recognize common disorders for those ethnic populations within your community. Recognition of cultural diversity helps you respect a client's uniqueness and provide higher-quality care.

INTEGRATION OF PHYSICAL EXAMINATION WITH NURSING CARE

You will learn to integrate an examination during routine client care. For example, you can assess the condition of body parts during a bed bath. Observe a client's gait and muscle strength while you assist with ambulation down a hallway. This practice makes more efficient use of your time.

SKILLS OF PHYSICAL ASSESSMENT

The five skills of physical assessment—inspection, palpation, percussion, auscultation, and olfaction—are used in a comprehensive examination.

Inspection

Inspection is the use of vision, hearing, and smell to distinguish normal from abnormal findings. It is important to know what is considered normal for clients of different age-groups. With experience you will recognize normal variations among clients. Inspection is a simple technique, and the quality of an inspection depends upon your willingness to spend time to be thorough and systematic. To inspect body parts accurately, follow these principles:
1. Make sure good lighting is available.
2. Position and expose body parts so that all surfaces can be viewed.
3. Inspect each area for size, shape, color, symmetry, position, and abnormalities.
4. If possible, compare each area inspected with the same area on the opposite side of the body.
5. Use additional light (e.g., a penlight) to inspect body cavities.
6. Do not hurry inspection. Pay attention to detail.

After inspection of a body part, findings may indicate the need for further examination. Palpation is often used with or after visual inspection.

Palpation

Palpation involves the use of the hands to touch body parts to make sensitive assessments. Palpation is used to examine all accessible parts of the body. For example, palpate the skin for temperature, moisture, texture, turgor, tenderness, and thickness. Palpate organs such as the liver for size, shape, tenderness, and absence of masses. You will use different parts of your hand to detect characteristics such as texture, temperature, and perception of movement.

Before palpating, help the client to relax and be comfortable because muscle tension during palpation impairs effective assessment. Have the client take slow, deep breaths and place the arms along the side of the body—these maneuvers enhance relaxation. Palpate tender areas last. Be sure to ask the client to point out the more sensitive areas and note any nonverbal signs of discomfort.

Warm hands, short fingernails, and a gentle approach are needed for this technique. Perform palpation slowly, gently, and deliberately. Light palpation of structures such as the abdomen determines areas of tenderness (Figure 12-1, *A*). Place your hand on the part to be examined and depress about 1 cm (½ inch). Examine tender areas further for potentially serious abnormalities. The sensation of touch is best preserved with light, intermittent pressure; heavy, prolonged pressure causes loss of sensitivity in your hand.

After light palpation, use deeper palpation to examine the condition of organs such as those in the abdomen (Figure 12-1, *B*). Depress the area being examined approximately 2 to 4 cm (1 to 2 inches) (Seidel and others, 1999). Caution is the rule. You should not try deep palpation without clinical supervision to avoid injuring a client. Deep palpation may be applied with one hand or both hands (bimanually). When using bimanual palpation, relax one hand (sensing hand) and place it lightly over the client's skin. Use the other hand (active hand) to apply pressure to the sensing hand. The lower hand does not exert pressure directly and thus retains the sensitivity needed to detect organ characteristics.

Use the most sensitive parts of the hand, the pads of the fingertips, to assess texture, shape, size, consistency, and pulsation (Figure 12-2, *A*). Temperature is best measured using the dorsum, or back, of the hand and fingers (Figure 12-2, *B*), where your skin is thinnest. The palm of the hand (Figure 12-2, *C*) is more sensitive to vibration. Measure position, consistency, and turgor by lightly grasping the body part with the fingertips (Figure 12-2, *D*).

You must not palpate without considering the client's condition. For example, if the client has a fractured rib, use extra care to locate the painful area. A vital artery is not palpated with pressure that obstructs blood flow.

Percussion

Percussion involves tapping the body with the fingertips to produce a vibration that travels through body tissues. The character of the sound determines the location, size, and density of underlying structures to verify abnormalities assessed by palpation and auscultation. This vibration is transmitted through the body tissues, and the character of the sound heard depends on the density of the underlying tissue. By knowing the way various densities influence sound, you can locate organs or masses, map their boundaries, and determine their size. An abnormal sound suggests a mass or substance such as air or fluid within an organ or body cavity. The skill of percussion requires dexterity and is usually reserved for advanced practitioners.

Auscultation

Auscultation involves listening to sounds made by body organs to detect variations from normal. You can hear some sounds without assistance, but you need a stethoscope for most of them. You must first learn the normal sounds made by the cardiovascular, respiratory, and gastrointestinal systems. You can recognize abnormal sounds after you become familiar with normal ones. You will become more proficient at auscultation by knowing the types of sounds arising from

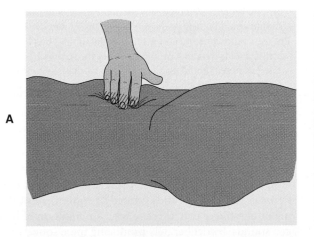
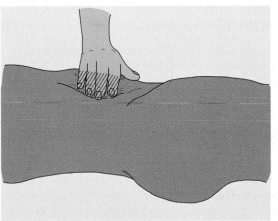

FIGURE **12-1**   **A,** During light palpation, gentle pressure against underlying skin and tissues can detect areas of irregularity and tenderness. **B,** During deep palpation, depress tissue to assess condition of underlying organs.

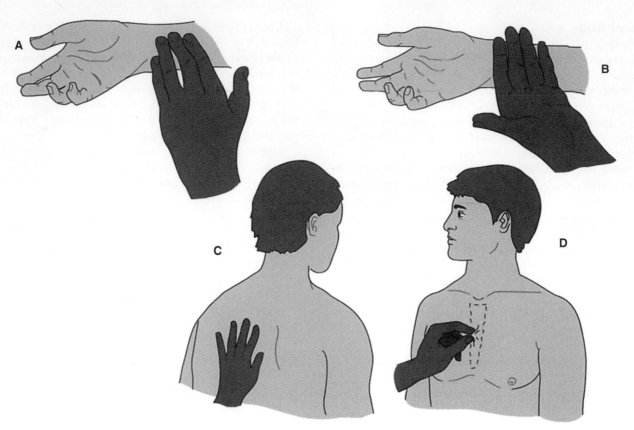

FIGURE 12-2   **A,** Radial pulse is detected with pads of fingertips, the most sensitive part of the hand. **B,** Dorsum of hand detects temperature variations in skin. **C,** The bony part of the palm at the base of the fingers detects vibrations. **D,** Skin is grasped with fingertips to assess turgor.

Exercises to Increase Familiarity With the Stethoscope   Box 12-1

Ensure that the earpieces follow the contour of the ear canals. Learn what fit is best for you by comparing amplification of sounds with the earpieces in both directions.

Place the earpieces in your ears with the tips of the earpieces turned toward the face. Lightly blow into the diaphragm. Again place the earpieces in your ears, this time with the ends turned toward the back of the head. Lightly blow into the diaphragm. After you have learned the right fit for the loudest amplification, wear the stethoscope the same way each time.

Put on the stethoscope, and lightly blow into the diaphragm. If the sound is barely audible, lightly blow into the bell. Sound is carried through only one part of the chestpiece at a time. If the sound is greatly amplified through the diaphragm, the diaphragm is in po-

sition for use. If the sound is barely audible through the diaphragm, the bell is in position for use. Rotation of the diaphragm and bell places the chestpiece in the desired position. Leave the diaphragm in position for the next exercise.

Place the diaphragm over the anterior part of your chest. Ask a friend to speak in a normal conversational tone. Environmental noise seriously detracts from hearing the noise created by body organs. When a stethoscope is used, the client and the examiner should remain quiet.

Put the stethoscope on, and gently tap the tubing. It is often difficult to avoid stretching or movement of the stethoscope's tubing. The examiner should be in a position so that the tubing hangs free. Moving or touching the tubing creates extraneous sounds.

---

each body structure and the location in which they can most easily be heard. You will also need to learn which areas do not normally emit sounds.

To auscultate correctly, you need to hear well, have a good stethoscope, and know how to use it properly. If you have a hearing disorder, you should use a stethoscope with greater sound amplification. Always place the stethoscope on skin, because clothing can obscure sound.

Chapter 11 describes the parts of the stethoscope and its general use. The bell is best for low-pitched sounds such as

vascular and certain heart sounds, and the diaphragm is best for high-pitched sounds such as bowel and lung sounds.

You must be familiar with the stethoscope before attempting to use it. Practice using the stethoscope with a friend. Extraneous sounds created by movement of the tubing or chestpiece can interfere with auscultation of body organ sounds. By deliberately producing these sounds, you can learn to recognize and disregard them during the actual examination (Box 12-1). Learn to recognize the following characteristics of sounds:

Assessment of Characteristic Odors		Table 12-1
Odor	Site or Source	Potential Causes
Alcohol	Oral cavity	Ingestion of alcohol
Ammonia	Urine	Urinary tract infection, renal failure
Body odor	Skin, particularly in areas where body parts rub together (e.g., under arms and breasts)	Poor hygiene, excess perspiration (hyperhidrosis), foul-smelling perspiration (bromidrosis)
Feces	Wound site	Wound abscess
	Vomitus	Bowel obstruction
	Rectal area	Fecal incontinence
Foul-smelling stools in infant	Stool	Malabsorption syndrome
Halitosis	Oral cavity	Poor dental and oral hygiene, gum disease
Sweet, fruity ketones	Oral cavity	Diabetic acidosis
Stale urine	Skin	Uremic acidosis
Sweet, heavy, thick odor	Draining wound	*Pseudomonas* (bacterial) infection
Musty odor	Casted body part	Infection inside cast
Fetid, sweet odor	Tracheostomy or mucus secretions	Infection of bronchial tree (*Pseudomonas* bacteria)

1. Frequency, or the number of sound wave cycles generated per second by a vibrating object. The higher the frequency, the higher the pitch of a sound and vice versa.
2. Loudness, or the amplitude of a sound wave. Auscultated sounds are described as loud or soft.
3. Quality, or the sounds of similar frequency and loudness from different sources. Terms such as *blowing* or *gurgling* describe the quality of sound.
4. Duration, or the length of time sound vibrations last. The duration of sound is short, medium, or long. Layers of soft tissue dampen the duration of sounds from deep internal organs.

Auscultation requires concentration and practice. Always consider the part of the body auscultated and the causes of the sounds. For example, the sounds you hear over the abdomen are caused by intestinal peristalsis. You would identify where the sound is best heard and how the sound is heard normally. Peristalsis is heard over all four abdominal quadrants as intermittent "tinkling" sounds. After understanding the cause and character of normal auscultated sounds, it becomes easier to recognize abnormal sounds and their origins.

Olfaction

While assessing a client, become familiar with the nature and source of body odors (Table 12-1). Olfaction helps to detect abnormalities not recognized by other means. For example, a client's cast should not have a sweet, heavy, thick odor indicative of an underlying infection. Findings from olfaction and other assessment skills allow you to detect serious abnormalities.

PREPARATION FOR EXAMINATION

Proper preparation of the environment, equipment, and client ensures a smooth examination with few interruptions. A disorganized approach when preparing for a physical examination can cause errors and incomplete findings.

Environment

A physical examination requires privacy. A well-equipped examination room is preferable, but often the examination occurs in the client's room. In the home, you may perform the examination in the client's bedroom. Adequate lighting is needed to illuminate body parts. Ideally an examination room is soundproof so clients feel comfortable discussing their conditions. Be sure to eliminate sources of noise, take precautions to prevent interruptions from others, and make sure the room is warm enough to maintain comfort.

Sometimes it is difficult to perform a complete examination when clients are in beds or on stretchers. Special examination tables make clients easily accessible and help them assume special positions. Carefully assist clients so they do not fall while getting on and off the table. Do not leave a confused, combative, or uncooperative client unsupervised on an examination table.

Examination tables are often hard and uncomfortable. When the client lies supine, the head of the table can be raised about 30 degrees. The client may also use a small pillow. When examining a client in bed, raise the bed to reach the client's body parts more easily.

Equipment

Wash your hands thoroughly before equipment preparation and the examination. Set up equipment so it is readily available and arranged in an order for easy use (Box 12-2). Equipment should be kept as warm as appropriate. The diaphragm of the stethoscope may be briskly rubbed between the hands before it is applied to the skin. Check all equipment to see that it functions properly. The ophthalmoscope and otoscope require good batteries and lightbulbs.

Client

PHYSICAL PREPARATION.   The client's physical comfort is vital for a successful examination. Before starting, ask if

Equipment and Supplies for Physical Assessment — Box 12-2

Cotton applicators	Scale with height
Cytobrush	measurement rod
Disposable pad	Specimen containers and
Drapes	microscope slides
Eye chart (e.g., Snellen	Sphygmomanometer
chart)	and cuff
Flashlight and spotlight	Stethoscope
Forms (e.g., physical,	Swabs or sponge forceps
laboratory)	Tape measure
Gloves (sterile or clean)	Thermometer
Gown for client	Tissues
Ophthalmoscope	Tongue depressor
Otoscope	Tuning fork
Papanicolaou smear slides	Vaginal speculum
Paper towels	Water-soluble lubricant
Percussion hammer	Wristwatch with second
Ruler	hand or digital display

the client needs to use the toilet. An empty bladder and bowel facilitate examination of the abdomen, genitalia, and rectum. Collection of urine or fecal specimens occurs at this time if they are ordered. Be sure to explain the proper method for collecting specimens and make sure each specimen is labeled properly.

Physical preparation involves being sure the client is dressed and draped properly. The client in the hospital will be wearing a simple gown. An outpatient will have to undress. If the examination is limited to certain body systems, it may not be necessary for the client to undress completely. Provide the client privacy and plenty of time during undressing. Walking into the room as the client undresses causes embarrassment. Drapes and gowns are made of linen or disposable paper. After clients have undressed and put on a gown, they should sit or lie down on the examination table with the drape over the lap or lower trunk. Make sure the client stays warm by eliminating drafts, controlling room temperature, and providing warm blankets. Routinely ask if the client is comfortable.

POSITIONING.   During the examination, ask the client to assume proper positions so body parts are accessible and clients stay comfortable. Table 12-2 lists the preferred positions for each part of the examination and contains figures illustrating these positions. Clients' abilities to assume positions will depend on their physical strength and degree of wellness. Be prepared to use alternative positions if the client is unable to assume the usual position needed for the examination. Many positions, such as the lithotomy and knee-chest position, are embarrassing and uncomfortable. Therefore clients should be kept in these positions no longer than necessary. Explain the positions, and assist clients in assuming them. Adjust the drapes to be sure the area to be examined is accessible and that no body part is unnecessarily exposed. A client may assume more than one position for the

same part of an examination. Be sure to use extra care when positioning older adults, as they are more prone to having disabilities and limitations.

PSYCHOLOGICAL PREPARATION.   Many clients may find an examination tiring or stressful, or they may experience anxiety about possible findings. A thorough explanation of the purpose and steps of each assessment lets clients know what to expect and what to do so they can cooperate. Keep explanations simple and in understandable terms. Clients should feel free to ask questions and mention any discomfort. As you examine each body system, give a more detailed explanation.

Your manner should be professional yet relaxed. A stiff, formal demeanor may inhibit the client's ability to communicate, but a too-casual style may fail to instill confidence (Seidel and others, 1999). When you and the client are of opposite gender, it may help to have a third person of the client's gender in the room. The presence of a third person assures the client that you will behave ethically. This person is also a witness to your conduct and the client's.

During the examination, watch the client's emotional responses. Observe whether the client's facial expression shows fear or concern and if body movements show anxiety. Remain calm, and explain each step clearly. It may be necessary to temporarily stop the examination and ask how the client feels. Do not force a client to continue. Postponing the examination may be best because the findings may be more accurate when the client can cooperate and relax. If fear results from misconceptions, clarify the purpose of the examination and how it is to be performed.

Assessment of Age-Groups

It is necessary to use different interview styles and approaches to examine clients of different age-groups. When assessing children, you must be sensitive and anticipate the child's reaction to the examination as a strange and unfamiliar experience. Routine pediatric examinations focus on health promotion and illness prevention, particularly for the care of well children who receive competent parenting and have no serious health problems (Wong and others, 1999). This examination focuses on growth and development, sensory screening, dental examination, and behavioral assessment. Children who are chronically ill or disabled, foster children, foreign-born, or adopted may require additional examinations. When examining children, the following tips assist in data collection:

1. Gather all or part of the histories on infants and children from parents or guardians.
2. Perform the examination in a nonthreatening area, and provide time for play to become acquainted.
3. Because parents may think they are being tested by the examiner, offer support during the examination and do not pass judgment.
4. Call children by their first name, and address the parents as "Mr." and "Mrs." rather than by their first names.
5. Use open-ended questions to allow parents to share more information and describe more of the children's problems.

Positions for Examination   Table 12-2

Position		Areas Assessed	Rationale	Limitations
Sitting		Head and neck, back, posterior thorax and lungs, anterior thorax and lungs, breasts, axillae, heart, vital signs, and upper extremities	Sitting upright provides full expansion of lungs and provides better visualization of symmetry of upper body parts.	Physically weakened client may be unable to sit. Examiner should use supine position with head of bed elevated instead.
Supine		Head and neck, anterior thorax and lungs, breasts, axillae, heart, abdomen, extremities, pulses	This is most normally relaxed position. It provides easy access to pulse sites.	If client becomes short of breath easily, examiner may need to raise head of bed.
Dorsal recumbent		Head and neck, anterior thorax and lungs, breasts, axillae, heart, abdomen	Position is used for abdominal assessment because it promotes relaxation of abdominal muscles.	Clients with painful disorders are more comfortable with knees flexed.
Lithotomy*		Female genitalia and genital tract	This position provides maximal exposure of genitalia and facilitates insertion of vaginal speculum.	Lithotomy position is embarrassing and uncomfortable, so examiner minimizes time that the client spends in it. Client is kept well draped.
Sims'*		Rectum and vagina	Flexion of hip and knee improves exposure of rectal area.	Joint deformities may hinder client's ability to bend hip and knee.
Prone		Musculoskeletal system	This position is used only to assess extension of hip joint.	This position is poorly tolerated in clients with respiratory difficulties.
Lateral recumbent		Heart	This position aids in detecting murmurs.	This position is poorly tolerated in clients with respiratory difficulties.
Knee-chest*		Rectum	This position provides maximal exposure of rectal area.	This position is embarrassing and uncomfortable.

*Clients with arthritis or other joint deformities may be unable to assume this position.

6. Interview older children, who can often provide details about their health history and severity of symptoms. This also allows you to observe parent-child interactions.
7. Treat adolescents as adults and individuals, because they tend to respond best when treated as such.
8. Remember that adolescents have the right to confidentiality. After talking with parents about historical information, speak alone with adolescents.

A comprehensive health assessment and examination of older adults should include physical data and a review of growth and development, family relationships, group involvement, and religious and occupational pursuits (Ebersole and Hess, 1998). An important part of health assessment involves analysis of basic activities of daily living (ADLs) (e.g., dressing, bathing, toileting, feeding, and continence) that are fundamental to independent living. In addition, the more complex instrumental ADLs (e.g., using the telephone, preparing meals, and managing money) are also assessed. Any examination of an older adult should also include an evaluation of mental status.

During the examination, you must recognize that with advancing age the body does not respond vigorously to injury or disease. Therefore older persons do not always exhibit the expected signs and symptoms (Lueckenotte, 1998). Characteristically, older adults have more blunted or atypical signs and symptoms.

Principles to use during examination of an older adult include the following:

1. Do not stereotype aging clients. Most are able to adapt to change and to learn about their health. Similarly, they are reliable historians.
2. Recognize that sensory or physical limitations can affect how quickly you are able to interview older adults and conduct examinations. Plan for more than one examination session. Sometimes it helps to give clients an initial health questionnaire before they come to a clinic or office (Ebersole and Hess, 1998).
3. Perform the examination with adequate space; this is especially important for clients with mobility aids such as a cane or walker.
4. During the examination use patience, allow for pauses, and observe for details. Recognize normalities of later life.
5. Older clients may find giving certain types of health information stressful. Illness is seen as a threat to independence and a step toward institutionalization.
6. Perform the examination near bathroom facilities if the client has an urgent need to void.
7. Be alert to signs of increasing fatigue such as sighing, grimacing, irritability, leaning against objects for support, and drooping of head and shoulders.

PHYSICAL EXAMINATION

Individual assessments for each body system constitute the physical examination. Clients with specific symptoms or needs require only portions of an examination. A complete health assessment follows the format of the health history (see Chapter 6). Obtain information from the history to focus attention on specific parts of the examination. For example, if the history shows that the client experiences difficulty in breathing, conduct an examination of the thorax and lungs more carefully. The examination supplements information from the history to confirm or refute the data.

The examination should be systematic and well organized so important assessments are not omitted. A head-to-toe approach includes all body systems and helps you anticipate each step. In an adult begin by assessing the head and neck, progressing methodically down the body to include all body systems. Inspect both sides of the body and compare for symmetry. If a client is seriously ill, examine the body system most at risk for being abnormal. If a client becomes fatigued, provide rest periods. Perform any painful procedures near the end of the examination. Record assessments in specific terms on a physical assessment form or in the nurses' notes. The use of common and accepted medical abbreviations helps to keep notes brief and concise.

General Survey

Assessment begins when you first meet the client. Determine the client's reasons and expectations for seeking health care. Initial data from the general survey begins with a review of the client's primary health problems. Make mental notes of the client's behavior and appearance. Begin the examination with the general survey that includes observing general appearance and measuring behavior, vital signs, height, and weight. The survey provides information about characteristics of an illness, a client's hygiene and body image, emotional state, recent changes in weight, and the client's developmental status. If you find any abnormalities or problems, closely assess the affected body system later.

General Appearance and Behavior

You can assess appearance and behavior while you prepare the client for the physical examination. The review of appearance and behavior includes the following:

1. *Gender and race.* A person's gender affects the type of examination performed and the manner in which assessments are made. Different physical features are related to gender and race. Certain illnesses are more likely affect a specific gender or race; for example, skin cancer is more common in lightly pigmented clients, pancreatic cancer is higher in African Americans, and cancer of the bladder is more common in men (American Cancer Society, 1998, 2001).
2. *Age.* Age influences normal physical characteristics and a person's ability to participate in some parts of the examination.
3. *Signs of distress.* There may be obvious signs or symptoms indicating pain, difficulty in breathing, or anxiety. These signs help to establish priorities regarding what to examine first.
4. *Body type.* Observe if a client appears trim and muscular, obese, or excessively thin. Body type can reflect level of health, age, and lifestyle.

5. *Posture.* Normal standing posture is an upright stance with parallel alignment of hips and shoulders. Normal sitting involves some degree of rounding of the shoulders. Observe whether the client has a slumped, erect, or bent posture. Posture may reflect mood or pain. Many older adults have a stooped, forward-bent posture, with hips and knees somewhat flexed and arms bent at the elbows, raising the level of the arms.

6. *Gait.* Observe the client walk into the room or along the bedside (if ambulatory). Note if movements are coordinated or uncoordinated. A person normally walks with arms swinging freely at the sides, with the head and face leading the body.

7. *Body movements.* Observe whether movements are purposeful. Note any tremors involving the extremities. Determine if any body parts are immobile.

8. *Hygiene and grooming.* Note the client's level of cleanliness by observing the appearance of the hair, skin, and fingernails. Note if the client's clothes are clean. Grooming may depend on the activities being performed just before the examination and the client's occupation. Also note amount and type of cosmetics used.

9. *Dress.* Culture, lifestyle, socioeconomic level, and personal preference affect the type of clothes worn. Note if the type of clothing worn is appropriate for temperature and weather conditions. Depressed or mentally ill persons may be unable to choose proper clothing. An older adult tends to wear extra clothing because of sensitivity to cold.

10. *Body odor.* An unpleasant body odor may result from physical exercise, poor hygiene, or certain disease conditions.

11. *Affect and mood.* Affect is a person's feelings as they appear to others. Mood or emotional state is expressed verbally and nonverbally. Note if verbal expressions match nonverbal behavior. Observe if mood is appropriate for the situation. Observe facial expressions while asking questions.

12. *Speech.* Normal speech is understandable and moderately paced. It shows an association with the person's thoughts. Note if the client talks rapidly or slowly. An abnormal pace may be caused by emotions or neurological impairment. Observe if the client speaks in a normal tone with clear inflection of words.

13. *Client abuse.* Abuse of children, women, and older adults is a growing health problem. It may be first suspected in clients who have suffered obvious physical injury or neglect (e.g., evidence of malnutrition or presence of bruising on the extremities or trunk). Assess for the client's fear of the spouse or partner, caregiver, parent, or adult child. Note if the partner or caregiver has a history of violence, alcoholism, or drug abuse. Is the person unemployed, ill, or frustrated in caring for the client? Most states mandate a report to a social service center if abuse or neglect is suspected. When abuse is suspected, interview the client in private. It is difficult to detect abuse because victims often will not complain or report that they are in an abusive situation. Clients are more likely to reveal any problems to you when the suspected abuser is absent from the room (Lynch, 1997). Table 12-3 summarizes clinical indicators of abuse.

14. *Substance abuse.* Health care providers' recognition of clients who abuse alcohol, prescribed medications, or illegal drugs is typically poor. Substance abuse affects all socioeconomic groups. A single visit to a clinic may not reveal the problem. Several visits often reveal behaviors that can be confirmed with a well-focused history and physical examination. Approach the client in a caring and nonjudgmental way because substance abuse involves both emotional and lifestyle issues. Clients to suspect for substance abuse include those listed in Box 12-3. When abuse is suspected, ask the following questions: Have you ever felt the need to CUT DOWN on your drinking or drug use? Have people ANNOYED you by criticizing your drinking or drug use? Have you ever felt bad or GUILTY about your drinking or drug use? Have you ever used or had a drink first thing in the morning as an EYE-OPENER to steady your nerves or feel normal? If two or more of the CAGE questions are positive, the nurse should strongly suspect abuse and consider how to motivate the client to seek treatment (Stuart and Laraia, 1998).

Vital Signs

Generally you will measure vital signs (see Chapter 11) before the physical examination. Positioning or moving the client can interfere with obtaining accurate values. You can also measure specific vital signs during individual body system assessments.

Height and Weight

Height and weight can reflect a person's general level of health. Weight is a routine measure during health screenings and visits to physicians' offices or clinics. Both height and weight are routine assessments during admission to a health care setting. Measuring an infant's or child's height and weight assesses their growth and development. In older adults, height and weight coupled with a nutritional assessment are important in determining cause and treatment for chronic disease and in assessing the older adult who has difficulty with feeding and other functional activities. Be sure to look for overall trends in height and weight changes.

A client's weight normally will vary daily because of fluid loss or retention. Assessments screen for abnormal weight changes. First, ask the client his or her current height and weight. Also assess weight gains or losses. A weight gain of 5 lb or 2.2 kg in a day may indicate fluid-retention problems. If a change exists, assess the amount; the period over which the change occurred; and a change in diet habits, appetite, prescription or over-the-counter drugs, or physical symptoms. Question whether the client has a concern with the weight change or the body shape.

Clinical Indicators of Abuse

Table 12-3

Physical Findings	Behavioral Findings
Child Sexual Abuse	
Vaginal or penile discharge	Problem in sleeping or eating
Blood on underclothing	Fear of certain people or places
Pain or itching in genital area	Play activities recreate the abuse situation
Genital injuries	Regressed behavior
Difficulty sitting or walking	Sexual acting out
Pain while urinating	Knowledge of explicit sexual matters
Foreign bodies in rectum, urethra, or vagina	Preoccupation with other's or own genitals
Venereal disease	
Domestic Abuse	
Injuries and trauma are inconsistent with reported cause	Attempted suicide
Multiple injuries involving head, face, neck, breasts, abdomen, and genitalia (black eyes, orbital fractures, broken nose, fractured skull, lip lacerations, broken teeth, strangulation marks)	Eating or sleeping disorders
	Anxiety
	Panic attacks
X-ray films show old and new fractures in different stages of healing	Pattern of substance abuse (follows physical abuse)
Burns	Low self-esteem
Human bites	Depression
	Sense of helplessness
	Guilt
	Increased forgetfulness
Older Adult Abuse	
Injuries and trauma are inconsistent with reported cause (e.g., cigarette burn, scratch, bruise, bite)	Dependent on caregiver
	Physically and/or cognitively impaired
Hematomas	Combative
Bruises at various stages of resolution	Wandering
Bruises, chafing, excoriation on wrist or legs (restraints)	Verbally belligerent
Burns	Minimal social support
Fractures inconsistent with cause described	
Dried blood	
Prolonged interval between injury and medical treatment	

Data from Berlinger JS: Why don't you just leave him? *Nursing 98* 28(4):34, 1998; Lynch SH: Elder abuse: what to look for, how to intervene, *Am J Nurs* 97(1):27, 1997; Pace H, Hoag-Apel CM: Stemming the tide of domestic violence, *Point of View Magazine* 33(3):12, 1996; and Shea CA and others: Breaking through the barriers to domestic violence intervention, *Am J Nurs* 97(6):26, 1997.

[handwritten annotation: Preferred first thing in Am. before breakfast / meds/breakfast]

Weigh clients at the same time of day, on the same scale, and in the same clothes. This allows for an objective comparison of subsequent weights. Accuracy of weight measurement is important because medical and nursing decisions may be based on changes. Clients capable of bearing their own weight use a standing scale. Calibrate a standard platform scale by moving the large and small weights to zero. Make the balance beam level and steady by adjusting the calibrating knob. The client stands on the scale platform and remains still. Move the largest weight to the 50-lb or 22.5-kg increment under the client's weight. Then adjust the smaller weight to balance the scale at the nearest $\frac{1}{4}$ lb or 0.1 kg (Seidel and others, 1999). Electronic scales are automatically calibrated each time they are used. Electronic scales automatically display weight within seconds.

Stretcher and chair scales are available for clients unable to bear weight. After being transferred to the scale, the client is lifted above the bed by a hydraulic device and the weight is measured on a balance beam or digital display. Caution must be used when transferring clients to and from the scales.

Always weigh infants in baskets or on platform scales. Remove the infant's clothing and weigh the infant in dry, disposable diapers. The weight can later be adjusted for the weight of the diaper, ensuring an accurate reading. Keep the room warm to prevent chills. A light cloth or paper placed on the scale's surface prevents cross infection from urine or feces. When placing infants in baskets or on platforms, hold a hand lightly above to prevent accidental falls. Measure weight in ounces and grams.

To measure the height of a weight-bearing client have the client remove his or her shoes. Place a paper towel on the scale platform so the feet remain clean. Have the client stand erect. The platform scale has a metal rod attached to the back of the scale; this swings out and over the crown of the client's head. Measure the client's height in inches or centimeters.

Position a non–weight-bearing client (such as an infant) supine on a firm surface. Portable devices are available that provide a reliable means to measure height. Place the infant on the device, having the parent hold the infant's head against the headboard. With the infant's legs straight at the

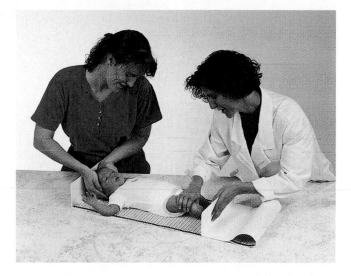

FIGURE **12-3**   Measure of infant length. (From Seidel HM and others: *Mosby's guide to physical examination,* ed 4, St. Louis, 1999, Mosby.)

knees, place the footboard against the bottom of the infant's feet (Figure 12-3). Record the infant's length to the nearest 0.5 cm or ¼ inch.

INTEGUMENT

The integument consists of the skin, nails, hair, and scalp. You may first inspect all skin surfaces or may assess the skin gradually as other body systems are examined. Use the assessment skills of inspection, palpation, and olfaction to assess the function and integrity of the integument.

Skin

Assessment of the skin can reveal changes in oxygenation, circulation, nutrition, local tissue damage, and hydration. In a hospital setting the majority of clients are older adults, debilitated clients, or young but seriously ill clients. There are significant risks for skin lesions resulting from trauma to the skin while administering care, from exposure to pressure during immobilization, or from reaction to medications used in treatment. Clients most at risk are the neurologically impaired; chronically ill; orthopedic clients; and clients with diminished mental status, poor tissue oxygenation, low cardiac output, and inadequate nutrition. In nursing homes and extended care facilities, clients may be at risk for many of the same problems, depending on their level of mobility and presence of chronic illness. Routinely assess the skin to look for primary or initial lesions that may develop. Without proper care, primary lesions can quickly worsen to become secondary

lesions that require more extensive nursing care. For example, development of a pressure ulcer can lengthen a hospital stay unless it is prevented or discovered early and treated properly.

The incidence of **melanoma,** an aggressive form of skin cancer, has increased about 4% every year since 1973 (American Cancer Society, 2000). In addition, the incidence of highly curable basal cell and squamous cell cancers is also increasing. Cutaneous malignancies are the most common neoplasms seen in clients. Incorporate a thorough skin assessment for all clients and educate them about self-examination (Box 12-4).

The condition of the client's skin reveals the need for nursing intervention. Use your assessment findings to determine abnormalities and the type of hygiene measures required to maintain integrity of the integument (see Chapter 26). Adequate nutrition and hydration become goals of therapy if an alteration in the status of the integument is identified.

You will need adequate illumination of the skin for accurate observations. The recommended choice is natural or halogen lighting. For detecting skin changes in the dark-skinned client, sunlight is the best choice (Talbot and Curtis, 1996). Room temperature may also affect skin assessment. A room that is too warm may cause superficial vasodilation, resulting in an increased redness of the skin. A cool environment may cause the sensitive client to develop cyanosis around the lips and nail beds (Talbot and Curtis, 1996).

Use disposable gloves for palpation if open, moist, or draining skin lesions are present. Because you will inspect all skin surfaces, the client must assume several positions. The examination includes inspecting the skin's color, moisture, temperature, texture, and turgor. Also note vascular changes, **edema,** and lesions. Carefully palpate abnormalities, and document your findings. Skin odors are usually noted in skinfolds, such as the axillae or under the female client's breasts.

HEALTH HISTORY. Before assessing the skin, ask the client about the presence of lesions, rashes, or bruises and determine whether the alterations can be linked to heat, cold, stress, exposure to toxic material or the sun, or new skin care

products. Also determine if there has been a recent change in skin color or trauma to the skin. If a client has been out in the sun, it is useful to know if a sunscreen has been worn. If not, the client will require education on ways to safeguard the skin. Also assess for history of allergies, use of topical medications, and a family history of serious skin disorders.

COLOR. Skin color varies from body part to body part and from person to person. Despite individual variations, skin color is usually uniform over the body. Table 12-4 lists common variations. Normal skin pigmentation ranges from ivory or light pink to ruddy pink in white skin and from light to deep brown or black in dark skin. Sun-darkened or darker skin is common around knees and elbows.

Basal cell carcinoma is most commonly seen in sun-exposed areas and frequently occurs in a background of sun-damaged skin. In older adults pigmentation increases unevenly, causing discolored skin. While inspecting the skin, you must be aware that color may be masked by cosmetics or tanning agents.

The assessment of color first involves areas of the skin not exposed to the sun, such as the palms of the hands. Note if the skin is unusually pale or dark. It is more difficult to note changes such as pallor or cyanosis in clients with dark skin. Usually color hues are best seen in the palms, soles of the feet, lips, tongue, and nail beds. Areas of increased color (hyperpigmentation) and decreased color (hypopigmentation) are common. Skin creases and folds are darker than the rest of the body in the dark-skinned client.

Inspect sites where abnormalities are more easily identified. For example, **pallor** is more easily seen in the face, buccal mucosa (mouth), conjunctivae, and nail beds. **Cyanosis** is best observed in the lips, nail beds, palpebral conjunctivae, and palms.

In recognizing pallor in the dark-skinned client, you would observe that normal brown skin appears to be

---

Client Teaching   Box 12-4

SKIN ASSESSMENT

- Instruct the client to conduct a monthly self-examination of the skin, noting moles, blemishes, and birthmarks.
- Tell the client to inspect all skin surfaces. Cancerous melanomas start as small, molelike growths that increase in size, change color, become ulcerated, and bleed. A simple ABCD rule (American Cancer Society, 2000) outlines warning signals:

  A is for **asymmetry.**

  B is for **border** irregularity; edges are ragged, notched, or blurred.

  C is for **color;** pigmentation is not uniform.

  D is for **diameter,** greater than 6 mm.
- Tell the client to report to a physician changes in skin lesions or a sore that does not heal.
- Instruct the client to prevent skin cancer by avoiding overexposure to the sun: wear wide-brimmed hat and long sleeves; apply sunscreens with SPF greater than or equal to 15 approximately 15 minutes before going into the sun and after swimming or perspiring; avoid tanning under direct sun between 10:00 AM and 3:00 PM; and do not use indoor sunlamps, tanning parlors, or tanning pills.
- Older adults and clients with certain chronic diseases tend to have delayed wound healing.
- Instruct the client to report any lesion that bleeds or fails to heal to a physician.
- To treat excessively dry skin, tell the client to avoid hot water, harsh soaps, and drying agents such as alcohol. Use a superfatted soap (e.g., Dove), and pat rather than rub the skin after bathing. Apply skin moisturizers regularly, and wear cotton clothing (Hardy, 1996).

Skin Color Variations   Table 12-4

Color	Condition	Causes	Assessment Locations
Bluish (cyanosis)	Increased amount of deoxygenated hemoglobin (associated with hypoxia)	Heart or lung disease, cold environment	Nail beds, lips, mouth, skin (severe cases)
Pallor (decrease in color)	Reduced amount of oxyhemoglobin	Anemia	Face, conjunctivae, nail beds, palms of hands
	Reduced visibility of oxyhemoglobin resulting from decreased blood flow	Shock	Skin, nail beds, conjunctivae, lips
Loss of pigmentation	Vitiligo	Congenital or autoimmune condition causing lack of pigment	Patchy areas on skin over face, hands, arms
Yellow-orange (jaundice)	Increased deposit of bilirubin in tissues	Liver disease, destruction of red blood cells	Sclera, mucous membranes, skin
Red (erythema)	Increased visibility of oxyhemoglobin caused by dilation or increased blood flow	Fever, direct trauma, blushing, alcohol intake	Face, area of trauma, sacrum, shoulders, other common sites for pressure ulcers
Tan-brown	Increased amount of melanin	Suntan, pregnancy	Areas exposed to sun: face, arms, areolae, nipples

yellow-brown and normal black skin appears to be ashen gray. Also assess the lips, nail beds, and mucous membranes for generalized pallor. If pallor is present, the mucous membranes will be ashen gray. Assessment of cyanosis in the dark-skinned client requires that you observe areas where pigmentation occurs the least (conjunctiva, sclera, buccal mucosa, tongue, lips, nail beds, and palms and soles). In addition, verify these findings with clinical manifestations (Talbot and Curtis, 1996).

The best site to inspect for **jaundice** (yellow-orange discoloration) is the client's sclera. Normal reactive hyperemia, or redness, is most often seen in regions exposed to pressure such as the sacrum, heels, and greater trochanter (Chapter 34).

Inspect for any patches or areas of skin color variation. Localized skin changes, such as pallor or **erythema** (red discoloration), may indicate circulatory changes. For example, an area of erythema may be caused by localized vasodilation resulting from sunburn or fever. In the dark-skinned client, erythema is not easily observed, so the area must be palpated for heat and warmth to note the presence of skin inflammation (Talbot and Curtis, 1996). An area of an extremity that appears unusually pale may result from an arterial occlusion or edema. It is important to ask if the client has noticed any changes in skin coloring.

A pattern of findings that is becoming more common is that associated with clients who are chemically dependent and are intravenous (IV) drug abusers. It may be difficult to recognize signs and symptoms after one examination. A client who takes repeated IV injections may have edematous, reddened, and warm areas along the arms and legs. This pattern suggests recent injections. Evidence of old injection sites appears as hyperpigmented and shiny or scarred areas. Table 12-5 summarizes additional physical findings associated with substance abuse.

MOISTURE.   The hydration of skin and mucous membranes helps to reveal body fluid imbalances, changes in the

Physical Findings of the Skin Indicative of Substance Abuse   Table 12-5

Body System	Commonly Associated Drug
Diaphoresis	Sedative hypnotic (including alcohol)
Spider angiomas	Alcohol, stimulants
Burns (especially fingers)	Alcohol
Needle marks	Opioids
Contusions, abrasions, cuts, scars	Alcohol, other sedative hypnotics
"Homemade" tattoos	Cocaine, IV opioids (prevents detection of injection sites)
Increased vascularity of face	Alcohol
Red, dry skin	Phencyclidine (PCP)

Modified from Caulken-Burnett I: Primary care screening for substance abuse, *Nurse Pract* 19(6):42, 1994; and Friedman L and others: *Source book of substance abuse and addiction,* Baltimore, 1996, Williams & Wilkins.

skin's environment, and regulation of body temperature. Moisture refers to wetness and oiliness. The skin is normally smooth and dry. Skinfolds such as the axillae are normally moist. Minimal perspiration or oiliness should be present (Seidel and others, 1999). Increased perspiration may be associated with activity, warm environments, obesity, anxiety, or excitement. Use ungloved fingertips to palpate skin surfaces and observe for dullness, dryness, crusting, and flaking. Flaking is the appearance of dandrufflike flakes when the skin surface is lightly rubbed. Scaling involves fishlike scales that are easily rubbed off the skin's surface. Both flaking and scaling are believed to indicate abnormally dry skin (Hardy, 1996). Excessively dry skin is common in older adults and persons who use excessive amounts of soap during bathing. Other factors causing dry skin include lack of humidity, exposure to sun, smoking, stress, excessive perspiration, and dehydration (Hardy, 1996). Excessive dryness can worsen existing skin conditions.

TEMPERATURE.   The temperature of the skin depends on the amount of blood circulating through the dermis. Increased or decreased skin temperature reflects an increase or decrease in blood flow. Localized erythema or redness of the skin often may be accompanied by an increase in skin temperature. A reduction in skin temperature reflects a decrease in blood flow. It is important to remember that if an examination room is cold, the client's skin temperature and color can be affected.

Accurately assess temperature by palpating the skin with the dorsum, or back, of the hand. Compare symmetrical body parts. Normally the skin is warm. Skin temperature may be the same throughout the body or may vary in one area. Always assess skin temperature in clients at risk for impaired circulation, such as after a cast application or vascular surgery. A stage I pressure ulcer could be identified early when noting warmth and erythema on an area of the skin.

TEXTURE.   The character of the skin's surface and the feel of deeper portions are its texture. Determine if the client's skin is smooth or rough, thin or thick, tight or supple, and indurated (hardened) or soft by stroking it lightly with the fingertips. The texture of the skin is normally smooth, soft, and flexible in children and adults. However, the texture is usually not uniform. The palms of the hands and soles of the feet tend to be thicker. In older adults the skin becomes wrinkled and leathery because of a decrease in collagen, subcutaneous fat, and sweat glands.

Localized changes may result from trauma, surgical wounds, or lesions. When you find irregularities in texture such as scars or **induration,** ask the client if a recent injury to the skin has occurred. Deeper palpation may reveal irregularities such as tenderness or localized areas of induration commonly caused by repeated injections.

TURGOR.   **Turgor** is the skin's elasticity, which can be diminished by edema or dehydration. Normally the skin loses its elasticity with age. To assess skin turgor, grasp a fold of

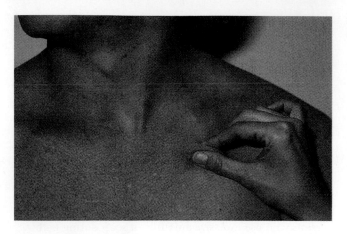

FIGURE **12-4**   Assessment of skin turgor.

skin on the back of the forearm or sternal area with the fingertips and release (Figure 12-4). Normally the skin lifts easily and snaps back immediately to its resting position. The skin stays pinched or tented when turgor is poor. The client with poor turgor does not have a resilience to the normal wear and tear on the skin. A decrease in turgor predisposes the client to skin breakdown.

VASCULARITY.   The circulation of the skin affects color in localized areas and the appearance of superficial blood vessels. With aging, capillaries become fragile. Localized pressure areas, found after a client has lain or sat in one position, appear reddened, pink, or pale (see Chapter 34). **Petechiae** are tiny, pinpoint-sized, red or purple spots on the skin caused by small hemorrhages in the skin layers. Petechiae may indicate serious blood-clotting disorders, drug reactions, or liver disease.

EDEMA.   Areas of the skin become swollen or edematous from fluid buildup in the tissues. Direct trauma and impairment of venous return are two common causes of edema. Inspect edematous areas for location, color, and shape. The formation of edema separates the skin's surface from the pigmented and vascular layers, masking skin color. Edematous skin also appears stretched and shiny. Palpate edematous areas to determine mobility, consistency, and tenderness. When pressure from your finger leaves an indentation in the edematous area, it is called *pitting edema*. To assess pitting edema, press the edematous area firmly with the thumb for several seconds and release. The depth of pitting, recorded in millimeters (Seidel and others, 1999), determines the degree of edema. For example, +1 edema equals 2 mm depth, and +2 edema equals 4 mm (see Figure 12-41, p. 254).

LESIONS.   The skin is normally free of lesions, except for common freckles or age-related changes such as skin tags or senile keratosis (thickening of skin), cherry angiomas (ruby red papules), and atrophic warts. Lesions may be primary (occurring as initial spontaneous manifestations of a pathological process), such as a wheal of an insect bite, or sec-

ondary (resulting from later formation of trauma to a primary lesion), such as a pressure ulcer. When you detect a lesion, inspect it for color, location, texture, size, shape, type (Box 12-5), grouping (e.g., clustered or linear), and distribution (localized or generalized). Observe any exudate for color, odor, amount, and consistency. Measure the size of the lesion by using a small, clear, flexible ruler, divided in centimeters. Measure lesions in height, width, and depth.

Palpation determines the lesion's mobility, contour (flat, raised, or depressed), and consistency (soft or hard). Palpate gently, covering the entire area of the lesion. If the lesion is moist or has draining fluid, wear gloves during palpation. Note if the client complains of tenderness during palpation. Cancerous lesions frequently undergo changes in color and size. Report abnormalities, especially lesions that have changed in character (e.g., color or size), to a physician for further examination.

Hair and Scalp

Good lighting allows you to inspect the condition and distribution of body hair and integrity of the scalp. Assessment of the hair occurs during all portions of the examination. Assess the distribution, thickness, texture, and lubrication of hair. In addition, inspect for infection or infestation of the scalp.

HEALTH HISTORY.   Ask questions such as the following: Has the client noted change in growth or loss of hair? Change in texture or color? What types of hair care products are used? Has the client recently been on chemotherapy (drugs that can cause hair loss) or taken vasodilators (minoxidil) for hair growth? Has the client noted changes in diet or appetite? If a client has a hairpiece, it should be removed if inspection of the scalp is essential.

INSPECTION.   During inspection explain that it may be necessary to separate parts of the hair to detect abnormalities. First inspect the distribution, thickness, texture, and lubrication of body hair. Hair is normally distributed evenly, is neither excessively dry nor oily, and is pliant. While separating sections of scalp hair, observe for characteristics of color and coarseness. Normal terminal hair is black, brown, red, yellow, or variations in shades of these colors. The hair is coarse or fine and shiny. Normal variations exist in the shape of hair fibers. Clients' hair may be straight, curly, spiral, or wavy. The hair of black persons is usually thicker and drier than the hair of whites.

In older adults, the hair becomes dull gray, white, or yellow. The hair also thins over the scalp, axillae, and pubic areas. Older men lose facial hair, whereas older women may develop hair on the chin and upper lip.

Changes may occur in the thickness, texture, and lubrication of scalp hair. Disturbances such as a febrile illness or scalp disease can result in hair loss. Conditions such as thyroid disease can alter the condition of the hair, making it fine and brittle. Baldness (**alopecia**) or thinning of the hair is usually related to genetic tendencies and endocrine disorders such as diabetes and even menopause. Poor nutrition can

Types of Primary Skin Lesions   Box 12-5

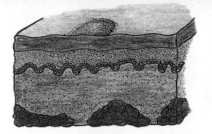

Macule: flat, nonpalpable change in skin color, smaller than 1 cm (e.g., freckle, petechia)

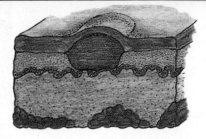

Papule: palpable, circumscribed, solid elevation in skin, smaller than 0.5 cm (e.g., elevated nevus)

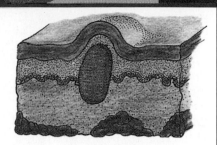

Nodule: elevated solid mass, deeper and firmer than papule, 0.2 to 0.5 cm (e.g., wart)

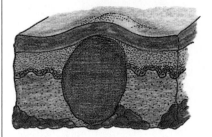

Tumor: solid mass that may extend deep through subcutaneous tissue, larger than 1 to 2 cm (e.g., epithelioma)

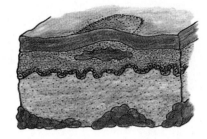

Wheal: irregularly shaped, elevated area or superficial localized edema, varies in size (e.g., hive, mosquito bite)

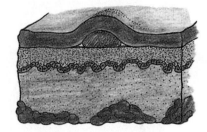

Vesicle: circumscribed elevation of skin filled with serous fluid, smaller than 0.5 cm (e.g., herpes simplex, chickenpox)

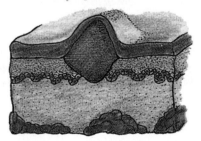

Pustule: circumscribed elevation of skin similar to vesicle but filled with pus, varies in size (e.g., acne, staphylococcal infection)

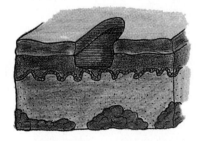

Ulcer: deep loss of skin surface that may extend to dermis and frequently bleeds and scars, varies in size (e.g., venous stasis ulcer)

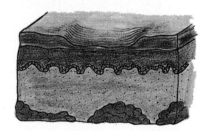

Atrophy: thinning of skin with loss of normal skin furrow with skin appearing shiny and translucent, varies in size (e.g., arterial insufficiency)

cause stringy, dull, dry, and thin hair. The hair is lubricated from the oil of sebaceous glands. Excessively oily hair is associated with androgen hormone stimulation. Dry, brittle hair occurs with aging and excessive use of chemical agents.

The amount of hair covering the extremities may be reduced as a result of aging and arterial insufficiency and is most commonly seen over the lower extremities. In women loss of hair should not be confused with shaven legs.

Inspect the scalp for lesions, which can easily go unnoticed in thick hair. The scalp is normally smooth and inelastic, with even coloration. By carefully separating strands of hair you can thoroughly examine the scalp for lesions. Note the characteristics of any scalp lesions. If lumps or bruises are found, ask if the client has experienced recent head trauma. Moles on the scalp are common. You should warn the client that combing or brushing can cause a mole to

bleed. Scaliness or dryness of the scalp is frequently caused by dandruff or psoriasis.

Careful inspection of hair follicles on the scalp and pubic areas may reveal lice or other parasites. Lice attach their eggs to hair. The head and body lice are tiny and have grayish white bodies. Crab lice have red legs. Lice eggs look like oval particles of dandruff. The lice themselves are difficult to see. Observe for bites or pustular eruptions in the follicles and in areas where skin surfaces meet, such as behind the ears and in the groin. The discovery of lice requires immediate treatment (Box 12-6).

Nails

The condition of the nails can reflect general health, state of nutrition, a person's occupation, and level of self-care. The most visible portion of the nails is the nail plate, the trans-

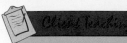

Box 12-6

HAIR AND SCALP ASSESSMENT

- Clients may require instruction about basic hygiene measures including shampooing and combing of the hair (see Chapter 26).
- Instruct clients who have head lice to shampoo thoroughly with pediculicide (shampoo available at drug stores) in cold water, comb thoroughly with fine-tooth comb (following product directions), and discard comb.
- After combing, remove any remaining nits or nit cases with tweezers or between the fingernails. A dilute solution of vinegar and water may help loosen nits.
- Instruct clients and parents about ways to reduce transmission of lice:

     Do not share personal care items with others.

     Vacuum all rugs, car seats, pillows, furniture, and flooring thoroughly and discard vacuum bag.

     Seal nonwashable items in plastic bags for 14 days if parents are unable to afford dry cleaning and do not have a vacuum.

     Use thorough hand washing.

     Launder all clothing, linen, and bedding in hot soap and water, and dry in a hot dryer for at least 20 minutes. Dry-clean nonwashable items.

     Do not use insecticide.

- Instruct the client that his or her partner must be notified if lice were sexually transmitted.
- Avoid physical contact with infested individuals and their belongings, especially clothing and bedding.

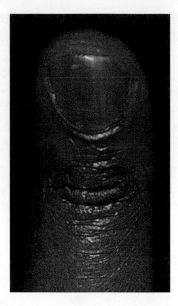

FIGURE **12-5** Pigmented bands in nail of client with dark skin. (From Seidel HM and others: *Mosby's guide to physical examination*, ed 4, St. Louis, 1999, Mosby.)

parent layer of epithelial cells covering the nail bed. The vascularity of the nail bed creates the nail's underlying color. The semilunar, whitish area at the base of the nail bed from which the nail plate develops is the lunula.

HEALTH HISTORY.   Before assessing the nails ask if the client has had any recent trauma. A blow to the nail can change the shape and growth of the nail, as well as loss of all or part of the nail plate. The client should also describe nail-care practices. Improper care can damage nails and cuticles. It is also important to find out if clients have acrylic nails or silk wraps, because these may be areas for fungal growth. Question whether the client has noticed changes in nail appearance or growth. Alterations may occur slowly over time. Knowing if the client has risks for nail or foot problems (e.g., diabetes, peripheral vascular disease, or older adulthood) will influence the level of hygienic care recommended.

INSPECTION AND PALPATION.   Inspect the nail bed color, the thickness and shape of the nail, the texture of the nail, and the condition of tissue around the nail. The nails are normally transparent, smooth, and convex, with surrounding cuticles smooth, intact, and without inflammation. In whites, nail beds are pink with translucent white tips. In dark-skinned clients, nail beds can be darkly pigmented with a blue or reddish hue. A brown or black pigmentation is normal with longitudinal streaks (Figure 12-5). Splinter hemorrhages can be caused by trauma, cirrhosis, diabetes mellitus,

and hypertension. Vitamin, protein, and electrolyte changes can cause various lines or bands to form on nail beds.

Nails normally grow at a constant rate, but direct injury or generalized disease can slow growth. With aging, the nails of the fingers and toes become harder and thicker. Longitudinal striations develop, and the rate of nail growth slows. Nails become more brittle, dull, and opaque and may turn yellow in older adults because of insufficient calcium. Also with age the cuticle becomes less thick and wide.

Inspection of the angle between the nail and nail bed normally reveals an angle of 160 degrees (Box 12-7). A larger angle and softening of the nail bed can indicate chronic oxygenation problems. Palpate the nail base to determine firmness and condition of circulation. The nail base is normally firm. To palpate, gently grasp the client's finger and observe the color of the nail bed. Next, apply gentle, firm, quick pressure with the thumb to the nail bed and release. As you apply pressure, the nail bed appears white or blanched; however, the pink color should return immediately on release of pressure. Failure of the pinkness to return promptly indicates circulatory insufficiency. An ongoing bluish or purplish cast to the nail bed occurs with cyanosis. A white cast or pallor results from anemia.

Calluses and corns are often found on the toes or fingers. A callus is flat and painless, resulting from thickening of the epidermis. Corns are caused by friction and pressure from shoes and are usually seen over bony prominences. During the examination instruct the client on proper nail care (Box 12-8).

HEAD AND NECK

An examination of the head and neck includes the head, eyes, ears, nose, mouth, pharynx, and neck (lymph nodes, carotid arteries, thyroid gland, and trachea). The carotid ar-

Abnormalities of the Nail Bed   Box 12-7

160 degrees — Normal nail: Approximately 160-degree angle between nail plate and nail

180 degrees — Clubbing: Change in angle between nail and nail base (eventually larger than 180 degrees); nail bed softening, with nail flattening; often, enlargement of fingertips
Causes: Chronic lack of oxygen: heart or pulmonary disease

180 degrees

Beau's lines: Transverse depressions in nails indicating temporary disturbance of nail growth (nail grows out over several months)
Causes: Systemic illness such as severe infection, nail injury

Koilonychia (spoon nail): Concave curves
Causes: Iron deficiency anemia, syphilis, use of strong detergents

Splinter hemorrhages: Red or brown linear streaks in nail bed
Causes: Minor trauma, subacute bacterial endocarditis, trichinosis

Paronychia: Inflammation of skin at base of nail
Causes: Local infection, trauma

Client Teaching   Box 12-8

NAIL ASSESSMENT
- Instruct the client to cut nails only after soaking them about 10 minutes in warm water. (Exception: Diabetic clients are warned against soaking nails.)
- Instruct the client to avoid using over-the-counter preparations to treat corns, calluses, or ingrown toenails.
- Tell the client to cut nails straight across and even with the tops of the fingers or toes. If the client has diabetes, tell the client to file rather than cut the nails.
- Instruct the client to shape nails with a file or emery board.
- If client is diabetic:
  - Wash feet daily in warm water. Inspect feet each day in good light, looking for dry places and cracks in the skin. Soften dry feet by applying a cream or lotion such as Nivea, Eucerin, or Alpha Keri.
  - Do not put lotion between the toes.
  - Caution client against using sharp objects to poke or dig under toenail or around the cuticle.
  - Have client see a podiatrist for treatment of ingrown toenails and nails that are thick or tend to split.

normally held upright and midline to the trunk. A horizontal jerking or bobbing may indicate a tremor. Holding the head tilted to one side may be an indication of unilateral hearing or visual loss. The skull is generally round with prominences in the frontal area anteriorly and the occipital area posteriorly. Local skull deformities are typically caused by trauma. In infants a large head may result from congenital anomalies or the accumulation of cerebrospinal fluid in the ventricles (**hydrocephalus**). Adults may have enlarged jaws and facial bones resulting from **acromegaly.** Palpate the skull for nodules or masses. Gentle rotation of the fingertips down the midline of the scalp and then along the sides of the head reveals abnormalities. Also note the client's facial features, looking at the eyelids, eyebrows, nasolabial folds, and mouth for shape and symmetry. It is normal for slight asymmetry to exist. If there is facial asymmetry, note if all features on one side of the face are affected or if only a portion of the face is involved. Various neurological disorders such as a facial nerve paralysis affect different nerves that innervate muscles of the face.

Eyes

Examination of the eye includes assessment of visual acuity, visual fields, and external and internal eye structures. Figure 12-6 shows a cross section of the eye. The assessment detects visual alterations and determines the level of assistance clients require when ambulating or performing self-care activities. Clients with visual problems may need special aids for reading teaching materials or instructions.

HEALTH HISTORY.   Determine if the client is at risk for partial or complete visual loss by reviewing history of eye disease (e.g., glaucoma or cataracts), eye trauma, diabetes, hypertension, or eye surgery. Assessment for common symp-

teries can also be assessed during the assessment of peripheral arteries. You need to understand each anatomical area and its normal function. Assessment of the head and neck uses inspection, palpation, and auscultation.

Head

HEALTH HISTORY.   The history allows you to screen for possible intracranial injury if necessary. Ask whether the client experienced recent trauma to the head or if neurological symptoms such as headache (note onset, duration, character, pattern, and associated symptoms), dizziness, seizures, poor vision, or loss of consciousness have occurred. The history also includes a review of the client's occupation, focusing on those clients who should wear safety helmets. In addition, ask if the client participates in contact sports, cycling, roller blading, or skateboarding.

INSPECTION AND PALPATION.   Inspect the client's head, noting the position, size, shape, and contour. The head is

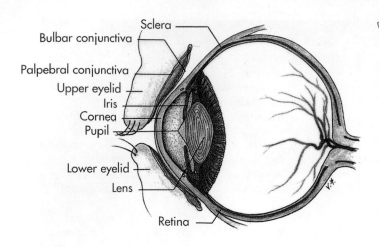

FIGURE **12-6** Cross section of eye.

EYE ASSESSMENT
- Tell clients that people under age 40 should have complete eye examinations every 3 to 5 years (or more often if family histories reveal risks such as diabetes or hypertension).
- Tell clients that people over age 40 should have eye examinations every 2 years to screen for conditions that may develop without client awareness (e.g., glaucoma).
- Tell clients that people over age 65 should have yearly eye examinations.
- Describe the typical symptoms of eye disease (see Chapter 35).
- Instruct older adults to take the following precautions because of normal visual changes: avoid driving at night, increase lighting in the home to reduce risk of falls, and paint the first and last steps of a staircase and the edge of each step in between a bright color to aid in depth perception.

toms of eye disease, such as eye pain, photophobia (sensitivity to light), burning, itching, excess tearing or crusting, diplopia (double vision), blurred vision, awareness of a "film" or "curtain" over the field of vision, floaters, flashing lights, or halos around lights, is critical. Review the client's occupational history, use of glasses or contact lenses, use of safety glasses at work and for hobbies, and regularity of visits to an ophthalmologist or optometrist (Box 12-9). Question the client about current medications, including eye drops or ointments. You should also determine whether there is a family history of eye disorders or disease.

VISUAL ACUITY. The assessment of visual acuity, the ability to see small details, tests central vision. The easiest way to assess visual acuity is to ask the client to read printed material under adequate lighting. If clients use glasses or contact lenses, they should wear them. You should know the language a client speaks and whether the client is literate. Asking the client to read aloud tests literacy. A client who has difficulty reading should consult an ophthalmologist or optometrist for further evaluation. If you are caring for a client who is unable to read clearly, assess if he or she can distinguish objects or light. Hold your hand 30 cm (1 foot) from the client's face, and instruct the client to count upraised fingers. To check light perception, shine a penlight into the eye and then turn the light off. If the client notes when the light is turned on or off, light perception is intact.

VISUAL FIELDS. As a person looks straight ahead, all objects in the periphery can normally be seen. To assess visual fields, have the client stand or sit 60 cm (2 feet) away, facing you at eye level. The client gently closes or covers one eye (e.g., the left) and looks at you directly opposite (client's left eye, your right eye). You close the opposite eye so that the field of vision is superimposed on that of the client. Move a finger equidistant at arm's length from you and the client outside the field of vision, then slowly bring it back into the visual field. Ask the client to tell you when he or she is able to see your finger. If you see the finger before the client does,

this reveals that a portion of the client's visual field is reduced. To test temporal field vision, the object should be slightly behind the client. (NOTE: You will be able to see the finger.) Repeat the procedure for each field of vision. The examination is only approximate and presumes that your visual fields are normal. Older adults commonly have loss of peripheral vision caused by changes in the lens.

EXTERNAL EYE STRUCTURES. To inspect external eye structures, stand directly in front of the client at eye level and ask the client to look at your face.

POSITION AND ALIGNMENT. Assess the position of the eyes in relation to one another. Normally they are parallel to each other. Bulging eyes (exophthalmos) usually indicate hyperthyroidism. The crossing of eyes (strabismus) results from neuromuscular injury or inherited abnormalities. Tumors or inflammation of the orbit can cause abnormal eye protrusion.

EYEBROWS. For the remainder of the examination the client removes contact lenses. Inspect the eyebrows for size, extension, texture of hair, alignment, and movement. Coarseness of hair and failure to extend beyond the temporal canthus may reveal hypothyroidism. If the brows are thinned, the client may pluck or wax the hair. Aging causes loss of the lateral third of the eyebrows. Have the client raise and lower the eyebrows. The brows should raise and lower symmetrically. An inability to move the eyebrows may indicate a facial nerve paralysis.

EYELIDS. Inspect the eyelids for position; color; condition of surface; condition and direction of lashes; and the client's ability to open, close, and blink. When the eyes are open in a normal position, the lids do not cover the pupil, and the sclera cannot be seen above the iris. The lids are also close to the eyeball. An abnormal drooping of the lid over the pupil is called **ptosis,** caused by edema or impairment of the third cranial nerve. In the older adult, ptosis results from a loss of elasticity that accompanies aging. Defects in the position of the lid margins may be observed. An older adult frequently has lid margins that turn out (**ectropion**) or in (**entropion**). An entropion may lead to the lashes of the lid irritating the conjunctiva and cornea, increasing risk of infection. The eyelashes are normally distributed evenly and curved outward away from the eye.

To inspect the surface of the upper lids, have the client close the eyes and then raise both eyebrows gently with the thumb and index finger. This stretches the skin. The lids are usually smooth and the same color as the skin. Redness indicates inflammation or infection. Lid edema may be caused by allergies or heart and kidney failure. If lesions are present, observe the size, shape, and distribution. Wear gloves if drainage is present.

The lids normally close symmetrically. Failure of lids to close exposes the cornea to drying. This condition is common in unconscious clients or those with facial nerve paralysis. While inspecting the lower lids, ask the client to open the eyes and observe the blink reflex. Normally a client blinks involuntarily and bilaterally as many as 20 times a minute. The blink reflex helps lubricate the cornea. Report absent or infrequent, rapid, or monocular (one-eyed) blinking.

LACRIMAL APPARATUS.   The lacrimal gland (Figure 12-7) is located in the upper, outer wall of the anterior part of the orbit and is responsible for tear production. Tears flow from the gland across the eye's surface to the lacrimal duct, which is located in the nasal corner or inner canthus of the eye. The lacrimal gland can be the site of tumors or infection and is inspected for edema and redness. Palpate the gland area gently to detect tenderness. Normally the gland cannot be felt. The nasolacrimal duct may become obstructed, blocking the flow of tears. Observe for evidence of excess tearing or edema in the inner canthus. Gentle palpation of the duct at the lower eyelid just inside the orbital rim may cause a regurgitation of tears.

CONJUNCTIVA AND SCLERA.   The bulbar conjunctiva covers the exposed surface of the eyeball up to the outer edge of the cornea. The sclera is seen under the bulbar conjunctiva and normally has the color of white porcelain in whites and light yellow in black-skinned clients. To view both structures, gently retract both lids simultaneously with thumb and index finger pressed against the lower and upper bony orbits. Wear gloves if there is crusty drainage on eyelid margins. A pair of new gloves should be worn to examine each eye to prevent cross contamination. For adequate exposure retract the eyelids without placing pressure directly on the eyeball. Ask the client to look up, down, and side to side. Inspect for color, texture, and lesions.

The palpebral conjunctiva is the delicate membrane lining the eyelids. Normally the conjunctiva is transparent, enabling you to view the tiny underlying blood vessels that give it a pink color. To inspect the palpebral conjunctiva, gently depress the lower lid. Often the client can depress the eyelid to facilitate examination. Note the conjunctiva's color and the presence of edema or lesions. A pale conjunctiva results

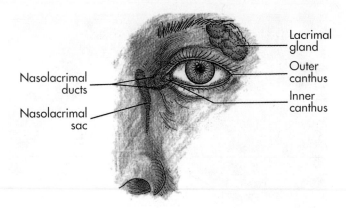

FIGURE **12-7**   Lacrimal apparatus.

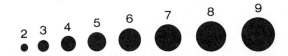

FIGURE **12-8**   Chart depicting pupillary size in millimeters.

from anemia, whereas a fiery red appearance is the result of inflammation (conjunctivitis). **Conjunctivitis** is highly contagious, and the crusty drainage that collects on eyelid margins can easily spread from one eye to the other.

CORNEA.   The cornea is the transparent, colorless portion of the eye covering the pupil and iris. From a side view, it looks like the crystal of a wristwatch. While the client looks straight ahead, inspect the cornea for clarity and texture while shining a penlight obliquely across the surface of the cornea. The cornea is normally shiny, transparent, and smooth. In older adults the cornea loses its luster. Any irregularity in the surface may indicate an abrasion or tear that requires further examination by a physician. Both conditions are quite painful. Note the color and details of the underlying iris. In an older adult the iris becomes faded. A thin, white ring along the margin of the iris, called an **arcus senilis,** is common with aging but is abnormal in anyone under age 40. To test for the corneal blink reflex, see Table 12-12, p. 273, in the cranial nerve function section of this chapter.

PUPILS AND IRISES.   Observe the pupils for size, shape, equality, accommodation, and reaction to light. The pupils are normally black, round, regular, and equal in size (3 to 7 mm in diameter) (Figure 12-8). Cloudy pupils indicate cataracts. Dilated or constricted pupils can result from neurological disorders or the effect of ophthalmic or certain systemic drugs. Pinpoint pupils are a common sign of opioid intoxication. When you shine a beam of light through the pupil and onto the retina, the third cranial nerve is stimulated and causes the muscles of the iris to constrict. Any abnormality along the nerve pathways from the retina to the iris alters the ability of the pupils to react to light. Changes in intracranial pressure, lesions along the nerve pathways, lo-

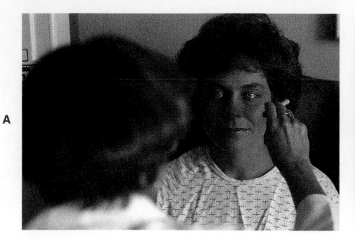
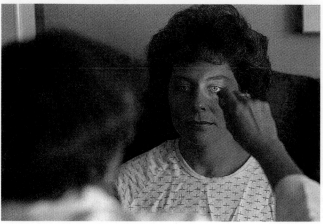

A   **B**

FIGURE **12-9**   **A,** To check pupil reflexes, first hold penlight to side of client's face. **B,** Illumination of pupil causes pupillary constriction.

cally applied eye drugs, and direct trauma to the eye may alter pupillary reaction.

Test pupillary reflexes (to light and accommodation) in a dimly lit room. While the client looks straight ahead, bring a penlight from the side of the client's face, directing the light onto the pupil (Figure 12-9). If the client looks at the light, there will be a false reaction to accommodation. A directly illuminated pupil constricts, and the opposite pupil constricts consensually. Observe the quickness and equality of the reflex. Repeat the examination for the opposite eye.

To test accommodation, ask the client to gaze at a distant object (the far wall) and then at a test object (finger or pencil) held by you approximately 10 cm (4 inches) from the bridge of the client's nose. The pupils normally converge and accommodate by constricting when looking at close objects. The pupil responses are equal. If assessment of pupillary reaction is normal in all tests, record the abbreviation **PERRLA** (pupils equal, round, reactive to light and accommodation).

INTERNAL EYE STRUCTURES.   The examination of internal eye structures is beyond the scope of a new graduate nurse's practice. Clients in greatest need of the examination are those with diabetes, hypertension, and intracranial disorders. By illuminating the internal eye structures with an **ophthalmoscope,** an examiner is able to view the optic disc, the integrity of retinal vessels, the presence of retinal lesions, and the appearance of the macula and fovea centralis.

Ears

The ear assessment determines the integrity of ear structures and hearing acuity. You will inspect and palpate external ear structures, inspect middle ear structures with the otoscope, and test the inner ear by measuring the client's hearing acuity. Assessment of clients with hearing impairment provides useful data for you in planning effective communication techniques.

HEALTH HISTORY.   The client's health history includes a review of risks for hearing problems (e.g., hypoxia at birth,

meningitis, intake of aspirin, ototoxic drugs, and exposure to noise), a history of ear surgery or trauma, and the client's current exposure to high noise levels. Determine if the client has ear pain, itching, discharge, **tinnitus, vertigo,** or change in hearing. Note behaviors indicative of hearing loss, such as failure to respond when spoken to, requests to repeat comments, leaning forward to hear, and a child's inattentiveness. If the client has had a recent hearing problem, determine the onset, contributing factors, and effect on ADLs. Also assess if the client wears a hearing aid and how the client normally cleans the ears.

AURICLES.   With the client sitting, inspect the position, color, size, shape, and symmetry of the auricle. Be sure to examine lateral and medial surfaces and surrounding tissue. The auricles are normally of equal size and level with each other. The upper point of attachment to the head is normally in a straight line with the outer canthus, or corner of the eye. Ears that are low set or at an unusual angle are a sign of chromosome abnormality (e.g., Down syndrome). The color is the same as the face without moles, cysts, deformities, or nodules. Redness is a sign of inflammation or fever. Extreme pallor can indicate frostbite. Palpate the auricles for texture, tenderness, swelling, and skin lesions. Auricles are normally smooth, firm, mobile, and without lesions. If the client complains of pain, gently pull the auricle and press on the tragus and palpate behind the ear over the mastoid process. If palpating the external ear increases the pain, an external ear infection is likely. If palpation of the auricle and tragus does not influence the pain, the client may have a middle ear infection. Tenderness in the mastoid area can indicate mastoiditis.

Inspect the opening of the ear canal for size and presence of discharge. If discharge is present, wear gloves during the examination. The meatus should not be swollen or occluded. A yellow, waxy substance called **cerumen** is common. Yellow or green foul-smelling discharge may indicate infection or a foreign body.

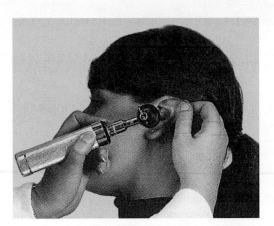

FIGURE **12-10** Otoscopic examination. (From Seidel HM and others: *Mosby's guide to physical examination,* ed 4, St. Louis, 1999, Mosby.)

EAR CANALS AND EARDRUMS.   The deeper structures of the external and middle ear can be observed only with the use of an **otoscope.** A special ear speculum attaches to the battery tube of the ophthalmoscope. For best visualization select the largest speculum that fits comfortably in the client's ear. Before inserting the speculum, check for foreign bodies in the opening of the auditory canal.

The client must avoid moving the head during the examination to avoid damage to the canal and tympanic membrane. Infants and young children often need to be restrained. Infants should lie supine with their heads turned to one side and their arms held securely at their sides. Young children can sit on their parents' laps with their legs held between the parents' knees.

Turn on the otoscope by rotating the dial at the top of the battery tube. To insert the speculum properly, ask the client to tip the head slightly to the opposite shoulder. Hold the handle of the otoscope in the space between the thumb and index finger, supported on your middle finger. This leaves the ulnar side of your hand to rest against the client's head, stabilizing the otoscope as it is inserted into the canal (Seidel and others, 1999). Two grips on the otoscope may be used. In one, you hold the battery tube along the client's neck with your fingers against the neck. In the other grip, lightly brace the inverted otoscope against the side of the client's head or cheek. Insert the scope while pulling the auricle upward and backward in the adult and older child (Figure 12-10). This maneuver straightens the ear canal. In infants pull the auricle back and down. Insert the speculum slightly down and forward, 1.0 or 1.5 cm ($\frac{1}{2}$ inch) into the ear canal.

Take care not to abrade the sensitive lining of the ear canal, which can be painful. The ear canal normally has little cerumen and is uniformly pink with tiny hairs in the outer third of the canal. Observe for color, discharge, scaling, lesions, foreign bodies, and cerumen. Normally cerumen is dry (light brown to gray and flaky) or moist (dark yellow or brown) and sticky. Dry cerumen occurs in Asians and Native Americans about 85% of the time (Seidel and others, 1999).

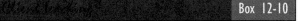

Box 12-10

EAR AND HEARING ASSESSMENT
- Instruct the client in the proper way to clean the outer ear (see Chapter 26), avoiding use of cotton-tipped applicators and sharp objects such as hairpins.
- Tell the client to avoid inserting pointed objects into the ear canal.
- Encourage clients over age 65 to have regular hearing checks. Explain that a reduction in hearing is a normal part of aging (see Chapter 35).
- Instruct family members of clients with hearing losses to avoid shouting and instead speak in low tones and to be sure the client can see the speaker's face.

A reddened canal with discharge is a sign of inflammation or infection. In older adults, accumulated cerumen is a common problem. Buildup of cerumen can create a mild hearing loss. During the examination ask the client how the ear canal is normally cleaned (Box 12-10). Caution the client on the danger of inserting pointed objects into the canal. The use of cotton-tipped applicators to clean the ears should be avoided because this causes impaction of cerumen deep in the ear canal.

The light from the otoscope allows visualization of the eardrum (tympanic membrane). Know the common anatomical landmarks and their appearance (Figure 12-11). Move the auricle to see the entire drum and its periphery. Because the eardrum is angled away from the ear canal, the light from the otoscope appears as a cone shape rather than a circle. The umbo is near the center of the drum, behind which is the attachment of the malleus. A knoblike structure at the top of the drum is created by the underlying short process of the malleus. Check carefully to be sure there are no tears or breaks in the membrane of the eardrum. The normal eardrum is translucent, shiny, and pearly gray. It is free from tears or breaks. A pink or red bulging membrane indicates inflammation. A white color reveals pus behind it. The membrane is taut, except for the small triangular pars flaccida near the top. If the tympanic membrane is blocked by cerumen, a warm water irrigation will safely remove the wax.

HEARING ACUITY.   You can often tell if the client has a hearing loss from a response to conversation. The three types of hearing loss are conduction, sensorineural, and mixed. A conduction loss involves an interruption of sound waves as they travel from the outer ear to the cochlea of the inner ear because they are not transmitted through the outer and middle ear structures. A sensorineural loss involves the inner ear, the auditory nerve, or the hearing center of the brain. Sound is conducted through the outer and middle ear structures, but the continued transmission of sound becomes interrupted at some point beyond the bony ossicles. A mixed loss involves a combination of conduction and sensorineural loss.

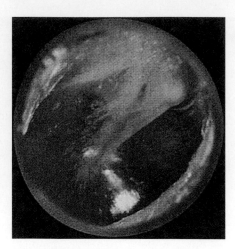

FIGURE 12-11 Normal tympanic membrane. (Courtesy Dr. Richard A. Buckingham, Abraham Lincoln School of Medicine, University of Illinois, Chicago.)

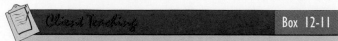

Box 12-11

NOSE AND SINUS ASSESSMENT
- Caution clients against overuse of over-the-counter nasal sprays, which can lead to "rebound," causing nasal inflammation and congestion.
- Instruct parents in care of children with nosebleeds: have child sit up and lean forward to avoid aspiration of blood; apply pressure to anterior nose with thumb and forefinger as child breathes through mouth; apply ice or a cold cloth to bridge of nose if pressure fails to stop bleeding.
- Instruct older adults to install smoke detectors on each floor of the home.
- Instruct older adults to always check dated labels on food to ensure against spoilage.

Clients working or living around loud noises are at risk for hearing loss. Older adults experience an inability to hear high-frequency sounds and consonants (e.g., *s, z, t,* and *g*). Deterioration of the cochlea and thickening of the tympanic membrane causes older adults to gradually lose hearing acuity. They are especially at risk for hearing loss caused by **ototoxicity** (injury to the auditory nerve) resulting from high maintenance doses of antibiotics (e.g., aminoglycosides).

To conduct a hearing assessment, have the client remove the hearing aid if worn. Note the client's response to questions. Normally the client should respond without excess requests to have you repeat questions. If hearing loss is suspected, check the client's response to the whispered voice. Test one ear at a time while the client occludes the other ear with a finger. Ask the client to gently move the finger up and down during the test. While standing 30 cm (1 foot) from the ear being tested, cover your mouth so the client is unable to read lips. After exhaling fully, whisper softly toward the unoccluded ear, reciting random numbers with equally accented syllables such as "nine-four-ten." If necessary, gradually increase voice intensity until the client correctly repeats the numbers. Then test the other ear for comparison. Seidel and others (1999) report that clients normally hear numbers clearly when whispered. A ticking watch may be used to test hearing acuity, but the spoken word allows for more accuracy and control in testing.

If a hearing loss is present, there are tests that can be performed by experienced practitioners using a tuning fork or audiometry.

Nose and Sinuses

Assess the integrity of the nose and sinuses by inspection and palpation. The client sits during the examination. A penlight allows for gross examination of each naris. A more detailed examination requires using a nasal speculum to inspect deeper nasal turbinates. You should not use a speculum unless a qualified practitioner is present.

HEALTH HISTORY. It is useful to know whether the client's health history indicates exposure to dust or pollutants, allergies, nasal obstruction, recent trauma, discharge, frequent infections, headaches, or postnasal drip. An assessment for a history of nosebleed (epistaxis) should include review of frequency, amount of bleeding, treatment, and difficulty stopping bleeding. Also determine whether the client has a history of using nasal spray or drops, including the amount, frequency, and duration of use (Box 12-11). Ask clients if they have been told that they snore or if they have difficulty breathing.

NOSE. When inspecting the external nose, observe the shape, size, skin color, and presence of deformity or inflammation. The nose is normally smooth and symmetrical, with the same color as the face. Recent trauma may have caused edema and discoloration. If swelling or deformities exist, gently palpate the ridge and soft tissue of the nose by placing one finger on each side of the nasal arch and gently moving fingers from the nasal bridge to the tip. Note any tenderness, masses, and underlying deviations. Nasal structures are usually firm and stable.

Air normally passes freely through the nose when a person breathes. To assess patency of the nares, place a finger on the side of the client's nose and occlude one naris. Ask the client to breathe with the mouth closed. Repeat the procedure for the other naris.

As you illuminate the anterior nares, inspect the mucosa for color, lesions, discharge, swelling, and evidence of bleeding. If discharge is present, apply gloves. Normal mucosa is pink and moist without lesions. Pale mucosa with clear discharge indicates allergy. A mucoid discharge indicates rhinitis. A sinus infection results in yellowish or greenish discharge. Habitual use of intranasal cocaine and opioids can cause puffiness and increased vascularity of the nasal mucosa. For the client with a nasogastric tube, check for local **excoriation** of the naris, characterized by redness and skin sloughing.

To view the septum and turbinates, have the client tip the head back slightly to give you a clearer view. Illuminate the

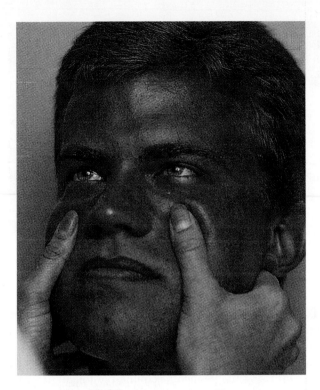

FIGURE **12-12** Palpation of maxillary sinuses.

septum and look for alignment, perforation, or bleeding. Normally the septum is close to the midline and thicker anteriorly than posteriorly. Normal mucosa is pink and moist, without lesions. A deviated septum can obstruct breathing and interfere with passage of a nasogastric tube. Perforation of the septum can occur after repeated use of intranasal cocaine. Note any polyps (tumorlike growths) or purulent drainage. Advanced, experienced clinicians use a nasal speculum for this procedure.

SINUSES.   The examination of the sinuses is limited to palpation. In cases of allergies or infection, the interior of the sinuses becomes inflamed and swollen. The most effective way to assess for tenderness is by externally palpating the frontal and maxillary facial areas (Figure 12-12). Palpate the frontal sinus by exerting pressure with the thumb up and under the client's eyebrow. Gentle upward pressure elicits tenderness easily if sinus irritation is present. Do not apply pressure to the eyes. If tenderness of sinuses is present, the sinuses may be transilluminated. This procedure, however, requires advanced experience.

Mouth and Pharynx

Assess the mouth and pharynx to detect signs of overall health, determine oral hygiene needs, and develop therapies for clients with dehydration, restricted intake, oral trauma, or oral airway obstruction. To assess the oral cavity use a penlight and tongue depressor or a single gauze square. Wear gloves when contacting mucous membranes. The client may sit or lie during the examination. The oral cavity may be assessed while administering oral hygiene.

HISTORY.   Determine if the client wears dentures or retainers and if they fit comfortably. An assessment of a recent change in appetite or weight may point to a problem with chewing or swallowing. Assess the client's dental hygiene practices and when the client last visited a dentist. To rule out risks for mouth and throat cancer, ask if the client smokes, chews tobacco, or smokes a pipe and consumes alcohol. Also assess for a history of pain or lesions of the mouth and pain with chewing. It helps to know if a tonsillectomy or adenoidectomy has been performed.

LIPS.   Inspect the lips for color, texture, hydration, contour, and lesions. With the client's mouth closed, view the lips from end to end. Normally they are pink, moist, symmetrical, smooth, and without lesions. Lip color in the dark-skinned client varies from pink to plum. Female clients should remove their lipstick before the examination. Pallor of the lips can be caused by anemia, with cyanosis caused by respiratory or cardiovascular problems. Any lesions such as nodules or ulcerations can be related to infection, irritation, or skin cancer.

MUCOSA.   To view the inner oral mucosa, have the client open the mouth slightly and gently pull the lower lip away from the teeth (Figure 12-13, *A*). Repeat this process for the upper lip. Inspect the mucosa for color, hydration, texture, and lesions such as ulcers, abrasions, or cysts. Normally the mucosa is a glistening pink. Varying shades of hyperpigmentation are normal in 10% of whites after age 50 and up to 90% of blacks by the same age. Any lesions are palpated with a gloved hand for tenderness, size, and consistency.

To inspect the buccal mucosa, ask the client to open the mouth and then gently retract the cheeks with a tongue depressor or gloved finger covered with gauze (Figure 12-13, *B*). A penlight illuminates the posterior mucosa. The surface of the mucosa must be viewed from right to left and top to bottom. Normal mucosa is glistening, pink, soft, moist, and smooth. For clients with normal pigmentation the buccal mucosa is a good site to inspect for jaundice and pallor. In older adults, the mucosa is normally dry because of reduced salivation. Thick white patches (**leukoplakia**) are often a precancerous lesion seen in heavy smokers and alcoholics. Palpate for any buccal lesions by placing the index finger within the buccal cavity and the thumb on the outer surface of the cheek.

GUMS AND TEETH.   Examine the gums or **gingivae** for color, edema, retraction, bleeding, and lesions. If a client wears dentures, irregularity or lesions of the gums can create discomfort and significantly impair the ability to chew. Ask the client to remove dentures for a complete assessment. Healthy gums are pink, moist, smooth, and tightly fit around each tooth. Blacks may have patchy pigmentation. In older adults the gums are usually pale. Using gloves, palpate the gums to assess for lesions, thickening, or masses. There should be no tenderness. Spongy gums that bleed easily indicate periodontal disease or vitamin C deficiency.

Ask the client to clench the teeth and smile to observe teeth occlusion. The upper molars should rest directly on the

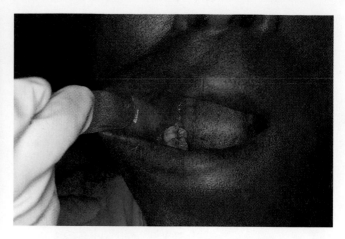

FIGURE **12-13** **A,** Inspection of inner oral mucosa of lower lip. **B,** Retraction allows for clear view of buccal mucosa.

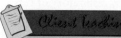

Box 12-12

MOUTH AND PHARYNX ASSESSMENT
- Discuss proper techniques for oral hygiene, including brushing and flossing.
- Explain the early warning signs of oral cancer, including a sore that bleeds easily and does not heel, a lump or thickening, and red or white patch on the mucosa that persists (American Cancer Society, 2000). Difficulty chewing and swallowing are late changes.
- Encourage regular dental examinations every 6 months for children, adults, and older adults.
- Identify older clients who have difficulty in chewing and changes in the teeth. Teach clients to eat soft foods and to cut food into small pieces.

lower molars, and the upper incisors slightly override the lower incisors. Note the position and alignment of teeth. Probe gently each tooth with a tongue blade when the client complains of any localized discomfort. The teeth are normally firmly set.

The quality of a client's dental hygiene is easily determined by inspecting the teeth (Box 12-12). To examine the posterior surface of the teeth, have the client open the mouth with lips relaxed. A tongue depressor may be needed to retract the lips and cheeks, especially when viewing the molars. Note the color of teeth and the presence of dental caries, tartar, and extraction sites. Normal healthy teeth are smooth, white, and shiny. A chalky white discoloration of the enamel is an early indication that caries are forming. Brown or black discolorations indicate formation of caries. A stained yellow color is from tobacco use, whereas coffee, tea, and colas cause a brown stain. In the older adult, loose or missing teeth are common because bone resorption increases. An older adult's teeth often feel rough when tooth enamel calcifies. Yellow and darkened teeth are also common in the older adult because of general wear and tear that exposes the darker underlying dentin.

TONGUE AND FLOOR OF MOUTH. Carefully inspect the tongue on all sides and the floor of the mouth. The client first relaxes the mouth and sticks the tongue out halfway. If the client protrudes the tongue too far, the gag reflex may be elicited. Using the penlight, examine the tongue for color, size, position, texture, movement, and coating or lesions. The tongue should appear medium or dull red in color, moist, slightly rough on the top surface, and smooth along the lateral margins. The tongue remains at midline. Ask the client to raise the tongue and move it from side to side. The tongue should move freely.

The undersurface of the tongue and floor of the mouth are highly vascular. Extra care is taken to inspect this area, a common site of origin for oral cancer lesions. The client lifts the tongue by placing its tip on the palate behind the upper incisors. Inspect for color, swelling, and lesions such as cysts. The ventral surface of the tongue is pink and smooth with large veins between the frenulum folds. To palpate the tongue ask the client to protrude the tongue and gently grasp its tip with a gauze square. While gently pulling the tongue to one side at a time, palpate its full length and base or floor of the mouth, noting any hardening or ulceration. The tongue should have a smooth, even texture and be free of lesions. Varicosities (swollen, tortuous veins) may be seen. Varicosities rarely cause problems but are common in the older adult.

PALATE. Have the client extend the head backward, holding the mouth open so that you can inspect the hard and soft palates. The hard palate, or roof of the mouth, is located anteriorly. The whitish hard palate should be dome shaped. The soft palate extends posteriorly toward the pharynx. It is normally light pink and smooth. Observe the palates for color, shape, texture, and extra bony prominences or defects. A bony growth, or **exostosis,** between the two palates is common.

PHARYNX. Perform an examination of the pharyngeal structures to rule out infection, inflammation, or lesions. Have the client tip the head back slightly, open the mouth

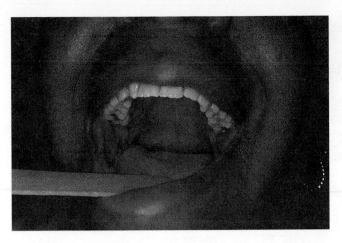

FIGURE **12-14** Tongue depressor allows view of pharynx and posterior soft palate.

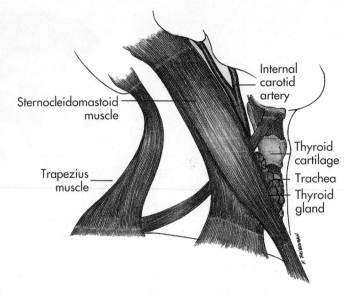

FIGURE **12-15** Anatomical position of major neck structures.

wide, and say "Ah" while you place the tip of a tongue depressor on the middle third of the tongue. Take care not to press the lower lip against the teeth (Figure 12-14). If the tongue depressor is placed too far anteriorly, the posterior part of the tongue mounds up, obstructing the view. Placing the tongue depressor on the posterior tongue elicits the gag reflex.

With a penlight, first inspect the uvula and soft palate. Both structures, which are innervated by the tenth cranial nerve (vagus), should rise centrally as the client says "Ah." Examine the anterior and posterior tonsillar pillars, and note the presence or absence of tonsillar tissue. The posterior pharynx is behind the pillars. Normally pharyngeal structures are smooth, pink, and well hydrated. Small irregular spots of lymphatic tissue and small blood vessels are normal. Note edema, petechiae (small hemorrhages), lesions, or exudate. Clients with chronic sinus problems frequently exhibit a clear exudate that drains along the wall of the posterior pharynx. Yellow or green exudate indicates infection. A client with a typical sore throat has a reddened and edematous uvula and tonsillar pillars with possible presence of yellow exudate.

Neck

Assessment of the neck includes assessing the neck muscles, lymph nodes of the head, carotid arteries, jugular veins, thyroid gland, and trachea (Figure 12-15). An examination of the carotid arteries and jugular veins can be deferred until you assess the vascular system. Inspect the neck to determine the integrity of neck structures and to examine the lymphatic system. An abnormality of superficial lymph nodes may reveal the presence of infection or malignancy. Examination of the thyroid gland and trachea also aids in ruling out malignancies. Examination is best performed with the client sitting.

HEALTH HISTORY.   Determine if the client has had a recent cold or infection or feels weak or fatigued. Screening for hypothyroidism and hyperthyroidism and risk factors for human immunodeficiency virus (HIV) infection may

be necessary. Also assess if the client has been exposed to radiation, toxic chemicals, or infection. Ask the client to describe any history of thyroid problems, head or neck injury, or pain of head and neck structures. Finally, ask if the client is taking thyroid medication or has a family history of thyroid disease.

NECK MUSCLES.   With the client sitting and facing you, inspect the gross neck structures. Observe for symmetry of neck muscles, alignment of the trachea, and any subtle fullness at the neck. Any distention or prominence of jugular veins and carotid arteries is abnormal. Ask the client to flex the neck with the chin to the chest, hyperextend the neck backward, and move the head laterally to each side and then sideways with the ear moving toward the shoulder. This tests the sternocleidomastoid and trapezius muscles. The neck should move freely without discomfort.

LYMPH NODES.   An extensive system of lymph nodes collects lymph from the head, ears, nose, cheeks, and lips (Figure 12-16). With the client's chin raised and head tilted slightly back, first inspect the area where lymph nodes are distributed and compare both sides. This position stretches the skin slightly over any possible enlarged nodes. Inspect visible nodes for edema, erythema, or red streaks. Nodes are not normally visible.

Use a methodical approach to palpate the lymph nodes to avoid overlooking any single node or chain. The client relaxes muscles and tissues by keeping the neck flexed slightly forward and, if needed, toward you. Palpate both sides of the neck for comparison. During palpation either face or stand to the side of the client for easy access to all nodes. Using the pads of the middle three fingers of each hand, gently palpate in a rotary motion over the nodes. Each node is checked methodically in the following sequence: occipital nodes at the base of the skull, postauric-

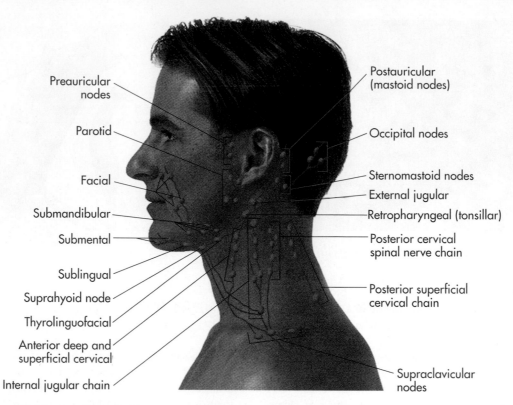

FIGURE **12-16**   Lymphatic drainage system of the head and neck. (From Seidel HM and others: *Mosby's guide to physical examination*, ed 4, St. Louis, 1999, Mosby.)

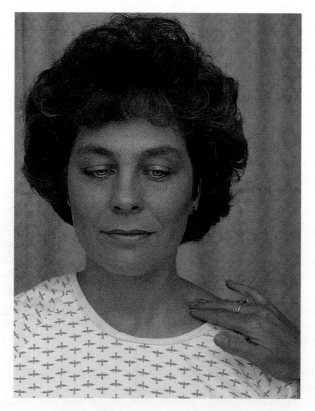

FIGURE **12-17**   Lymph node palpation.

ular nodes over the mastoid, preauricular nodes just in front of the ear, retropharyngeal nodes at the angle of the mandible, submandibular nodes, and submental nodes in the midline behind the mandibular tip. Try to detect enlargement, and note the location, size, shape, surface characteristics, consistency, mobility, tenderness, and warmth of the nodes. If the skin is mobile, move the skin over the area of the nodes (Figure 12-17) (Seidel and others, 1999). It is important to press underlying tissue in each area and not simply move the fingers over the skin. However, if excessive pressure is applied, small nodes are missed and palpable nodes are obliterated.

To palpate supraclavicular nodes ask the client to bend the head forward and relax the shoulders. You may have to hook the index and third finger over the clavicle, lateral to the sternocleidomastoid muscle, to palpate these nodes. The deep cervical nodes can be palpated only with your fingers hooked around the sternocleidomastoid muscle.

Normally lymph nodes are not easily palpable. Lymph nodes that are large, fixed, inflamed, or tender indicate a problem such as local infection, systemic disease, or neoplasm (Seidel and others, 1999). Tenderness almost always indicates inflammation (Box 12-13). A problem involving a lymph node of the head and neck may mean an abnormality in the mouth, throat, abdomen, breasts, thorax, or arms. These are the areas drained by the head and neck nodes.

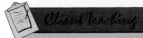

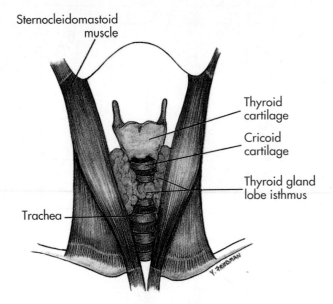

FIGURE **12-18**   Thyroid gland.

THYROID GLAND.   The thyroid gland lies in the anterior lower neck, in front of and to both sides of the trachea. The gland is fixed to the trachea with the isthmus overlying the trachea and connecting the two irregular, cone-shaped lobes (Figure 12-18). Inspect the lower neck over the thyroid gland for obvious masses and symmetry. Offer the client a glass of water and while observing the neck, have the client swallow. This maneuver helps to visualize an abnormally enlarged thyroid gland. More-experienced nurses can examine the thyroid by palpating for more subtle masses; this technique will not be discussed here.

TRACHEA.   The trachea is a part of the upper airway that can be directly palpated. It is normally located in the midline above the suprasternal notch. Masses in the neck or mediastinum and pulmonary abnormalities can cause displacement laterally. The client may sit or lie down during palpation. Determine the position of the trachea by palpating at the suprasternal notch, slipping the thumb and index fingers to each side. Note if the finger and thumb are shifted laterally. Forceful pressure must not be applied to the trachea because this may elicit a cough.

THORAX AND LUNGS

Examination of the thorax and lungs includes an in-depth look at ventilatory and respiratory functions of the lungs. If the lungs are affected by disease, other body systems are also affected. For example, reduced oxygenation can cause changes in mental alertness because of the brain's sensitivity to lowered oxygen levels. This data is used from all body systems to determine the nature of pulmonary alterations.

Before assessing the thorax and lungs, you must be familiar with the landmarks of the chest (Figure 12-19). These landmarks help you locate findings and use assessment skills correctly. The client's nipples, angle of Louis, suprasternal notch, costal angle, clavicles, and vertebrae are key landmarks that provide a series of imaginary lines for sign identification. You should keep a mental image of the location of the lobes of the lung and the position of each rib (Figure 12-20). The proper orientation to anatomical structures ensures a thorough assessment of the anterior, lateral, and posterior thorax.

Locating the position of each rib is critical to visualizing the lobe of the lung being assessed. The angle of Louis, at the

junction between the manubrium and the body of the sternum, is the starting point for locating the ribs anteriorly. Knowing that the second rib extends from the angle makes it easy to locate and palpate the intercostal spaces (between the ribs) in succession. The spinous process of the third thoracic vertebra and the fourth, fifth, and sixth ribs serve to locate the lobes of the lung laterally (Figure 12-21). The lower lobes project laterally and anteriorly.

Posteriorly the tip or inferior margin of the scapula lies approximately at the level of the seventh rib. After the seventh rib is identified, you can count upward to locate the third thoracic vertebra and align it with the inner borders of the scapula to locate the posterior lobes (Figure 12-22).

The examination requires the client to be undressed to the waist, with good lighting. The examination begins with the client sitting for assessment of the posterior and lateral chest. The client may sit or lie for assessment of the anterior chest.

Health History

A complete health history includes determining if the client has a history of tobacco or marijuana use, including number of years smoked, age started, number of cigarettes or cigars daily, and length of time since smoking stopped. To screen for warning signals of lung cancer, ask if the client has a persistent cough, sputum production, chest pain, or recurrent attacks of pneumonia or bronchitis. Asking the client about symptoms of **orthopnea,** shortness of breath, **dyspnea** during exertion or at rest, and poor activity tolerance can reveal cardiopulmonary problems. A client's risk for having lung disease is further assessed by reviewing presence of pollutants in the work environment or at home and reviewing the client's family history for cancer, tuberculosis, allergies, or chronic obstructive pulmonary disease.

Tuberculosis is on the increase in the United States. Be alert for clients at risk, including persons with HIV infection, sub-

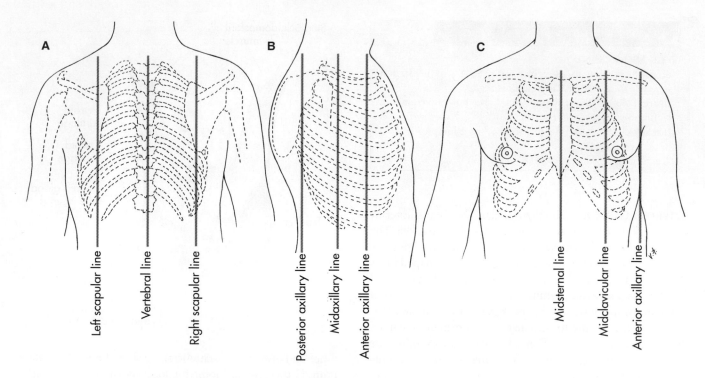

FIGURE **12-19**   Anatomical chest wall landmarks. **A,** Posterior chest. **B,** Lateral chest. **C,** Anterior chest.

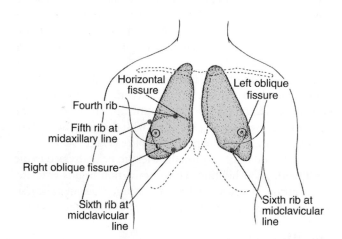

FIGURE **12-20**   Anterior position of lung lobes in relation to anatomical landmarks.

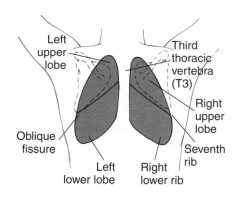

FIGURE **12-22**   Posterior position of lung lobes in relation to anatomical landmarks.

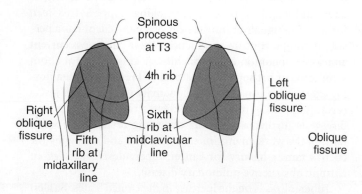

FIGURE **12-21**   Lateral position of lung lobes in relation to anatomical landmarks.

stance abusers, residents of nursing homes, low-income individuals, and recent immigrants to the United States (Haney and others, 1996; Hopkins and Schoener, 1996). Evaluate at-risk clients and those who exhibit symptoms of persistent cough, hemoptysis, unexplained weight loss, fatigue, anorexia, night sweats, and fever for tuberculosis and/or HIV infection.

The history also includes assessment of allergies to airborne irritants, foods, drugs, or chemical substances. It is important to learn if a client has had a pneumonia or influenza vaccine and a tuberculosis test. The very young, very old, and those with chronic respiratory problems are at increased risk for disease. If the client has not been vaccinated, educate the individual on the need for vaccination to protect against illnesses.

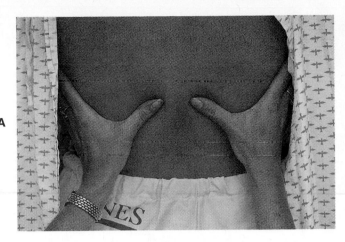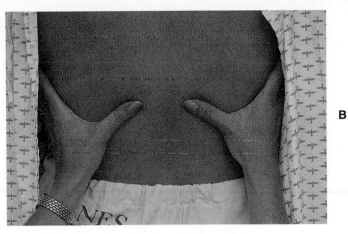

FIGURE **12-23**   **A,** Position of hands for palpation of posterior thorax excursion. **B,** When the client inhales, the movement of chest excursion separates the thumbs.

Posterior Thorax

Begin examination of the posterior thorax by observing for any signs or symptoms in other body systems that may indicate pulmonary problems. Reduced mental alertness, nasal flaring, somnolence, and cyanosis are examples of signs assessed during other portions of the examination that can indicate oxygenation problems. Inspect the posterior thorax by observing the shape and symmetry of the chest from the client's back and front. Note the anteroposterior diameter. Body shape or posture can significantly impair ventilatory movement. Normally the chest contour is symmetrical, with the anteroposterior diameter one third to one half the size of the transverse or side-to-side diameter. Aging and chronic lung disease are characterized by a barrel-shaped chest (anteroposterior diameter equals transverse). Infants have an almost round shape. Abnormal contours are caused by congenital and postural alterations. A client may lean over a table or splint the side of the chest because of a breathing problem. Splinting or holding the chest wall because of pain causes a client to bend toward the affected side. Such a posture impairs ventilatory movement.

Standing at a midline position behind the client, look for deformities, position of the spine, slope of the ribs, retraction of the intercostal spaces during inspiration, and bulging of the intercostal spaces during expiration. The spine is normally straight, and scapulae normally are symmetrical and closely attached to the chest wall. The spine normally is straight without lateral deviation. Posteriorly, the ribs tend to slope across and down. The ribs and intercostal spaces are easier to see in a thin person. Normally no bulging or active movement occurs within the intercostal spaces during breathing. Bulging indicates that the client is using great effort to breathe.

You may also assess the rate and rhythm of breathing at this time (see Chapter 11). Observe the thorax as a whole. The thorax normally expands and relaxes with equality of movement bilaterally. In healthy adults the normal respiratory rates vary from 12 to 20 respirations per minute.

Palpation of the posterior thorax assesses further characteristics. Palpate the thoracic muscles and skeleton for lumps, masses, pulsations, and unusual movement. If pain or tenderness is noted, avoid deep palpation. Fractured rib fragments could be displaced against vital organs. Normally the chest wall is not tender. If you detect a suspicious mass or swollen area, lightly palpate it for size, shape, and typical qualities of a lesion.

To measure chest excursion or depth of breathing, stand behind the client and place the thumbs along the spinal processes at the tenth rib, with the palms lightly contacting the posterolateral surfaces. Place your thumbs about 5 cm (2 inches) apart, pointing toward the spine and fingers pointing laterally (Figure 12-23, *A*). Press the hands toward the spine so that a small skinfold appears between the thumbs. Do not slide the hands over the skin. Instruct the client to take a deep breath after exhaling. Note movement of the thumbs (Figure 12-23, *B*). Chest excursion should be symmetrical, separating the thumbs 3 to 5 cm ($1\frac{1}{4}$ to 2 inches). Reduced chest excursion may be caused by pain, postural deformity, or fatigue. In older adults, chest excursion normally declines because of costal cartilage calcification and respiratory muscle atrophy.

During speech the sound created by the vocal cords is transmitted through the lung to the chest wall. The sound waves create vibrations that can be palpated externally. These vibrations are called **tactile fremitus** or **vocal fremitus.** The buildup of mucus secretions, the collapse of lung tissue, or the presence of lung lesions can block the vibrations from reaching the chest wall. This technique is used by more experienced nurses.

Auscultation assesses the movement of air through the tracheobronchial tree and detects mucus or obstructed airways. Normally air flows through the airways in an unobstructed pattern. Recognizing the sounds created by normal air flow allows for detection of sounds caused by airway obstruction.

Place the diaphragm of the stethoscope over the posterior chest wall between the ribs. The client folds the arms in front of the chest and keeps the head bent forward while taking slow, deep breaths with the mouth slightly open. Listen to an entire inspiration and expiration at each position of the

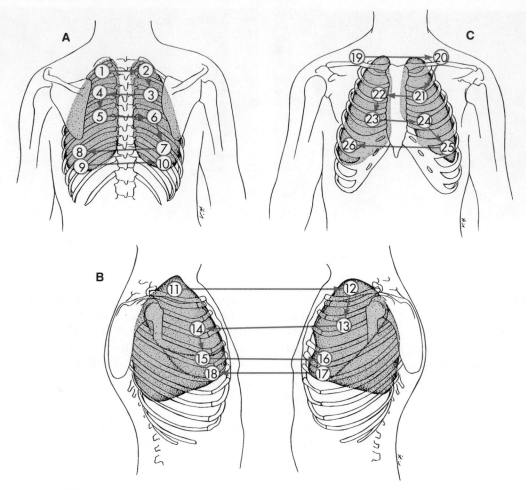

FIGURE **12-24**   **A** to **C,** A systematic pattern (posterior-lateral-anterior) is followed for auscultation.

stethoscope (Figure 12-24, *A*). If sounds are faint, as with an obese client, ask the client to breathe harder and faster temporarily. Breath sounds are much louder in children because of their thin chest walls. In children the bell works best because of a child's small chest. Use a systematic pattern comparing the sounds in one region on one side of the body with sounds in the same region on the opposite side.

Auscultate for normal breath sounds and abnormal sounds (**adventitious sounds**). Normal breath sounds differ in character, depending on the area being auscultated. Sounds normally heard over the posterior thorax include bronchovesicular and vesicular sounds. Bronchovesicular sounds are medium-pitched blowing sounds normally heard posteriorly between the scapulae. The sounds have equal inspiratory and expiratory phases. The character of bronchovesicular sounds is related to the larger underlying airways. Vesicular sounds are heard over the periphery of the lungs. The sounds are created by air moving through the smaller airways. Vesicular sounds are soft, breezy, and low pitched, and the inspiratory phase is about three times longer than the expiratory phase.

Abnormal sounds result from air passing through moisture, mucus, or narrowed airways. They can also result from alveoli suddenly reinflating or from an inflammation be-

tween the pleural linings of the lung. Adventitious sounds often occur superimposed over normal sounds. The four types of adventitious sounds are **crackles, rhonchi, wheezes,** and **pleural friction rub.** Each sound is caused by a specific entity and is characterized by typical auditory features (Table 12-6). During auscultation note the location and characteristics of the sounds and listen for the absence of breath sounds (found in clients with collapsed or surgically removed lobes).

Lateral Thorax

Usually you extend the assessment of the posterior thorax to the lateral sides of the chest (Figure 12-24, *B*). The client sits during the lateral chest examination. Also have the client raise the arms to improve access to lateral thoracic structures. Use inspection, palpation, and auscultation skills. Excursion cannot be assessed laterally. Normally the breath sounds heard are vesicular.

Anterior Thorax

Inspect the anterior thorax for the same features as the posterior thorax. The client sits or lies down with the head elevated. Observe the accessory muscles of breathing: sternocleidomastoid, trapezius, and abdominal muscles. The accessory muscles move little with normal passive breathing.

Adventitious Sounds — Table 12-6

Sound	Site Asculated	Cause	Character
Crackles	Are most commonly heard in dependent lobes: right and left lung bases	Random, sudden reinflation of groups of alveoli; disruptive passage of air	Fine crackles are high-pitched fine, short, interrupted crackling sounds heard during end of inspiration, usually not cleared with coughing. Moist crackles are lower, more moist sounds heard during middle of inspiration; not cleared with coughing. Coarse crackles are loud, bubbly sounds heard during inspiration, not cleared with coughing
Rhonchi (sonorous wheeze)	Are primarily heard over trachea and bronchi; if loud enough, can be heard over most lung fields	Muscular spasm, fluid, or mucus in larger airways, causing turbulence	Are loud, low-pitched, rumbling coarse sounds heard most often during inspiration or expiration; may be cleared by coughing
Wheezes (sibilant wheeze)	Can be heard over all lung fields	High-velocity airflow through severely narrowed bronchus	Are high-pitched, continuous musical sounds like a squeak heard continuously during inspiration or expiration; usually louder on expiration; do not clear with coughing
Pleural friction rub	Is heard over anterior lateral lung field (if client is sitting upright)	Inflamed pleura, parietal pleura rubbing against visceral pleura	Has dry, grating quality heard best during inspiration; does not clear with coughing; heard loudest over lower lateral anterior surface

Data from Basfield-Holland ES: Assessing pulmonary status: it's more than listening to breath sounds, *Nursing 97* 27(8):32, 1997; and Seidel HM and others: *Mosby's guide to physical examination*, ed 4, St. Louis, 1999, Mosby.

When a client requires effort to breathe as a result of strenuous exercise or disease (Box 12-14), the accessory muscles and abdominal muscles contract. Some clients may produce a grunting sound.

Observe the width of the costal angle. It is usually larger than 90 degrees between the two costal margins. Respiratory rate and rhythm are more often assessed anteriorly (see Chapter 11). The male client's respirations are usually diaphragmatic, whereas the female's are more costal.

Palpate the anterior thoracic muscles and skeleton for lumps, masses, tenderness, or unusual movement. The sternum and xiphoid are relatively inflexible. To measure chest excursion anteriorly, place your thumbs along the costal margin parallel 6 cm (2½ inches) apart with the palms touching the anterolateral chest. Push the thumbs toward the midline to create a skinfold. As the client inhales deeply, the thumbs should normally separate approximately 3 to 5 cm (1¼ to 2 inches), with each side expanding equally.

Auscultation of the anterior thorax also follows a systematic pattern (Figure 12-24, C). The client should sit, if possible, to maximize chest expansion. Give special attention to the lower lobes, where mucous secretions commonly gather. Bronchovesicular and vesicular sounds are heard above and below the clavicles and along the lung periphery. An additional normal breath sound, a bronchial sound, can be heard over the trachea. Bronchial sounds are loud, high pitched,

LUNG ASSESSMENT

- Explain the risk factors for chronic lung disease and lung cancer, including cigarette smoking, history of smoking for over 20 years, exposure to environmental pollution, and radiation exposure from occupational, medical, and environmental sources. Residential radon exposure may also increase risk, especially for cigarette smokers. Exposure to sidestream cigarette smoke increases risk for nonsmokers.
- Share brochures on lung cancer from the American Cancer Society with client and family.
- Discuss the warning signs of lung cancer, such as a persistent cough, sputum streaked with blood, chest pains, and recurrent attacks of pneumonia or bronchitis.
- Counsel older adults on benefits of receiving influenza and pneumonia vaccinations because of a greater susceptibility to respiratory infection.
- Persons at risk for tuberculosis who visit clinics or health care centers should be referred for skin testing.
- Instruct clients with chronic obstructive pulmonary disease in coughing and pursed-lip–breathing exercises.

and hollow sounding, with expiration lasting longer than inspiration (3:2 ratio).

HEART

Compare your assessment of heart function with findings from the vascular examination. Alterations in either system may be manifested as changes in the other. A client with signs and symptoms of heart problems may have a life-threatening condition requiring immediate attention. In this case, you quickly act and conduct only portions of the examination that are absolutely necessary. When a client is more stable, you will conduct a more thorough examination.

Assess cardiac function through the anterior thorax. You should form a mental image of the heart's exact location (Figure 12-25). In the adult the heart is located in the center of the chest (precordium) behind and to the left of the sternum, with a small section of the right atrium extending to the right of the sternum. The base of the heart is the upper portion, and the apex is the bottom tip. The surface of the right ventricle comprises most of the heart's anterior surface. A section of the left ventricle shapes the left anterior side of the apex. The apex actually touches the anterior chest wall at approximately the fourth to fifth intercostal space along the midclavicular line. This is known as the apical impulse.

An infant's heart is positioned more horizontally. The apex of the heart is at the third or fourth intercostal space, just to the left of the midclavicular line. By the age of 7 years a child's apical impulse is in the same location as the adult's. In tall, slender persons the heart hangs more vertically and is positioned more centrally. With increased stockiness and shortness, the heart tends to lie more to the left and horizontally (Seidel and others, 1999).

To assess heart function, the cardiac cycle and the physiological signs of each event must be understood (Figure

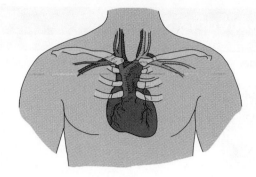

FIGURE **12-25** Anatomical position of the heart.

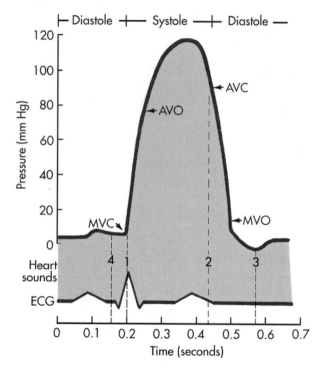

FIGURE **12-26** Cardiac cycle. *MVC,* Mitral valve closes; *AVO,* aortic valve opens; *AVC,* aortic valve closes, *MVO,* mitral valve opens.

12-26). The heart normally pumps blood through its four chambers in a methodical, even sequence. Events on the left side occur just before those on the right. As the blood flows through each chamber, valves open and close, pressures within chambers rise and fall, and chambers contract. Each event creates a physiological sign. Both sides of the heart function in a coordinated fashion.

There are two phases to the cardiac cycle: systole and diastole. During systole the ventricles contract and eject blood from the left ventricle into the aorta and from the right ventricle into the pulmonary artery. During diastole the ventricles relax and the atria contract to move blood into the ventricles and fill the coronary arteries.

Heart sounds occur in relation to physiological events in the cardiac cycle. As systole begins, ventricular pressure rises and closes the mitral and tricuspid valves. Valve closure

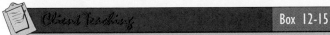

Box 12-15

HEART ASSESSMENT
- Explain the risk factors for heart disease, including high dietary intake or saturated fat or cholesterol, lack of regular aerobic exercise, smoking, excess weight, stressful lifestyle, hypertension, and family history of heart disease.
- Refer clients (appropriate) to resources available for controlling or reducing risks (e.g., nutritional counseling, exercise class, stress reduction programs).
- Recommend reduction in dietary intake of cholesterol and saturated fats. The National Institutes of Health recommends a daily intake of total fat less than 30% of calories, saturated fatty acids less than 10% of calories, and cholesterol less than 300 mg/100 ml.
- Encourage clients to have regular measurements of blood pressure and blood cholesterol and triglycerides.
- Clients who have known angina may benefit from taking a daily low dose of aspirin. Consult physician before starting therapy.

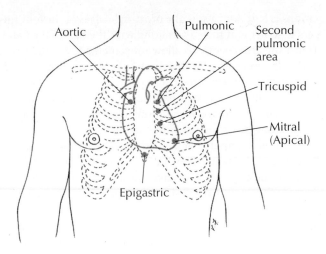

FIGURE **12-27**   Anatomical sites for assessment of cardiac function.

causes the first heart sound (S_1), often described as "lub." The ventricles then contract, and blood flows through the aorta and pulmonary circulation. After the ventricles empty, ventricular pressure falls below that in the aorta and pulmonary artery. This allows the aortic and pulmonary valves to close, causing the second heart sound (S_2), described as "dub." As ventricular pressure continues to fall, it drops below that of the atria. The mitral and tricuspid valves reopen to allow ventricular filling. Rapid ventricular filling may create a third heart sound (S_3). This is heard more often in children and young adults. An S_3 can also be heard as an abnormality in adults over 30 years of age. A fourth heart sound (S_4) may be heard when the atria contract to enhance ventricular filling. The S_4 is not normally heard in adults but may be heard in healthy older adults, children, and athletes. Because S_4 may also indicate an abnormal condition, it should be reported to a physician.

Health History

The health history should focus on risk factors for cardiovascular disease (Box 12-15). Assess the client's history of smoking, alcohol intake, caffeine intake, use of prescriptive and recreational drugs, exercise habits, and dietary patterns including fat and sodium intake. Does the client have a stressful lifestyle? If so, what are the physical demands or emotional stresses? It is important to know if the client takes medications for cardiovascular function (e.g., antidysrhythmics or antihypertensives). Also assess for signs and symptoms suggestive of heart disease, including chest pain or discomfort, **palpitations,** excess fatigue, cough, dyspnea, edema of the feet, cyanosis, fainting, or orthopnea. If the client reports chest pain, determine if it is cardiac in nature; anginal pain is usually a deep pressure or ache that is substernal and diffuse, radiating to one or both arms, the neck, or the jaw. Determine whether the client has preexisting diabetes, lung disease, obesity, or hypertension. Finally, assess the client's personal and family history for heart disease.

Inspection and Palpation

Use the skills of inspection and palpation simultaneously. The examination begins with the client supine and the upper body elevated 45 degrees because clients with heart disease frequently suffer shortness of breath while lying flat. Stand at the client's right side. The client must not talk, especially when you auscultate heart sounds. Good lighting in the room is essential.

Direct your attention to the anatomical sites best suited for assessment of cardiac function. The sternal angle or angle of Louis can be felt as a ridge in the sternum approximately 2 inches below the sternal notch. Slip your fingers along the angle on each side of the sternum to feel the adjacent ribs. The intercostal spaces are just below each rib. The second intercostal space allows for identification of each of the six anatomical landmarks (Figure 12-27). The second intercostal space on the right is the aortic area, and the left second intercostal space is the pulmonic area. Deeper palpation is needed to feel the spaces in obese or heavily muscled clients. After locating the pulmonic area, move your fingers down the client's left sternal border to the third intercostal space, called the second pulmonic area. The tricuspid area is located at the fourth left intercostal space along the sternum. To find the apical area or **point of maximal impulse (PMI),** locate the fifth intercostal space just to the left of the sternum and move your fingers laterally to the left midclavicular line. Locate the apical area with the palm of the hand, or your fingertips. Normally at the apical impulse the apical pulse is a light tap felt in an area 1 to 2 cm ($1\frac{1}{2}$ inches) in diameter at the apex. Another landmark is the epigastric area at the tip of the sternum. It is typically used to palpate for aortic abnormalities.

As you locate the six anatomical landmarks of the heart, each area is inspected and palpated. Look for the appearance of pulsations, viewing each area over the chest at an angle to the side. Normally no pulsations can be seen except perhaps at the apical impulse in thin clients or at the epigastric area as a result of abdominal aortic pulsation. Palpation for pulsations is best done using the proximal halves of the four fingers together and then alternating with the ball of the hand. Touch the areas gently to allow movements to lift the hand. Normally no pulsations or vibrations can be felt in the second, third, or fourth intercostal spaces. A vibration is caused by loud murmurs. If you palpate pulsations or vibrations, time their occurrence in relation to systole or diastole by auscultating heart sounds simultaneously.

The apical impulse or PMI should be felt easily. If not, have the client turn onto the left side, moving the heart closer to the chest wall. Estimate the size of the heart by noting the diameter of the PMI and its position relative to the midclavicular line. In cases of serious heart disease, the cardiac muscle enlarges, with the PMI found to the left of the midclavicular line. The PMI may be difficult to find in older adults because the chest deepens in its anteroposterior diameter. It may also be difficult to find in muscular or overweight clients. An infant's PMI is usually at the third or fourth intercostal space. It is easy to palpate because of the child's thin chest wall.

Auscultation

Auscultation of the heart detects normal heart sounds, extra heart sounds, and **murmurs.** Concentration is needed to detect the low-intensity sounds caused by valve closure. To begin auscultation eliminate all sources of room noise and ex-

plain the procedure to relieve the client's anxiety. Follow a systematic pattern beginning with the aortic area and inching the stethoscope along each of the six landmarks. Be sure you hear the complete cycle (lub-dub) of heart sounds clearly at each location. Then repeat the sequence using the bell of the stethoscope. You may ask the client to assume three different positions during the examination (Figure 12-28):

- Sitting up and leaning forward (good for all areas and to hear high-pitched murmurs)
- Supine (good for all areas)
- Left lateral recumbent (good for all areas; best position to hear low-pitched sounds in diastole)

You must learn to identify the first (S_1) and second (S_2) heart sounds. At normal rates, S_1 occurs after the long diastolic pause and preceding the short systolic pause. S_1 is high pitched, dull in quality, and heard best at the apex. If you have difficulty hearing S_1, it can be timed in relation to the carotid pulse. It occurs just before the carotid pulsation. S_2 follows the short systolic phase and precedes the long diastolic phase. It is heard best at the aortic area.

Auscultate for rate and rhythm after both sounds can be heard clearly. Each combination of S_1 and S_2 or "lub-dub" counts as one heartbeat. Count the rate for 1 minute, and listen for the interval between S_1 and S_2, and then the time between S_2 and the next S_1. A regular rhythm involves regular intervals of time between each sequence of beats. There is a

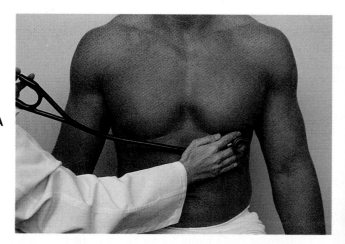
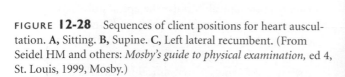
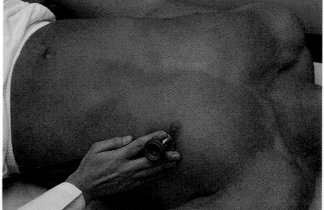
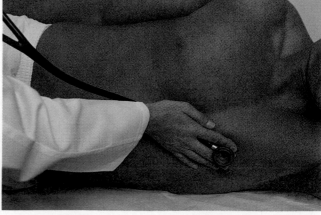

FIGURE **12-28** Sequences of client positions for heart auscultation. **A,** Sitting. **B,** Supine. **C,** Left lateral recumbent. (From Seidel HM and others: *Mosby's guide to physical examination,* ed 4, St. Louis, 1999, Mosby.)

distinct silent pause between S_1 and S_2. Failure of the heart to beat at regular successive intervals is a **dysrhythmia.** Some dysrhythmias can be life threatening.

When the heart rhythm is irregular, compare apical and radial pulse rates to determine if a pulse deficit exists. Auscultate the apical pulse first, and then immediately assess the radial pulse (one examiner technique). When two examiners are available, the apical and radial rates are assessed at the same time. Compare the two rates. When a client has a pulse deficit, the radial pulse is slower than the apical because ineffective contractions fail to send pulse waves to the periphery. Report a difference in pulse rates to the physician immediately.

Extra heart sounds and murmurs may be assessed at each auscultatory site. Assess these low-pitched sounds (such as S_3 and S_4 gallops, clicks, or rubs) using the bell of the stethoscope. Presence of these sounds usually indicates a pathologic condition and should be reported immediately. This portion of the examination is typically reserved for advanced practice nurses.

VASCULAR SYSTEM

Examination of the vascular system includes measuring the blood pressure (see Chapter 11) and assessing the integrity of the peripheral vascular system. Use the skills of inspection, palpation, and auscultation. Portions of the vascular examination may be performed during other body system assessments.

Health History

The history includes determining if the client has leg cramps, numbness or tingling in the extremities, or the continual sensation of cold hands or feet. These signs and symptoms may indicate vascular disease. Also learn if the client has noted swelling or cyanosis of the feet, ankles, or hand or pain in the feet or legs. If the client has leg pain or cramps, ask if symptoms are aggravated by walking or standing for long periods or during sleep. This question helps to clarify if the problem is musculoskeletal or vascular in nature. For example, arterial occlusion can create muscle ischemia or claudication. This particular type of pain is a dull ache and cramping, usually appearing during sustained exercise and disappearing after a short rest. Musculoskeletal pain is not generally relieved when exercise ends. You should also ask if clients wear tight-fitting garters or hosiery and sit or lie in bed with their legs crossed. These activities can impair venous return. The history includes a review of the client's medical history for heart disease, hypertension, phlebitis, diabetes, or varicose veins. Finally, risk factors assessed earlier for smoking, exercise, and nutritional problems are important when assessing the vascular system.

Carotid Arteries

When the left ventricle pumps blood into the aorta, pressure waves are transmitted through the arterial system. The carotid artery reflects heart function better than peripheral arteries, because its pressure correlates with that of the aorta.

The carotid artery supplies oxygenated blood to the head and neck (Figure 12-29) and is protected by the overlying sternocleidomastoid muscle.

To examine the carotid arteries, have the client sit or lie supine with the head of the bed elevated 15 to 30 degrees. Examine one carotid artery at a time. If you occlude both arteries simultaneously during palpation, the client could lose consciousness as a result of inadequate circulation to the brain. Do not palpate or massage the carotid arteries vigorously because the carotid sinus is in the upper third of the neck. The sinus sends impulses along the vagus nerve. Its stimulation can cause a reflex drop in heart rate and blood pressure, which causes **syncope** or circulatory arrest. This can be a particular problem for older adults.

Begin inspection of the neck for obvious pulsation of the artery. Have the client turn the head slightly away from the artery being examined. Sometimes you can see the wave of the pulse. An absent pulse wave can indicate arterial occlusion (blockage) or **stenosis** (narrowing).

To palpate the pulse, ask the client to look straight ahead or turn the head slightly to the side being examined. Turning relaxes the sternocleidomastoid muscle. Slide the tips of your index and middle fingers around the medial edge of the sternocleidomastoid muscle. Gently palpate to avoid occlusion of circulation (Figure 12-30).

The normal carotid pulse is localized rather than diffuse. As a strong pulse, the carotid has a thrusting quality. As the client breathes, no change occurs. Rotation of the neck or a shift from a sitting to a supine position should not change the carotid's quality. Both carotid arteries should be equal in pulse rate, rhythm, and strength and should be equally elastic. Diminished or unequal carotid pulsations may indicate **atherosclerosis** or other forms of arterial disease.

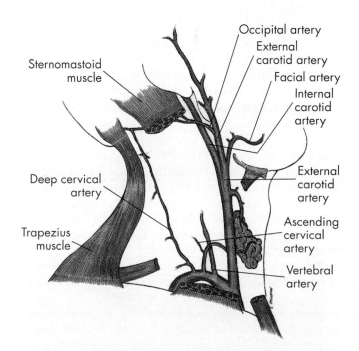

FIGURE **12-29** Anatomical position of carotid artery.

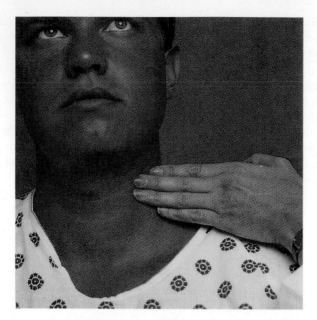

FIGURE **12-30** Palpation of the internal carotid artery.

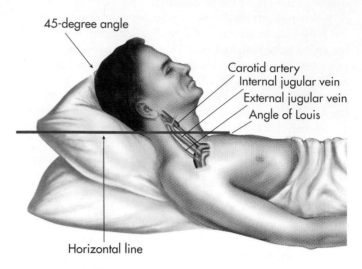

FIGURE **12-31** Position of client to assess jugular vein distention. (From Thompson JM and others: *Mosby's clinical nursing,* ed 5, St. Louis, 2001, Mosby.)

The carotid is the most commonly auscultated pulse. Auscultation is especially important for middle-age or older adults or clients suspected of having cerebrovascular disease. When the lumen of a blood vessel is narrowed, its blood flow is disturbed. As blood passes through the narrowed section, a turbulence is created, causing a blowing or swishing sound. The blowing sound is called a **bruit** (pronounced "brew-ee"). Place the bell of the stethoscope over the carotid artery at the base of the neck and move it gradually toward the jaw. Ask clients to hold their breath for a moment so that breath sounds do not obscure a bruit. Normally no sound is heard during carotid auscultation. If you hear a bruit, gently palpate the artery lightly for a **thrill** (palpable bruit).

Jugular Veins

The most accessible veins for examination are the internal and external jugular veins in the neck. Both veins drain bilaterally from the head and neck into the superior vena cava. The external jugular lies superficially and can be seen just above the clavicle. The internal jugular lies deeper, along the carotid artery. Normally when a client lies in the supine position, the external jugular distends and becomes easily visible. In contrast, the jugular veins normally flatten when the client is in a sitting or standing position. A client with heart disease, however, may have distended jugular veins when sitting.

As an entry-level nurse you can learn to assess for jugular venous distention. Inspect the client's jugular veins in the supine position (normally veins protrude), when standing (normally veins are flat), and when sitting at a 45-degree angle (jugular veins distended only if client has right-sided heart failure) (Figure 12-31). The specific measurement of jugular venous pressure is completed by an advanced practitioner.

Peripheral Arteries

The most accurate assessment of peripheral arteries involves palpation over arteries that are close to the body surface and lie over bones. An arterial pulsation is a bounding wave of blood that diminishes in intensity with increasing distance from the heart (Seidel and others, 1999).

Assess the arterial pulses in the extremities to determine sufficiency of the entire arterial circulation. Factors such as coagulation disorders, local trauma or surgery, constricting casts or bandages, and systemic disease such as diabetes or arteriosclerosis can impair circulation to the extremities. Discuss risk factors for circulatory problems with the client (Box 12-16).

Examine each peripheral artery using the distal pads of your second and third fingers. The thumb may help anchor the brachial and femoral artery. Apply firm pressure, but avoid occluding a pulse. When a pulse is difficult to find, it may help to vary pressure and feel all around the pulse site. Be sure not to palpate your own pulse.

Routine vital signs usually include assessment of the rate and rhythm of the radial artery, because it is easily accessible (see Chapter 11). Count the pulse for either 30 seconds or a full minute, depending on the character of the pulse. With palpation the pulse wave is normally felt at regular intervals. When an interval is interrupted by an early, late, or missed beat, the pulse rhythm is irregular. In emergencies the carotid artery is chosen because it is accessible and closest to the heart and thus most useful in evaluating heart activity. To check local circulatory status of tissues, palpate the peripheral arteries long enough to note that a pulse is present.

Assess each peripheral artery for elasticity of vessel wall, strength, and equality. The arterial wall is normally elastic, making it easily palpable. After the artery is depressed, it will spring back to shape when pressure is released. An abnormal artery may be described as hard, inelastic, or calcified.

The strength of a pulse is a measurement of the force with which blood is ejected against the arterial wall. Some examiners use a rating from 0 (zero) to 4+ (Seidel and others, 1999):

0   Absent, not palpable
1+ Pulse is diminished, barely palpable
2+ Easily palpable, normal pulse
3+ Full, increased pulse
4+ Bounding, cannot be obliterated

Measure all peripheral pulses for equality and symmetry. Compare the left radial pulse with that of the right, the left brachial pulse with that of the left radial, and so on. Lack of symmetry may indicate impaired circulation such as a localized obstruction or an abnormally positioned artery.

In the upper extremities the brachial artery channels blood to the radial and ulnar arteries of the forearm and hand. If circulation in this artery becomes blocked, the hands will not receive adequate blood flow. If circulation in the radial or ulnar arteries becomes impaired, the hand will still receive adequate perfusion. An interconnection between the radial and ulnar arteries guards against arterial occlusion (Figure 12-32).

To locate pulses in the arm, have the client sit or lie down. You will find the radial pulse along the radial side of the forearm at the wrist. In a thin individual a groove is formed lateral to the flexor tendon of the wrist. The radial pulse can be felt with light palpation in the groove (Figure 12-33). The ulnar pulse is on the opposite side of the wrist and feels less prominent (Figure 12-34). Palpate the ulnar pulse only when you expect arterial insufficiency to the hand.

To palpate the brachial pulse, find the groove between the biceps and triceps muscle above the elbow at the antecubital fossa (Figure 12-35). The artery runs along the medial side of the extended arm. Palpate the artery with the fingertips of your first three fingers in the muscle groove.

The femoral artery is the primary artery in the leg, delivering blood to the popliteal, posterior tibial, and dorsalis pedis arteries (Figure 12-36). An interconnection between the posterior tibial and dorsalis pedis arteries guards against

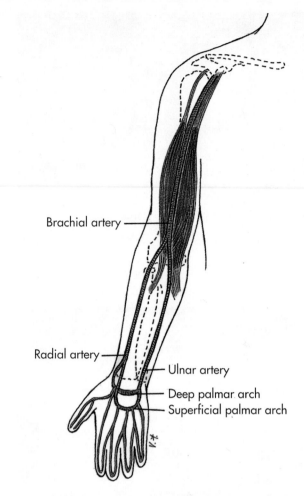

Brachial artery

Radial artery

Ulnar artery

Deep palmar arch

Superficial palmar arch

FIGURE **12-32** Anatomical positions of brachial, radial, and ulnar arteries.

local arterial occlusion. Find the femoral pulse with the client lying down with the inguinal area exposed (Figure 12-37). The femoral artery runs below the inguinal ligament, midway between the symphysis pubis and the anterosuperior iliac spine. You may need to use deep palpation to feel the pulse. Bimanual palpation is effective in obese clients. Place your fingertips of both hands on opposite sides of the pulse site. A pulsatile sensation can be felt as the fingertips are pushed apart by the arterial pulsation.

The popliteal pulse runs behind the knee (Figure 12-38). The client should slightly flex the knee with the foot resting on the examination table. The client may also assume a prone position with the knee slightly flexed. Instruct the client to keep leg muscles relaxed. Palpate with the fingers of both hands deeply into the popliteal fossa, just lateral to the midline. The popliteal pulse is difficult to locate.

With the client's foot relaxed locate the dorsalis pedis pulse. The artery runs along the top of the foot in a line with the groove between the extensor tendons of the great toe and first toe (Figure 12-39). You can often find the pulse by placing your fingertips between the great and first toe and slowly inching up the foot. This pulse may be congenitally absent.

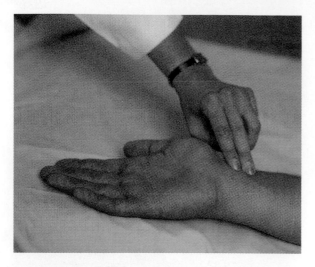

FIGURE 12-33   Palpation of radial pulse.

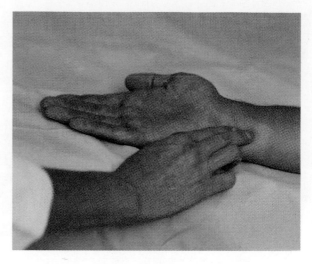

FIGURE 12-34   Palpation of ulnar pulse.

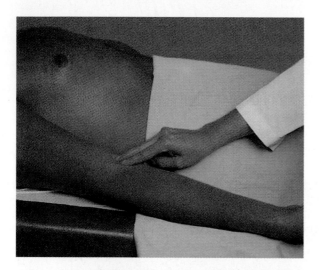

FIGURE 12-35   Palpation of brachial pulse.

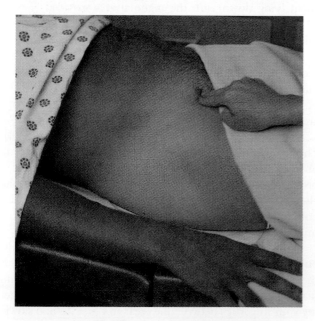

FIGURE 12-37   Palpation of femoral pulse.

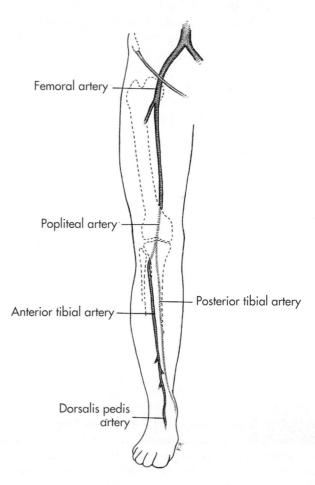

Femoral artery

Popliteal artery

Anterior tibial artery

Posterior tibial artery

Dorsalis pedis artery

FIGURE 12-36   Anatomical position of femoral, popliteal, dorsalis pedis, and posterior tibial arteries.

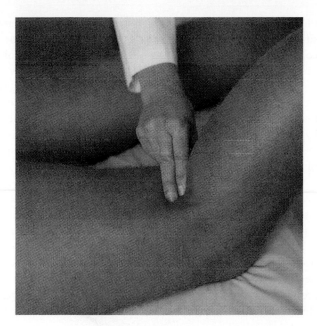

FIGURE **12-38**   Palpation of popliteal pulse.

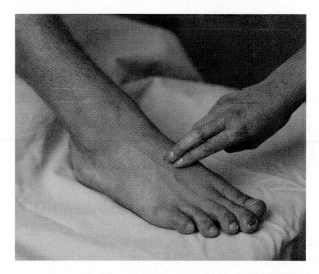

FIGURE **12-39**   Palpation of dorsalis pedis pulse.

The posterior tibial pulse is found on the inner side of each ankle (Figure 12-40). Place your fingers behind and below the client's medial malleolus (ankle bone). The artery is easily located with the client's foot relaxed and slightly extended.

ULTRASOUND STETHOSCOPES.   If you have difficulty palpating a pulse, an ultrasound stethoscope is a useful tool that amplifies sounds of a pulse wave. Apply a thin layer of transmission gel to the client's skin at the pulse site or directly onto the transducer tip of the probe. Turn the volume control "on" and place the tip of the probe at a 45- to 90-degree angle on the skin. Move the probe until hearing a pulsating "whooshing" sound that indicates that arterial blood flow is present.

Tissue Perfusion

The condition of the skin, mucosa, and nail beds offers useful data about the status of circulatory blood flow. Examine the face and upper extremities first, looking at the color of skin, mucosa, and nail beds. The presence of cyanosis requires special attention. Central cyanosis, which indicates poor arterial oxygenation, may be caused by heart disease. It can be noted by a bluish discoloration of the lips, mouth, and conjunctivae. Peripheral cyanosis, which indicates peripheral vasoconstriction, is noted by blue lips, earlobes, and nail beds. When cyanosis is present, consult with a physician to have laboratory testing of oxygen saturation to determine severity of the problem. Examination of the nails involves inspection for **clubbing,** a bulging of the tissues at the nail base. Clubbing is caused by insufficient oxygenation at the periphery resulting from conditions such as congenital heart disease and chronic emphysema.

Inspect the lower extremities for changes in color, temperature, and condition of the skin indicating either arterial

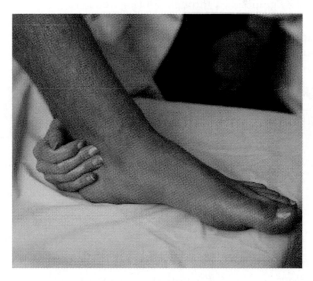

FIGURE **12-40**   Palpation of posterior tibial pulse.

or venous alterations (Table 12-7). This is a good time to ask the client about history of pain in the legs. If an arterial occlusion is present, the client has signs resulting from absence of blood flow. Pain will be distal to the occlusion. The three P's characterize an occlusion—pain, pallor, and pulselessness. Venous congestion causes tissue changes indicating inadequate circulatory flow back to the heart.

During examination of the lower extremities, you also inspect skin and nail texture; hair distribution on the lower legs, feet, and toes; venous pattern; and scars, pigmentation, or ulcers. The absence of hair growth over the legs may indicate circulatory insufficiency. Do not be mislead by shaven lower legs. Also, many men have less hair around the calves because of tight-fitting dress socks or jeans. Chronic recurring ulcers of the feet or lower legs are a serious sign of circulatory insufficiency and require a physician's intervention.

Peripheral Veins

Assess the status of the peripheral veins by asking the client to assume sitting and standing positions. Assessment includes inspection and palpation for varicosities, peripheral edema, and phlebitis. Varicosities are superficial veins that become dilated, especially when legs are in a dependent position. They are common in older adults because the veins normally fibrose, dilate, and stretch. They are also common in people who stand for prolonged periods. Varicosities in the anterior or medial part of the thigh and the posterolateral part of the calf are abnormal.

Dependent edema around the feet and ankles can be a sign of venous insufficiency or right-sided heart failure. Dependent edema is common in older adults and persons who spend a lot of time standing (e.g., nurses, waitresses, and security guards). To assess for pitting edema use your thumb to press firmly 1 to 2 seconds and then release over the medial malleolus or the shins. A depression left in the skin indicates edema. The severity of the edema is characterized by grading +1 through +4 (Figure 12-41).

Phlebitis is an inflammation of a vein that occurs commonly after trauma to the vessel wall, infection, immobilization, or prolonged insertion of IV catheters (see Chapter 14).

Phlebitis promotes clot formation, a potentially dangerous situation because a clot within a deep vein of the leg can become dislodged and travel through the heart, causing a pulmonary embolus. To assess for phlebitis inspect the calves for localized redness, tenderness, and swelling over vein sites. Gentle palpation of calf muscles reveals tenderness and firmness of the muscle. You may also check for Homans' sign by supporting the leg while dorsiflexing the foot. If phlebitis is present in the lower leg, forceful dorsiflexion of the foot often causes pain in the calf.

Lymphatic System

Assess the lymphatic drainage of the lower extremities during examination of the vascular system or during the female or male genital examination. The legs are drained by superficial and deep lymph nodes, but only two groups of superficial nodes are palpable. With the client supine, palpate the area of the superior superficial nodes in the groin area (Figure 12-42). Then move your fingertips toward the inner

Signs of Venous and Arterial Insufficiency		Table 12-7
Assessment Criterion	Venous	Arterial
Color	Normal or cyanotic	Pale; worsened by elevation of extremity; dusky red when extremity lowered
Temperature	Normal	Cool (blood flow blocked to extremity)
Pulse	Normal	Decreased or absent
Edema	Often marked	Absent or mild
Skin changes	Brown pigmentation around ankles	Thin, shiny skin; decreased hair growth; thickened nails

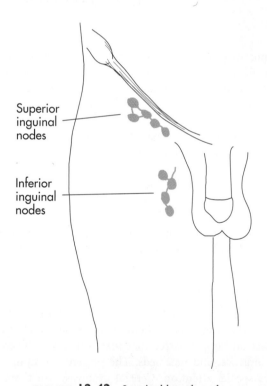

FIGURE **12-42** Inguinal lymph nodes.

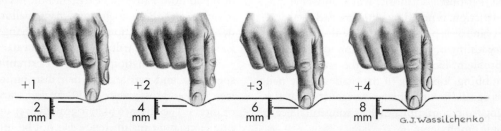

FIGURE **12-41** Assessing for pitting edema. (From Seidel HM and others: *Mosby's guide to physical examination,* ed 4, St. Louis, 1999. Mosby.)

thigh, feeling for any palpable inferior nodes. Use a firm but gentle pressure when palpating over each lymphatic chain. Multiple nodes are not normally palpable, although a few soft, nontender nodes are not unusual. Enlarged, hardened, tender nodes can reveal potential sites of infection or metastatic disease.

BREASTS

It is important to examine the breasts of female and male clients. A small amount of glandular tissue, a potential site for the growth of cancer cells, is located in the male breast. In contrast, the majority of the female breast is glandular tissue.

Female Breasts

New cases of breast cancer affected 180,800 (approximately one in every nine) women in the United States in 2000 (American Cancer Society, 2001). The disease is second to lung cancer as the leading cause of death in women with cancer. Early detection is the key to cure. A major responsibility for you is to teach clients health behaviors such as breast self-examination (BSE) (Box 12-17). Studies suggest a minority of women actually perform BSE. You should know factors that increase the likelihood of a woman performing BSE.

If the client already performs a self-examination, assess the method she uses and the time she does the examination in relation to her menstrual cycle. The best time for a self-examination is on the last day of the menstrual period, when the breast is no longer swollen or tender from hormone elevations. If the woman is postmenopausal, she should check her breasts on the same day each month. The pregnant woman also must check her breasts on a monthly basis.

Older women may require special attention when reviewing the need for BSE. Many older women are limited by fixed incomes and thus fail to pursue regular clinical breast examination and mammography. Unfortunately, many older women ignore changes in their breasts, assuming they are a part of aging. In addition, physiological factors can affect the ease with which older women can perform BSE. Musculoskeletal limitations, diminished peripheral sensation, reduced eyesight, and changes in joint range of motion can limit palpation and inspection abilities. The nurse should find resources for older women, including free screening programs. Often family members can be taught to perform examinations.

The American Cancer Society (2001) recommends the following guidelines for the early detection of breast cancer:
1. BSE should be performed monthly by women 20 years of age and older.
2. An examination by a physician should be performed every 3 years from ages 20 to 40, and yearly for women over 40.
3. Women with a family history of breast cancer should have a yearly physician's examination.
4. Asymptomatic women should have a screening mammogram by age 40; women age 40 and over should have a mammogram annually.
5. For women age 35 or over with a history of breast cancer, a yearly examination is recommended.

The client's history should alert you to any signs of breast disease and normal development changes. Because of this glandular structure, the breast undergoes changes during a woman's life. Knowledge of these changes (Box 12-18) helps you complete an accurate assessment.

HEALTH HISTORY. A history can reveal risk factors for breast cancer, including women over age 40; women with a personal or family history of breast cancer; early-onset menarche (before age 12) or late-age menopause (after age 50); and women who have never had children, who gave birth to their first child after age 30, or who have not breast-fed their infants. A history should also determine whether a client (both sexes) has signs and symptoms of breast cancer such as a lump, thickening, pain, or tenderness of the breast; discharge, distortion, retraction, or scaling of the nipple; or change in breast size. Determine the client's use of medications such as oral contraceptives, digitalis, diuretics, steroids, estrogen, or foods high in fat. Assess the client's caffeine intake to review risk factors for fibrocystic disease. Ask if the client performs monthly BSE. If so, determine the time of month she performs the examination in relation to her menstrual cycle. Have the client describe or demonstrate the method used. If the client reports a breast mass, perform a symptom analysis.

INSPECTION. Have the client remove the top gown or drape to allow simultaneous visualization of both breasts. The client may stand or sit with her arms hanging loosely at her sides. If possible, place a mirror in front of the client during inspection so she can see what to look for when performing a self-examination. To recognize abnormalities, the client must be familiar with the normal appearance of her breasts.

Describe observations or findings in relation to imaginary lines that divide the breast into four quadrants and a tail. The lines cross at the center of the nipple. Each tail extends outward from the upper outer quadrant (Figure 12-43).

Inspect the breasts for size and symmetry. Normally the breasts extend from the third to the sixth ribs, with the nipple at the level of the fourth intercostal space. It is common for one breast to be smaller. However, a difference in size may be caused by inflammation or a mass. As the woman becomes older, the ligaments supporting the breast tissue weaken, causing the breasts to sag and the nipples to lower.

Observe the contour or shape of the breasts and note masses, flattening, retraction, or dimpling. Breasts vary in shape from convex to pendulous or conical. Retraction or dimpling results from invasion of underlying ligaments by tumors. The ligaments fibrose and pull the overlying skin inward toward the tumor. Edema also changes the contour of the breasts. To bring out the presence of retraction or changes in the shape of the breasts, ask the client to assume three positions: raise arms above the head, press hands against the hips, and extend arms straight ahead while sitting and leaning forward. Each maneuver causes a contraction of

Breast Self-Examination

Box 12-17

Breast self-examination (BSE) should be done once a month so that you become familiar with the usual appearance and feel of your breasts. Familiarity makes it easier to notice any changes in the breast from one month to another. Early discovery of a change from what is "normal" is the main idea behind BSE.

If you menstruate, the best time to do BSE is the last day of your menstrual cycle, when your breasts are least likely to be tender or swollen. If you no longer menstruate, pick a day, such as the first day of the month, to remind yourself it is time to do BSE.

Here is how to do BSE:

1. Stand before a mirror. Inspect both breasts for anything unusual, such as any discharge from the nipples, puckering, dimpling, or scaling of the skin.

    The next two steps are designed to emphasize any change in the shape or contour of your breasts. As you do them, you should be able to feel your chest muscles tighten.

2. Watching closely in the mirror, clasp hands behind your head and press hands forward.

3. Next, press hands firmly on hips and bow slightly toward your mirror as you pull your shoulders and elbows forward.

Some women do the next part of the examination in the shower. Fingers glide over soapy skin, making it easy to appreciate the texture underneath.

4. Raise your left arm. Use three or four fingers of your right hand to explore your left breast firmly, carefully, and thoroughly. Beginning at the outer edge, press the flat part of your fingers in small circles, moving the circles slowly around the breast. Gradually work toward the nipple. Be sure to cover the entire breast. Pay special attention to the area between the breast and the armpit, including the armpit itself. Feel for any unusual lump or mass under the skin.

5. Gently squeeze the nipple and look for a discharge. Repeat the exam on your right breast.

6. Steps 4 and 5 should be repeated lying down. Lie flat on your back, left arm over your head and a pillow or folded towel under your left shoulder. This position flattens the breast and makes it easier to examine. Use the same circular motion described earlier.

    Repeat on your right breast.

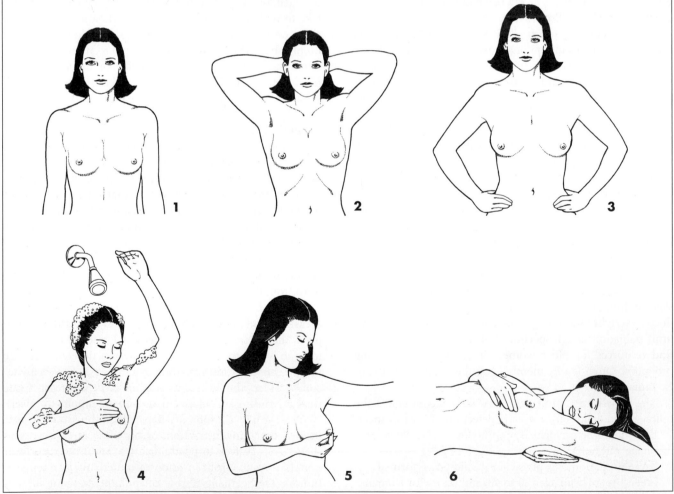

From Seidel HM and others: *Mosby's guide to physical examination*, ed 4, St. Louis, 1999, Mosby.

Normal Changes in the Breast During a Woman's Life Span   Box 12-18

PUBERTY (8 TO 20 YEARS)*

Breasts mature in five stages. One breast may grow more rapidly than the other. The ages at which changes occur and rate of developmental progression vary.

Stage 1 (Preadolescent)

This stage involves elevation of the nipple only.

Stage 2

The breast and nipple elevate as a small mound, and the areolar diameters enlarge.

Stage 3

There is further enlargement and elevation of the breast and areola, with no separation of contour.

Stage 4

The areola and nipple project into the secondary mound above the level of the breast (may not occur in all girls).

Stage 5 (Mature Breast)

Only the nipple projects, and the areola recedes (may vary in some women).

YOUNG ADULTHOOD (20 TO 30 YEARS)

Breasts reach full (nonpregnant) size. Shape is generally symmetrical. Breasts may be unequal in size.

PREGNANCY

Breast size gradually enlarges to two to three times the previous size. Nipples enlarge and may become erect. Areolae darken and diameters increase. Superficial veins become prominent. A yellowish fluid (colostrum) may be expelled from the nipples.

MENOPAUSE

Breasts shrink. Tissue becomes softer, sometimes flabby.

OLDER ADULTHOOD

Breasts become elongated, pendulous, and flaccid as a result of glandular tissue atrophy. The skin of the breasts tends to wrinkle, appearing loose and flabby.

Nipples become smaller, flatter, and lose erectile ability.[†] Nipples may invert because of shrinkage and fibrotic changes.[‡]

Data from:
*Wong D and others: *Whaley and Wong's nursing care of infants and children,* ed 6, St. Louis, 1999, Mosby.
[†]Seidel HM and others: *Mosby's guide to physical examination,* ed 4, St. Louis, 1999, Mosby.
[‡]Ebersole P, Hess P: *Toward healthy aging,* ed 5, St. Louis, 1998, Mosby.

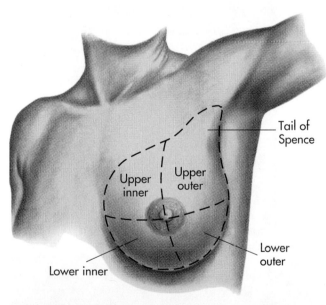

FIGURE **12-43** Quadrants of the left breast and axillary tail of Spence. (From Seidel HM and others: *Mosby's guide to physical examination,* ed 4, St. Louis, 1999, Mosby.)

the pectoral muscles, which will accentuate the presence of any retraction.

Carefully inspect the skin for color; venous pattern; and presence of edema, lesions, or inflammation. Lift each breast when necessary to observe lower and lateral aspects for color and texture changes. The breasts are the color of neighboring skin, and venous patterns are the same bilaterally. Venous patterns are more easily seen in thin clients or pregnant women. Women with large breasts often have redness and excoriation of the undersurface caused by rubbing of skin surfaces.

Inspect the nipple and areola for size, color, shape, discharge, and the direction the nipples point. The normal areolae are round or oval and nearly equal bilaterally. Color ranges from pink to brown. In light-skinned women the areola turns brown during pregnancy and remains dark. In dark-skinned women the areola is brown before pregnancy (Seidel and others, 1999). Normally the nipples point in symmetrical directions, are everted, and have no drainage. If the nipples are inverted, ask if this has been a lifetime history. A recent inversion or inward turning of the nipple may indicate an underlying growth. Rashes or ulcerations are not normal on the breast or nipples. Note any bleeding or discharge from the nipple. Clear yellow discharge 2 days after childbirth is common. While inspecting the breasts, explain the characteristics seen. The client must be taught the significance of abnormal signs or symptoms.

PALPATION.   Palpation allows you to determine the condition of underlying breast tissue and lymph nodes. Breast tissue consists of glandular tissue, fibrous supportive ligaments, and fat. Glandular tissue is organized into lobes that end in ducts opening onto the nipple's surface. The largest portion of glandular tissue is in the upper outer quadrant and tail of each breast. Suspensory ligaments connect to skin and fascia underlying the breast to support the breast and maintain its upright position. Fatty tissue is located superficially and to the sides of the breast.

A large proportion of lymph from the breasts drains into axillary lymph nodes. If cancerous lesions **metastasize** or spread, the nodes commonly become involved. You must learn the location of supraclavicular, infraclavicular, and axillary nodes (Figure 12-44). The axillary nodes drain lymph from the chest wall, breasts, arms, and hands. A tumor of one breast may involve nodes on the opposite side, as well as those on the same side.

To palpate lymph nodes have the client sit with arms at her sides and muscles relaxed. While facing the client and standing on the side being examined, support the client's arm in a flexed position and abduct the arm from the chest wall. Place your free hand against the client's chest wall and high in the axillary hollow (Figure 12-45). With your fingertips press gently down over the surface of the ribs and muscles. Palpate the axillary nodes with your fingertips gently rolling soft tissue. Palpate four areas of the axilla at the edge of the pectoralis major muscle along the anterior axillary line, the chest wall in the midaxillary area, the upper part of the humerus, and the anterior edge of the latissimus dorsi muscle along the posterior axillary line. Normally lymph nodes are not palpable. A palpable node feels like a small mass that may be hard, tender, and immobile. Also palpate

along the upper and lower clavicular ridges. Reverse the procedure for the client's other side.

It may be difficult for the client to learn to palpate for lymph nodes. Lying down with the arm abducted makes the area more accessible. Instruct your client to use her left hand for the right axillary and clavicular areas and vice versa. You can take the client's fingertips and move them in the proper fashion.

Palpation of breast tissue is best performed with the client lying supine and one arm behind the head (alternating with each breast). The supine position allows the breast tissue to flatten evenly against the chest wall. The client should raise her hand and place it behind the neck to further stretch and position breast tissue evenly (Figure 12-46, *A*). Place a small pillow or towel under the client's shoulder blade to further position breast tissue.

The consistency of normal breast tissue varies widely. The breasts of a young client are firm and elastic. In an older

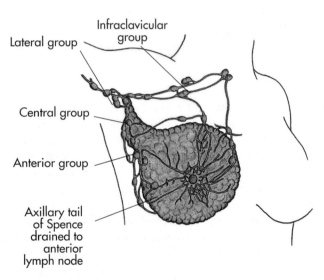

FIGURE **12-44** Anatomical position of axillary and clavicular lymph nodes.

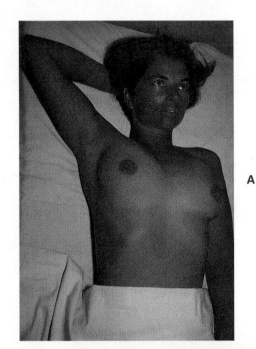

A

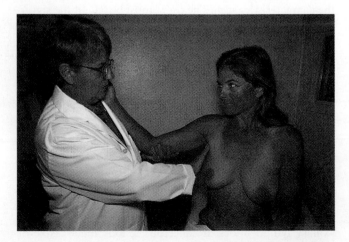

FIGURE **12-45** Support the client's arm while palpating axillary lymph nodes.

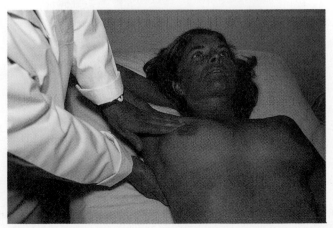

B

FIGURE **12-46** A, Client lies flat with arm abducted and hand under head to help flatten breast tissue evenly over the chest wall. B, Palpate each breast in systematic fashion.

client the tissue may feel stringy and nodular. The client's familiarity with the texture of her own breasts is most important. This familiarity is gained through monthly BSE (Box 12-19).

If the client complains of a mass, examine the opposite breast first to ensure an objective comparison of normal and abnormal tissue. Use the pads of your first three fingers to compress breast tissue gently against the chest wall, noting tissue consistency (Figure 12-46, *B*). Perform palpation systematically in one of three ways: *(A)* using a vertical technique with the fingers moving up and down each quadrant; *(B)* clockwise or counterclockwise, forming small circles with the fingers along each quadrant and the tail; or *(C)* palpating from center of the breast in a radial fashion, returning to the areola to begin each spoke (Fig. 12-47). Whatever approach is used, you must be sure to cover the entire breast and tail, directing attention to any areas of tenderness. When palpating large, pendulous breasts, use a bimanual technique. Support the inferior portion of the breast in one hand while you use your other hand to palpate breast tissue against the supporting hand.

During palpation note the consistency of breast tissue. It normally feels dense, firm, and elastic. With menopause, breast tissue shrinks and becomes softer. The lobular feel of glandular tissue is normal. The lower edge of each breast may feel firm and hard. This is the normal inframammary ridge and is not a tumor. It may help to move the client's hand so she can feel normal tissue variations. Palpate abnormal masses to determine location in relation to quadrants, diameter in centimeters, shape (e.g., round or discoid), consistency (soft, firm, or hard), tenderness, mobility, and discreteness (clear or unclear borders). Cancerous lesions are hard, fixed, nontender, irregular in shape, and usually unilateral.

A common benign condition of the breast is **fibrocystic breast disease.** This condition is characterized by bilateral lumpy, painful breasts and sometimes nipple discharge. Symptoms are more apparent during the menstrual period. When palpated, the cysts (lumps) are soft, well differentiated, and moveable. Deep cysts may feel hard.

Give special attention to palpating the nipple and areola. Palpate the entire surface gently. Use your thumb and index finger to compress the nipple, and note any discharge. As you examine the nipple and areola, the nipple may become erect with wrinkling of the areola. These changes are normal.

After completing the examination, have the client demonstrate self-palpation. Observe the client's technique, and emphasize the importance of a systematic approach. Urge the client to see her physician if she discovers an abnormal mass during monthly self-examination.

Male Breasts
Examination of the male breast is relatively easy. Inspect the nipple and areola for nodules, edema, and ulceration. An enlarged male breast may result from obesity or glandular en-

---

Client Teaching   Box 12-19

FEMALE BREAST ASSESSMENT
- Have the client perform return demonstration of BSE, and offer the opportunity to ask questions.
- Explain recommended frequency of mammography and assessment by a health care provider.
- Discuss signs and symptoms of breast cancer.
- Discuss signs and symptoms of fibrocystic disease.
- Inform a woman who is obese or who has a family history of breast cancer that she is at higher risk for the disease (American Cancer Society, 2000). Encourage dietary changes, including limiting meat consumption to well-trimmed, lean beef, pork, or lamb; removing skin from cooked chicken before eating it; selecting tuna and salmon packed in water and not oil; and using low-fat dairy products.
- Encourage the client to reduce intake of caffeine. Although controversial, decreasing caffeine intake is believed to reduce symptoms of fibrocystic disease.

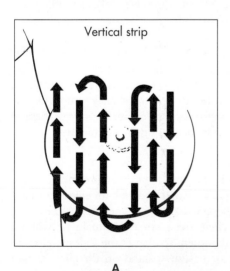

A

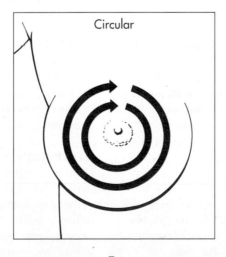

B

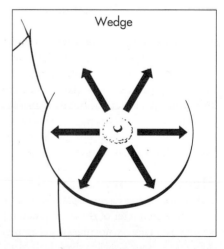

C

FIGURE **12-47** Various methods for breast palpation. **A,** Palpate from top to bottom in vertical strips. **B,** Palpate in concentric circles. **C,** Palpate out from the center in wedge sections. (From Seidel HM and others: *Mosby's guide to physical examination,* ed 4, St. Louis, 1999, Mosby. In Belcher A: *Cancer nursing,* St. Louis, 1992, Mosby.)

largement. Breast enlargement in young males may result from steroid use. Fatty tissue feels soft, whereas glandular tissue is firm. Use the same techniques to palpate for masses used in examination of the female breast. Because male breast cancer is relatively rare, routine self-examinations are unnecessary.

ABDOMEN

The abdominal examination can be complex because of the organs located within and near the abdominal cavity. The organs are assessed anteriorly and posteriorly. A system of landmarks helps to map out the abdominal region. The xiphoid process (tip of the sternum) is the upper boundary of the anterior abdominal region. The symphysis pubis delineates the lower boundary. By dividing the abdomen into four imaginary quadrants (Figure 12-48, *A*), you can refer to assessment findings and record them in relation to each quadrant. Posteriorly the kidneys, located from the T12 to L3 vertebrae, are protected by the lower ribs and heavy back muscles. The costovertebral angle formed by the last rib and vertebral column is a landmark used during palpation of the kidney.

The examination includes an assessment of structures of the lower gastrointestinal (GI) tract in addition to the liver, stomach, kidneys, and bladder. Abdominal pain is one of the most common symptoms clients will report when seeking medical care. An accurate assessment requires matching client history data with a careful assessment of the location of physical symptoms.

During the abdominal examination, the client must be relaxed. A tightening of abdominal muscles hinders palpation. Ask the client to void before beginning. Be sure the room is warm, and drape the client's upper chest and legs. The client lies supine or in a dorsal recumbent position with the arms at the sides and knees slightly bent. Small pillows can be placed beneath the knees. If the client places the arms under the head, the abdominal muscles may tighten. Proceed calmly and slowly, being sure there is adequate lighting. Expose the abdomen from just above the xiphoid process down to the symphysis pubis. Warm hands and stethoscope further promote relaxation. Ask the client to report pain and point out areas of tenderness. Assess tender areas last.

The order for an abdominal examination differs slightly from previous assessments. The nurse begins with inspection and then auscultation. By using auscultation before palpation, there is less chance of altering the frequency and character of bowel sounds. During the examination you may need a tape measure and marking pen.

Health History

Ask whether the client has abdominal or low back pain and assess the character of the pain in detail (see Chapter 29). Also review the client's normal bowel habits and stool character. Ask if the client uses laxatives. Determine if the client has had abdominal surgery, trauma, or diagnostic tests of the GI tract. Signs and symptoms of belching, difficulty swallowing, flatulence, bloody emesis (**hematemesis**), black tarry stools (**me-**

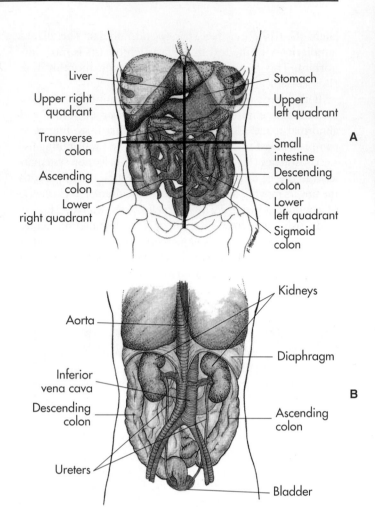

FIGURE **12-48**   **A,** Anterior view of abdomen divided by quadrants. **B,** Posterior view of abdominal sections.

lena), heartburn, diarrhea, or constipation may reveal a pattern of a problem. Also ask if the client has had a recent weight change or intolerance to diet. If the client takes antiinflammatory drugs (e.g., aspirin, ibuprofen, or steroids) and antibiotics, there may be risk for GI upset or bleeding. Inquire about a family history of cancer, kidney disease, alcoholism, hypertension, or heart disease. Assess the client's usual intake of alcohol. Also determine if the female client is pregnant and note her last menstrual period. Review the client's history for risk factors of hepatitis B virus exposure. Finally, ask the client to locate tender areas before beginning the examination.

Inspection

Make it a habit to observe the client during routine care activities. Note the client's posture and look for evidence of abdominal splinting, lying with the knees drawn up, or moving restlessly in bed. A client free from abdominal pain will not stoop or splint the abdomen. To inspect the abdomen for abnormal movement or shadows, stand on the client's right side and inspect the abdomen from above. By sitting down to look across the abdomen, you assess abdominal contour. Direct the examination light over the abdomen.

Inspect the skin over the abdomen for color, scars, venous patterns, lesions, and **striae** (stretch marks). The skin is subject to the same color variations as the rest of the body. Venous patterns are normally faint, except in thin clients. Artificial openings may indicate drainage sites resulting from surgery or an ostomy. Scars reveal evidence of past trauma or surgery that may have created permanent changes in underlying organ anatomy. Bruising may indicate accidental injury, physical abuse, or a type of bleeding disorder. Ask if the client self-administers injections (e.g., insulin or heparin). Unexpected findings include generalized color changes such as jaundice or cyanosis. A glistening taut appearance indicates ascites.

Inspection continues with the umbilicus. Note the position; shape; color; and presence of inflammation, discharge, or protruding masses. A normal umbilicus is flat or concave with the color the same as surrounding skin. Inspect for contour, symmetry, and surface motion of the abdomen, noting any masses, bulging, or distention. A flat abdomen forms a horizontal plane from the xiphoid process to the symphysis pubis. A round abdomen protrudes in a convex sphere from a horizontal plane. A concave abdomen appears to sink into the muscular wall. Each of these findings is normal if the shape of the abdomen is symmetrical. In older adults there is often an overall increased distribution of adipose tissue.

The presence of masses on only one side, or asymmetry, may indicate an underlying pathological condition. Observe the contour of the abdomen while asking the client to take a deep breath and hold it. The contour should remain smooth and symmetrical. To evaluate abdominal musculature, have the client raise the head. This position causes superficial abdominal wall masses, hernias, and muscle separations to become more apparent.

Intestinal gas, tumor, or fluid in the abdominal cavity may cause distention (swelling). When distention is generalized, the entire abdomen protrudes. The skin often appears taut, as if it were stretched over. When gas causes distention, the flanks do not bulge. However, if fluid is the source of the problem, such as in ascites, the flanks bulge. Ask the client to roll onto one side. A protuberance forms on the dependent side if fluid is the cause of the distention. Ask the client if the abdomen feels unusually tight. Be careful not to confuse distention with obesity. In obesity the abdomen is large, rolls of adipose tissue are often present along the flanks, and the client does not complain of tightness in the abdomen. If you expect abdominal distention, measure the girth of the abdomen by placing a tape measure around the abdomen at the level of the umbilicus. Consecutive measurements will show any increase or decrease in distention. Use a marking pen to indicate where the tape measure was applied.

Next inspect for movement. Normally men breathe abdominally and women breathe more costally. If the client has severe pain, respiratory movement is diminished, and the client tightens abdominal muscles to guard against the pain. Also observe for peristaltic movement or aortic pulsation by looking across the abdomen from the side. These movements may be seen in thin clients; otherwise no movement is present.

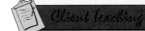

Client Teaching   Box 12-20

ABDOMINAL ASSESSMENT
- Explain factors that promote normal bowel elimination, such as diet, regular exercise, limited use of over-the-counter drugs causing constipation, establishment of a regular elimination schedule, and a good fluid intake (see Chapter 32). Stress importance for older adults.
- Caution clients about dangers of excessive use of laxatives or enemas.
- Instruct clients to have acute abdominal pain evaluated by a health care provider.
- If the client has chronic pain, explain measures used for pain relief (e.g., relaxation exercises, positioning) (see Chapter 29).
- Instruct the client about warning signs of colon cancer, including bleeding from the rectum, black or tarry stools, blood in the stool, and a change in bowel habits (constipation or diarrhea).

Auscultation

Auscultate the abdomen to listen to the bowel sounds of normal intestinal **peristalsis** and to detect vascular sounds. Clients with GI tubes connected to suction must have them temporarily turned off before beginning the examination. Place the warmed diaphragm of the stethoscope lightly over each of the four quadrants. Ask the client not to speak. Normally air and fluid move through the intestines, creating soft gurgling or clicking sounds that occur irregularly 5 to 35 times per minute (Seidel and others, 1999). Sounds may last $1\frac{1}{2}$ seconds to several seconds. It normally takes 5 to 20 seconds to hear a bowel sound. However, it may take 5 minutes of continuous listening before determining bowel sounds are absent. Auscultate all four quadrants to be sure no sounds are missed. The best time to auscultate is between meals. Sounds are generally described as normal, audible, absent, hyperactive, or hypoactive.

Absent sounds indicate cessation of GI motility that may result from late-stage bowel obstruction, **paralytic ileus,** or **peritonitis.** Hyperactive sounds are loud, "growling" sounds called **borborygmi,** which indicate increased GI motility. Inflammation of the bowel, anxiety, bleeding, excess ingestion of laxatives, and reaction of the intestines to certain foods cause increased motility (Box 12-20).

Bruits indicate narrowing of major blood vessels and disruption of blood flow. Presence of bruits in the abdominal area can reveal **aneurysms** or stenotic vessels. Use the bell of the stethoscope to auscultate in the epigastric region and each of the four quadrants. Normally there are no vascular sounds over the aorta (midline through the abdomen) or femoral arteries (lower quadrants). Report a bruit immediately to a physician.

Palpation

Palpation primarily detects areas of abdominal tenderness, abnormal distention, or masses. As you become more skilled, you will learn to palpate for specific organs such as the liver. Light and deep palpation are used.

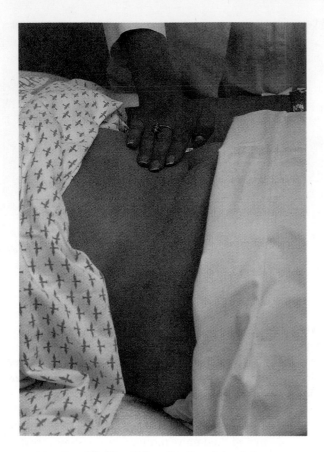

FIGURE **12-49**   Light palpation of the abdomen.

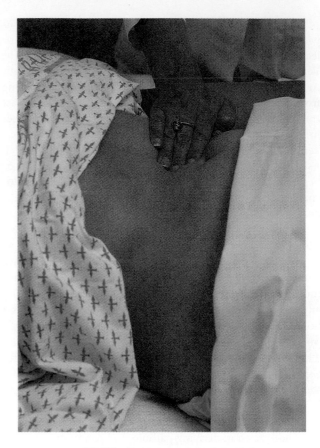

FIGURE **12-50**   Deep palpation of the abdomen.

Perform light palpation over each abdominal quadrant. Initially avoid areas previously identified as problem spots. Lay the palm of your hand with fingers extended and approximated lightly on the abdomen. Explain the maneuver to the client and then with the palmar surface of your fingers depress 1.3 cm (½ inch) in a gentle dipping motion (Figure 12-49). Avoid quick jabs and use smooth, coordinated movements. For ticklish clients, first place your hand under the client's abdomen until palpation is tolerated. Feel for muscular resistance, tenderness, and superficial organs or masses. While palpating, observe the client's face for signs of discomfort. The abdomen is normally smooth with consistent softness and nontender without masses. The older adult often lacks abdominal tone.

With experience you can perform deep palpation (Figure 12-50) to delineate abdominal organs and to detect less-obvious masses. A qualified examiner must assist until you become skilled in the technique. Short fingernails are needed. It is important for the client to be relaxed while your hands are depressed approximately 2.5 to 7.5 cm (1 to 3 inches) into the abdomen. Deep palpation is never used over a surgical incision or over extremely tender organs. It is also unwise to use deep palpation on abnormal masses. Deep pressure may cause tenderness in the healthy client over the cecum, sigmoid colon, and aorta and in the midline near the xiphoid process (Seidel and others, 1999).

Survey each quadrant systematically. Palpate masses for size, location, shape, consistency, tenderness, pulsation, and mobility. If you note tenderness, check for rebound tenderness. This test may be performed by pressing your hand slowly and deeply into the involved area and then let go quickly. If pain is elicited with the release of the hand, the test is positive. Rebound tenderness occurs in clients with peritoneal irritation such as in appendicitis; pancreatitis; or any peritoneal injury causing bile, blood, or enzymes to enter the peritoneal cavity.

To assess aortic pulsation, palpate with the thumb and forefinger of one hand deeply into the upper abdomen just left of the midline. Normally a pulsation is transmitted forward. If there is enlargement of the aorta from an aneurysm (localized dilation of a vessel wall), the pulsation expands laterally. Do not palpate a pulsating abdominal mass. In obese clients it may be necessary to palpate with both hands, one on each side of the aorta.

FEMALE GENITALIA

Examination of the female genitalia, including external and internal sex organs, can be embarrassing to the client unless a calm, relaxed approach is used. The gynecological examination is one of the most difficult experiences for adolescents. Cultural background may further add to apprehension. For example, female Mexican-Americans have a strong social value that women do not expose their bodies to men or even to other women. Provide a thorough explanation as to the reason for the procedures used in the examination.

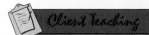

FEMALE GENITALIA ASSESSMENT

- Instruct the client about the purpose and recommended frequency of Papanicolaou (Pap) smears and gynecological examinations. Explain that the Pap smear is painless and should be performed annually with a pelvic examination for women who are sexually active or who are over age 18 (unless three consecutive tests are normal and physician recommends less-frequent screening).
- Counsel clients with STDs about diagnosis and treatment.
- Instruct on genital self-examination: Using a mirror, position self to examine the area covered by the pubic hair. Spread the hair apart, looking for bumps, sores, or blisters. Also, look for any warts, which may appear as small, bumpy spots and that enlarge to fleshy, cauliflower-like lesions. Next, spread the outer vaginal lips apart and look at the clitoris for bumps, blisters, sores, or warts. Also look at both sides of the inner vaginal lips. The area around the urinary and vaginal opening should be inspected for bumps, blisters, sores, or warts.
- Explain warning signs of STDs: pain or burning on urination, pain in the pelvic area, bleeding between menstruation, an itchy rash around the vagina, and vaginal discharge (different from usual).
- Teach measures to prevent STDs (e.g., male partner's use of condoms, restricting number of sexual partners, avoidance of sex with persons who have several other partners, perineal hygiene measures).
- Tell clients with STDs that they must inform their sexual partner of the need for an examination.
- Reinforce the importance of perineal hygiene (as appropriate).

The lithotomy position assumed during the examination is an added source of embarrassment. Comfort is achieved through correct positioning and draping. Be sure to explain each portion of the examination in advance so that clients can anticipate your actions. Adolescents may choose to have parents present in the examination room.

A client may require a complete examination, including assessing external genitalia and performing a vaginal examination, or the nurse may examine external genitalia while performing routine hygiene measures or preparing to insert a urinary catheter. An examination should be a part of each woman's preventive health care, because uterine and ovarian cancer cause more deaths than any other cancer of the female reproductive system (American Cancer Society, 2000).

Adolescents and young adults should be examined because of the growing incidence of sexually transmitted diseases (STDs). The average age of menarche among young girls has declined, and the majority of male and female teenagers are sexually active by age 19 (Wong and others, 1999). Rectal and anal assessments are easily combined with this examination because the client can assume a lithotomy or dorsal recumbent position.

Health History

The history reviews the client's previous illnesses or surgeries involving reproductive organs, including STDs. A review of the menstrual history includes age at menarche, frequency and duration of cycle, character of flow, presence of **dysmenorrhea,** pelvic pain, dates of last two menstrual periods, and premenstrual symptoms. You also assess for signs of bleeding, vaginal discharge, or pain outside the normal menstrual period or after menopause. A review of the client's obstetrical history is also valuable. Ask your client if she has symptoms of genitourinary problems such as burning during urination, frequency, urgency, nocturia, hematuria, incontinence, or stress incontinence.

Ask the client to describe her obstetrical history, including each pregnancy and history of abortions or miscarriages. Also question the client about current and past contraceptive practices and problems encountered. It is important to determine if your client uses safe sex practices. Discuss risks of STDs and HIV infection. Determine if the client has signs and symptoms of vaginal discharge, painful or swollen perianal tissues, or genital lesions. Also review a client's risk for developing cervical, endometrial, or ovarian cancer (Box 12-21).

Preparing the Client

As a beginning nurse, your responsibility will be assisting the client's primary health care provider with the examination. This examination is best performed with the client lying on an examination table, or it may be performed with the client in bed with the legs supported with pillows or bath blankets. The following equipment is needed for a complete examination: examination table with stirrups; vaginal speculum of correct size; adjustable light source; sink; clean, disposable gloves; glass microscopic slides; plastic spatula and/or Cytobrush; and specimen bottles with fixative spray (hairspray).

Equipment must be ready before the examination begins. Ask the client to empty her bladder so that urine is not accidentally expelled during the examination. Often it is necessary to collect a urine specimen. Assist the client to the lithotomy position, in bed or on an examination table, for an external genitalia assessment. Assist the client into stirrups if a speculum examination is to be performed. Have the woman stabilize each foot in a stirrup and then have her slide the buttocks down to the edge of the examining table. Place your hand at the edge of the table and instruct the client to move until touching the hand. The client's arms should be at her sides or folded across the chest to prevent tightening of abdominal muscles.

A woman suffering from pain or deformity of the joints may be unable to assume a lithotomy position. In this situation, it may be necessary to have the client abduct only one leg or to have another assist in separating the client's thighs. The side-lying position may also be used with the client on the left side and the right thigh and knee drawn up to her chest.

A square drape or sheet is given to the client. She holds one corner over her sternum, the adjacent corners fall over each knee, and the fourth corner falls over the perineum. After the examination begins, lift the drape over the perineum. The male examiner should always have a female in attendance during the examination. A female examiner may prefer to work alone but should have a female attendant if the client is particularly anxious or emotionally unstable.

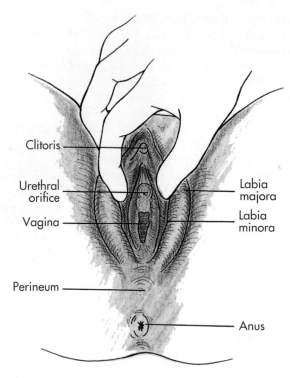

FIGURE 12-51   Female external genitalia.

External Genitalia

The perineal area must be well illuminated. Apply gloves on both hands. The perineum is extremely sensitive and tender; do not touch the area suddenly without warning the client. It is best to touch the neighboring thigh first before advancing to the perineum.

While sitting at the end of the examination table or bed, inspect the quantity and distribution of hair growth. Preadolescents have no pubic hair. During adolescence hair grows along the labia, becoming darker, coarser, and curlier. In an adult, hair grows in a triangle over the female perineum and along the medial surface of the thighs. Hair should be free of nits and lice.

Inspect surface characteristics of the labia majora. The skin of the perineum is smooth, clean, and slightly darker than other skin. The mucous membranes appear dark pink and moist. The labia majora may be gaping or closed and appear dry or moist. They are usually symmetrical. After childbirth the labia majora are separated, causing the labia minora to become more prominent. When a woman reaches menopause, the labia majora become thinned. With advancing age they become **atrophied.** The labia majora are normally without inflammation, edema, lesions, or lacerations.

To inspect the remaining external structures, use your nondominant hand and gently place the thumb and index finger inside the labia minora and retract the tissues outward (Figure 12-51). Be sure to have a firm hold to avoid repeated retraction against the sensitive tissues. Use your other hand to palpate the labia minora between the thumb and second finger. On inspection the labia minora are normally thinner than the labia majora, and one side may be larger. The tissue should feel soft on palpation and without tenderness. The

size of the clitoris is variable, but it normally does not exceed 2 cm in length and 0.5 cm in diameter. Look for atrophy, inflammation, or adhesions. If inflamed, the clitoris will be a bright cherry red. In young women it is a common site for syphilitic lesions or **chancres,** which appear as small open ulcers that drain serous material. Older women may have malignant changes that result in dry, scaly, nodular lesions.

Inspect the urethral orifice carefully for color and position. It is normally intact and without inflammation. The urethral meatus is anterior to the vaginal orifice and is pink. It may appear as a small slit or pinhole opening just above the vaginal canal. Note any discharge, polyps, or fistulas.

Inspect the vaginal introitus next for inflammation, edema, discoloration, discharge, and lesions. Normally the introitus is a thin vertical slit or a large orifice. The tissue is moist. In women who have had several children, the opening to the vaginal canal may extend upward, blocking the view of the urethra. While inspecting the vaginal orifice or introitus, notice the condition of the hymen, which is just inside the introitus. In the virgin the hymen may restrict the opening of the vagina. Only remnants of the hymen remain after sexual intercourse.

Inspect the anus looking for lesions and hemorrhoids (see rectal examination). After completion of the external examination, dispose of your gloves and offer your client perineal hygiene.

Clients who are at risk for contracting STDs should learn to perform a genital self-examination (see Box 12-21). The purpose of the examination is to detect any signs or symptoms of STDs. Many persons do not know they have an STD, and some STDs can remain undetected for years.

Speculum Examination of Internal Genitalia

An examination of internal genitalia requires much skill and practice. It is performed by advanced practice nurses and primary care providers. Beginning students will more than likely only observe the procedure or assist the examiner by helping the client with positioning, handing off specimen supplies, and comforting the client.

The examination involves use of a plastic or metal speculum, consisting of two blades and an adjustable thumbscrew. The speculum is inserted into the vagina to assess the vaginal walls and cervix for cancerous lesions and other abnormalities. During the examination a **Papanicolaou (Pap) smear** is collected to test for cervical and vaginal cancer. This examination will not be discussed here.

MALE GENITALIA

An examination of the male genitalia assesses the integrity of the external genitalia, inguinal ring, and canal. Because the incidence of STDs in adolescents and young adults is high, an assessment of the genitalia should be a routine part of any health maintenance examination for this age-group. Use a calm, gentle approach to lessen the client's anxiety. The position and exposure obtained during the examination can be embarrassing. It often helps to minimize the client's anxiety by offering explanations of each step of the examination so the client can anticipate all actions. Manipulate the genitalia

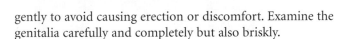

MALE GENITALIA ASSESSMENT
Box 12-22

- Counsel clients with STDs about diagnosis and treatment.
- Teach measures to prevent STDs:
  Use of condoms
  Avoiding sex with infected partners
  Restricting number of sexual partners
  Avoiding sex with persons who have multiple partners
  Using regular perineal hygiene
- Tell clients with STDs that sexual partners must be informed of the need to have an examination.
- Instruct client to seek treatment as soon as possible if partner becomes infected with an STD.
- Instruct clients on how to perform genital self-examination (Box 12-23).

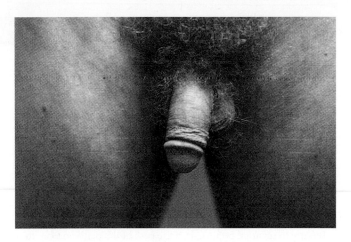

FIGURE **12-52**   Normal male genitalia (circumcised). (From Seidel HM and others: *Mosby's guide to physical examination*, ed 4, St. Louis, 1999, Mosby.)

gently to avoid causing erection or discomfort. Examine the genitalia carefully and completely but also briskly.

Health History

Assess the client's normal urinary pattern, including frequency of voiding; character and volume of urine; daily fluid intake; and symptoms of burning, urgency and frequency, difficulty starting stream, and hematuria. The history also includes a review of previous surgery or illness involving urinary or reproductive organs, including STDs. The client's sexual history and use of safe sex habits will alert you to any risks for HIV or other STDs. A client's sexual performance can be influenced by a number of disorders; thus ask if the client has difficulty achieving erection or ejaculation. Also review medications that might influence sexual performance, including diuretics, sedatives, antihypertensives, and tranquilizers. Ask if the client has noted penile pain or swelling, lesions of the genitalia, or urethral discharge (signs and symptoms of STDs). The client's knowledge of testicular self-examination will guide you in health teaching (Box 12-22). Ask the client if he has noticed heaviness or painless enlargement of a testis or irregular lumps (warning signs of testicular cancer). Finally, if the client reports an enlargement in the inguinal area, assess if it is intermittent or constant; associated with straining or lifting; painful; and whether pain is affected by coughing, lifting, or straining at stool (signs and symptoms indicative of inguinal hernia).

Sexual Maturity

The examination begins by having the client void. The examination room should be warm. The client lies supine with the chest, abdomen, and lower legs draped, or the client may also stand during the examination. Apply disposable gloves. First, note the sexual maturity of the client by observing the size and shape of the penis and testes; the size, color, and texture of scrotal skin; and the character and distribution of pubic hair. The testes first increase in size in preadolescence. During this time there is no pubic hair. By the end of puberty, the testes and penis enlarge to

adult size and shape and scrotal skin darkens and becomes wrinkled. With puberty, hair is coarse and abundant in the pubic area. The penis has no hair, and the scrotum has scant amounts. Also inspect the skin covering the genitalia for lice, rashes, excoriations, or lesions. Normally the skin is clear, without lesions.

Penis

To inspect penile surfaces thoroughly you must manipulate the genitalia or have the client assist. Inspect the corona, prepuce (foreskin), glans, urethral meatus, and shaft (Figure 12-52). In uncircumcised males retract the foreskin to reveal the glans and urethral meatus. The foreskin should retract easily. A bit of white, cheesy smegma may have collected under this foreskin. In the circumcised male, the glans is exposed; in either case, the glans should look smooth and pink along all surfaces. Observe for discharge, lesions, edema, and inflammation. The urethral meatus is slitlike and normally positioned at the tip of the glans. In some congenital conditions the meatus is displaced along the penile shaft. The area between the foreskin and glans is a common site for venereal lesions.

Gentle compression of the glans between your thumb and index finger opens the meatus to allow inspection for discharge, lesions, and edema. (The client may perform this maneuver.) Normally the opening is glistening and pink without discharge. Palpate any lesion gently to note tenderness, size, consistency, and shape. When you complete inspection of the glans, pull the foreskin down to its original position. Continue by inspecting the entire shaft of the penis, including the undersurface, looking for any lesions, scars, or areas of edema. Palpate the shaft between the thumb and first two fingers to detect localized areas of hardness or tenderness. A client who has lain in bed for a prolonged time may develop dependent edema in the penile shaft. It is important for any male client to learn to perform a genital self-examination to detect signs and symptoms of STDs. Many people who have an STD do not know it. A self-examination should be a routine part of self-care (Box 12-23).

Male Genital Self-Examination

Box 12-23

All men 15 years and older should perform this examination monthly using the following steps:

GENITAL EXAMINATION

Perform the examination after a warm bath or shower when the scrotal sac is relaxed.

Stand naked in front of a mirror, hold the penis in your hand, and examine the head. Pull back the foreskin if uncircumcised.

Inspect and palpate the entire head of the penis in a clockwise motion, looking carefully for any bumps, sores, or blisters. Look also for any bumpy warts (see the illustration).

Look at the opening at the end of the penis for discharge.

Look along the entire shaft of the penis for the same signs.

Be sure to separate pubic hair at the base of the penis and carefully examine the skin underneath.

TESTICULAR SELF-EXAMINATION

Look for swelling or lumps in the skin of the scrotum while looking in the mirror.

Use both hands, placing the index and middle fingers under the testicles and the thumb on top (see the illustration).

Gently roll the testicle, feeling for lumps, thickening, or a change in consistency (hardening).

Find the epididymis (a cordlike structure on the top and back of the testicle; it is not a lump).

Feel for small, pea-sized lumps on the front and side of the testicle. The lumps are usually painless and are abnormal.

Call your physician if you find a lump.

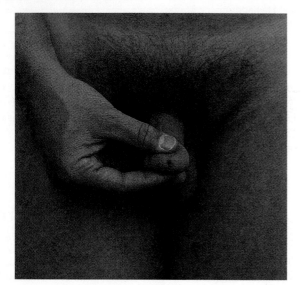
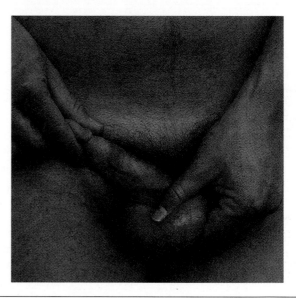

Illustrations from Seidel HM and others: *Mosby's guide to physical examination*, ed 4, St. Louis, 1999, Mosby.

Scrotum

Be especially cautious while inspecting and palpating the scrotum because the structures that lie within the scrotal sac are very sensitive. The scrotum is a saclike structure divided internally into halves. Each half contains a testicle, epididymis, and the vas deferens, which travels upward into the inguinal ring. The left testicle is normally lower than the right. Inspect the size, color, shape, and symmetry of the scrotum while observing for lesions or edema.

Gently lift the scrotum to view the posterior surface. The scrotal skin is usually loose, and the surface is coarse. The skin color is often more deeply pigmented than body skin. Tightening or loss of wrinkling may reveal edema. The size of the scrotum normally changes with temperature variations because its dartos muscle contracts in cold and relaxes in warm temperature. Lumps in the scrotal skin are commonly sebaceous cysts.

Testicular cancer is a solid tumor commonly found in young men ages 18 to 34 years. Early detection is critical. Clients must learn to perform testicular self-examinations (see Box 12-23). Explain this technique while examining the client. While the client retracts the penis upward, gently palpate the testes and epididymis between the thumb and first two fingers (Figure 12-53).

Note the size, shape, and consistency of tissue, and ask if the client feels any tenderness. The testes should be sensitive but not tender. The underlying testicles are normally ovoid and approximately 2 by 4 cm ($\frac{4}{5}$ by $1\frac{3}{5}$ inches) in size. The testes feel smooth and rubbery and are free from nodules. The epididymis is resilient. In the older adult the testicles decrease in size and are less firm during palpation. The most common symptoms of testicular cancer are a painlesss enlargement of one testis and appearance of a palpable small, hard lump about the size of a pea on the front or side of the testicle.

Continue to palpate the vas deferens separately as it forms the spermatic cord toward the inguinal ring, noting nodules or swelling. It normally feels smooth and discrete.

Inguinal Ring and Canal

The external inguinal ring provides the opening for the spermatic cord to pass into the inguinal canal. The canal forms a passage through the abdominal wall, a potential site for her-

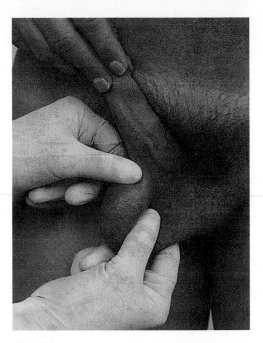

FIGURE **12-53**   Palpating contents of scrotal sac. (From Seidel HM and others: *Mosby's guide to physical examination*, ed 4, St. Louis, 1999. Mosby.)

RECTAL AND ANAL ASSESSMENT

- Discuss the American Cancer Society's guidelines (2000) for early detection of colorectal cancer:
    Digital rectal examination performed yearly after age 40
    Stool blood slide test (guaiac test) performed yearly after age 50
    Proctosigmoidoscopy (flexible) involving visual inspection of the rectum and lower colon with a hollow, lighted tube, performed by a physician every 3 to 5 years after age 50, on the advice of a physician
    Know the warning signs of colorectal cancer
- Discuss dietary planning to reduce fat and increase fiber content.
- Warn clients against problems caused by overuse of laxatives, cathartic medications, codeine, or enemas.
- Discuss with male clients the American Cancer Society's guidelines (2000) for early detection of prostatic cancer:
    Digital rectal examination performed annually after age 40
    Men age 50 and over should have an annual prostate-specific antigen (PSA) blood test
    If either test is suspicious, prostate ultrasound may be performed
    Know the warning signs of prostate cancer

Box 12-24

nia formation. A **hernia** is a protrusion of a portion of intestine through the inguinal wall or canal. An intestinal loop may even enter the scrotum. The client stands during this portion of the examination.

During inspection ask the client to strain or bear down. The maneuver will help to make a hernia more visible. Look for obvious bulging in the inguinal area.

Complete the examination by palpating for inguinal lymph nodes. Small, nontender, mobile horizontal nodes may normally be found. Any abnormality may indicate local or systemic infection or malignant disease.

RECTUM AND ANUS

A good time to perform the rectal examination is after the genital examination. The procedure can be uncomfortable, so explaining all steps helps the client relax. Usually the examination is not performed on young children or adolescents. The examination can detect colorectal cancer in its early stages. In men the rectal examination can also detect prostatic tumors.

Health History

The history includes review of the client's personal history of colorectal cancer, polyps, or inflammatory bowel disease. If the client is over age 40, ask if the client has ever had a rectal examination or proctosigmoidoscopy. Ask the client about symptoms of bleeding from the rectum, black or tarry stools (melena), rectal pain, or change in bowel habits, all of which are indicative of colorectal cancer. The client's dietary habits, including intake of high-fat foods or deficient fiber content, may be linked to colon cancer. To screen male clients for

possible prostate cancer ask if your client has experienced weak or interrupted urine flow; an inability to urinate; difficulty in starting or stopping the urinary stream; polyuria; nocturia; hematuria; dysuria; or continuing pain in the lower back, pelvis, or upper thighs. Also review the client's use of laxatives, cathartics, codeine, or iron preparations, which can cause elimination problems (Box 12-24).

Inspection

Female clients may remain in the dorsal recumbent position following genitalia examination, or they may assume a side-lying (Sims') position. Men are best examined by having the client stand and bend over forward with the hips flexed and upper body resting across the examination table. A nonambulatory client can be examined in Sims' position. Use disposable gloves.

Using your nondominant hand gently retract the buttocks to view the perianal and sacrococcygeal areas. Perianal skin is smooth and more pigmented and coarser than skin overlying the buttocks. Inspect anal tissue for skin characteristics, lesions, external **hemorrhoids** (dilated veins that appear as reddened skin protrusions), ulcers, inflammation, rashes, or excoriation. Anal tissues are moist and hairless, and the anus is held closed by the voluntary sphincter. Next, ask the client to bear down as though having a bowel movement. Any internal hemorrhoids or fissures will appear at this time. Use clock referents (e.g., 12 o'clock or 5 o'clock) to describe the location of findings. There normally is no protrusion of tissue.

Digital Palpation

Digital palpation is used to examine the anal canal and sphincters. In male clients, the prostate gland is palpated to

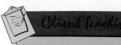

MUSCULOSKELETAL SYSTEM ASSESSMENT

- Instruct the client about correct postural alignment. Consult with a physical therapist to provide the client with exercises for improving posture.
- To reduce bone demineralization, instruct older adults about a proper exercise program (e.g., walking) to be followed three or more times a week. Also encourage intake of calcium to meet the recommended daily allowance. Increased vitamin D will aid calcium absorption.
- Recommendations for calcium supplements are 1000 mg before and 1500 mg after menopause.
- Explain to clients with low back pain that they can benefit from modification of worker risk factors (e.g., lifting heavy weights, use of protective equipment), regular aerobic exercise, exercises that strengthen the back and increase trunk flexibility, and learning how to lift properly.
- Instruct the client on use of assistive devices (e.g., zippers on clothing instead of buttons, elevation of chairs to minimize bending of knees and hips) when he or she is unable to perform ADLs.
- Instruct older adults and those with osteoporosis on proper body mechanics and range of motion and moderate weight-bearing exercises (e.g., swimming, walking) to minimize trauma and subsequent bone fractures.
- Instruct older clients to pace activities to compensate for loss in muscle strength.

rule out enlargement. This portion of the examination is usually reserved for advanced practitioners.

MUSCULOSKELETAL SYSTEM

The musculoskeletal assessment can be done as a separate examination or integrated with other parts of the total physical examination. This system may also be assessed while performing other nursing care measures such as bathing or positioning. The assessment of musculoskeletal integrity is especially important when the client reports pain or loss of function in a joint or muscle. Frequently, muscular disorders are the result of neurological disease. For this reason a neurological assessment is often conducted simultaneously.

While examining the client's musculoskeletal function, you visualize the anatomy of bone and muscle placement and joint structure. Joints vary in their degree of mobility. Some, as in the knee, are freely moveable. The spinal vertebrae are examples of slightly moveable joints. For a complete examination expose the muscles and joints so that they are free to move. Depending on the muscle groups being assessed, the client assumes a sitting, supine, prone, or standing position.

Health History

A history includes the client's description of any problems in bone, muscle, or joint function, including history of recent falls, trauma, lifting heavy objects, fractures, and bone or joint disease. Ask the client to point out locations of any alterations. It is useful to assess the client's normal activity pattern, including the type of exercise routinely performed (Box 12-25). Also assess the nature and extent of pain or stiffness and determine if a musculoskeletal problem affects the client's ability to perform ADLs and participate in social activities. Determine if the client is involved in competitive sports (particularly involving collision and contact), fails to warm up adequately, is in poor physical condition, or had a rapid growth spurt (adolescents). Review the client's history for **osteoporosis** risk factors, including heavy alcohol use; cigarette smoking; constant dieting; calcium intake less than 500 mg daily; thin and light body frame; nulliparous; menopause before age 45; postmenopause; family history of osteoporosis; or white, Asian, or Native American, or northern European ancestry.

General Inspection

Observe the client's gait and posture when entering the examination room. When a client is unaware of your observation, gait is more natural. Later a more formal test has the client walk in a straight line away from you. Note how the client walks, sits, and rises from a sitting position. Normally clients walk with arms swinging freely at the sides and the head leading the body. Older adults walk with smaller steps and a wider base of support. Note foot dragging, limping, shuffling, and the position of the trunk in relation to the legs.

Observe the client from the side in a standing position. The normal standing posture is an upright stance with parallel alignment of the hips and shoulders (Figure 12-54). There should be an even contour of the shoulders, level scapulae and iliac crests, alignment of the head over the gluteal folds, and symmetry of extremities. Looking sideways at the client, note the normal cervical, thoracic, and lumbar curves. The head is held erect. As the client sits, some degree of rounding of the shoulders is normal. Older adults tend to assume a stooped, forward-bent posture, with hips and knees somewhat flexed and arms bent at the elbows, raising the level of the arms (Ebersole and Hess, 1998). Common postural abnormalities include kyphosis, lordosis, and scoliosis. **Kyphosis,** or hunchback, is an exaggeration of the posterior curvature of the thoracic spine. This postural abnormality is common in the older adult. **Lordosis,** or swayback, is an increased lumbar curvature. A lateral spinal curvature is called **scoliosis.** Loss of height is frequently the first clinical sign of osteoporosis, in which height loss occurs in the trunk as a result of vertebral fracture and collapse (Galsworthy and Wilson, 1996). Although a small amount of height loss is to be expected with aging, if the amount of loss is greater than expected, osteoporosis is likely. As men and women age, they are more likely to have osteoporotic fractures of the forearms, hips, and vertebrae (Kessenich and Rosen, 1996).

During general inspection look at the extremities for overall size, gross deformity, bony enlargement, alignment, and symmetry. There should be bilateral symmetry in length, circumference, alignment, and position and number-

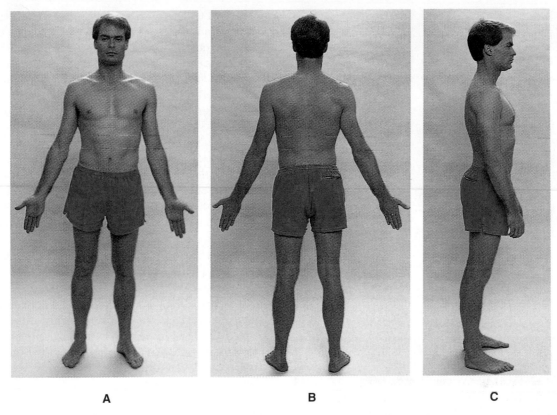

A   B   C

FIGURE **12-54**   Inspection of overall body posture. **A,** Anterior view. **B,** posterior view. **C,** lateral view. (From Seidel HM and others: *Mosby's guide to physical examination*, ed 4, St. Louis, 1999, Mosby.)

Terminology for Normal Range-of-Motion Positions		Table 12-8
Term	Range of Motion	Examples of Joints
Flexion	Movement decreasing angle between two adjoining bones; bending of limb	Elbow, fingers, knee
Extension	Movement increasing angle between two adjoining bones	Elbow, knee, fingers
Hyperextension	Movement of body part beyond its normal resting extended position	Head
Pronation	Movement of body part so that front or ventral surface faces downward	Hand, forearm
Supination	Movement of body part so that front or ventral surface faces upward	Hand, forearm
Abduction	Movement of extremity away from midline of body	Leg, arm, fingers
Adduction	Movement of extremity toward midline of body	Leg, arm, fingers
Internal rotation	Rotation of joint inward	Knee, hip
External rotation	Rotation of joint outward	Knee, hip
Eversion	Turning of body part away from midline	Foot
Inversion	Turning of body part toward midline	Foot
Dorsiflexion	Flexion of toes and foot upward	Foot
Plantar flexion	Bending of toes and foot downward	Foot

ing of skinfolds (Seidel and others, 1999). A general review pinpoints areas requiring specialized assessment.

Palpation

Apply gentle palpation to all bones, joints, and surrounding muscles during a complete examination. In the case of a focused assessment, only an involved area needs to be examined. Note any heat, tenderness, edema, or resistance to pressure. The client should feel no discomfort when you apply palpation. Muscles should be firm.

Range-of-Joint Motion

Ask the client to put each major joint and its muscle groups through full range of motion (ROM) (Table 12-8). The examination includes comparison of both active and passive ROM. To assess ROM passively, ask the client to relax and then passively move the joints until the end of range is felt. Compare the same body parts for equality in movement. Do not force a joint into a painful position. You must know the normal range of each joint and the extent to which the client's joints can be moved. Ideally the client's normal range

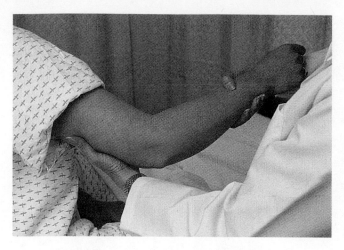

FIGURE 12-55 Assess muscle tone when moving the extremity passively.

is assessed to determine a baseline for assessing later change. Joints should be free from stiffness, instability, swelling, or inflammation. There should be no discomfort when you apply pressure to bones and joints. In older adults joints often become swollen and stiff, with reduced ROM resulting from cartilage erosion and fibrosis of synovial membranes. If a joint appears swollen and inflamed, palpate it for warmth.

Muscle Tone and Strength

Assess muscle strength and tone during ROM measurement. Note muscle tone, the slight muscular resistance felt as you passively move the relaxed extremity through its ROM. Ask the client to allow an extremity to relax or hang limp. This is often difficult, particularly if the client feels pain in the extremity. Support the extremity and grasp each limb, moving it through the normal ROM (Figure 12-55). Normal tone causes a mild, even resistance to passive movement through the entire range.

If a muscle has increased tone, or **hypertonicity,** sudden passive movement of a joint is met with considerable resistance. Continued movement eventually causes the muscle to relax. A muscle that has little tone (**hypotonicity**) feels flabby. The involved extremity hangs loosely in a position determined by gravity.

For assessment of muscle strength the client assumes a stable position. The client performs maneuvers demonstrating strength of major muscle groups (Table 12-9). Compare symmetrical muscle pairs for strength, based on a grading scale of 0 to 5 (Table 12-10). The arm on the dominant side is normally stronger than the arm on the nondominant side. In the older adult a loss of muscle mass causes bilateral weakness, but muscle strength remains greater in the dominant arm or leg.

Examine each muscle group. Ask the client first to flex the muscle to be examined and then to resist when you apply opposing force against that flexion. It is important to not allow the client to move the joint. Gradually increase pressure to a muscle group (e.g., elbow extension). The client resists the pressure you apply by attempting to move against resistance (e.g., elbow flexion). The client resists until instructed to stop. As you vary the amount of pressure applied, the joint moves. If a weakness is identified, compare the size of the muscle with its opposite counterpart by measuring the circumference of the muscle body with a tape measure. A muscle that has atrophied (reduced in size) may feel soft and baggy when palpated.

Maneuvers to Assess Muscle Strength	Table 12-9
Muscle Group	Maneuver
Neck (sternocleido-mastoid)	Place hand firmly against client's upper jaw. Ask client to turn head laterally against resistance.
Shoulder (trapezius)	Place hand over midline of client's shoulder, exerting firm pressure. Have client raise shoulders against resistance.
Elbow	
Biceps	Pull down on forearm as client attempts to flex arm.
Triceps	As client's arm is flexed, apply pressure against forearm. Ask client to straighten arm.
Hip	
Quadriceps	When client is sitting, apply downward pressure to thigh. Ask client to raise leg up from table.
Gastrocnemius	Client sits, holding shin of flexed leg. Ask client to straighten leg against resistance.

Muscle Strength			Table 12-10
	Scales		
Muscle Function Level	Grade	% Normal	Lovett Scale
No evidence of contractility	0	0	0 (zero)
Slight contractility, no movement	1	10	T (trace)
Full range of motion, gravity eliminated*	2	25	P (poor)
Full range of motion with gravity	3	50	F (fair)
Full range of motion against gravity, some resistance	4	75	G (good)
Full range of motion against gravity, full resistance	5	100	N (normal)

From Barkauskas VH and others: *Health and physical assessment,* ed 2, St. Louis, 1998, Mosby.
*Passive movement.

NEUROLOGICAL SYSTEM

An assessment of neurological function alone can be quite time consuming. For efficiency, integrate neurological measurements with other parts of the physical examination. Cranial nerve function can be tested during the survey of the head and neck. Observe mental and emotional status during the initial interview.

Many variables must be considered when deciding the extent of the examination. A client's level of consciousness influences the ability to follow directions. General physical status influences tolerance to assessment. The client's chief complaint also helps to determine the need for a thorough neurological assessment. If the client complains of headache or a recent loss of function in an extremity, a complete neurological review is needed. Special equipment is required, including reading material, vials of aromatic substances (e.g., vanilla extract and coffee), opposite tip of cotton swab or tongue blade broken in half, Snellen eye chart, penlight, vials of sugar or salt, tongue blade, two test tubes (one containing hot water, the other containing cold), cotton balls or cotton-tipped applicators, tuning fork, and reflex hammer.

Health History

Gather a history that includes a screening for symptoms of headache, seizures, tremors, dizziness, vertigo, numbness or tingling of body parts, visual changes, weakness, pain, or changes in speech. The presence of any symptom then requires a more detailed review (e.g., onset, severity, precipitating factors, or sequence of events). Review the client's use of analgesics, alcohol, sedatives, hypnotics, antipsychotics, antidepressants, nervous system stimulants, or recreational drugs.

Mini-Mental State Examination Sample Questions	Box 12-26

Orientation to time
  "What is the date?"
Registration
  "Listen carefully. I am going to say three words. You say them back after I stop.
  Ready? Here they are . . .
  HOUSE (pause), CAR (pause), LAKE (pause). Now repeat those words back to me."
  [Repeat up to 5 times, but score only the first trial.]
Naming
  "What is this?" [Point to a pencil or pen.]
Reading
  "Please read this and do what it says." [Show examinee the words on the stimulus form.]
  CLOSE YOUR EYES

Reproduced by special permission of the Publisher, Psychological Assessment Resources, Inc., 16204 North Florida Avenue, Lutz, Florida 33549, from Mini Mental State Examination, by Marshal Folstein and Susan Folstein, Copyright 1975, 1998, 2001 by MiniMental, LLC, Inc. Published 2001 by Psychological Assessment Resources, Inc. Further reproduction is prohibited without permission of PAR, Inc. The MMSE can be purchased from PAR, Inc. by calling (800) 331-8378 or (813) 968-3003.

Also ask the client's family if they have noticed any recent changes in the client's behavior (e.g., increased irritability, mood swings, memory loss, or change in energy level). Ask about any noticeable changes in vision, hearing, smell, taste, and touch. A history of head or spinal cord trauma, meningitis, congenital anomalies, neurological disease, or psychiatric counseling will focus your assessment of select findings. If an older adult client displays sudden acute confusion (delirium), review history for drug toxicity, serious infections, metabolic disturbances, heart failure, and severe anemia.

Mental and Emotional Status

A great deal can be learned about mental capacities and emotional state by interacting with the client. You can ask questions during an examination to gather data and observe the appropriateness of emotions and thoughts. There are special assessment tools designed to assess a client's mental status. The Mental Status Questionnaire (MSQ) developed by Kahn and others (1960) is a 10-item instrument and a widely used tool. The Mini-Mental State Examination (MMSE) is another assessment instrument developed by Folstein and colleagues (1975) that measures client's orientation and cognitive function. Box 12-26 offers examples of questions found on the MMSE. A maximum score on the MMS is 30. Clients with scores of 21 or less generally reveal cognitive impairment requiring further evaluation.

To ensure an objective assessment you must consider the client's cultural and educational background, values, beliefs, previous experiences, and current level of coping. Such factors influence response to questions. An alteration in mental or emotional status may reflect a disturbance in cerebral functioning. The cerebral cortex controls and integrates intellectual and emotional functioning. Primary brain disorders, medications, and metabolic changes are examples of factors that may change cerebral function.

Level of Consciousness

A person's level of consciousness exists along a continuum from full awakeness, alertness, and cooperation to unresponsiveness to any form of external stimuli. Converse with the client, asking questions about events involving the client or concerns about any health problem. A fully conscious client responds to questions quickly, and ideas are expressed logically. With a lowering of the client's consciousness, you use the Glasgow Coma Scale (GCS) for an objective measurement of consciousness on a numerical scale (Table 12-11). The client must be as alert as possible before testing. Caution is needed in using the scale if a client has sensory losses (e.g., vision or hearing).

The GCS allows you to evaluate a client's neurological status over time. The higher the score, the better the client's neurological function. Ask short, simple questions, such as "What is your name?" or "Where are you?" Also ask the client to follow simple commands, such as "Move your toes."

If the client's consciousness is lowered to the point of being unable to follow commands, try to elicit a response by applying firm pressure with your thumb over the root of the client's fingernail. The normal response to painful stimuli is withdrawal of the body part from the stimulus.

Glasgow Coma Scale   Table 12-11

Action	Response	Score
Eyes open	Spontaneously	④
	To speech	3
	To pain	2
	None	1
Best verbal response	Oriented	⑤
	Confused	4
	Inappropriate words	3
	Incomprehensible sounds	2
	None	1
Best motor response	Obeys commands	⑥
	Localized pain	5
	Flexion withdrawal	4
	Abnormal flexion	3
	Abnormal extension	2
	Flaccid	1
	TOTAL SCORE	⑮

Behavior and Appearance

Behaviors, moods, hygiene, grooming, and choice of dress reveal pertinent information about mental status. You must remain perceptive of the client's mannerisms and actions during the entire physical assessment. Note both nonverbal and verbal behaviors. Does the client respond appropriately to directions? Does the client's mood vary with no apparent cause? Does the client show concern about appearance? Is the client's hair clean and neatly groomed, and are the nails trim and clean? The client should behave in a manner expressing concern and interest in the examination. The client should make eye contact with you and express appropriate feelings that correspond to the situation. Normally the client's appearance will show some degree of personal hygiene.

Choice and fit of clothing may reflect socioeconomic background or personal taste rather than deficiency in self-concept or self-care. Avoid being judgmental, and focus assessments on the appropriateness of clothing for the weather. Older adults may neglect their appearance because of a lack of energy, finances, or reduced vision.

Language

Normal cerebral function allows a person to understand spoken or written words and to express the self through written words or gestures. Observe the client's voice inflection, tone, and manner of speech. The client's voice should have inflections, be clear and strong, and increase in volume appropriately. Speech should be fluent. When communication is clearly ineffective (e.g., omission or addition of letters and words, misuse of words, or hesitations), assess for **aphasia.** Injury to the cerebral cortex may result in aphasia.

The two types of aphasia are sensory (or receptive) and motor (or expressive). With receptive aphasia a person cannot understand written or verbal speech. With expressive aphasia a person understands written and verbal speech but cannot write or speak appropriately when attempting to communicate. A client may suffer a combination of receptive and expressive aphasia. Assessment requires that you ask the client to name familiar objects when pointing at them. You may also ask the client to respond to simple verbal commands, such as "Stand up." Finally, you may ask the client to read a simple sentence out loud. Normally a client names objects correctly, follows commands, and reads sentences correctly.

Intellectual Function

Intellectual function includes memory, knowledge, abstract thinking, and judgment. Testing each aspect of function involves a specific technique. However, because cultural and educational background influences the ability to respond to test questions, you should not ask questions related to concepts or ideas with which the client is unfamiliar.

MEMORY.   Assess immediate recall and recent and remote memory. Immediate recall is reflected in the ability of the client to repeat a series of numbers in the order they are presented or in reverse order. Clients can normally recall five to eight digits forward or four to six digits backward.

Ask if the client's memory can be tested. Then state clearly and slowly the name of three unrelated objects. After you say all three, ask the client to repeat each. Continue until the client is successful. Then, later in the assessment, ask the client to repeat the three words again. The client should be able to identify the three words. Another test for recent memory involves asking the client to recall events occurring during the same day (e.g., what was eaten for breakfast). Information may need to be validated with a family member.

To assess past memory, you may ask the client to recall the maiden name of the client's mother, a birthday, or a special date in history. It is best to ask open-ended questions rather than simple yes-or-no questions. A client should have immediate recall of such information. With older adults you should not interpret a hearing loss as confusion. Good communication techniques are necessary throughout the examination to ensure the client clearly understands all the directions and testing.

KNOWLEDGE.   You can assess the client's knowledge by asking how much is known about the illness or the reason for hospitalization. By assessing a client's knowledge, you determine the client's ability to learn or understand. If there is an opportunity to teach information, test the client's mental status by asking for feedback during a follow-up visit.

ABSTRACT THINKING.   Interpreting abstract ideas or concepts reflects the capacity for abstract thinking. A higher level of intellectual functioning is required for an individual to explain common sayings such as "A stitch in time saves nine" or "Don't count your chickens before they're hatched." Note whether the client's explanations are relevant and concrete. The client with altered mentation will probably interpret the phrase literally or will merely rephrase the words.

JUDGMENT.   Judgment requires a comparison and evaluation of facts and ideas to understand their relationships and to form appropriate conclusions. Attempt to measure the

Cranial Nerve Function and Assessment

Table 12-12

Number	Name	Type	Function	Method
I	Olfactory	Sensory	Sense of smell	Ask client to identify different nonirritating aromas such as coffee and vanilla.
II	Optic	Sensory	Visual acuity	Use Snellen chart or ask client to read printed material while wearing glasses.
III	Oculomotor	Motor	Extraocular eye movement	Assess directions of gaze.
			Pupil constriction and dilation	Measure pupil reaction to light reflex and accommodation.
IV	Trochlear	Motor	Upward and downward movement of eyeball	Assess directions of gaze.
V	Trigeminal	Sensory and motor	Sensory nerve to skin of face	Lightly touch cornea with wisp of cotton. Assess corneal reflex. Measure sensation of light pain and touch across skin of face.
			Motor nerve to muscles of jaw	Palpate temples as client clenches teeth.
VI	Abducens	Motor	Lateral movement of eyeballs	Assess directions of gaze.
VII	Facial	Sensory and motor	Facial expression	As client smiles, frowns, puffs out cheeks, and raises and lowers eyebrows, look for asymmetry.
			Taste	Have client identify salty or sweet taste on front of tongue.
VIII	Auditory	Sensory	Hearing	Assess ability to hear spoken word.
IX	Glossopharyngeal	Sensory and motor	Taste	Ask client to identify sour or sweet taste on back of tongue.
			Ability to swallow	Use tongue blade to elicit gag reflex.
X	Vagus	Sensory and motor	Sensation of pharynx	Ask client to say "Ah." Observe palate and pharynx movement.
			Movement of vocal cords	Assess speech for hoarseness.
XI	Spinal accessory	Motor	Movement of head and shoulders	Ask client to shrug shoulders and turn head against passive resistance.
XII	Hypoglossal	Motor	Position of tongue	Ask client to stick out tongue to midline and move it from side to side.

client's ability to make logical decisions with questions such as "Why did you decide to seek health care?" or "What would you do if you suddenly became ill at home?" Normally a client can make logical decisions.

Cranial Nerve Function

All 12 cranial nerves or a single nerve or related group of nerves may be assessed. A dysfunction in one nerve reflects an alteration at some point along the distribution of the cranial nerve. Measurements used to assess the integrity of organs within the head and neck also assess cranial nerve function. A complete assessment involves testing the 12 cranial nerves in order of their number. To remember the order of the nerves, this simple phrase can be used: "On old Olympus' towering tops a Finn and German viewed some hops." The first letter of each word in the phrase is the same as the first letter of the names of the cranial nerves listed in order (Table 12-12).

Sensory Function

The sensory pathways of the central nervous system conduct the sensations of pain, temperature, position, vibration, and crude and finely localized touch. Different nerve pathways relay the various types of sensations. Most clients require only a quick screening of sensory function, unless there are symptoms of reduced sensation, motor impairment, or paralysis.

Normally a client has sensory responses to all stimuli tested. Sensations are felt equally on both sides of the body in all areas. Perform all sensory testing with the client's eyes closed so that the client is unable to see when or where a stimulus strikes the skin (Table 12-13). Then apply stimuli in a random, unpredictable order to maintain the client's attention and to prevent detection of a predictable pattern. The client tells you when, what, and where each stimulus is felt. You compare symmetrical areas of the body while applying stimuli to the arms, trunk, and legs.

Motor Function

An assessment of motor function includes measurements made during the musculoskeletal examination. In addition, cerebellar function is determined. The cerebellum coordinates muscular activity, maintains balance and equilibrium, and helps to control posture. Clients with any degree of motor dysfunction are at risk for injury (Box 12-27).

BALANCE.   Assess balance by asking the client to stand with the feet together and arms at the sides, with eyes open and closed. Standing close to the client prevents an accidental fall.

Assessment of Sensory Nerve Function

Table 12-13

Function	Equipment	Method	Precautions
Pain	Broken tongue blade or wooden end of cotton applicator	Ask client to voice when dull or sharp sensation is felt. Alternately apply sharp and blunt ends of tongue blade to skin's surface. Note areas of numbness or increased sensitivity.	Remember that areas where skin is thickened, such as heel or sole of foot, may be less sensitive to pain.
Temperature	Two test tubes, one filled with hot water and the other with cold	Touch skin with tube. Ask client to identify hot or cold sensation.	Omit test if pain sensation is normal.
Light touch	Cotton ball or cotton-tipped applicator	Apply light wisp of cotton to different points along skin's surface. Ask client to voice when sensation is felt.	Apply at areas where skin is thin or more sensitive (e.g., face, neck, inner aspect of arms, top of feet and hands).
Vibration	Tuning fork	Apply stem of vibrating fork to distal interphalangeal joint of fingers and interphalangeal joint of great toe, elbow, and wrist. Have client voice when and where the vibration is felt.	Be sure client feels vibration and not merely pressure.
Position		Grasp finger or toe, holding it by its sides with thumb and index finger. Alternate moving finger or toe up and down. Ask client to state when finger is up or down. Repeat with toes.	Avoid rubbing adjacent appendages as finger or toe is moved. Do not move joint laterally; return to neutral position before moving again.
Two-point discrimination	Two broken tongue blades	Lightly apply one or both tongue blade tips simultaneously to skin's surface. Ask client if one or two pricks are felt. Find the distance at which client can no longer distinguish two points.	Apply blade tips to same anatomical site (e.g., fingertips, palm of hand, upper arms). Minimum distance at which client can discriminate two points varies (2 to 8 mm on fingertips).

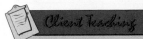

Box 12-27

NEUROLOGICAL SYSTEM ASSESSMENT

- Explain to family or friends the implications of any behavioral or mental impairment shown by the client.
- If the client has sensory or motor impairments, explain measures to ensure safety (e.g., use of ambulation aids, use of safety bars in bathrooms or on stairways).
- Teach older adults to plan enough time to complete tasks because reaction time is slowed.
- Teach older adults to observe skin surface for areas of trauma because their perception of pain is reduced.

Slight swaying of the body is expected in Romberg's test. A loss of balance (positive Romberg) causes a client to fall to the side.

COORDINATION.   To avoid confusion, you should demonstrate each coordination assessment maneuver and then have the client repeat it while you observe for smoothness and balance in the client's movement. In older adults normally slow reaction time may cause movements to be less rhythmical.

To assess fine motor function, have the client extend the arms out to the sides and touch each forefinger alternately to the nose (first with eyes open, then with eyes closed). Normally the client alternately touches the nose smoothly. Performing rapid, rhythmical, alternating movements demonstrates coordination in the upper extremities. While sitting, the client begins by patting the knees with both hands. Then the client alternately turns up the palm and back of the hands while continuously patting. The maneuver should be done smoothly and regularly with increasing speed.

Test lower extremity coordination with the client lying supine, legs extended. Place your hand at the ball of the client's foot. The client taps your hand with the foot as quickly as possible. Test each foot for speed and smoothness. The feet do not normally move as rapidly or evenly as the hands.

Reflexes

Reflex testing assesses the integrity of sensory and motor pathways of the reflex arc and specific spinal cord segments. When a muscle and tendon are stretched, nerve impulses travel along afferent nerve pathways to the dorsal horn of the spinal cord segment. Impulses synapse and travel to the efferent motor neuron in the spinal cord. A motor nerve then sends the impulses back to the muscle, causing the reflex response. Practice is needed to test reflexes accurately.

The two categories of normal reflexes are deep tendon reflexes, elicited by mildly stretching a muscle and tapping a tendon, and cutaneous reflexes, elicited by stimulating the skin superficially. Reflexes are graded as follows:

0   No response
1+   Low normal with slight muscle contraction
2+   Normal with visible muscle twitch and movement of the arm or leg
3+   Brisker than normal; may not indicate disease

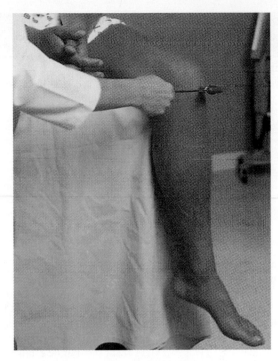

FIGURE **12-56**   Position for testing patellar tendon reflex. Lower leg will normally extend.

4+   Hyperactive and very brisk; often associated with spinal cord disorders

When reflexes are being assessed, the client relaxes as much as possible to avoid voluntary movement or muscle tensing. Position the limbs to slightly stretch the muscle being tested. Hold the reflex hammer loosely between your thumb and fingers so it can swing freely. Then tap the tendon briskly (Figure 12-56). Compare the symmetry of the reflex from one side of the body to the other. Reflexes are graded based on the degree of response. In older adults reflexes are normally slowed. Table 12-14 summarizes common deep tendon and cutaneous reflexes.

AFTER THE EXAMINATION

You may record findings from the physical assessment during the examination or at the end. Special forms are available to record data. Review all findings before assisting the client with dressing in case of a need to recheck any information or gather additional data. Physical assessment findings are integrated into the plan of care.

After completing the assessment, give the client time to dress. The hospitalized client may need help with hygiene and returning to bed. When the client is comfortable, it helps to share a summary of the assessment findings. If the findings have revealed serious abnormalities such as a highly irregular heart rate, the client's physician should be consulted before any findings are revealed. It is the physician's responsibility to make definitive medical diagnoses. You can explain the type of abnormality found and the need for the physician to conduct an additional examination.

Assessment of Common Reflexes

Table 12-14

Type	Procedure	Normal Reflex
Deep Tendon Reflexes		
Biceps	Flex client's arm up to 45 degrees at elbow with palms down. Place your thumb in antecubital fossa at base of biceps tendon and your fingers over the biceps muscle. Strike triceps tendon with reflex hammer.	Flexion of arm at elbow
Triceps	Flex client's arm at the elbow, holding arm across chest, or hold upper arm horizontally and allow lower arm to go limp. Strike triceps tendon just above elbow.	Extension at elbow
Patellar	Have client sit with legs hanging freely over side of table or chair, or have client lie supine and support knee in a flexed 90-degree position. Briskly tap patellar tendon just below patella.	Extension of lower leg
Achilles	Have client assume same position as for patellar reflex. Slightly dorsiflex client's ankle by grasping toes in palm of your hand. Strike Achilles tendon just above heel at the ankle malleolus.	Plantar flexion of foot
Cutaneous Reflexes		
Plantar	Have client lie supine with legs straight and feet relaxed. Take handle end of reflex hammer, and stroke lateral aspect of sole from heel to ball of foot, curving across ball of foot toward big toe.	Plantar flexion of all toes
Gluteal	Have client assume side-lying position. Spread buttocks apart, and lightly stimulate perineal area with cotton applicator.	Contraction of anal sphincter
Abdominal	Have client stand or lie supine. Stroke abdominal skin with base of cotton applicator over lateral borders of rectus abdominus muscle toward midline. Repeat test in each abdominal quadrant.	Contraction of rectus abdominus muscle with pulling of umbilicus toward stimulated side

Support staff may be delegated to clean the examination area. Infection-control practices are used in removing materials or instruments soiled with potentially infectious wastes. If the client's bedside was the site for the examination, clear away soiled items from the bedside table and makes sure the bed linen is dry and clean. The client may appreciate a clean gown and the opportunity to wash the face and hands. Afterward, be sure to wash your hands.

Check to be sure the recording of the assessment is complete. If entry of items into the assessment form was delayed, enter them at this time to avoid forgetting important information. If entries were made periodically during the examination, review them for accuracy and thoroughness. Communicate significant findings to appropriate medical and nursing personnel, either verbally or in the client's written care plan.

The client often needs a number of ancillary examinations such as x-ray film examinations, laboratory tests, or ultrasonography after a physical examination. The tests provide additional screening information to rule out and to help diagnose specific abnormalities found during the examination. You should explain the purpose of these tests and the sensations that the client can expect.

Key Terms

acromegaly, p. 231
adventitious sounds, p. 244
alopecia, p. 228
aneurysms, p. 261
aphasia, p. 272
arcus senilis, p. 233
atherosclerosis, p. 249
atrophied, p. 264
auscultation, p. 217
basal cell carcinoma, p. 226
borborygmi, p. 261
bruit, p. 250
cerumen, p. 234

chancres, p. 264
clubbing, p. 253
conjunctivitis, p. 233
crackles, p. 244
cyanosis, p. 226
dysmenorrhea, p. 263
dyspnea, p. 241
dysrhythmia, p. 249
ectropion, p. 233
edema, p. 225
entropion, p. 233
erythema, p. 227
excoriation, p. 236
exostosis, p. 238
fibrocystic breast disease, p. 259

gingivae, p. 237
hematemesis, p. 260
hemorrhoids, p. 267
hernia, p. 267
hydrocephalus, p. 231
hypertonicity, p. 270
hypotonicity, p. 270
induration, p. 227
inspection, p. 216
jaundice, p. 227
kyphosis, p. 268
leukoplakia, p. 237
lordosis, p. 268
melanoma, p. 225
melena, p. 260

Key Concepts

- Baseline assessment findings reflect the client's functional abilities when you first assess the client and serve as the basis for comparison with subsequent assessment findings.
- Assessment data are used to make nursing diagnoses, select appropriate nursing interventions, and evaluate the outcomes of nursing care.
- Physical assessment of a child or infant requires that you apply principles of physical growth and development.
- You should recognize that the normal process of aging affects physical findings collected from an older adult.
- Integrate client teaching throughout the examination to help clients learn about health promotion and disease prevention.
- You can use time more efficiently by integrating physical assessment with routine nursing care.
- Inspection requires good lighting, full exposure of the body part, and a careful comparison of the part with its counterpart on the opposite side of the body.
- Palpation involves the use of parts of the hand to detect different types of physical characteristics.
- Use auscultation to assess the character of sounds created in various body organs.
- Perform a physical examination only after proper preparation of the environment and equipment and after preparing the client physically and psychologically.
- Throughout the examination keep the client warm, comfortable, and informed of each step of the assessment process.

- The client assumes various positions during the physical examination to provide greater accessibility of body parts and to increase accuracy in assessment.
- A competent examiner learns to be systematic while combining assessments of different body systems simultaneously.
- Information from the history helps you to focus on body systems likely to be affected.
- When assessing a seriously ill client, concentrate on the body systems most likely to be affected.
- Accuracy in assessing the thorax, heart, and abdomen is enhanced by creating a mental image of internal organs in relation to external anatomical landmarks.
- When assessing heart sounds, imagine events occurring during the cardiac cycle.
- Never palpate the carotid arteries simultaneously.
- When examining a woman's breasts, explain the techniques for breast self-examination.
- The abdominal assessment differs from other portions of the examination in that auscultation follows inspection.
- During assessment of the genitalia, explain the technique for genital self-examination.
- Assessment of musculoskeletal function can be easily conducted when observing the client ambulate or participate in other active movements.
- Assess mental and emotional status by interacting with the client throughout the examination.
- At the end of the examination provide for the client's comfort and then complete a detailed review of physical assessment findings.

Critical Thinking Activities

1. A 32-year-old client entering a neighborhood clinic exhibits the following symptoms: frequent productive cough, fatigue, decreased appetite, and persistent fever. What focused assessment should you conduct?
2. You are performing an abdominal assessment and observe a pulsating midline abdominal mass. What is your next line of action?
3. What physical examination techniques do you use during the following situations: evaluating a client's oral hygiene, a client with a cast on the lower leg, a client found on the floor, and a client reporting abdominal pain?
4. An older adult woman with reduced visual acuity would have difficulty performing what aspect of breast self-examination?
5. You are visiting a 75-year-old black male 1 week postoperatively to assess peripheral vascular status following a femoral-popliteal bypass graft for arterial insufficiency. What assessment data do you obtain?

Review Questions

1. The first technique you employ when conducting a client's physical examination is:
   1. palpation.
   2. inspection.
   3. percussion.
   4. auscultation.

2. To assess the client's posterior tibial pulse, you would palpate:
   1. behind the knee.
   2. over the lateral malleolus.
   3. in the groove behind the medial malleolus.
   4. lateral to the extensor tendon of the great toe.

3. The main reason you auscultate before palpation of the client's abdomen is to:
   1. prevent distortion of vascular sounds.
   2. prevent distortion of the bowel sounds.
   3. determine any areas of tenderness or pain.
   4. allow the client to relax and be comfortable.

4. To correctly palpate the client's skin for temperature, you will use the:
   1. base of your hands.
   2. fingertips of your hands.
   3. dorsal surface of your hands.
   4. palmar surface of your hands.

5. To assess a client's superficial lymph nodes, you would:
   1. deeply palpate using entire hand.
   2. deeply palpate using a bimanual technique.
   3. lightly palpate using a bimanual technique.
   4. gently palpate using the pads of your index and middle fingers.

6. To spread the breast tissue evenly over the chest wall during an examination, you ask the client to lie supine with:
   1. hands clasped just above the umbilicus.
   2. both arms overhead with palms upward.
   3. the dominant arm straight alongside the body.
   4. the ipsilateral arm overhead with a small pillow under the shoulder.

7. In assessing for chronic tissue hypoxia, you assess for clubbing. To perform the examination, you:
   1. inspects for bulging of tissues at the nail base.
   2. palpate the chest wall for vibrations while the client says "99."
   3. compare the anteroposterior diameter of the chest with the lateral diameter of the chest.
   4. observe the amount of time it takes for normal color to return to fingernail after pressure has been applied for a few seconds.

8. In performing a breast assessment on a female client, you teach the client that it is especially important to palpate the upper outer quadrant of breast tissue because this area is:
   1. the largest area of the breast.
   2. more prone to calcifications.
   3. where most breast tumors are located.
   4. where most lymph nodes are located.

9. You are teaching the client to inspect all skin surfaces and to report pigmented skin lesions that:
   1. are symmetrical.
   2. have irregular borders.
   3. are uniform in color.
   4. are less than 6 mm in diameter.

10. The client is being assessed for range-of-joint movement. You ask the client to move the arm away from the body, evaluating the movement of:
    1. flexion.
    2. extension.
    3. abduction.
    4. adduction.

11. During a thoracic examination, you place your thumbs along the spinal processes at the tenth rib, with the palms lightly contacting the client's posterolateral surfaces. As the client deep breathes, you evaluate symmetry. This technique is known as:
    1. vocal fremitus.
    2. tactile fremitus.
    3. diaphragmatic excursion.
    4. lateral thoracic excursion.

12. The client's respiratory assessment reveals bilateral high pitches, continuous musical sounds heard loudest upon expiration. The nurse interprets these sounds as:
    1. normal.
    2. crackles.
    3. rhonchi.
    4. wheezes.

13. When inspecting the client's anterior thorax, you observe for:
    1. presence of fremitus.
    2. presence of breath sounds.
    3. movement of the diaphragm.
    4. symmetry of chest excursion.

14. When auscultating the adult client's thorax, you would:
    1. instruct the client to take deep, rapid breaths.
    2. instruct the client to breathe in and out through the nose.
    3. use the bell of the stethoscope held lightly against the chest.
    4. use the diaphragm of the stethoscope held firmly against the chest.

15. You are auscultating the client's lung fields. The systematic pattern you use for comparison is:
    1. side to side.
    2. top to bottom.
    3. anterior to posterior.
    4. interspace to interspace.

16. You are teaching a client how to perform a testicular self-examination. You should tell the client:
    1. "Contact your physician if you feel a painless pea-sized nodule."
    2. "The testes are normally round, moveable, and have a lumpy consistency."
    3. "The best time to do a testicular self-examination is before your bath or shower."
    4. "Perform a testicular self-examination every week to detect signs of testicular cancer."

17. When testing sensory pathways, you:
    1. use a predictable order.
    2. perform each test quickly.
    3. compare symmetrical areas.
    4. ensure that the client's eyes remain open.

18. You ask the client to interpret the saying "Don't count your chickens before they're hatched." The client's response reveals:
    1. judgment.
    2. knowledge.
    3. association.
    4. abstract reasoning.

19. You ask the client to smile, frown, and raise and lower the eyebrows; these actions test cranial nerve number:
    1. VII – facial.
    2. V – trigeminal.
    3. III – oculomotor.
    4. XII – hypoglossal.
20. You used the reflex hammer to test the client's patellar tendon reflex and graded it a 3+. A 3+ reflex is:
    1. normal.
    2. hyperactive.
    3. low normal.
    4. brisker than normal.
21. The client had surgery 24 hours ago. After listening for 30 seconds at a site below and to the right of the umbilicus, you are unable to hear bowel sounds. The best assessment of this situation is that:
    1. the client has gastritis.
    2. you need to listen longer.
    3. the client has a partial bowel obstruction.
    4. you are not listening in the right place.
22. To examine for hernias you ask the client to:
    1. jump in place.
    2. lift a heavy object.
    3. strain or bear down.
    4. assume the prone position.
23. While auscultating heart sounds, you document that S_1 is heard best at the apex. This sound correlates with closure of the:
    1. aortic and mitral valves.
    2. mitral and tricuspid valves.
    3. aortic and pulmonic valves.
    4. tricuspid and pulmonic values.
24. You are conducting the general survey of an adult client. The general survey includes:
    1. appearance and behavior.
    2. measurement of vital signs.
    3. observing specific body systems.
    4. conducting a detailed health history.
25. When conducting an otoscopic examination on an infant, you:
    1. release the auricle once the speculum is in place.
    2. use the largest speculum to see all the landmarks.
    3. pull the auricle up and back before inserting the speculum.
    4. pull the auricle down and back before inserting the speculum.

References

American Cancer Society: *1998 Cancer facts and figures,* New York, 1998, The Society.

American Cancer Society: *2001 Cancer facts and figures,* New York, 2001, The Society.

Barkauskas VH and others: *Health and physical assessment,* ed 2, St. Louis, 1998, Mosby.

Basfield-Holland ES: Assessing pulmonary status: it's more than listening to breath sounds, *Nursing 97* 27(8):32, 1997.

Berlinger JS: Why don't you just leave him? *Nursing 98* 23(4):34, 1998.

Caulker-Burnett I: Primary care screening for substance abuse, *Nurse Pract* 19(6):42, 1994.

Ebersole P, Hess P: *Toward healthy aging,* ed 5, St. Louis, 1998, Mosby.

Folstein MF and others: Mini-mental state: a practical method for grading the cognitive state of patients for the clinician, *J Psychiatr Res* 12:189, 1975.

Friedman L and others: *Source book of substance abuse and addiction,* Baltimore, 1996, Williams & Wilkins.

Galsworthy T, Wilson P: Osteoporosis: it steals more than bone, *Am J Nurs* 96(6):27, 1996.

Haney PE and others: Tuberculosis makes a comeback, *AORN J* 63(4):705, 1996.

Hardy M: What can you do about your patient's dry skin? *J Gerontol Nurs* 22(5):10, 1996.

Hopkins ML, Schoener L: Tuberculosis and the elderly living in long-term care facilities, *Geriatr Nurs* 17(1):27, 1996.

Kahn RL and others: Brief objective measures for the determination of mental status in the aged, *Am J Psychiatry* 117:326, 1960.

Kessenich CR, Rosen CJ: Osteoporosis implications for elderly men, *Geriatr Nurs* 17(4):171, 1996.

Lueckenotte A: *Pocket guide to gerontologic assessment,* ed 3, St. Louis, 1998, Mosby.

Lynch SH: Elder abuse: what to look for, how to intervene, *Am J Nurs* 97(1):27, 1997.

Master S, Terpstra J: Recognition and diagnosis. In Schnoll SH and others: *Prescribing drugs with abuse liability,* Richmond, Va, 1992, DSAM, MCV-VCU.

Pace H, Hoag-Apel CM: Stemming the tide of domestic violence, *Point of View Magazine* 33(3):12, 1996.

Seidel HM and others: *Mosby's guide to physical examination,* ed 4, St. Louis, 1999, Mosby.

Shea CA and others: Breaking through the barriers to domestic violence intervention, *Am J Nurs* 97(6):26, 1997.

Stuart G, Laraia M: *Stuart and Sundeen's principles and practice of psychiatric nursing,* ed 6, St. Louis, 1998, Mosby.

Talbot L, Curtis L: The challenges of assessing skin indicators in people of color, *Home Healthc Nurse* 14(3):167, 1996.

Thompson JM and others: *Mosby's clinical nursing,* ed 5, St. Louis, 2001, Mosby.

Wong DL and others: *Whaley and Wong's nursing care of infants and children,* ed 6, St. Louis, 1999, Mosby.

13

Administering Medications

Objectives

- Define the key terms listed.
- Discuss the nurse's legal responsibilities in medication prescription and administration.
- Describe the physiological mechanisms of medication action, including absorption, distribution, metabolism, and excretion of medications.
- Differentiate toxic, idiosyncratic, allergic, and side effects of medications.
- Discuss developmental factors that influence pharmacokinetics.
- Discuss factors that influence medication actions.
- Discuss methods of educating a client about prescribed medications.
- Describe the roles of the pharmacist, physician, and nurse in medication administration.
- Describe factors to consider when choosing routes of medication administration.
- Correctly calculate a prescribed medication dosage.
- Discuss factors to include in assessing a client's needs for and response to medication therapy.
- List the five rights of medication administration.
- Correctly prepare and administer subcutaneous, intramuscular, and intradermal injections; intravenous medications; oral and topical skin preparations; eye, ear, and nose drops; vaginal instillations; rectal suppositories; and inhalants.

*C*lients with acute or chronic alterations in their health may use a variety of medications. A medication is a substance used in the diagnosis, treatment, relief, or prevention of health alterations. No matter where clients receive their health care—as the nurse—you play an essential role in medication administration, teaching, and evaluation of the effectiveness of medications in restoring or maintaining health. Your role in medication administration differs based on the setting of the client-nurse interaction.

In the primary care setting, the client often self-administers medications. In this setting you are responsible for evaluating the effects of the medications on the client's health status, teaching the client about medications and their side effects, ensuring client compliance with medication regimens, and evaluating the client's medication administration technique. In the acute care setting, much time is spent administering medications to clients. Before discharge, you must ensure that clients are adequately prepared to administer their medications when they return to the community. In the home, clients usually administer their own medications. When clients cannot administer their own medications, family caregivers may be responsible for doing so. You must assess the effect the medications have in restoring or maintaining health as well as provide continued education to the client, family, or caregiver in all aspects of medication administration.

▌SCIENTIFIC KNOWLEDGE BASE

Because medication administration is essential to nursing practice, you need to be knowledgeable about the actions and effects of the medications you give to clients. To safely and accurately administer medications, you must have an understanding of pharmacokinetics (the movement of drugs in the human body), growth and development, nutrition, and mathematics.

Application of Pharmacology in Nursing Practice

NAMES.   A medication may have as many as three different names. A medication's chemical name provides an exact description of the medication's composition and molecular structure. Chemical names are rarely used in clinical practice. An example of a chemical name is *N*-acetyl-*para*-aminophenol, which is commonly known as Tylenol. The manufacturer who first develops the medication gives the generic or nonproprietary name, with United States Adopted Name Council (USANC) approval. Acetaminophen is an example of a generic name. It is the generic name for Tylenol. The generic name becomes the official name that is listed in publications such as the *United States Pharmacopeia* (USP). The trade or brand name (e.g., Tylenol) is the name under which a manufacturer markets a medication. The trade name has the symbol ® at the upper right of the name, indicating that the manufacturer has copyrighted the medication's name. You will find medications under a variety of different names. Because medications often have similar spellings and may sound similar, be careful to obtain the exact name and spelling for a particular medication (Goucher, 2000).

CLASSIFICATION.   Medications with similar characteristics are grouped into classifications. Medication classification indicates the effect of the medication on a body system, the symptoms the medication relieves, or the medication's desired effect. Usually each class contains more than one medication that can be prescribed for a type of health problems. For example, clients who have type 2 diabetes often take oral medications to lower their blood sugar. This class of medication is called *oral hypoglycemic agents*. There are more than eight different types of oral hypoglycemic agents. The physical and chemical composition of medications within a class may be slightly different. A health care provider chooses a particular oral hypoglycemic medication based on client characteristics, cost, efficacy, dosing frequency, or experience with the medication. A medication may also be part of more than one class. For example, aspirin is an analgesic, an antipyretic, and an antiinflammatory medication.

MEDICATION FORMS.   Medications are available in a variety of forms or preparations. The form of the medication determines its route of administration. Many medications are made in several forms, such as tablets, capsules, elixirs, and suppositories. When administering a medication, be certain to use the proper form (Table 13-1).

Medication Legislation and Standards

GOVERNMENTAL REGULATION OF MEDICATIONS. The role of the U.S. government in regulation of the pharmaceutical industry is to protect the health of the people by ensuring that medications are safe and effective. The first U.S. law to regulate medications was the Pure Food and Drug Act. This law simply requires all medications to be free of impure products. Subsequent legislation has set standards related to safety, potency, and efficacy. Enforcement of medication laws rests with the Food and Drug Administration (FDA) by ensuring that all medications on the market undergo vigorous review before they are allowed to be dispensed to the public.

In 1993 the FDA instituted the MedWatch program. This voluntary program encourages nurses and other health care professionals to report when a medication, product, or medical event causes serious harm to a client. A MedWatch form is available to report such events.

State and local medication laws must conform to federal laws. Individual states may have stricter controls than the federal government.

HEALTH CARE INSTITUTIONS AND MEDICATION LAWS. Health care institutions establish individual policies that must meet federal, state, and local regulations. The size of an institution, the types of services it provides, and the types of professional personnel it employs influence these policies. Institutional policies are often more restrictive than governmental controls. An institution is concerned primarily with

Forms of Medication — Table 13-1

Form	Description
Caplet	Solid dosage for oral use; shaped like a capsule and coated for ease of swallowing.
Capsule	Solid dosage form for oral use; medication in a powder, liquid, or oil form and encased by a gelatin shell; capsule colored to aid in product identification.
Elixir	Clear fluid containing water and/or alcohol; designed for oral use; usually has a sweetener added.
Enteric-coated	Tablet for oral use is coated with materials that do not dissolve in the stomach; coatings dissolve in the intestine, where medication is absorbed.
Extract	Concentrated drug form made by removing the active portion of a drug from its other components (e.g., a fluid extract is a drug made into a solution from a vegetable source).
Glycerite	Solution of drug combined with glycerin for external use; contains at least 50% glycerin.
Intraocular disk	A small, flexible oval consisting of two soft, outer layers and a middle layer containing medication. When moistened by ocular fluid, it releases medication for up to 1 week.
Liniment	Preparation usually containing alcohol, oil, or soapy emollient that is applied to skin.
Lotion	Drug in liquid suspension applied to protect skin.
Ointment (salve)	Semisolid preparation, thicker and stiffer than ointment; absorbed through skin more slowly than ointment.
Paste	Semisolid preparation, thicker and stiffer than ointment; absorbed through skin more slowly than ointment.
Pill	Solid dosage form containing one or more drugs, shaped into globules, ovoids, or oblong shapes; true pills are rarely used; they have been replaced by tablets.
Solution	Liquid preparation that may be used orally, parenterally, externally, or inhaled; can also be instilled into a body organ or cavity (e.g., bladder irrigations); contains water with one or more dissolved compounds; must be sterile for parenteral use.
Suppository	Solid dosage form mixed with gelatin and shaped in form of pellet for insertion into body cavity (rectum or vagina); melts when it reaches body temperature, releasing drug for absorption.
Suspension	Finely divided drug particles dispersed in a liquid medium; when suspension is left standing, particles settle to the bottom of the container; commonly an oral medication and is not to be given intravenously.
Sustained-release	Solid dosage form that contains small particles of the drug coated with material that requires a varying amount of time to dissolve.
Syrup	Medication dissolved in a concentrated sugar solution; may contain flavoring to make drug more palatable.
Tablet	Powdered dosage form compressed into hard disks or cylinders; in addition to primary drug, contains binders (adhesive to allow powder to stick together), disintegrators (to promote tablet dissolution), lubricants (for ease of manufacturing), and fillers (for convenient tablet size).
Transdermal disk or patch	Medication contained within semipermeable membrane disk or patch, which allows medication to be absorbed through skin slowly over long periods.
Tincture	Alcohol or water-alcohol drug solution.
Troche (lozenge)	Flat, round dosage form containing drug, flavoring, sugar, and mucilage; dissolves in mouth to release drug.

preventing health problems resulting from medication use. A common institutional policy is the automatic discontinuation of narcotic analgesics after a set number of days. Although a prescriber may reorder the medication, this policy helps to control unnecessarily prolonged medication therapy.

MEDICATION REGULATIONS AND NURSING PRACTICE. State **nurse practice acts** have the most influence over nursing practice by defining the scope of a nurse's professional functions and responsibilities. In general, most practice acts are purposefully broad so as not to limit the professional responsibilities of the nurse. Institutions and agencies may interpret specific actions allowed under the acts, but they cannot modify, expand, or restrict the act's intent. The primary intent of the state nurse practice acts is to protect the public from unskilled, undereducated, and unlicensed nurses.

You are responsible for following legal provisions when administering controlled substances or narcotics, which are controlled through federal and state guidelines. Violations of the Controlled Substances Act are punishable by fines, im-

prisonment, and loss of nurse licensure. Hospitals and other health care institutions have policies for the proper storage and distribution of narcotics (Box 13-1).

NONTHERAPEUTIC MEDICATION USE. Some people use medications for purposes other than their intended effect. Factors such as peer pressure, curiosity, and the pursuit of pleasure may be motivators for nontherapeutic medication use. Problems with medication use are not limited to heroin, cocaine, and other street drugs.

You have ethical and legal responsibilities to understand the problems of persons using medications improperly. When caring for clients with suspected **medication abuse** or **medication dependence,** be aware of your values and attitudes about the willful use of potentially harmful substances. You cannot develop therapeutic relationships with clients if personal values interfere with acceptance or understanding of their needs. Knowing the physical, psychological, and social changes resulting from medication abuse allows you to identify clients with medication problems.

Guidelines for Safe Narcotic Administration and Control   Box 13-1

Keep all narcotics in a locked, secure place (e.g., cabinet or computerized medication cart).

During an institution's change of shift, a nurse going off duty counts all narcotics with a nurse coming on duty. Both nurses sign the narcotic record, indicating the count is correct.

Discrepancies in narcotic counts are reported immediately.

A record is kept each time a narcotic is dispensed. The record includes the client's name, date, time of drug administration, name of drug, and dosage. If a paper record is kept, the nurse dispensing the drug must sign the record. If the medication is dispensed through a computerized system, the computer records the nurse's name.

An ongoing record of narcotics used and remaining is kept.

If part of a controlled substance must be wasted, a second nurse must witness the disposal of the unused portion. Both nurses must record their names on the narcotic record.

Health professionals also misuse medications. Stress in the workplace, personal problems, and the strong desire to perform well are some factors that may cause nurses to misuse medications. You must recognize and understand the problems of colleagues who abuse medications. Many programs are available to assist these nurses toward recovery. These programs may be offered through the institution's employees' assistance program (EAP), the state board of nursing, or community agencies. *Stop Apr. 25*

Pharmacokinetics as the Basis of Medication Actions

For a medication to be therapeutically useful, it must be taken into a client's body; absorbed and distributed to cells, tissues, or a specific organ; and alter physiological functions. **Pharmacokinetics** is the study of how medications enter the body, reach their site of action, are metabolized, and exit the body (McKenry and Salerno, 2000). Knowledge of pharmacokinetics is used when timing medication administration, selecting the route of administration, judging the client's risk for alterations in medication action, and evaluating the client's response.

ABSORPTION.   **Absorption** refers to passage of medication molecules into the blood from the site of administration. Factors that influence medication absorption are the route of administration, ability of the medication to dissolve, blood flow to the site of administration, body surface area, and lipid solubility of the medication.

ROUTE OF ADMINISTRATION.   Medications can be administered by various routes. Each route has a different rate of absorption. When medications are placed on the skin, absorption is slow because of the physical makeup of the skin. Medications placed on the mucous membranes and in respiratory airways are quickly absorbed, because these tissues contain many blood vessels. Because orally administered

medications must pass through the gastrointestinal (GI) tract to be absorbed, the overall rate of absorption may be slowed. Intravenous (IV) injection produces the most rapid absorption, because this route provides immediate access to the systemic circulation.

ABILITY OF THE MEDICATION TO DISSOLVE.   The ability of an oral medication to dissolve depends largely on its form of preparation. Solutions and suspensions are already in a liquid state and are absorbed more readily than tablets or capsules. Acidic medications pass through the gastric mucosa rapidly, whereas medications that are basic are not absorbed before reaching the small intestine.

BLOOD FLOW TO THE AREA OF ABSORPTION.   The blood supply to the site of administration determines how quickly a drug is absorbed. Sites with rich blood supplies absorb medications more quickly.

BODY SURFACE AREA.   When a medication is in contact with a large surface area, the medication will be absorbed at a faster rate. This explains why the majority of medications are absorbed in the small intestine rather than the stomach.

LIPID SOLUBILITY OF THE MEDICATION.   Medications that are highly lipid soluble are absorbed easier because they readily cross the cell membrane, which is made of a lipid layer.

Another factor that may affect absorption of a medication is the presence of food in the stomach. Some oral medications are absorbed quicker on an empty stomach, whereas other medications are unaffected by gastric contents. In addition, some medications may interfere with the absorption of each other if given at the same time. Know the factors that may alter or impair absorption of the medications that have been prescribed for your clients. This knowledge ensures that all prescribed medications are administered at the correct time to allow for correct absorption of the drug.

DISTRIBUTION.   After a medication is absorbed, it is distributed within the body to tissues and organs and ultimately to its specific site of action. The rate and extent of distribution depend on the physical and chemical properties of medications and the physiology of the person taking the medication.

CIRCULATION.   Once a medication enters the bloodstream, it is carried throughout the tissue and organs of the body. How fast it gets there depends on the vascularity of the various tissues and organs. When conditions exist that limit blood flow or intended sites of action are poorly perfused, the distribution of a medication is inhibited. For example, solid tumors have poor blood supply and may not respond to therapy intended to destroy them.

MEMBRANE PERMEABILITY.   To be distributed to an organ, a medication must pass through all the biological membranes of that organ. Some membranes may serve as barriers to the passage of medications. For example, the blood-brain barrier allows only fat-soluble medications to pass into the brain and cerebrospinal fluid. Therefore central nervous system (CNS) infections require treatment with antibiotics injected directly into the subarachnoid space in the spinal cord. Older clients may experience adverse effects (e.g., confusion) as a result of the change in the permeability of the blood-brain barrier, with easier passage of fat-soluble medications. The placental membrane is a nonselective barrier to medications. Fat-soluble and non–fat-soluble agents may cross the placenta and produce fetal deformities, respiratory depression, and, with narcotic abuse, withdrawal symptoms.

PROTEIN BINDING.   The degree to which medications bind to serum proteins, such as albumin, affects medication distribution. Most medications bind to protein to some extent. When medications bind to albumin, they cannot exert any pharmacological activity. The unbound, or "free," medication is the active form of the medication. Older adults or clients with liver disease or malnutrition have decreased albumin in the bloodstream. Because more medication may be unbound in these clients, they are at risk for an increase in medication activity, toxicity, or both.

METABOLISM.   After a medication reaches its site of action, it becomes metabolized. **Biotransformation** occurs under the influence of enzymes that **detoxify,** degrade (break down), and remove biologically active chemicals. Most biotransformation occurs within the liver, although the lungs, kidneys, blood, and intestines also metabolize medications. The liver is especially important because its specialized structure oxidizes and transforms many toxic substances. The liver degrades many harmful chemicals before they become distributed to the tissues. If a decrease in liver function occurs, such as with aging or liver disease, a medication may be eliminated more slowly, resulting in an accumulation of the medication. If the organs that metabolize medications are altered, clients are at risk for medication toxicity.

EXCRETION.   After medications are metabolized, they exit the body through the kidneys, liver, bowel, lungs, and exocrine glands. The chemical makeup of a medication determines the organ of excretion. Gaseous and volatile compounds, such as nitrous oxide and alcohol, exit through the lungs. Deep breathing and coughing (see Chapter 36) help the postoperative client to eliminate anesthetic gases more rapidly. The exocrine glands excrete lipid-soluble medications. When medications exit through sweat glands, the skin may become irritated. The nurse assists the client in good hygiene practices (see Chapter 26) to promote cleanliness and skin integrity.

If a medication is excreted through the mammary glands, there is a risk that a nursing infant will ingest the chemicals. Mothers should check on the safety of any medication used while breast-feeding.

The GI tract is another route for medication excretion. Many medications enter the hepatic circulation to be broken down by the liver and excreted into the bile. After chemicals enter the intestines through the biliary tract, they may be reabsorbed by the intestines. Factors that increase peristalsis (e.g., laxatives, enemas) accelerate medication excretion through the feces, whereas factors that slow peristalsis (e.g., inactivity, improper diet) may prolong a medication's effects.

The kidneys are the main organs for medication excretion. Some medications escape extensive metabolism and exit unchanged in the urine. Other medications must undergo biotransformation in the liver before being excreted by the kidney. If renal function declines, a client is at risk for medication toxicity. If the kidney cannot adequately excrete a medication, it may be necessary to reduce the dose. Maintenance of an adequate fluid intake (50 ml/kg/day) promotes proper elimination of medications for the average adult.

Types of Medication Action

Medications vary considerably in the way they act and their types of action. Factors other than characteristics of the medication also influence medication actions. A client may not respond in the same way to each successive dose of a medication. Likewise, the same medication dosage may cause very different responses in different clients. Box 13-2 lists important variables that influence medication action.

THERAPEUTIC EFFECTS.   The **therapeutic effect** is the expected or predictable physiological response a medication causes. Each medication has a desired therapeutic effect for which it is prescribed. For example, nitroglycerin is used to reduce the cardiac workload and increase myocardial oxygen supply, thus decreasing or eliminating chest pain. A single medication may have many therapeutic effects. For example, aspirin is an analgesic, antipyretic, and anti-inflammatory, and it reduces platelet aggregation (clumping). It is important to know the expected therapeutic effect for each medication your clients receive. This will allow you to properly teach the client about the medication's intended effect and to evaluate the effectiveness of the medication.

SIDE EFFECTS.   A **side effect** occurs when a medication causes predictable, unintended, secondary effects. Side effects may be harmless or injurious. If the side effects are serious enough to negate the beneficial effects of a medication's therapeutic action, the medication is usually discontinued. Clients often stop taking medications because of side effects.

ADVERSE EFFECTS.   **Adverse effects** are generally considered severe responses to medication. For example, a client may become comatose when a drug is ingested. When adverse responses to medications occur, the prescriber must discontinue the medication. Some adverse effects are unexpected effects that were not discovered during drug testing. When this situation occurs, health care providers are obligated to report the adverse effect to the FDA.

Factors Influencing Drug Actions   Box 13-2

GENETIC DIFFERENCES

A person's genetic makeup can influence drug metabolism. Members of a family may share sensitivity to a medication.

PHYSIOLOGICAL VARIABLES

Gender, age, body weight, nutritional status, and disease states all affect drug actions.

Hormonal differences between men and women affect drug metabolism.

Children require lower drug doses than adults. The changes accompanying aging alter the influence of drugs.

There is a direct relationship between the amount of medication administered and the amount of body tissue in which it is distributed.

Diseases that impair the function of organs responsible for normal pharmacokinetics also impair drug action.

ENVIRONMENTAL CONDITIONS

Stress and the exposure to heat and cold affect drug actions. Clients receiving vasodilators, for example, require lower drug dosages in warm weather.

The setting in which a drug is administered can influence a client's reaction. If a person is alone or isolated, more pain medication may be needed than if he or she is in a room with other clients.

PSYCHOLOGICAL FACTORS

A client's attitude, reaction to the meaning of a drug, and the nurse's behavior affect drug actions. If a client understands and accepts the need for a drug and if it is administered with a supportive behavior, the drug's effect is enhanced.

DIET

Drug and nutrient interactions can alter a drug's action or the effect of a nutrient. For example, mineral oil decreases the absorption of fat-soluble vitamins.

Proper drug metabolism relies on good nutrition.

TOXIC EFFECTS.   Toxic effects may develop after prolonged intake of a medication or when a medication accumulates in the blood because of impaired metabolism or excretion. Excess amounts of a medication within the body may have lethal effects, depending on the medication's action. Sometimes, antidotes are available to treat specific types of medication toxicity. For example, a client experiencing toxic effects of morphine may have severe respiratory depression. In this case, you would give Narcan to reverse the toxic effects of the morphine.

IDIOSYNCRATIC REACTIONS.   Medications may cause unpredictable effects, such as **idiosyncratic reactions in which a client overreacts or underreacts to a medication or has a reaction different from normal. For example, a child receiving an antihistamine (e.g., Benadryl) may become extremely agitated or excited instead of drowsy.

ALLERGIC REACTIONS.   Allergic reactions are also unpredictable responses to a medication. A client can become sensitized immunologically to the initial dose of a medication. With repeated administration, the client develops an allergic response to the medication, its chemical preservatives, or a metabolite. The medication or chemical acts as an antigen, triggering the release of the body's antibodies. A client's **medication allergy** may be mild or severe. Allergic symptoms vary, depending on the individual and the medication. Common, mild allergy symptoms are summarized in Table 13-2. Severe or **anaphylactic reactions** are characterized by sudden constriction of bronchiolar muscles, edema of the pharynx and larynx, and severe wheezing and shortness of breath. Antihistamines, epinephrine, and bronchodilators may be used to treat anaphylactic reactions.

In anaphylaxis a client may also become severely hypotensive, necessitating emergency resuscitation measures. A client with a known history of an allergy to a

Mild Allergic Reactions   Table 13-2

Symptom	Description
Urticaria (hives)	Raised, irregularly shaped skin eruptions with varying sizes and shapes; have reddened margins and pale centers
Eczema (rash)	Small, raised vesicles that are usually reddened; often distributed over entire body
Pruritus	Itching of skin; accompanies most rashes
Rhinitis	Inflammation of mucous membranes lining nose; causes swelling and clear, watery discharge

medication should avoid reexposure and wear an identification bracelet or medal (Figure 13-1) that alerts health care providers to the allergy if the client is unconscious when receiving medical care.

MEDICATION INTERACTIONS.   When one medication modifies the action of another medication, a **medication interaction occurs. A medication may potentiate or diminish the action of other medications and may alter the way in which another medication is absorbed, metabolized, or eliminated from the body. When two medications have a **synergistic effect,** the effect of the two medications combined is greater than the effects of the medications when given separately. For example, alcohol is a CNS depressant that has a synergistic effect on antihistamines, antidepressants, barbiturates, and narcotic analgesics.

A medication interaction is not always undesirable. Often a physician orders combination medication therapy to create a medication interaction for the client's therapeutic benefit. For example, a client with moderate hypertension typically receives several medications, such as di-

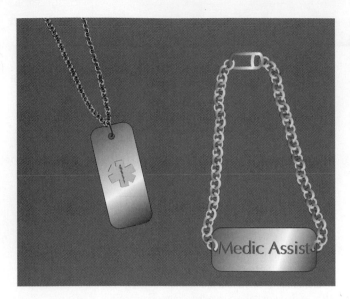

FIGURE 13-1   Identification bracelet and medal.

| Common Dosage Administration Schedule | Table 13-3 |
Abbreviation	Meaning
AC, ac	Before meals
ad lib	As desired
BID, bid	Twice per day
h	Hour
HS, hs	Hour of sleep
PC, pc	After meals
prn	Whenever there is a need
qAM	Every morning, every AM
qd, od	Every day
qh	Every hour
q2h	Every 2 hours
q4h	Every 4 hours
q6h	Every 6 hours
q8h	Every 8 hours
QID, qid	4 times per day
QOD, qod	Every other day
stat	Give immediately
TID, tid	3 times per day

uretics and vasodilators, that act together to control blood pressure.

MEDICATION DOSE RESPONSES.   A medication undergoes absorption, distribution, metabolism, and excretion after it is given. Except when administered intravenously, medications take time to enter the bloodstream.

All medications have a **serum half-life,** which is the time it takes for excretion to lower the serum medication **concentration** by half. To maintain a therapeutic plateau, the client must receive regular fixed doses. For example, it has been shown that pain medications are most effective when they are given "around the clock" rather than when the client intermittently complains of pain. In this way an almost constant level of pain medication is maintained. After an initial medication dose, the client receives each successive dose when the previous dose reaches its half-life.

You and the client must adhere to prescribed doses and dosage intervals. Table 13-3 lists common dosage schedules used in acute care settings. When teaching clients about dosage schedules, use language that is familiar to the client. For example, when teaching a client about twice-daily medication dosing, instruct the client to take the medication in the morning and again in the evening. Knowledge of the time intervals of medication action will help you anticipate a medication's effect. With this knowledge, you can instruct the client when to expect a response. Table 13-4 lists common terms associated with medication actions.

Routes of Administration

The route prescribed for administering a medication depends on the medication's properties and desired effect and on the client's physical and mental condition (Table 13-5). You should collaborate with the prescriber in determining the best route for a client's medication. For example, you are caring for a client who has 650 mg of acetaminophen or-

| Terms Associated With Medication Actions | Table 13-4 |
Term	Meaning
Onset	Time it takes after a drug is administered for it to produce a response
Peak	Time it takes for a drug to reach its highest effective concentration
Trough	Minimum blood serum concentration of a drug reached just before the next scheduled dose
Duration	Time during which the drug is present in a concentration great enough to produce a response
Plateau	Blood serum concentration of a drug reached and maintained after repeated fixed doses

dered by mouth over 4 hours as needed for a temperature greater than 38.0° C (100.4° F). Your client has a temperature of 38.5° C (101.2° F), is vomiting, and is unable to tolerate oral fluids. Knowing your client cannot tolerate oral medications at this time, you consult with the prescriber and have the medication changed to a rectal suppository.

ORAL ROUTES.   The oral route is the easiest and the most commonly used. Medications are given by mouth and swallowed with fluid. Oral medications have a slower onset of action and a more prolonged effect than parenteral medications. Clients generally prefer the oral route.

SUBLINGUAL ADMINISTRATION.   Some medications are designed to be readily absorbed after being placed under the tongue to dissolve (Figure 13-2). A medication given by the **sublingual** route should not be swallowed or chewed,

Factors Influencing Choice of Administration Routes   Table 13-5

Advantages	Disadvantages
Oral, Buccal, Sublingual Routes	
Routes are convenient and comfortable for client.	These routes are avoided when client has alterations in GI function
Routes are economical.	(e.g., nausea, vomiting), reduced motility (after general anesthesia or
Medications may produce local or systemic effects.	bowel inflammation), gastric suction, surgical resection of portion
Routes rarely cause anxiety for client.	of GI tract, and reduced ability to swallow.
	Oral medications may irritate lining of GI tract, discolor teeth, or have
	unpleasant taste.
SQ, IM, IV, ID Routes	
Routes provide means of administration when oral drugs are	There is risk of introducing infection, drugs are expensive, and these
contraindicated.	routes are avoided in clients with bleeding tendencies.
More rapid absorption occurs than with topical or oral routes.	There is risk of tissue damage with SQ injections.
IV infusion provides drug delivery when client is critically ill.	IM and IV routes are dangerous because of rapid absorption.
If peripheral perfusion is poor, IV route is preferred over	These routes cause considerable anxiety in many clients, especially
injections.	children.
Skin	
Topical	
Topical skin applications primarily provide local effect.	Extensive applications may be bulky and cause difficulty in maneuvering.
Route is painless.	Clients with skin abrasions are at risk for rapid drug absorption and
Limited side effects occur.	systemic effects.
Transdermal	
Transdermal applications provide prolonged systemic effects,	Application leaves oily or pasty substance on skin and may soil clothing.
with limited side effects.	
Mucous Membranes*	
Therapeutic effects are provided by local application to in-	Mucous membranes are highly sensitive to some drug concentrations.
volved sites.	Insertion of rectal and vaginal medication often causes embarrassment.
Aqueous solutions are readily absorbed and capable of caus-	Client with ruptured eardrum cannot receive irrigations.
ing systemic effects.	Rectal suppositories are contraindicated if client has had rectal surgery
Mucous membranes provide route of administration when	or if active rectal bleeding is present.
oral drugs are contraindicated.	
Inhalation	
Inhalation provides rapid relief for local respiratory problems.	Some local agents can cause serious systemic effects.
Route provides easy access for introduction of general anes-	
thetic gases.	

*Includes eyes, ears, nose, vagina, rectum, buccal and sublingual routes.

or the desired effect will not be achieved. Nitroglycerin is commonly given by the sublingual route. The client should not take a drink until the medication is completely dissolved.

BUCCAL ADMINISTRATION.   Administration of a medication by the **buccal** route involves placing the solid medication in the mouth and against the mucous membranes of the cheek until the medication dissolves (Figure 13-3). Teach clients to alternate cheeks with each subsequent dose to avoid mucosal irritation and not to chew or swallow the medication or to take any liquids with it. A buccal medication acts locally on the mucosa or systemically as it is swallowed in a person's saliva.

PARENTERAL ROUTES.   **Parenteral administration** involves injecting a medication into body tissues. The four major parenteral routes are as follows:

1. **Subcutaneous (SQ):** injection into tissues just below the dermis of the skin
2. **Intramuscular (IM):** injection into a muscle
3. **Intravenous (IV):** injection into a vein
4. **Intradermal (ID):** injection into the dermis just under the epidermis

Some medications may be administered into body cavities through other routes, including epidural, intraperitoneal, intrathecal or intraspinal, intracardiac, intrapleural, intra-arterial, intraosseous, and intra-articular routes. Nurses with advanced training or in advanced practice may administer medications by these routes. Medication routes such as intracardiac or intra-articular are usually limited to physician administration. Regardless of who actually administers the medication by these routes, you are responsible for monitoring the integrity of the system of medication delivery, understanding the therapeutic value of the medication, and evaluating the client's response to the therapy.

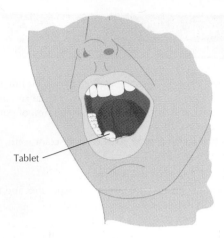

FIGURE **13-2**   Sublingual administration of a tablet.

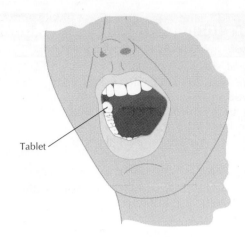

FIGURE **13-3**   Buccal administration of a tablet.

TOPICAL ADMINISTRATION.   Medications applied to the skin and mucous membranes generally have local effects. Topical medication is applied to the skin by painting or spreading it over an area, applying moist dressings, soaking body parts in a solution, or giving medicated baths. Systemic effects can occur if a client's skin is thin, if the medication concentration is high, or if contact with the skin is prolonged.

Some medications (e.g., nitroglycerin, Catapres, estrogens) have systemic effects because they are applied topically by a **transdermal disk** or patch. The disk secures the medicated ointment to the skin. These topical applications may be applied for as little as 12 hours or as long as 7 days.

Medications can be applied to mucous membranes in a variety of ways, including the following:

1. By directly applying a liquid or ointment (e.g., eye drops, gargling, swabbing the throat)
2. By inserting a medication into a body cavity (e.g., placing a suppository in rectum or vagina, inserting medicated packing into vagina)
3. By instilling fluid into body part or cavity (e.g., ear drops, nose drops, bladder or rectal **instillation** [fluid is retained])
4. By irrigating a body cavity (e.g., flushing eye, ear, vagina, bladder, or rectum with medicated fluid [fluid is not retained])
5. By spraying a medication into a body cavity (e.g., instillation into nose and throat)

INHALATION ROUTE.   The deeper passages of the respiratory tract provide a large surface area for medication absorption. Medications can be administered through the nasal passages, oral passage, or tubes that have been placed into the client's mouth to the trachea (Figure 13-4). Medications that are administered by the **inhalation** route are readily absorbed and work rapidly because of the rich vascular alveolar-capillary network present in the pulmonary tissue. Inhaled medications may have local or systemic effects.

INTRAOCULAR ROUTE.   **Intraocular** medication delivery involves inserting a medication similar to a contact lens into

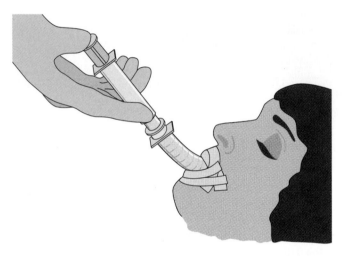

FIGURE **13-4**   Medication being instilled through endotracheal tube using the syringe method.

the client's eye. The eye medication disk has two soft outer layers that have medication enclosed in them. The disk is inserted into the client's eye, much like a contact lens. The disk can remain in the client's eye for up to 1 week. Pilocarpine, a medication used to treat glaucoma, is the most common medication disk used.

Systems of Medication Measurement

The proper administration of a medication requires the ability to compute medication doses accurately and measure medications correctly. A careless mistake in placing a decimal point or adding a zero to a dose can lead to a fatal error. Check the dose before giving a medication.

The metric, apothecary, and household systems of measurement are used in medication therapy. Most nations, including Canada, use the metric system as their standard of measurement. Although the U.S. Congress has not officially adopted the metric system, most health professionals in the United States use it. **Prescriptions** to be self-administered are often written in household measures for clients. The **apothecary system** is rarely used.

METRIC SYSTEM.   As a decimal system, the **metric system** is the most logically organized. Metric units can easily be converted and computed through simple multiplication and division. Each basic unit of measurement is organized into units of 10. In multiplication, the decimal point moves to the right; in division, the decimal moves to the left. For example:

$$10.0 \text{ mg} \times 10 = 100.0 \text{ mg}$$
$$10.0 \text{ mg} \div 10 = 1.0 \text{ mg}$$

The basic units of measurement in the metric system are the meter (length), liter (volume), and gram (weight). For medication calculations, only the volume and weight units are used. In the metric system, lower-case or upper-case letters are used to designate units:

Gram = g or Gm
Liter = l or L
Milligram = mg
Milliliter = ml

A system of Latin prefixes designates subdivision of the basic units: deci- ($^1/_{10}$ or 0.1), centi- ($^1/_{100}$ or 0.01), and milli- ($^1/_{1000}$ or 0.001). Greek prefixes designate multiples of the basic units: deka- (10), hecto- (100), and kilo- (1000). When writing medication doses in metric units, fractions or multiples of a unit are used. Fractions are always in decimal form:

500 mg or 0.5 g, not $^1/_2$ g
10 ml or 0.01 L, not $^1/_{100}$ L

When fractions are used, a zero is always placed in front of the decimal to prevent error (National Coordinating Council for Medication Error Reporting and Prevention [NCCMERP], 1999).

HOUSEHOLD MEASUREMENTS.   Household units of measure are familiar to most people. The disadvantage with household measures is their inaccuracy. Household utensils, such as teaspoons and cups, often vary in size. Scales to measure pints or quarts are often not well calibrated. Household measures include drops, teaspoons, tablespoons, and cups for volume and pints and quarts for weight. Although pints and quarts are considered household measures, they are also used in the apothecary system.

The advantages of household measurements are their convenience and familiarity. When the accuracy of a medication dose is not critical, it is safe to use household measures. For example, many over-the-counter (OTC) medications can safely be measured by this method. Table 13-6 gives common equivalents from each measurement unit.

SOLUTIONS.   The nurse uses solutions of various concentrations for **injections, irrigations,** and **infusions.** A **solution** is a given mass of solid substance dissolved in a known volume of fluid or a given volume of liquid dissolved in a known volume of another fluid. When a solid is dissolved in a fluid, the concentration is in units of mass per units of volume (e.g., g/ml, g/L, mg/ml). A concentration of a solution

Equivalents of Measurement   Table 13-6

Metric	Apothecary	Household
1 ml	15-16 minims (♏)	15 drops (gtt)
4-5 ml	1 fluidram (f℈)	1 teaspoon (tsp)
16 ml	4 fluidrams (f℈)	1 tablespoon (tbsp)
30 ml	1 fluid ounce (f℥)	2 tablespoons (tbsp)
240 ml	8 fluid ounces (f℥)	1 cup (c)
480 ml (approximately 500 ml)	1 pint (pt)	1 pint (pt)
960 ml (approximately 1 L)	1 quart (qt)	1 quart (qt)
3840 ml (approximately 5 L)	1 gallon (gal)	1 gallon (gal)

may also be expressed as a percentage. A 10% solution, for example, is 10 g of solid dissolved in 100 ml of solution. A proportion also expresses concentrations. A $^1/_{1000}$ solution represents a solution containing 1 g of solid in 1000 ml of liquid or 1 ml of liquid mixed with 1000 ml of another liquid.

Clinical Calculations

To administer medications safely, it is necessary to understand basic arithmetic to calculate medication dosages, mix solutions, and perform a variety of other activities. This is important because medications are not always dispensed in the unit of measure in which they are ordered. Medication companies package and bottle certain standard equivalents. For example, the physician may order 250 mg of a medication that is available only in grams. You are responsible for converting available units of volume and weight to the desired doses. Therefore you should be aware of approximate equivalents in all major measurement systems.

CONVERSIONS WITHIN ONE SYSTEM.   Converting measurements within one system is relatively easy. In the metric system, division or multiplication is used. For example, to change milligrams to grams, divide by 1000 or move the decimal 3 points to the left:

1000 mg = 1 g
350 mg = 0.35 g

To convert liters to milliliters, multiply by 1000 or move the decimal 3 points to the right:

1 L = 1000 ml
0.25 L = 250 ml

To convert units of measurement within the apothecary or household system, you must know the equivalent. For example, when converting fluid ounces to quarts, you must know that 32 ounces is the equivalent of 1 quart. To convert 8 ounces to a quart measurement, divide 8 by 32 to get the equivalent, $^1/_4$ or 0.25 quart.

CONVERSION BETWEEN SYSTEMS.   Frequently, the proper dose of a medication is determined by converting weights or volumes from one system of measurement to another. Often, metric units must be converted to equivalent household measures for use at home. To make actual medication calculations, it is necessary to work with units in the same measurement system. Tables of equivalent measurements are available in all health care institutions. The pharmacist is also a good resource.

Before making a conversion, compare the measurement system available with what was ordered. For example, Robitussin, 30 ml, is ordered for your client. To provide proper instruction to the client, "ml" must be converted to a common household measurement. By referring to a table, such as Table 13-6, p. 289, you determine that 30 ml = 2 tablespoons. Therefore you instruct the client to take 2 tablespoons of Robitussin.

DOSAGE CALCULATIONS.   Many formulas can be used to calculate medication dosages. The following basic formula can be applied when preparing solid or liquid forms:

$$\frac{\text{Dose ordered}}{\text{Dose on hand}} \times \text{Amount on hand} = \text{Amount to administer}$$

The dose ordered is the amount of medication prescribed. The dose on hand is the weight or volume of medication available in units supplied by the pharmacy. It may be expressed on the medication label as the contents of a tablet or capsule or as the amount of medication dissolved per unit volume of liquid. The amount on hand is the basic unit or quantity of the medication that contains the dose on hand. For solid medications, the amount on hand may be one capsule. The amount of liquid on hand may be 1 ml or 1 L. The amount to administer is the actual amount of available medication the nurse will administer. The amount to administer is always expressed in the same unit as the amount on hand.

Example 1.   Your client is to receive Demerol, 50 mg IM (dose ordered). The medication is available only in ampules containing 100 mg (dose on hand) in 1 ml (amount on hand). You apply the formula as follows:

$$\frac{50 \text{ mg}}{100 \text{ mg}} \times 1 \text{ ml} = 0.5 \text{ ml (amount to administer)}$$

After working the equation, you would know to prepare 0.5 ml in a syringe.

Example 2.   The physician orders 0.125 mg PO of digoxin. The medication is available in tablets containing 0.25 mg. You apply the formula as follows:

$$\frac{0.125 \text{ mg}}{0.25 \text{ mg}} \times 1 \text{ tablet} = 0.5 \text{ tablets (amount to administer)}$$

Therefore you would administer ½ tablet.

Example 3.   The order states, "Erythromycin suspension 250 mg PO." The pharmacy delivers 100-ml bottles with the labels stating, "5 ml contains 125 mg of erythromycin." You apply the formula as follows:

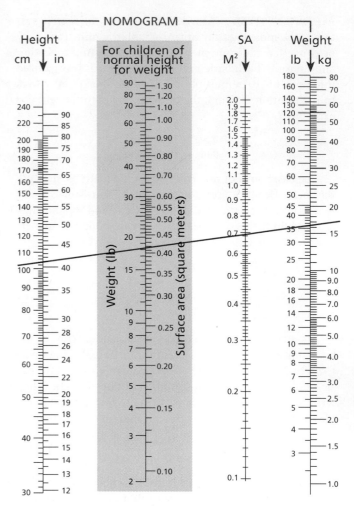

FIGURE **13-5**   West nomogram for estimation of surface areas in children. A straight line is drawn between height and weight. The point where the line crosses the surface area column is the estimated body surface area. (From Behrman RE, Vaughan VC, editors: *Nelson textbook of pediatrics,* ed 13, Philadelphia, 1987, WB Saunders; modified from data of Boyd E, by West CD.)

$$\frac{250 \text{ mg}}{125 \text{ mg}} \times 5 \text{ ml} = 10 \text{ ml (amount to administer)}$$

PEDIATRIC DOSAGES.   Calculating children's medication dosages requires caution. Children are unable to metabolize many medications as readily as adults. The child's body size also requires smaller dosages. Most medication references list the normal ranges for pediatric dosages.

The most accurate method of calculating pediatric dosages is based on a child's body surface area. Body surface area is estimated by the child's height and weight. A standard nomogram (e.g., the West nomogram) can be used for estimation of a child's body surface area (Figure 13-5).

To calculate a pediatric dose, a formula that reflects the ratio of the child's body surface area compared with the body surface area of an average adult (1.7 square meters [m^2]) is used:

$$\text{Child's dose} = \frac{\text{Surface area of child}}{1.7 \text{ m}^2} \times \text{Normal adult dose}$$

Dangerous Abbreviations

Table 13-7

Abbreviation	Intended Meaning	Common Error
U	Units	Mistaken as a zero or a four (4) resulting in overdose. Also mistaken for "cc" (cubic centimeters) when poorly written.
μg	Micrograms	Mistaken for "mg" (milligrams) resulting in a tenfold overdose.
Q.D.	Latin abbreviation for every day	The period after the "Q" has sometimes been mistaken for an "I," and the drug has been given "QID" (four times daily) rather than daily.
QOD	Latin abbreviation for every other day	Misinterpreted as "QD" (daily) or "QID" (four times daily). If the "O" is poorly written, it looks like a period or "I."
SC or SQ	Subcutaneous	Mistaken as "SL" (sublingual) when poorly written.
TIW	Three times a week	Misinterpreted as "three times a day" or "twice a week."
D/C	Discharge; also discontinue	Patient's medications have been prematurely discontinued when D/C (intended to mean "discharge") was misinterpreted as "discontinue," because it was followed by a list of drugs.
HS	Half strength	Misinterpreted as the Latin abbreviation "HS" (hour of sleep).
cc	Cubic centimeters	Mistaken as "U" (units) when poorly written.
AU, AS, AD	Latin abbreviation for both ears; left ear; right ear	Misinterpreted as the Latin abbreviation "OU" (both eyes); "OS" (left eye); "OD" (right eye).

Prescribers should not use vague instructions such as "Take as directed" or "Take/Use as needed" as the sole direction for use. Specific directions to the patient are useful to help reinforce proper medication use, particularly if therapy is to be interrupted for a time. Clear directions are a necessity for the dispenser to (1) check the proper dose for the patient and (2) enable effective patient counseling.

In summary, the council recommends:

Don't Wait . . . Automate!

When In Doubt, Write It Out!

When In Doubt, Check It Out!

Lead, Don't Trail!

For example, ampicillin is ordered for a child weighing 12 kg. The normal adult dose for ampicillin is 250 mg. The West nomogram shows that a child weighing 12 kg has a surface area of 0.54 m^2. Using this information, you calculate the appropriate child's dose:

$$\frac{0.54 \text{ m}^2}{1.7 \text{ m}^2} \times 250 \text{ mg} = 75 \text{ mg of ampicillin}$$

Administering Medications

You do not have sole responsibility for medication administration. The prescriber (e.g., physician, advanced practice nurse) and pharmacist also help to ensure the right medication gets to the right client. However, you are accountable for knowing what medications are prescribed, their therapeutic and nontherapeutic effects, and the client's needs and abilities.

PRESCRIBER'S ROLE.   The physician or advanced practice nurse prescribes the client's medications. The prescriber writes an order on a form in the client's medical record, in an order book, on a legal prescription pad, or through a computer terminal. Where allowed, a prescriber may also order a medication by telephone or by giving a verbal order.

If a telephone or verbal order is received, the nurse who took the order writes the name of the prescriber ordering the medication followed by the nurse's signature. The prescriber must countersign the order at a later time, usually within 24 hours after the order is made.

Institutional policies vary regarding the personnel who can take verbal or telephone orders. Generally, nursing students cannot take medication orders. No medication is to be given without an order.

Common abbreviations are often used when writing orders. The abbreviations indicate dosage frequencies or times, routes of administration, and special information for giving the medication (see Table 13-3, p. 286). However, the National Coordinating Council for Medication Error Reporting and Prevention (NCCMERP, 1999) recommends that abbreviations not be used when writing medication orders because of the high number of medication errors that occur related to the use of abbreviations. Table 13-7 lists abbreviations that are associated with a high incidence of medication errors. These abbreviations should not be used; rather, they should be written out.

TYPES OF ORDERS IN ACUTE CARE AGENCIES.   Four common types of medication orders are based on the frequency and/or urgency of medication administration.

STANDING ORDERS.   A standing order is carried out until the physician cancels it by another order or until a prescribed number of days elapse. A standing order may indicate a final

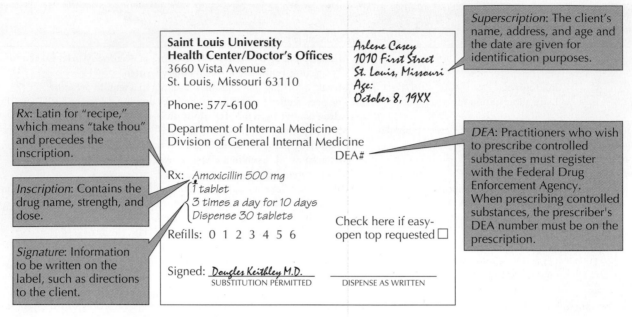

Saint Louis University
Health Center/Doctor's Offices
3660 Vista Avenue
St. Louis, Missouri 63110

Phone: 577-6100

Department of Internal Medicine
Division of General Internal Medicine
                              DEA#

Rx: Amoxicillin 500 mg
     1 tablet
     3 times a day for 10 days
     Dispense 30 tablets

Refills: 0 1 2 3 4 5 6

Signed: _Douglas Keithley M.D._
         SUBSTITUTION PERMITTED

DISPENSE AS WRITTEN

Arlene Casey
1010 First Street
St. Louis, Missouri
Age:
October 8, 19XX

Check here if easy-
open top requested ☐

Rx: Latin for "recipe," which means "take thou" and precedes the inscription.

Inscription: Contains the drug name, strength, and dose.

Signature: Information to be written on the label, such as directions to the client.

Superscription: The client's name, address, and age and the date are given for identification purposes.

DEA: Practitioners who wish to prescribe controlled substances must register with the Federal Drug Enforcement Agency. When prescribing controlled substances, the prescriber's DEA number must be on the prescription.

FIGURE 13-6 Example of a medication prescription. (Courtesy Saint Louis University Medical Center, St. Louis.)

date or number of dosages. Many institutions have policies for automatically discontinuing standing orders. The following are examples of standing orders:

Tetracycline, 500 mg PO q6h, and Decadron, 10 mg PO qd, × 5 days

PRN ORDERS.   The physician may order a medication to be given only when a client requires it. This is a prn order. Objective assessment, subjective assessment, and nursing discretion are used in determining whether the client needs the medication. Often the physician sets minimum intervals for the time of administration. This means the medication cannot be given any more frequently than what is prescribed. Examples of prn orders include the following:

Morphine sulfate, 10 mg IM q3-4h prn for incisional pain, and Maalox, 30 ml prn for heartburn

When prn medications are administered, document the assessment data used to decide to give the medication and the time of medication administration. Frequently evaluate the effectiveness of the medication, and record findings in the appropriate record.

SINGLE (ONE-TIME) ORDERS.   A prescriber will often order a medication to be given only once at a specified time. This is common for preoperative medications or medications given before diagnostic examinations. For example:

Versed, 25 mg IM on call to OR

STAT ORDERS.   A stat order signifies that a single dose of a medication is to be given immediately and only once. Stat

orders are often written for emergencies when the client's condition changes suddenly. For example:

Give Apresoline, 10 mg IM stat.

Some conditions change the status of a client's medication orders. For example, surgery automatically cancels all a client's preoperative medications (see Chapter 36). Because the client's condition changes after surgery, the prescriber must write new orders. When a client is transferred to another health care agency or a different service within a hospital or is discharged, the prescriber should review the medications and write new orders as indicated.

PRESCRIPTIONS.   Prescriptions are written for clients who are to take medications outside the hospital. The prescription includes more detailed information than a regular order, because the client must understand how to take the medication and when to refill the prescription if necessary. The parts of a prescription are included in Figure 13-6.

PHARMACIST'S ROLE.   The pharmacist prepares and distributes prescribed medications. Pharmacists may also assess the medication plan and evaluate the client's medication-related needs. The pharmacist is responsible for filling prescriptions accurately and for being sure that prescriptions are valid.

DISTRIBUTION SYSTEMS.   Systems for storing and distributing medications vary. Pharmacists provide the medications, but nurses distribute medications to clients. Institutions providing nursing care have special areas for stocking and dispensing medications, such as special medication rooms, portable locked carts, computerized medication cabinets, and

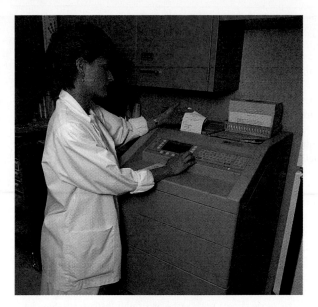

FIGURE **13-7**   Computer-controlled medication dispensing system.

individual storage units in clients' rooms. Medication storage areas must be locked when unattended.

UNIT DOSE.   The unit-dose system uses portable carts containing a drawer with a 24-hour supply of medications for each client. The unit dose is the ordered dose of medication the client receives at one time. Each tablet or capsule is wrapped separately. At a designated time each day, the pharmacist refills the drawers in the cart with a fresh supply. The cart also contains limited amounts of prn and stock medications for special situations. The unit-dose system is designed to reduce the number of medication errors and saves steps in dispensing medications.

COMPUTER-CONTROLLED DISPENSING SYSTEMS.   Computer-controlled dispensing systems are used successfully throughout the United States (Figure 13-7). They are especially useful for the delivery and control of **narcotics.** Each nurse has a security code, allowing access to the system. In these systems, the client's name and the desired medication, dosage, and route are selected. The system delivers the medication to the nurse, records it, and charges it to the client.

NURSE'S ROLE.   The administration of medications to clients requires knowledge and a set of skills that are unique to nursing. Responsibilities of medication administration include assessing the client's ability to self-administer medications, determining whether a client should receive a medication at a given time, administering medications correctly, and monitoring the effects of prescribed medications. Client and family education about proper medication administration and monitoring is an integral part of the nurse's role, which should never be delegated to assistive personnel.

CRITICAL THINKING
Synthesis

Critical thinking is extremely important in the administration of medications. Factors that contribute to the need for critical thinking during this process include the growing number of medications readily available to clients, the acute and complex nature of client problems, higher acuity levels in acute care settings, and reductions in nursing and pharmacy staff. The skill of medication administration requires the synthesis of all factors that might influence a client's reaction to prescribed medications. This requires more than the knowledge of the medication's classification, desired effect, and common side effects (Cook, 1995). You must conduct an ongoing synthesis of knowledge, experience, attitudes, and standards in order to apply the nursing process appropriately when administering medications.

KNOWLEDGE.   Knowledge from many disciplines is used when administering medications. It is this knowledge that helps you understand why a particular medication has been prescribed for a client and how this medication will alter the client's physiology so as to exert its therapeutic effect. For example, in physiology you may have learned that potassium is a major intracellular iron. When a client does not have enough potassium in the body, the client may experience signs and symptoms that are associated with hypokalemia, such as dysrhythmias or weakness. In these cases, medications are prescribed to restore the client's potassium level to normal. Knowledge about child development indicates that children often perceive medication administration as a negative experience. Principles from child development are used to ensure that the child cooperates with medication administration.

EXPERIENCE.   As a nursing student, you may have limited experience with medication administration as it applies to professional practice. However, clinical experience provides you with the opportunity to use the nursing process and learn how it applies to medication administration. As you gain experience in medication administration, psychomotor skills (e.g., the preparation and actual administration of a medication) become more refined. As you acquire experience in observing clients' responses to medication, you will become more competent in anticipating and evaluating the effects of medications.

ATTITUDES.   To administer medications safely to clients, certain critical thinking attitudes are essential. When you administer a medication to a client, you accept the responsibility that the medication or the nursing actions in administering it will not harm the client in any way. You are responsible for knowing that the medication that is ordered for the client is the correct medication and the correct dose. You are held accountable for administering an ordered medication that is obviously inappropriate for the client. Because of this, you should be familiar with the therapeutic effect, usual dosage,

Ways to Prevent Drug Administration Errors   Table 13-8

Precaution	Rationale
Read drug labels carefully.	Many products come in similar containers, colors, and shapes.
Question administration of multiple tablets or vials for single dose.	Most doses are one or two tablets or capsules or one single-dose vial. Incorrect interpretation of order may result in excessively high dose.
Be aware of drugs with similar names.	Many drug names sound alike (e.g., digoxin and digitoxin, Keflex and Keflin, Orinase and Ornade).
Check decimal point.	Some drugs come in quantities that are multiples of one another (e.g., Coumadin in 2.5- and 25-mg tablets, Thorazine in 30- and 300-mg Spansules).
Question abrupt and excessive increases in dosages.	Most dosages are increased gradually so that physician can monitor therapeutic effect and response.
When new or unfamiliar drug is ordered, consult resource.	If prescriber is also unfamiliar with drug, there is greater risk of inaccurate dosages being ordered.
Do not administer drug ordered by nickname or unofficial abbreviation.	Many prescribers refer to commonly ordered medications by nicknames or unofficial abbreviations. If nurse or pharmacist is unfamiliar with name, wrong drug may be dispensed and administered.
Do not attempt to decipher illegible writing.	When in doubt, ask prescriber. Unless nurse questions order that is difficult to read, chance of misinterpretation is great.
Know clients with same last names. Also have clients state their full names. Check name bands carefully.	It is common to have two or more clients with same or similar last names. Special labels on Kardex or medication book can warn of potential problem.
Do not confuse equivalents.	When in a hurry, it may be easy to misread equivalents (e.g., milligram instead of milliliter).

anticipated changes in laboratory data, and side effects of all medications that are administered. You are also responsible for ensuring that clients have been properly informed about all aspects of self-administration.

You must demonstrate accountability and act responsibly in professional practice by acknowledging when errors in professional practice occur. Most errors made by nurses are medication errors. A **medication error** is any event that could cause or lead to a client receiving inappropriate medication therapy or failing to receive appropriate medication therapy. Most medication errors occur when routine procedures, such as checking dosage calculations or deciphering illegible handwriting without consulting the prescriber, are not followed (NCCMERP, 1999b). When an error occurs, it should be acknowledged immediately and reported to the appropriate hospital personnel (e.g., nurse manager, physician). Measures to counteract the effects of the error may be necessary. You are also responsible for completing an incident report describing the nature of the incident (see Chapter 3). Table 13-8 summarizes methods to prevent errors in medication administration.

Institutional policy may place limitations on your ability to administer certain types of medications, by certain routes, or in certain units of the health care setting. Most settings have nursing procedure manuals that outline policies to define the classes of medications nurses employed by the agency may and may not administer.

STANDARDS.   Standards are those actions that ensure safe nursing practice. To ensure safe medication administration, you should be aware of the five rights of medication administration:
1. The right medication
2. The right dose
3. The right client
4. The right route
5. The right time

RIGHT MEDICATION.   When medications are first ordered, compare the medication recording form or computer orders with the physician's written orders. When administering medications, compare the label of the medication container with the medication form three times: (1) before removing the container from the drawer or shelf, (2) as the amount of medication ordered is removed from the container, and (3) before returning the container to storage (NCCMERP, 1999c). With unit-dose packaged medications, the medication's label is checked before opening at the client's bedside. Never prepare medications from unmarked containers or containers with illegible labels. At home, clients should keep medications in their original labeled containers.

Only administer medications you prepare. The nurse who administers the medication is responsible for any errors related to that medication. If a client questions a medication, it is important not to ignore these concerns. An alert client will know whether a medication is different from those received before. In most cases, the client's medication order has been changed; however, the client's questions might reveal an error. You should withhold the medication until it can be rechecked against the prescriber's orders.

RIGHT DOSE.   The unit-dose system is designed to minimize errors. When a medication must be prepared from a larger volume or strength than needed or when the prescriber orders a system of measurement different from what the pharmacist supplies, the chance of error increases. When

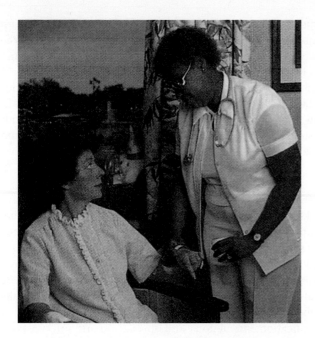

FIGURE 13-8   Before administering any medications, the nurse checks the client's identification and allergy bracelets.

performing medication calculations or conversions, have another qualified nurse check the calculated doses.

After calculating dosages, prepare the medication using standard measurement devices. Graduated cups, syringes, and scaled droppers can be used to measure medications accurately. At home, clients should use kitchen measuring spoons rather than teaspoons and tablespoons, which vary in volume.

When it is necessary to break a scored tablet, the break should be even. A tablet may be cut in half by using a knife edge or by using a cutting device. Tablets that do not break evenly are discarded. The two halves are given in successive doses if the second half was repackaged and labeled.

Sometimes a tablet is crushed so it can be mixed in food. The crushing device should always be cleaned completely before the tablet is crushed. Remnants of previously crushed medications may increase a medication's concentration or result in the client receiving a portion of an unprescribed medication. Crushed medications should be mixed with very small amounts of food or liquid. The client's favorite foods or liquids should not be used because a medication may alter their taste and decrease the client's desire for them.

RIGHT CLIENT. An important step in administering medications safely is being sure the medication is given to the right client. It is difficult to remember every client's name and face. To identify a client correctly, check the medication administration form against the client's identification bracelet (Figure 13-8) and ask the client to state his or her name. If an identification bracelet becomes illegible or is missing, acquire a new one for the client. When asking the client's name, ask the client to state his or her full name.

RIGHT ROUTE. If a prescriber's order does not designate a route of administration, consult the prescriber. Likewise, if the specified route is not the recommended route, alert the prescriber immediately.

When you administer injections, precautions are necessary to ensure that the medications are given correctly. It is also important to prepare injections only from preparations designed for parenteral use. The injection of a liquid designed for oral use can produce local complications, such as a sterile abscess or fatal systemic effects. Medication companies label parenteral medications "for injectable use only."

RIGHT TIME. You must know why a medication is ordered for certain times of the day and whether the time schedule can be altered. For example, two medications are ordered, one q8h (every 8 hours) and the other tid (3 times per day). Both medications are to be given 3 times within a 24-hour period. The prescriber intends the q8h medication to be given around the clock to maintain therapeutic blood levels of the medication. In contrast, the tid medication is given during the waking hours. Each institution has a recommended time schedule for medications ordered at frequent intervals.

The prescriber often gives specific instructions about when to administer a medication. A preoperative medication to be given on call means that you are to administer the medication when the operating room staff members tell you they are coming to get the client for surgery. A medication ordered PC (after meals) is to be given within 30 minutes after a meal when the client has a full stomach. A stat medication is to be given immediately.

Medications that must act at certain times are given priority. For example, insulin should be given at a precise interval before a meal. All routinely ordered medications should be given within 30 minutes of the times ordered (30 minutes before or after the prescribed time).

Some medications require your clinical judgment in determining the proper time for administration. A prn sleeping medication should be administered when the client is prepared for bed or at a time appropriate for maximum benefit. Also, use nursing judgment when administering prn analgesics. For example, you may need to obtain a stat order from the prescriber if the client requires a medication before the prn interval has elapsed. Document whenever you call the client's health care provider to obtain a change in a medication's order.

At home a client may have to take several medications throughout the day. Help plan schedules based on preferred medication intervals and the client's daily schedule. For clients who have difficulty remembering when to take medications, make a chart that lists the times when each medication is to be taken or prepare a special container to hold each timed dose.

Professional standards influence the activities of medication administration. The American Nurses Association's (ANA's) *Standards of Nursing Practice* (see Chapter 2), based on the nursing process, also applies to the activity of med-

Nurses' Six Rights for Safe Medication Administration   Box 13-3

1. The right to a complete and clearly written order
2. The right to have the correct drug route and dose dispensed
3. The right to have access to information
4. The right to have policies on medication administration
5. The right to administer medications safely and to identify problems in the system
6. The right to stop, think, and be vigilant when administering medications

From Cook MC: Nurses' six rights for safe medication administration, *Massachusetts Nurs* 69(6):8, 1999.

ication administration. Other professional nursing standards may also apply. For example, the Massachusetts Nurses Association developed a list of the six rights for nurses who administer medications (Box 13-3).

MAINTAINING CLIENTS' RIGHTS. In accordance with the *Patient's Bill of Rights* (see Chapter 3) and because of the potential risks related to medication administration, a client has the right to:

1. Be informed of medication name, purpose, action, and potential undesired effects
2. Refuse a medication regardless of the consequences
3. Have qualified nurses or physicians assess a medication history, including allergies
4. Be properly advised of the experimental nature of medication therapy and to give written consent for its use
5. Receive labeled medications safely without discomfort in accordance with the five rights of medication administration (see section on medication delivery)
6. Receive appropriate supportive therapy in relation to medication therapy
7. Not receive unnecessary medications

NURSING PROCESS

Assessment

To determine the need for and potential response to medication therapy, you assess many factors.

HISTORY. Before administering medications, obtain or review the client's medical history. A client's medical history may provide indications or contraindications for medication therapy. Disease or illness may place clients at risk for adverse medication effects. For example, if a client has a gastric ulcer, compounds containing aspirin will increase the likelihood of bleeding. Long-term health problems require specific medications. This knowledge will help you anticipate the medications your client requires. A client's surgical history may indicate use of medications. For example, after a thyroidectomy a client may require hormone replacement.

HISTORY OF ALLERGIES. All members of the health care team must be informed of the client's history of allergies to medications and foods. Many medications have ingredients found in food sources. For example, if your client is allergic to shellfish, the client may be sensitive to any product containing iodine, such as Betadine or dyes used in radiological testing. In an acute care setting, clients may wear identification bands listing medications to which they are allergic. All allergies and the type of reaction should be noted on the client's admission notes, medication records, and history and physical.

MEDICATION HISTORY. Assess what medications the client takes, including the length of time the drug has been taken, current dosage schedule, and whether the client has experienced ill effects. In addition, drug data are reviewed, including action, purpose, normal dosages, routes, side effects, and nursing implications for administration and monitoring. Be sure that the smallest possible dose is ordered, especially when caring for older adults or children. Also, be aware of medication interactions and special nursing interventions needed for medication administration. Often, several references must be consulted to gather needed information. Pharmacology textbooks, nursing journals, the *Physicians' Desk Reference (PDR)*, medication package inserts, and pharmacists are valuable resources. You are responsible for knowing as much as possible about each medication given.

DIET HISTORY. An effective dosage schedule is planned around normal eating patterns and food preferences. Some medications interact with food. Clients who take these medications need to be taught to avoid those foods that interact with medications.

CLIENT'S PERCEPTUAL OR COORDINATION PROBLEMS. For a client with perceptual or coordination limitations, self-administration may be difficult. Assess the client's ability to prepare doses (e.g., open containers, fill syringes) and take medications (e.g., perform self-injection, instill eyedrops) correctly. If the client is unable to self-administer medications, you may need to assess whether family or friends will be available to assist.

CLIENT'S CURRENT CONDITION. The ongoing physical or mental status of a client may affect whether a medication is given or how it is administered. Assess a client carefully before giving any medication. For example, the client's blood pressure should be checked before giving an antihypertensive. Assessment findings also serve as a baseline in evaluating the effects of medication therapy.

CLIENT'S ATTITUDE ABOUT MEDICATION USE. The client's attitude about medications may reveal a level of medication dependence or drug avoidance. Clients may not express their feelings about taking a particular medication, particularly if dependence is a problem. Observe the client's behavior for evidence of medication dependence or avoidance. The client's cultural beliefs about Western med-

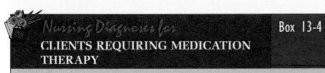

icine can also interfere with medication compliance (see Chapter 16).

CLIENT'S KNOWLEDGE AND UNDERSTANDING OF MEDICATION THERAPY.   The client's knowledge and understanding of medication therapy influence the willingness or ability to follow a medication regimen. Unless a client understands a medication's purpose, the importance of regular dosage schedules and proper administration methods, and the possible side effects, compliance is unlikely. Questions that assess knowledge of a medication includes the following: What is it for? How is it taken? When is it taken? What side effects have there been? Has the client ever stopped taking doses? Is there anything else the client does not understand and would like to know about the medication? If the client cannot afford medications, discuss financial resources.

CLIENT'S LEARNING NEEDS.   On assessment, you may discover the need to explain the action and purpose of medications, expected side effects, correct administration techniques, and ways to help the client to remember the medication regimen. In addition, clients might require instruction on ways to adjust a medication schedule to their lifestyle. If a client has been placed on a newly prescribed medication, instruction may need to be more involved.

Nursing Diagnosis

Assessment provides data about the client's condition, ability to self-administer medications, and medication use patterns, which can be used to determine actual or potential problems with medication therapy. Certain data are defining characteristics, which when clustered together reveal nursing diagnoses (Box 13-4). For example, a client's admission of missing a dose may indicate noncompliance regarding a medication regimen. Once the diagnosis is selected, identify the related factor. The related factors of inadequate resources versus lack of knowledge require different interventions. If the client's noncompliance is related to inadequate finances, collaborate with family members, social workers, or community agencies to help a client receive necessary medications. If the related factor is lack of knowledge, implement a teaching plan with follow-up.

Planning

Organize nursing activities to ensure the safe administration of medications. Hurrying to give clients medications can lead to errors. Plan to teach clients about their medications while you are administering medications. Collaborate with the client's family or friends when you provide instruction. Family members can reinforce the importance of medication regimens in the home setting. When clients are hospitalized, do not postpone instruction until the day of discharge. For the client to understand medications and self-administration guidelines, there must be time for questions and discussion. Early planning is critical.

In the community, ensure that the client knows where and how to obtain medications and that the client can read medication labels. Whether a client attempts self-administration or you assume responsibility for administering medications, the following goals and expected outcomes must be met:

1. Client and family understand medication therapy.
2. Client gains therapeutic effect of the prescribed medications without discomfort or complications.
3. Client has no complications related to the route of administration.
4. Medications are safely administered.

Implementation

HEALTH PROMOTION ACTIVITIES.   In promoting or maintaining the client's health, identify factors that may improve or diminish well-being. Health beliefs, personal motivations, socioeconomic factors, and habits (e.g., smoking) can influence the client's compliance with the medication regimen. Several nursing interventions can promote adherence to a medication regimen. These include teaching the client and family about the benefit of a medication and the knowledge needed to take it correctly, integrating the client's health beliefs and cultural practices into the treatment plan, and making referrals to community resources if the client is unable to afford, or cannot get out to obtain, necessary medications.

CLIENT AND FAMILY TEACHING.   Unless a client is properly informed about medications, he or she may take the medications incorrectly or not at all. Provide information about the purpose of medications and their actions and effects. Many health care institutions offer easy-to-read education sheets on specific types of medications. A client must know how to take a medication properly and the effects if he or she fails to do so. For example, after receiving a prescription for an antibiotic, a client must understand the importance of taking the full prescription. Failure to do this can lead to a worsening of the condition, as well as the development of bacteria resistant to the medication.

When your clients depend on daily injections, they must learn to prepare and administer an injection correctly using aseptic technique. Family members or friends should be taught to give injections in case the client becomes ill or physically unable to handle a syringe. Provide specially designed equipment such as syringes with enlarged calibrated scales for easier reading or braille-labeled medication vials for clients with visual alterations.

Clients must be aware of the symptoms of medication side effects or toxicity. For example, clients taking anticoagulants need to know to notify the physician immediately when signs of bleeding or bruising develop. Inform family members of medication side effects, such as changes in behavior, because they are often the first persons to recognize such effects. Your clients are better able to cope with problems caused by medications if they understand how and when to act. All clients should learn the basic guidelines for medication safety. These guidelines ensure the proper use and storage of medications in the home (Box 13-5).

ACUTE CARE ACTIVITIES.   In the acute care setting, expert nursing observation and documentation of responses to medications are essential. Several nursing interventions are critical to provide safe and effective medication administration when a medication order is received.

RECEIVING MEDICATION ORDERS.   A medication order is required for any medication to be administered to a client. The medication order must contain all the elements in Box 13-6. If the medication order is incomplete, contact the prescriber to verify the order. Some medication orders can be given verbally or by telephone by the prescriber to the nurse. A verbal order is a medication or treatment order received in the presence of the prescriber. Verbal orders are entered into the client's medical record and transcribed the same way as if the prescriber wrote the order himself or herself. Telephone orders are medication or treatment orders given to the nurse over the phone by the prescriber, generally after the prescriber has been updated about a change in the client's condition. Institutional policy regarding the receiving, recording, and transcription of verbal and telephone orders must be followed. Generally, verbal and telephone orders must be signed by the provider within 24 hours. When the prescriber is present, a verbal order is discouraged and the order should be written. As a student, you are prohibited from receiving verbal and telephone orders.

CORRECT TRANSCRIPTION AND COMMUNICATION OF ORDERS. Write the physician's complete order on the appropriate medication form, called a medication administration record (MAR). The MAR must include the client's name, room, and bed number as well as the names, dosages, frequencies, and routes of administration for each medication. Each time a medication dosage is prepared, refer to the medication form. When transcribing orders, ensure the names, dosages, and symbols are legible. Any illegible transcriptions must be clarified and rewritten.

In some institutions, a computer printout lists all currently ordered medications with dosage information (Figure 13-9). Orders are entered directly into the computer, preventing the need for transcription of orders. The same printout may be used to record medications given.

All transcribed orders must be checked against the original order for accuracy and thoroughness by a registered nurse. If an order seems incorrect or inappropriate, consult the prescriber. When you give the wrong medication or an incorrect dose, you are legally responsible for the error.

ACCURATE DOSAGE CALCULATION AND MEASUREMENT. Calculate each dose when preparing medications. To avoid calculation errors, pay close attention to the process of calculation, and avoid interference from other nursing activities. If you are in doubt about the accuracy of your calculation or are calculating a new or unusual dose, ask another nurse to double-check your calculations against the prescriber's order. If you are administering a liquid medication, be sure to use a standard measuring container.

CORRECT ADMINISTRATION.   Before administering a medication to a client, verify the client's identity by looking at the client's identification band and asking the client to state his

Room: 3700-03

Patient: PDM, Pharmacy
Birth: 11/30/79 Admit: 01/01/00
MRN: 2000403 Acct: 900015
A Doctor: Jim Smith

Age: 20 y Ht: 5 ft 2 in Wt: 125.2 lbs
Metric: Ht: 1 m 57 cm Wt: 56.79 kg

Saint Francis Medical Center

MEDICATION ADMINISTRATION RECORD

Date: 01/18/00 – 01/19/00

ADEs/Nondrug allergies: Latex – Zosyn – Amoxicillin – Insulins – Darvocet – Lugols soln. – Antihi +

Medication	0800	0900	1000	1100	1200	1300	1400	1500	1600	1700	1800	1900	2000	2100	2200	2300	2400	0100	0200	0300	0400	0500	0600	0700
P00014 Bacitracin ointment AKA: Bacitracin ointment Dose: Apply STRGH: 30 gm/tube TID Topical: Right lower leg For external use only Testing			RL 10																					
P00029 Insulin/human regular AKA: Humulin R Dose: 15 units Strgh: 1 ml = 100 units AC SQ	RL 0730																							
P00030 Fexofenadine 60 mg/psuedo 120 mg AKA: Allegra–D Sr Tab Dose: 1 tab STRGH: 60/120/tab BID Oral Auto Sub: 1 Allegra–D Tab bid For Claritin–D 12 hr and 24 hr Per P&T Comm			RL 10																					
P00036 Aspirin AKA: Aspirin 325 mg Tab Dose: 2 tab 650 mg STRGH: 325 mg/tab Q3–4h Oral Testing						RL 1315																		
P00039 Haloperidol tablet AKA: Haldol 0.5 mg tab Dose: 1 mg STRGH: 1 mg/tab QHS Oral																								
P00035 Zolpidem AKA: Ambien 5 mg tab Dose: 5 mg STRGH: 5/tab QHS PRN Oral MR × 1 Testing																								
	0800	0900	1000	1100	1200	1300	1400	1500	1600	1700	1800	1900	2000	2100	2200	2300	2400	0100	0200	0300	0400	0500	0600	0700

Circle = Dose not given
Initials = Dose given
Deltoid = R.D., L.D.
Vastus Lateralis = R.V.L., L.V.L.
Lower Abdominal = R.L.A., L.L.A.
Anterior Gluteal = R.A.G., L.A.G.
Posterior Gluteal = R.P.G., L.P.G.

Page: 01 (continued)

Initials and signature Rita Lassater RL	**Initials and signature**	**Initials and signature**
Initials and signature	**Initials and signature**	**Initials and signature**
Initials and signature	**Initials and signature**	**Initials and signature**

FIGURE 13-9 Example of medication administration record (MAR). (Courtesy OSF Saint Francis Medical Center, Peoria, Ill.)

or her name. Use aseptic technique and proper procedures when handling and giving medications. Some medications require an assessment before they can be administered (e.g., assessing heart rate before giving a cardiac glycoside).

RECORDING MEDICATION ADMINISTRATION. After administering a medication, you record it immediately on the appropriate record form (see Figure 13-9, p. 299). **Never chart a medication before administering it.** Recording immediately after administration prevents errors.

The recording of a medication includes the name of the medication, dosage, route, and exact time of administration. Agency policies may also require that you record the location of an injection.

If a client refuses a medication or is undergoing tests or procedures that result in a missed dose, explain why the medication was not given in the nurse's notes. Some agencies require the prescribed administration time to be circled on the medication record when a dose is missed.

RESTORATIVE CARE ACTIVITIES. Because of the numerous types of restorative care settings, medication administration activities vary. You may need to administer all medications to clients with functional limitations. However, in the home health and rehabilitation settings, your client usually administers his or her own medications. Regardless of the type of medication activity, you remain responsible for

medication instruction. You are also responsible for monitoring compliance with medications and determining the effectiveness of medications that have been prescribed.

SPECIAL CONSIDERATIONS FOR ADMINISTERING MEDICATIONS TO SPECIFIC AGE-GROUPS. A client's developmental level is a factor in the way you administer medications. Knowledge of your client's developmental needs helps you anticipate responses to medication therapy.

INFANTS AND CHILDREN. Children vary in age; weight; surface area; and the ability to absorb, metabolize, and excrete medications. Children's medication dosages are lower than those of adults, so special caution is needed when preparing medications for them. Medications are usually not prepared and packaged in standardized dose ranges for children. Preparing an ordered dosage from an available amount requires careful calculation.

A child's parents often are valuable resources for determining the best way to give the child medications. Sometimes it is less traumatic for the child if a parent gives the medication while you supervise. Tips for administering medications to children are summarized in Box 13-7.

OLDER ADULTS. Older adults also require special consideration during medication administration (Box 13-8). In addition to physiological changes of aging (Figure 13-10), behavioral and economic factors influence an older person's use of medications.

Polypharmacy. **Polypharmacy** means that your client is taking many medications, prescribed or not, in an attempt to treat several disorders simultaneously. When this occurs,

---

Tips for Administering Medications to Children — Box 13-7

ORAL MEDICATIONS

Liquids are safer to swallow to avoid aspiration.

Offer juice, a soft drink, or a frozen juice bar after a drug is swallowed.

A carbonated beverage poured over finely crushed ice reduces nausea.

When mixing drugs with palatable flavorings, such as syrup or honey, use only a small amount. The child may refuse to take all of a larger mixture.

Avoid mixing medications in foods or liquids the child enjoys because the child may then refuse them.

A plastic disposable syringe is the most accurate device for preparing liquid dosages. Cups, teaspoons, and droppers are inaccurate.

When administering liquid medications, a spoon, plastic cup, or syringe without a needle is useful.

INJECTIONS

Be very careful when selecting IM injection sites. Infants and small children have underdeveloped muscles.

Children can be unpredictable and uncooperative. Have someone available to hold a child if needed.

Always awaken a sleeping child before giving an injection.

Distracting the child with conversation or a toy may reduce pain perception.

Give the injection quickly, and do not fight with the child.

A lidocaine ointment may be applied to an injection site before the injection to reduce the pain perception during the injection.

Gerontological Nursing Practice — Box 13-8

- Space oral medications so that not more than one or two are taken at one time.
- Have client drink a little fluid before taking oral medications to ease swallowing.
- Encourage the client to drink at least 5 or 6 ounces of fluid after taking medications to ensure that the medications have left the esophagus and are in the stomach and to speed absorption of the medication.
- If the client has difficulty swallowing a large capsule or tablet, ask the physician to substitute a liquid medication if possible. Cutting the tablet in half or crushing it and placing it in applesauce or fruit juice may distort the action of some medications, reduce the dose, or cause choking or aspiration of particles of medication or applesauce.
- Teach alternatives to medications if approved by the prescriber, such as proper diet instead of vitamins, exercise instead of laxatives, bedtime snacks instead of hypnotics, weight reduction, and limited salt or fats in diet instead of antihypertensive agents.

Modified from Ebersole P, Hess P: *Toward healthy aging: human needs and nursing response,* ed 5, St. Louis, 1998, Mosby.

there is a high risk of medication interactions with other medications and with foods that the client may eat. There is also an increased risk of the client having an adverse reaction to the medications.

Self-Prescribing of Medications.   Older adults can experience a variety of symptoms (e.g., pain, constipation, insomnia, indigestion). All these symptoms are amenable to OTC medications. Many of these OTC preparations have ingredients that, when used inappropriately, may cause undesirable side effects or adverse reactions or may be contraindicated in the client's condition.

Misuse of Medications.   Misuse includes overuse, underuse, erratic use, and contraindicated use of medications. Clients of all ages may misuse medications. However, there is a greater risk of this with older adults.

Noncompliance.   Noncompliance is defined as a deliberate misuse of medication. Up to 50% of clients with chronic illness do not take their medications as prescribed (Seal, 2000). In older adults, the reason for noncompliance is

often physical or mental deterioration or an inability to afford medications. Carefully assess the medications your client takes and compare them with what was prescribed for the client. If noncompliance is detected, investigate contributing factors and work with the client to develop a medication regimen the client can follow. Box 13-9 provides interventions that may help promote medication compliance.

 ## Evaluation

Your client's response to medications is evaluated on an ongoing basis. This requires that you know the therapeutic action, side effects, and nursing implications of each medication. A change in your client's condition can be physiologically related to health status or may result from medications or both. The goal of safe and effective medication administration involves a careful evaluation of the client's response to therapy and ability to assume responsibility for self-care.

Many different measures can be used to evaluate client responses to medications: direct observation of behavior or response, rating scales (e.g., pain scale) and checklists, and oral questioning. The type of measurements used varies with the

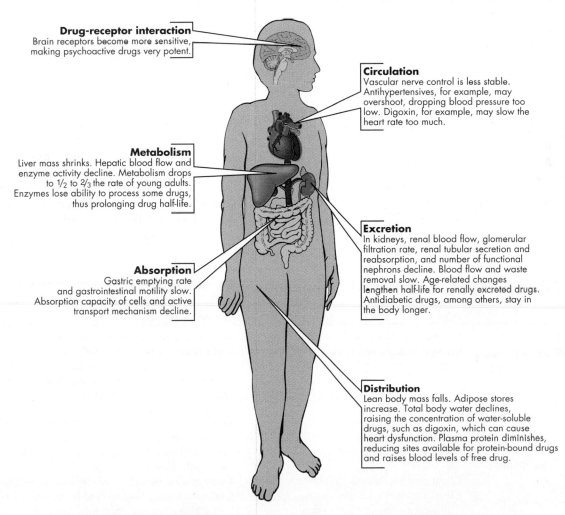

Drug-receptor interaction
Brain receptors become more sensitive, making psychoactive drugs very potent.

Circulation
Vascular nerve control is less stable. Antihypertensives, for example, may overshoot, dropping blood pressure too low. Digoxin, for example, may slow the heart rate too much.

Metabolism
Liver mass shrinks. Hepatic blood flow and enzyme activity decline. Metabolism drops to 1/2 to 2/3 the rate of young adults. Enzymes lose ability to process some drugs, thus prolonging drug half-life.

Excretion
In kidneys, renal blood flow, glomerular filtration rate, renal tubular secretion and reabsorption, and number of functional nephrons decline. Blood flow and waste removal slow. Age-related changes lengthen half-life for renally excreted drugs. Antidiabetic drugs, among others, stay in the body longer.

Absorption
Gastric emptying rate and gastrointestinal motility slow. Absorption capacity of cells and active transport mechanism decline.

Distribution
Lean body mass falls. Adipose stores increase. Total body water declines, raising the concentration of water-soluble drugs, such as digoxin, which can cause heart dysfunction. Plasma protein diminishes, reducing sites available for protein-bound drugs and raises blood levels of free drug.

FIGURE **13-10**   The effects of aging on drug metabolism. (From Lewis SM and others: *Medical-surgical nursing,* ed 5, St. Louis, 2000, Mosby.)

action being evaluated, the reading skill and knowledge level of the client, and the client's cognitive and psychomotor ability. One type of measurement commonly used is a physiological measure. Examples of physiological measures are blood pressure, heart rate, and visual acuity. Client statements can also be used as evaluative measures. Table 13-9 contains examples of goals, expected outcomes, and corresponding evaluative measures.

ORAL ADMINISTRATION

The easiest and most desirable way to administer medications is by mouth (Skill 13-1). Clients usually are able to ingest or self-administer oral medications with a minimum of problems. Most tablets and capsules should be swallowed and administered with approximately 60 to 100 ml of fluid (as allowed). However, there may be situations that contraindicate

---

Nursing Interventions to Improve Compliance With Medications   Box 13-9

Establish a therapeutic nurse-client relationship.
Involve the client in deciding dosage schedule and regimen for drug preparation.
Simplify the medication regimen as much as possible.
Encourage use of generic prescriptions and limit use of OTC medications.
Educate clients so they can make informed decisions about medications.
Educate clients about expected side effects of medications and how to reduce, eliminate, or manage the side effects.
Review the client's medications regularly, and consult with the prescriber if unnecessary or duplicate medications are prescribed or if discrepancies exist between what the client should be taking and what the client is actually taking.

From Ryan AA: Medication compliance and older people: a review of the literature, *Int J Nurs Stud* 36:153, 1999.

---

the client's ability to receive medications by mouth. Table 13-5 (p. 287) summarizes the primary contraindications to giving oral medications. An important precaution to take when administering any oral preparation is to protect clients from aspiration. Aspiration occurs when food, fluid, or medication intended for GI administration is inadvertently administered into the respiratory tract. Evaluate your client's ability to swallow before administering oral medications. When there is a risk of aspiration, you can use certain interventions (Box 13-10). Properly positioning the client is essential in preventing aspiration. When possible, place the client in a seated position. You can also place the client in the side-lying position when your client's swallow, gag, and cough reflexes are intact. If your client has difficulty swallowing, consult appropriate personnel (e.g., speech therapist) for a swallow evaluation before administering oral medications. You may have to give medications through a nasogastric or feeding tube if the client cannot tolerate taking medications by mouth. Box 13-11 summarizes guidelines for administering medications through gastric tubes.

TOPICAL MEDICATION APPLICATIONS

Topical medications are medications applied locally, most often to intact skin. They can be in the form of lotions, pastes, or ointments (see Table 13-1, p. 282). They can also be applied to mucous membranes.

Skin Applications

Because many locally applied medications, such as lotions, pastes, and ointments, can create systemic and local effects, wear gloves and use applicators when administering them. Sterile technique is indicated if the client has an open wound.

Skin encrustation and dead tissues harbor microorganisms and block contact of medications with the tissues to be treated. Therefore clean the skin thoroughly before applying topical medications (McConnell, 1998b).

Text continued on p. 307

Example Evaluations for Client Goals   Table 13-9

Goal	Expected Outcomes	Evaluative Measure With Example
Client and family understand drug therapy.	Client and family describe information about drug, dosage, schedule, purpose, and adverse effects.	Written measurement: Have client write out medication schedule for a 24-hour period. Oral questioning: Ask client to describe purpose, dosage, and adverse effects of each prescribed medication.
	Client and family identify situations that require medical intervention.	Oral questioning: Have family describe what to do when a client has adverse effects from a medication.
	Client and family demonstrate appropriate administration technique.	Direct observation: Have client demonstrate filling of an insulin syringe and self-injection.
Client safely self-administers medications.	Client follows prescribed treatment regimen.	Anecdotal notes: Have family keep log of client's compliance with therapy for 1 week.
	Client performs techniques correctly.	Direct observation: Observe client instill eye drops.
	Client identifies available resources for obtaining necessary medication.	Oral questioning: Ask family to identify how to contact local pharmacy or community clinic for necessary medications.

Skill 13-1

ADMINISTERING ORAL MEDICATIONS

DELEGATION CONSIDERATIONS

Administering medications by the oral route requires problem solving and knowledge application unique to professional nursing. For this procedure delegation to unlicensed personnel is not appropriate. Assistive personnel should be instructed about potential side effects of medications and to report their occurrence.

EQUIPMENT

- Disposable medication cups
- Glass of water, juice, or preferred liquid
- Drinking straw
- Pill-crushing or pillating device (optional)
- MAR or computer printout

STEPS	RATIONALE
1. Assess for any contraindications to client receiving oral medication: Is client suffering from nausea and vomiting? Was client diagnosed as having bowel inflammation or reduced peristalsis? Has client had recent GI surgery? Does client have gastric suction? Check the client's swallow, cough, and gag reflexes.	Alerations in GI function interfere with drug absorption, distribution, and excretion. Clients with GI suction might not receive benefit from the medication because it may be suctioned from the GI tract before it can be absorbed. Giving medications to clients who cannot swallow increases the risk of aspiration.
2. Assess client's medical history, history of allergies, medication history, and diet history. Client's food and drug allergies should be listed on each page of the MAR and prominently displayed on the client's medical record.	Identifies potential food and drug interaction. Reflects client's need for medications. Effective communication of allergies is essential for all health care providers to provide safe, effective care.
3. Gather and review assessment and laboratory data that may influence drug administration.	Physical examination or laboratory data may contraindicate drug administration.

- **Critical Decision Point**

  If there are any contraindications to client receiving oral medications, or if in doubt about client's ability to swallow oral medications, temporarily withhold medication and notify prescriber.

STEPS	RATIONALE
4. Assess client's knowledge regarding health and medication usage.	Determines client's need for medication education and assists in identifying client's adherence to drug therapy at home. Assessment may reveal drug use problems, such as drug tolerance, abuse, addiction, or dependency.
5. Assess client's preferences for fluids. Maintain ordered fluid restriction (when applicable).	Fluids ease swallowing and facilitate absorption from the GI tract. Fluid restrictions must be maintained.
6. Check accuracy and completeness of each MAR or computer printout with prescriber's written medication order. Check client's name, drug name and dosage, route of administration, and time for administration.	The order sheet is the most reliable source and only legal record of drugs client is to receive.
7. Prepare medications:	
a. Wash hands.	Reduces transfer of microorganisms.
b. If medication cart is used, move it outside client's room.	Organization of equipment saves time and reduces error.
c. Unlock medicine drawer or cart.	Medications are safeguarded when locked in cabinet or cart.
d. Prepare medications for one client at a time. Keep all pages of MARs or computer printouts for one client together.	Prevents preparation errors.
e. Select correct drug from stock supply or unit-dose drawer. Compare label of medication with MAR or computer printout (see illustration).	Reading label and comparing it with transcribed order reduce errors.
f. Check expiration date on all medications.	Medications used past their expiration date may be inactive, less effective, or harmful to client.
g. Calculate drug dose as necessary. Double-check calculation.	Double checking reduces risk of error.
h. When preparing narcotics, check narcotic record for previous drug count and compare with supply available.	Controlled substance laws require careful monitoring of dispensed narcotics.

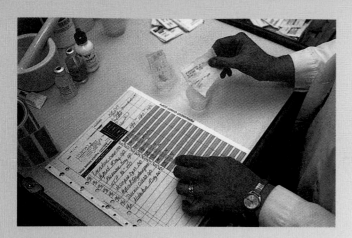

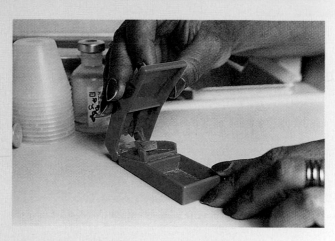

STEP 7E Check the label of the medication with the transcribed medication order.

STEP 7I Place tablet in pillating device, and cut in half.

i. To prepare tablets or capsules from a floor stock bottle, pour required number into bottle cap and transfer medication to medication cup. Do not touch medication with fingers. Return extra tablets or capsules to bottle. Medications that need to be broken to administer half the dosage can be broken, using a gloved hand, or cut with a pillating device (see illustration). Tablets that are to be broken in half must be prescored. Prescored tablets are identified by a manufactured line that traverses the center of the tablet.

Maintains clean technique required of medication administration. Tablets that are prescored can be split to ensure accurate dose is given to client.

j. To prepare unit-dose tablets or capsules, place packaged tablet or capsule directly into medicine cup. (Do not remove wrapper; see illustration.)

Wrapper maintains cleanliness of medications and identifies drug name and dosage.

k. All tablets or capsules to be given to client at same time may be placed in one medicine cup. Medications requiring preadministration assessments (e.g., pulse rate, blood pressure) should be placed in separate cups.

Keeping medications that require preadministration assessments separate from others makes it easier for you to remember to make special assessments and withhold drugs as necessary.

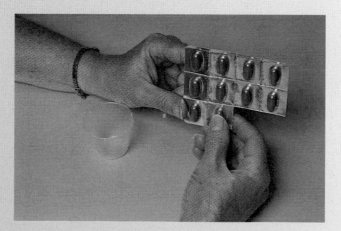

STEP 7J Place tablet into medicine cup without removing wrapper.

STEPS	RATIONALE
l. If client has difficulty swallowing and liquid medications are not an option, use a pill-crushing device, such as a mortar and pestle, to grind pills. If a pill-crushing device is not available, place tablet between two medication cups and grind with a blunt instrument. Mix ground tablet in small amount of soft food (custard, applesauce).	Large tablets can be difficult to swallow. Ground tablet mixed with palatable soft food is usually easier to swallow.

- **Critical Decision Point**
  Not all drugs can be crushed (e.g., capsules, enteric-coated drugs). Consult pharmacist when in doubt.

STEPS	RATIONALE
m. To prepare liquids:	
(1) Gently shake container. Remove bottle cap from container and place cap upside down or open the unit-dose container. If unit-dose container has correct amount to administer, no further preparation is necessary.	Shaking container ensures medication is mixed before administration. Placing cap of bottle upside down prevents contamination of inside of cap.
(2) Hold bottle with label against palm of hand while pouring.	Spilled liquid will not soil or fade label.
(3) Hold medication cup at eye level and fill to desired level (see illustration a). Scale should be even with fluid level at its surface or base of meniscus, not edges. Volumes less than 10 ml should be drawn up in syringe without needle (see illustration b).	Ensures accuracy of measurement.
(4) Discard any excess liquid into sink. Wipe lip and neck of bottle with paper towel.	Prevents contamination of bottle's contents and prevents bottle cap from sticking.
(5) Liquid medications packaged in single-dose cups need not be poured into medicine cups. They can be administered directly from the single-dose cup.	Avoids unnecessary manipulation of dose.
(6) For small doses of liquid medications, draw liquid into a calibrated oral syringe, with needle attached.	This technique is more accurate for measuring small doses of liquid medications.
n. Check expiration date on all medications.	Medications used past expiration date may be inactive or harmful to client.
o. When preparing narcotics, check narcotic record for previous drug count and compare with supply available.	Controlled substance laws require careful monitoring of dispensed narcotics.

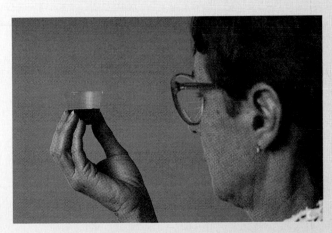

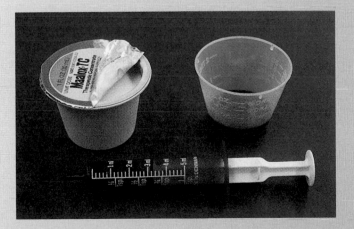

STEP 7M(3)A Pour the desired volume of liquid so that base of meniscus is level with line on scale.

STEP 7M(3)B Use needleless syringe to draw up volumes under 10 ml.

STEPS	RATIONALE
p. Compare MAR or computer printout with prepared drug and container.	Reading label second time reduces error.
q. Return stock containers or unused unit-dose medications to shelf or drawer, and read label again.	Third check of label reduces administration errors.
r. Do not leave drugs unattended.	Nurse is responsible for safekeeping of drugs.
8. Administering medications:	
a. Take medications to client at correct time.	Medications are administered within 30 minutes before or after prescribed time to ensure intended therapeutic effect. Stat or single-order medications should be given at time ordered.
b. Identify client by comparing name on MAR or computer printout with name on client's identification bracelet (see Figure 13-8, p. 295). Ask client to state name.	Identification bracelets are made at time of client's admission and are most reliable source of identification.

• *Critical Decision Point*
Client identification bracelets that are missing, illegible, or faded must be replaced.

STEPS	RATIONALE
c. Explain purpose of each medication and its action to client. Allow client to ask any questions about drugs.	Client has right to be informed about medication therapy. Questions may indicate need for education or noncompliance with therapy.
d. Assist client to sitting position. Use side-lying position if sitting is contraindicated.	Sitting position prevents aspiration during swallowing (Galvan, 2001).
e. Administer medication:	
(1) **For tablets:** Client may wish to hold solid medications in hand or cup before placing in mouth.	Client can become familiar with medications by seeing each drug.
(2) Offer water or juice to help client swallow medications. Give cold carbonated water if available and not contraindicated.	Choice of fluid promotes client's comfort and can improve fluid intake. Carbonated water helps passage of tablet through esophagus.
(3) **For sublingual medications:** Have client place medication under tongue and allow it to dissolve completely. Caution client against swallowing tablet whole (see Figure 13-2, p. 288).	Drug is absorbed through blood vessels of undersurface of tongue. If swallowed, drug is destroyed by gastric juices or rapidly detoxified by liver so that therapeutic blood levels are not attained.
(4) **For buccal medications:** Have client place medication in mouth against mucous membranes of the cheek until it dissolves (see Figure 13-3, p. 288). Avoid administering liquids until buccal medication has dissolved.	Buccal medications act locally on mucosa or systemically as they are swallowed in saliva.
(5) Caution client against chewing or swallowing lozenges.	Drug acts through slow absorption through oral mucosa, not gastric mucosa.
(6) **For powdered medications:** Mix with liquids at bedside, and give to client to drink.	When prepared in advance, powdered drugs may thicken and even harden, making swallowing difficult.
(7) Give effervescent powders and tablets immediately after dissolving.	Effervescence improves unpleasant taste of drug and often relieves GI problems.
f. If client is unable to hold medications, place medication cup to the lips and gently introduce each drug into the mouth, one at a time. Do not rush.	Administering single tablet or capsule eases swallowing and decreases risk of aspiration.
g. If tablet or capsule falls to the floor, discard it and repeat preparation.	Drug is contaminated when it touches floor.
h. Stay until client has completely swallowed each medication. Ask client to open mouth if uncertain whether medication has been swallowed.	You are responsible for ensuring that client receives ordered dosage. If left unattended, client may not take dose or may save drugs, causing risk to health.
i. For highly acidic medications (e.g., aspirin), offer client nonfat snack (e.g., crackers) if not contraindicated by client's condition.	Reduces gastric irritation.
j. Assist client in returning to comfortable position.	Maintains client's comfort.

STEPS	RATIONALE
k. Dispose of soiled supplies, and wash hands.	Reduces transmission of microorganisms.
l. Record administration of medication on MAR or computer printout. Return MAR or computer printout to appropriate file for next administration time.	Timely recording reduces medication errors. Computer printouts or MARs are used as reference for when next dose is due. Loss can lead to administration error.
m. Replenish stock, such as cups and straws, return cart to medicine room, and clean work area.	Clean working space assists other staff in completing duties efficiently.
9. Evaluate client's response to medications at times that correlate with the medication's onset, peak, and duration.	Evaluates drug's therapeutic benefit and can detect onset of side effects or allergic reactions.

UNEXPECTED OUTCOMES AND RELATED INTERVENTIONS

- Client exhibits adverse effects (side effect, toxic effect, allergic reaction).
  - Symptoms such as urticaria, rash, **pruritus,** rhinitis, and wheezing may indicate allergic reaction.
  - Always notify prescriber and pharmacy when the client exhibits adverse effects. Withhold further doses.
- Client refuses medication.
  - Explore reasons why client does not want medication.
  - Educate if misunderstandings of medication therapy are apparent.

- Do not force client to take medication.
- Clients have the right to refuse treatment.
- If client continues to refuse medication despite education, record why the drug was withheld on client's chart and notify prescriber.

RECORDING AND REPORTING

- Record administration of oral medications on MAR, using your initials or signature.
- Record the reason any drug is withheld and follow agency's policy for proper recording.

Interventions to Prevent Aspiration of Medications in Clients With Dysphagia   Box 13-10

Allow the client to self-administer medications if possible.

Position client in an upright, seated position if possible.

If the client has unilateral weakness, place the medication in the stronger side of the mouth.

Administer medications one at a time, ensuring that each medication is properly swallowed before the next one is introduced.

Thicker liquids are often easier to tolerate. Regular liquids should be thickened or fruit nectars offered to enhance swallowing.

Straws decrease the amount of control the client has over the amount of fluid taken into the mouth. Therefore do not have the client use a straw.

Time medications to coincide with meals if appropriate.

Give medications at times when the client is well rested and awake.

If dysphagia is severe, explore alternative routes of administration.

Modified from Galvan TJ: Dysphagia: going down and staying down, *Am J Nurs* 101(1):37, 2001.

Procedural Guidelines for   Box 13-11
GIVING MEDICATIONS THROUGH A NASOGASTRIC TUBE, G-TUBE, J-TUBE, OR SMALL-BORE FEEDING TUBE

1. Investigate and use alternative routes of medication administration if possible (e.g., transdermal, rectal).
2. Avoid complicated medication regimens that frequently interrupt enteral feedings.
3. Be sure the medication is compatible with the enteral feeding before administering medications. If the medication is incompatible with the feeding, stop the feeding 1 to 2 hours before the medication is given, and restart the feeding 1 to 2 hours after the medication is given. **Never** add medications directly to the tube feeding.
4. Administer medications in a liquid form (suspension, elixir, solution) when possible to prevent obstruction of the tube.
5. Before crushing medications, be sure they can be crushed. Buccal, sublingual, enteric-coated, or sustained-release medications cannot be crushed.
6. Dissolve crushed tablets, gelatin capsules, and powders in 15 to 30 ml of warm water. Dissolve and administer each medication separately, flushing with 15 to 30 ml of water between each medication. Unless contraindicated, the total amount of liquid volume administered to the client for each medication should be approximately 60 ml.
7. Do not give whole or undissolved medications through the feeding tube.
8. Continually evaluate the client's response to medication therapy. If the desired effect is not achieved, a different medication or route of administration may be indicated because of problems with drug bioavailability when given by the enteral route.

Modified from Gilbar PJ: A guide to enteral drug administration in palliative care, *J Pain Symptom Manage* 17(3):197, 1999.

When applying ointments or pastes, spread the medication evenly over the involved surface. A gauze dressing may need to be applied over the medication to prevent soiling of clothes and wiping away of the medication. Each type of medication should be applied according to directions to ensure proper penetration and absorption. Lotions and creams are spread lightly onto the skin's surface, because rubbing may cause irritation. A liniment is applied by rubbing it gently but firmly into the skin. A powder is dusted lightly to cover the affected area with a thin layer. Before and during any application, assess the skin thoroughly. Note the area applied, name of medication, and condition of skin on the MAR.

Nasal Instillation

Clients with nasal sinus alterations may receive medications by spray, drops, or tampons (Skill 13-2). The most commonly administered form of nasal instillation is decongestant spray or drops, used to relieve symptoms of sinus congestion and colds. Caution your client to avoid abuse of nose drops and sprays, because overuse can lead to rebound nasal congestion. In addition, when excess decongestant solution is swallowed, serious systemic effects may develop, especially in children. Saline drops are safer as a decongestant for children than

nasal preparations that contain sympathomimetics (e.g., Afrin, Neo-Synephrine).

It is easier to have the client self-administer sprays, because the client can control the spray and inhale as it enters the nasal passages. If clients use nasal sprays repeatedly, observe the nares for irritation. Severe nosebleeds are usually treated with packing or nasal tampons, which are treated with epinephrine, to reduce blood flow. Usually a physician places nasal tampons.

Eye Instillation

Common medications used by clients are eye drops and ointments, including OTC preparations (e.g., Visine, Murine). Many clients receive prescribed **ophthalmic** medications for eye conditions such as glaucoma or after cataract extraction. A large percentage of clients receiving eye medications are older adults. Age-related problems, including poor vision, hand tremors, and difficulty grasping or manipulating small containers, affect the ease with which older adults can self-administer eye medications. Educate your clients and their family members about the proper techniques for administering eye medications (Skill 13-3). Evaluate the client and family's ability to self-administer

Text continued on p. 314

Skill 13-2

ADMINISTERING NASAL INSTILLATION

DELEGATION CONSIDERATIONS

Administration of nasal drops and ointments requires problem solving and knowledge application unique to professional nursing. For this procedure delegation to assistive personnel is not appropriate. Assistive personnel should be instructed about potential side effects of medications and to report their occurrence.

EQUIPMENT

- Prepared medication with clean dropper or spray container
- Facial tissue
- Small pillow (optional)
- Washcloth (optional)
- Gloves (if client has extensive nasal drainage)
- MAR or computer printout

STEPS	RATIONALE
1. For nasal drops, determine which sinus is affected by referring to medical record.	Affects client's position during drug instillation.
2. Assess client's history of hypertension, heart disease, diabetes mellitus, and hyperthyroidism.	These conditions can contraindicate use of decongestants that stimulate CNS. Side effects of transient hypertension, tachycardia, palpitations, and headache may occur.
3. Inspect condition of nose and sinuses. Palpate sinuses for tenderness.	Provides baseline to monitor effects of medication. Presence of discharge interferes with drug absorption.
4. Assess client's knowledge regarding use of nasal instillations and technique for instillation and willingness to learn self-administration.	Indicates need for medication teaching. Level of motivation influences teaching approach.
5. Check client's identification bracelet, and ask name.	Ensures right client receives drug.
6. Explain procedure to client regarding positioning and sensations to expect, such as burning or stinging of mucosa, or choking sensation as medication trickles into throat.	Helps client anticipate experience of procedure to reduce anxiety.
7. Wash hands. Arrange supplies and medications at bedside. Apply gloves if client has nasal drainage.	Reduces transmission of microorganisms and prevents exposure to body fluids (NIOSH, 1999).
8. Instruct client to clear or blow nose gently unless contraindicated (e.g., risk of increased intracranial pressure or nosebleeds).	Removes mucus and secretions that can block distribution of medication.

9. Administer nasal drops:
    a. Assist client to supine position and position head properly:

    Positions provide access to nasal passages.

        (1) For access to posterior pharynx, tilt client's head backward.
        (2) For access to ethmoid or sphenoid sinus, tilt head back over edge of bed or place small pillow under client's shoulder and tilt head back (see illustration).
        (3) For access to frontal or maxillary sinus, tilt head back over edge of bed or pillow with head turned toward side to be treated (see illustration).

    Position allows medication to drain into affected sinus.

    b. Support client's head with nondominant hand.

    Prevents straining of neck muscles.

    c. Instruct client to breathe through mouth.

    Mouth breathing reduces chance of aspirating nasal drops into trachea and lungs.

    d. Hold dropper 1 cm (½ inch) above nares, and instill prescribed number of drops toward midline of ethmoid bone (see illustration from step 9a[2]).

    Avoids contamination of dropper. Instilling toward ethmoid bone facilitates distribution of medication over nasal mucosa.

    e. Have client remain in supine position 5 minutes.

    Prevents premature loss of medication through nares.

    f. Offer facial tissue to blot runny nose, but caution client against blowing nose for several minutes.

    Allows maximal amount of medication to be absorbed.

10. Assist client to a comfortable position after drug is absorbed.

    Restores comfort.

11. Dispose of soiled supplies in proper container, and wash hands.

    Maintains neat, orderly environment. Reduces spread of microorganisms.

12. Observe client for onset of side effects 15 to 30 minutes after administration.

    Drugs absorbed through mucosa can cause systemic reaction.

13. Ask if client is able to breathe through nose after decongestant administration. May be necessary to have client occlude one nostril at a time and breathe deeply.

    Determines effectiveness of decongestant medication.

14. Reinspect condition of nasal passages for swelling or irritation between instillations.

    Condition of mucosa reveals response to medication.

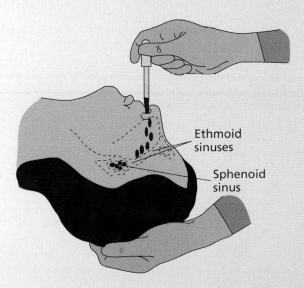

STEP 9a(2) Position for instilling nose drops into ethmoid or sphenoid sinus.

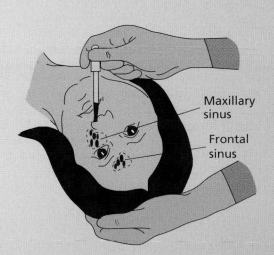

STEP 9a(3) Position for instilling nose drops into frontal and maxillary sinus.

STEPS	RATIONALE
15. Ask client to review risks of overuse of decongestants and methods for administration.	Feedback ensures that client can self-administer drugs properly.
16. Have client demonstrate self-medication with next dose.	Feedback demonstrates learning.

UNEXPECTED OUTCOMES AND RELATED INTERVENTIONS
- Client begins wheezing or displays other signs of allergic reaction to drug.
  - Follow institutional policy or guidelines for appropriate response to allergic reactions.
  - Notify client's health care provider immediately.
- Client is unable to breathe easily through nasal passages. Mucosa appears swollen, and congestion is unrelieved.
  - Client may be experiencing rebound effect. Stop medication use, and notify prescriber.
- Nasal mucosa remains inflamed and tender with discharge from nares.
  - Inflammatory or infectious process remains. May need to consider alternative therapy.
- Client complains of sinus headache. Sinuses remain congested.
  - May need to consider alternative therapy.

- Client is unable to explain technique and risks of drug therapy.
  - Further explanation is required.
- Client is unable to self-administer medication.
  - Reinstruction is necessary.

RECORDING AND REPORTING
- Record medication administration, including drug name, concentration, number of drops, nostril into which drug was instilled, and time of administration.
- Record client's response in nurse's notes.
- Report any unusual systemic effects to nurse in charge or physician.

Skill 13-3
ADMINISTERING OPHTHALMIC MEDICATIONS

DELEGATION CONSIDERATIONS
The skill of administering eye medications should not be delegated to assistive personnel. Assistive personnel should be instructed about potential side effects of medications and to report their occurrence. In addition, assistive personnel should be notified if vision impairment is possible after administration of eye medications.

EQUIPMENT
- Medication bottle with sterile eye dropper or ointment tube or medicated intraocular disk
- Cotton ball or tissue
- Washbasin filled with warm water and washcloth if eyes have crust or drainage
- Eye patch and tape (optional)
- Clean gloves
- MAR or computer printout

STEPS	RATIONALE
1. Review prescriber's medication order for number of drops (if a liquid) and eye (right = O.D.; left = O.S.; both = O.U.) to receive medication.	Ensures correct administration of medication.
2. Assess condition of external eye structures. (May also be done just before drug instillation.)	Provides baseline to later determine if local response to medications occurs. Also indicates need to clean eye before drug application.
3. Determine whether client has any known allergies to eye medications. Also ask if client has allergy to latex.	Protects client from risk of allergic drug response. If client has a latex allergy, use nonlatex gloves.
4. Determine whether client has any symptoms of visual alterations.	Certain eye medications act to either lessen or increase these symptoms. You must be able to recognize change in client's condition.
5. Assess client's level of consciousness and ability to follow directions.	If client becomes restless or combative during procedure, a greater risk of accidental eye injury exists.

STEPS	RATIONALE
6. Assess client's knowledge regarding drug therapy and desire to self-administer medication.	Client's level of understanding may indicate need for health teaching. Motivation influences teaching approach.
7. Assess client's ability to manipulate and hold equipment necessary for eye medication (e.g., dropper, tube of ointment, intraocular disk).	Reflects client's ability to self-administer drug.
8. Check client's identification bracelet, and ask name.	Ensures correct client receives medication.
9. Explain procedure to client before and during procedure.	Relieves anxiety about medication being instilled into eye.
10. Wash hands and arrange supplies at bedside; apply clean gloves.	Reduces transmission of microorganisms and follows CDC recommendations to prevent accidental exposure to body fluids (NIOSH, 1999).
11. Ask client to lie supine or sit back in chair with head slightly hyperextended.	Position provides easy access to eye for medication instillation and minimizes drainage of medication through tear duct.

- *Critical Decision Point*

  If the client has a cervical spine injury, do not hyperextend the neck.

12. If crusts or drainage is present along eyelid margins or inner canthus, gently wash away. Soak crusts that are dried and difficult to remove by applying damp washcloth or cotton ball over eye for a few minutes. Always wipe clean from inner to outer canthus.	Crusts or drainage harbors microorganisms. Soaking allows easy removal and prevents pressure from being applied directly over eye. Cleansing from inner to outer canthus avoids entrance of microorganisms into lacrimal duct.
13. Hold cotton ball or clean tissue in nondominant hand on client's cheekbone just below lower eyelid.	Cotton or tissue absorbs medication that escapes eye.
14. With tissue or cotton resting below lower lid, gently press downward with thumb or forefinger against bony orbit	Technique exposes lower conjunctival sac. Retraction against bony orbit prevents pressure and trauma to eyeball and prevents fingers from touching eye.
15. Ask client to look at ceiling.	Action retracts sensitive cornea up and away from conjunctival sac and reduces stimulation of blink reflex.
16. Administer ophthalmic medication.	
a. To instill eye drops:	
(1) With dominant hand resting on client's forehead, hold filled medication eye dropper or ophthalmic solution approximately 1 to 2 cm (½ to ¾ inch) above conjunctival sac (see illustration).	Helps prevent accidental contact of eye dropper with eye structures, thus reducing risk of injury to eye and transfer of infection to dropper. Ophthalmic medications are sterile.
(2) Drop prescribed number of medication drops into conjunctival sac.	Conjunctival sac normally holds 1 or 2 drops. Provides even distribution of medication across eye.
(3) If client blinks or closes eye or if drops land on outer lid margins, repeat procedure.	Therapeutic effect of drug is obtained only when drops enter conjunctival sac.
(4) After instilling drops, ask client to close eye gently.	Helps to distribute medication. Squinting or squeezing of eyelids forces medication out of conjunctival sac (McConnell, 1998a).

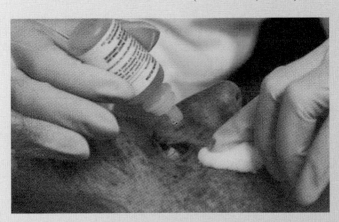

STEP 16A(1)   Hold eye dropper above conjunctival sac.

STEPS	RATIONALE
(5) When administering drugs that cause systemic effects, apply gentle pressure with your finger and clean tissue on the client's nasolacrimal duct for 30 to 60 seconds.	Prevents overflow of medication into nasal and pharyngeal passages. Prevents absorption into systemic circulation.
b. To instill eye ointment:	
(1) Ask client to look at ceiling.	Action retracts sensitive cornea up and away from conjunctival sac and reduces stimulation of blink reflex.
(2) Holding ointment applicator above lower lid margin, apply thin stream of ointment evenly along inner edge of lower eyelid on conjunctiva (see illustration) from the inner canthus to outer canthus.	Distributes medication evenly across eye and lid margin.
(3) Have client close eye and roll eye behind closed eyelid.	Further distributes medication without traumatizing eye (McConnell, 1999).
c. To administer intraocular disk:	
(1) Application:	
(a) Open package containing the disk. Apply gloves. Gently press your fingertip against the disk so that it adheres to your finger. Position the convex side of the disk on your fingertip (see illustration).	Allows you to inspect disk for damage or deformity.
(b) With your other hand, gently pull the client's lower eyelid away from the eye. Ask client to look up.	Prepares conjunctival sac for receiving medicated disk.
(c) Place the disk in the conjunctival sac so that it floats on the sclera between the iris and lower eyelid (see illustration).	Ensures delivery of medication.
(d) Pull the client's lower eyelid out and over the disk (see illustration).	Ensures accurate medication delivery.

- **Critical Decision Point**
  You should not be able to see the disk at this time. Repeat Step 4 if you can see the disk.

STEPS	RATIONALE
(2) Removal:	
(a) Wash hands, and put on gloves.	Prevents transfer of microorganisms and follows CDC recommendations to prevent accidental exposure to body fluids (NIOSH, 1999).
(b) Explain procedure to client.	Relieves anxiety about manipulation of disk in eye.
(c) Gently pull down on the client's lower eyelid.	Exposes intraocular disk.

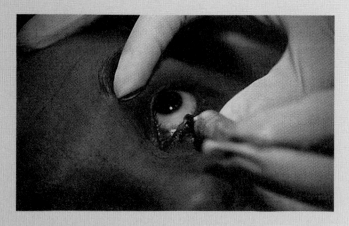

STEP 16B(2) Apply ointment along lower eyelid.

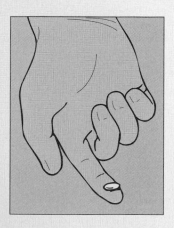

STEP 16C(1)A Gently position the convex side of the disk against your fingertip.

STEPS   RATIONALE

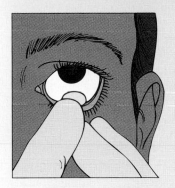

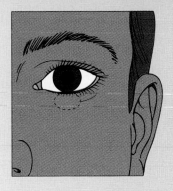

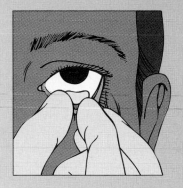

STEP 16C(1)(C) Place disk in the conjunctival sac between the iris and lower eyelid.

STEP 16C(1)(D) Gently pull lower eyelid over the disk.

STEP 16C(2)(D) Carefully pinch the disk to remove it from client's eye.

     (d) Using your forefinger and thumb of your opposite hand, pinch the disk and lift it out of the client's eye (see illustration).

17. If excess medication is on eyelid, gently wipe it from inner to outer canthus.

Promotes comfort and prevents trauma to eye.

18. If client had eye patch, apply clean one by placing it over affected eye so entire eye is covered. Tape securely without applying pressure to eye.

Clean eye patch reduces chance of infection.

19. If client receives more than one eye medication to the same eye at the same time, wait at least 5 minutes before administering the next medication.

Allows medication to absorb and avoids interaction between medications (Patient's Library, 2000).

20. If client receives eye medication to both eyes at the same time, use a different tissue or cotton ball with each eye.

Prevents cross contamination between eyes (McConnell, 1999).

21. Remove gloves, dispose of soiled supplies in proper receptacle, and wash hands.

Maintains neat environment at bedside and reduces transmission of microorganisms.

22. Note client's response to instillation; ask if any discomfort was felt.

Determines if procedure was performed correctly and safely.

23. Observe response to medication by assessing visual changes and noting any side effects.

Evaluates effects of medication.

24. Ask client to discuss drug's purpose, action, side effects, and technique of administration.

Determines client's level of understanding.

25. Have client demonstrate self-administration of next dose.

Provides feedback regarding competency with skill.

UNEXPECTED OUTCOMES AND RELATED INTERVENTIONS

- Client cannot instill drops without supervision.
  - Reinforce teaching, and allow client to self-administer drops as much as possible to enhance confidence.
  - If client cannot self-administer drops, teach others, such as family members, to instill drops into the client's eye.
- Client displays signs of allergic reaction (e.g., tearing, reddened sclera) or systemic response (e.g., bradycardia) to medication.
  - Hold medication, and speak with prescriber.

- Follow institutional policy or guidelines for reporting of adverse or allergic reaction to medications.

RECORDING AND REPORTING

- Record drug, concentration, number of drops, time of administration, and eye (left, right, or both) that received medication on MAR.
- Record appearance of eye in nurse's notes.

through a return demonstration of the procedure. Showing clients each step of the procedure for instilling eye drops can improve their compliance. Apply the following principles when administering eye medications:

1. Avoid instilling any form of eye medication directly onto the cornea. The cornea of the eye is richly supplied with pain fibers and thus very sensitive to anything applied to it.
2. Avoid touching the eyelids or other eye structures with eye droppers or ointment tubes. The risk of transmitting infection from one eye to the other is high.
3. Use eye medication only for the client's affected eye.
4. Never allow a client to use another client's eye medications.

Some medications are administered by an intraocular disk (see Skill 13-3, p. 310). Intraocular medicated disks resemble a contact lens. The medication is placed onto the conjunctival sac where it remains in place for up to 1 week. Teach your client receiving medications in this way to monitor for adverse reactions to the disk as well as methods of insertion and removal.

Ear Instillation

Internal ear structures are very sensitive to temperature extremes. Failure to instill ear drops or irrigating fluid at room temperature may cause vertigo (severe dizziness) or nausea. Although the structures of the outer ear are not sterile, sterile drops and solutions are used in case the eardrum is ruptured. The entrance of nonsterile solutions into middle ear structures could result in infection. If the client has ear drainage, check with the physician to be sure the client does not have a ruptured eardrum before instilling ear drops. Never occlude the ear canal with the dropper or irrigating syringe. Forcing medication into an occluded ear canal creates pressure that may injure the eardrum. When administering medications into the ear, straighten the ear canal properly to allow medications to reach the deeper, external ear structures. Box 13-12 provides guidelines for administering ear drops and ear irrigations and describes how to straighten the ear canal for children and for adults.

Vaginal Instillation

Vaginal medications are available as suppositories, foams, jellies, or creams. Suppositories come individually packaged and may be stored in a refrigerator to prevent them from melting. After a suppository is inserted into the vaginal cavity, body temperature causes it to melt and be distributed and absorbed. Foams, jellies, and creams are administered with an applicator or inserter (Figure 13-11). A suppository is given with a gloved hand in accordance with Standard precautions (Figure 13-12). Clients often prefer administering their own vaginal medications and should be given privacy. After instillation of the medication, your client may wish to wear a perineal pad to collect drainage. Because vaginal medications are often given to treat infection, discharge may be foul-smelling. Aseptic technique should be followed, and your client should be offered frequent opportunities to maintain perineal hygiene (see Chapter 26).

Rectal Instillation

Rectal suppositories are thinner and more bullet-shaped than vaginal suppositories. The rounded end prevents anal trauma during insertion. Rectal suppositories contain medications that exert local effects, such as promoting defecation, or systemic effects, such as reducing nausea. Rectal suppositories may be stored in the refrigerator until administered.

During administration, place the suppository past the internal anal sphincter and against the rectal mucosa. Otherwise, the suppository may be expelled before it can dissolve and be absorbed into the mucosa. You will feel the sphincter relaxing around the finger when you administer the suppository. Suppositories should not be forced into a mass of fecal material. You may need to clear the rectum with a small cleansing enema before a suppository can be inserted.

ADMINISTERING MEDICATIONS BY INHALATION

Medications administered with handheld inhalers are dispersed through an aerosol spray, mist, or powder that penetrates lung airways. The alveolar-capillary network absorbs medications rapidly. **Metered-dose inhalers (MDIs)** are usually designed to produce local effects, such as bronchodilation. However, some medications can create serious systemic side effects.

Clients who receive medications by inhalation frequently have a chronic respiratory disease, such as chronic asthma, emphysema, or bronchitis. Medications given by inhalation provide these clients with control of airway obstruction. Therefore they must learn about inhaled medications and how to administer them safely (Skill 13-4).

ADMINISTERING MEDICATIONS BY IRRIGATION

Medications may be used to irrigate or wash out a body cavity and are delivered through a stream of solution. Irrigations most commonly use sterile water, saline, or antiseptic solutions on the eye, ear, throat, vagina, and urinary tract. If there is a break in the skin or mucosa, aseptic technique is used. When the cavity to be irrigated is not sterile, as is the case with the ear canal (see Box 13-12, p. 315) or vagina, clean technique is acceptable. Irrigations can cleanse an area, instill a medication, or apply hot or cold to injured tissue.

PARENTERAL ADMINISTRATION OF MEDICATIONS

Parenteral administration of medications is the administration of medications by injection. When medications are administered this way, it is an invasive procedure that must be performed using aseptic techniques (Box 13-13). After a

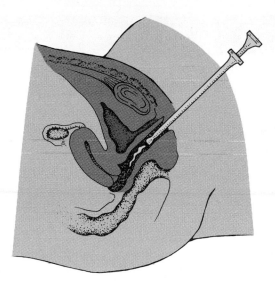

FIGURE **13-11**   Instillation of medication in vaginal canal.

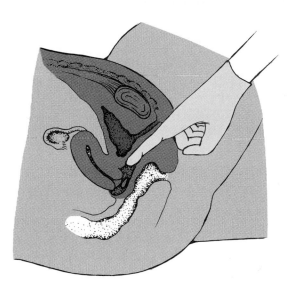

FIGURE **13-12**   Insertion of a suppository into the vaginal canal.

needle pierces the skin, there is risk of infection. Each type of injection requires certain skills to ensure that the medication reaches the proper location. The effects of a parenterally administered medication can develop rapidly, depending on the rate of medication absorption. Therefore you must closely observe the client's response to the medication.

Equipment
A variety of syringes and needles are available, each designed to deliver a certain volume of a medication to a specific type of tissue. Use nursing judgment when determining the syringe or needle that will be most effective.

SYRINGES.   Syringes have a cylindrical barrel with a close-fitting plunger and a tip designed to fit the hub of a hypodermic needle. Syringes in general are classified as being Luer-lok or non–Luer-lok. This name is based on the design

---

Procedural Guidelines for   **Box 13-12**
ADMINISTERING EAR MEDICATIONS

EAR DROPS
1. Place client in side-lying position if not contraindicated by client's condition, with ear to be treated facing up. The client may also sit in a chair or at the bedside.
2. Straighten ear canal by pulling auricle down and back for children or upward and outward for adults.
3. Instill prescribed drops holding dropper 1 cm ($^1/_2$ inch) above ear canal (see illustration).

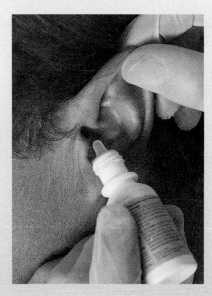

4. Ask client to remain in side-lying position for 2 to 3 minutes. Apply gentle massage or pressure to tragus of ear with finger.
5. If a cotton ball is to be placed into the outermost part of ear canal, do not press cotton ball into the canal. Remove cotton after 15 minutes.

EAR IRRIGATIONS
1. Assess the tympanic membrane or review medical record for history of eardrum perforation, which contraindicates ear irrigation.
2. Assist client into sitting or lying position with head tilted or turned toward affected ear. Place towel under client's head and shoulder, and have client hold basin under affected ear.
3. Fill irrigating syringe with solution (approximately 50 ml) at room temperature.
4. Gently grasp auricle, and straighten ear by pulling it down and back for children or upward and outward for adults.
5. Slowly instill irrigating solution by holding tip of syringe 1 cm ($^1/_2$ inch) above opening of ear canal. Allow fluid to drain out during instillation. Continue until canal is cleansed or all solution is used.

---

on the syringe's tip. Luer-lok syringes (Figure 13-13, *A*) require special needles, which are twisted onto the tip and lock themselves in place. This design prevents the inadvertent removal of the needle. Non–Luer-lok syringes (Figure 13-13, *B* to *D*) require needles that slip onto the tip.

To fill the syringe, pull the plunger outward while the needle tip remains immersed in the prepared solution. To maintain sterility, you can touch the outside of the syringe

Skill 13-4
USING METERED-DOSE INHALERS

DELEGATION CONSIDERATIONS
The skill of administering MDI medications should not be delegated to assistive personnel. Assistive personnel should be instructed about potential side effects of medications and to report their occurrence. In addition, the care provider should report paroxysmal coughing, ineffective breathing patterns, and other respiratory difficulties.

EQUIPMENT
- MDI with medication canister
- Aerochamber (optional)
- Facial tissues (optional)
- Wash basin or sink with warm water
- Paper towel
- MAR or computer printout

STEPS	RATIONALE
1. Assess client's ability to hold, manipulate, and depress canister and inhaler.	Approximately 5 to 10 pounds of pressure must be used to activate the aerosol. Any impairment of grasp or presence of hand tremors, such as those related to effects of aging or chronic respiratory disease, interferes with client's ability to depress canister within inhaler.
2. Assess client's readiness to learn: client asks questions about medication, disease, or complications; requests education in use of inhaler; is mentally alert; participates in own care.	Influences client's motivation to understand explanations and actively participate in teaching process.
3. Assess client's ability to learn: client should not be fatigued, in pain, or in respiratory distress; assess level of understanding of technical vocabulary terms.	Mental or physical limitations affect client's ability to learn and methods nurse uses for instruction.
4. Assess client's knowledge and understanding of disease and purpose and action of prescribed medications.	Knowledge of disease and medications is essential for client to realistically understand use of inhaler.
5. Determine drug schedule and number of inhalations prescribed for each dose.	Influences explanations nurse provides for use of inhaler.
6. If previously instructed in self-administration of inhaled medicine, assess client's technique in using an inhaler.	Nurse's instruction may require only simple reinforcement, depending on client's level of dexterity.
7. Help client into a comfortable position, such as sitting in chair in hospital room or sitting at kitchen table in home.	Client will be more likely to remain receptive of nurse's explanations.
8. Check client's identification bracelet, and ask name.	Ensures correct client receives medication.
9. Explain procedure to client. Be specific if client wishes to self-administer drug. Explain where and how to set up in the home.	Makes client a participant in care and minimizes anxiety.
10. Provide adequate time for teaching session.	Prevents interruptions. Instruction should occur when client is receptive.
11. Wash hands, and arrange equipment needed.	Reduces transfer of microorganisms and saves time.
12. Have client manipulate inhaler, canister, and spacer device. Explain and demonstrate how canister fits into inhaler.	Client must be familiar with how to use equipment.
13. Explain what metered dose is, and warn client about overuse of inhaler, including drug side effects.	Client must not arbitrarily administer excessive inhalations because of risk of serious side effects. If drug is given in recommended doses, side effects are uncommon.
14. **To administer inhaled dose of medication (demonstrate steps when possible):**	Use of simple, step-by-step explanations allows client to ask questions at any point during procedure.

- *Critical Decision Point*
  If a corticosteroid and bronchodilator are ordered for the same time, the bronchodilator should be used first to open the airway and allow the corticosteroid to be absorbed better (Gazarian, 1997).

a. Remove mouthpiece cover from inhaler.	
b. Shake inhaler well.	Ensures fine particles are aerosolized.
c. Have client take a deep breath and exhale.	Prepares the client's airway to receive the medication.

d. Instruct the client to position the inhaler in one of two ways:

(1) Open lips and place inhaler in mouth with opening toward back of throat (see illustration).

(2) Position the device 1 to 2 inches from the mouth (see illustration).

Directs aerosol spray toward airway.

Positioning the mouthpiece 1 to 2 inches from the mouth is considered the best way to deliver the medication because the spray is more fully dispersed.

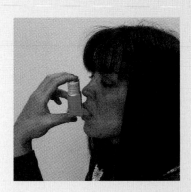

STEP 14D(1)   One technique for use of the inhaler. The client opens lips and places inhaler in mouth with opening toward back of throat.

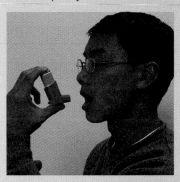

STEP 14D(2)   One technique for use of the inhaler. The client positions the mouthpiece 1 to 2 inches from the mouth. This is considered the best way to deliver the medication.

e. With the inhaler properly positioned, have client hold inhaler with thumb at the mouthpiece and the index finger and middle finger at the top. This is called a three-point or lateral hand position.

MDIs work best when clients use a three-point or lateral hand position to activate canisters.

f. Instruct client to tilt head back slightly, inhale slowly and deeply through mouth, and depress medication canister fully.

Medication is distributed to airways during inhalation. Inhalation through mouth rather than nose draws medication more effectively into airways.

• *Critical Decision Point*

If inhaled dry powder capsules are used, client should close mouth tightly around mouthpiece of inhaler and inhale rapidly.

g. Hold breath for approximately 10 seconds.

Allows tiny drops of aerosol spray to reach deeper branches of airways.

h. Exhale through pursed lips.

Keeps small airways open during exhalation.

15. To administer inhaled dose of medication using a spacer such as an aerochamber (demonstrate when possible):

a. Remove mouthpiece cover from MDI and mouthpiece of aerochamber.

Inhaler fits into end of aerochamber.

b. Insert MDI into end of aerochamber.

Aerochamber is a spacer that traps medication released from the MDI; the client then inhales the drug from the device. These devices deposit up to 80% more medication in the lungs rather than in the oropharynx.

c. Shake inhaler well.

Ensures fine particles are aerosolized.

d. Place aerochamber mouthpiece in mouth, and close lips. Do not insert beyond raised lip on mouthpiece. Avoid covering small exhalation slots with the lips (see illustration).

Medication should not escape through mouth.

e. Breathe normally through aerochamber mouthpiece.

Allows client to relax before delivering medication.

f. Depress medication canister, spraying one puff into aerochamber.

Emits spray that allows finer particles to be inhaled. Large droplets are retained in aerochamber.

g. Breathe in slowly and fully.

Ensures particles of medication are distributed to deeper airways.

STEPS	RATIONALE

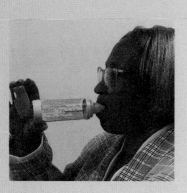

STEP 15D   Have client place mouthpiece in mouth and close lips, being careful to keep exhalation slots exposed.

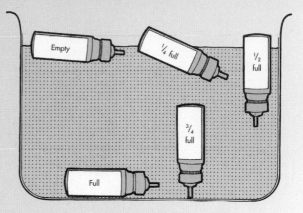

STEP 21   A simple method of estimating amount left in the inhalant canister is to place it in a container filled with water. The position the canister takes in the water demonstrates the amount of inhalant remaining.

STEPS	RATIONALE
h. Hold full breath for 10 to 15 seconds.	Ensures full drug distribution.
16. Instruct client to wait at least 1 minute between inhalations or as ordered by prescriber.	Drugs must be inhaled sequentially. First inhalation opens airways and reduces inflammation. Second or third inhalation penetrates deeper airways.

• *Critical Decision Point*
If a corticosteroid was used, have client rinse mouth with water or salt water after inhalation to reduce risk of fungal infection. Also teach client to inspect oral cavity daily for redness, sores, or white patches. Abnormal assessment findings should be reported to the client's health care provider (Gazarian, 1997).

STEPS	RATIONALE
17. Explain that client may feel gagging sensation in throat caused by droplets of medication on pharynx or tongue.	Results when inhalant is sprayed and inhaled incorrectly.
18. Instruct client in removing medication canister and cleaning inhaler in warm water.	Accumulation of spray around mouthpiece can interfere with proper distribution during use.
19. Have client explain and demonstrate steps in use of inhaler.	Return demonstration provides feedback for measuring client's learning.
20. Ask client to explain medication schedule, side effects, and when to call health care provider.	Understanding of schedule and medication improves likelihood of compliance with therapy.
21. Teach client how to determine fullness of canisters, using displacement in water (see illustration).	Helps client determine when to reorder prescription.
22. After medication instillation, assess client's respirations and auscultate lungs.	Determines status of breathing pattern and adequacy of ventilation.

UNEXPECTED OUTCOMES AND RELATED INTERVENTIONS
- Client needs a bronchodilator more than every 4 hours.
  - May indicate respiratory problems; reassessment of type of medication and delivery methods needed.
- Client experiences cardiac dysrhythmias, especially if receiving beta-adrenergics.
  - If client experiences symptoms with the dysrhythmias (e.g., light-headedness, syncope), withhold all further doses of medication. Discuss with prescriber.
- Client may not be able to self-administer medication properly.
  - Alternative delivery routes or methods may need to be explored.

- Client experiences paroxysms of coughing.
  - Aerosolized particles irritate posterior pharynx. Notify prescriber; may need to reassess type of medication or delivery method.

RECORDING AND REPORTING
- Document in nurse's notes what skills were taught and client's ability to perform skills.
- Record time when client used MDI (amount of puffs).
- Report any undesirable effects from medication.

Sto5

SSto5

barrel and the handle of the plunger, but do not touch the tip or inside of the barrel, the hub, the shaft of the plunger, and the needle (Figure 13-14).

Syringes come in a number of sizes, ranging from 0.5 to 60 ml. It is unusual to use a syringe larger than 5 ml for an injection. A 2- to 3-ml syringe is usually adequate for IM and SQ injections. Large syringes are used to administer certain IV medications, add medications to IV solutions, and irrigate wounds or drainage tubes. Some syringes may come prepackaged with a needle attached. However, you may need to change the needle based on the route of administration and the size of the client.

The tuberculin syringe (see Figure 13-13, *B*) has a long, thin barrel with a preattached thin needle. The syringe is calibrated in sixteenths of a minim and hundredths of a milliliter and has a capacity of 1 ml. Tuberculin syringes are used to prepare small amounts of medications. They may also be used for ID and SQ injections.

Insulin syringes (see Figure 13-13, *C* and *D*) hold 0.3 to 1 ml and are calibrated in units. Most insulin syringes are U-100s, designed for use with U-100 strength insulin. Each milliliter of solution contains 100 units of insulin.

NEEDLES.   Sometimes needles come attached to syringes. Other needles come packaged individually to allow flexibility in selecting the right needle for a client. Needles are disposable, with most made of stainless steel.

The needle has three parts: the hub, which fits onto the tip of a syringe; the shaft, which connects to the hub; and the bevel or slanted tip (see Figure 13-14, p. 320). The tip of a needle, or the bevel, is always slanted. The bevel creates a narrow slit when injected into tissue and quickly closes when the needle is removed to prevent leakage of medication, blood, or serum. Long beveled tips are sharp and narrow, which minimizes discomfort when entering tissue used for SQ or IM injections.

Needles vary in length from $^1/_4$ to 3 inches (Figure 13-15). The needle length you choose depends on the client's size and weight and the route of administration. A child or slender adult generally requires a shorter needle. Longer needles

(1 to $1^1/_2$ inches) are used for IM injections, and shorter needles ($^3/_8$ to $^5/_8$ inch) are used for SQ injections. As the needle gauge gets smaller, the needle diameter becomes larger (see Figure 13-15). The selection of a gauge depends on the viscosity of fluid to be injected or infused. The rationale for needle selection is included in each skill.

DISPOSABLE INJECTION UNITS.   Disposable, single-dose, prefilled syringes are available for some medications. With these syringes, you do not have to prepare medication dosages, except perhaps to expel portions of unneeded medications.

The Tubex and Carpoject injection systems include reusable plastic syringes that hold prefilled, disposable, sterile cartridge-needle units (Figure 13-16). The cartridge is placed into the syringe and secured, following package directions. Check for air bubbles in the syringe before administering the medication to the client. To expel excess medication, advance the plunger, as in a regular syringe. Another type of injection system involves screwing a plungerlike device into the end of a prefilled vial containing a needle. After the medication is given, discard the entire unit in a receptacle. This design reduces the risk of needle-stick injuries.

Preparing an Injection From an Ampule

Ampules contain single doses of medication in a liquid. Ampules are available in many sizes, from 1 ml to 10 ml or more (Figure 13-17, *A*). An ampule is made of glass with a constricted, prescored neck that must be snapped off to allow access to the medication. A colored ring around the neck indicates where the ampule is prescored to be broken easily. Aspiration of the medication into a syringe occurs easily with a filter needle and syringe. Filter needles are used when preparing medications from glass ampules to prevent glass

Preventing Infection During an Injection   Box 13-13

To prevent contamination of solution in an ampule, quickly draw the medication into the syringe. Do not allow the ampule to stand open.

Do not allow the needle to touch a contaminated surface (e.g., outer edges of ampule or vial, outer surface of needle cap, your hands, the counter top).

Avoid touching the length of the plunger or inner part of the barrel. Keep tip of syringe covered with cap or needle.

Wash skin soiled with dirt, drainage, or feces with soap and water. Use friction and a circular motion while cleaning with an antiseptic swab. Swab from center of site, and move outward in a 2-inch radius.

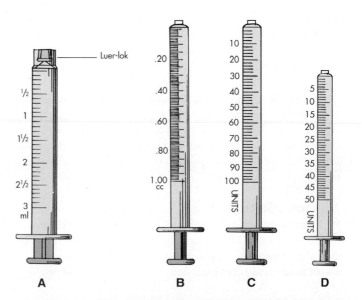

FIGURE **13-13**   Types of syringes. **A,** Luer-lok syringe marked in 0.1 (tenths). **B,** Tuberculin syringe marked in 0.01 (hundredths) for doses less than 1 ml. **C,** Insulin syringe marked in units (100). **D,** Insulin syringe marked in units (50).

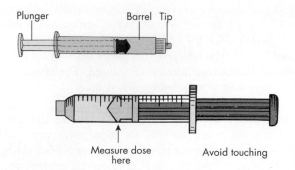

Plunger   Barrel Tip

Measure dose   Avoid touching
here

FIGURE **13-14**   Parts of a syringe.

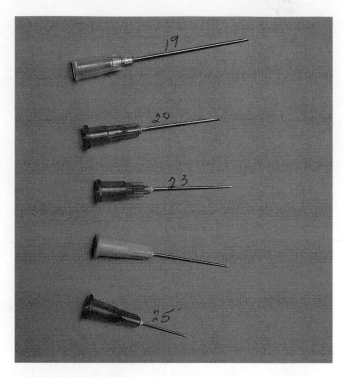

FIGURE **13-15**   Hypodermic needles *(top to bottom):* 19 gauge, $1^{1}/_{2}$-inch length; 20 gauge, 1-inch length; 23 gauge, 1-inch length; and 25 gauge, $^{5}/_{8}$-inch length.

particles from being drawn into the syringe with the medication (Meister, 1998).

Preparing an Injection From a Vial

A vial is a single-dose or multidose container that has a rubber seal at the top (see Figure 13-17, *B*). A metal cap protects the seal until it is ready to use. Vials contain liquid or dry forms of medications. Medications that are unstable in solution are packaged dry. The vial label specifies the solvent or diluent used to dissolve the medication and the amount of diluent needed to prepare a desired medication concentration. Normal saline and sterile distilled water are solutions commonly used to dissolve medications.

Unlike the ampule, the vial is a closed system, and air must be injected into it to permit easy withdrawal of the solution. Failure to inject air when withdrawing solution creates a vacuum within the vial that makes withdrawal difficult (Skill 13-5).

To prepare a powdered medication, the amount of diluent or solvent recommended on the vial's label is prepared in the syringe. Inject the diluent into the vial in the same manner as injecting air into the vial. Most powdered medications dissolve easily, but it may be necessary to withdraw the needle to mix the contents thoroughly. Gently shake or roll the vial between your hands to dissolve the powdered medication. Reinsert the needle to draw up the dissolved medication. After mixing multidose vials, place a label that includes the date and time of mixing and the concentration of medication per milliliter on the vial. Multidose vials may require refrigeration after the contents are reconstituted.

Mixing Medications

If two medications are compatible, it is possible to mix them in one injection. Most nursing units have charts that list common compatible medications. If there is any uncertainty about medication compatibilities, consult a pharmacist.

MIXING MEDICATIONS FROM A VIAL AND AN AMPULE. The medication from the vial is prepared first. Then, using the same syringe and needle, withdraw the medication from the ampule.

MIXING MEDICATIONS FROM TWO VIALS.   Use the following principles when mixing medications from two vials:
1. Do not contaminate one medication with another.
2. Ensure the final dosage is accurate.
3. Maintain aseptic technique.

Only one syringe is needed to mix medications from two vials (Figure 13-18). Aspirate the volume of air equivalent to the first medication's dose (vial A) into the syringe. Inject the air into vial A, making sure the needle does not touch the solution. Withdraw the needle from vial A, and aspirate air that is equivalent to the second medication's dose (vial B) into the syringe. Inject the volume of air into vial B, and immediately withdraw the medication in vial B into the syringe. Then insert the needle into vial A, being careful not to push the plunger and expel the medication within the syringe into the vial. Withdraw the desired amount of medication from vial A into the syringe. After the correct dose is prepared, withdraw the needle from vial A and apply a new needle, suitable for injection.

Insulin Preparation

Insulin is the hormone used to treat diabetes mellitus. It must be administered by injection, because it is broken down and destroyed in the GI tract. In the United States and Canada, the medication is available in 100 units per milliliter of solution. When preparing insulin, the correct syringe must be used; a 100-unit scaled syringe is used to prepare 100-unit insulin.

Text continued on p. 325

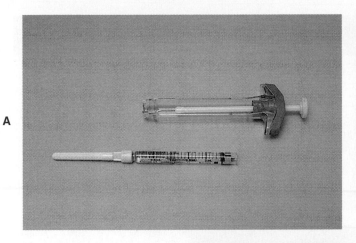

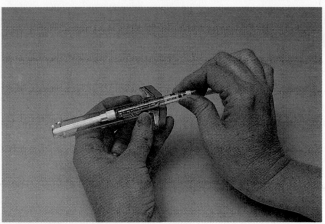

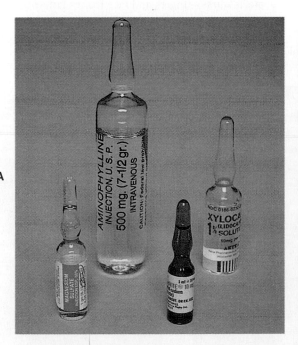

FIGURE **13-16**   **A,** Carpoject syringe and prefilled sterile cartridge with needle. **B,** Assembling the Carpoject. **C,** Cartridge locks at needle end; plunger screws into opposite end.

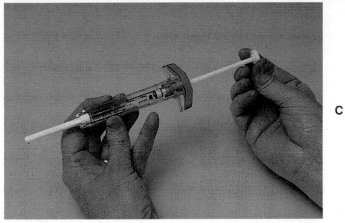

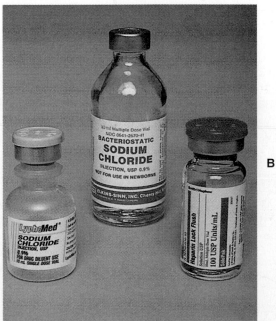

FIGURE **13-17**   **A,** Medication in ampules. **B,** Medication in vials. Rubber top must be cleansed with alcohol with vial is opened or when it is reused.

Skill 13-5
PREPARING INJECTIONS

DELEGATION CONSIDERATIONS

Preparing injections from ampules and vials requires problem solving and knowledge application unique to professional nursing. For this procedure, delegation to assistive personnel is not appropriate.

EQUIPMENT

Medication in an Ampule
- Syringe, needle, and filter needle
- Small gauze pad or alcohol swab

Medication in a Vial
- Syringe and two needles (filter needle if indicated)
- Small gauze pad
- Diluent (e.g., normal saline or sterile water) (if indicated)

Both
- MAR or computer printout

STEPS	RATIONALE
1. Check client's name and drug name, dosage, route of administration, and time of administration.	Ensures correct administration of medication.
2. Review pertinent information related to medication, including action, purpose, side effects, and nursing implications.	Allows you to administer drug properly and to monitor client's response.
3. Assess client's body build, muscle size, and weight if giving SQ or IM medication.	Determines type and size of syringe and needles for injection.
4. Wash hands and assemble supplies.	Reduces transmission of microorganisms and saves nursing time.
5. Check medication order or MAR against label on medication.	Ensures correct medication and dose are prepared.
6. Prepare medication:	
A. Ampule Preparation:	
(1) Tap top of ampule lightly and quickly with finger until fluid moves from neck of ampule (see illustration).	Dislodges any fluid that collects above neck of ampule. All solution moves into lower chamber.
(2) Place small gauze pad around neck of ampule (see illustration).	Placing pad around neck of ampule protects fingers from trauma as glass tip is broken off.
(3) Snap neck of ampule quickly and firmly away from hands (see illustration).	Protects nurse's fingers and face from shattering glass.

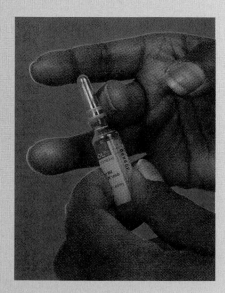

STEP 6A(1) Tapping ampule moves fluid down neck.

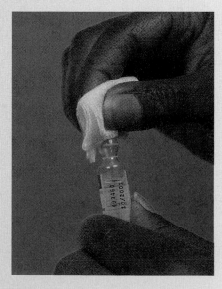

STEP 6A(2) Gauze pad placed around neck of ampule.

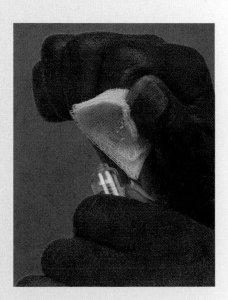

STEP 6A(3) Snapping neck away from hands.

STEPS	RATIONALE
(4) Draw up medication quickly, using a filter needle long enough to reach bottom of ampule.	System is open to airborne contaminants. Needle must be long enough to access medication for preparation. Filter needles are used to filter out any fragments of glass (Beyea and Nicoll, 1995).
(5) Hold ampule upside down, or set it on a flat surface. Insert filter needle into center of ampule opening (see illustrations). Do not allow needle tip or shaft to touch rim of ampule.	Broken rim of ampule is considered contaminated. When ampule is inverted, solution dribbles out if needle tip or shaft touches rim of ampule.
(6) Aspirate medication into syringe by gently pulling back on plunger.	Withdrawal of plunger creates negative pressure within syringe barrel, which pulls fluid into syringe.
(7) Keep needle tip under surface of liquid. Tip ampule to bring all fluid within reach of the needle.	Prevents aspiration of air bubbles.
(8) If air bubbles are aspirated, do not expel air into ampule.	Air pressure may force fluid out of ampule and medication will be lost.
(9) To expel excess air bubbles, remove needle from ampule. Hold syringe with needle pointing up. Tap side of syringe to cause bubbles to rise toward needle. Draw back slightly on plunger, and then push plunger upward to eject air. Do not eject fluid.	Withdrawing plunger too far will remove it from barrel. Holding syringe vertically allows fluid to settle in bottom of barrel. Pulling back on plunger allows fluid within needle to enter barrel so fluid is not expelled. Air at top of barrel and within needle is then expelled.
(10) If syringe contains excess fluid, use sink for disposal. Hold syringe vertically with needle tip up and slanted slightly toward sink. Slowly eject excess fluid into sink. Recheck fluid level in syringe by holding it vertically.	Medication is safely dispersed into sink. Position of needle allows medication to be expelled without flowing down needle shaft. Rechecking fluid level ensures proper dose.
(11) Cover needle with its safety sheath or cap. Replace filter needle with regular needle.	Minimizes needle sticks. Filter needles cannot be used for injection.

B. **Vial Containing a Solution:**

(1) Remove cap covering top of unused vial to expose sterile rubber seal. If a multidose vial has been used before, cap is already removed. Firmly and briskly wipe surface of rubber seal with alcohol swab and allow it to dry.	Vial comes packaged with cap that cannot be replaced after seal removal. Not all drug manufacturers guarantee that caps of unused vials are sterile (Posey and Long, 1996). Therefore caps must be swabbed with alcohol before preparing medication. Allowing alcohol to dry prevents needle from being coated with alcohol and mixing with medication.

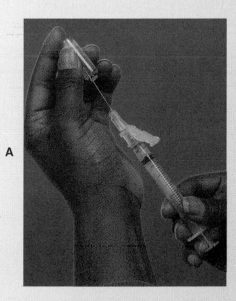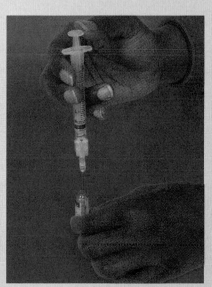

STEP 6A(6)   **A,** Medication aspirated with amplue inverted. **B,** Medication aspirated with ampule on flat surface.

STEPS	RATIONALE
(2) Pick up syringe and remove needle cap. Pull back on plunger to draw amount of air into syringe equivalent to volume of medication to be aspirated from vial.	Air must first be injected into vial to prevent buildup of negative pressure in vial when aspirating medication.
(3) With vial on flat surface, insert tip of needle through center of rubber seal (see illustration). Apply pressure to tip of needle during insertion.	Center of seal is thinner and easier to penetrate. Using firm pressure prevents coring of rubber seal, which could enter vial or needle.
(4) Inject air into the vial's air space, holding on to plunger. Hold plunger with firm pressure; plunger may be forced backward by air pressure within the vial.	Air must be injected before aspirating fluid. Injecting into vial's air space prevents formation of bubbles and inaccuracy in dosage.
(5) Invert vial while keeping firm hold on syringe and plunger (see illustration). Hold vial between thumb and middle fingers of nondominant hand. Grasp end of syringe barrel and plunger with thumb and forefinger of dominant hand to counteract pressure in vial.	Inverting vial allows fluid to settle in lower half of container. Position of hands prevents forceful movement of plunger and permits easy manipulation of syringe.
(6) Keep tip of needle below fluid level.	Prevents aspiration of air.
(7) Allow air pressure from the vial to fill syringe gradually with medication. If necessary, pull back slightly on plunger to obtain correct amount of solution.	Positive pressure within vial forces fluid into syringe.
(8) When desired volume has been obtained, position needle into vial's air space; tap side of syringe barrel carefully to dislodge any air bubbles. Eject any air remaining at top of syringe into vial.	Forcefully striking barrel while needle is inserted in vial may bend needle. Accumulation of air displaces medication and causes dosage errors.
(9) Remove needle from vial by pulling back on barrel of syringe.	Pulling plunger rather than barrel causes plunger to separate from barrel, resulting in loss of medication.
(10) Hold syringe at eye level, at 90-degree angle, to ensure correct volume and absence of air bubbles. Remove any remaining air by tapping barrel to dislodge any air bubbles (see illustration). Draw back slightly on plunger; then push plunger upward to eject air. Do not eject fluid.	Holding syringe vertically allows fluid to settle in bottom of barrel. Pulling back on plunger allows fluid within needle to enter barrel so fluid is not expelled. Air at top of barrel and within needle is then expelled.

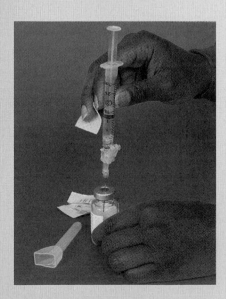

STEP 6B(3)   Insert adapter through center of vial diaphragm (with vial flat on table).

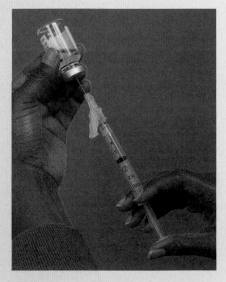

STEP 6B(5)   Withdraw fluid with vial inverted.

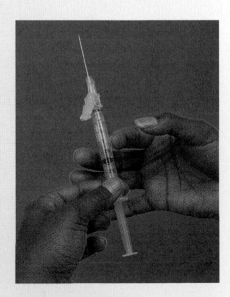

STEP 6B(10)   Hold syringe upright, tap barrel to dislodge air bubbles.

STEPS	RATIONALE
(11) If medication is to be injected into client's tissue, change needle to appropriate gauge and length according to route of medication.	Inserting needle through a rubber stopper may dull beveled tip. New needle is sharper. Because no fluid is along shaft, needle will not track medication through tissues.
(12) For multidose vial, make label that includes date of opening vial and your initials.	Ensures that future doses will be prepared correctly. Some drugs must be discarded after certain number of days after opening a vial.

C. Vial Containing a Powder (Reconstituting Medications):

(1) Remove cap covering vial of powdered medication and cap covering vial of proper diluent. Firmly swab both caps with alcohol swab, and allow to dry.	Not all drug manufacturers guarantee that caps of unused vials are sterile (Posey and Long, 1996). Allowing alcohol to dry prevents needle from being coated with alcohol and mixing with medication.
(2) Draw up diluent into syringe following Steps 6B(2) through 6B(10).	Prepares diluent for injection into vial containing powdered medication.
(3) Insert tip of needle through center of rubber seal of vial of powdered medication. Inject diluent into vial. Remove needle.	Diluent begins to dissolve and reconstitute medication.
(4) Mix medication thoroughly. Roll in palms. Do not shake.	Ensures proper dispersal of medication throughout solution.
(5) Reconstituted medication in vial is ready to be drawn into new syringe. Read label carefully to determine dose after reconstitution.	Once diluent has been added, concentration of medication (mg/ml) determines dose to be given.

• *Critical Decision Point*
Some institutions require that medications prepared for parenteral medication be verified for accuracy by another nurse (Zimmerman and Pierce, 1998). Check institutional guidelines before administering medication.

7. Dispose of soiled supplies. Place broken ampule and/or used vials and used needle in puncture-proof and leak-proof container. Clean work area, and wash hands.	Proper disposal of glass and needle prevents accidental injury to staff. Controls transmission of infection.

UNEXPECTED OUTCOMES AND RELATED INTERVENTIONS

- Air bubbles remain in syringe.
  - Expel air from syringe, and add medication to syringe until correct dose is prepared.
- Incorrect dose is prepared.
  - Discard prepared dose. Prepare corrected new dose.

Insulin is classified by rate of action, including rapid, intermediate, and long-acting. A client with diabetes may require more than one type of insulin. For example, by receiving a rapid-acting (regular) and an intermediate-acting (NPH) insulin, a client receives more sustained control of blood sugar over 24 hours.

Regular insulin is a clear solution that acts rapidly and can be given either subcutaneously or intravenously. Other types of insulin are cloudy because of the addition of a protein, which slows absorption. These slower-acting insulin preparations can only be given subcutaneously.

Insulin is ordered by specific dosage at select times or by a sliding scale. A sliding scale dictates a certain dosage based on the client's blood sugar level. For example, your client's sliding scale insulin order reads as follows: Give 5 units of regular insulin SQ for blood sugar between 150 and 200, 10 units of regular insulin for blood sugar between 200 and 275, and call for blood sugars higher than 275. For example, if your client's blood sugar is 199, follow the sliding scale and give the client 5 units of regular insulin.

Before mixing different types of insulin, rotate each vial at least 1 minute between both hands. This resuspends the modified insulin preparations and helps to warm the medication. Insulin vials should not be shaken. Shaking causes bubbles to form, which take up space in a syringe and alter the dosage.

When mixing two types of insulin in a syringe, prepare the regular (clear) insulin first to prevent the regular insulin from becoming contaminated with the longer-acting

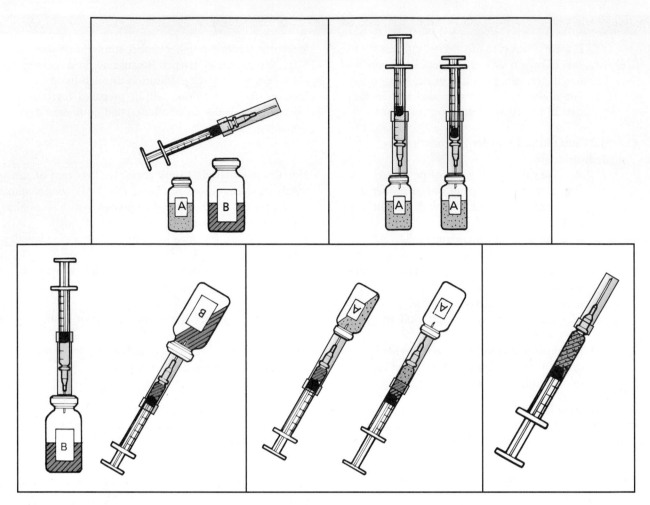

FIGURE **13-18**   Steps in mixing medications from two vials.

(cloudy) insulin. Box 13-14 describes guidelines used for mixing two kinds of insulin in the same syringe.

Administering Injections

Each injection route differs based on the type of tissues into which the medication is injected. The characteristics of the tissues influence the rate of medication absorption, which influences the onset of medication action. Before injecting a medication, you should know the volume of the medication to administer, the medication's characteristics and viscosity, and the location of anatomical structures underlying injection sites (Skill 13-6).

Failure to select an injection site in relation to anatomical landmarks can result in nerve or bone damage during needle insertion. If the syringe is not aspirated before injecting a medication, the medication may accidentally be injected directly into an artery or vein. Injecting too large a volume of medication for the site selected causes extreme pain and may result in local tissue damage.

Many clients, particularly children, fear injections. Clients with serious or chronic illnesses often are given several injections daily. You may be able to minimize the client's discomfort in the following ways:

1. Use a sharp-beveled needle in the smallest suitable length and gauge.
2. Position the client as comfortably as possible to reduce muscular tension.
3. Select the proper injection site, using anatomical landmarks.
4. Divert the client's attention from the injection through conversation.
5. Insert the needle quickly and smoothly to minimize tissue pulling.
6. Hold the syringe steady while the needle remains in tissues.
7. Inject the medication slowly and steadily.

SUBCUTANEOUS INJECTIONS.   SQ injections involve injecting medications into the loose connective tissue under the dermis (see Skill 13-6). Because SQ tissue is not as richly supplied with blood as the muscles, medication absorption is somewhat slower than with IM injections.

The best SQ injection sites include the outer posterior aspect of the upper arms, the abdomen from below the costal margins to the iliac crests, and the anterior aspects of the thighs (Figure 13-19). The site most frequently recommended for heparin injections is the abdomen (Figure

Procedural Guidelines for   Box 13-14
Mixing Two Kinds of Insulin in One Syringe

Clients whose blood sugars are well controlled on a mixed-insulin dose should maintain their individual routine when preparing and administering their insulin.

Insulin should not be mixed with any other medications or diluent unless approved by the prescriber.

Rapid-acting insulins that are mixed with NPH or Ultralente insulins should be injected within 15 minutes before a meal.

Short-acting and Lente insulins should not be mixed unless the client's blood sugars are currently under control with this mixture.

Phosphate-buffered insulins (e.g., NPH) should not be mixed with Lente insulins.

To mix insulin, follow these steps:

1. Using an insulin syringe, inject air, equal to the dose of cloudy insulin to be administered, into the cloudy vial. Do not let the tip of the needle touch the insulin.
2. Remove the syringe from the vial of cloudy insulin.
3. With the same syringe, inject air, equal to the dose of clear insulin to be administered, into the clear vial and withdraw the correct dose into the syringe.
4. Remove the syringe from the clear insulin, and dispel air bubbles to ensure accurate dosing.
5. Place the needle of the syringe back into the cloudy vial, and withdraw the correct dose.

Modified from American Diabetes Association: Insulin administration: clinical practice recommendations, *Diabetes Care* 20(1S):46S, 1997.

13-20). Other sites include the scapular areas of the upper back and the upper ventral or dorsal gluteal areas. Choose an injection site that is free of skin lesions, bony prominences, and large underlying muscles or nerves.

The SQ tissues of the upper arm, anterior and lateral portions of the thigh, buttocks, and abdomen are sites recommended for insulin injection. Rotating injections within the same body part for a sequence of injections provides more consistency in the absorption of insulin. For example, if the morning insulin is injected into the client's arm, then a subsequent injection should also be given in the arm. The rate of absorption is another factor in site selection for insulin administration. The abdomen has the quickest absorption rate, followed by the arms, thighs, and buttocks (American Diabetes Association, 1997).

Only small doses (0.5 to 1 ml) of water-soluble medications should be given subcutaneously because the tissue is sensitive to irritating solutions and large volumes of medications. Collection of medications within the tissues can cause sterile abscesses, which appear as hardened, painful lumps under the skin.

A client's body weight indicates the depth of the SQ layer. Therefore the needle length and angle of insertion are based on weight. Generally a 25-gauge $\frac{5}{8}$-inch needle inserted at a 45-degree angle (Figure 13-21) or a $\frac{1}{2}$-inch needle inserted at a 90-degree angle deposits medications into the SQ tissue of a normal-size client. A child may require only a $\frac{1}{2}$-inch

Skill 13-6
Administering Injections

DELEGATION CONSIDERATIONS

Administering injections requires problem solving and knowledge application unique to professional nursing. For this procedure delegation to assistive personnel is not appropriate. Assistive personnel should be instructed to report any unexpected drug reactions as soon as possible.

EQUIPMENT

- Proper-size syringe and needle:

Site	Size of Syringe	Needle Size
SQ	0.3-3 ml	25-27 gauge, $\frac{3}{8}$-$\frac{5}{8}$ inch
IM (adult)	2-3 ml	21-25 gauge, 1-1$\frac{1}{2}$ inch (need 2 needles) ?
IM (infant or child)	0.5-1 ml	21-25 gauge, 1 inch (need 2 needles) ?
ID	1 ml tuberculin	26-27 gauge, preattached needle

- Small gauze pad
- Alcohol swab
- Vial or ampule of medication or skin test solution
- Disposable gloves

STEPS	RATIONALE
For all injections:	
1. Review physician's medication order for client's name, drug name, dose, time, and route of administration.	Ensures safe and correct administration of medication.
2. Assess client's history of allergies and know substances client is allergic to and normal allergic reaction.	Certain substances have similar compositions; clients should not receive a medication if they have a known allergy to a medication.

|

STEPS	RATIONALE
3. Check date of expiration for medication vial or ampule.	Drug potency may increase or decrease when outdated.
4. Observe verbal and nonverbal responses toward receiving injection.	Injections can be painful. Clients may have anxiety, which can increase pain.
5. Assess for contraindications:	
a. For subcutaneous injections: Assess for factors such as circulatory shock or reduced local tissue perfusion. Assess adequacy of client's adipose tissue.	Reduced tissue perfusion interferes with drug absorption and distribution. Physiological changes of aging or client illness may influence the amount of SQ tissue a client possesses. This influences methods for administering injections.
b. For intramuscular injections: Assess for factors such as muscle atrophy, reduced blood flow, or circulatory shock.	Atrophied muscle absorbs medication poorly. Factors interfering with blood flow to muscles impair drug absorption.

• *Critical Decision Point*
Because of documented adverse effects of IM injections, other routes of medication injection are safer (Beecroft and Kongelbeck, 1994). Consider calling prescriber for alternate route of medication administration.

STEPS	RATIONALE
6. Aseptically prepare correct medication dose from ampule or vial (see Skill 13-5, p. 322). Check carefully. Be sure all air is expelled.	Ensures that medication is sterile. Preparation techniques differ for ampule and vial.
7. Identify client by checking identification arm band and asking client's name. Compare with MAR.	Ensures correct client receives ordered drug.
8. Explain steps of procedure, and tell client injection will cause a slight burning or sting.	Helps minimize client's anxiety.
9. Close room curtain or door.	Provides privacy.
10. Wash hands thoroughly and apply clean disposable gloves.	Reduces transfer of microorganisms.
11. Keep sheet or gown draped over body parts not requiring exposure.	Respects dignity of client while area to be injected is exposed.
12. Select appropriate injection site. Inspect skin surface over sites for bruises, inflammation, or edema.	Injection sites should be free of abnormalities that may interfere with drug absorption. Sites used repeatedly can become hardened from lipohypertrophy (increased growth in fatty tissue). Do not use an area that is bruised or has signs associated with infection.
a. SQ: Palpate sites for masses or tenderness. Be sure needle is correct size by grasping skinfold at site, with thumb and forefinger. Measure fold from top to bottom. Needle should be one-half length.	SQ injections can be inadvertently given in the muscle, especially in the abdomen and thigh sites (Peragallo-Dittko, 1997). Appropriate size of needle ensures that medication will be injected in the SQ tissue.
b. IM: Note integrity and size of muscle, and palpate for tenderness or hardness. Avoid these areas. If injections are given frequently, rotate sites.	The ventrogluteal site is the preferred site for children older than 7 months and adults unless there are contraindications to this site. In infants younger than 7 months, the vastus lateralis should be used (Beyea and Nicoll, 1995).
c. ID: Note lesions or discolorations of forearm. Select site three or four fingerwidths below antecubital space and one handwidth above wrist. If forearm cannot be used, inspect the upper back. If necessary, sites for SQ injections may be used (Workman, 1999).	An ID injection site should be free of discolorations or hair so that results of skin test can be seen and interpreted correctly.
13. Assist client to comfortable position:	
a. SQ: Have client relax arm, leg, or abdomen, depending on site chosen for injection.	Relaxation of site minimizes discomfort.
b. IM: Position client depending on site chosen (e.g., sit, or lie flat, on side, or prone).	Reduces strain on muscle and minimizes discomfort of injections.
c. ID: Have client extend elbow and support it and forearm on flat surface.	Stabilizes injection site for easiest accessibility.
d. Talk with client about subject of interest.	Distraction reduces anxiety.

STEPS	RATIONALE

- **Critical Decision Point**

Ensure that client's position is not contraindicated by medical condition.

14. Relocate site using anatomical landmarks.	Injection into correct anatomical site prevents injury to nerves, bones, and blood vessels.
15. Cleanse site with an antiseptic swab. Apply swab at center of the site and rotate outward in a circular direction for about 5 cm (2 inches) (see illustration).	Mechanical action of swab removes secretions containing microorganisms.
16. Hold swab or gauze between third and fourth fingers of nondominant hand.	Gauze or swab remains readily accessible when needle is withdrawn.
17. Remove needle sheath or cap from needle by pulling it straight off.	Preventing needle from touching sides of cap prevents contamination.
18. Hold syringe between thumb and forefinger of dominant hand:	
a. SQ: Hold as dart, palm down (see illustration).	Quick, smooth injection requires proper manipulation of syringe parts.
b. IM: Hold as dart, palm down.	
c. ID: Hold bevel of needle pointing up.	With bevel up, medication is less likely to be deposited into tissues below dermis.
19. Administer injection:	
A. Subcutaneous:	
(1) For average-size client, spread skin tightly across injection site or pinch skin with nondominant hand.	Needle penetrates tight skin easier than loose skin. Pinching skin elevates SQ tissue and may desensitize area.
(2) Inject needle quickly and firmly at 45- to 90-degree angle. Then release skin, if pinched.	Quick, firm insertion minimizes discomfort. (Injecting medication into compressed tissue irritates nerve fibers.) Correct angle prevents accidental injection into muscle.
(3) For obese client, pinch skin at site and inject needle at 90-degree angle below tissue fold.	Obese clients have fatty layer of tissue above SQ layer.

- **Critical Decision Point**

Aspiration after injecting an SQ medication is not necessary. Piercing a blood vessel in an SQ injection is very rare (Peragallo-Dittko, 1997).

(4) Inject medication slowly (see illustration).	Minimizes discomfort.

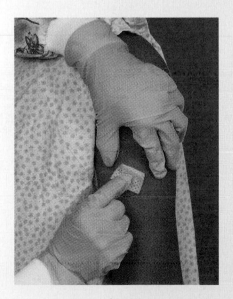

STEP 15   Cleanse site with circular motion.

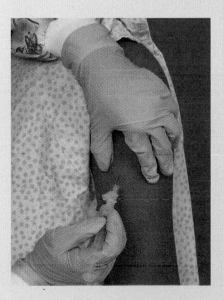

STEP 18A   Hold syringe as if grasping a dart.

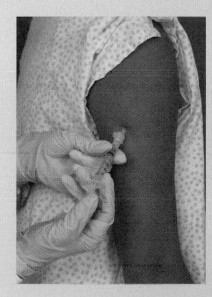

STEP 19A(4)   Inject medication slowly.

B. **Intramuscular:**

(1) Position hand or hands at proper anatomical landmarks and pull skin down with nondominant hand to administer in a Z-track. Inject needle quickly at 90-degree angle into muscle.

Z-track creates zigzag path through tissues that seals needle track to avoid tracking of medication. A quick, dartlike injection reduces discomfort. Z-track injections should be used for all IM injections (Beyea and Nicoll, 1995).

(2) If client's muscle mass is small, grasp body of muscle between thumb and fingers (Workman, 1999).

Ensures that medication reaches muscle mass (Wong and others, 1999).

(3) After needle pierces skin, grasp lower end of syringe barrel with nondominant hand to stabilize syringe. Continue to hold skin tightly with nondominant hand. Move dominant hand to end of plunger. Do not move syringe.

Smooth manipulation of syringe reduces discomfort from needle movement. Skin must remain pulled until after drug is injected to ensure Z-track administration.

(4) Pull back on plunger 5 to 10 seconds. If no blood appears, inject medication slowly.

Aspiration of blood into syringe indicates IV placement of needle. Slow injection reduces pain and tissue trauma (Beyea and Nicoll, 1995).

- *Critical Decision Point*

If blood appears in syringe, remove needle, dispose of medication and syringe properly, and prepare another dose of medication for injection.

(5) Wait 10 seconds.

Allows time for medication to absorb into muscle before removing syringe.

C. **Intradermal:**

(1) With nondominant hand, stretch skin over site with forefinger or thumb.

Needle pierces tight skin more easily.

(2) With needle almost against client's skin, insert it slowly at a 5- to 15-degree angle until resistance is felt. Then advance needle through epidermis to approximately 3 mm ($\frac{1}{8}$ inch) below skin surface. Needle tip can be seen through skin.

Ensures needle tip is in dermis.

(3) Inject medication slowly. Normally, resistance is felt. If not, needle is too deep; remove and begin again.

Slow injection minimizes discomfort at site. Dermal layer is tight and does not expand easily when solution is injected.

(4) While injecting medication, note that small bleb (approximately 6 mm [$\frac{1}{2}$ inch]) resembling mosquito bite appears on skin surface (see illustration).

Bleb indicates medication is deposited in dermis.

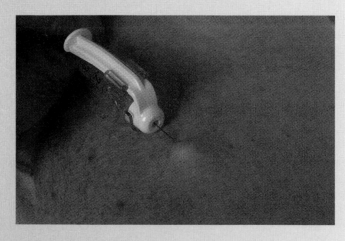

STEP 19C(4)   Injection creates a small bleb.

STEPS	RATIONALE
20. Withdraw needle while applying alcohol swab or gauze gently over site.	Support of tissue around injection site minimizes discomfort during needle withdrawal. Dry gauze may minimize discomfort associated with alcohol on nonintact skin.
21. Apply gentle pressure. Do not massage site. Apply bandage if needed.	Massage can damage underlying tissue. Massage of ID site may disperse medication into underlying tissue layers and alter test results.
22. Assist client to comfortable position.	Gives client sense of well-being.
23. Discard uncapped needle or needle enclosed in safety shield and attached syringe into puncture- and leak-proof receptacle.	Prevents injury to client and health care personnel. Recapping needles increases risk of needle-stick injury (NIOSH, 1999).
24. Remove disposable gloves and wash hands.	Reduces transmission of microorganisms.
25. Stay with client, and observe for any allergic reactions.	Severe anaphylactic reaction is characterized by dyspnea, wheezing, and circulatory collapse.
26. Return to room, and ask if client feels any acute pain, burning, numbness, or tingling at injection site.	Continued discomfort may indicate injury to underlying bones or nerves.
27. Inspect site, noting any bruising or induration.	Bruising or induration indicates complication associated with injection. Document findings, and notify health care provider. Provide warm compress to site.
28. Observe client's response to medication at times that correlate with the medication's onset, peak, and duration.	IM medications are rapidly absorbed. Adverse effects of parenteral medications may develop rapidly. Evaluate effect of medication based on the medication's onset, peak, and duration of action.
29. Ask client to explain purpose and effects of medication.	Evaluates client's understanding of information taught.
30. *For ID injections,* use skin pencil and draw circle around perimeter of injection site. Read site within appropriate amount of time, designated by type of medication or skin test given.	Pencil mark makes site easy to find. The results of skin testing are determined at various times, based on the type of medication used or the type of skin testing completed. Refer to the manufacturer's directions to determine when to read the test's results.

UNEXPECTED OUTCOMES AND RELATED INTERVENTIONS
- Raised, reddened, or hard zone (induration) forms around ID test site.
  - Notify client's health care provider.
  - Document sensitivity to injected allergen or positive test if tuberculin skin testing was completed.
- Hypertrophy of skin develops from repeated SQ injections.
  - Do not use this site for future injections.
  - Instruct client not to use site for 6 months.
- Client develops signs and symptoms of allergy or side effects.
  - Follow institutional policy or guidelines for appropriate response to adverse drug reactions.
  - Notify client's health care provider immediately.

- Client complains of localized pain, numbness, or tingling or burning at injection site.
  - Potential injury to nerve or tissues may have occurred.
  - Assess injection site.
  - Document findings.
  - Notify client's health care provider.

RECORDING AND REPORTING
- Chart medication dose, route, site, time, and date given in medication record.
- Report any undesirable effects from medication to prescriber.
- Record client's response to medications in nurse's notes.

needle. If the client is obese, the tissue is pinched, and a needle long enough to insert through fatty tissue at the base of the skinfold must be used. The preferred needle length is one half the width of the skinfold. With this method the angle of insertion may be between 45 and 90 degrees. Thin clients may have insufficient tissue for SQ injections. The upper abdomen is the best site for injection with this type of client.

Insulin syringes generally come with 26- to 29-gauge needles. Generally, insulin should be injected at a 90-degree angle. However, if you are giving an injection to a thin adult or a child, you may need to pinch the skin and inject at a 45-degree angle to avoid giving the injection in the muscle (American Diabetes Association, 1997).

INTRAMUSCULAR INJECTIONS. The IM route provides faster medication absorption than the SQ route because of a muscle's greater vascularity. There is less danger of causing tissue damage when medications enter deep muscle, but the risk

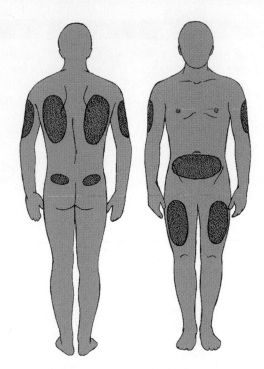

FIGURE **13-19** Sites recommended for SQ injections.

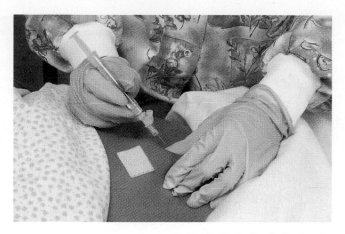

FIGURE **13-20** Giving SQ heparin in the abdomen.

of inadvertently injecting medications directly into blood vessels exists. A longer and heavier-gauge needle is used to pass through SQ tissue and penetrate deep muscle tissue (see Skill 13-6, p. 327). Weight and the amount of adipose tissue influence needle size selection. An obese client may require a needle 3 inches long, whereas a thin client may only require a ½- to 1-inch needle (Beyea and Nicoll, 1995; Workman, 1999).

The angle of insertion for an IM injection is 90 degrees (see Figure 13-21). Muscle is less sensitive to irritating and viscous drugs. A normal, well-developed client can tolerate as much as 4 ml of medication in larger muscles, such as the gluteus medius (Beyea and Nicoll, 1995). Children, older adults, and thin clients can tolerate only 2 ml of an IM injection. Small children and older infants (e.g., under the age of 2 years) should receive no more than 1 ml of medication (Wong and others, 1999).

Assess the muscle before giving an injection. The muscle should be free of tenderness. Repeated injections in the same muscle can cause severe discomfort. With the client relaxed, palpate the muscle to rule out any hardened lesions. Help the client assume a comfortable position to minimize discomfort during an injection.

SITES. When selecting an IM site, consider the following: Is the area free of infection or necrosis? Are there local areas of bruising or abrasions? What is the location of underlying bones, nerves, and major blood vessels? What volume of medication is to be administered? Each site has certain advantages and disadvantages (Box 13-15).

Ventrogluteal. The ventrogluteal muscle involves the gluteus medius and minimus and is a safe site for all

clients. Research has shown that injuries such as fibrosis, nerve damage, abscess, tissue necrosis, muscle contraction, gangrene, and pain have been associated with all the common IM sites except the ventrogluteal site (Beyea and Nicoll, 1995). The ventrogluteal site is the preferred injection site for adults and anyone over 7 months old (Beyea and Nicoll, 1996).

Locate the muscle by placing the heel of the hand over the greater trochanter of the client's hip with the wrist perpendicular to the femur. Use the right hand for the left hip and the left hand for the right hip. Point your thumb toward the client's groin with your index finger pointed to the anterosuperior iliac spine. Point your middle finger back along the iliac crest toward the buttock. Your index finger, the middle finger, and the iliac crest form a V-shaped triangle. The injection site is the center of the triangle (Figure 13-22). The client may lie on the side or back. Flexing of the knee and hip helps the client relax this muscle.

Vastus Lateralis. The vastus lateralis muscle is another injection site used in adults and children. The muscle is thick and well developed, is located on the anterior lateral aspect of the thigh, and extends in an adult from a handbreadth above the knee to a handbreadth below the greater trochanter of the femur (Figure 13-23). The middle third of the muscle is the suggested site for injection. The width of the muscle usually extends from the midline of the thigh and the midline of the thigh's outer side. With young children or cachectic clients, grasp the body of the muscle during injection to be sure that the medication is deposited in muscle tissue. To help relax the muscle, have the client lie flat with the knee slightly flexed or assume a sitting position.

Deltoid. Because the radial and ulnar nerves and brachial artery lie within the upper arm along the humerus (Figure 13-24, *A*), this site should be used only for small medication volumes or when other sites are inaccessible because of dressings or casts. Locate the deltoid muscle by fully exposing the client's upper arm and shoulder and having the client relax the

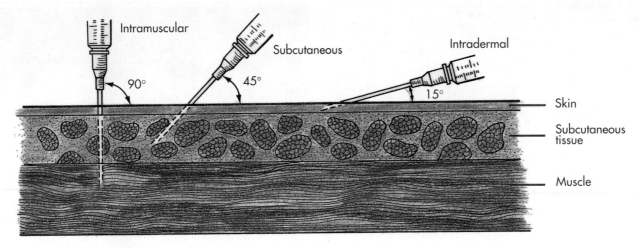

FIGURE **13-21**   Comparison of angles of insertion for IM (90 degrees), SQ (45 degrees), and ID (15 degrees) injections.

Characteristics of Intramuscular Sites

Box 13-15

VASTUS LATERALIS
Lacks major nerves and blood vessels
Rapid drug absorption

VENTROGLUTEAL
A deep site, situated away from major nerves and blood vessels
Less chance of contamination in incontinent clients or infants
Easily identified by prominent bony landmarks

DELTOID
Easily accessible but muscle not well developed in most clients
Used for small amounts of drugs
Not used in infants or children with underdeveloped muscles
Potential for injury to radial and ulnar nerves or brachial artery

arm at the side and flex the elbow. Do not roll up a tight-fitting sleeve. The client may sit, stand, or lie down (see Figure 13-24, *B*). Palpate the lower edge of the acromion process, which forms the base of a triangle in line with the midpoint of the lateral aspect of the upper arm. The injection site is in the center of the triangle, about 2.5 to 5 cm (1 to 2 inches) below the acromion process (see Figure 13-24, *A*). You may also locate the site by placing four fingers across the deltoid muscle, with the top finger along the acromion process. The injection site is then three fingerwidths below the acromion process.

TECHNIQUE IN INTRAMUSCULAR INJECTIONS

Z-Track Method. It is recommended that when giving IM injections, the **Z-track injection** method be used to minimize irritation by sealing the medication in muscle tissue (Beyea and Nicoll, 1995). Choose an IM site, preferably in a larger, deeper muscle such as the ventrogluteal muscle. Apply a new needle to the syringe after preparing the medication so that no solution remains on the outside needle shaft. Pull the overlying skin and SQ tissues approximately 2.5 to 3.5 cm (1 to 1½ inches) laterally to the side with the ulnar side of the

nondominant hand (McConnell, 1999). Hold the skin in this position until the injection is administered. After preparing the site with an antiseptic swab, inject the needle deep into the muscle. Slowly inject the medication if there is no blood return on aspiration. Keep the needle inserted for 10 seconds to allow the medication to disperse evenly (McConnell, 1999). Then release the skin after withdrawing the needle. This leaves a zigzag path that seals the needle track where tissue planes slide across each other (Figure 13-25). The medication cannot escape from the muscle tissue.

INTRADERMAL INJECTIONS.   ID injections are usually used for skin testing (e.g., tuberculin screening, allergy tests). Because these medications are potent, they are injected into the dermis, where blood supply is reduced and medication absorption occurs slowly. A client may have a severe anaphylactic reaction if the medications enter the circulation too rapidly.

You must be able to assess the injection site for changes in color and tissue integrity. Therefore choose an ID site that is lightly pigmented, free of lesions, and relatively hairless. The inner forearm and upper back are ideal locations.

To administer an injection intradermally, use a tuberculin or small syringe with a short (¼ to ½ inch), fine-gauge (26 or 27) needle. The angle of insertion for an ID injection is 5 to 15 degrees (see Figure 13-21). As you inject the medication, a small bleb resembling a mosquito bite should appear on the skin's surface (see Skill 13-6, p. 327). If a bleb does not appear or if the site bleeds after needle withdrawal, there is a good chance the medication entered SQ tissues. In this case, test results will not be valid.

SAFETY IN ADMINISTERING MEDICATIONS BY INJECTION

NEEDLELESS DEVICES.   Between 600,000 and 1 million accidental needle-stick and sharps injuries occur annually in health care settings (American Nurses Association, 1999). These injuries commonly occur when needles are recapped, IV lines and needles are mishandled, or stray

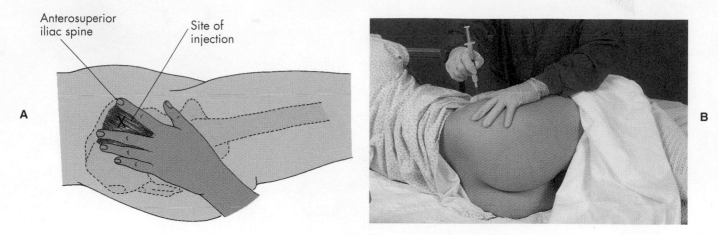

FIGURE 13-22   **A,** Landmarks for ventrogluteal site. **B,** Locating IM injection for ventrogluteal site.

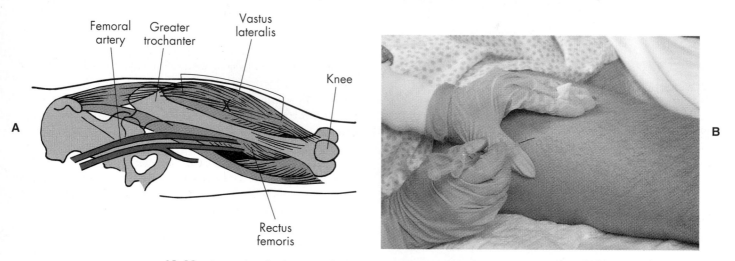

FIGURE 13-23   **A,** Landmarks for vastus lateralis site. **B,** Giving IM injection in vastus lateralis muscle.

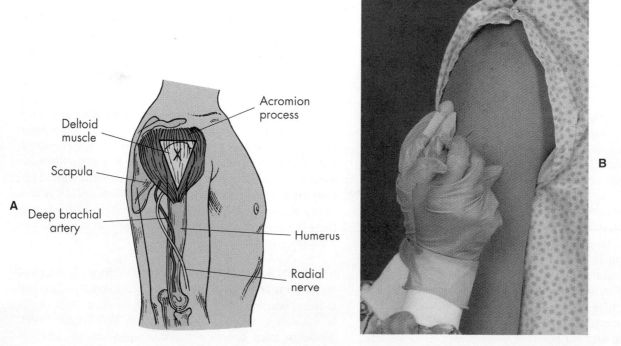

FIGURE 13-24   **A,** Landmarks for deltoid site. **B,** Giving IM injection in deltoid muscle.

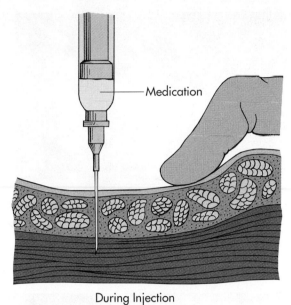

Medication

During Injection

Injection tract seals
as skin is released

Skin

Subcutaneous
tissue

Muscle

Medication

After release

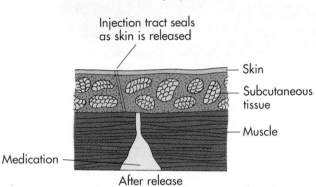

FIGURE **13-25** Z-Track method of injection prevents deposit
of medication into sensitive tissues.

needles are left at a client's bedside. The risk of exposure of
health care workers to blood-borne pathogens has led to
the development of "needleless" devices or special needle-
safety devices.

Special syringes are designed with a sheath or guard that
covers the needle after it is withdrawn from the skin (Figure
13-26). The needle is immediately covered, eliminating the
chance for a needle-stick injury. The syringe and sheath are
disposed of together in a receptacle. "Needleless" devices
should be used whenever possible to reduce the risk of needle-
stick injuries (OSHA, 2001).

Needles and other instruments considered "sharps" are
always disposed of into clearly marked, appropriate containers (Figure 13-27). Containers should be puncture-proof
and leak-proof. Never force a needle into a full needle-
disposal receptacle, and never place used needles and syringes in a wastebasket, in your pocket, on a client's meal
tray, or at the client's bedside. Box 13-16 summarizes recommendations for the prevention of needle-stick injuries.

Intravenous Administration

Medications are administered intravenously by the following
methods:

1. As mixtures within large volumes of IV fluids
2. By injection of a bolus, or small volume, of medication
   through an existing IV infusion line or intermittent venous access (heparin or saline lock)
3. By piggyback infusion of a solution containing the prescribed medication and a small volume of IV fluid
   through an existing IV line

In all three methods the client has either an existing IV
infusion line or an IV access site, such as an intermittent infusion (heparin or saline lock). In most institutions, policies
and procedures identify the medications that nurses are allowed to administer intravenously. These policies are based
on the medication, capability and availability of staff, and
type of monitoring equipment available.

Chapter 14 describes the technique for performing venipuncture and establishing continuous IV fluid infusions.
Medication administration is only one reason for supplying
IV fluids. IV fluid therapy is used primarily for fluid replacement in clients unable to take oral fluids and as a means of
supplying electrolytes and nutrients.

When using any method of IV medication administration, observe clients closely for symptoms of adverse reactions. After a medication enters the bloodstream, it begins
to act immediately, and there is no way to stop its action.
Therefore avoid errors in dose calculation and preparation. Follow the five rights of safe medication administration, understand the desired action and side effects of the
medication, and document the medication according to
agency policy. If the medication has an antidote, have it
available during administration. When administering potent medications, assess vital signs before, during, and after the infusion.

Administering medications by the IV route has advantages. Often the IV route is used in emergencies when a fast-
acting medication must be delivered quickly. The IV route is
also best when it is necessary to establish constant therapeutic blood levels. Some medications are highly alkaline and irritating to muscle and SQ tissue. These medications cause
less discomfort when given intravenously.

LARGE-VOLUME INFUSIONS.   Of the three methods of
administering IV medications, mixing medications in large
volumes of fluids is the safest and easiest. Medications are diluted in large volumes (500 ml or 1000 ml) of compatible IV
fluids, such as normal saline or lactated Ringer's solution
(Skill 13-7). In most institutions the pharmacist adds medications to the primary container of IV solution to ensure
asepsis. Because the medication is not in a concentrated
form, the risk of side effects or fatal reactions is lessened
when infused over the prescribed time frame. Vitamins and
potassium chloride are two types of medications commonly
added to IV fluids. However, there is a danger with continuous infusion. If the IV fluid is infused too rapidly, the client
may suffer circulatory fluid overload.

INTRAVENOUS BOLUS.   An IV bolus involves introducing
a concentrated dose of a medication directly into the sys-

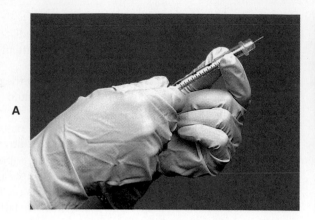
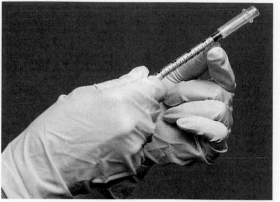

FIGURE **13-26**   Needle with plastic guard to prevent needle sticks. **A,** Position of guard before injection. **B,** After injection, the nurse locks the guard in place, covering the needle.

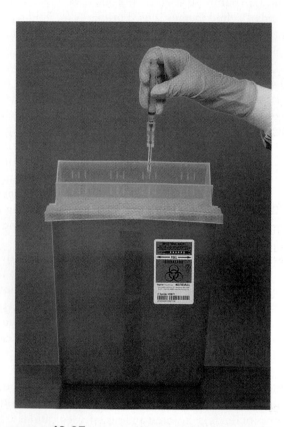

FIGURE **13-27**   Sharps disposal using only one hand.

temic circulation (Box 13-17). Because a bolus requires only a small amount of fluid to deliver the medication, it is an advantage when the amount of fluid the client can take is restricted. The IV bolus is the most dangerous method for administering medications because there is no time to correct errors. In addition, a bolus may cause direct irritation to the lining of blood vessels. Before administering a bolus, confirm placement of the IV line. Never give an IV medication if the insertion site appears puffy or edematous or the IV fluid does not flow at the proper rate. Accidental injection of a medication into the tissues around a vein can cause pain, sloughing of tissues, and abscesses.

Recommendations for the Prevention of Needle-Stick Injuries

Box 13-16

Avoid using needles when effective needleless systems or Sharps with Engineered Sharps Injury Protections (SESIP) safety devices are available.

Do not recap any needle.

Plan safe handling and disposal of needles before beginning the procedure.

Immediately dispose of needles, needleless systems, and SESIP into puncture-proof and leak-proof sharps disposal containers.

Maintain an exposure control plan (ECP) that includes:
- Assessment and implementation of innovations in procedures and technological developments to reduce risks of exposure to contaminated sharps
- Documentation of consideration and use of appropriate, commercially available, and effective safer devices
- Selection of devices that do not jeopardize client or employee safety or are determined to be medically inadvisable
- Documentation of input from employees in ECP as to methods to reduce exposure
- Annual reexamination of ECP

Maintain a sharps injury log that includes:
- Type and brand of device involved in the incident
- Location of the incident (e.g., department or work area)
- Description of the incident
- Maintains privacy of the employees who have had sharps injuries

From Occupational Safety and Health Administration (OSHA). Occupational exposure to bloodborne pathogens; needlestick and other sharps injuries; final rule. *Federal Register,* CFR 29, part 1910 (*Federal Register* #66:5317-5325), January 18, 2001. National Institute for Occupational Safety and Health (NIOSH): NIOSH alert preventing needle-stick injuries in health care settings, NIOSH Publications Dissemination, DHHS (NIOSH); Publication No. 2000-108, November, 1999.

Skill 13-7
ADDING MEDICATIONS TO INTRAVENOUS FLUID CONTAINERS

DELEGATION CONSIDERATIONS

Adding medications to IV fluid containers requires problem solving and knowledge application unique to professional nursing. For this procedure delegation to assistive personnel is not appropriate. (In some institutions the pharmacist may add drugs to primary containers of IV solutions to ensure asepsis.)

EQUIPMENT

- Vial or ampule of prescribed medication
- Syringe of appropriate size (1 to 20 ml)
- Sterile needle (1 to 1½ inch, 19 to 21 gauge) with special filters if indicated
- Correct diluent if indicated (e.g., sterile water, normal saline)
- Sterile IV fluid container (bag or bottle, 25 to 1000 ml in volume)
- Alcohol or antiseptic swab
- Label to attach to IV bag or bottle
- MAR or computer printout

STEPS	RATIONALE
1. Check physician's order to determine type of IV solution to use and type of medication and dosage.	Client's overall physical condition dictates type of IV solution used. Ensures safe and accurate drug administration.
2. Collect information necessary to administer drug safely, including action, purpose, side effects, normal dose, time of peak onset, and nursing implications.	Allows you to give drug safely and to monitor client's response to therapy.
3. When more than one medication is to be added to IV solution, assess for compatibility of medications.	Drugs often are incompatible when mixed together. Chemical reactions that occur result in clouding or crystallization of IV fluids. Check institutional policy for drug compatibility list.
4. Assess client's systemic fluid balance, as reflected by skin hydration and turgor, body weight, pulse, and blood pressure.	Danger of continuous IV infusions, especially in older adults or children, is that fluids may infuse too rapidly, causing circulatory overload (Powers, 1999; Wong and others, 1999).
5. Assess client's history of drug allergies.	IV administration of drugs causes rapid effects. Allergic response can be immediate.
6. Assess IV insertion site for signs of infiltration or phlebitis (see Chapter 14).	An intact, properly functioning site ensures medication is given safely.
7. Assess client's understanding of purpose of drug therapy.	May reveal need for education.
8. Wash hands thoroughly.	Reduces transfer of microorganisms.
9. Assemble supplies in medication room.	Ensures procedure will be orderly, with less likelihood of contaminating supplies.
10. Prepare prescribed medication from vial or ampule (see Skill 13-5, p. 322).	Ensures accurate delivery of medication.
11. Add medication to new container (usually done in medication room or at medication cart):	
a. *Solutions in a bag:* Locate medication injection port on plastic IV solution bag. Port has small rubber stopper at end. Do not select port for the IV tubing insertion or air vent.	Medication injection port is self-sealing to prevent introduction of microorganisms after repeated use.
b. *Solutions in bottles:* Locate injection site on IV solution bottle, which is often covered by a metal or plastic cap.	Accidental injection of medication through main tubing port or air vent can alter pressure within bottle and cause fluid leaks through air vent. Cap seals bottle to maintain its sterility.
c. Wipe off port or injection site with alcohol or antiseptic swab (see illustration).	Reduces risk of introducing microorganisms into bag during needle insertion.
d. Remove needle cap or sheath from syringe, and insert needle of syringe through center of injection port or site; inject medication (see illustration).	Insertion of needle into sides of port may produce leak and lead to fluid contamination.
e. Withdraw syringe from bag or bottle.	Withdrawal automatically self-seals the injection port, preventing introduction of microorganisms.
f. Mix medication and IV solution by holding bag or bottle and turning it gently end to end.	Allows even distribution of medication.

STEPS	RATIONALE
g. Complete medication label with name and dose of medication, date, time, and your initials. Stick it on bottle or bag. *Optional (check institution's policy): Apply a flow strip that identifies the time the solution was hung and intervals indicating fluid levels (see illustration).*	Label can be easily read during infusion of solution and informs nurses and physicians of contents of bag or bottle. Do **not** use felt-tip markers on plastic surfaces. The ink can penetrate the plastic and leak into the IV solution.
12. Bring assembled items to client's bedside.	Organization reduces errors.
13. Identify client by reading identification band and asking name. Compare with MAR.	Ensures correct client receives ordered medication.
14. Prepare client by explaining that medication is to be given through existing IV line or one to be started. Explain that no discomfort should be felt during drug infusion. Encourage client to report symptoms of discomfort.	Most IV medications do not cause discomfort when diluted. However, potassium chloride can be irritating. Pain at insertion site may be early indication of infiltration.
15. Regulate infusion at ordered rate.	Prevents rapid infusion of fluid.

- *Critical Decision Point*

  Some medications (e.g., potassium chloride) can cause serious adverse reactions, including fatal cardiac dysrhythmias. These medications should be infused on an IV pump. Check institutional guidelines or policies indicating which IV medications require administration on an IV pump.

16. Add medication to existing container:

- *Critical Decision Point*

  Because there is no way to know exactly how much IV fluid is in an existing hanging IV container, there is no way to determine the exact concentration of the medication in the IV solution. Therefore it is recommended that medications should be added to new IV fluid containers whenever possible.

a. Check volume of solution remaining in bottle or bag.	Proper minimal volume (see drug insert) is needed to dilute medication adequately.

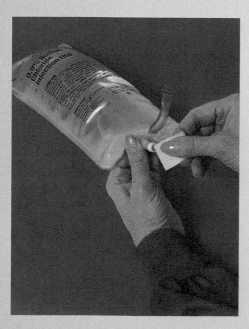

STEP 11C   Cleanse injection port with antiseptic swab.

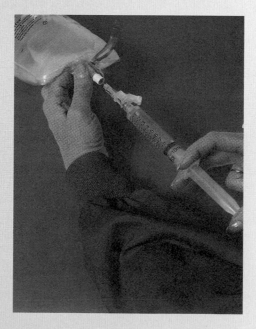

STEP 11D   Inject medication through port.

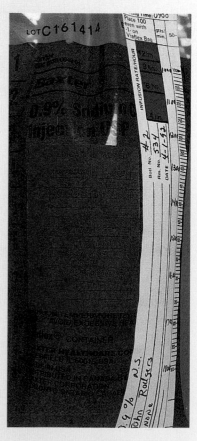

STEP 11G   Affix label to IV bag.

STEPS	RATIONALE
b. Close off IV infusion clamp.	Prevents medication from directly entering circulation as it is injected into bag or bottle.
c. Wipe off medication injection port with an alcohol or antiseptic swab.	Mechanically removes microorganisms that could enter container during needle insertion.
d. Remove needle cap or sheath from syringe, insert syringe needle through injection port, and inject medication.	Injection port is self-sealing and prevents fluid leaks.
e. Withdraw syringe from bag or bottle.	Self-seals medication port.
f. Lower bag or bottle from IV pole, and gently mix. Rehang bag.	Ensures medication is evenly distributed.
g. Complete medication label, and stick it to bag or bottle.	Informs nurses and physicians of contents of bag or bottle.
h. Regulate infusion to desired rate.	Prevents rapid infusion of fluid.
17. Properly dispose of equipment and supplies. Do not cap needle of syringe. Specially sheathed needles are discarded as a unit with needle covered.	Proper disposal of needle prevents injury to nurse and client. Capping of needles increases risk of needle-stick injuries.
18. Wash hands.	Reduces transmission of microorganisms.
19. Observe client for signs or symptoms of drug reaction.	IV medications can cause rapid effects.
20. Observe for signs and symptoms of fluid volume excess.	Rapid uncontrolled infusion can cause circulatory overload.
21. Periodically return to client's room to assess IV insertion site and rate of infusion.	Over time IV site may become infiltrated or needle malpositioned. Flow rate may change according to client's position or volume left in container.
22. Observe for signs or symptoms of IV infiltration.	Infiltrated drugs can injure tissue.

UNEXPECTED OUTCOMES AND RELATED INTERVENTIONS

- Client has adverse or allergic reaction to medication.
  - Follow institutional policy or guidelines for appropriate response to and reporting of adverse drug reactions.
  - Notify client's health care provider immediately.
- Client develops signs of fluid volume overload (e.g., abnormal breath sounds, shortness of breath, intake greater than output).
  - Circulatory regulation may be compromised.
  - Stop IV infusion.
  - Notify client's health care provider immediately.
- IV site becomes swollen, warm, reddened, and tender to touch (see Chapter 14).
  - Indicates phlebitis.
  - Stop IV infusion.
  - Discontinue IV infusion.
  - Treat IV site as indicated by institutional policy.

- Insert new IV site if continuation of IV therapy is indicated.
- IV site becomes cool, pale, and swollen (see Chapter 14).
  - Indicates signs of infiltration.
  - Some IV medications are extremely harmful to subcutaneous tissue.
  - Provide IV extravasation care (e.g., inject phentolamine [Regitine] around the IV infiltration site) as indicated by institutional policy, or use a medication reference or manual, or consult a pharmacist to determine appropriate follow-up care.

RECORDING AND REPORTING

- Record solution and medication added to parenteral fluid on appropriate form.
- Report any adverse effects to client's health care provider, and document adverse effects according to institutional policy.

The rate of administration of an IV bolus medication is usually determined by the amount of medication that can be given each minute. Look up each medication to determine the recommended concentration and rate of administration. The purpose for which a medication is prescribed and any potential adverse effects related to the rate or route of administration must be considered when giving a medication by IV push.

VOLUME-CONTROLLED INFUSIONS.   Another way of administering IV medications is through small amounts (25 to 100 ml) of compatible IV fluids. The fluid is in a secondary fluid container separate from the primary fluid bag. The container connects directly to the primary IV line or to separate tubing that inserts into the primary line. Different types of containers used include volume-control administration sets (e.g., Volutrol, Pediatrol), piggyback and/or tandem sets, and mini-infusers. Using volume-controlled infusions has the following advantages:

1. Medications are diluted and infused over longer time intervals (e.g., 30 to 60 minutes), reducing risks to the client associated with IV push.
2. Medications (e.g., antibiotics) that are stable for a limited time in solution can be administered.
3. IV fluid intake is controlled.

1. Verify physician's order for type of medication to be administered, dosage, and route.
2. Wash hands.
3. Prepare a syringe with ordered medication and two syringes with saline. Carefully read package directions or medication manual for proper dilution of medication.
4. Carefully check client's identification by looking at arm band and asking name.
5. Assess IV insertion site for signs of infiltration or phlebitis. If present, restart IV line or intermittent IV access in another site before administering medication.
6. If needleless system is not available, attach a small-gauge needle (22 to 25 gauge) to each syringe.
7. Apply gloves.
8. To administer IV push through an IV lock:
   - Clean injection port with antiseptic swab.
   - Insert syringe filled with saline into cap of IV saline lock.
   - Flush lock with 2 ml saline.
   - Insert syringe filled with medication into IV access, and administer over time recommended by institutional guidelines or medication manual. Use a watch with a second hand to time infusion.
   - Flush lock with the same amount of saline used before medication was given. Be sure to flush lock at the same rate of medication administration to avoid giving client a bolus of the medication.
   - In some institutions, the lock is flushed with heparin. The concentration and amounts of heparin used vary based on

the type of IV site. Refer to institutional guidelines if heparin is to be used.
9. To give IV push through an IV line:
   - Be sure medication is compatible with IV fluids. If the medication is incompatible with the IV fluids, you may be able to temporarily stop the medication infusion and give the IV push medication as if it were being given through an IV lock, after flushing the line well with saline. However, not all medications (e.g., heparin, cardiac medications) can be stopped temporarily. In these cases, start a new IV lock and use this site for medication administration.
   - If IV medication and fluids are compatible, select injection port closest to client and cleanse with antiseptic swab.
   - Administer medication over time recommended by institutional policy or medication manual, using a watch with a second hand. You can temporarily pinch the IV tubing as you inject the medication, but be sure to allow the IV fluids to flow during times you are not giving the medication to allow the medication to get to the client.
10. Dispose of gloves, and wash hands.
11. Observe client closely for adverse reactions as the drug is administered and for several minutes after giving the medication.
12. Place syringes in proper container.
13. Record drug, dosage, route, and time administered on MAR.
14. Note adverse reactions in the client's chart, and notify the client's caregiver if necessary.

PIGGYBACK. A piggyback is a small (25 to 250 ml) IV bag or bottle connected to a short tubing line that connects to the *upper* Y-port of a primary infusion line or to an intermittent venous access (Figure 13-28). The piggyback tubing is a microdrip or macrodrip system (see Chapter 14). The set is called a piggyback because the small bag or bottle is set higher than the primary infusion bag or bottle. In the piggyback setup, the main line does not infuse when the piggybacked medication is infusing. The port of the primary IV line contains a back-check valve that automatically stops flow of the primary infusion once the piggyback infusion flows. After the piggyback solution infuses and the solution within the tubing falls below the level of the primary infusion drip chamber, the back-check valve opens and the primary infusion begins to flow again.

TANDEM. A tandem setup is a small (25 to 100 ml) IV bag or bottle connected to a short tubing line to the *lower* Y-port of a primary infusion line or to an intermittent venous access. The tandem set is placed at the same height as the primary infusion bag or bottle. In the tandem setup, the tandem and the main line infuse simultaneously. The tandem setup must be monitored closely. If the tandem setup is not immediately clamped when the medication is infused, the IV solution from the primary line will back up into the tandem line.

VOLUME-CONTROL ADMINISTRATION. Volume-control administration sets (e.g., Volutrol, Buretrol, Pediatrol) are small (50 to 150 ml) containers that attach just below the primary infusion bag or bottle. The set is attached and filled in a manner similar to that used with a regular IV infusion. However, the priming filling of the set is different, depending on the type of filter (floating valve or membrane) within the set. Follow package directions for priming sets (Skill 13-8).

MINI-INFUSION PUMP. The mini-infusion pump is battery operated and delivers medications to be given in very small amounts of fluid (5 to 60 ml) within controlled infusion times using standard syringes (Skill 13-8).

INTERMITTENT VENOUS ACCESS. An intermittent venous access (commonly called a heparin lock or saline lock) is an IV catheter with a small "well" or chamber covered by a rubber cap (Figure 13-29). Special rubber-seal injection caps can be inserted into most IV catheters (see Chapter 14). Advantages to intermittent venous access include the following:
1. Cost savings resulting from the omission of continuous IV therapy

2. Saves nurses' time by eliminating constant monitoring of IV flow rates
3. Increased mobility, safety, and comfort for client by eliminating the need for a continuous IV line

After an IV bolus or piggyback medication has been administered through an intermittent venous access, the access must be flushed with a solution to keep it patent. Generally, saline is effective as a flush solution. Some institutions require the use of heparin. Be sure to check and follow institutional policies regarding the care and maintenance of the IV site.

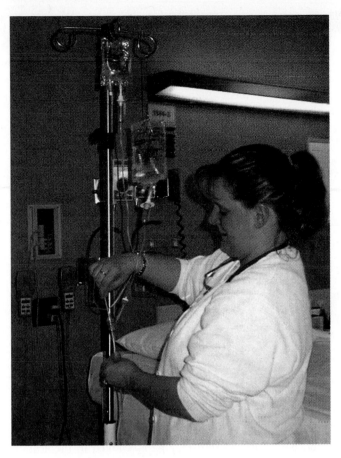

FIGURE **13-28**   Piggyback setup.

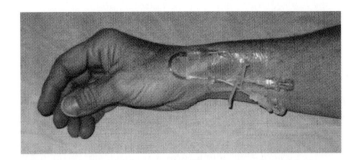

FIGURE **13-29**   Intermittent lock covered with a rubber diaphragm.

Skill 13-8

ADMINISTERING INTRAVENOUS MEDICATIONS BY PIGGYBACK, INTERMITTENT INTRAVENOUS INFUSION SETS, AND MINI-INFUSION PUMPS

DELEGATION CONSIDERATIONS
Administering medications by IV piggyback, intermittent infusion, and mini-infusion pumps requires problem solving and knowledge application unique to professional nursing. For this procedure delegation is not appropriate. Assistive personnel should be instructed to report any unexpected drug reactions or reported discomfort at infusion site as soon as possible.

EQUIPMENT
PIGGYBACK, TANDEM, OR MINI-INFUSION PUMP
- Medication prepared in 5- to 250-ml, labeled infusion bag or syringe
- Short microdrip or macrodrip IV tubing set
- Needleless device or stopcocks if available
- Needles (21 or 23 gauge, only if stopcocks or other needleless methods are not available)

- Mini-infusion pump if indicated
- Adhesive tape (optional)
- Antiseptic swab
- IV pole or rack
- MAR or computer printout

VOLUME-CONTROL ADMINISTRATION SET
- Volutrol or Burette
- Infusion tubing (may have needleless system attachment)
- Syringe (1 to 20 ml)
- Vial or ampule of ordered medication
- Antiseptic swab
- IV pole or rack
- Medication label
- MAR or computer printout

STEPS	RATIONALE
1. Check physician's order to determine type of IV solution to be used, type of medication, dose, route, and time of administration.	Client's overall physical condition dictates type of IV solution used. Ensures safe and accurate drug administration.

STEPS	RATIONALE
2. Collect information necessary to administer drug safely, including action, purpose, side effects, normal dose, time of peak onset, and nursing implications.	Allows you to give drug safely and to monitor client's response to therapy.
3. Assess compatibility of drug with existing IV solution.	Drugs that are incompatible with IV solutions may result in clouding or crystallization of solution in IV tubing, which may harm the client.

- *Critical Decision Point*
  Never administer IV medications through tubing that is infusing blood, blood products, or parenteral nutrition solutions.

STEPS	RATIONALE
4. Assess patency of client's existing IV infusion line (see Chapter 14).	IV line must be patent and fluids must infuse easily for medication to reach venous circulation effectively.

- *Critical Decision Point*
  If the client's IV site is saline locked, cleanse the port with alcohol and assess the patency of the IV line by flushing the IV line with 2 to 3 ml of sterile normal saline. Attach appropriate IV tubing to the saline lock, and administer the medication via piggyback, tandem, mini-infusion, or volume-control administration set. When the infusion is completed, disconnect the tubing, cleanse the port with alcohol, and flush the IV line with 2 to 3 ml sterile normal saline. Maintain sterility of IV tubing between intermittent infusions.

STEPS	RATIONALE
5. Assess IV insertion site for signs of infiltration or phlebitis: redness, pallor, swelling, or tenderness on palpation.	Confirmation of placement of IV needle or catheter and integrity of surrounding tissues ensure medication is administered safely.
6. Assess client's history of drug allergies.	Effects of medications can develop rapidly after IV infusion. Nurse should be aware of clients at risk.
7. Assess client's understanding of purpose of drug therapy.	May reveal need for education.
8. Assemble supplies at bedside. Prepare client by informing client that medication will be given through IV equipment.	Drug preparation usually is not required. Infusion tubing and bag of medication may be assembled in medication room or client's room. Allows client to understand procedure and minimizes anxiety.
9. Wash hands.	Reduces transmission of microorganisms.
10. Check client's identification by looking at arm band and asking client's name.	Ensures drug is administered to correct client.
11. Explain purpose of medication and side effects to client, and explain that medication is to be given through existing IV line. Encourage client to report symptoms of discomfort at site.	Keeps client informed of planned therapies. Clients who can verbalize pain at the IV site can help detect IV infiltrations early, lessening damage to surrounding tissues.
12. Administer infusion:	
A. Piggyback or Tandem Infusion:	
(1) Connect infusion tubing to medication bag (see Chapter 14). Allow solution to fill tubing by opening regulator flow clamp. Once tubing is full, close clamp and cap end of tubing.	Infusion tubing should be filled with solution and free of air bubbles to prevent air embolus.
(2) Hang piggyback medication bag above level of primary fluid bag. (Hook may be used to lower main bag.) Hang tandem infusion at same level as primary fluid bag (see illustration).	Height of fluid bag affects rate of flow to client.

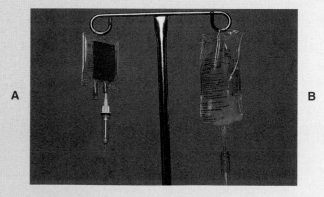

STEP 12A(2)   **A,** IV medication bag. **B,** Main IV infusion fluid.

(3) Connect tubing of piggyback or tandem infusion to appropriate connector on primary infusion line:

(a) *Stopcock:* Wipe off stopcock port with alcohol swab, and connect tubing. Turn stopcock to open position.

Stopcock eliminates need for needle.

(b) *Needleless system:* Wipe off needleless port of IV tubing, and insert tip of piggyback or tandem infusion tubing (see illustration).

The CDC strongly recommends needleless connections to prevent accidental needle-stick injuries (NIOSH, 1999). Establishes route for IV medication to enter main IV line.

(c) *Needle system:* Connect sterile needle to end of piggyback or tandem infusion tubing, remove cap, cleanse injection port on main IV line, and insert needle through center of port. Secure by taping connection.

Prevents introduction of miroorganisms during needle insertion.

(4) Regulate flow rate of medication solution by adjusting regulator clamp. (Infusion times vary. Refer to medication reference or institutional policy for safe flow rate.)

Provides slow, safe infusion of medication and maintains therapeutic blood levels.

(5) After medication has infused, check flow regulator on primary infusion. The primary infusion should automatically begin to flow after the piggyback or tandem solution is empty.

Back-check valve on piggyback stops flow of the primary infusion until medication infuses. The tandem and primary infusions flow together until the tandem set empties. Checking flow rate ensures proper administration of IV fluids.

(6) Regulate main infusion line to desired rate if necessary.

Infusion of piggyback may interfere with the main line infusion rate.

(7) Leave IV piggyback bag and tubing in place for future drug administration or discard in appropriate containers.

Establishment of secondary line produces route for microorganisms to enter main line. Repeated changes in tubing increase risk of infection transmission (check institutional policy).

B. Mini-infusion Administration:

(1) Connect prefilled syringe to mini-infusion tubing.

Special tubing designed to fit syringe delivers medication to main IV line.

(2) Carefully apply pressure to syringe plunger, allowing tubing to fill with medication.

Ensures tubing is free of air bubbles to prevent air embolus.

(3) Place syringe into mini-infusion pump (follow product directions). Be sure syringe is secure (see illustration).

Correct placement is necessary for proper infusion.

(4) Connect mini-infusion tubing to main IV line.

(a) *Stopcock:* Wipe off stopcock port with alcohol swab, and connect tubing. Turn stopcock to open position.

Stopcock reduces risk of needle-stick injuries.

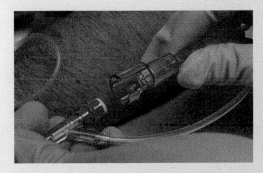 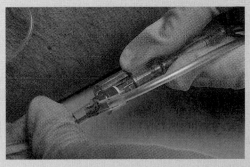

STEP 12A(3)(B) For the needleless system, insert tip of piggyback or tandem infusion tubing into port.

STEPS	RATIONALE

(b) *Needleless system:* Wipe off needleless port of IV tubing, and insert tip of the mini-infusion tubing.

Needlesless system reduces risk of needle-stick injuries.

(c) *Needle system:* Connect sterile needle to mini-infusion tubing, remove cap, cleanse injection port on main IV line or saline lock, and insert needle through center of port. Consider placing tape where IV tubing enters port to keep connection secured.

Cleansing reduces transmission of microorganisms.

(5) Hang infusion pump with syringe on IV pole alongside main IV bag. Set pump to deliver medication within time recommended by institutional policy, a pharmacist, or a medication reference manual. Press button on pump to begin infusion.

Pump automatically delivers medication at safe, constant rate based on volume in syringe.

(6) After medication has infused, check flow regulator on primary infusion. The infusion should automatically begin to flow once the pump stops. Regulate main infusion line to desired rate as needed. (note: If stopcock is used, turn off mini-infusion line.)

Maintains patency of primary IV line.

C. **Volume-control Administration Set (e.g., Volutrol):**

(1) Prepare medication from vial or ampule (see Skill 13-5, p. 322).

Ensures medication is sterile.

(2) Fill Volutrol with desired amount of fluid (50 to 100 ml) by opening clamp between Volutrol and main IV bag (see illustration).

Small volume of fluid dilutes IV medication and reduces risk of too-rapid infusion.

(3) Close clamp, and check to be sure clamp on air vent of Volutrol chamber is open.

Prevents additional leakage of fluid into Volutrol. Air vent allows fluid in Volutrol to exit at regulated rate.

(4) Clean injection port on top of Volutrol with antiseptic swab.

Prevents introduction of microorganisms during needle insertion.

(5) Remove needle cap or sheath, and insert syringe needle through port, then inject medication (see illustration). Gently rotate Volutrol between hands.

Rotating mixes medication with solution in Volutrol to ensure equal distribution.

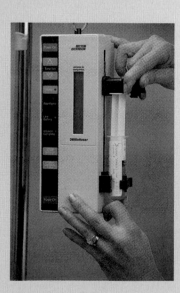

STEP 12B(3)   Ensure syringe is secure after placing it into mini-infusion pump.

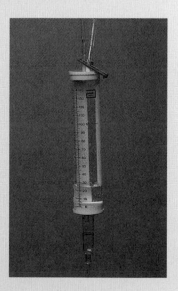

STEP 12C(2)   Fill with desired amount of fluid by opening clamp between Volutrol and main IV bag.

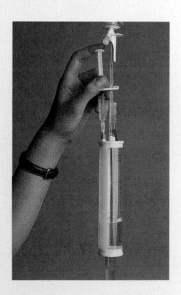

STEP 12C(5)   Inject medication into device.

Steps	Rationale
(6) Regulate IV infusion rate to allow medication to infuse in time recommended by institutional policy, a pharmacist, or a medication reference manual.	For optimal therapeutic effect, drug should infuse in prescribed time interval.
(7) Label Volutrol with name of drug, dosage, total volume including diluent, and time of administration.	Alerts nurses to drug being infused. Prevents other medications from being added to Volutrol.
(8) Dispose of uncapped needle or needle enclosed in safety shield and syringe in proper container.	Prevents accidental needle sticks.
13. Observe client for signs of adverse reactions.	IV medications act rapidly.
14. During infusion, periodically check infusion rate and condition of IV site.	IV must remain patent for proper drug administration. Development of infiltration necessitates discontinuing infusion.
15. Ask client to explain purpose and side effects of medication.	Evaluates client's understanding of instruction.

Unexpected Outcomes and Related Interventions

- Client develops adverse drug reaction.
  - Stop medication infusion immediately.
  - Follow institutional policy or guidelines for appropriate response and reporting of adverse drug reactions.
  - Notify client's health care provider of adverse effects immediately.
- Medication does not infuse over desired period.
  - Determine reason (e.g., improper calculation of flow rate, malpositioning of IV needle at insertion site, infiltration)
  - Take corrective action as indicated.
- IV site becomes swollen, warm, reddened, and tender to touch (see Chapter 14). Indicates phlebitis.
  - Stop IV infusion.
  - Discontinue IV infusion.
  - Treat IV site as indicated by institutional policy.
  - Insert new IV site if continuation of therapy is indicated.

- IV site becomes cool, pale, and swollen (see Chapter 14). Indicates signs of infiltration.
  - Some IV medications are extremely harmful to SQ tissue.
  - Provide IV extravasation care (e.g., injecting phentolamine [Regitine] around IV infiltration site) as indicated by institutional policy or use a medication reference or consult a pharmacist to determine appropriate follow-up care.

Recording and Reporting

- Record drug, dose, route, and time administered on MAR or computer printout.
- Record volume of fluid in medication bag or Volutrol on intake and output form.
- Report any adverse reactions to client's health care provider.

Key Terms

absorption, p. 283
adverse effects, p. 284
allergic reactions, p. 285
anaphylactic reactions, p. 285
apothecary system, p. 288
biotransformation, p. 284
buccal, p. 287
concentration, p. 286
detoxify, p. 284
idiosyncratic reaction, p. 285
infusions, p. 289
inhalation, p. 288
injections, p. 289
instillation, p. 288

intradermal (ID), p. 287
intramuscular (IM), p. 287
intraocular, p. 288
intravenous (IV), p. 287
irrigations, p. 289
medication abuse, p. 282
medication allergy, p. 285
medication dependence, p. 282
medication error, p. 294
medication interaction, p. 285
metered-dose inhalers (MDIs), p. 314
metric system, p. 289
narcotics, p. 293
nurse practice acts, p. 282
ophthalmic, p. 308
parenteral administration, p. 287

pharmacokinetics, p. 283
polypharmacy, p. 300
prescriptions, p. 288
pruritus, p. 307
serum half-life, p. 286
side effect, p. 284
solution, p. 289
subcutaneous (SQ), p. 287
sublingual, p. 286
synergistic effect, p. 285
therapeutic effect, p. 284
toxic effect, p. 285
transdermal disk, p. 288
Z-track injection, p. 333

Key Concepts

- Learning medication classifications improves understanding of nursing implications for administering medications with similar characteristics.
- All controlled substances are handled according to strict procedures that account for each medication.
- You apply understanding of the physiology of medication action when timing administration, selecting routes, initiating actions to promote medication efficacy, and observing responses to medications.
- The older adult's body undergoes structural and functional changes that alter medication actions and influence the manner in which nurses provide medication therapy.
- Children's medication doses are computed on the basis of body surface area or weight.
- Medications given parenterally are absorbed more quickly than medications administered by other routes.
- Each medication order should include the client's name, dosage, route, and time of administration, and the prescriber's signature.
- A medication history reveals allergies, medications a client is taking, and the client's compliance with therapy.
- The five rights of medication administration ensure accurate preparation and administration of medication doses.
- Only administer medications you prepare, and never leave medications unattended.
- Document medications immediately after administration.
- Use clinical nursing judgment when determining the best time to administer prn medications.
- Report medication errors immediately.
- When preparing medications, check the medication container label against the MAR or computer printout three times.
- The Z-track method for IM injections protects SQ tissues from irritating parenteral fluids.
- Failure to select injection sites by anatomical landmarks may lead to tissue, bone, or nerve damage.

Critical Thinking Activities

1. You are working with a critical care nurse who has been floated to your unit. You observe this nurse drawing up 0.25 mg of digoxin into a 3-ml syringe. The nurse does not dilute the medication and is preparing to give this medication by IV bolus. You tell her that neither you nor any other nurse has given digoxin by IV bolus. She tells you that she does almost every day. How would you intervene in this situation? What rationale would you use to justify your position?
2. Fifteen minutes after you have hung an IV antibiotic, the client is itching. You determine that the client may be having an allergic reaction to the antibiotic. What steps would you take immediately and why?
3. You have prepared an IM injection for your client. You did not assess the client before preparing the medication.

You draw the medication up in a syringe with a 1½ inch, 25-gauge needle. When you arrive to give the injection, you find that the client is cachectic and has very little muscle mass. How would you proceed with your assessment and intervention? Give your rationale.

4. You are caring for an older woman in her home. She takes digoxin (Lanoxin), 0.25 mg every day; warfarin (Coumadin), 2.5 mg once daily; and lorazepam (Ativan), 2 mg at bedtime. On previous home visits, she has been oriented. Today, you find that she is confused and cannot put sentences together. When you look in her bathroom, you find all her pills are dumped out of their bottles and are spread out on her bath towels. When you ask her about the pills, she states, "I was just counting them to see how many were left." What might explain her confusion? What do you need to assess? Explain how you would proceed in this situation. What would you need to teach your client?

Review Questions

1. A client receiving an antihypertensive medication is complaining of postural hypotension. This is an example of:
   1. a side effect.
   2. a toxic effect.
   3. an allergic reaction.
   4. an idiosyncratic reaction.
2. A client is requesting Tylenol (acetaminophen) for a headache, but there is no order for this medication. The nurse should:
   1. tell the client he does not have an order for Tylenol.
   2. notify the client's physician and acquire an order for Tylenol.
   3. tell the client he will have to wait until the physician comes to see him.
   4. give the Tylenol now and notify the physician that Tylenol was given when he makes rounds.
3. A client is receiving a medication that has a serum half-life of 4 days. The nurse will teach the client that:
   1. the medication will need to be taken every 4 days.
   2. the client will not experience adverse effects until the client has been on the medication for 4 days.
   3. the client will probably experience effects of the drug for 4 days after the client stops taking the medication.
   4. the client will have to receive the medication intravenously for 4 days in order to achieve an effective serum concentration.
4. A client is being discharged with nitroglycerin sublingually as needed for angina. The nurse knows the client understands medication teaching when the client states:
   1. It will take a long time for this medication to work.
   2. I should put the tablet under my tongue and not swallow it.

3. I should drink 8 ounces of water whenever I take this medication.
4. I should alternate cheeks when I take multiple doses of this medication.
5. A client is to receive an IM injection of morphine sulfate. The client is 5 feet, 10 inches tall and weighs 185 pounds. The nurse plans to administer the injection in the ventrogluteal muscle. The most appropriate needle size to use for this injection is:
   1. 20 gauge, 1 inch.
   2. 23 gauge, ⅝ inch.
   3. 25 gauge, ½ inch.
   4. 22 gauge, 1½ inch.
6. The client has a gastric tube. There is an order for you to give the client 0.25 mg of digoxin. The bottle of digoxin has 60 ml of digoxin. Each ml has 50 μg of digoxin. The nurse should give:
   1. 5 ml.
   2. 50 ml.
   3. 0.5 ml.
   4. 0.05 ml.
7. The client has an order for 2 tablespoons of milk of magnesia. The nurse, converting this to the metric system, would give the client:
   1. 2 ml.
   2. 5 ml.
   3. 16 ml.
   4. 30 ml.
8. The nurse is having difficulty reading a physician's order for a medication. The nurse knows the physician is very busy and does not like to be called. The nurse should:
   1. call a pharmacist to interpret the order.
   2. call the physician and have the order verified.
   3. consult the nursing care manager to help interpret the order.
   4. talk to the unit secretary on the floor who is good at reading the physician's handwriting.
9. A client is being discharged with insulin injections. The nurse knows the client understands how to give his injections when he states:
   1. I can give my shots in the same place, all the time.
   2. I need to take my shot about 15 minutes before I sit down to eat.
   3. I should draw the cloudy insulin into the syringe before the clear insulin.
   4. I should check my blood sugars 4 times each day and whenever I feel hypoglycemic.
10. A client is receiving an enteral feeding through a G-tube. He is to receive a medication that is incompatible with the feeding. The nurse should:
    1. get a liquid form of the medication from the pharmacy.
    2. not give the medication until checking with the prescriber.
    3. stop the feedings for at least 1 hour before and 1 hour after giving the medication.
    4. flush the G-tube with 60 ml of water, give the medication, and flush the G-tube with another 60 ml of water before restarting the feeding.
11. A client is to receive cephalexin (Keflex), 500 mg PO. The pharmacy has sent 250 mg tablets. The nurse should give:
    1. ½ tablet.
    2. 1 tablet.
    3. 1½ tablets.
    4. 2 tablets.

References

American Diabetes Association: Insulin administration: clinical practice recommendations, *Diabetes Care* 20(1S):46S, 1997.

American Nurses Association: *Nursing facts about needlestick injuries,* 1999. Retrieved 1/25/01 from the World Wide Web at http://www.nursingworld.org/readroom/fsneedle.htm.

Beecroft PC, Kongelbeck RS: How safe are intramuscular injections? *AACN Clin Issues* 5(4):207, 1994.

Behrman RE, Vaughan VC, editors: *Nelson textbook of pediatrics,* ed 13, Philadelphia, 1987, WB Saunders

Beyea SC, Nicoll LH: Administration of medication via the intramuscular route: an integrative review of the literature and research-based protocol for the procedure, *Appl Nurs Res* 8(1):23, 1995.

Beyea SC, Nicoll LH: Back to basics: administering IM injections the right way, *Am J Nurs* 96(1):34, 1996.

Cook MC: Nurses' six rights for safe medication administration, *Massachusetts Nurse* 69(6):8, 1999.

Cook PR: Using critical thinking skills to improve medication administration, *MEDSURG Nurs* 4(4):309, 1995.

Ebersole P, Hess P: *Toward healthy aging: human needs and nursing response,* ed 5, St. Louis, 1998, Mosby.

Galvan TJ: Dysphagia: going down and staying down, *Am J Nurs* 101(1):37, 2001.

Gazarian PK: The direct route for asthma therapy: teaching your patient to use a metered-dose inhaler, *Nursing 97* 27(10):52, 1997.

Gilbar PJ: A guide to enteral drug administration in palliative care, *J Pain Symptom Manage* 17(3):197, 1999.

Goucher A: Looks alike, sounds alike, *Massachusetts Nurse* 70(4):4, 2000.

Lewis SM and others: *Medical-surgical nursing,* ed 5, St. Louis, 2000, Mosby.

McConnell EA: Instilling eye ointment, *Nursing 98* 29(8):14, 1998a.

McConnell EA: Applying transdermal ointments, *Nursing 98* 29(10):30, 1998b.

McConnell EA: Administering a Z-track IM injection, *Nursing 99* 29(1):26, 1999.

McKenry LM and Salerno E: *Mosby's pharmacology in nursing,* ed 20, St. Louis, 2000, Mosby.

Meister FL: Ask the experts, *Crit Care Nurse* 18(4):97, 1998.

National Coordinating Council for Medication Error Reporting and Prevention (NCCMERP): *Recommendations to correct error-prone aspects of prescription writing,* 1996a. Retrieved 1/25/01 from the World Wide Web at http://www.nccmerp.org/rec_960904.htm.

NCCMERP: *Recommendations to reduce errors related to administration of drugs,* 1999b. Retrieved 1/25/01 from the World Wide Web at http://nccmerp.org/rec_990629.htm.

NCCMERP: *National Coordinating Council announces medication administration recommendations to prevent errors,* 1999c. Retrieved 1/25/01 from the World Wide Web at http://www.nccmerp.org/rel_990916.htm.

National Institute for Occupational Safety and Health (NIOSH): NIOSH alert: preventing needlestick injuries in health care settings, *NIOSH Publications Dissemination,* DHHS (NIOSH) Publication No. 2000-108, Nov 1999.

Occupational Safety and Health administration (OSHA). (January 18, 2001) Occupational exposure to bloodborne pathogens; needlestick and other sharp injuries; final rule. *Federal Register,* CFR 29, part 1910(66:5317-5325).

Patient's Library: Usign eye drops, *RN* 63(4):230, 2000.

Peragallo-Dittko V: Rethinking subcutaneous injection technique, *Am J Nurs* 97(5):71, 1997.

Posey D, Long B: Always swab the stopper on vials before each use, *RN* 59(2):9, 1996.

Powers FA: Your elderly patient needs I.V. therapy . . . can you keep her safe? *Nursing 99* 99(7):14, 1999.

Ryan AA: Medication compliance and older people: a review of the literature, *Int J Nurs Stud* 36:153, 1999.

Seal R: How to promote drug compliance in the elderly, *Community Nurse* 6(1):41, 2000.

Wong DL and others: *Whaley and Wong's nursing care of infants and children,* ed 6, St. Louis, 1999, Mosby.

Workman B: Safe injection techniques, *Nurs Standard* 13(39): 47, 1999.

Zimmerman PG, Pierce B: Double-checking medications, *J Emerg Nurs* 24(6):586, 1998.

Fluid, Electrolyte, and Acid-Base Balance

Objectives

- Define key terms.
- Describe the basic physiological mechanism responsible for maintaining fluid and electrolyte balance.
- Describe the processes involved in acid-base balance.
- Discuss common disturbances in fluid, electrolyte, and acid-base balances.
- Discuss variables that affect fluid, electrolyte, and acid-base balances.
- Discuss clinical assessments for fluid, electrolyte, and acid-base imbalances.
- List and discuss appropriate nursing interventions for clients with fluid, electrolyte, and acid-base imbalances.
- Describe procedures for initiating and maintaining fluid balance.
- Discuss complications of intravenous therapy.
- Describe the procedure for initiating a blood transfusion and the complications of blood therapy.
- Identify appropriate nursing interventions that can be delegated by the nurse.

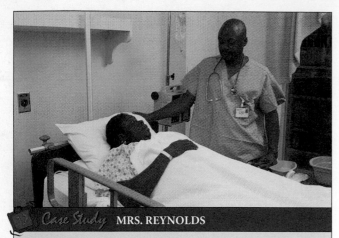

Case Study   MRS. REYNOLDS

Susan Reynolds, a 42-year-old black married accountant, has just been admitted to the medical-surgical unit with a history of nausea, loss of appetite for 3 days, and vomiting and diarrhea for 2 days. She feels her symptoms are related to "bad food" she must have had on her recent business trip. Past medical history includes hypertension controlled by Lasix 40 mg once a day and a no-salt-added diet. After obtaining a blood sample for electrolytes, complete blood count, and an electrocardiogram (ECG), the doctor has admitted her for observation and has ordered that she have nothing by mouth (NPO) and have an intravenous (IV) infusion of 0.45% normal saline at 125 ml/hr inserted. She is also ordered to be on intake and output (I&O) recordings and vital signs every 4 hours, with daily weights.

Robert is a junior nursing student assigned to Mrs. Reynolds. He is 35 years old, married with three young children, and a former paramedic. Although this is somewhat of a career change for him, after two semesters of medical-surgical nursing he has enjoyed each rotation and he is sure a career in nursing is for him.

*F*luid, electrolyte, and acid-base balances within the body are necessary to maintain health and function in all body systems. These are maintained by the intake and output of water and electrolytes, their distribution in the body, and the regulation of renal and pulmonary function. Imbalances may result from many factors, including illnesses, altered fluid intake, or prolonged episodes of vomiting or diarrhea. Acid-base balance is necessary for many physiological processes. Imbalances can alter respiration, metabolism, cardiovascular and renal function, and the functioning of the central nervous system.

▋ SCIENTIFIC KNOWLEDGE BASE

Water is the largest single component of the body; 60% of the average 30-year-old adult male and 50% of the average female weight is fluid. A healthy, mobile, well-oriented adult is usually capable of maintaining normal fluid, electrolyte, and acid-base balances because of the body's adaptive physiological mechanisms.

Distribution of Body Fluids

Body fluids are distributed in two distinct compartments, one containing **intracellular fluid (ICF)** and the other ex-

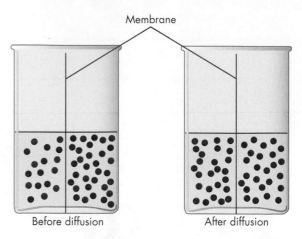

FIGURE **14-1**   Diffusion across a semipermeable membrane. (From Lewis SM and others: *Medical-surgical nursing: assessment and management of clinical problems,* ed 5, St. Louis, 1999, Mosby.)

tracellular fluid (ECF). ICF comprises all fluid within body cells. This fluid contains dissolved solutes essential to fluid and electrolyte balance and metabolism. In adults approximately 40% of body weight is ICF (Beare and Myers, 1998).

ECF is all fluid outside a cell, which is divided into two smaller compartments: **interstitial** and **intravascular fluids.** Interstitial fluid is the fluid between cells and outside the blood vessels, whereas intravascular fluid is blood plasma. Other extravascular fluids are the lymph, transcellular, and organ fluids (McCance and Huether, 1998). ECF makes up about 20% of the total body weight.

Composition of Body Fluids

Body fluid contains substances that are sometimes called minerals or salts but are technically known as electrolytes (Christensen and Kockrow, 1999). An **electrolyte** is an element or compound that, when dissolved in water or another **solvent,** separates into **ions** and is able to carry an electric current. Positively charged electrolytes are **cations.** Negatively charged electrolytes are **anions.** Although the accumulation of electrolytes differs in ECF and ICF, the total number of anions and cations in each fluid compartment should be the same. Electrolytes are commonly measured in **milliequivalents per liter (mEq/L).**

Movement of Body Fluids

Fluids and electrolytes constantly shift from compartment to compartment to meet a variety of metabolic needs. The movement of fluids depends on cell membrane permeability.

Diffusion (Figure 14-1) is a process in which a **solute** (gas or substance) in a **solution** moves from an area of higher concentration to an area of lower concentration, evenly distributing the solute in the solution. For example, when you pour a small amount of cream into a cup of black coffee, the cream mixes or diffuses through the whole cup of coffee. The difference in the two concentrations is known as a **concentration gradient.** Fluids and electrolytes diffuse across cellular membranes. For a substance to cross the membrane, the membrane must be permeable to it.

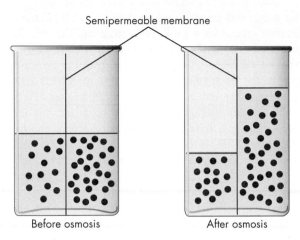

FIGURE **14-2**   Osmosis through a semipermeable membrane. (From Lewis SM and others: *Medical-surgical nursing: assessment and management of clinical problems,* ed 5, St. Louis, 1999, Mosby.)

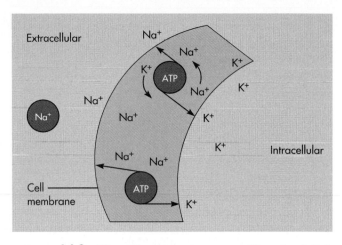

FIGURE **14-3**   The sodium-potassium pump. (From Lewis SM and others: *Medical-surgical nursing: assessment and management of clinical problems,* ed 5, St. Louis, 1999, Mosby.)

Osmosis is the movement of water across a semipermeable membrane from an area of lower concentration to one that has a higher concentration (Figure 14-2). Osmosis equalizes the concentration of molecules (ions) on each side of the membrane. Boiling a hot dog is an example of osmosis. The concentration of molecules inside the hot dog is greater than in water. The water passes through the hot dog skin, which is a semipermeable membrane, in an attempt to equalize the number of molecules on both sides of the membrane. Finally, when the hot dog can hold no more water, the skin, or semipermeable membrane, ruptures (Christensen and Kockrow, 1999).

When you have a more concentrated solution on one side of a selectively permeable membrane and a less concentrated solution on the other side, there is a pull called **osmotic pressure** that draws the water through the membrane to the more concentrated side. When the solutions on both sides of the semipermeable membrane have established equilibrium, or are equal in concentration, they are isotonic. The measure of a solution's ability to create osmotic pressure and thus affect the movement of water is termed **osmolality.** Changes in extracellular osmolality may result in changes in both ECF and ICF volume.

Osmolarity, another term used to describe the concentration of solutions, reflects the number of molecules in a liter of solution and is measured in milliosmoles per liter (mOsm/L). Solutions are classified as **hypertonic, isotonic,** or **hypotonic.** Hypertonic (a solution of higher osmotic pressure) solutions pull fluid from cells; isotonic (a solution of same osmotic pressure) solutions expand the body's fluid volume without causing a fluid shift from one compartment to another; and hypotonic (a solution of lower osmotic pressure) solutions move into the cells, causing them to enlarge. Each of these actions occurs through osmosis.

Diffusion and osmosis are passive processes that do not require energy from the body's cells. **Active transport** is the movement of molecules or ions "uphill" against osmotic pressures to areas of higher concentration. An example of active transport found in the body is the sodium-potassium-ATPase

pump, which moves sodium to the outside of the cell and then returns potassium to the inside of the cell (Figure 14-3).

Hydrostatic pressure is the force of the fluid pressing outward against a surface. When there is a difference in the hydrostatic pressure on two sides of a membrane, water and diffusible solutes move out of the solution that has the higher hydrostatic pressure. This process is called **filtration.** At the arterial end of the capillary, the hydrostatic pressure is greater than the **colloid osmotic pressure** (oncotic pressure), causing fluid and diffusible solutes to move out of the capillary into the interstitial space. At the venous end, the colloid osmotic pressure **(oncotic pressure),** or pull, is greater than the hydrostatic pressure, and fluids and some solutes move into the capillary from the interstitial space. The excess fluid and solutes remaining in the interstitial space are returned to the intravascular compartment by the lymph channels. The pressure at the capillary bed is called colloid osmotic pressure because blood plasma proteins are not allowed to pass freely because the capillary membrane is impermeable to proteins (colloids). This activity enhances the osmotic pressure by forcing the blood proteins to stay within the capillary.

Regulation of Body Fluids

Homeostasis is the process by which body fluids are maintained in a balance. Body fluids are regulated by fluid intake, hormonal controls, and fluid output. In health the body readily responds to disturbances in fluids and electrolytes to prevent or repair damage.

FLUID INTAKE.   Fluid intake is regulated primarily through the thirst mechanism, a major factor influencing fluid intake. The thirst-control center is located in the hypothalamus. The **osmoreceptors** continually monitor the serum osmotic pressure, and when osmolality increases, the hypothalamus is stimulated and a person becomes thirsty. Eating food that is salty can increase the osmotic pressure of the body fluids and stimulate the thirst mechanism. Increased plasma osmolality can occur with any condition that interferes with the oral ingestion of fluids, or it can occur with the intake of hypertonic

Adult Average Daily Fluid Gains and Losses			Table 14-1
Fluid Gains	(ml)	Fluid Losses	(ml)
Oral fluids	1100-1400	Kidneys	1200-1500
Solid foods	800-1000	Skin	500-600
Metabolism	300	Lungs	400
		Gastrointestinal	100-200
TOTAL GAINS	2200-2700	TOTAL LOSSES	2200-2700

fluids. The hypothalamus will also be stimulated when excess fluid is lost, and **hypovolemia** occurs, as in excessive vomiting and hemorrhage.

The average adult's fluid intake (Table 14-1) is about 2200 to 2700 ml per day; oral intake accounts for 1100 to 1400 ml, solid foods about 800 to 1000 ml, and oxidative metabolism 300 ml daily (Horne and others, 1997). Water oxidation (oxidative metabolism) is the by-product of cellular metabolism of ingested solid foods. Fluid intake requires an alert state. Infants, clients with neurological or psychological problems, and some older adults are unable to perceive or respond to the thirst mechanism; they are at risk for **dehydration.**

HORMONAL REGULATION. Antidiuretic hormone **(ADH)** stored in the posterior pituitary gland is released in response to changes in the blood osmolarity. ADH prevents diuresis, thus causing the body to save water. The osmoreceptors in the hypothalamus are stimulated when there is an increase in the osmolarity, thus causing release of ADH. The ADH works directly on the renal tubules and collecting ducts to make them more permeable to water. This in turn causes water to return to the systemic circulation, diluting the blood and decreasing its osmolarity. The client will experience a decrease in urinary output as the body tries to compensate. When the blood has been sufficiently diluted, the osmoreceptors stop the release of ADH.

Aldosterone is released by the adrenal cortex in response to increased plasma potassium levels or as a part of the renin-angiotensin-aldosterone mechanism to counteract hypovolemia. It acts on the distal portion of the renal tubule to increase the reabsorption (saving) of sodium and the secretion and excretion of potassium and hydrogen. Because sodium retention leads to water retention, the release of aldosterone acts as a volume regulator (Horne and others, 1997).

Renin, an enzyme, responds to decreased renal perfusion secondary to a decrease in extracellular volume. Renin acts to produce angiotensin I, which causes some vasoconstriction. However, **angiotensin** I almost immediately becomes reduced by an enzyme that converts angiotension I into angiotensin II. Angiotensin II then causes massive selective vasoconstriction of many blood vessels and relocates and increases the blood flow to the kidney, improving renal perfusion. In addition, angiotensin II also stimulates the release of aldosterone.

FLUID OUTPUT REGULATION. Fluid output (see Table 14-1) occurs through four organs of water loss: the kidneys,

skin, lungs, and gastrointestinal (GI) tract. The kidneys are the major regulatory organs of fluid balance. They receive approximately 180 L of plasma to filter each day and produce 1200 to 1500 ml of urine. Water loss from the skin is regulated by the sympathetic nervous system, which activates sweat glands. Water loss from the skin can be a sensible or insensible loss. An average of 500 to 600 ml of sensible and insensible fluid is lost via the skin each day (Horne and others, 1997). **Insensible water loss** is continuous and is not perceived by the person. **Sensible water loss** occurs through excess perspiration and can be perceived by the client or by the nurse through inspection. The amount of sensible perspiration is directly related to the stimulation of the sweat glands.

The lungs expire about 400 ml of water daily. This insensible water loss may increase in response to changes in respiratory rate and depth. In addition, devices for giving oxygen can increase insensible water loss from the lungs.

Under normal conditions, the GI tract accounts for only 100 to 200 ml of fluid loss each day, yet it plays a vital role in fluid regulation because it is the site of nearly all fluid gain. In disease, however, the GI tract may become a site of major fluid loss because approximately 3 to 6 L of isotonic fluid is secreted into and reabsorbed out of the GI tract daily.

Regulation of Electrolytes

CATIONS. Major cations within the body fluids include sodium (Na^+), potassium (K^+), calcium (Ca^{++}), and magnesium (Mg^{++}). Cations interchange when one cation leaves the cell and is replaced by another. This occurs because cells tend to maintain electrical neutrality.

SODIUM REGULATION. Sodium is the most abundant cation (90%) in ECF. Sodium ions are the major contributors to maintaining water balance through their effect on serum osmolality, nerve impulse transmission, regulation of acid-base balance, and participation in cellular chemical reactions (McCance and Huether, 1998). Sodium is regulated by dietary intake and aldosterone secretion. The normal extracellular sodium concentration is 135 to 145 mEq/L.

POTASSIUM REGULATION. Potassium is the predominant intracellular cation; only 2% is located in ECF. It regulates many metabolic activities and is necessary for glycogen deposits in the liver and skeletal muscle, transmission and conduction of nerve impulses, normal cardiac rhythms, and skeletal and smooth muscle contraction (McCance and Huether, 1998). The normal range for serum potassium concentrations is 3.5 to 5 mEq/L. Potassium is regulated by dietary intake and renal excretion. The body does not conserve potassium well, so any condition that increases urine output will result in a decreased serum potassium.

CALCIUM REGULATION. Calcium is stored in bone, plasma, and body cells. Ninety-nine percent of calcium is located in bone, and only 1% is located in ECF. Approximately 50% of calcium in the plasma is bound to protein, primarily albumin, and 40% is free ionized calcium. Normal serum ionized calcium is 4 to 5 mEq/L. Normal total calcium is 8.5 to 10.5 mg/dl. Calcium is necessary for bone and teeth formation, blood clotting, hormone secretion, cell membrane integrity, cardiac conduction, transmission of nerve impulses, and muscle contraction.

MAGNESIUM REGULATION. Magnesium is essential for enzyme activities, neurochemical activities, and cardiac and skeletal muscle excitability. Plasma concentrations of magnesium range from 1.5 to 2.5 mEq/L. Serum magnesium is regulated by dietary intake, renal mechanisms, and actions of parathyroid hormone (PTH).

ANIONS. The three major anions of body fluids are chloride (Cl^-), bicarbonate (HCO_3^-), and phosphate (PO_4^{-3}), ions.

CHLORIDE REGULATION. Chloride is the major anion in ECF. The transport of chloride follows sodium. Normal concentrations of chloride range from 95 to 108 mEq/L. Serum chloride is regulated by dietary intake and the kidneys. A person with normal renal function who has a high chloride intake will excrete a higher amount of urine chloride.

BICARBONATE REGULATION. Bicarbonate is the major chemical base buffer within the body. The bicarbonate ion is found in ECF and ICF. The bicarbonate ion is an essential component of the carbonic acid–bicarbonate buffering system essential to acid-base balance. The kidneys regulate bicarbonate. Normal arterial bicarbonate levels range between 22 and 26 mEq/L; venous bicarbonate is measured as carbon dioxide content, and the normal value is 24 to 30 mEq/L.

PHOSPHORUS-PHOSPHATE REGULATION. Nearly all the phosphorus in the body exists in the form of phosphate (PO_4^{-3}), which assists in the regulation of acid-base regulation. Phosphate and calcium help to develop and maintain bones and teeth. Generally calcium and phosphate are inversely proportional; if one rises, the other falls. Phosphate also promotes normal neuromuscular action and participates in carbohydrate metabolism. Phosphate is normally absorbed through the GI tract. It is regulated by dietary intake, renal excretion, intestinal absorption, and PTH. The normal serum level is 2.5 to 4.5 mg/dl.

Regulation of Acid-Base Balance

Metabolic processes maintain a steady balance between acids and bases for optimal functioning of cells. Arterial pH is an indirect measurement of hydrogen ion (H^+) concentration (i.e., the greater the concentration of H^+ ions, the more acidic the solution and the lower the pH; the lower the concentration of H^+ ions, the more alkaline the solution and the higher the pH). pH is also a reflection of the balance between carbon dioxide (CO_2), which is regulated by the lungs, and bicarbonate (HCO_3^-), a base regulated by the kidneys. Acid-base balance exists when the net rate at which the body produces acids or bases equals the rate at which acids or bases are excreted. This balance results in a stable concentration of hydrogen ions (H^+) in body fluids that is expressed as the pH value. Normal hydrogen ion level is necessary to maintain cell membrane integrity and the speed of cellular enzymatic reactions. A pH value of 7 is neutral; below 7 is acid, and above 7 is alkaline. Normal values in arterial blood range from 7.35 to 7.45.

The three general types of acid-base regulators within the body are chemical (the carbonic acid–bicarbonate buffer system), biological (the absorption and release of hydrogen ions by cells), and physiological buffering systems (the lungs and the kidneys). A **buffer** is a substance or a group of substances that can absorb or release H^+ to correct an acid-base imbalance.

Disturbances in Electrolyte, Fluid, and Acid-Base Balance

Disturbances in electrolyte, fluid, or acid-base balances seldom occur alone and can disrupt normal body processes. When there is a loss of body fluids because of burns, illnesses, or trauma, the client is also at risk for electrolyte imbalances. In addition, some untreated electrolyte imbalances (e.g., potassium loss) result in acid-base disturbances.

ELECTROLYTE IMBALANCES

SODIUM IMBALANCES. Hyponatremia is a lower-than-normal concentration of sodium in the blood (serum), which can occur with a net sodium loss or net water excess (Table 14-2). Clinical treatment depends on the cause and whether it is associated with a normal, decreased, or increased ECF volume. The usual situation is a loss of sodium without a loss of fluid, and this results in a decrease in the osmolality of ECF. The body initially adapts by reducing water excretion and thus sodium excretion to maintain serum osmolality at near-normal levels. As the sodium loss continues, the body preserves the blood and interstitial (tissue) volume. As a result, the sodium in ECF becomes diluted.

Hypernatremia is a greater-than-normal concentration of sodium in ECF that can be caused by excess water loss or overall sodium excess (see Table 14-2). When the cause of hypernatremia is increased aldosterone secretion, sodium is retained and potassium is excreted. When hypernatremia occurs, the body attempts to conserve as much water as possible through renal reabsorption.

POTASSIUM IMBALANCES. Hypokalemia is one of the most common electrolyte imbalances in which an inadequate amount of potassium circulates in ECF (see Table 14-2, p. 354). When severe, hypokalemia can affect cardiac conduction and function. Because the normal amount of serum potassium is so small, there is little tolerance for fluctuations. The most common cause is the use of potassium-wasting diuretics such as thiazide and loop diuretics.

Hyperkalemia is a greater-than-normal amount of potassium in the blood. Severe hyperkalemia produces marked cardiac conduction abnormalities. The primary cause of hyperkalemia is renal failure because any decrease in renal

Electrolyte Imbalances
Table 14-2

Causes	Signs and Symptoms
Hyponatremia Kidney disease resulting in salt wasting Adrenal insufficiency GI losses Increased sweating Use of diuretics, especially when combined with low-sodium diet Pyschogenic polydipsia Syndrome of inappropriate ADH (SIADH)	*Physical examination:* apprehension, personality change, postural hypotension, postural dizziness, abdominal cramping, nausea and vomiting, diarrhea, tachycardia, convulsions and coma, and fingerprints remaining on sternum after palpation *Laboratory findings:* serum sodium level <135 mEq/L, serum osmolality <280 mOsm/kg, and urine specific gravity <1.010 (if not caused by SIADH)
Hypernatremia Ingestion of large amounts of concentrated salt solutions Iatrogenic administration of hypertonic saline solution parenterally Excess aldosterone secretion Diabetes insipidus Increased sensible and insensible water loss Water deprivation	*Physical examination:* thirst, dry and flushed skin, dry and sticky tongue and mucous membranes, fever, agitation, convulsions, restlessness, and irritability *Laboratory findings:* serum sodium levels >145 mEq/L, serum osmolality >295 mOsm/kg, and urine specific gravity >1.030 (if not caused by diabetes insipidus)
Hypokalemia Use of potassium-wasting diuretics Diarrhea, vomiting, or other GI losses Alkalosis Excess aldosterone secretion Polyuria Extreme sweating Excessive use of potassium-free intravenous (IV) solutions Treatment of diabetic ketoacidosis with insulin	*Physical examination:* weakness and fatigue, decreased muscle tone, intestinal distention, decreased bowel sounds, ventricular dysrhythmias, paresthesias, and weak, irregular pulse *Laboratory findings:* serum potassium level <3.5 mEq/L and ECG abnormalities (e.g., ventricular dysrhythmias)*
Hyperkalemia Renal failure Fluid volume deficit Massive cellular damage such as from burns and trauma Iatrogenic administration of large amounts of potassium intravenously Adrenal insufficiency Acidosis, especially diabetic ketoacidosis Rapid infusion of stored blood Use of potassium-sparing diuretics	*Physical examination:* anxiety, dysrhythmias, paresthesias, weakness, abdominal cramps, and diarrhea *Laboratory findings:* serum potassium level >5.3 mEq/L and ECG abnormalities (bradycardia, heart block, dysrhythmias); eventually QRS pattern widens and cardiac arrest occurs*
Hypocalcemia Rapid administration of blood transfusions containing citrate Hypoalbuminemia Hypoparathyroidism Vitamin D deficiency Pancreatitis Alkalosis	*Physical examination:* numbness and tingling of fingers and circumoral region, hyperactive reflexes, positive Trousseau's sign (carpopedal spasm with hypoxia), positive Chvostek's sign (contraction of facial muscles when facial nerve is tapped), tetany, muscle cramps, and pathological fractures (chronic hypocalcemia) *Laboratory findings:* serum calcium level <4.0 mEq/L or 8.5 mg/100 ml and ECG abnormalities
Hypercalcemia Hyperparathyroidism Malignant neoplastic disease Paget's disease Osteoporosis Prolonged immobilization Acidosis	*Physical examination:* anorexia, nausea and vomiting, weakness, lethargy, low back pain (from kidney stones), decreased level of consciousness, personality changes, and cardiac arrest *Laboratory findings:* serum calcium level >5 mEq/L or 10.5 mg/100 ml; x-ray examination showing generalized osteoporosis, widespread bone cavitation, radiopaque urinary stones; elevated blood urea nitrogen (BUN) level >25 mg/100 ml and elevated creatinine level >1.5 mg/100 ml caused by fluid volume deficit (FVD) or renal damage caused by urolithiasis; and ECG abnormalities

Electrolyte Imbalances—cont'd	Table 14-2
Causes	**Signs and Symptoms**
Hypomagnesemia	
Inadequate intake: malnutrition and alcoholism	*Physical examination:* muscular tremors, hyperactive deep tendon reflexes,
Inadequate absorption: diarrhea, vomiting, nasogastric drainage, fistulas; diseases of small intestine	confusion and disorientation, dysrhythmias, and positive Chvostek's sign and Trousseau's sign
Excessive loss resulting from thiazide diuretics	*Laboratory findings:* serum magnesium level <1.5 mEq/L
Aldosterone excess	
Polyuria	
Hypermagnesemia	
Renal failure	*Physical examination:* physical findings that are more frequent in acute elevations in magnesium levels: hypoactive deep tendon reflexes, decreased
Excess oral or parenteral intake of magnesium	depth and rate of respirations, hypotension, and flushing
	Laboratory findings: serum magnesium level >2.5 mEq/L

*Data from Horne MM and others: *Mosby's pocket guide series: fluid, electrolyte, and acid-base balance,* ed 3, St. Louis, 1997, Mosby.

function diminishes the amount of potassium the kidney can excrete.

CALCIUM IMBALANCES. Hypocalcemia represents a drop in serum and/or ionized calcium. It can result from several illnesses, some of which directly affect the thyroid and parathyroid glands (see Table 14-2). Another cause is renal insufficiency (kidneys unable to excrete phosphorus, causing the phosphorus level to rise and the calcium level to decline). Signs and symptoms can be related to the physiological role of serum calcium in neuromuscular function.

Hypercalcemia is an increase in the total serum concentration of calcium and/or ionized calcium. Hypercalcemia is frequently a symptom of an underlying disease resulting in excess bone resorption with release of calcium.

MAGNESIUM IMBALANCES. Disturbances in magnesium levels are summarized in Table 14-2. Symptoms are the result of changes in neuromuscular excitability.

CHLORIDE IMBALANCES. Hypochloremia occurs when the serum chloride level falls below normal. Vomiting or prolonged and excessive nasogastric or fistula drainage can result in hypochloremia because of the loss of hydrochloric acid. The use of loop and thiazide diuretics also increases chloride excretion as sodium is excreted. When serum chloride levels fall, metabolic alkalosis results while the body adapts by increasing reabsorption of the bicarbonate ion to maintain electrical neutrality.

Hyperchloremia occurs when the serum chloride level rises above normal, which usually occurs when the serum bicarbonate value falls or sodium level rises. Hypochloremia and hyperchloremia rarely occur as single disease processes but are commonly associated with acid-base imbalance. There is no single set of symptoms associated with these two alterations.

FLUID DISTURBANCES. The basic types of fluid imbalances are isotonic and osmolar. Isotonic deficit and excess exist when water and electrolytes are either gained or lost in equal proportions. In contrast, osmolar imbalances are losses or excesses of only water so that the concentration (osmolality) of the serum is affected. Table 14-3 lists the causes and symptoms of common fluid disturbances.

ACID-BASE IMBALANCES. Arterial blood gas (ABG) analysis is the best way of evaluating acid-base balance. When we measure ABG levels, we look at six components: pH, $PaCO_2$, PaO_2; oxygen saturation, base excess, and HCO_3^-. Deviation from a normal value will indicate that the client is experiencing an acid-base imbalance.

pH. pH measures H^+ ion concentration in body fluids. Even a slight change can be potentially life threatening. An increase in concentration of hydrogen ions (H^+) makes a solution more acidic; a decrease makes the solution more alkaline. The normal arterial blood pH value is 7.35 to 7.45 (acidic is less than 7.35, and alkalotic is more than 7.45).

$PaCO_2$. $PaCO_2$ is the partial pressure of carbon dioxide in arterial blood and is a reflection of the depth of pulmonary ventilation. Normal range is 35 to 45 mm Hg. A $PaCO_2$ of less than 35 mm Hg indicates that hyperventilation has occurred. As rate and depth of respiration increase, more carbon dioxide is exhaled and the carbon dioxide concentration decreases. A $PaCO_2$ of more than 45 mm Hg indicates hypoventilation. As rate and depth of respiration decrease, less carbon dioxide is exhaled and more is retained, increasing the concentration of carbon dioxide.

PaO_2. PaO_2 is the partial pressure of oxygen in arterial blood. It has no primary role in acid-base regulation if it is within normal limits. A PaO_2 less than 60 mm Hg can lead to anaerobic metabolism, resulting in lactic acid production and metabolic acidosis. There is a normal decline in PaO_2 in older adults. Hypoxemia may cause hyperventilation, resulting in respiratory alkalosis. Normal range is 80 to 100 mm Hg.

Fluid Disturbances
Table 14-3

Causes	Signs and Symptoms
Isotonic Imbalances	
FLUID VOLUME DEFICIT (FVD)—WATER AND ELECTROLYTES LOST IN EQUAL OR ISOTONIC PROPORTIONS	
Losses from the GI system, such as from diarrhea, vomiting, or drainage from fistulas or tubes	*Physical examination:* postural hypotension, tachycardia, dry mucous membranes, poor skin turgor, thirst, confusion, rapid weight loss, slow vein filling, lethargy, oliguria, weak pulse
Loss of plasma or whole blood, such as with burns or hemorrhage	*Laboratory findings:* urine specific gravity >1.025, increased hematocrit level >50%, and increased BUN level >25 mg/100 ml (hemoconcentration)
Excessive perspiration	
Fever	
Decreased oral intake of fluids	
Use of diuretics	
FLUID VOLUME EXCESS (FVE)—WATER AND SODIUM RETAINED IN ISOTONIC PROPORTIONS	
Congestive heart failure	*Physical examination:* rapid weight gain, edema (especially in dependent areas), hypertension, polyuria (if renal mechanisms are normal), neck vein distention, increased venous pressure, crackles in lungs
Renal failure	
Cirrhosis of the liver	
Increased serum aldosterone and steroid levels	*Laboratory findings:* decreased hematocrit level <38% and decreased BUN level <10 mg/100 ml (hemodilution)
Excessive sodium intake or administration	
Osmolar Imbalances	
HYPEROSMOLAR IMBALANCE—DEHYDRATION	
Diabetes insipidus	*Physical examination:* dry and sticky mucous membranes, flushed and dry skin; thirst, elevated body temperature, irritability, convulsions, coma
Interruption of neurologically driven thirst drive	*Laboratory findings:* increased serum sodium level >145 mEq/L and increased serum osmolality >295 mOsm/kg
Diabetic ketoacidosis	
Osmotic diuresis	
Administration of hypertonic parenteral fluids or tube-feeding formulas	
HYPOOSMOLAR IMBALANCE—WATER EXCESS	
Syndrome of Inappropriate Secretion of Antidiuretic Hormone (SIADH)	*Physical examination:* decreased level of consciousness, convulsions, coma
Excess water intake	*Laboratory findings:* decreased serum sodium level <135 mEq/L and decreased serum osmolality <280 mOsm/kg

OXYGEN SATURATION. Saturation is the point at which hemoglobin is saturated by oxygen (O_2). It can be affected by changes in temperature, pH, and $PaCO_2$. The normal range is 95% to 100%.

BASE EXCESS. Base excess is the amount of blood buffer (hemoglobin and bicarbonate) that exists. A high value indicates alkalosis, and a low value indicates acidosis. The normal range is ±2.

BICARBONATE. Serum bicarbonate (HCO_3^-) is the major renal component of acid-base balance and is excreted and reproduced by the kidneys to maintain a normal acid-base environment. The normal range is 22 to 26 mEq/L. Less than 22 mEq/L usually indicates metabolic acidosis, and more than 26 mEq/L indicates metabolic alkalosis.

TYPES OF ACID-BASE IMBALANCES. The four primary types of acid-base imbalance are respiratory acidosis, respiratory alkalosis, metabolic acidosis, and metabolic alkalosis (Table 14-4).

Respiratory acidosis is marked by an increased arterial carbon dioxide concentration ($PaCO_2$), excess carbonic acid (H_2CO_3), and an increased hydrogen ion concentration (decreased pH). With respiratory acidosis the cerebrospinal fluid and brain cells become acidic, causing neurological changes. Hypoxemia occurs because of respiratory depression, resulting in further neurological impairments. Electrolyte changes such as hyperkalemia and hypercalcemia may accompany the acidosis.

Respiratory alkalosis is marked by decreased $PaCO_2$ and increased pH. Like respiratory acidosis, respiratory alkalosis can begin outside the respiratory system (e.g., anxiety with hyperventilation) or within the respiratory system (e.g., initial phase of an asthma attack).

Metabolic acidosis results because of the high acid content of the blood, which also causes a loss of sodium bicarbonate. In an attempt to identify the cause of the metabolic acidosis, an analysis of serum electrolytes to detect an anion gap may be helpful. **Anion gap** reflects unmeasurable anions present in plasma and is calculated by subtracting the sum of chloride and bicarbonate from the amount of plasma sodium concentration.

Metabolic alkalosis is marked by the heavy loss of acid from the body or by increased levels of bicarbonate. The most common cause is vomiting.

NURSING KNOWLEDGE BASE

Fluid and electrolyte imbalances may affect anyone regardless of age, sex, color, or religion. Infants, severely ill adults, disoriented or immobile clients, and older adults are frequently at greater risk because of their inability to

Acid-Base Imbalances
Table 14-4

Causes	Signs and Symptoms
Respiratory Acidosis	
HYPOVENTILATION RESULTING FROM PRIMARY RESPIRATORY PROBLEMS	
Atelectasis (obstruction of small airways often caused by retained mucus)	*Physical examination:* confusion, dizziness, lethargy, headache, ventricular dysrhythmias, warm and flushed skin, muscular twitching, convulsions, and coma
Pneumonia	
Cystic fibrosis	*Laboratory findings:* arterial blood gas alterations pH <7.35, $PaCO_2$ >45 mm Hg, PaO_2 <80 mm Hg, and bicarbonate level normal (if uncompensated) or >26 mEq/L (if compensated)
Respiratory failure	
Airway obstruction	
Chest wall injury	
HYPOVENTILATION RESULTING FROM FACTORS OUTSIDE OF THE RESPIRATORY SYSTEM	
Drug overdose with a respiratory depressant	
Paralysis of respiratory muscles caused by various neurological alterations	
Head injury	
Obesity	
Respiratory Alkalosis	
HYPERVENTILATION RESULTING FROM PRIMARY RESPIRATORY PROBLEMS	
Asthma	*Physical examination:* dizziness, confusion, dysrhythmias, tachypnea, numbness and tingling of extremities, convulsions, and coma
Pneumonia	
Inappropriate mechanical ventilator settings	*Laboratory findings:* arterial blood gas alterations: pH >7.45, $PaCO_2$ <35 mm Hg, PaO_2 normal, and bicarbonate level normal (if short lived or uncompensated) or <22 mEq/L (if compensated)
HYPERVENTILATION RESULTING FROM FACTORS OUTSIDE OF THE RESPIRATORY SYSTEM	
Anxiety	
Hypermetabolic states	
Disorders of the central nervous system (head injuries, infections)	
Salicylate overdose	
Metabolic Acidosis	
HIGH ANION GAP	*Physical examination:* headache, lethargy, confusion, dysrhythmias, tachypnea with deep respirations, abdominal cramps, and flushed skin
Starvation	
Diabetic ketoacidosis	*Laboratory findings:* arterial blood gas alterations: pH <7.35, $PaCO_2$ normal (if uncompensated) or <35 mm Hg (if compensated), PaO_2 normal or increased (with rapid, deep respirations), bicarbonate level <22 mEq/L, and oxygen saturation normal
Renal failure	
Lactic acidosis from heavy exercise	
Use of drugs (methanol, ethanol, formic acid, paraldehyde, aspirin)	
NORMAL ANION GAP	
Renal tubular acidosis	
Diarrhea	
Metabolic Alkalosis	
Excessive vomiting	*Physical examination:* dizziness; dysrhythmias; numbness and tingling of fingers, toes, and circumoral region; muscle cramps; tetany
Prolonged gastric suctioning	
Hypokalemia or hypercalcemia	*Laboratory findings:* arterial blood gas alterations: pH >7.45, $PaCO_2$ normal (if uncompensated) or >45 mm Hg (if compensated), PaO_2 normal, and bicarbonate level >26 mEq/L
Excess aldosterone	
Use of drugs (steroids, sodium bicarbonate, diuretics)	

respond independently to the early warnings of a developing problem. Over time, the body's compensatory mechanisms cannot maintain fluid and electrolyte or acid-base balance adequately, and the client's health becomes compromised. The severity and long-term effects on the client's health will influence a client's ability to return to a state of optimal functioning. Prolonged or severe compromises may lead to irreversible chronic health problems that not only may change the lifestyle of the client but may also have an impact on caregiver(s), guardians, parents, families, and/or friends.

CRITICAL THINKING
Synthesis

A client's condition can change very quickly with a fluid and electrolyte imbalance. Multiple factors can be involved; therefore you need to realize that clinical decision making using the nursing process includes a synthesis of knowledge, experience, attitudes, and intellectual and professional standards to provide safe, quality care.

KNOWLEDGE. To provide care for the client with a fluid and electrolyte or acid-base imbalance you need to use previously learned nursing knowledge and related knowledge acquired in anatomy, physiology, pharmacology, and/or chemistry courses. It is important to consider any and all factors that might have contributed to a client's health problem. For example, a client's dehydration might have been caused by decreased fluid intake from a loss of appetite from a flu virus, or dizziness when getting out of bed may be related to a fluid loss and subsequent orthostatic hypotension. In these examples synthesizing previous learned knowledge about hypotension and fluid volume loss would help you plan and provide appropriate client care.

EXPERIENCE. Professional experience assists you when caring for clients with fluid and electrolyte or acid-base imbalances. Understanding the relationship between clients' clinical signs and symptoms helps you to identify and make appropriate clinical decisions when similar signs and symptoms are presented again with new clients. Reflecting back on client care experiences makes you more adept at problem solving in the future.

ATTITUDES. An example of two attitudes to use when caring for clients with fluid and electrolyte and acid-base imbalance are accountability and integrity. Accountability is important when performing vital signs, documenting I&O, or calculating IV flow rates. Data must be accurate. Integrity is necessary when supporting clients' need for privacy during voiding or defecation or attempting to minimize a client's embarrassment because of the malodorous vomitus and diarrhea.

STANDARDS. The use of IV therapy for a client experiencing an alteration in fluid and electrolyte or acid-base balance is standard nursing practice. You should be familiar with the standards of care involved in appropriately establishing, maintaining, monitoring, and discontinuing IV lines and fluid therapy. The standards of the Infusion Nurses Society are incorporated throughout this chapter. In addition, standards for infection control must be applied for invasive procedures such as IV therapy.

NURSING PROCESS

 ## Assessment

You need to understand the importance of fluid, electrolyte, and acid-base balance to homeostasis. By gathering assessment data you will identify clients at risk and identify all appropriate nursing diagnoses.

NURSING HISTORY. The nursing assessment begins with a client history, which is designed to reveal any risk factors or preexisting conditions that may cause or contribute to a disturbance of fluid and electrolytes and acid-base balance. Explore with the client any factors that may cause a disturbance, and integrate the information with knowledge of fluid volume regulation, electrolyte concentration, and acid-base regulation.

First consider the client's age. Infants and young children have a greater need for water and are more vulnerable to alteration in fluid volume. They have a greater fluid intake and output relative to their size (Wong and others, 1999). They are thus at greater risk for **fluid volume deficit (FVD)** and hyperosmolar imbalance because body water loss is proportionately greater per kilogram of weight. Children ages 2 through 12 have less stable regulatory responses to imbalance. In the event of high fevers or diarrhea, children have a narrow range of tolerance for severe fluid or electrolyte alterations. Adolescents have an increased metabolism and increased water production with girls having greater fluid changes because of hormonal changes.

Older adults experience a number of age-related changes that can affect fluid and electrolyte and acid-base balance. These changes include a reduction in body water, a diminished thirst sensation, decreased glomerular filtration, and a change in normal concentration of electrolytes (Ignatavicius and others, 1999). In addition, older adults are at risk for decreased excretion of medication, which can cause metabolic or respiratory acidosis. In the presence of sodium depletion or overload the older adult may be unable to maintain homeostasis. The changes in lung function that accompany aging can lead to respiratory acidosis and the inability to compensate for metabolic acidosis.

Chronic disease (e.g., cancer, congestive heart failure [CHF], and renal disease) becomes a focus of the nursing history. When clients have chronic disease, review the normal pathologic findings of such conditions to understand how fluid and electrolyte and acid-base status may be affected. It is also important to determine how long the client has suffered with the disease and the type of treatment currently being administered. In addition to chronic health problems, determine if the client has a history of GI alterations (e.g., diarrhea, vomiting, or colostomy), nasogastric suctioning, or intestinal drainage. Any condition that results in the loss of GI fluids predisposes the client to dehydration and a variety of electrolyte disturbances.

Recent surgery, head and chest trauma, and second- or third-degree burns are conditions that place clients at high risk for fluid and electrolyte alterations. The stress response of surgery causes fluid balance changes in the second to fifth postoperative day. Aldosterone, glucocorticoids, and ADH are increasingly secreted, causing sodium and chloride retention, potassium excretion, and decreased urinary output.

Certain environmental factors must also be included in the nursing history. Clients who have vigorously exercised or who have become exposed to temperature extremes may have clinical signs of fluid and electrolyte alterations. Exposure to environmental temperatures exceeding 28° to 30° C (82.4° to 86° F) results in excessive sweating with weight loss. A body weight loss over 7% decreases the ability of the cooling mechanism to conserve water.

A client's current dietary history is also an important component of nursing assessment. Recent changes in appetite or the ability to chew and swallow can affect nutritional status and fluid intake. Dieting can lead to acidosis because rapid water loss can lead to hyperosmolar fluid imbalance.

Lifestyle factors should also be included in the client's history. If a client already has preexisting medical risks, a history of smoking or alcohol consumption can further impair the client's ability to adapt to acid-base alterations. Alcohol and tobacco use can ultimately cause respiratory depression, which can result in respiratory acidosis.

A final category to include in the assessment is a history of medication use (Box 14-1). If the assessment reveals a medication that is likely to cause an electrolyte or acid-base disorder, you will need to closely examine the client's laboratory blood tests and determine if the client has taken the correct dosage as prescribed.

PHYSICAL EXAMINATION.   A thorough examination is necessary, because fluid and electrolyte or acid-base disturbances can affect all body systems (see Chapter 12). While examining each system, carefully consider the signs and symptoms to expect as a result of any imbalance (Table 14-5). For example, an examination of the oral cavity will likely reveal signs of dehydration if you suspect the client is experiencing a fluid loss. Table 14-6 is an example of a focused client assessment for a fluid and electrolyte evaluation.

MEASURING FLUID INTAKE AND OUTPUT.   Measuring and recording all liquid I&O during a 24-hour period is an important part of the client's assessment database for fluid and electrolyte balance. It is important to note trends in the I&O (e.g., a gradually decreasing urine output can indicate that the body is trying to adapt to an FVD or hyperosmolar fluid imbalance). Accurate I&O measurements identify both clients at risk for and clients who are experiencing fluid, electrolyte, and acid-base disturbances. You can delegate measurement of I&O to assistive personnel. Stress the importance of accuracy and reporting of findings.

For clients in health care settings, you may initiate I&O measurement without a physician's order when you believe the client is at risk for an imbalance. Generally I&O is routinely measured for clients after surgery, clients whose conditions are unstable, clients who have a temperature elevation, clients on fluid restriction, and clients who are receiving diuretic or IV therapy. You should also measure I&O for any client with chronic cardiopulmonary or renal illnesses and clients whose health status has deteriorated.

Oral intake includes all liquids taken by mouth, such as gelatin, ice cream, soup, juice, and water. Liquid intake also includes fluid given through nasogastric or jejunostomy feeding tubes, liquids given as IV fluids (including both continuous infusions and intermittent IV piggybacks), and blood or its components. Liquid output includes urine, diar-

Box 14-1   Medications That Cause Fluid and Electrolyte and Acid-Base Disturbances

Diuretics—metabolic alkalosis and hypokalemia

Steroids—metabolic alkalosis

Potassium supplements—GI disturbances, including intestinal and gastric ulcers and diarrhea

Respiratory center depressants such as opioid analgesics may decrease rate and depth of respirations, resulting in respiratory acidosis

Antibiotics—nephrotoxicity (e.g., vancomycin, methicillin, aminoglycosides), hyperkalemia and/or hypernatremia (e.g., azlocillin, carbenicillin, piperacillin, ticarcillin, Unasyn)

Calcium carbonate (Tums)—mild metabolic alkalosis with nausea and vomiting

Magnesium hydroxide (Milk of Magnesia)—hypokalemia

Nonsteroidal antiinflammatory drugs—nephrotoxicity

Modified from MckEnry LM, Salerno E: *Mosby's pharmacology in nursing*, ed 21, St. Louis, 2000, Mosby.

rhea, vomitus, gastric suction, and drainage from postsurgical wounds or other tubes.

Ambulatory clients' urinary output is recorded after each trip to the bathroom. Instruct these clients to save their urine in a graduated container so that you can record the amount, or clients may be instructed to measure and record their own output. When a client has an indwelling Foley catheter, drainage tube, or suction, that output is recorded at the end of each nursing shift or more frequently (e.g., every hour) as the client's condition requires. You should measure, not estimate, I&O.

Taking I&O measurements is a procedure requiring help from the client and family. Explain the reasons that measurements are needed, and instruct the client and family to not empty any container with voided fluid but to ask you to do so. A client using a toilet should be instructed to use a calibrated "hat" or insert, which attaches to the rim of the toilet bowl (Figure 14-4). After each urination ask the client to notify you so you can measure, record, and empty the urine and rinse the insert. Occasionally clients may also be instructed to measure and record their own output. It is important for the client to have good vision and motor skills to ensure accuracy.

Occasionally clients receive a specific amount of a liquid medication every 1 to 2 hours. A client receiving tube feedings may receive numerous liquid medications, and water may be used to flush the tube with the medications. Over a 24-hour period these liquids can amount to a significant intake and should always be recorded on the I&O record. Recording I&O is essential for obtaining an accurate database. This information helps to maintain an ongoing evaluation of the client's hydration status to prevent severe imbalances.

LABORATORY STUDIES.   Review the client's laboratory test results to obtain further objective data about fluid, electrolyte, and acid-base balances (Box 14-2). These tests include serum and urinary electrolyte levels, hematocrit, blood

Physical and Behavioral Nursing Assessment for Fluid, Electrolyte, and Acid-Base Imbalances

Table 14-5

Assessment	Imbalance
Weight Changes	
2%-5% loss	Mild fluid volume deficit (FV)
5%-15% loss	Moderate to severe FVD
>15% loss	Death
2% gain	Mild fluid volume excess (FVE)
5%-8% gain	Moderate to severe FVE
Head	
History:	
Headache	FVD, metabolic or respiratory acidosis, metabolic alkalosis
Dizziness	FVD, respiratory acidosis or alkalosis, hyponatremia
Observation:	
Irritability	Metabolic or respiratory alkalosis, hyperosmolar imbalance, hypernatremia, hypokalemia
Lethargy	FVD, metabolic acidosis or alkalosis, respiratory acidosis, hypercalcemia
Confusion, disorientation	FVD, hypomagnesemia, metabolic acidosis, hypokalemia
Eyes	
Inspection:	
Sunken, dry conjunctivae, decreased or absent tearing	FVD
Periorbital edema, papilledema	FVE
History:	
Blurred vision	FVE
Throat and Mouth	
Inspection:	
Sticky, dry mucosa and lips, decreased salivation	FVD, hypernatremia
Cardiovascular System	
Inspection:	
Flat neck veins	FVD
Distended neck veins	FVE
Dependent body parts: legs, sacrum, back	
Slow venous filling	FVD
Palpation:	
Edema (dependent body parts: back, sacrum, legs)	FVE
Dysrhythmias (also noted as ECG changes)	Metabolic acidosis, respiratory alkalosis and acidosis, potassium imbalance, hypomagnesemia
Increased pulse rate	Metabolic alkalosis, respiratory acidosis, hyponatremia, FVD, FVE, hypomagnesemia
Decreased pulse rate	Metabolic alkalosis, hypokalemia
Weak pulse	FVD, hypokalemia
Decreased capillary filling	FVD
Bounding pulse	FVE
Auscultation:	
Blood pressure (BP) low or without orthostatic changes	FVD, hyponatremia, hyperkalemia, hypermagnesemia
Third heart sound	FVE
Hypertension	FVE
Respiratory System	
Inspection:	
Increased rate	FVE, respiratory alkalosis, metabolic acidosis
Dyspnea	FVE
Auscultation:	
Crackles	FVE

Data from Horne M and others: *Mosby's pocket guide series; fluid, electrolyte, and acid-base balance,* ed 3, St. Louis, 1997, Mosby.

Physical and Behavioral Nursing Assessment for Fluid, Electrolyte, and Acid-Base Imbalances—cont'd	Table 14-5
Assessment	**Imbalance**

Gastrointestinal System

History:	
Anorexia	Metabolic acidosis
Abdominal cramps	Metabolic acidosis
Inspection:	
Sunken abdomen	FVD
Distended abdomen	Third-space syndrome
Vomiting	FVD, hypercalcemia, hyponatremia
Diarrhea	Hyponatremia
Auscultation:	
Hyperperistalsis with diarrhea, or hypoperistalsis	FVD, hypokalemia

Renal System

Inspection:	
Oliguria or anuria	FVD, FVE
Diuresis (if kidneys are normal)	FVE
Increased urine specific gravity	FVD

Neuromuscular System

Inspection:	
Numbness, tingling	Metabolic alkalosis, hypocalcemia, potassium imbalances
Muscle cramps, tetany	Hypocalcemia, metabolic or respiratory alkalosis
Coma	Hyperosmolar or hypoosmolar imbalances, hyponatremia
Tremors	Respiratory acidosis, hypomagnesemia
Palpation:	
Hypotonicity	Hypokalemia, hypercalcemia
Hypertonicity	Hypocalcemia, hypomagnesemia, metabolic alkalosis
Percussion:	
Decreased or absent deep tendon reflexes	Hypercalcemia, hypermagnesemia
Increased or hyperactive deep tendon reflexes	Hypocalcemia, hypomagnesemia

Skin

Body temperature:	
Increased	Hypernatremia, hyperosmolar imbalance, metabolic acidosis
Decreased	FVD
Inspection:	
Dry, flushed	FVD, hypernatremia, metabolic acidosis
Palpation:	
Inelastic skin turgor, cold, clammy skin	FVD

Example of a Focused Client Assessment		Table 14-6
Factors to Assess	**Questions and Approaches**	**Physical Assessment Strategies**
Vital signs	Ask client about experiencing dizziness when changing positions.	When client gets out of bed, assess for orthostatic hypotension.
	Ask if client feels a "racing heart rate."	Palpate client's pulse or ascultate heart rate.
Intake and output	Ask client about usual I&O patterns.	Evaluate client's 24- and/or 36-hour I&O amount.
	Ask client to specify if there has been a significant increase or decrease in I&O.	Inspect client's urine and vomitus or diarrhea if applicable.
	Determine cause of the I&O change.	Obtain a baseline weight, and monitor weight daily.
Skin turgor	Ask client about skin, dryness, or swelling.	Inspect client's skin, palpate for turgor and edema.
	Determine if client has experienced any itching or changes in the skin, and have client explain.	Inspect for any skin changes.

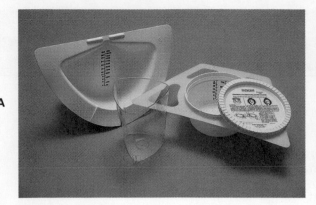

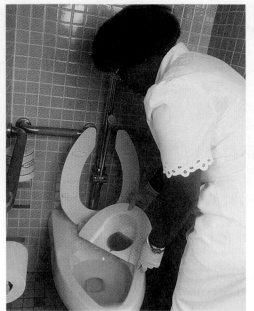

FIGURE **14-4** **A,** Graduated measuring containers. *Clockwise from left to right:* "hat" receptacle, specimen, and measurement container. **B,** Nurse emptying collected urine.

Laboratory Data for Fluid, Electrolyte, and Acid-Base Imbalances   Box 14-2

FLUID AND ELECTROLYTES

Altered concentrations of sodium, potassium, magnesium, calcium, phosphates, chloride, and bicarbonate (venous CO_2 concentrations)

Increase in hematocrit, BUN, sodium, and osmolality in serum (related to loss of ECF fluid or gain of solutes)

Decrease in hematocrit, BUN, sodium, and osmolality in serum (related to gain of ECF fluid or loss of solutes)

Concentrated urine demonstrated by urine specific gravity >1.030

Dilute urine demonstrated by a specific gravity <1.012

METABOLIC ALKALOSIS

pH >7.45

$PaCO_2$ normal or >45 mm Hg if lungs are compensating

PaO_2 normal

O_2 saturation (SaO_2) normal

HCO_3^- >26 mEq/L

K^+ <3.5 mEq/L

METABOLIC ACIDOSIS

pH <7.35

$PaCO_2$ normal or <35 mm Hg if lungs are compensating

PaO_2 normal

SaO_2 normal

HCO_3^- <22 mEq/L

K^+ >5.3 mEq/L

K^+ <3.5 mEq/L

RESPIRATORY ALKALOSIS

pH >7.45

$PaCO_2$ <35 mm Hg

PaO_2 normal

SaO_2 normal

HCO_3^- normal

K^+ <3.5 mEq/L

RESPIRATORY ACIDOSIS

pH <7.35

$PaCO_2$ >45 mm Hg

PaO_2 normal or <80 mm Hg, depending on cause of acidosis

SaO_2 normal or <95%, depending on cause of acidosis

HCO_3^- normal if early respiratory acidosis or 26 mEq/L if kidneys are compensating

K^+ >5.3 mEq/L

---

creatinine level, blood urea nitrogen (BUN) levels, urine specific gravity, and ABG readings. Serum electrolytes are measured to determine the hydration status, the electrolyte concentration of the blood plasma, and acid-base balance. The frequency with which these electrolytes are measured depends on the severity of the client's illness. Serum electrolyte tests are routinely performed on any client entering a hospital to screen for alterations and to serve as a baseline for future comparisons.

The complete blood count (CBC) is a determination of the number and type of red and white blood cells per cubic millimeter of blood. As long as a client is not anemic, the hematocrit can be an indication of the hydration status of the client. The hematocrit will increase (become more con-

centrated) in situations where fluid is lost, whereas it will decrease in situations in which fluid is excessively retained in the vascular space.

Blood creatinine levels measure kidney function. Creatinine is a normal by-product of muscle metabolism and is excreted by the kidneys at fairly constant levels, regardless of factors such as fluid intake, diet, or exercise. Therefore it provides a measure of renal function that is relatively independent of the hydration status of the client or the client's dietary intake. BUN is the amount of nitrogenous substance present in the blood as urea. It is a rough indicator of kidney function.

Serum osmolality measures the concentration of the plasma. The osmolality will decrease when the client has hy-

Laboratory Profile: Acid-Base Assessment   Table 14-7

	Normal Range for Adults		
Test	Arterial	Venous	Significance of Abnormal Findings
pH	7.35-7.45	7.32-7.43	Increased: metabolic alkalosis, loss of gastric fluids, decreased potassium intake, diuretic therapy, fever, salicylate toxicity
>90 years age	7.25-7.45		Decreased: metabolic or respiratory acidosis, ketosis, renal failure, starvation, diarrhea, hyperthyroidism
PaO_2 (mm Hg)	83-108		Increased: increased ventilation, oxygen therapy, exercise
>90 years age	>50		Decreased: respiratory depression, high altitude, carbon monoxide poisoning, decreased cardiac output
$PaCO_2$ (mm Hg)	35-48	41-55	Increased: respiratory acidosis, emphysema, pneumonia, cardiac failure, respiratory depression
			Decreased: respiratory alkalosis, excessive ventilation, diarrhea
Bicarbonate	22-26	24-29	Increased: bicarbonate therapy, metabolic alkalosis
(mEq/L or mmol/L)			Decreased: metabolic acidosis, diarrhea, pancreatitis
Lactate (mg/100 ml)	<11.3	8.1-15.3	Increased: hypoxia, exercise, insulin infusion, alcoholism, pregnancy
			Decreased: fluid overload

From Ignatavicius DD and others: *Medical-surgical nursing across the health care continuum*, ed 3, St. Louis, 1999, Mosby.
$PaCO_2$, Partial pressure of arterial carbon dioxide; PaO_2, partial pressure of arterial oxygen.

poosmolar fluid imbalance (water excess) or hyponatremia. Decreased serum osmolality results in the movement of fluid into body cells (cellular edema) by osmosis. The osmolality will increase with a hyperosmolar fluid imbalance (water deficit) or hypernatremia or other gains of solutes such as glucose. This will result in the movement of fluid out of body cells into the interstitial space (cellular shrinkage). Both cellular edema and shrinkage disrupt normal cell processes.

The urine specific gravity test measures the urine's degree of concentration and evaluates the ability of the kidneys to conserve or excrete water. The specific gravity normally ranges between 1.010 and 1.025.

ABG analysis provides information on the status of acid-base balance and the effectiveness of ventilatory function in providing normal oxygen–carbon dioxide exchange (Table 14-7). You should understand that an ABG result is evaluated in a systematic approach. First, the pH is examined; a value less than 7.35 is considered acidic and greater than 7.45 is considered alkalotic. Next, the $PaCO_2$ is checked; the pH and $PaCO_2$ should move in opposite directions (e.g., as pH increases, the $PaCO_2$ should decrease). The HCO_3^- (bicarbonate) is then examined, and it is important to remember that the pH and HCO_3^- should move in the same direction. If the $PaCO_2$ and the HCO_3^- are both abnormal, then the value that corresponds more closely to the pH is examined. The value that more closely corresponds to the pH and deviates more from the norm usually points to the primary disturbance responsible for altering the pH.

CLIENT EXPECTATIONS.   Fluid and electrolyte or acid-base disturbance can be either insidious or acute. If a client is alert enough to discuss care with you, a review of expectations may reveal short-term needs (e.g., provision of comfort from nausea or IV placement) or long-term needs (e.g., understanding how to prevent alterations from occurring in the future). The client must be able to understand the impli-

Case Study SYNTHESIS IN PRACTICE

Robert reviews Mrs. Reynolds's clinical condition. The nursing history found in the medical record reveals that Mrs. Reynolds's loss of appetite, episodes of diarrhea, and continued use of Lasix (a non–potassium-sparing diuretic) for hypertension have placed her at risk for a fluid and electrolyte imbalance. The cause of her GI symptoms is unclear, although the physician plans further diagnostic tests. Robert reviews the physiology of potassium as an electrolyte and studies the pathologic findings of potassium excess and deficiency. He also reads recommendations in his pharmacology text on how to minimize the risk of hypokalemia when diuretics are taken. Robert anticipates the need to be able to perform a concise physical assessment of this client tomorrow and to be prepared to manage and monitor her IV therapy. He knows that client education will eventually be important for this client because her therapy for hypertension will likely continue.

Just a few weeks ago, Robert cared for a client with ulcerative colitis. Although Mrs. Reynolds's condition is different, both clients had diarrhea. Robert knows that Mrs. Reynolds will require careful monitoring of I&O, as well as stabilization of GI function. The lessons learned from his previous client will help Robert to be more alert should Mrs. Reynolds's clinical condition change under his care.

Robert knows the importance of being accountable in completing an examination, assessing and documenting I&O, assessing vital signs, and administering medications in a timely manner. A well-organized approach to Mrs. Reynolds's care will minimize the chance of errors being made.

Robert checks the policy and procedure manual at the institution he is assigned to for an IV therapy protocol. He has reviewed the new standards for dressing changes and is familiar with the new technique.

cations of fluid and electrolyte or acid-base changes to be able to express expectations of care. Clients' trust in you is strengthened through your competent response to sudden changes in clients' condition and through communication with clients and/or family members. Keeping them abreast

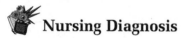

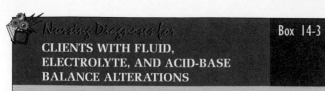	Box 14-3

CLIENTS WITH FLUID, ELECTROLYTE, AND ACID-BASE BALANCE ALTERATIONS

- Breathing pattern, ineffective
- Cardiac output, decreased
- Fluid volume, deficient
- Fluid volume, excess
- Fluid volume, risk for deficient
- Fluid volume, risk for imbalanced
- Gas exchange, impaired
- Oral mucous membrane, impaired
- Skin integrity, impaired
- Skin integrity, risk for impaired
- Therapeutic regimen management, ineffective
- Therapeutic regimen management, ineffective community
- Therapeutic regimen management, ineffective family
- Tissue integrity, impaired
- Tissue perfusion, ineffective

of the changes and the interventions will allow them to be active participants in their care.

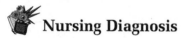 **Nursing Diagnosis**

When caring for clients with suspected fluid, electrolyte, and acid-base imbalances, it is important that you be skilled in using critical thinking to formulate nursing diagnoses (Box 14-3). The assessment data that establish the risk for or the actual presence of a nursing diagnosis in these areas may be subtle. For example, relevant assessment data for the nursing diagnosis *deficient fluid volume* could include any combination of the following: insufficient oral intake, weight loss, dry skin and mucous membranes, decreased skin turgor, decreased blood pressure, and increased heart rate. The serum sodium and osmolality could be elevated. The urine could be dark, with an elevated specific gravity. The volume of the urine could be decreasing over a period of days.

In addition to the accurate clustering of assessment data, you must precisely identify the related factor for the nursing diagnosis to plan appropriate nursing care. For example, for the nursing diagnosis *deficient fluid volume* the related factor could be diarrhea or vomiting. If the related factor were diarrhea, nursing interventions would include administering ordered antidiarrheal medications, providing oral fluids containing electrolytes and glucose, and teaching the client to use careful hand washing and to avoid dairy products. In contrast, if the related factor were vomiting, you might administer antiemetics, or remove sights and odors that could induce nausea, and provide a small amount of fluids containing electrolytes. When choosing which nursing diagnosis is appropriate, it is important that you analyze the defining characteristics carefully. It is also necessary to prioritize the client's needs based on the diagnostic findings.

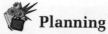 **Planning**

GOALS AND OUTCOMES.   During planning work with the client to establish goals and expected outcomes for each nursing diagnosis. Each goal should be measurable and achievable. While planning care for the client it is important that you collaborate as much as possible with the client and family. The family can be particularly helpful in identifying subtle changes in a client's behavior associated with any imbalances (e.g., anxiety, confusion, and irritability). For those clients with acute disturbances, discharge planning should begin early. In the acute care setting anticipating the needs of the client and family can help make the transition to home or a long-term care setting have fewer disruptions. For example, a client might be discharged home with IV therapy. In this situation it is important that you determine the knowledge and skills of the family member or friend who is to assume caregiving responsibilities and make a referral to home IV therapy as soon as possible. When creating a care plan for a client, remember to take into consideration the client's personal preferences and available resources (see care plan). Planning care for a client also requires you to collaborate closely with other members of the health care team, such as the physician, the dietitian, or perhaps a pharmacist. Generally the physician will direct the treatment of any fluid and electrolyte or acid-base alteration. The dietitian can be a valuable resource in recommending food sources to either increase or reduce intake of certain electrolytes. Chapter 30 describes various therapeutic diets (e.g., low sodium). The pharmacy and pharmacist can offer a wealth of information regarding a client's medication, the potential side effects, and over-the-counter medication to be avoided.

SETTING PRIORITIES.   The client's clinical condition determines which of the diagnoses takes the greatest priority. Many nursing diagnoses in the area of fluid and electrolyte and acid-base balance are of highest priority, because the consequences for the client can be serious or even life threatening.

Consultation with the client's physician may assist in setting realistic time frames for the goals of care, particularly when the client's physiological status is unstable. While the client is unstable you will be responsible for most of the direct client care that involves the administration of medications, IV and/or oxygen therapy, and hemodynamic assessments. As the client becomes stable, you can safely delegate daily weights, I&O, and direct physical client care. It is important that you establish a rapport of open communication with assistive personnel, as with any member of the interdisciplinary team, and collaborate in meeting the specific needs of your client.

CONTINUITY OF CARE.   As a client moves from one health care setting to another or to their home, it is important that a plan for continuity of care is established. Regimens that are initiated at one setting should be continued at the next setting until completed. For example, a client who is instructed to continue monitoring I&O will

Case Study Nursing Care Plan FLUID AND ELECTROLYTE IMBALANCE

ASSESSMENT

Mrs. Reynolds's vital signs are temperature 99.6° F, **pulse 100** and regular, **blood pressure 110/60** with no changes when the client stands. The client's skin is intact, without discoloration, but **turgor is decreased.** Inspection of **mucous membranes** shows them to be **dry,** with thick mucus. Respirations were 18 and nonlabored with bilateral breath sounds clear to auscultation. Bowel sounds were present in all four quadrants but hyperactive before one loose bowel movement this morning. The perianal area is slightly reddened. Mrs. Reynolds has had no nausea or vomiting since yesterday and only two loose stools since midnight. Twenty-four-hour intake equaled 2450 ml, with output of 2200 ml **(urine output was only 1000 ml).** Mrs. Reynolds voids without difficulty, with **dark yellow urine.** Robert also reviewed laboratory results: **hematocrit 44%** (suggesting hypovolemia); potassium 3.6 mEq/L and sodium 138 mEq/L (both low normal because of prolonged vomiting and diarrhea). Mrs. Reynolds's ECG showed a normal sinus rhythm, and her admission **weight** of 143 lb was **down** only **1 lb** this morning. The client's Lasix is on hold this morning pending the next potassium level.

*Defining characteristics are shown in bold type.

NURSING DIAGNOSIS

Fluid volume deficit related to excessive diarrhea, vomiting, and use of potassium-wasting diuretic.

PLANNING

GOAL	EXPECTED OUTCOMES
Client's fluid and electrolyte levels will return to normal limits by discharge.	Mucous membranes will be moist, and skin turgor will recoil normally within 48 hours.
	Blood pressure will remain within 10% of baseline during position changes within 24 hours.
	Urine output will equal intake within 48 hours.
	Hematocrit, potassium, and sodium levels will return to normal ranges within 48 hours.

IMPLEMENTATION

STEPS	RATIONALE
1. Monitor and maintain IV fluids (0.45% normal saline) at 125 ml/hour.	Replacement of body fluid restores blood volume and normal serum electrolyte levels; use of hypotonic fluid allows fluid to move into body cells, relieving cellular dehydration.
2. Administer as ordered bismuth subsalicylate (Pepto Bismol) for diarrhea.	Pepto Bismol is indicated as an antidiarrheal to inhibit GI secretions, stimulate absorption of fluid and electrolytes, inhibit intestinal inflammation, and suppress the growth of *Helicobacter pylori* (McKenry and Salerno, 2001).
3. Provide comfort measures: oral hygiene every 2 hours while awake or as client desires, lip balm to lips, A&D ointment to perianal area.	Local hydration lubrication keep mucous membranes moist and intact.
4. Monitor I&O and vital signs every 8 hours.	Documents progress of treatment regimen.
5. Begin client teaching regarding types of foods that offer source of potassium.	Lasix is a potassium-wasting diuretic. Body cannot store potassium, thus requiring diet supplements rich in potassium (Christensen and Kockrow, 1999).

EVALUATION

- Inspect oral mucous membranes.
- Palpate skin turgor.
- Auscultate blood pressure with client lying, sitting, and standing.
- Measure urine output, and note color of urine with each void.
- Monitor daily laboratory test results.

---

need to be taught how to properly measure and document fluid intake and output. Once a client's discharge has been ordered, it is important that you identify what resources are available for the client. Most health care facilities have a health care team that will assist you in creating appropriate discharge plans for your client. The client's family or significant other and community resources should be evaluated to identify whether they meet the specific needs of your client. For the most part no client should ever be discharged without the capability of continuing his or her regimens and hence the opportunity to return to a state of optimal functioning.

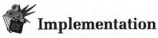

Implementation

HEALTH PROMOTION.   Health promotion activities in the area of fluid, electrolyte, and acid-base imbalances focus primarily on client teaching. Clients and caregivers need to recognize risk factors for these imbalances and implement appropriate preventive measures. For example, parents of infants need to understand that GI losses can quickly lead to serious imbalances; therefore when vomiting or diarrhea occur in the infant, the parent needs to recognize the risk and promptly seek health care to restore normal balance. Even the healthy adult is at risk for developing imbalances when subjected to elevated environmental temperatures. Advise active adults to supplement their fluid loss from perspiration by increasing oral fluids such as water, maintaining adequate environmental ventilation, and refraining from excessive activity during this period of time.

Clients with chronic health alterations are at high risk for developing changes in their fluid, electrolyte, and acid-base balance. They need to understand their own risk factors and measures to take to avoid imbalances. For example, the client with renal failure must avoid excess intake of fluid, sodium, potassium, and phosphorus. Through diet education these clients learn the types of foods to avoid and the volume of fluid they are permitted daily. Clients with chronic diseases need to be made aware of early signs and symptoms of fluid, electrolyte, and acid-base imbalances. For example, a client with heart disease should be instructed to obtain an accurate body weight each day at the approximate same time and to inform the physician of significant changes of weight from one day to another. Increase in weight, shortness of breath, orthopnea, and dependent edema are all associated with fluid retention.

ACUTE CARE. A client with fluid and electrolyte or acid-base imbalance in the acute care setting can be seriously ill. You as the nurse will be expected to manage complex technical skills in the care of your client.

DAILY WEIGHT AND INTAKE AND OUTPUT MEASUREMENT. When implementing specific measures to increase or reduce fluid, two nursing interventions are necessary: daily weight and I&O measurements. Weigh clients with fluid and electrolyte alterations daily. Daily weights are the single most important indicator of fluid status (Horne and others, 1997). Weight should be obtained at the same time each day on a scale that has been calibrated with the client wearing approximately the same clothes. Have the client void before weighing. If a bed scale is used, always apply the same number of bedsheets.

I&O records provide additional information about fluid balance. I&O measurements, when examined for trends, can indicate whether excess fluid volume is excreted in the form of urine or whether excretion of fluids through the kidneys has diminished. The I&O is not as accurate as daily weights in assessing daily fluid balance.

ENTERAL REPLACEMENT OF FLUIDS. Oral replacement of fluids and electrolytes is appropriate as long as the client is not so physiologically unstable that oral fluids cannot be replaced rapidly. Oral replacement of fluids is contraindicated when the client is vomiting, has a mechanical obstruction of the GI tract, is at risk for aspiration, or has impaired swallowing. Clients unable to tolerate solid foods may still be able to ingest fluids.

When replacing fluids by mouth in a client with a fluid deficit, it is wise to choose fluids with adequate calories and electrolyte content (e.g., fruit juices, gelatin, and replacements like Pedialyte and Gastrolyte). However, it is important to remember that liquids containing lactose, caffeine, or low-sodium content may not be appropriate when the client has diarrhea.

A feeding tube may be appropriate when the client's GI tract is healthy but the client cannot ingest fluids (e.g., after oral surgery or with impaired swallowing). Fluids can also be replaced through a gastrostomy or jejunostomy feeding tube, or they can be administered via a small-bore nasogastric feeding tube (Chapter 30).

RESTRICTION OF FLUIDS. Clients who retain fluids and have **fluid volume excess (FVE)** require restricted fluid intake. Fluid restriction is often difficult for clients, particularly if they take drugs that dry the oral mucous membranes or if they breathe through the mouth. You will need to explain the reason fluids are restricted. In addition, the client needs to know the amount of fluid permitted orally and should understand that ice chips, gelatin, and ice cream are considered fluid. The client should help to decide the amount of fluid with each meal, between meals, before bed, and with medications. Frequently clients on fluid restriction can swallow a number of pills with as little as 1 oz (30 ml) of liquid.

A good rule of thumb for fluid restrictions is to allow half of the allotted total oral fluids between 7 AM and 3 PM, the period when clients usually are more active, receive two meals, and take most of their oral medications. An additional two fifths of the allotted total fluid is permitted between 3 PM and 11 PM. This permits fluids with meals and evening visitors. Between 11 PM and 7 AM, the remainder is permitted. It is equally as important that you make sure that clients receive the type of fluids they like best (unless contraindicated). Clients on fluid restriction require mouth care frequently to moisten mucous membranes, to decrease the chance of mucosal drying and cracking, and to achieve comfort.

PARENTERAL REPLACEMENT OF FLUIDS AND ELECTROLYTES. Fluid and electrolytes may be replaced through infusion of fluids directly into the bloodstream. Parenteral replacement includes **total parenteral nutrition (TPN),** IV fluid and electrolyte therapy (crystalloids), and blood and blood component (colloids) administration.

Standard precautions for infection control (Chapter 10) must be practiced when administering parenteral fluids to minimize the risk of exposure to the human immunodeficiency virus (HIV), the cause of acquired immunodeficiency syndrome (AIDS), hepatitis B virus (HBV), and other infectious diseases. Know the policy and procedure of parenteral infusions at the institution where you practice.

Vascular Access Devices.   **Vascular access devices** are catheters, cannulas, or infusion ports designed for long-term repeated access to the vascular system. These devices are more effective than peripherally placed catheters for administering medications and solutions that are irritating to veins and for the delivery of long-term IV therapy. Increased use of central venous catheters and implanted infusion ports requires you to be educated in the care of these devices.

Total Parenteral Nutrition.   TPN is a nutritionally adequate hypertonic solution consisting of glucose and other nutrients and electrolytes given through an indwelling peripheral or central IV catheter. TPN is used as an intervention in severe cases of malnutrition (see Chapter 30).

Intravenous Therapy.   The goal of IV fluid administration is to correct or prevent fluid and electrolyte disturbances. It allows for direct access to the vascular system, permitting the infusion of continuous fluids over a period of time. IV fluid therapy must be continuously regulated because of continual changes in the client's fluid and electrolyte balance. When IV fluid administration is required, you should know the correct ordered solution, equipment needed, and procedures required to initiate an infusion, regulate the infusion rate, maintain the system, identify and correct problems, and discontinue the infusion.

ADMINISTRATION OF INTRAVENOUS THERAPY

Types of Solutions.   Many prepared IV solutions are available for use (Table 14-8). IV solutions fall into the following categories: isotonic, hypotonic, and hypertonic.

In general, isotonic fluids are used most commonly for extracellular volume replacement (e.g., FVD after prolonged vomiting). The decision to use a hypotonic or hypertonic solution is based on the client's specific fluid and electrolyte imbalance. For example, the client with a hypertonic fluid imbalance will generally receive a hypotonic IV to dilute the ECF and rehydrate the cells. All IV fluids should be given carefully, especially hypertonic solutions, because these pull fluid into the vascular space by osmosis, resulting in an increased vascular volume that can lead to pulmonary edema, particularly in clients with heart or renal failure. Isotonic solutions are those that have the same effective osmolality as body fluids and are effectively used to mimic the body's fluid loss in the absence of imbalance, for example, when supporting the client during a surgical procedure.

Certain additives, most commonly vitamins and potassium chloride (KCl), are frequently added to IV solutions. A physician's order includes the IV solution and required additives plus the volume and prescribed infusion time. For example:

Bottle #1: 1000 ml $D_5^1/_2$ NS with 20 mEq KCl and 1 ampule of multivitamins at 125 ml/hr

Clients with normal renal function who are receiving nothing by mouth should have potassium added to IV solutions.

Intravenous Solutions		Table 14-8
Solution	Concentration	Other Names
Dextrose in Water Solutions		
Dextrose 5% in water*	Isotonic	D_5W
Dextrose 10% in water	Hypertonic	$D_{10}W$
Saline Solutions		
0.45% sodium chloride (half normal saline)	Hypotonic	$^1/_2$ NS 0.45% NS
0.9% sodium chloride† (normal saline)	Isotonic	NS 0.9% NS 0.9% NaCl
3%-5% sodium chloride	Hypertonic	3%-5% NS 3%-5% NaCl
Dextrose in Saline Solutions		
Dextrose 5% in 0.9% sodium chloride	Hypertonic	$D_5$0.9% NaCl $D_5$0.9% NS D_5NS
Dextrose 5% in 0.45% NaCl sodium chloride	Hypertonic	$D_5$0.45% NaCl $D_5$0.45% NS $D_5^1/_2$ NS
Multiple Electrolyte Solutions		
Lactated Ringer's‡	Isotonic	LR
Dextrose 5% in lactated Ringer's	Hypertonic	D_5LR

*Dextrose is quickly metabolized, leaving free water to be distributed evenly in all fluid compartments (Horne and others, 1997).
†Although it is isotonic because the total concentration of electrolytes equals plasma concentration, it contains 154 mEq of both sodium and chloride, which is a higher concentration of these electrolytes than is found in the plasma, which can cause FVE (Metheny, 2000).
‡Contains sodium, potassium, calcium, chloride, and lactate.

The body cannot conserve potassium, and even when the serum level falls, the kidneys continue to excrete potassium. If there is no potassium intake orally or parenterally, hypokalemia can develop quickly. Conversely, you must verify that the client has adequate urine output before administering an IV solution containing potassium, because hyperkalemia can quickly develop. *However, under no circumstances can potassium chloride (KCl) be given IV push. A direct IV infusion of KCl is fatal.*

Equipment.   Correct selection and preparation of IV equipment assists in safe and quick placement of an IV line. Because fluids are instilled into the bloodstream, sterile technique is necessary; you must therefore have all equipment organized and at the bedside. IV equipment includes catheters or needles, tourniquet, gloves, dressings, solution containers, various types of tubing, and IV pumps or volume-control devices. Intravenous catheters come in gauges (e.g., 19 gauge, 21 gauge). The larger the gauge size, the smaller is the catheter.

Different types of tubing are used to administer medications or IV fluids. A solution given rapidly needs to be infused with macrodrip tubing, which delivers large drops

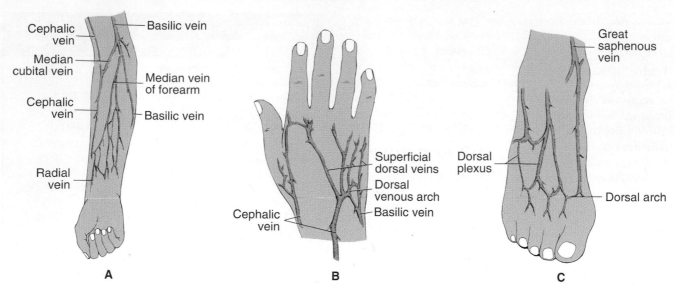

FIGURE **14-5**   Common IV sites. **A,** Inner arm. **B,** Dorsal surface of hand. **C,** Dorsal surface of foot (used for children only).

(standard drop size is 10 or 15 gtt/ml depending on the manufacturer) so that a rapid rate can be maintained. In contrast, microdrip tubing provides a standard drop size of 60 gtt/ml. Microdrip tubing allows precise regulation of IV fluids even at slow rates. In addition, clients may require IV extension tubing to increase mobility or to facilitate changes in position. IV pumps or volume-control devices are used with children, with clients with renal or cardiac failure, or with critically ill clients to prevent sudden uncontrolled rapid infusion of large volumes of fluid.

Initiating the Intravenous Line.   After collecting equipment at the bedside, prepare to insert an IV line by assessing the client for a **venipuncture** site. A venipuncture is a technique in which a vein is punctured through the skin by a sharp rigid stylet (e.g., butterfly needle), an over-the-needle catheter [ONC], or a needle attached to a syringe. Common peripheral IV puncture sites include the hand and the arm (Figure 14-5, *A* and *B*). The use of the foot (Figure 14-5, *C*) for an IV site is common with pediatric clients but is avoided in the adult because of the danger of thrombophlebitis (Pearson, 1996). When you assess the client for potential venipuncture sites for IV infusion, you should consider conditions and contraindications that exclude certain sites. Because very young children and older adults have fragile veins, you should avoid sites that are easily moved or bumped, such as the dorsal surface of the hand. Box 14-4 describes special considerations for initiating IV therapy in older adult clients.

Venipuncture is contraindicated in a site that has signs of infection, infiltration, or thrombosis. An infected site is red, tender, swollen, and possibly warm to the touch. Exudate may be present. An infected site is not used because of the danger of introducing bacteria from the skin surface into the bloodstream. Avoid using an extremity with a vascular (dialysis) graft or fistula or on the same side as a mastectomy. IVs should be placed at the most distal point when possible. Using a distal site first allows for the use of proximal sites later if the client would need a venipuncture site change.

Large intravenous catheters placed into a central vein such as the subclavian vein are used to deliver large volumes of fluids and TPN or to administer irritating medications. Although these catheters are inserted by physicians, you will be responsible for maintaining them.

When veins are fragile or collapse, venipuncture becomes extremely difficult, but it is also a life-saving measure. For these difficult clients, an experienced practitioner should perform venipuncture. The general purposes of venipuncture are to collect a blood specimen, to instill a medication, to start an IV fluid infusion, or to inject a radiopaque or radioactive tracer for special examinations. Skill 14-1 describes venipuncture for IV fluid infusion.

A **peripherally inserted central catheter (PICC)** line provides an alternative intravenous access when the client requires intermediate-length venous access greater than 7 days to 3 months. Using sterile technique, PICC catheters are inserted through a vein in the antecubital fossa and advanced until the tip enters the central venous system. PICC lines may remain in place longer than a peripheral line because there is less risk for infiltration and phlebitis because IV fluids and medication are diluted into the greater amount of blood flow present in the larger veins. PICCs can be used to infuse IV fluids, parenteral nutrition, blood and blood products, and medications such as antibiotics. The smaller-sized catheters cannot be used to infuse blood, blood products, and total parenteral nutrition, and not all PICC lines can be used to draw blood. It is important to check the policy and the product used at your agency before caring for a client with a PICC line (Perry and Potter, 2001). A primary responsibility of the nurse is to keep the sterile dressing intact and to maintain patency of the IV line.

Regulating the Infusion Flow Rate.   After an IV infusion is secured and the line is patent, you must regulate the rate of infusion according to the physician's orders (Skill 14-2). An infusion rate that is too slow can lead to further cardiovascular and circulatory collapse in a critically ill client who has FVD or hyperosmolar imbalance or who is in shock. An IV that is running too slowly can also become clotted off more easily. An infusion rate that is too rapid can result in FVE. Calculate the infusion rate to prevent too-slow or too-rapid administration of IV fluids. The minimal rate used to keep a vein open and patent is about 10 to 15 ml/hr using a microdrip infusion set.

Infusion devices will assist you in maintaining a correct flow rate of IV fluids; many electronic infusion devices record the volume of the fluid infused. An **infusion pump** is designed to deliver a measured amount of fluid over a period of time (e.g., 125 ml/hr). The pump has an electronic drop sensor and an alarm that will sound if drops are not detected at the appropriate rate. There are alarms to alert the nurse to increased system pressure that can occur from a variety of factors (e.g., kinking of IV tubing, infiltration of fluid into surrounding tissue, and clotting off of the IV).

A second type of infusion device is an IV controller (i.e., Dial-a-Flow) that delivers small amounts of fluid with the aid of gravity. The rate of infusion with an IV controller depends on the height of the IV fluid container, IV tubing size, and fluid viscosity. The IV controller is less precise than the IV pump in delivering IV fluids with precision. With either device, the client requires close monitoring to verify the correct infusion of the IV solution and to detect the occurrence of any complication.

Patency of the IV needle or catheter means that there are no clots at the tip of the needle or catheter and that the catheter or needle tip is not against the vein wall. A blocked catheter or needle can affect the rate of infusion of the IV fluids. IV flow rates can also be affected by the patency of the IV needle or catheter, infiltration, a knot or kink in the tubing, the height of the solution, and the position of the client's extremity. You can assess patency by lowering the IV bag below the level of the IV insertion site and observing for a blood return. If no blood return occurs and fluid does not flow easily from the drip chamber when the roller clamp is opened, several problems may exist: a too-tight IV dressing may be impeding the flow, a clot may be occluding the cannula of the HIV catheter, or the catheter tip may be occluded against the wall of the vein. The tubing and area around the insertion site should be inspected for anything that could obstruct the flow of IV fluids. A knot or kink in the tubing can decrease the flow rate. Occasionally the tubing is kinked under a dressing, which requires you to remove the dressing to locate the problem. The flow rate frequently resumes after the tubing is straightened. The client may also occlude the tubing by lying or sitting on it. The height of the IV bag can also affect flow rates. Raising the bag usually increases the rate because of increased hydrostatic pressure.

The position of the extremity, particularly at the wrist or elbow, can decrease flow rates. Occasionally the use of an arm board helps to keep the joint extended and provides some protection to the site. Sometimes it is more comfortable for the client to have an infusion started in a new location rather than dealing with a site that causes problems. However, before discontinuing the infusion hampered by an extremity position, you should start the infusion in another site to verify that the client has other accessible veins.

An infiltration may be present when the insertion site is cool, clammy, swollen, and in some cases painful. An infiltration occurs when the needle or catheter has dislodged from the vein and is in the subcutaneous space. When an infiltration occurs, the IV line must be discontinued and a new line inserted. Factors that alter IV flow rates can occur with any client at any time. When caring for a client with an infusion, you should assess the site and the infusion rate at least every hour.

Text continued on p. 385

Skill 14-1

INITIATING INTRAVENOUS THERAPY

DELEGATION CONSIDERATIONS

The skill of initiating peripheral intravenous therapy should not be delegated to assistive personnel.

EQUIPMENT

- Correct IV solution (with time tape attached).
- Proper IV access devices for venipuncture (will vary with client's body size and reason for IV fluid administration).
- IV start kit (available in some agencies): may contain a sterile drape to place under the client's arm, cleansing and antiseptic preparations, dressings, and a small roll of sterile tape.
- Saline lock (optional).
- Administration set (choice depends on type of solution and rate of administration; infants and children require microdrip tubing, which provides 60 gtt/ml)

- 0.22-μmm filter (if required by agency policy or if particulate matter is likely)
- Extension tubing
- Transparent dressing or 2 × 2 gauze.
- Prepping agent: alcohol, povidone-iodine, or chlorhexidine cleansing swabs or sticks
- Disposable gloves
- Tourniquet (can be a source of contamination; use a single-use product)
- Flush solution (e.g., normal saline or heparin flush solution).
- Arm board (optional)

STEPS	RATIONALE
1. Review physician's order for type and amount of IV fluid and rate of fluid administration. In addition, follow five rights of medication administration (see Chapter 13).	An order requesting the initiation of a peripheral IV access and administration of an IV solution must be made by a physician before the implementation of this procedure.

- *Critical Decision Point*

  In most medical facilities, physicians do not write an order to "initiate peripheral access" or "perform venipuncture." "Start IV" may be written followed by the exact IV therapy order. The order to perform the venipuncture is implied. If the order is confusing or in question, clarify with the physician before proceeding.

STEPS	RATIONALE
2. Assess for clinical factors/conditions that will respond to or be affected by IV fluid administration:	Provides baseline to determine effect IV fluids have on client's fluid and electrolyte balance.
a. Peripheral edema—can be rated for severity by assessing pitting over bony prominences (see Chapter 12).	Indicates expanded interstitial volume. This is usually most evident in dependent areas (i.e., feet and ankles). Fluid overload will worsen edema.
b. Greater than 2% increase or decrease in body weight	Daily weights document fluid retention or loss. Change in body weight of 1 kg corresponds to 1 L of fluid retention or loss (Horne and Swearingen, 1997).
c. Dry skin and mucous membranes	May signal fluid volume excess.
d. Distended neck veins	Suggests fluid volume excess.
e. Blood pressure changes	Elevated blood pressure may indicate volume excess due to increase in stroke volume. Decreased blood pressure may indicate fluid volume deficit due to a decrease in stroke volume.
f. Irregular pulse rhythm; increased pulse rate	Rhythm changes may occur with potassium, calcium, and/or magnesium abnormalities; rate change may occur with fluid volume deficit.
g. Auscultation of crackles or rhonchi in lungs	May signal fluid buildup in the lungs due to fluid volume excess.
h. Inelastic skin turgor (after pinching, fails to return to normal position within 3 seconds)	With fluid volume deficit, the pinched skin stays elevated for several seconds.

- *Critical Decision Point*

  This is a less reliable indicator for older adults because their skin has lost elasticity naturally as a result of aging.

STEPS	RATIONALE
i. Anorexia, nausea, and vomiting	May occur with acute fluid volume deficit or fluid volume excess.
j. Thirst	Symptomatic of fluid volume deficit.

STEPS	RATIONALE
k. Decreased urine output	During dehydration, kidney attempts to restore fluid balance by reducing urine production. Average daily adult urine output is 1500 ml; urine output of less than 400 ml/24 hr (oliguria) signals the retention of metabolic wastes (Horne and Swearingen, 1997).
l. Behavioral changes (e.g., restlessness, confusion)	May occur with fluid volume deficit or acid-base imbalance.
3. Assess client's previous or perceived experience with IV therapy and arm placement preference.	Determines level of emotional support and instruction needed.
4. Obtain information from drug reference books or pharmacist about composition of IV fluids, purposes of administration, potential incompatibilities, and side effects to monitor for.	This allows detection of an inadvisable IV fluid order and helps to determine priority assessments.
5. Determine if client is to undergo any planned surgeries or is to receive blood infusion later.	Allows you to anticipate and place large-sized catheter (e.g., 18 or 16 gauge) for fluid infusion and to avoid placement in area that will interfere with medical procedures.
6. Assess for the following risk factors: child or older adult; presence of heart failure or renal failure, skin lesions, infection, low platelet count or receiving anticoagulants.	Persons at extremes in age develop fluid imbalances more rapidly because they have a proportionately larger extracellular fluid volume; persons with heart failure cannot adapt to sudden increases in vascular volume, and persons with renal failure cannot eliminate excess extracellular fluid. Skin lesions or infection may influence choice of access site. Low platelets or use of anticoagulants increase client's risk for bleeding from IV site.
7. Assess laboratory data and client's history of allergies.	May reveal information that affects insertion of devices, such as fluid volume deficit or allergy to iodine, adhesive, or latex.
8. Prepare client and family by explaining the procedure, its purpose, and what is expected of client. Also explain sensations client is to expect.	Cognitive and sensory information decrease anxiety and help to promote cooperation.
9. Assist client to comfortable sitting or supine position with bed raised to nurse's level.	
10. Wash hands.	Reduces transmission of infection.
11. Organize equipment on clean, clutter-free bedside stand or over-bed table.	Reduces risk of contamination and accidents.
12. Change client's gown to the more easily removed gown with snaps at the shoulder, if available.	Use of a special IV gown facilitates safe removal of the gown once IV has been inserted.
13. Open sterile packages using sterile aseptic technique (see Chapter 10)	Maintains sterility of equipment and reduces spread of microorganisms.
14. Prepare IV infusion tubing and solution.	
a. Check IV solution, using five rights of medication administration (see Chapter 13). Make sure prescribed additives, such as potassium and vitamins, have been added. Check solution for color, clarity, and expiration date. Check bag for leaks, which is best if done before reaching the bedside.	IV solutions are medications and should be carefully checked to reduce risk of error. Solutions that are discolored, contain particles, or are expired are not to be used. Leaky bags present an opportunity for infection and must not be used.
b. Open infusion set, maintaining sterility of both ends of tubing. Many sets allow for priming of tubing without removal of end cap.	Prevents bacteria from entering infusion equipment and bloodstream.
c. Place roller clamp (see illustration) about 2 to 5 cm (1 to 2 inches) below drip chamber and move roller clamp to "off" position (see illustration).	Close proximity of roller clamp to drip chamber allows more accurate regulation of flow rate. Moving clamp to "off" prevents accidental spillage of IV fluid on client, nurse, bed, or floor.

STEPS	RATIONALE
d. Remove protective sheath over IV tubing port on plastic IV solution bag (see illustration).	Provides access for insertion of infusion tubing into solution.
e. Insert infusion set into fluid bag or bottle. Remove protector cap from tubing insertion spike, not touching spike, and insert spike into opening of IV bag (see illustration). Cleanse rubber stopper on bottled solution with antiseptic, and insert spike into black rubber stopper of IV bottle.	Flat surface on the top of bottled solution may contain contaminants, whereas opening to plastic bag is recessed. Prevents contamination of bottled solution during insertion of spike.

- **Critical Decision Point**
  Do not touch spike because it is sterile. If contamination occurs (e.g., spike is accidently dropped on the floor), then discard that IV tubing and obtain a new one.

STEPS	RATIONALE
f. Prime infusion tubing by filling with IV solution: (1) Compress drip chamber and release, allowing it to fill one-third to one-half full (see illustration).	Ensures tubing is cleared of air before connection with IV site. Creates suction effect; fluid enters drip chamber to prevent air from entering tubing.

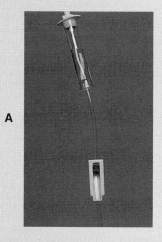 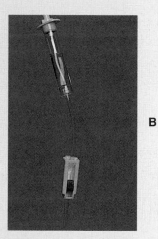

A   B

STEP 14C   A, roller clamp in open position. **B,** roller clamp in closed position.

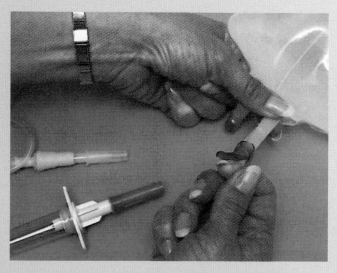

STEP 14D Removing protective sheath from IV bag port.

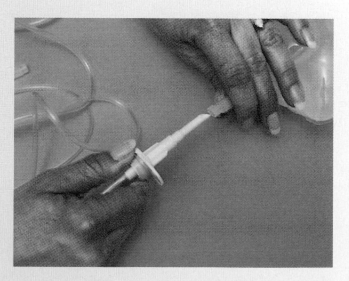

STEP 14E Inserting spike into IV bag.

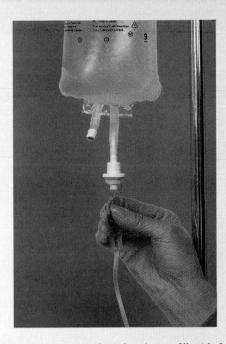

STEP 14F Squeezing drip chamber to fill with fluid.

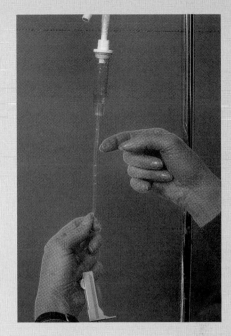

STEP 14H Removing air bubbles from tubing.

g. Remove protector cap on end of tubing (some tubing can be primed without removal) and slowly release roller clamp to allow fluid to travel from drip chamber through tubing to needle adapter. Return roller clamp to "off" position after tubing is primed (filled with IV fluid).

Slow fill of tubing decreases turbulence and chance of bubble formation. Removes air from tubing and permits tubing to fill with solution. Closing the clamp prevents accidental loss of fluid.

h. Be certain tubing is clear of air and air bubbles. To remove small air bubbles, firmly tap IV tubing where air bubbles are located. Check entire length of tubing to ensure that all air bubbles are removed (see illustration). If multiple port tubing is used, turn ports upside down and tap to fill and remove air.

Large air bubbles can act as emboli.

• *Critical Decision Point*
An extra extension tubing may be added to IV tubing to allow for more length, which will enable client to move more freely while still keeping IV line stable.

i. Replace cap protector on end of infusion tubing.

Maintains system sterility.

15. Option: Prepare heparin or normal saline lock for infusion:

a. If a loop or short extension tubing is needed because of an awkward IV site placement, use sterile technique to connect the IV plug to the loop of short extension tubing. Inject 1 to 3 ml normal saline through the plug and through the loop or short extension tubing. Keeps ends sterile until ready to attach to IV device.

Removes air to prevent introduction into the vein. Do the same with the saline plug.

16. Apply disposable gloves. Eye protection and mask may be worn (see agency policy) if splash or spray of blood is possible.

Reduces transmission of microorganisms. Decreases exposure to HIV, hepatitis, and other blood-borne organisms (Centers for Disease Control and Prevention [CDC], 1996b) and prevents spraying of blood on nurse's mucous membranes.

• *Critical Decision Point*
Gloves are not absolutely required to assess accessible veins but must be applied before insertion.

STEPS	RATIONALE
17. Identify accessible vein for placement of IV catheter or needle. Apply flat tourniquet around arm above antecubital fossa (see illustration) or 4 to 6 inches (10 to 15 cm) above proposed insertion site. Do not apply tourniquet too tightly to avoid injury or bruising to skin. Check for presence of radial pulse. Try applying tourniquet on top of a thin layer of clothing such as a gown sleeve. It may become necessary to remove tourniquet and move lower down arm. Consider eliminating tourniquet, apply it loosely, or reduce tourniquet time in older adults (Ellenberger, 1999).	Tourniquet impedes venous return but should not occlude arterial flow. If vein cannot be found in antecubital fossa, move down along arm to locate vessel in lower arm or hand.

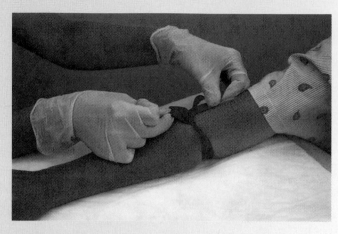

STEP 17   Tourniquet placed on arm for initial vein selection.

STEPS	RATIONALE
18. Select the vein for IV insertion. The cephalic, basilic, and median cubital are preferred in adults.	
a. Use the most distal site in the nondominant arm, if possible.	Venipuncture should be performed distal to proximal, which increases the availability of other sites for future IV therapy.
b. Avoid areas that are painful to palpation.	
c. Select a vein large enough for catheter placement.	Prevents interruption of venous flow while allowing adequate blood flow around the catheter.
d. Choose a site that will not interfere with client's activities of daily living (ADLs) or planned procedures.	Keeps client as mobile as possible.
e. Palpate the vein by pressing downward and noting the resilient, soft, bouncy feeling as the pressure is released. Always use the same fingers to palpate.	Use of the same finger causes a development of sensitivity to better assess the vein's condition (Perucca and Micek, 1993).
f. If possible, place extremity in dependent position.	Permits venous dilation and visibility.
g. Select well-dilated vein. Methods to foster venous distention include:	
(1) Stroking the extremity from distal to proximal below the proposed venipuncture site.	Increases the volume of blood in the vein at the venipuncture site.
(2) Having client alternately open and close the fist.	Muscle contraction increases the amount of blood in the extremity.
(4) Applying warmth to the extremity for several minutes, for example, with a warm washcloth.	Increases blood supply and fosters venous dilation.

• *Critical Decision Point*
Vigorous friction and multiple tapping of the veins, especially in older adults, may cause hematoma and/or venous constriction (Whitson, 1996).

STEPS	RATIONALE
h. Avoid sites distal to previous venipuncture site, veins in antecubital fossa or inner wrist, sclerosed or hardened veins, infiltrate site or phlebotic vessels, bruised areas, and areas of venous valves.	Such sites can cause infiltration of newly placed IV catheter and excessive vessel damage.
i. Avoid fragile dorsal veins in older adult clients and vessels in an extremity with compromised circulation (e.g., in cases of mastectomy, dialysis graft, or paralysis).	Venous alterations can increase risk of complications (e.g., infiltration and decreased catheter dwell time).
19. Release tourniquet temporarily and carefully. Clip arm hair with scissors.	Restores blood flow while preparing for venipuncture. Hair impedes venipuncture or dressing adherence.

STEPS	RATIONALE

- **Critical Decision Point**
  Do not shave area. Shaving may cause microabrasions and predispose to infection.

20. Place needle adapter end of infusion set nearby on sterile gauze or sterile towel.	Permits smooth, quick connection of infusion to IV needle once vein is punctured.
21. (If area of insertion appears to need cleansing, use soap and water first.) Then cleanse insertion site using friction and a circular motion (middle to outward) with antiseptic prep solution; refrain from touching the cleansed site; allow the site to dry for at least 2 minutes (povidone or chlorhexidine) or 60 seconds (alcohol).	Touching the cleansed area would introduce organisms from your hand to the site. Drying prevents chemical reactions between agents and allows time for maximum microbicidal activity of agents (Baranowski, 1993).
22. Place tourniquet 10 to 12 cm (4 to 5 inches) above anticipated insertion site (see illustration). Check presence of distal pulse.	Diminished arterial flow prevents venous filling. The pressure of the tourniquet should cause the vein to dilate.
23. Perform venipuncture. Anchor vein below site by placing thumb over vein and by stretching the skin against the direction of insertion 2 to 3 inches (5 to 7.5 cm) distal to the site (see illustration). Warn client of a sharp, quick stick.	Stabilizes vein for needle insertion. Places needle parallel to vein. When vein is punctured, risk of puncturing posterior vein wall is reduced.

     a. *Over-the-needle catheter (ONC):* Insert with bevel up at 20- to 30-degree angle slightly distal to actual site of venipuncture in the direction of the vein.

     b. *IV catheter with safety device:* Insert using same position as for ONC (see illustration).

     c. *Butterfly needle:* Hold needle at 20- to 30-degree angle with bevel up slightly distal to actual site of venipuncture.

- **Critical Decision Point**
  Only one needle/catheter should be utilized for each attempt at insertion.

24. Look for blood return through flashback chamber of catheter, or tubing of butterfly needle, indicating that needle has entered vein (see illustration). Lower catheter until almost flush with skin. Advance catheter another $1/4$ inch into vein and then loosen stylet. Continue to hold skin taut and advance catheter into vein until hub rests at venipuncture site. *Do not reinsert the stylet once it is loosened.* (If available, advance the safety device by using push-off tab to thread the catheter; see illustration.) Advance butterfly needle until hub rests at venipuncture site.	Increased venous pressure from tourniquet increases backflow of blood into catheter or tubing. Reinsertion of the stylet can cause catheter breakage in the vein.

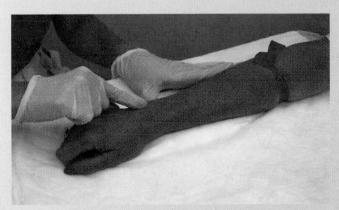

STEP 22   Placement of tourniquet above anticipated insertion site.

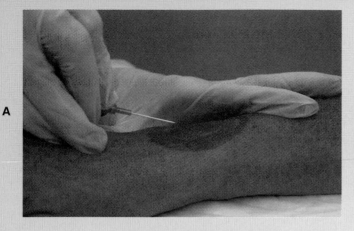
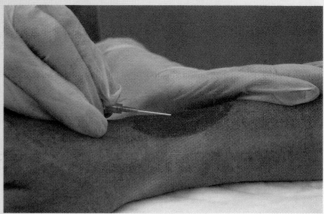

STEP 23B **A,** Illustration of IV catheter with bevel angled 20 to 30 degrees above vein. **B,** IV catheter tip enters vein.

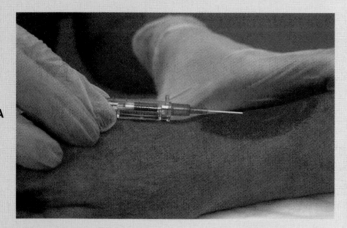
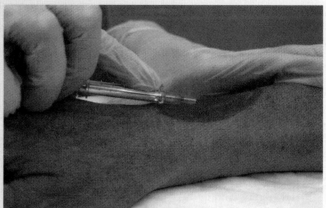

STEP 24 **A,** Blood return indicates catheter placed inside vein. **B,** Advance catheter into vein using one-handed technique with needle guard sliding over introducer.

- **Critical Decision Point**
  No more than three attempts at initiating the IV access should be made by a single nurse.

25. Stabilize catheter/needle with one hand and release tourniquet with other (see illustration). Apply gentle but firm pressure with index finger of nondominant hand 1¼ inches (3 cm) above the insertion site (see illustration). Keep a needle stable. Remove the stylet of ONC. Do not recap the stylet. For a safety device, slide the catheter off the stylet while gliding the protective guard over the stylet. A click indicates the device is locked over the stylet. (NOTE: techniques will vary with each IV device.)

   Permits venous flow, reduces backflow of blood, and allows connection with administration set with minimal blood loss.

26. Quickly connect needle adapter of infusion tubing set (see illustration) or the heparin/saline lock adapter to hub of catheter or butterfly tubing. Do not touch point of entry of needle adapter.

   Prompt connection of infusion set maintains patency of vein and prevents risk of exposure to blood. Maintains sterility.

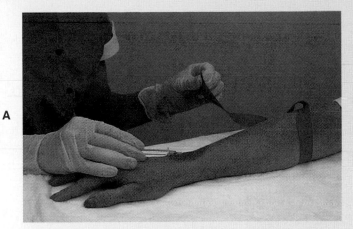

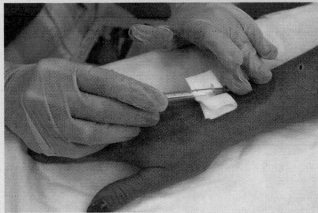

STEP 25 **A,** Stabilize catheter with one hand and release tourniquet with other. **B,** Apply pressure above insertion site while preparing to attach infusion tubing.

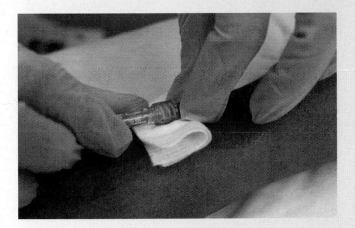

STEP 26   Connect IV tubing adapter to ONC catheter hub.

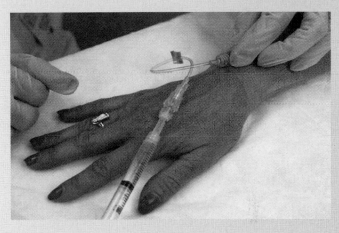

STEP 27   Syringe containing saline flush connected to heparin lock injection cap.

27. *Intermittent infusion:* Hold the sterile heparin/saline lock firmly with nondominant hand. Insert prefilled syringe containing flush solution into injection cap (see illustration). Flush slowly with flush solution. Withdraw the syringe while still flushing.

"Positive-pressure flushing" allows fluid to displace the removed needle, creates positive pressure in the catheter, and prevents reflux of blood during flushing. Stabilizing the cannula prevents accidental withdrawal or dislodgement.

28. *Continuous infusion:* Begin infusion by slowly opening the slide clamp or adjusting the roller clamp of the IV tubing.

Initiates flow of fluid through IV catheter, preventing clotting of device.

• *Critical Decision Point*
  Be sure to calculate rate so as not to infuse IV solution too rapidly or too slowly.

29. Tape or secure catheter needle (procedures can differ; follow agency policy):
   a. Transparent dressing: secure catheter with nondominant hand while preparing to apply dressing.

Prevents accidental dislodgement of catheter.

b. Sterile gauze dressing: Place narrow piece (½ inch) of sterile tape under catheter hub with sticky side up and cross tape over catheter hub (see illustrations). Place tape only on the catheter, never over the insertion site. Secure site to allow easy visual inspection. Avoid applying tape around the arm.

Prevents accidental removal of catheter from vein. Prevents back-and-forth motion, which can irritate the vein and introduce bacteria on the skin into the vein. Adhesive tape is a potential source of bacteria (Redelmeier and Livesley, 1999). Sterile tape should be used close to IV site.

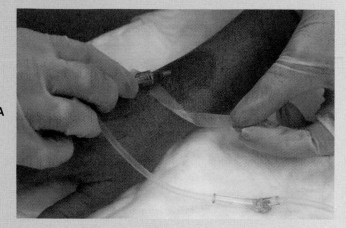
A

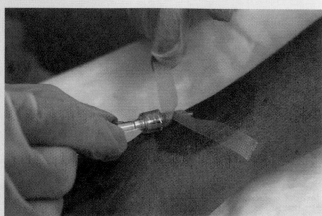
B

STEP 29B   **A,** Slide tape under ONC catheter hub. **B,** Cross tape ends over hub.

30.   Apply sterile dressing over site.
   A. Transparent Dressing
      (1) Carefully remove adherent backing. Apply one edge of dressing, and then gently smooth remaining dressing over IV site, leaving connection between IV tubing and catheter hub uncovered (see illustration). Curl a loop of tubing alongside the arm, and place a second piece of tape directly over the tubing, securing the tubing.

Occlusive dressing protects site from bacterial contamination. Connection between administration set and hub needs to be uncovered to facilitate changing the tubing if necessary. CDC (1996a) no longer recommends application of antimicrobial ointment to catheter site.

   B. Sterile Gauze Dressing
      (1) Fold a 2 × 2 gauze in half and cover with a 1-inch–wide tape extending about an inch from each side. Place under the tubing/catheter hub junction. Curl a loop of tubing alongside the arm, and place a second piece of tape directly over the tubing and padded 2 × 2, securing tubing in two places (see illustration).

Tape on top of gauze makes it easier to access hub/tubing junction. Gauze pad elevates hub off skin to prevent pressure area. Securing loop of tubing reduces risk of dislodging catheter.

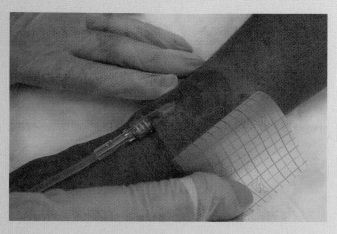

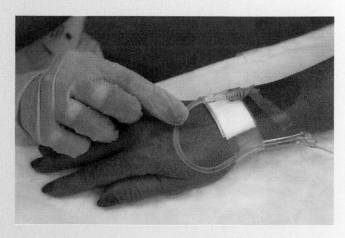

STEP 30 A(1)   Apply transparent dressing over IV site and catheter.

STEP 30B(1)   Place folded 2 × 2 gauze under catheter hub junction and secure loop of tubing with tape.

(2) Place 2 × 2 gauze pad over insertion site and catheter hub. Secure all edges with tape. Do not cover connection between IV tubing and catheter hub.

31. For IV fluid administration recheck flow rate to correct drops per minute (see Skill 14-2).

Manipulation of catheter during dressing application may alter flow rate. Maintains correct rate of flow for IV solution. Flow can fluctuate so it must be checked at intervals if accuracy.

32. Write date and time of IV placement, catheter/needle gauge size on dressing.

Provides immediate access to data as to when IV was inserted and when subsequent dressing changes are needed.

33. Dispose of sheathed stylet or other sharps in appropriate sharps container. Discard supplies. Remove gloves and wash hands.

Reduces transmission of microorganisms and protects staff from infection and injury.

34. Instruct client in how to move about in and out of bed without dislodging IV catheter.

35. Peripheral IV access should be changed every 72 hours (INS, 2000) or per physician orders or more frequently if complications occur. CDC (2001) allows for replacement every 96 hours.

Incidence of complications may be higher when peripheral IV is allowed to remain in a vein over 72 hours. However, Homer and Holmes (1998) studied 722 clients with peripheral IV catheters and found that restarting catheters at 72 hours did not reduce the risk of complication when compared to simply continuing therapy with original catheter.

36. When solution has less than 100 ml remaining, present nursing shift should have new solution at client's bedside and slow flow rate.

This reduces risk of solution emptying during change-of-shift report.

37. Observe client every 1 to 2 hours:
    a. Check if correct amount of IV solution has infused by looking at time tape on IV bag or by checking infusion pump record.

Correct administration of fluid volume prevents fluid imbalance.

    b. Count drip rate (if gravity drip) or check rate on infusion pump.

Accurate monitoring of drip rate further ensures correct volume administration.

    c. Check patency of IV catheter or needle: briefly compress cannulated vein proximal to site. Observe for slowing or momentary cessation of IV rate.

Compression results in mechanical obstruction of vein. When IV catheter is patent, compression results in slowing or cessation of flow rate. No change in flow rate may indicate infiltration.

• *Critical Decision Point*
If IV is positional, fluid will run less slowly or stop depending on position of client's arm. Instruct client to position arm to maintain flow; if this continues, IV may have to be restarted.

    d. Observe client during compression of vessel for signs of discomfort.

Tenderness can be early sign of phlebitis.

    e. Inspect insertion site, note color (e.g., redness or pallor). Inspect for presence of swelling. Palpate temperature of skin above dressing.

Redness of inflammation along with tenderness and warmth indicate vein inflammation or phlebitis. Swelling above insertion site and cool temperature may indicate infiltration of fluid into tissues.

38. Observe client every hour to determine response to therapy (e.g., I&O, weights, vital signs, postprocedure assessments).

IV fluids and additives are given to maintain or restore fluid and electrolyte balance. If I&O, weights, or vital signs change unexpectedly, fluid volume alterations can be serious.

STEPS	RATIONALE
UNEXPECTED OUTCOMES AND RELATED INTERVENTIONS	• If bleeding occurs around venipuncture site and catheter is within vein, gauze dressing may be applied over site. Eventually, IV may need to be discontinued.
■ Fluid volume deficit (FVD) as manifested by decreased urine output, dry mucous membranes, hypotension, tachycardia.	• Blood on the dressing can result when the administration set becomes disconnected from the catheter's hub. When blood appears on the dressing, verify that the system is intact and change the dressing.
• Notify physician; may require readjustment of infusion rate.	
■ Fluid volume excess (FVE) as manifested by crackles in the lungs, shortness of breath, edema.	**RECORDING AND REPORTING**
• Reduce IV flow rate if symptoms appear, and notify physician.	■ Record in nurses' notes number of attempts at insertion, type of fluid, insertion site by vessel, flow rate, size and type catheter or needle, and when infusion was begun. A special parenteral therapy flow sheet may be used.
■ Electrolyte imbalances as manifested by abnormal serum electrolyte levels, changes in mental status, alterations in neuromuscular function, changes in vital signs, and other manifestations.	■ If an electronic infusion device is used, document type and rate of infusion. Include the number on the pump.
• Notify physician. Additives in IV or type of IV fluid may be adjusted.	■ Record client's response to IV fluid, amount infused, and integrity and patency of system every 4 hours or according to agent policy.
■ Infiltration as indicated by swelling and possible pitting edema, pallor, coolness, pain at insertion site, possible decrease in flow rate (Table 14-9, p. 385).	■ Report to oncoming nursing staff: type of fluid, flow rate, status of venipuncture site, amount of fluid remaining in present solution, expected time to hang next IV bag or bottle, and any side effects.
• Stop infusion and discontinue IV. Elevate affected extremity. Restart new IV if continued therapy is necessary.	■ Report to physician adverse reactions such as pulmonary congestion, shock, or thrombophlebitis.
■ Phlebitis is indicated by pain, increased skin temperature, erythema along path of vein (Table 14-10, p. 385).	
• Stop infusion and discontinue IV. Restart new IV if continued therapy is necessary.	
• Place moist warm compress over area of phlebitis.	
■ Bleeding occurs at venipuncture site. Bleeding from vein is usually slow, continuous seepage. Common in clients who have received heparin or have a bleeding disorder or if the IV site is over bend in arm/hand.	

Skill 14-2
REGULATING INTRAVENOUS FLOW RATE

DELEGATION CONSIDERATIONS
The skill of regulating intravenous flow rate should not be delegated to assistive personnel. Assistive personnel should be instructed to report if electronic infusion device alarm sounds.

EQUIPMENT
• Watch with second hand
• Paper and pencil
• IV infusion pump (optional)
• Volume-control device (optional)

STEPS	RATIONALE
1. Check client's medical record for correct solution and additives. Follow five rights of medication administration (Chapter 13). Usual order includes solution for 24 hours, usually divided into 2 or 3 L. Occasionally, IV order contains only 1 L to keep vein open (KVO). Record also shows time over which each liter is to infuse.	Five rights prevent medication administration error.
2. Observe for patency of IV line and catheter or needle:	For fluid to infuse at proper rate, IV line and needle must be free of kinks, knots, and clots.
a. Open drip regulator and observe for rapid flow of fluid from solution into drip chamber, then close drip regulator to prescribed rate.	Rapid flow of fluid into drip chamber indicates patency of IV line. Closing drip chamber to prescribed rate prevents fluid overload.

STEPS	RATIONALE
b. Compress cannulated vein slightly proximal to end of catheter and observe drip chamber.	Compression will temporarily cause cessation of drops from drip chamber, indicating catheter or needle is in vein. If fluid continues to drip, infiltration may be present and further assessment is needed.
3. Check client's knowledge of how positioning of IV site affects flow rate.	Fosters client participation in maintaining most effective position of arm with IV equipment. Position or setting of control clamp or infusion device drip rate should be done only by health care provider.
4. Verify with client how venipuncture site feels; for example, determine if there is pain or burning.	Pain or burning may be early indication of phlebitis. Includes client in decision making.
5. Have paper and pencil to calculate flow rate.	The beginning student is unfamiliar with IV fluid rates and should use mathematical calculations to obtain correct rate.
6. Know calibration (drop factor) in drops per milliliter (gtt/ml) of infusion set: *Microdrip:* 60 gtt/ml *Macrodrip* (Metheny, 2000): Abbott: 15 gtt/ml Travenol: 10 gtt/ml McGaw: 15 gtt/ml	Microdrip tubing, also called pediatric tubing, universally delivers 60 gtt/ml and is used when small or very precise volumes are to be infused. However, there are different commercial parenteral administration sets for macrodrip tubing. Macrodrip tubing should be used when large quantities or fast rates are necessary.

• *Critical Decision Point*
Know which company's infusion set an agency uses.

7. Select one of the following formulas to calculate flow rate after determining ml/hr.

> ml/hr = total infusion (ml)/hours of infusion
> (a) ml/hr/60 min = ml/min
> (b) Drop factor × ml/min = drops/min
> *or*
> (c) ml/hr × drop factor/60 min = drops/min

	Once hourly rate has been determined, these formulas give correct flow rate.
8. Read physician's orders, and follow five rights for correct solution and proper additives.	IV fluids are medications; following five rights decreases chance of medication error.
9. Intravenous fluids are usually ordered for 24-hour period, indicating how long each liter of fluid should run; for example, IV order for client is: *Bottle 1:* 1000 ml D_5W with 20 mEq KCl to run 8 hours *Bottle 2:* 1000 ml D_5W with 20 mEq KCl to run 8 hours *Bottle 3:* 1000 ml D_5W with 20 mEq KCl to run 8 hours *Total 24-hour IV intake:* 3000 ml	Determines volume of fluid that should infuse hourly.

• *Critical Decision Point*
It is common for physicians to write an abbreviated IV order such as: "D_5W with 20 mEq KCl 125 ml/hr continuous." This order implies that the IV should be maintained at this rate until order has been written for IV to be discontinued.

10. Determine hourly rate by dividing volume by hours, for example:	Provides even infusion of fluid over prescribed hourly rate.

> 1000 ml/8 hr = 125 ml/hr

or if 3 L is ordered for 24 hours

> 3000 ml/24 hr = 125 ml/hr

STEPS	RATIONALE
11. Place marked adhesive tape or commercial fluid indicator tape on IV bottle or bag next to volume markings (see illustration)	Time taping IV bag gives nurse visual cue as to whether fluids are being administered over correct period of time. Time tapes should be used for all IV infusions, including those on therapies infused via electronic infusion devices (EIDs).

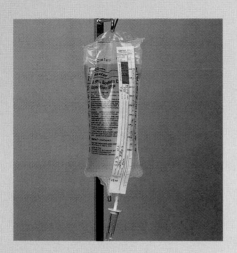

STEP 11   IV fluid bag with time tape.

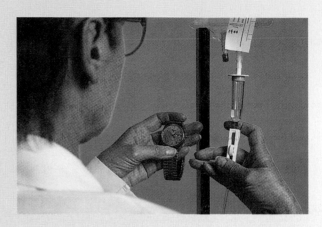

STEP 13   Nurse counts drops infusing.

- *Critical Decision Point*
  Avoid drawing directly on IV bags with felt-tip pens or permanent markers because the ink could contaminate the solution (Millam, 1992).

12. After hourly rate has been determined, calculate minute rate based on drop factor of infusion set. Microdrip infusion set has a drop factor of 60 gtt/ml. Regular drip or macrodrip infusion set used in this example has drop factor of 20 gtt/ml. Using formula (see Step 7), calculate minute flow rates: Bottle 1:1000 ml with 20 mEq KCl over 8 hours.	Allows nurse to calculate minute flow rate based on this formula:
Microdrip:	
125 ml/hr × 60 gtt/ml = 7500 gtt/hr 7500 gtt ÷ 60 minutes = 125 gtt/min	When using microdrip, milliliters per hour always equals gtt per minute.
Macrodrip:	
125 ml/hr × 20 gtt/ml = 2500 gtt/hr 2500 gtt ÷ 60 minutes = 41 gtt/min	
Volume is multiplied by drop factor, and the product is divided by time (in minutes).	
13. Determine flow rate by counting drops in drip chamber for 1 minute by watch, then adjust roller clamp to increase or decrease rate of infusion (see illustration).	Determines if fluids are administered too slowly or too fast.
14. Follow this procedure for infusion controller or pump: a. Place electronic eye on drip chamber below origin of drop and above fluid level in chamber, or consult manufacturer's directions for setup of the infusion (see illustration). If a controller is used, ensure that IV bag is 36 inches above IV site.	Electronic eye counts number of drops flowing from administration set to ensure that proper rate infuses. IV controller works by gravity.

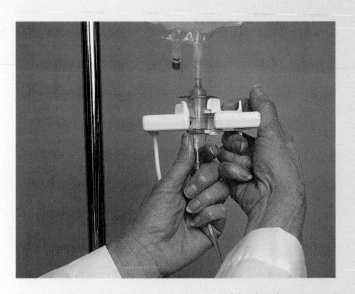

STEP 14A   Place electronic eye on drip chamber.

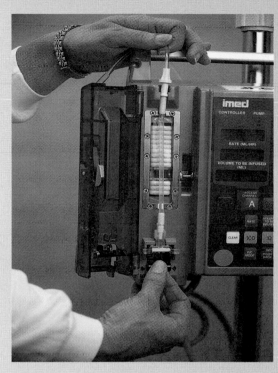

STEP 14B   Place infusion tubing inside infusion pump control box.

STEPS	RATIONALE
b. IV infusion tubing is placed into chamber of control device in direction of flow (i.e., portion of tubing nearest IV bag at top and portion of tubing nearest client at bottom) (see illustration). Consult manufacturer's directions for use of pump (see illustration). Secure portion of tubing through "air in line" alarm system. Turn on pump and select rate per hour and total volume to be infused. Close door to control chamber.	Infusion pumps move fluid by compressing and milking IV tubing, thus propelling fluid through tubing.

• *Critical Decision Point*
Special infusion tubing is required for some pumps. Check agency equipment and associated policies.

STEPS	RATIONALE
c. Open drip regulator completely while infusion controller or pump is in use.	Ensures that pump freely regulates infusion rate.
d. Monitor infusion rates and IV site for infiltration according to agency policy. Rate of infusion should be checked by watch, even when infusion pump is used.	Infusion controllers or pumps are not infallible and do not replace frequent, accurate nursing evaluation. Infusion pumps may continue to infuse IV fluids after an infiltration has begun.
e. Assess patency of system when alarm sounds.	Alarm indicates that electronic eye has not noted precise number of drops from drip chamber. Alarm on infusion pump can be triggered by empty solution bag or bottle, kink in tubing, closed drip regulator, infiltrated or clotted needle, and/or air in the tubing.
15. Follow this procedure for a volume-control device:	
a. Place volume-control device between IV bag and insertion spike of infusion set (see illustration).	Reduces risk of sudden increases in fluid volume.

STEPS	RATIONALE
b. Place 2 hours' allotment of fluid into device.	Prevents IV line from running dry if nurse does not return in exactly 60 minutes. In addition, if there is accidental increase in flow rate, client receives at most only a 2-hour allotment of fluid.
c. Assess system at least hourly; add fluid to volume-control device. Regulate flow rate.	Maintains patency of system.
16. Monitor IV infusion at least every hour, noting volume of IV fluid infused and rate.	Ensures correct volume infuses over prescribed time period.
17. Observe client for signs of overhydration or dehydration to determine response to therapy and restoration of fluid and electrolyte balance.	Signs and symptoms of dehydration or overhydration warrant changing rate of fluid infused.
18. Evaluate for signs of infiltration: inflammation at site, clot in catheter, or kink or knot in infusion tubing.	Prevents decrease or cessation of flow rate.

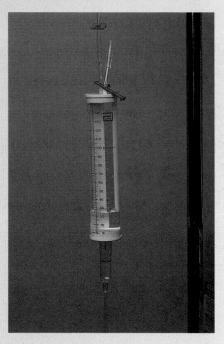

STEP 15   Volume-control device.

UNEXPECTED OUTCOMES AND RELATED INTERVENTIONS

- Sudden infusion of large volume of solution occurs with client having symptoms of dyspnea, crackles in the lung, and increased urine output, indicating fluid overload.
  - Slow infusion to KVO rate, and notify physician immediately. New IV orders will be required. Client may require diuretics.
- IV fluid bag runs empty with subsequent loss of IV line patency.
  - IV will be restarted.
- The IV infusion is slower than ordered.
  - Check client for positional change that might affect rate, height of IV bag, kinking of tubing.
- An infiltration may be developing at IV site. Check condition of site.
- If volume infused is deficient, consult physician for new order to provide necessary fluid volume.

RECORDING AND REPORTING

- Record rate of infusion, drops per minute, and millilieters per hour in nurses' notes or parenteral fluid form every 4 hours or according to agency policy.
- Immediately record in nurses' notes any new IV fluid rates.
- Document use of any electronic infusion device or controlling device and number on that device.
- At change of shift or when leaving on break, report rate of infusion to nurse in charge or next nurse assigned to care for client.

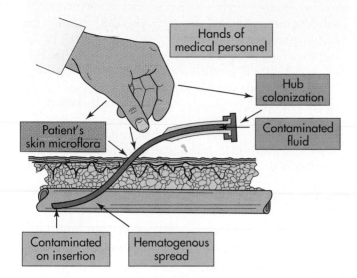

FIGURE **14-6** Potential sites for contamination of an intravascular device.

From Infusion Nurses Society: Intravenous nursing standards of practice, *J Infusion Nurs* 23(6S):S57, 2000.

Infiltration Scale — Table 14-9

Grade	Clinical Criteria
0	No symptoms
1	Skin blanched Edema less than 1 inch in any direction Cool to touch With or without pain
2	Skin blanched Edema 1 to 6 inches in any direction Cool to touch With or without pain
3	Skin blanched, translucent Gross edema greater than 6 inches in any direction Cool to touch Mild to moderate pain Possible numbness
4	Skin blanched, translucent Skin tight, leaking Skin discolored, bruised, swollen Gross edema greater than 6 inches in any direction Deep pitting tissue edema Circulatory impairment Moderate to severe pain Infiltration of any amount of blood product, irritant, or vesicant

Phlebitis Scale — Table 14-10

Grade	Clinical Criteria
0	No clinical symptoms
1	Erythema at access site with or without pain
2	Pain at access site with erythema and/or edema
3	Pain at access site with erythema and/or edema Streak formation Palpable venous cord
4	Pain at access site with erythema and/or edema Streak formation Palpable venous cord greater than 1 inch in length Purulent drainage

From Infusion Nurses Society: Infusion nursing standards of practice, *J Infusion Nurs* 23(6S):S56, 2000.

Children, older adults, clients with severe head trauma, and clients susceptible to volume overload must be protected from sudden increases in infusion volumes. You need to understand that when certain IV controller devices are opened, the IV fluid will infuse rapidly. If this is not controlled, an excessive amount of solution can infuse. Sudden increases can occur accidentally. For example, a restless client may loosen the roller clamp with a sudden movement and increase the flow rate, or the flow rate may be accidentally increased if the client ambulates. A sudden increase in IV infusion rate causes a rapid increase in vascular volume, which can make the client critically ill or even cause death. Volume-control devices can prevent sudden excessive increases in the volume of IV solution infused.

Maintaining the System. After the IV line is in place and the flow rate is regulated, you need to maintain the system. This is achieved by (1) keeping the system sterile; (2) changing solutions, tubing, and site dressings; and (3) assisting the client with self-care activities so as to not disrupt the system.

You will play an important role in maintaining the integrity of an IV to prevent infection from developing. Figure 14-6 demonstrates the potential sites for contamination of an intravascular device. The procedure for IV insertion is designed to minimize the client's microflora on the skin and to reduce contamination by insertion. The other factors are controlled through conscientious ongoing use of infection-control principles. This begins with the use of thorough hand washing before and after you handle any component of the IV system.

The integrity of the IV system must always be maintained. Never disconnect a tubing because it becomes tangled or because it might be more convenient in positioning or moving a client. If a client needs more room to maneu-

ver, extension tubing can be added to an IV line. Stopcocks are available for connecting more than one IV solution to a single IV access site. An IV tubing should be inserted into each port on a stopcock; otherwise the port should be plugged with a sterile cap. Do not allow a port to remain exposed to air.

IV tubing also contains injection ports through which needleless syringe tips or needles can be inserted for medication injection. An injection port must be cleaned thoroughly with 70% alcohol or povidone-iodine solution before accessing the system (Pearson, 1996). Clients receiving IV therapy over several days will require frequent changing of solutions. It is important for you to organize tasks so that this can be done in plenty of time before the solution runs out and possibly becomes clotted. The Centers for Disease Control and Prevention (CDC) (Pearson, 1996) has no recommendations for the hang time of IV fluids; however, you should refer to the policies of the agency where you practice. To prevent entry of bacteria into the bloodstream, sterility must be maintained during tubing and solution changes. Skill 14-3 reviews steps for changing IV solutions.

Generally IV tubing administration sets can remain sterile for 72 hours (Pearson, 1996). The exception is tubing containing blood, blood products, and lipid emulsions, which are more likely to promote bacterial growth. It is recommended to change tubing each time a new IV bag or bottle is being hung (see Skill 14-3). Consult the agency policy where you practice. The dressings over IV sites are applied to reduce the entrance of bacteria into the insertion site. The two forms of dressings are transparent and gauze. Transparent dressings reliably secure the IV device, allow continuous visual inspection of the IV site, become less easily soiled or moistened, and require less frequent changes than standard gauze (Pearson, 1996). Either form of dressing must be changed when the IV device is removed or replaced or when the dressing becomes, loosened, or soiled. Agency policy may require an IV dressing to be changed every 48 to 72 hours (Skill 14-4, p. 390).

To prevent the accidental disruption of an IV system, you may need to assist the client with hygiene, comfort measures, meals, and ambulation. Because a client with an infusion in the arm finds it difficult to meet hygiene needs, you should help or delegate someone to help with bathing and changing gowns. It helps to use a gown specifically made with snaps along the top sleeve seam to facilitate changing the gown without disturbing the venipuncture site. Regular gowns are changed for maximum arm mobility and speed by following these six steps:

1. Remove the sleeve of the gown from the arm without the IV.
2. Remove the sleeve of the gown from the arm with the IV.
3. Remove the IV bottle or bag from its stand and pass it and the tubing through the sleeve. (If this involves removing the tubing from an IV pump, use the roller clamp to slow the infusion to prevent the accidental infusion of a large volume of solution or medication).
4. Place the IV bottle or bag and tubing through the sleeve of the clean gown and hang it on its stand. (If the IV is connected to a pump, resemble and open the roller clamp. Turn the pump on.)
5. Place the arm with the IV through the gown sleeve.
6. Place the arm without the IV through the gown sleeve. (Breaking the integrity of an IV line to change a gown leads to contamination.)

The client with an arm or a hand infusion is able to walk, unless contraindicated. A walking IV pole (a standard IV pole with wheels) is needed. Place the pole next to the involved arm and instruct the client to hold on to the pole with the involved hand and to push it while walking. You should assess the equipment to make sure that the IV bag is at the proper height, that there is no tension on the tubing, and that the flow rate is correct. Once the client returns to bed instruct the client to report any blood in the tubing, a stoppage in the flow, or increased discomfort. IV catheters and drugs, especially antibiotics and potassium, can cause discomfort and burning sensations at the IV site. Reassure clients that occasional discomfort is normal. Sometimes discomfort is relieved by repositioning the extremity, but occasionally it is necessary to start a new IV line in a larger vein.

COMPLICATIONS OF INTRAVENOUS THERAPY.   An **infiltration** occurs when IV fluids enter the subcutaneous space around the venipuncture site. This is manifested as swelling (from increased tissue fluid) and pallor (caused by decreased circulation) around the venipuncture site. Fluid may be flowing through the IV line at a decreased rate or may have stopped flowing. Pain may also be present and usually results from edema and increases proportionately as the infiltration continues.

When infiltration occurs, the infusion must be discontinued and, if IV therapy is still necessary, the catheter or needle is reinserted into another extremity. To reduce discomfort, raise the extremity, which promotes venous drainage, to help decrease the edema. Then it helps to wrap the extremity in a warm towel for 20 minutes, which increases circulation and reduces pain and edema. Heat therapy may be repeated 3 to 4 times during the day.

Phlebitis is an inflammation of the vein. Signs and symptoms include pain, increased skin temperature over the vein, and, in some instances, redness traveling along the path of the vein. Selected risk factors include the type of catheter material, chemical irritation of additives and drugs given IV, and the anatomical position of the catheter. When phlebitis develops, the IV line must be discontinued and a new line inserted in another vein. Warm, moist heat on the site of phlebitis can offer some relief to the client. Phlebitis can be dangerous, because blood clots (thrombophlebitis) can occur and in some cases may result in emboli. The routine removal and rotation of IV sites prevent phlebitis. The CDC recommends replacing peripheral venous catheters and rotating sites every 48 to 72 hours (Pearson, 1996).

An additional complication of IV therapy is FVE. This occurs when IV fluids have infused too rapidly. The assessment findings include shortness of breath, crackles in the lungs, and tachycardia. In the event of these clinical signs, slow the rate of infusion, raise the head of the bed, assess the client's vital signs, and notify the physician.

DISCONTINUING INTRAVENOUS INFUSIONS.   Discontinuing an infusion is necessary after the prescribed amount of fluid has been infused, when an infiltration occurs, if phlebitis is present, or if the infusion catheter or needle develops a clot at its tip. Discontinue an infusion by first

Text continued on p. 393

Skill 14-3

CHANGING INTRAVENOUS SOLUTION AND INFUSION TUBING

DELEGATION CONSIDERATIONS

The skill of changing IV solutions and tubing should not be delegated to assistive personnel.

EQUIPMENT

IV Infusion

• Bottle/bag of IV solution as ordered by physician
• Time tape
• Infusion tubing
• 0.22 μmm filter and extension tubing (if necessary)
• Antiseptic prep (alcohol, povidone-iodine, or chlorhexidine)

Heparin Flush

• Injection cap, loop, or short extension tubing (if necessary)

Normal Saline Flush

• Syringes
• 2 sterile 2 × 2 gauze pads
• Tape
• Disposable nonsterile gloves

STEPS	RATIONALE
Changing IV Solution	
1. Check physician's orders for type of fluid and infusion rate.	Ensures the correct solution will be used.
2. If order is written for keep vein open (KVO) or to keep open (TKO), note date and time when solution was last changed.	A hang time is no longer recommended by the CDC (Pearson, 1996) to ensure sterility of solutions in bag or bottle. Refer to agency policy.
3. Determine the compatibility of all IV fluids and additives by consulting appropriate literature or the pharmacy.	Incompatibilities can cause physical, chemical, and therapeutic client changes.
4. Determine client's understanding of need for continued IV therapy.	Reveals need for client instruction.
5. Assess patency of current IV access site.	If patency is not verified, a new IV access site may be needed. Notify physician.
6. Have next solution prepared at least 1 hour before needed. If prepared in pharmacy, be sure it has been delivered to the client's hospital unit. Check that solution is correct and properly labeled. Check solution expiration date.	Adequate planning reduces risk of clot formation in vein caused by empty IV bag. Checking prevents medication error.
7. Check client's identification by checking arm bracelet and asking client to state name.	Ensures correct solution is administered to correct client.
8. Prepare to change solution when about 50 ml of fluid remains in bottle or bag.	Prevents air from entering tubing and vein from clotting from lack of flow.
9. Prepare client and family by explaining the procedure, its purpose, and what is expected of client.	Decreases anxiety and promotes cooperation.
10. Be sure drip chamber is at least half full.	Provides fluid to vein while bag is changed.
11. Wash hands.	Reduces transmission of microorganisms.
12. Prepare new solution for changing. If using plastic bag, remove protective cover from IV tubing port. If using glass bottle, remove metal cap and metal and rubber disks.	Permits quick, smooth, and organized change from old to new solution.
13. Move roller clamp to stop flow rate.	Prevents solution remaining in drip chamber from emptying while changing solutions.
14. Remove old IV fluid container from IV pole.	Brings work to nurse's eye level.
15. Quickly remove spike from old solution bag or bottle and, without touching tip, insert spike into new bag or bottle.	Reduces risk of solution in drip chamber running dry and maintains sterility.

• *Critical Decision Point*

  If spike is contaminated, a new IV tubing set is required. Sterile IV tubing is good for 72 hours.

16. Hang new bag or bottle of solution.	Gravity assists with delivery of fluid into drip chamber.
17. Check for air in tubing. If bubbles form, they can be removed by closing the roller clamp, stretching the tubing downward, and tapping the tubing with the finger (the bubbles rise in the fluid to the drip chamber). For a larger amount of air, insert syringe into a port below	Reduces risk of air embolus. Use of an air-eliminating filter also reduces this risk.

STEPS	RATIONALE
the air and aspirate the air into the syringe. Swab port with alcohol and allow to dry before inserting syringe into port. Reduce air in tubing by priming slowly instead of allowing a wide-open flow.	
18. Make sure drip chamber is one-third to one-half full. If the drip chamber is too full, pinch off tubing below the drip chamber, invert the container, squeeze the drip chamber, hang up the bottle, and release the tubing.	Reduces risk of air entering tubing.
19. Regulate flow to prescribed rate.	Maintains measures to restore fluid balance and deliver IV fluid as ordered.
20. Observe client for signs of overhydration or dehydration to determine response to IV fluid therapy.	Provides ongoing evaluation of client's fluid and electrolyte status.
21. Observe IV system for patency and development of complications (e.g., infiltration or phlebitis).	Provides ongoing evaluation of IV system.

Changing IV Tubing

STEPS	RATIONALE
22. Determine when new infusion set is needed:	The CDC (Pearson, 1996) recommends tubing change no more often than 72-hour intervals.
a. Agency policy will indicate frequency of routine change for IV administration sets and heparin flushes.	
b. Puncture of infusion tubing.	Punctured tubing results in fluid leakage and bacterial contamination.
c. Contamination of tubing.	Contamination of tubing allows entry of bacteria into client's bloodstream.
d. Occlusions in existing tubing. Such occlusions can occur after infusion of packed red cells, whole blood, albumin, other blood components, or administration of incompatible mixtures.	Whole blood or blood component product can occlude or partially occlude tubing because viscous solutions adhere to walls of tubing and decrease the size of the lumen.
23. Prepare client and family by explaining the procedure, its purpose, and what is expected of client.	Decreases anxiety, promotes cooperation, and prevents sudden movement of extremity, which could dislodge IV needle or catheter.
24. Wash hands.	Reduces transmission of microorganisms.
25. Open new infusion set and connect filter and/or extension tubing, keeping protective coverings over infusion spike and end of tubing.	Provides nurse with ready access to new infusion set and maintains sterility of infusion set.
26. Apply nonsterile, disposable gloves.	Reduces risk of exposure to HIV, hepatitis, and other blood-borne bacteria (CDC, 1987; Garner, 1996).
27. If IV catheter hub or needle is not visible, remove IV dressing. Hold catheter or needle hub securely with nondominant hand. Do not remove tape securing catheter or needle to skin.	Catheter hub must be accessible to provide smooth transition when removing old and inserting new tubing.
28. For IV infusion:	
a. Move roller clamp on new IV tubing to "off" position.	Prevents spillage of solution after bag or bottle is spiked.
b. Slow rate of infusion by regulating drip rate on old tubing. Be sure rate is at KVO rate.	Prevents complete infusion of solution that remains in tubing, which can increase risk of occlusion of IV catheter or needle.
c. With old tubing in place, compress drip chamber and fill chamber.	Provides surplus of fluid in drip chamber so there is enough fluid to maintain IV patency while changing tubing.
d. Remove old tubing from solution and hang or tape drip chamber on IV pole 36 inches above IV pole.	Allows fluid to continue to flow through IV catheter while nurse is preparing new tubing.
e. Place insertion spike of new tubing into old solution bag opening and hang solution bag on IV pole.	Permits flow of fluid from solution into new infusion tubing.

• *Critical Decision Point*
If spike becomes contaminated, a new tubing set is required.

STEPS	RATIONALE
f. Compress and release drip chamber on new tubing; slowly fill drip chamber one-third to one-half full.	Allows drip chamber to fill and promotes rapid, smooth flow of solution through new tubing.

STEPS	RATIONALE
g. Slowly open roller clamp, remove protective cap from needle adapter (if necessary), and flush tubing with solution. Replace cap.	Removes air from tubing and replaces it with fluid.
h. Turn roller clamp on old tubing to "off" position.	Prevents spillage of fluid as tubing is removed from needle hub.
29. For saline/heparin lock:	
a. If a new loop or short extension tubing is needed because of an awkward IV site placement, use sterile technique to connect the new injection cap to the loop or tubing.	
b. Swab injection cap with alcohol. Insert syringe with 1 to 3 ml saline, and inject through the injection cap into the loop or short extension tubing.	Removes air to prevent introduction into the vein.
30. Stabilize hub of catheter or needle, and apply pressure over vein just above insertion site. Gently disconnect old tubing (see illustration *A*). Maintain stability of hub and quickly insert adapter of new tubing or saline lock into hub (see illustrations *B* and *C*).	Prevents accidental displacement of catheter or needle. Prevents clot formation in catheter or needle and backflow of blood.

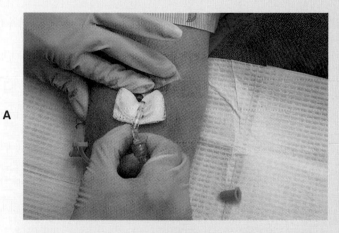

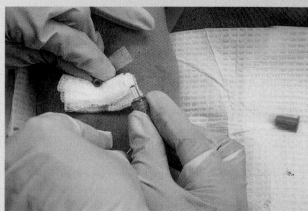

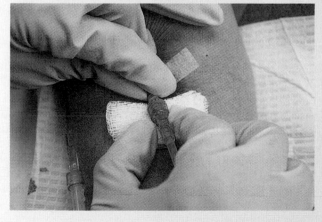

STEP 30 **A,** Stabilize IV catheter while disconnecting old tubing. **B,** Insert tip of new tubing into IV catheter hub. **C,** Be sure tubing tip is firmly inserted into hub.

STEPS	RATIONALE
31. Open roller clamp on new tubing. Allow solution to run rapidly for 30 to 60 seconds.	Permits IV solution to enter catheter to prevent catheter occlusion.
32. Regulate IV drip rate (see Skill 14-2) according to physician's orders and monitor rate hourly.	Maintains infusion flow at prescribed rate.
33. If necessary, apply new dressing. Secure tubing to extremity with tape.	Reduces risk of bacterial infection from skin.
34. Discard old tubing in proper container.	Reduces accidental transmission of microorganisms.
35. Remove and dispose of gloves. Wash hands.	Reduces transmission of microorganisms.

STEPS	RATIONALE
36. Evaluate flow rate hourly, and observe connection site for leakage.	Maintains prescribed rate of flow of IV fluid and determines if fit is secure.
37. Observe client for signs of overhydration or dehydration.	Determines response to IV fluid therapy.

UNEXPECTED OUTCOMES AND RELATED INTERVENTIONS

- Flow rate is incorrect; client receives too little or too much fluid.
  - Readjust infusion rate to ordered rate; evaluate client for adverse effects; notify physician.
- Flow of IV fluid is decreased or absent.
  - Assess IV infusion system for patency.
  - Recalibrate drip rate on new tubing.
  - Assess IV site for infiltration.

RECORDING AND REPORTING

- Record amount and type of fluid infused and amount and type of new fluid according to agency policy. A special flow sheet may be used for parenteral fluids.
- Record changing of tubing and solution on client's record. A special parenteral therapy flow sheet may be used.
- Mark a piece of tape or preprinted label with date and time of tubing change, and attach to tubing below the level of drip chamber.

Skill 14-4
CHANGING A PERIPHERAL INTRAVENOUS DRESSING

DELEGATION CONSIDERATIONS

The skill of changing a peripheral intravenous dressing should not be delegated to assistive personnel. Assistive personnel caring for clients with peripheral IVs should be instructed to report if a client complains of moistness or loosening of an IV dressing.

EQUIPMENT
- Povidone-iodine swab stick
- Alcohol swab stick
- Adhesive remover (if needed)
- Strips of sterile, precut tape
- Disposable gloves

For Transparent Dressing
- Sterile transparent dressing

For Gauze Dressing
- Sterile 2 × 2 gauze pad or
- Sterile 4 × 4 gauze pad

STEPS	RATIONALE
1. Determine when dressing was last changed. Many institutions require nurse to write date and time on dressing and date the device was first placed.	Provides information regarding length of time that present dressing has been in place. In addition, you are able to plan for dressing change.
2. Observe present dressing for moisture and intactness.	Moisture is medium for bacterial growth and renders dressing contaminated. Nonadhering dressing increases risk of bacterial contamination to venipuncture site or displacement of IV catheter.
3. Observe IV system for proper functioning or complications: current flow rate, presence of kinks in infusion tubing or IV catheter. Palpate the catheter site through the intact dressing for subjective complaints of pain or burning.	Unexplained decrease in flow rate requires nurse to investigate placement and patency of IV catheter. Pain can be associated with both phlebitis and infiltration.
4. Inspect exposed catheter site for inflammation and swelling.	Inflammation indicates phlebitis. Swelling indicates infiltration, with fluid infusing into surrounding tissues. These signs require removal of IV catheter.
5. Monitor body temperature.	Elevated temperature may be related to infection at IV site.
6. Assess client's understanding of the need for continued IV infusion.	Reveals need for client instruction.
7. Explain procedure and purpose to client and family. Explain that affected extremity must be held still and how long procedure will take.	Decreases anxiety, promotes cooperation, and gives client time frame around which personal activities can be planned.
8. Wash hands. Apply disposable gloves.	Reduces transmission of microorganisms. Infections related to IV therapy are most often caused by catheter hub contamination, so careful technique must be used throughout the dressing change. Gloves reduce your risk of exposure to HIV, hepatitis, and other blood-borne viruses or bacteria.

STEPS	RATIONALE
9. Remove tape, gauze, and/or transparent dressing from old dressing one layer at a time, leaving tape that secures IV needle or catheter in place. Be cautious if catheter tubing becomes tangled between two layers of dressing. When removing transparent dressing, hold catheter hub and tubing with nondominant hand.	Prevents accidental displacement of catheter or needle.
10. Observe insertion site for signs and/or symptoms of infection, namely redness, swelling, and exudate.	Presence of infection indicates need to discontinue IV at current site.
11. If infiltration, phlebitis, or clot occur or if ordered by physician, discontinue infusion.	
12. If IV is infusing properly, gently remove tape securing needle or catheter. Stabilize needle or catheter with one hand. Use adhesive remover to cleanse skin and remove adhesive residue, if needed.	Exposes venipuncture site. Stabilization prevents accidental displacement of catheter or needle. Adhesive residue decreases ability of new tape to adhere tightly to skin.

- *Critical Decision Point*
  Keep one finger over catheter at all times until tape is replaced for security. It may help to have another staff member assist.

13. Using friction and circular motion, cleanse peripheral IV insertion site with alcohol, povidone-iodine solution and/or chlorhexidine (see illustration), starting at insertion site and working outwards, creating concentric circles. Allow each solution to dry for 2 minutes.	Circular motion prevents cross contamination from skin bacteria near venipuncture site. Povidone-iodine is a topical antiinfective that reduces skin surface bacteria; the solution must be dry to be effective in reducing microbial counts (Baranowski, 1993).

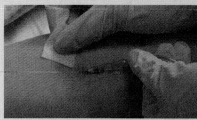

STEP 13   Cleanse insertion site with alcohol swab.

14. Tape or secure catheter.	
a. Applying gauze dressing: Place a narrow piece ($\frac{1}{2}$ inch) of tape under hub of catheter with adhesive side up and cross tape over hub. Place tape only on the catheter, never over the insertion site.	
b. Applying transparent dressing: Secure catheter with nondominant hand while preparing to apply dressing.	

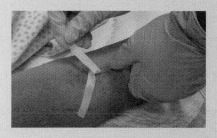

STEP 14A   Cross-over sterile tape to secure IV catheter.

- *Critical Decision Point*
  Do not tape over connection of access tubing or port to IV catheter.

15. Apply sterile dressing over site:	
A. Sterile Gauze Dressing	
(1) Fold a 2 × 2 gauze in half and cover with a 1-inch–wide piece of tape extending about an inch from each side. Place gauze under the tubing/catheter hub junction (see illustration A). Curl a loop of tubing alongside the arm and place a second piece of tape directly over the padded 2 × 2, securing tubing in two places (see illustration B).	Gauze prevents pressure of catheter hub against skin. Securing loop of tubing reduces risk of dislodging catheter from accidental pull.
(2) Place another 2 × 2 gauze pad over the venipuncture site and catheter hub. Secure all edges with tape. Do not cover connection between IV tubing and catheter hub.	Access to catheter hub is needed in times of emergency and when changing tubing.

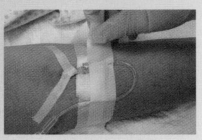

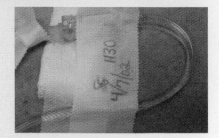

STEP 15(1) **A,** Place a folded 2 × 2 gauze under catheter hub. **B,** Secure dressing and loop of IV tubing.

STEP 18 Date and time on dressing change.

Steps	Rationale
B. Transparent Dressing	
(1) Carefully remove adherent backing. Apply one edge of dressing, and then gently smooth remaining dressing over IV site, leaving end of catheter hub uncovered.	Secures catheter and provides tight dressing seal.
16. Remove and discard gloves.	
17. Anchor IV tubing with additional pieces of tape if necessary. When using transparent dressing, avoid placing tape over dressing.	Prevents accidental displacement of IV needle or catheter or separation of IV tubing from needle adapter.
18. Place date and time of dressing change and size and gauge of catheter directly on dressing.	Documents dressing change.
19. Discard equipment and wash hands.	Reduces transmission of microorganisms.
20. Observe IV flow rate, and compare with rate at time dressing change began.	Validates that IV is patent and functioning correctly.
21. Monitor client's body temperature.	Elevated temperature indicates an infection that may be associated with bacterial contamination of the venipuncture site.

UNEXPECTED OUTCOMES AND RELATED INTERVENTIONS

- IV catheter or needle is infiltrated, as evidenced by decreased flow rate or edema, pallor, or decreased temperature around insertion site.
  - Stop infusion and discontinue IV. Restart new IV in other extremity if continued therapy is necessary. Elevate affected extremity.
- Phlebitis is present, as evidenced by erythema and tenderness along vein pathway.
  - Stop infusion and discontinue IV. Restart new IV in other extremity if continued therapy is necessary.
  - Apply warm moist compress to area of phlebitis.
- IV catheter or needle is accidentally removed.
  - Restart IV if continued therapy is needed.
- Client has an elevated temperature.
  - Notify physician. IV may be removed and restarted. Client will be evaluated for source of infection.

- Insertion site is red and/or edematous and/or painful and/or has presence of exudate, indicating infection at venipuncture site.
  - IV is discontinued. Antibiotic therapy may begin.
  - Apply warm moist compress to area of inflammation.

RECORDING AND REPORTING

- Record in nurses' notes time IV dressing was changed and type of dressing used. Include patency of system and description of venipuncture site.
- Report to nurse in charge or oncoming nursing shift that dressing was changed and any significant information about integrity of system.
- Report to physician any complications.

applying disposable gloves and carefully removing the tape and dressing that is in place. Always stabilize the IV when removing the dressing to minimize client discomfort. Move the roller clamp to the "off" position to prevent spillage of IV fluid, and apply a sterile 2 × 2 gauze pad over the venipuncture site. Using the other hand, withdraw the catheter needle by pulling straight back away from the puncture site (Figure 14-7). Elevate the extremity and apply pressure to the site for 1 to 2 minutes to control bleeding and prevent hematoma formation. Clients who have received heparin require longer pressure because of the action of heparin on blood-clotting mechanisms. If necessary, use alcohol or soap and water to remove dried blood or other drainage. You may need to apply a bandage over the venipuncture site if you believe a small amount of seepage is occurring. You should then record the amount of fluid infused and the time of the discontinuation. Do not forget to go back and check a venipuncture site after you have discontinued an IV, especially if you had to apply a bandage over the wound.

BLOOD REPLACEMENT. Blood replacement or transfusion is the IV administration of whole blood or a component such as plasma, packed red blood cells (RBCs), or platelets. The objectives for blood transfusions include (1) to increase circulating blood volume after surgery, trauma, or hemorrhage; (2) to increase the number of RBCs and to maintain hemoglobin levels in clients with severe anemia; and (3) to provide selected cellular components as replacement therapy (e.g., clotting factors, platelets, or albumin).

Blood Groups and Types. The most important grouping for transfusion purposes is the ABO system, which includes A, B, O, and AB blood types. The determination of blood groups is based on the presence or absence of A and B red cell antigens. Individuals with A antigens, B antigens, or no antigens belong to groups A, B, and O respectively. The person with A and B antigens has AB blood.

Individuals with type A blood naturally produce anti-B antibodies in their plasma. Similarly, type B individuals naturally produce anti-A antibodies. An individual with type O has neither type A nor type B antigen and thus is considered a universal donor. A type AB individual produces neither antibody, which is why type AB individuals can be universal recipients and receive any type of blood. In the event blood that is mismatched with the client's blood is transfused, a **transfusion reaction** occurs. The transfusion reaction is an antigen-antibody reaction and can range from a mild response to severe anaphylactic shock and could be fatal.

Another consideration when matching for blood transfusions is the Rh factor, an antigenic substance in the erythrocytes of most people. A person with the factor is Rh positive, whereas a person without it is Rh negative.

Autologous Transfusion. **Autologous transfusion** (autotransfusion) is the collection and reinfusion of a client's own blood. The blood for an autologous transfusion can be obtained by having the client make preoperative donation weeks before the scheduled procedure, depending on the type of surgery and the ability of the client to maintain an acceptable hematocrit. The blood is tested for HIV and HBV. An autologous transfusion can also be obtained during perioperative blood salvage (e.g., during vascular and orthopedic surgery, organ transplant surgery, and traumatic injuries) and reinfused during the surgery. Blood can also be salvaged postoperatively from mediastinal and chest-tube drains and after joint and spinal surgery. Autologous transfusions are safer for the client because they decrease the risk of complications such as mismatched blood and exposure to blood-borne infectious agents.

BLOOD TRANSFUSIONS. Transfusing blood or blood components is a nursing procedure. It is your responsibility to assess the client before, during, and after the transfusion and for regulation of the transfusion. If the client has an IV line already in place, assess the venipuncture site for signs of infection or infiltration and patency. Determine whether the venipuncture was performed with an 18- or 19-gauge catheter. If a smaller-sized (larger gauge) catheter is present, the IV will likely be restarted. The larger catheter is needed because blood is thicker and stickier than IV fluids. The tubing for blood administration has an in-line filter (Figure 14-8). The tubing should be filled with 0.9% normal saline to prevent **hemolysis** of RBCs.

Information obtained from the client before the transfusion establishes whether the client knows the reason for the blood transfusion and whether the client has ever had a previous transfusion or transfusion reaction. A client who has had a transfusion reaction is usually at no greater risk for a reaction with a subsequent transfusion. However, the client may be anxious about the transfusion, requiring nursing intervention. Before giving a transfusion, check if the client has signed an informed consent. Then explain the procedure to the client and instruct him or her to report any side effects (e.g., chills, dizziness, or fever) once the transfusion begins.

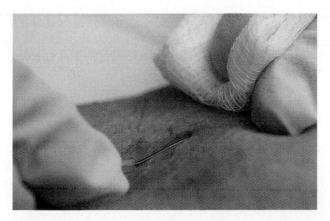

FIGURE **14-7**   IV catheter is withdrawn slowly, keeping catheter parallel to vein.

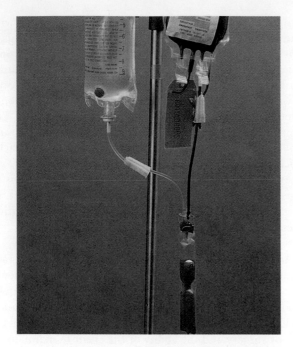

FIGURE **14-8** Tubing for blood administration has an in-line filter.

Nursing Interventions for Blood Transfusion Reaction   Box 14-5

1. If a blood reaction is suspected, STOP the transfusion immediately.
2. Keep the IV line open by "piggybacking" 0.9% normal saline directly into the IV line.
3. Do not turn off the blood and simply turn on the 0.9% normal saline that is connected to the Y-tubing infusion set. This would cause blood remaining in the Y tubing to infuse into the client. Even a small amount of mismatched blood can cause a major reaction.
4. Have the physician notified immediately.
5. Remain with the client, observing signs and symptoms and monitoring vital signs as often as every 5 minutes.
6. Prepare to administer emergency drugs such as antihistamines, vasopressors, fluids, and steroids per physician order.
7. Prepare to perform cardiopulmonary resuscitation.
8. Obtain a urine specimen, and send it to the laboratory.
9. Save the blood container, tubing, attached labels, and transfusion record, and return them to the laboratory.
10. Document the transfusion reaction, how it was treated, and the outcome.

Because of the danger of transfusion reactions, it is very important to use precautions in administering blood or blood products. Obtain the client's baseline vital signs before the transfusion begins. This data will allow you to determine when changes in vital signs occur, which can indicate that a transfusion reaction is developing. To ensure that the right client receives the correct type of blood or blood product, a thorough procedure is used to check the identity of the blood products, the client, and the compatibility of the blood and the client. Although you are not involved in the blood labeling process, you are responsible for determining that the blood delivered to the client corresponds to the client's blood type listed in the medical record. Two registered nurses or one registered nurse and a licensed practical nurse (see agency policy) must together check the label on the blood product against the client's identification number, blood group, and complete name. If even a minor discrepancy exists, the blood should not be given and the blood bank is immediately notified.

Initiation of a transfusion begins slowly to allow for the early detection of a transfusion reaction. Maintain the infusion rate, monitor for side effects, assess the client's vital signs, and promptly record all findings. It is important that you stay with the client during the first 15 minutes, the time when a reaction is most likely to occur. After that time you will need to continue to monitor the client and obtain vital signs periodically during the transfusion as directed by agency policy. If a transfusion reaction is anticipated or suspected, STOP the transfusion immediately, obtain vital signs, and notify the physician.

The rate of transfusion is usually specified in the physician's orders. Ideally a unit of whole blood or packed RBCs is transfused in 2 hours. This time can be lengthened to 4 hours if the client is at risk for FVE. Beyond 4 hours there is a risk of the blood becoming contaminated.

When clients have a severe blood loss such as with hemorrhage, they may receive rapid transfusions through a central venous pressure catheter. A blood-warming device is often necessary, because the tip of the central venous pressure catheter lies in the superior vena cava, above the right atrium. Rapid administration of cold blood can result in cardiac dysrhythmia.

Transfusion Reactions. A transfusion reaction is a systemic response by the body to incompatible blood. Causes include red cell incompatibility or allergic sensitivity to the components of the transfused blood or to the potassium or citrate preservative in the blood. Blood transfusion can also result in the transmission of infectious disease. A second category of reactions includes diseases transmitted by infected blood donors who are asymptomatic. Diseases transmitted through transfusions are malaria, hepatitis, and AIDS. Because all units of blood collected must undergo serological testing and screening for HIV and HBV, the risk of acquiring blood-borne infections from blood transfusions is reduced.

Circulatory overload is a risk when a client receives massive whole blood or packed RBC transfusions for massive hemorrhagic shock or when a client with normal blood volume receives blood. Clients particularly at risk for circulatory overload are older adults and those with cardiopulmonary diseases. Blood transfusion reactions are life threatening, but prompt nursing intervention can maintain the client's physiological stability (Box 14-5).

INTERVENTIONS FOR ACID-BASE IMBALANCES. Nursing interventions to promote acid-base balance support prescribed

HOME INTRAVENOUS THERAPY
- Explain to client and caregiver the importance of IV therapy in maintaining hydration and access for the delivery of medications.
- Emphasize the risks involved when the IV system is not kept sterile.
- Be sure the client and/or caregiver is able to manipulate the required equipment.
- Instruct client or caregiver in how to change IV solutions, tubing, and dressing when they become soiled or dislodged. (NOTE: The home health nurse may be able to visit frequently enough to perform scheduled tubing and dressing changes.)
- Instruct client and caregiver about signs and symptoms of infiltration, phlebitis, and infection and to notify the home health nurse immediately.
- Instruct client and caregiver to notify the home health nurse if the infusion slows or stops or if blood is seen in the tubing.
- Teach client with caregiver's assistance how to ambulate, perform hygiene, and participate in other activities of daily living without dislodging or disconnecting catheter and tubing.
- Instruct client and caregiver how to properly dispose of used infusion equipment.

medical therapies and are aimed at reversing the acid-base imbalance that exists. Such imbalances can be life threatening and require rapid correction. It is important that you maintain a functional IV line and frequently check the physician's orders for new medications or fluids. Prescribed drugs, such as insulin or sodium bicarbonate, fluid and electrolyte replacement, and oxygen supportive therapy should be given promptly.

In addition, you will need to monitor the client closely for changes in acid-base balance. Any client with acid-base disturbances usually needs repeated ABG analysis. This procedure involves obtaining arterial blood samples for analysis of hydrogen ion concentration.

Arterial Blood Gases.   ABG determination requires the removal of a sample of blood from an artery to assess the client's acid-base status and the adequacy of ventilation and oxygenation. Arterial blood is drawn from a peripheral artery (usually the radial) or from an arterial line inserted by a physician. In some agencies, registered nurses are responsible for radial artery punctures. After the specimen is obtained, care is taken to prevent air from entering the syringe because this will affect the blood gas analysis. To reduce metabolism of cells, the syringe is submerged in crushed ice and transported immediately to the laboratory. It is necessary to apply pressure to the puncture site for at least 5 minutes to reduce the risk of a hematoma formation. A longer period of time is needed if the client is on anticoagulant medications. The radial pulse is reassessed after pressure has been removed.

CONTINUING CARE.   After experiencing acute alterations in fluid and electrolyte or acid-base balance, clients

often require ongoing maintenance to prevent a recurrence of health alterations. Older adults and the chronically ill require special considerations to prevent complications from developing.

HOME INTRAVENOUS THERAPY.   IV therapy is often continued in the home setting for clients requiring long-term hydration, parenteral nutrition, or long-term medication administration. A home IV therapy nurse will work closely with the client to ensure that a sterile IV system is maintained and that complications can be avoided or recognized promptly. Box 14-6 summarizes client education guidelines for home IV therapy.

NUTRITIONAL SUPPORT.   Most clients who have had electrolyte disorders or metabolic acid-base disturbances require ongoing nutritional support. Depending on the type of disorder, certain fluids or food may be encouraged or restricted. If clients are still responsible for preparing their own meals, they should learn to look at the lists of the nutrient content of foods and to read the labels of commercially prepared foods.

MEDICATION SAFETY.   Numerous drugs contain constituents or create potential side effects that can alter fluid and electrolyte balance. Clients with chronic disease who are receiving multiple medications and those with renal or liver disorders are at significant risk for alterations to develop. Client and family education is essential to providing information regarding potential side effects or over-the-counter medication to avoid. Review all medications with clients, and encourage them to consult with their local pharmacist each time they try a new over-the-counter medication.

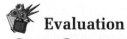

Evaluation

CLIENT CARE.   The evaluation of a client's clinical status is especially important if an acute alteration in fluid and electrolyte or acid-base disturbance exists (Box 14-7). The client's condition can change very quickly, and you must be able to recognize the signs and symptoms of impending problems by integrating the client's presenting clinical status, the effects of the present treatment regimen, and the potential causative agent. The client's assessment is ongoing, and therapies that are initiated are evaluated for their effectiveness. For example, assessment of heart rate and rhythm, muscle tone, bowel sounds, and peripheral sensation can detect if a client with hypokalemia is showing signs of improvement. The physical signs and symptoms of hypokalemia should begin to disappear or lessen in intensity if the hypokalemia is being managed.

For clients with less acute alterations, evaluation likely occurs over a longer period of time. In this situation the evaluation may be focused more on behavioral changes (e.g., the client's ability to follow dietary restrictions and medication schedules). The family's ability to anticipate alterations

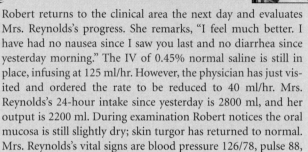

Outcome Evaluation for MRS. REYNOLDS   Box 14-7

Nursing Action	Client Response/Finding	Achievement of Outcome
Inspect oral mucous membranes. Assess skin turgor.	Mucous membranes are moist. Skin recoil is sluggish.	Fluid status improving; continue to support hydration.
Auscultate blood pressure (BP) with Mrs. Reynolds lying, sitting, and standing.	Mrs. Reynolds does not experience any changes in BP while changing positions.	Orthostatic hypotension has improved. Continue to encourage Mrs. Reynolds to get up slowly.
Measure urine output, and note color of urine with each void.	Mrs. Reynolds's urinary output is approximately equal to intake. Urine is dark amber.	I&O appears to have improved. Fluid intake needs to be encouraged. Urine is still dark in color.
Monitor daily laboratory tests results.	Hematocrit and electrolyte levels are all within normal limits.	Laboratory results appear to indicate an improvement. Mrs. Reynolds will need to be encouraged to increase potassium in her diet.

Case Study   EVALUATION

Robert returns to the clinical area the next day and evaluates Mrs. Reynolds's progress. She remarks, "I feel much better. I have had no nausea since I saw you last and no diarrhea since yesterday morning." The IV of 0.45% normal saline is still in place, infusing at 125 ml/hr. However, the physician has just visited and ordered the rate to be reduced to 40 ml/hr. Mrs. Reynolds's 24-hour intake since yesterday is 2800 ml, and her output is 2200 ml. During examination Robert notices the oral mucosa is still slightly dry; skin turgor has returned to normal. Mrs. Reynolds's vital signs are blood pressure 126/78, pulse 88, and respirations 18. She is afebrile. The serum potassium level drawn at 6 AM was 4.0.

Robert tells Mrs. Reynolds he is pleased with her progress. He prepares her breakfast, during which she receives her first soft foods since entering the hospital. Robert plans time to discuss with Mrs. Reynolds the information she has learned from their discussion about food sources for potassium. Robert asks, "After discussing the importance of potassium in your diet, tell me what food you would select that might include potassium." Mrs. Reynolds is again able to identify six different sources of potassium that she would be able to routinely include in her diet.

DOCUMENTATION NOTE

Client denies nausea and reports feeling better. No diarrhea stool since yesterday morning. On inspection, oral mucosa remains dry, without lesions or inflammation. Skin turgor is normal. Bowel sounds are normal in all four quadrants, and abdomen is soft to palpation. IV of 0.45% normal saline is infusing in left forearm at 125 ml/hr, without tenderness or inflammation at site. Client is able to identify six food sources for potassium to include in her diet. Client left resting comfortably, out of bed in a chair, family at the bedside. Will continue to monitor.

and prevent problems from recurring is also an important element to evaluate.

The client's level of progress determines whether you need to continue or revise the plan of care. It is more than likely that you will need to communicate with the other members of the health care team about interventions that have and have not been successful. If goals are not met as a result of the failure to meet expected outcomes, you may have to increase the frequency of an intervention (e.g., provide more fluids to a dehydrated client), introduce a new therapy (e.g., initiate insertion of an IV), or discontinue a therapy (e.g., consult with physician in discontinuing a diuretic). Once outcomes have been met, you can resolve the nursing diagnosis and focus on other priorities.

CLIENT EXPECTATIONS.   Routinely review if you have met the client's expectations of care. For example, ask the client, "Tell me if I have helped you feel more comfortable." If the client's concerns involve having a better understanding of a chronic problem, you may need to evaluate the client's satisfaction with instruction. Often the client's level of satisfaction with care also depends on your success in involving family and friends. If the client has concerns about returning home or to a different care setting, it is important to evaluate if the client feels prepared for the transition from acute care. Acknowledge these fears and concerns, and give honest and clear explanations.

Listening attentively to your clients and their families or significant others will assist you in planning and providing appropriate care. Often they are fearful of potential dangers that exist and the sense they have of not knowing what to expect. Providing them with opportunities to ask questions and seek affirmation is part of the nursing care you will deliver.

Key Terms

active transport, *p. 351*
aldosterone, *p. 352*
angiotensin, *p. 352*

anion gap, *p. 356*
anions, *p. 350*
antidiuretic hormone (ADH), *p. 352*
autologous transfusion, *p. 393*
buffer, *p. 353*

cations, *p. 350*
colloid osmotic pressure, *p. 351*
concentration gradient, *p. 350*
dehydration, *p. 352*
diffusion, *p. 350*

Key Concepts

- Body fluids are distributed in ECF and ICF compartments.
- Body fluids are composed of electrolytes, cells, and water.
- Body fluids are regulated through fluid intake, output, and hormonal regulation.
- Volume disturbances include isotonic and osmolar deficits and excesses.
- Electrolytes are regulated by dietary intake and hormonal controls.
- Chronic and serious illnesses increase the risk of fluid, electrolyte, and acid-base imbalances.
- Clients who are very young or very old are at greater risk for fluid, electrolyte, and acid-base imbalances.
- Assessment for fluid, electrolyte, and acid-base alterations includes the nursing history; physical and behavioral assessment; measurements of I&O; daily weights; and specific laboratory data such as measurement of serum osmolality, serum electrolytes, BUN, urine specific gravity, and ABG levels.
- FVD and osmolar imbalances can be corrected by enteral or parenteral administration of fluid.
- Common complications of IV therapy include infiltration, phlebitis, infection, FVE, and bleeding at the infusion site.
- Blood transfusions are given to replace fluid volume loss from hemorrhage, to treat anemia, or to replace coagulation factors.
- Administration of blood or blood products requires you to follow a specific procedure to identify transfusion reactions quickly.
- In addition to transfusion reactions, the risks of transfusion include hyperkalemia, hypocalcemia, FVE, and infection.
- Treatment for electrolyte disturbances includes dietary and pharmacological interventions.
- Acid-base balance depends on the hydrogen ion concentration in the blood.
- Acid-base imbalances are buffered by chemical, biological, and physiological buffering systems, especially the lungs and kidneys.
- The body's chemical buffering system responds first to acid-base abnormalities.
- Respiratory acidosis is characterized by increased carbon dioxide and hydrogen ion concentrations.
- Respiratory alkalosis is characterized by decreased carbon dioxide and hydrogen ion concentrations.
- Metabolic acidosis is characterized by a decrease in bicarbonate level and increase in hydrogen ion concentration.
- Metabolic alkalosis is characterized by an increase in bicarbonate level and decrease in hydrogen ion concentration.
- The goals of therapy for acid-base imbalances are to treat the underlying illness and to restore the arterial pH to normal.

Critical Thinking Activities

1. Mr. St. John is admitted to the hospital after his wife found him confused, with an increase in his breathing and a fever. She states, "He has had a terrible cold for 2 weeks now." His temperature is 102° F, heart rate 110, respirations 30, and blood pressure 128/64. His serum electrolyte levels are within normal limits, and his ABG analysis reveals the following: pH 7.25, PO_2 88, PCO_2 55, and HCO_3^- 24. What does Mr. St. John's ABG analysis indicate? Why would the physician order a chest x-ray examination for Mr. St. John? If left untreated, could Mr. St. John's problem be life threatening?

2. Justin is receiving IV fluids because he is NPO after surgery earlier today. His IV fluid order is 1000 ml lactated Ringer's with 20 mEq KCl to run over 8 hours. What IV tubing should be used to administer these fluids in terms of drop size? The nurse hangs a new bag of IV fluids at 5 PM. At 8 PM, the nurse notes that 375 ml has infused from the bag. Are these fluids on time?

3. While starting an IV, Alexandra begins to advance the ONC and notes that the area immediately around the insertion site is swelling. What should she do?

Review Questions

1. A client has been admitted to the hospital with a history of gastroenteritis for 3 days. Her arterial blood gas levels on admission are pH 7.31, $PaCO_2$ 35; HCO_3^- 17, and PaO_2 90. You correctly understand this client's acid-base imbalance is:
   1. metabolic acidosis.
   2. respiratory acidosis.
   3. metabolic alkalosis.
   4. respiratory alkalosis.

2. A 20-year-old student is seen at the college's health center complaining of the feeling of difficulty catching his breath and dizziness. You note that his respiratory rate is elevated and that he appears anxious. Your next action would be to:
   1. call 911.
   2. obtain a past drug history.
   3. have him take slow deep breaths in a brown paper bag.
   4. speak with the roommate to learn what happened before this incident.

3. A client with a history of hypertension who has been taking a non–potassium-sparing diuretic is seen at her physician's office for a routine checkup. The nurse practitioner learns that she has been experiencing fatigue and muscle weakness for the last few weeks but attributes these symptoms to the recent flu shot. The laboratory test you would expect is for levels of:
   1. CO_2 protein.
   2. sodium and chloride.
   3. potassium and blood glucose.
   4. hemoglobin and hematocrit.

4. The client at greatest risk for fluid volume excess is a:
   1. 20-year-old client with a 3-year history of diabetes mellitus.
   2. 86-year-old client with a fractured pelvis scheduled for surgery.
   3. 49-year-old client with second-degree burns on the hands and feet.
   4. 60-year-old client with a recent diagnosis of congestive heart failure.

5. While planning care for a client with a history of respiratory acidosis, the nursing diagnosis you would include is:
   1. anxiety related to stress.
   2. ineffective breathing pattern related to hyperventilation.
   3. impaired gas exchange related to inadequate ventilation.
   4. high risk for injury related to nervous system excitability.

6. A client has the following arterial blood gas levels: pH 7.55, $PaCO_2$ 22, and HCO_3^- 24. You would expect the physician to order:
   1. oxygen at 2 L.
   2. sodium bicarbonate 1 amp every 12 hours.
   3. potassium chloride 20 mEq in $\frac{1}{2}$ normal saline.
   4. respiratory exercises to reduce the client's respiratory rate.

7. When providing for a client's hydration status, you would initiate:
   1. providing a variety of fluids at frequent intervals.
   2. seven glasses of ice chips every 3 to 4 hours.
   3. fluids when the client express the sensation of thirst.
   4. a new intake and output flow sheet with each nursing shift.

8. A client is seen at a local health clinic complaining of dry mucous membranes, a 3-day history of vomiting, and feeling light-headed when getting out of bed this morning. You understand correctly that the client's feeling of light-headedness is known as:
   1. supine hypotension.
   2. adapted hypotension.
   3. orthostatic hypotension.
   4. situational hypotension.

References

Baranowski L: Central venous access device: current technologies, users, and management strategies, *J Intraven Nurs* 16(3):167, 1993.

Beare PG, Myers JL: *Adult health nursing*, ed 3, St. Louis, 1998, Mosby.

Centers for Disease Control and Prevention: Recommendations for prevention of HIV in health care settings, *MMWR Morb Mortal Wkly Rep* 36 (suppl 25):35, 1987.

Centers for Disease Control and Prevention: Guidelines for prevention of intravascular device-related infections, *Infect Control Hosp Epidemiol* 17(7):438, 1996a.

Centers for Disease Control and Prevention: Hospital Infection Control Practices Advisory Committee: Guidelines for isolation precautions in hospitals, *Am J Infect Control* 24:24, 1996b.

Christensen B, Kockrow E: *Foundations of nursing*, ed 3, St. Louis, 1999, Mosby.

Ellenberger A: Starting an IV line. *Nursing 99,* March, 56-59, 1999.

Garner J: Guideline for isolation precautions in hospitals, *Infect Control Hosp Epidemiol* 17(1):53, 1996.

Homer LD, Holmes KR: Risks associated with 72- and 96-hour peripheral intravenous catheter dwell times, *J Intraven Nurs* 21(5):301, 1998.

Horne MM, Swearingen PL: *Mosby's pocket guide series: fluid, electrolyte, and acid-base balance*, ed 3, St. Louis, 1997, Mosby.

Ignatavicius DD and others: *Medical-surgical nursing across the health care continuum*, ed 3, St. Louis, 1999, Mosby.

Intravenous Nurses Society: Intravenous nursing standards of practice, *J Intraven Nurs* 21(15):535, 1998.

Infusion Nurses Society: Infusion nursing standards of practice, *J Intraven Nurs* 23(65):556, 2000.

Lewis SM and others: *Medical-surgical nursing: assessment and management of clinical problems*, ed 5, St. Louis, 1999, Mosby.

McCance KL, Huether SE: *Pathophysiology: the biologic basis for disease in adults and children*, ed 2, St. Louis, 1998, Mosby.

McKenry LM, Salerno E: *Pharmacology in nursing*, ed 21, St. Louis, 2001, Mosby.

Metheny N: *Fluid and electrolyte balance: nursing considerations*, ed 4, Philadelphia, 2000, Lippincott.

Meyer-Gaspar P: Water intake of nursing home residents, *J Gerontol Nurs* 25(4):23, 1999.

Millam DA: Starting IVs: How to develop your venipuncture experience, *Nursing* 22(9):33, 1992.

O'Grady and others: Draft guidelines for the preventin of intravascular catheter-related infections, Healthcare Infection Control Practices Advisory Committee, CDC, 2001. htp://www.cdc.gov/ncidod/hip/IV.

Pearson ML: Hospital Infection Control Practices Advisory Committee: Guideline for prevention of intravascular-device–related infections, *Infect Control Hosp Epidemiol* 17(7):438, 1996.

Perucca R, Micek J: Treatment of infusion related phlebitis: review and nursing protocol, *J Intraven Nurs* 16:5, 286, 1993.

Perry A, Potter P: *Clinical Nursing Skills and Techniques*, ed 5, St. Louis, 2001, Mosby.

Redelmeier DA, Livesley NJ: Adhesive tape and intravenous catheter associated infections, *J Gen Intern Med,* 14:373, 1999.

Whitson M: Intravenous therapy in the older adult: special needs and considerations, *J Intraven Nurs* 19:251, 1996.

Wong D and others: *Whaley and Wong's nursing care of infants and children*, ed 6, St. Louis, 1999, Mosby.

Caring in Nursing Practice

Objectives

- Define key terms.
- Discuss the role that caring plays in building a nurse-client relationship.
- Compare and contrast theories on the concept of caring.
- Describe ways to convey caring through communication.
- Discuss the potential implications when nurses' and clients' perceptions of caring might differ.
- Describe how providing presence can be applied when performing a nursing procedure.
- Describe the therapeutic benefit of listening to clients' stories.
- Explain the relationship between knowing a client and clinical decision making.

CLINICAL SCENARIO

Mrs. Levine has terminal ovarian cancer and has been having trouble with low back pain. Sue, her nurse, comes to her room and takes the hand lotion from her bedside stand. Sue puts a lot of lotion on her hands, warns Mrs. Levine that it might feel cold—apologizing for it—and gently massages the client's lower back. As Sue performs the massage she speaks to Mrs. Levine, offering gentle encouragement and spending time just listening to what Mrs. Levine has to say. Sue knows that Mrs. Levine does not talk about her feelings easily and uses the back rub to give the client a chance to talk. Once the massage is finished, Sue assists Mrs. Levine in finding a comfortable position in bed.

In this clinical scenario, Sue demonstrates an act of **caring** through her words and actions. Caring is central to nursing practice, but perhaps it has never been more important because the health care environment seems to become more hectic and fast paced day by day. The pressure and time constraints characteristic of most health care settings can create the risk of nurses' and other health professionals' becoming cold and indifferent to clients and their needs. Technological advances often come first in health care, with little regard for the interpersonal connections that are critical in therapeutic client relationships. Benner and Wrubel (1989) warn that technological advances can be dangerous and inappropriate without a context of skillful and compassionate care. It is time to value and embrace the caring practices and expert knowledge that are an important part of nursing practice.

THEORETICAL VIEWS ON CARING

Caring is a universal phenomenon that influences the way we think, feel, and behave in relation to one another. Caring in nursing has been studied from a variety of philosophical and ethical perspectives since the time of Florence Nightingale. A number of nursing scholars have developed theories on caring because of its importance not only to the practice of nursing, but also to the existence of humankind. This chapter does not detail all of the theories on caring, but it should help beginning nurses understand that caring is at the heart of a nurse's ability to work with people in a respectful and therapeutic way.

Caring Is Primary

Benner and Wrubel (1989) suggest that caring is a basic way of being in the world. After spending considerable time studying the clinical stories of expert nurses, Benner (1984) describes the essence of excellent nursing practice, which is caring. Caring means that persons, events, projects, and things matter to people. It is a word for being connected. Because caring determines what matters to a person, it describes a wide range of involvements, from parental love to friendship, from caring for one's work to caring for one's pet, to caring for and about one's clients. Our ability to care reveals what is stressful for each of us and the available options we have for coping. If something does not matter to an individual, it will not likely create stress or the need for coping. For example, if you as a nurse have little concern for a client suffering severe pain, the experience will not likely direct you to take timely, compassionate action. Benner and Wrubel (1989) note: "Caring creates possibility." Personal concern for some person or thing provides motivation and direction for people. The personal concern of caring in nursing practice allows nurses to help clients to recover in the face of illness, to give meaning to that illness, and to maintain or reestablish connection. Caring makes nurses notice which interventions are successful, and this concern then guides future caregiving activities.

Clients are not all the same. Each brings a different background of experiences, values, and cultural perspectives to a health care encounter. Caring is always specific and relational for each nurse-client meeting. As you acquire more nursing experience, you will learn that caring helps you to focus on the client for whom you care. Caring facilitates your ability to know a client, allowing you to recognize a client's problems, to find solutions, and to implement those solutions (Benner and Wrubel, 1989).

In addition to their work in understanding caring, Benner and Wrubel (1989) describe the relationship between health, illness, and disease. Health is not the absence of illness, nor is illness identical with disease. Health is a state of being that people define in relation to their own values, personality, and lifestyle. Health exists along a continuum (see Chapter 1). Illness is the experience of loss or dysfunction, whereas disease is the manifestation of an abnormality at the cellular, tissue, or organ level. A client may have a disease (e.g., arthritis or diabetes) but not experience the sense of being ill. An individual does not seek health care until there is a disruption, loss, or concern. For example, a client may have had diabetes for a number of years but not sense being ill until the disease begins to cause serious visual impairment, threatening the ability to work. Illness therefore has meaning within the context of the person's life. Any symptoms a person feels are experienced as interruptions or a health worry.

Benner and Wrubel (1989) argue that since illness is the human experience of loss or dysfunction, any treatment or intervention given without consideration of its meaning to the individual is likely to be worthless. Expert nurses understand the difference between health, illness, and disease. Through caring relationships, nurses learn to listen to clients' stories about their illness so that an understanding of the meaning of illness can be obtained. With this understanding, therapeutic, client-centered care can be provided.

The Essence of Nursing and Health

From a **transcultural** perspective Madeleine Leininger (1978) describes the concept of care as the essence and dominant domain that distinguishes nursing from other health disciplines. Care is an essential human need, necessary for the health and survival of all individuals. Care, unlike cure, is oriented to assisting an individual or group in improving a human condition. Acts of caring refer to the direct or indirect **nurturant** and skillful activities, processes, and decisions that assist people in ways that are empathetic, compassionate, and supportive and that are dependent on the needs, problems, and values of the individual being assisted. Leininger's studies (1988) of numerous cultures around the world have found that care is essential for well-being, health, growth, survival, and facing handicaps or death. Care is vital to recovery from illness and to the maintenance of healthy life practices.

Leininger (1988) stresses the importance of nurses' understanding both universal and nonuniversal folk and professional caring behaviors to be effective in the care of clients. Even though human caring is a universal phenomenon, the expressions, processes, and patterns of caring vary among cultures. For example, the Papua New Guinean people of Melanesia value surveillance and protection as basic elements of care, whereas Southern rural African-Americans in the United States value concern and support as care. Caring is very personal, and thus its expression will differ for each client. For caring to achieve cure, you as a nurse must learn those culturally specific behaviors that reflect human care processes for clients in different cultures (see Chapter 16).

Transpersonal Caring

Clients and their families should be able to expect a high quality of human interaction from nurses. Unfortunately, many of the conversations that occur between clients and their nurses are very brief and oftentimes disconnected. Watson's theory of caring (1979, 1988) describes a consciousness that allows nurses to raise questions about what it means to be a nurse, to be ill, and to be caring and healing. Watson's transpersonal caring theory (1988) rejects the disease orientation to health care and places care before cure. Caring therefore becomes the ethical standard by which nursing care is measured. Caring preserves human dignity in a cure-dominated health care system.

In Watson's view, caring becomes almost spiritual. A nurse communicates caring-healing through the conscious-ness of the nurse to the individual being cared for (Watson, 1988). Caring-healing consciousness takes place during a single caring moment between nurse and client. An interconnectedness forms between the one cared for and the one caring. Both the nurse and the client are influenced by the transaction, for better or for worse. The caring-healing consciousness can promote healing and release a person's own inner power and resources.

Swanson's Theory of Caring

In the development of her caring theory, Swanson (1991) conducted interviews with three different groups: women who had miscarried, parents and professionals in a newborn intensive care unit, and socially at-risk mothers who had received long-term, public health intervention. All groups were in a perinatal (before, during, or after the birth of a child) situation or context and had experienced the phenomenon of caring. Each group was asked questions about how caring was experienced or expressed in their situation. Swanson's theory of caring is a composite of the three studies. The theory describes caring as consisting of five processes (Table 15-1). Swanson defines caring as a nurturing way of relating to a valued other toward whom one feels a personal sense of commitment and responsibility. The theory supports the claim that caring is a central nursing phenomenon but not necessarily unique to nursing practice.

The contributions by Swanson (1991) are valuable in providing direction for how to develop useful and effective caring strategies. Each of the caring processes has definitions and subdimensions that serve as the basis for nursing interventions. For example, if a caring-based nurse counseling

Swanson's Theory of Caring   Table 15-1

Caring Process	Definitions	Subdimensions
Knowing	Striving to understand an event as it has meaning in the life of the other	Avoiding assumptions Centering on the one cared for Assessing thoroughly Seeking cues Engaging the self or both
Being with	Being emotionally present to the other	Being there Conveying ability Sharing feelings Not burdening
Doing for	Doing for the other as he or she would do for the self if it were at all possible	Comforting Anticipating Performing skillfully Protecting Preserving dignity
Enabling	Facilitating the other's passage through life transitions (e.g., birth, death) and unfamiliar events	Informing/explaining Supporting/allowing Focusing Generating alternatives Validating/giving feedback
Maintaining belief	Sustaining faith in the other's capacity to get through an event or transition and face a future with meaning	Believing in/holding in esteem Maintaining a hope-filled attitude Offering realistic optimism "Going the distance"

From Swanson K: Empirical development of a middle-range theory of caring, *Nurs Res* 40(3):161, 1991.

program for at-risk mothers were developed, the researcher would develop strategies to help nurses learn how to know and be with clients, based on the subdimensions of caring. Future research is needed to determine if Swanson's caring theory applies to other populations of clients.

Summary of Theoretical Views

There are common themes in nursing caring theories. Caring is highly relational. The nurse and the client enter into a relationship that is much more than one person simply "doing tasks for" another. There is a mutual give-and-take that develops as nurse and client begin to know and care for one another. Frank (1998) described a personal situation when he was suffering from cancer: "What I wanted when I was ill, was a mutual relationship of persons who were also clinician and client." It was important for Frank to be seen as one of two fellow human beings, not the dependent client being cared for by the expert technical clinician.

Caring may seem highly invisible at times when a nurse and client enter a relationship of respect, concern, and support. The nurse's empathy and compassion become a natural part of every client encounter. However, when caring is absent, it becomes very obvious. For example, if you show disinterest or choose to avoid a client's request for assistance, your inaction will quickly convey an uncaring attitude. Benner and Wrubel (1989) relate the story of one expert clinical nurse specialist who learned from a client what caring is all about: "I felt that I was teaching him a lot, but actually he taught me. One day he said to me (probably after I had delivered some well-meaning technical information about his disease), 'You are doing an OK job, but I can tell that every time you walk in that door you are walking out.'"

Clients can quickly tell when you fail to relate to them. In contrast, when caring is practiced, the client senses a commitment on your part and is willing to enter into a relation-ship that allows you to gain an understanding of the client and his or her experience of illness. In a study of oncology clients, one participant described a nurse's caring as "putting the heart in it" and "having an investment" that makes "clients feel that you are with them" (Radwin, 2000). Caring allows you to become a coach and partner rather than a detached provider of nursing care.

Another common theme is understanding the context of the person's life and illness. It is difficult to show caring to other individuals without gaining an understanding of who they are and their perception of their illness. With experience you will appreciate the value of learning about the client's situation: How was the illness first recognized? How did the client feel? How does the illness affect the client's daily life practices? What values and beliefs influence the client's response? Knowing the context of a client's illness helps you as the nurse to choose and individualize interventions that will actually help the client. This approach will be more successful than simply selecting interventions on the basis of the client's symptoms or disease process.

CLIENTS' PERCEPTIONS OF CARING

Swanson's theory of caring (1991) is an excellent beginning to understanding the behaviors and processes that characterize caring. Other researchers have studied caring from clients' perceptions (Table 15-2). The identification of those behaviors that clients perceive as caring helps to emphasize what clients expect from their caregivers. Clients have always valued nurses' effectiveness in performing tasks, but clearly clients also value the affective dimension of nursing care (Williams, 1997). Establishing a reassuring presence, recognizing an individual as unique, and keeping a close, attentive eye on the client are recurrent caring behaviors that researchers have identified. All clients are unique; however,

Nursing Care Behavior (as Perceived by Clients)			Table 15-2
Riemen (1986)		Brown (1986)	Radwin (2000)
Perceptions of Female Clients	Perceptions of Male Clients	Perceptions of Hospitalized Adult Clients	Perceptions of Cancer Clients
Responding to client's uniqueness	Being physically present so client feels valued	Providing a reassuring presence	Expressing concern
Being perceptive and supportive of client's concerns	Returning voluntarily without being called	Providing information	Being nurturant
Being physically present	Making client feel comfortable, relaxed, and secure	Demonstrating professional knowledge and skill	Remembering the client
Having attitudes and displaying behaviors that make client feel valued as a human being	Attending to comfort and needs of client before doing tasks	Assisting with pain	Individualization—selecting therapies more likely to feel nurturing
Return to client voluntarily without being asked	Using a kind, soft, pleasant, gentle voice and attitude	Taking more time than actually needed	Being attentive
Showing concern that is comforting and relaxing		Promoting autonomy	
Using a soft, gentle voice		Recognizing individual qualities and needs	
Invoking feelings of security		Keeping client under watch	
Invoking feelings in client of wanting to reciprocate			

understanding common behaviors that clients associate with caring will help you learn to express caring in practice.

The study of clients' perceptions is important because health care organizations place great emphasis on client satisfaction (see Chapter 2). What clients experience in their interactions with institutional services and health care professionals, and what they think of that experience, will determine how clients use the health care system and how they will benefit from it (Gerteis and others, 1993). When clients sense that health care providers are interested in them as people, it is likely clients will be more willing to follow recommendations and therapeutic plans. Williams (1997) studied the relationship between clients' perceptions of four dimensions of caring (physical, interpretive, spiritual, and sensitive) and their satisfaction with nursing care. Clients indicated that they were most satisfied when they perceived nurses to be caring. Sensitive caring was the strongest predictor of client satisfaction. As institutions look for ways of improving client satisfaction, creating an environment of caring is a necessary and worthwhile goal. Clients' satisfaction with nursing care is the most important factor in their decision to return to a hospital (Risser, 1975; Bader, 1988).

As you begin your clinical practice, it is important to consider how clients perceive caring and what are the best approaches to providing care. The behaviors that researchers have associated with caring offer an excellent starting point. But it is also important to understand clients and their unique expectations. Researchers have learned that clients and nurses often differ in their perceptions of caring (Mayer, 1987). For that reason you must build a relationship that allows you to know what is important to the client. A client who is fearful of having an intravenous (IV) catheter inserted may benefit more if you acquire assistance from a staff member who can quickly and skillfully insert the catheter than if you attempt to relieve anxiety through a lengthy description of the procedure. Knowing who clients are will help you to select those caring approaches that are most appropriate to the clients' needs.

CARING IN NURSING PRACTICE

It is impossible to prescribe ways for you to become a caring professional. There is disagreement as to whether caring can be taught or is more fundamentally a way of being in the world. For those who find caring a normal part of their life, caring is a product of their culture, values, beliefs, experiences, and relationships with others. Persons who do not experience care in their lives often find it difficult to act in caring ways. As nurses deal with health and illness in their practice, they grow in the ability to care. Expert nurses understand the differences and relationships among health, illness, and disease and become able to see clients in their own context, to interpret their needs, and to offer caring acts that improve clients' health. Caring is not a separate act that you perform. Caring is embedded within each encounter and each action that you share with a client.

Providing Presence

To provide presence is to have a person-to-person encounter that conveys a closeness and sense of security. The ability to provide presence, to be with another person in a way that acknowledges one's shared humanity, is at the core of nursing as a caring practice (Benner and Wrubel, 1989). Presence is more than mere physical presence, although the physical closeness is important. Presence also represents being "in tune" with each other, an awareness of each individual's uniqueness (Simons, 1987).

Eye contact, body language, voice tone, listening, and having a positive and encouraging attitude are all part of establishing presence. Openness and understanding are a result of providing presence. You convey the message that the client's experience matters to you (Swanson, 1991). In the opening clinical scenario in which Sue provides her client a massage, Sue's gentle encouragement and willingness to listen conveyed a presence that allowed the client to express her feelings. Being able to establish presence with a client enhances your ability to learn from the client. As a result your ability to provide adequate and appropriate nursing care is strengthened each time you are with the client.

It is especially important to establish presence when clients are experiencing stressful events or situations. Awaiting a doctor's report of test results, preparing for an unfamiliar procedure, and planning for a return home after serious illness are just a few examples of events in the course of a person's illness that can create unpredictability and dependency on care providers. You presence can help to allay anxiety and fear related to stress. Giving reassurance and thorough explanations about a procedure, remaining at the client's side, and coaching the client through the experience all convey a presence that is invaluable to the client's well-being.

Comforting

Clients face situations that can be embarrassing, frightening, painful, and exhausting. Whatever the feeling or symptom, clients look to nurses to provide comfort. **Comforting** provides both an emotional and physical calm.

The use of touch is one comforting approach whereby you reach out to clients to communicate concern and support. Touch may involve holding a client's hand, giving a back massage, or gently positioning a body part. Because touch can convey many messages, you must use it with discretion.

Comforting also involves the skillful and gentle performance of a nursing procedure. An expert nurse learns that any procedure is more effective when it is administered carefully and in consideration of any client concern. If a client is anxious about having a procedure, such as the insertion of a nasogastric tube, you afford comfort by offering an explanation of the procedure that answers the client's questions and concerns. Some clients dislike lengthy explanations, so it is important to know what the client wishes to learn about the procedure. In addition, comfort is associated with your expressed confidence in being able to perform the procedure safely and successfully. For example, the confidence you show when preparing supplies, positioning the client, and gently manipulating and inserting the nasogastric tube helps the client to relax and feel more at ease. Throughout a procedure talk quietly with the client to provide reassurance and support.

Chapters 26 and 29 review principles of hygiene and comfort. Both chapters describe measures that can be used to comfort a client. However, it is not simply the "doing for" that is comforting; rather, it is a comforting approach that should be emphasized. For example, a client who is undergoing chemotherapy may suffer fatigue and have ulcerative lesions of the mouth. Anyone can provide mouth care. However, for the mouth care to be comforting, choose a time, outside of a routine, that best meets the client's needs. Perhaps time the mouth care to coincide with 30 minutes after an analgesic has been administered. Provide gentle, cleansing mouth care, dim the room lights, reposition the client, and offer some encouraging words to allow the client to rest peacefully.

Listening

Caring involves an interpersonal interaction that is much more than two persons simply talking back and forth. In a caring relationship you learn to establish trust, open lines of communication, and listen to what the client has to say (Figure 15-1). Listening is key because it can convey your full attention and interest. Listening to the meaning of what a client says helps create a mutual relationship.

When individuals become ill, there usually is a story about the meaning of their illness. Any critical or chronic illness affects a client's life choices and decisions. Being able to tell that story helps the client break the distress of illness. To tell a story one needs a listener. Frank (1998) described his own feelings during his experience with cancer, emphasizing the need to be able to express what he needed. The personal concerns that are part of a client's illness story determine what is at stake for the client. Caring for a client enables you to be a participant in the client's life. You must be able to give clients your undivided, full attention while their stories are told. Listening should not be simply a task, but instead a gift; otherwise its efficacy is lost (Frank, 1998).

When an ill person chooses to tell his or her story, it involves reaching out to another human being. Telling the story implies a relationship that can develop only if the clinician exchanges personal stories as well. Frank (1998) argues that professionals do not routinely take seriously their own need to be known as part of a clinical relationship. Yet, unless the professional acknowledges this need, there is no reciprocal relationship, only an interaction (Campo, 1997). There is pressure on the clinician to know as much as possible about the client without allowing a relationship to develop, but this isolates the clinician from the client. By contrast, in knowing and being known each supports the other (Frank, 1998). As a clinician you will hear and share a variety of stories from clients. To show that you are listening, you may tell parts of your own stories but do so in response to the ill person's story. For example, when a client tells a story about how the client's family is reacting to his or her illness, you might choose to share a personal family story that enforces a sense of hope as to how a family is able to cope with illness. To give the gift of listening is to appreciate receiving the gift of a client's story and to then share a part of yourself.

Learning to listen to a client is sometimes difficult. It is easy to become distracted by the tasks at hand and colleagues shouting instructions. However, the time you take to listen (and listen effectively) is worthwhile both in the information gained and in the strengthening of the nurse-client relationship. Listening involves paying attention to the individual's words and tone of voice and entering the client's world. By observing the expressions and body language of the client, you can find cues to help assist the client in exploring ways to achieve greater peace, to take action, or to do whatever a situation requires (Hungelmann and others, 1996). Chapter 8 discusses additional listening techniques.

Knowing the Client

One of the five caring processes described by Swanson (1991) is knowing the client. To know a client means that you must avoid assumptions, center on the client, and engage in a caring relationship with the client that reveals information and cues that facilitate critical thinking and clinical judgment. Knowing is a central aspect of nursing practice that develops in the everyday practical work of client care: getting a grasp of the client, getting situated into what is occurring clinically, and understanding the client's situation in context of the illness and the effects it has on the client's life (Tanner and others, 1993). The concept comprises both the nurse's understanding of a specific client and the nurse's ability to then select appropriate nursing interventions (Radwin, 1995). Knowing the client is at the core of clinical decision making. It is always specific to what can be known in the nurse-client-family interaction and clinical context (Tanner and others, 1993). The mutuality that develops from establishing a caring relationship helps you to better know the client as a unique individual and to then choose the most appropriate and effective nursing therapies.

The caring relationship, coupled with your growing knowledge and experience, provide a rich source of meaning when there are clinical changes in a client. Expert nurses develop the ability to detect changes in clients' conditions almost effortlessly. A nurse learns to recognize particular responses and patterns: the effect of a slight change

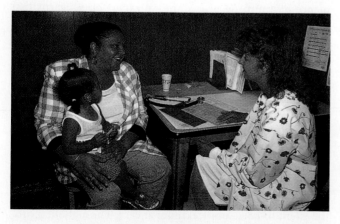

FIGURE 15-1 Nurse listening to client.

in an antihypertensive drug on a client's blood pressure, the effect of physical turning on the client's heart rate, and the avoidance of conversation as a client's pain increases. Clinical decision making involves various aspects of knowing the client: responses to therapies, routines, and habits, coping resources, physical capacities and endurance, and body typology and characteristics (Tanner and others, 1993). Additional factors that the experienced nurse knows about clients are their experiences, behaviors, feelings, and perceptions (Radwin, 1995). When clinical decisions are made accurately in the context of knowing a client well, improved client outcomes will result. Swanson-Kaufman (1986) notes that when care is based on knowing the client, it is perceived by clients as personalized, comforting, supportive, and healing.

Knowing a client is much more than simply gathering data about the client's clinical signs and condition. Although this information must be gathered, success in knowing the client lies in the relationship that is established. To know a client is to enter into a caring, social process that results in a "bonding" whereby the client comes to feel known by you (Lamb and Stempel, 1994). The bonding then sets the stage for the relationship to evolve into "working" and "changing" phases in which you can help the client to become involved in personal care and to accept help when needed.

Spiritual Caring

Remen (1988) suggests that healing is not a matter of mechanism, such as treatments or medications, but rather a work of spirit. It is an individual's intrinsic spirit that seems to be a factor in the healing process. Spiritual health is achieved when a person finds a balance between personal life values, goals, and belief systems and those of others. Research has shown a link between spirit, mind, and body. An individual's beliefs and expectations can and do have effects on the person's physical well-being (Coe, 1997).

Establishing a caring relationship with a client involves an interconnectedness between the nurse and the client. This is the reason why Watson (1979) describes the caring relationship in a spiritual sense. Spirituality offers a sense of connectedness as well, intrapersonally (connected with oneself), interpersonally (connected with others and the environment), and transpersonally (connected with the unseen, God, or a higher power). When a caring relationship is established, the client and the nurse come to know one another and move toward a healing relationship by:

1. Mobilizing hope for the client and for the nurse
2. Finding an interpretation or understanding of illness, symptoms, or emotions that is acceptable to the client
3. Assisting the client in using social, emotional, or spiritual resources

Chapter 17 describes in detail the significance that spirituality plays in an individual's health.

Family Care

People inhabit their worlds in an involved way. Each individual experiences life through relationships with others. Caring for an individual therefore cannot occur in isolation from that person's family. As a nurse, it is important for you to know the family almost as thoroughly as you know a client (Figure 15-2). The family is an important resource. Success with interventions often depends on the family's willingness to share information about the client, their acceptance and understanding of therapies, whether the interventions fit with the family's daily practices, and whether the family can support and deliver the therapies recommended.

Mayer (1986) identified 10 nurse caring behaviors that were perceived as most helpful by families of clients with cancer (Box 15-1). Ensuring the client's well-being and helping the family to become active participants are critical for family members. Although specific to families of clients with cancer, the behaviors offer useful guidelines for developing caring relationships with all families. Early in the nurse-client relationship, ask who are members of the client's family and what their roles are in the client's life. Showing the family that you care about the client creates an openness that enables a relationship to form with them. Caring for the family takes into consideration the context of the client's illness and the stress it imposes on all members.

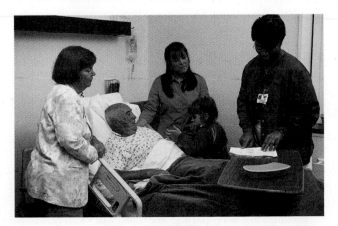

FIGURE 15-2 Nurse discusses client's health care needs with family.

Nurse Caring Behaviors as Perceived by Families   Box 15-1

Being honest
Giving clear explanations
Keeping family members informed
Trying to make the client comfortable
Showing interest in answering questions
Providing necessary emergency care
Assuring the client that nursing services will be available
Answering family members' questions honestly, openly, and willingly
Allowing clients to do as much for themselves as possible
Teaching the family how to keep the client physically comfortable

Data from Mayer DK: Cancer patients' and families' perceptions of nurse caring behaviors, *Top Clin Nurs* 8(2):63, 1986.

THE CHALLENGE OF CARING

Caring is a motivating force for people to become nurses, and it becomes the source of satisfaction when nurses know they have made a difference in their clients' lives. It is becoming more of a challenge to care in today's health care system. Being a part of the helping professions is difficult and demanding. Nurses are given less time to spend with clients, making it much harder to know who they are. Leininger (1988) notes that advanced technology also threatens human concerns. A reliance on technology and cost-effective health care strategies and efforts to standardize and refine work processes all undermine the nature of caring. Too often clients become just numbers, with their real needs either overlooked or ignored.

Morrison (1989) surveyed nurses' perceptions about themselves as professional carers. Although the study involved only a small number of experienced nurses, the results posed some interesting questions for all nurses. The nurses were asked to compare "themselves" with an "ideal self" in regard to eight different characteristics: compassionate, safe, selfish, lacking awareness, empathetic, insecure, tolerant, and kind. Any differences between perceptions of "themselves" and the "ideal self" suggested a need for personal change. The study found discrepancies, with nurses perceiving themselves as lacking certain skills within their caring role. Morrison described various reasons that might explain the discrepancies. The nurses might have set unrealistic expectations for themselves, making it difficult to live up to standards. The group also might have lacked appropriate training or knowledge for the caring role. Most important, the system of values prevalent within their "organizational culture" might have differed from the values held by the nurses working in that organization. When organizations fail to reinforce and provide ways for nurses to practice caring, nurses are less likely to meet their personal expectations.

Recently the Tri-Council for Nursing (2001), an organization representing an alliance of the American Nurses Association (ANA), National League for Nursing (NLN), American Organization of Nurse Executives (AONE), and American Association of Colleges of Nursing (AACN), has recommended strategies to reverse the current nursing shortage. A number of the strategies can potentially create work environments that enable nurses to demonstrate more caring behaviors. The strategies include introducing greater flexibility into the work environment structure, rewarding experienced nurses who serve as mentors, improving nurse staffing, and providing nurses with sufficient autonomy over their practice in all settings.

Human beings cannot be treated like machines or robots if health care is to make a positive difference in their lives. Instead, health care must become more humanizing. As a professional, you play an important role in making care an integral part of health care. This begins by making caring a part of the philosophy and environment in the workplace. Incorporating care concepts into standards of nursing care establishes the guidelines for professional conduct. Finally, you must be committed to caring and be willing in your day-to-day practice to establish relationships with clients and families that afford personal, compassionate, and meaningful nursing care.

Key Terms

caring, *p. 400*
comforting, *p. 403*
nurturant, *p. 400*
transcultural, *p. 400*

Key Concepts

- According to Benner, *caring* is a word for being connected and is the essence of excellent nursing practice.
- Because illness is the human experience of loss or dysfunction, any treatment or intervention given without consideration of its meaning to the individual is likely to be worthless.
- Leininger stresses the importance of understanding that even though human caring is universal, the patterns and expressions of caring vary among cultures.
- Watson's transpersonal caring theory rejects the disease orientation to health care and places care before cure.
- Swanson's theory of caring includes five caring processes: knowing, being with, doing for, enabling, and maintaining belief.
- Caring is highly relational, involving a mutual give-and-take between you and the client.

- To care for another individual, you must understand the context of the person's life and illness.
- Clients' perceptions of nurses' caring include establishing a reassuring presence, recognizing an individual as unique, and keeping a close, attentive eye on the client.
- Clients tend to be more satisfied with nursing care when they perceive that nurses care.
- Knowing a client allows you to select caring approaches appropriate to the client's needs.
- When you establish presence, eye contact, body language, voice tone, listening, and having a positive and encouraging attitude act together to create openness and understanding.
- Comforting involves the use of touch and the skillful and gentle performance of nursing care procedures.
- Listening involves paying attention to an individual's words and tone of voice and entering into his or her frame of reference.

- Knowing the client is at the core of the process by which nurses make clinical decisions.
- When clinical decisions are made in the context of knowing a client well, improved client outcomes will result.
- You demonstrate caring by helping family members become active participants in a client's care.

Critical Thinking Activities

1. Lindsey is a student nurse assigned to care for Mrs. Lowe, a 62-year-old client being treated for lymphoma (cancer of the lymph nodes). The charge nurse informs Lindsey that the nurse who does intravenous procedures will be up shortly to insert a long-term, percutaneous intravascular catheter for Mrs. Lowe's chemotherapy. This is the first day Lindsay has cared for Mrs. Lowe, but she has learned that the client has not had an intravenous line previously. In what way can Lindsay express caring for Mrs. Lowe during the procedure?
2. During your next clinical practicum, select a client to talk with for at least 15 to 20 minutes. Ask the client to tell you about his or her illness. Review the skills of listening in this chapter and in Chapter 8. Immediately after your discussion, reflect on the discussion with the client and answer the following questions: What do you believe the client was trying to tell you about the illness? Why was it important for the client to share this story? What did you do that made it easy or difficult for the client to talk with you? Would you rate yourself a good listener? If not, why not? If so, explain.
3. The next time you are assigned to a clinical agency, ask to read the agency's philosophy and standards of care documents. Does the language in the documents convey a caring environment for practice.

Review Questions

1. As part of your work in a teen pregnancy clinic you talk with a young teenage client about her experience in relationships with young men. The teen faces how to talk with her boyfriend about the use of a condom during intercourse. You respond to the teen, "From what you have told me, I think you know how to talk with your boyfriend. Tell me how you would explain the need for him to wear a condom." This is an example of:
   1. knowing.
   2. enabling.
   3. doing for.
   4. maintaining belief.
2. You enter a client's room, greet the client, and check the IV medications infusing into the client's arm. You increase the rate of the IV and wait a few minutes after checking vital signs to see if the client's behavior changes in any way. Your combined actions are an example of:
   1. knowing.
   2. presence.
   3. listening.
   4. doing for.
3. A client has been diagnosed as having early stages of a neurological disease. The client must undergo a lumbar puncture for a test of the spinal fluid. It is a painful procedure involving the insertion of a needle into the spinal fluid canal. You help to turn the client onto the client's side, lower your head, and speak into the client's ear while coaching the client on how to breathe slowly and deeply during the needle insertion. You are demonstrating:
   1. enabling.
   2. comforting.
   3. conveying hope.
   4. providing presence.
4. When you change a client's wound dressing, you drape the client to expose only the wound and change the dressing without soiling the bed linen or pulling the skin unnecessarily. This series of actions exhibits:
   1. enabling.
   2. nurturing.
   3. doing for.
   4. comforting.
5. When you are able to demonstrate culturally specific behaviors that express caring, you are applying the theory of caring developed by:
   1. Benner.
   2. Radwin.
   3. Swanson.
   4. Leininger.

References

Bader MM: Nursing care behaviors that predict patient satisfaction, *J Nurs Qual Assur* 2:11, 1988.

Benner P: *From novice to expert,* Menlo Park, Calif, 1984, Addison-Wesley.

Benner P, Wrubel J: *The primacy of caring: stress and coping in health and illness,* Menlo Park, Calif, 1989, Addison-Wesley.

Brown L: The experience of care: patient perspectives, *Top Clin Nurs* 8(2):56, 1986.

Campo R: *The poetry of healing: a doctor's education in empathy, identification, and desire,* New York, 1997, WW Norton.

Coe RM: The magic of science and the science of magic: an essay on the process of healing, *J Health Soc Behav* 38(3):1, 1997.

Frank AW: Just listening: narrative and deep illness, *Fam Syst Health* 16(3):197, 1998.

Gerteis M and others: What patients really want, *Health Manage Q* 15:2, 1993.

Hungelmann J and others: Focus on spiritual well-being: harmonious interconnectedness of mind-body-spirit—use of the JAREL spiritual well-being scale, *Geriatr Nurs* 17(6):262, 1996.

Lamb G, Stempel G: Nursing case management from the client's view: growing as insider-expert, *Nurs Outlook* 42(7):7, 1994.

Leininger M: *Transcultural nursing: concepts, theories and practices,* New York, 1978, John Wiley & Sons.

Leininger M: *Care: the essence of nursing and health,* Detroit, 1988, Wayne State University Press.

Mayer DK: Cancer patients' and families' perceptions of nurse caring behaviors, *Top Clin Nurs* 8(2):63, 1986.

Mayer DK: Oncology nurses' versus cancer patients' perceptions of nurse caring behaviors: a replication study, *Oncol Nurs Forum* 14(3):48, 1987.

Morrison P: Nursing and caring: a personal construct theory study of some nurses' self-perceptions, *J Adv Nurs* 14:421,1989.

Radwin L: Knowing the patient: a process model for individualized interventions, *Nurs Res* 44:364, 1995.

Radwin L: Oncology patients' perceptions of quality nursing care, *Res Nurs Health* 23:179, 2000.

Remen RN: Spirit: resource for. healing, *Noetic Sci Rev,* p 61, autumn 1988.

Riemen DJ: The essential structure of a caring interaction: doing phenomenology. In Munhall PL, Oiler CJ: *Nursing research: a qualitative perspective,* Norwalk, Conn, 1986, Appleton-Century-Crofts.

Risser NL: Development of an instrument to measure patient satisfaction with nurses and nursing care in primary care settings, *Nurs Res* 24:45, 1975.

Simons JE: Science update: patients' and nurses' perception of caring, *Res Rev* 4:2, 1987.

Swanson KM: Empirical development of a middle-range theory of caring, *Nurs Res* 40(3):161, 1991.

Swanson-Kauffman K: Caring in the instance of unexpected early pregnancy loss, *Top Clin Nurs* 8(2):37, 1986.

Tanner C and others: The phenomenology of knowing the patient, *Image J Nurs Sch* 25:273, 1993.

Tri-Council for Nursing: Tri-Council for Nursing Policy Statement, January 31, 2001, NLNupdate@nln.org.

Watson MJ: *Nursing: the philosophy and science of caring,* Boston, 1979, Little, Brown.

Watson MJ: New dimensions of human caring theory, *Nurs Sci Q* 1:175, 1988.

Williams SA: The relationship of patients' perceptions of holistic nurse caring to satisfaction with nursing care, *J Nurs Care Qual* 11(5):15, 1997.

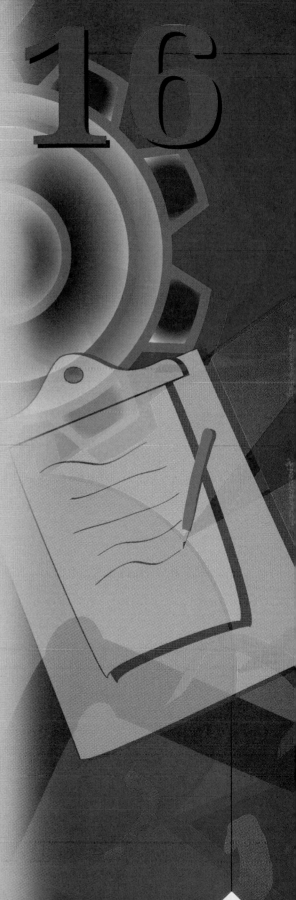

Cultural Diversity

Objectives

- Describe the communication problems encountered when caring for clients and families from multicultural backgrounds.
- Describe culturally sensitive nursing care.
- Identify types of health care practices, including folk beliefs, that may have significant impact on wellness, illness, and health-seeking behaviors of persons from various cultural groups.
- Describe biological variations present in individuals and families from different racial backgrounds.
- Discuss ways to develop cognitive and psychomotor skills needed to provide culturally competent care.
- Discuss the term *cultural stereotyping* and its relevance to rendering culturally competent care.

The United States is rapidly becoming a diverse, multicultural society. This is evidenced by the changes in the 2000 census and the projections for the next 30 years. In 1998 the majority (70.9%) of the U.S. population were of white European descent, 12.9% were African-American, 11.4% were Hispanic-American, 4.1% were Asian-American, and 0.9% were Native American Indian (U.S. Department of Commerce, Bureau of Census, 2000). It is projected that by the year 2020 only 53% of the U.S. population will be white of European descent. It is further projected that by the year 2021 the number of Asian-Americans and Hispanic-Americans will triple, whereas the number of African-Americans will double (U.S. Department of Commerce, Bureau of Census, 2000).

Given the increasing diversity of the population, you as a nurse need to develop an understanding about culture and how it relates to competent client care. There is no magic formula for the delivery of culturally competent and appropriate care because there is as much variation within certain races and cultural or ethnic groups as there is across cultural groups. However, as an informed nurse, you can take into account the significance of culture and approach your clients with a more informed perspective. Transcultural nursing represents and reflects the need for respect and acknowledgment of the wholeness of all human beings (Figure 16-1). It is essential to remember that regardless of race, ethnicity, culture, or cultural heritage, every human being is culturally unique.

TRANSCULTURAL NURSING

Transcultural nursing is client centered, providing culturally competent care to clients from various ethnic and cultural backgrounds. To understand transcultural nursing, you must understand key concepts such as culture, ethnicity, race, and stereotyping.

Culture is a patterned behavioral response that develops over time as a result of patterning the mind through social and religious structures and intellectual and artistic works. It is shaped by values, beliefs, norms, and practices that are shared by members of the same cultural group. Culture guides our thinking, doing, and being and becomes patterned expressions of who we are. These expressions are passed down from one generation to the next.

Ethnicity is frequently and perhaps incorrectly used to mean race. The term *ethnicity* includes more than biological identification. Ethnicity in its broadest sense refers to groups whose members share a common social and cultural heritage that is passed on to successive generations. For example, ethnic traditions regarding celebration of holidays and traditional garments of the Orthodox Jewish faith are passed from generation to generation. The most important characteristic of ethnicity is that members of an ethnic group feel a sense of identity.

In contrast to the term *ethnicity* is the term **race,** which is related to biology. Members of a particular group share distinguishing physical features such as skin color, bone structure, or blood group. For example, members of American Indian tribes have similar facial features, as do

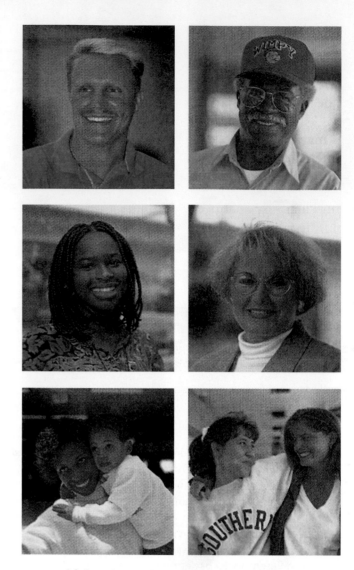

FIGURE 16-1   Ethnic and cultural diversity makes health care challenging and rewarding. (From Birchenall J: *Mosby's textbook for the home care aide,* St. Louis, 1997, Mosby.)

members of Asian cultures. Ethnic and racial groups can and do overlap because in many cases the biological and cultural similarities reinforce one another (Bullough and Bullough, 1982).

Stereotyping is the assumption that all people in a similar cultural, racial, or ethnic group are alike and share exactly the same values and beliefs. Examples of stereotyping include assigning an African-American nurse to provide hair care for an African-American client simply because of ethnicity and race or making the assumption that all Jewish clients maintain dietary restrictions. It is important to know the practices and beliefs of your diverse clients to provide culturally sensitive care.

Every individual is culturally unique, and you are no exception. Therefore avoid projecting your own cultural uniqueness. Carefully identify your personal **cultural values** and beliefs, and then separate them from the client's beliefs and values. To deliver culturally sensitive care, remember that each individual is unique and a product of past experiences, beliefs, and values that have been learned and passed down from one generation to the next.

The more you know about your clients' cultural beliefs and values, the more culturally sensitive will be the care you provide. You will be better prepared to provide a caring presence and approach to any nursing interventions (Chapter 15). Continually assess and evaluate each client's responses, and never assume that all individuals within a specific cultural group will think and behave in a similar manner. The goal of transcultural nursing is the discovery of culturally relevant facts about the client to provide culturally appropriate and competent care.

CULTURE AND HEALTH CARE

In the broadest sense, health may be viewed as a balance between the individual and the environment. Health practices such as eating nutritiously or subscribing to preventive health services available in the community are all believed to have a positive effect on the individual, who in turn can positively affect the environment (Spector, 1996). Perceptions of health and illness are shaped by cultural factors (Table 16-1). How one experiences and copes with illness is very individual. You must incorporate both personal and cultural reactions of the client to illness, disease, and discomfort to give culturally appropriate nursing care. Just as culture influences health-related behavior, it also has a profound effect on expectations and perceptions of illness. As a direct result of cultural shaping, individuals vary in health care behaviors, health status, and health-seeking attitudes.

Communication

Communication and culture are closely intertwined. Communication is the means by which culture is transmitted and preserved. Culture influences how feelings are expressed and what verbal and nonverbal expressions are appropriate. Sensitivity to cultural communication patterns is needed to accurately assess and intervene in caring for clients from all cultures. The potential for misunderstanding your client increases when you and the client are from different ethnic, racial, or cultural groups. Although the most significant variations occur when two people speak different languages, difficulties can also be encountered when you and client speak variations in English.

Whether you relate to the client in an interview setting, during the process of client care, in a more informal level on the hospital unit, or in a clinic, following the guidelines in Box 16-1 will increase the likelihood that your nurse-client relationship will be positive.

Cultural Health Practices

Cultural health practices can be categorized as beneficial, neutral, or harmful. Beneficial cultural health practices are those practices that are viewed as beneficial to the client's health status, even though they can differ vastly from modern scientific practices. You should actively encourage the use of these practices among and across cultural groups. For example, some Mexican-Americans may subscribe to the theory of hot and cold. For these clients, headaches may have a causative agent that is believed to have a hot or cold quality. If the causative agent is believed to have a hot quality, then cold herbs may be placed on the person's head to absorb the heat (Giger and Davidhizar, 1999).

Neutral cultural health practices have no measurable effect on the health status of an individual. Although some health care practitioners may consider neutral health practices irrelevant, remember that such practices may be extremely important to your client because they may be linked to beliefs that are closely integrated with an individual's behavior. For example, Southeast Asian women believe that sitting in a door frame or on a step will complicate labor. Therefore, when in waiting or examination rooms, these women will avoid sitting near a door (Giger and Davidhizar, 1999).

Be aware of practices that are harmful. For example, a Canadian study noted that women of the Canadian Native population did not participate in routine gynecological screening and their mortality from cervical cancer was higher than that of the general population (Hilsop and others, 1992). In this example, you would teach the client about the benefits of routine screening, and assist the client in blending cultural beliefs with contemporary screening practices.

Always identify the client's health practices and respect them. Unless these practices are harmful, incorporate them into the client's individualized plan of care. One of the most prevalent types of cultural health practices is folk medicine.

FOLK MEDICINE.   **Folk medicine** is the use of herbs, plants, minerals, and animal substances to prevent and treat illnesses. Folk medicine is practiced in a variety of countries and cultural groups. Folk remedies have usually been passed down from generation to generation. Many of the remedies are herbal, and the customs and rituals related to the use of herbs vary among cultural groups.

Some religious groups (e.g., Jehovah's Witnesses and Christian Scientists) have specific guidelines concerning health care behaviors, including the giving and receiving of health care. Religious experiences are based on cultural beliefs and may include such experiences as blessings from spiritual leaders, apparitions of dead relatives, and even miracle cures. Healing power based on religion may also be found in animate and inanimate objects. Religion can and does dictate social, moral, and dietary practices that are designed to assist an individual in maintaining a healthy balance and play a vital role in illness prevention.

COMMON CULTURAL GROUPS AND HEALTH CARE PRACTICES
African-Americans

Some of the health problems noted particularly in African-Americans are thought to be the result of varying genetic pools and hereditary immunity. However, many of these problems have been found to be more closely associated with economic status than with race. Three intervening and reinforcing variables include poverty, discrimination, and social and psychological barriers. These variables are

Cross-Cultural Examples of Cultural Phenomena Affecting Nursing Care

Table 16-1

Nations of Origin	Communication	Space	Time Orientation	Social Organization	Environmental Control	Biological Variations
Asian China Hawaii Philippines Korea Japan Southeast Asia (Laos, Cambodia, Vietnam)	National language preference Dialects, written characters Use of silence Nonverbal and contextual cuing	Noncontact people	Present	Family; hierarchical structure, loyalty Devotion to tradition Many religions, including Taoism, Buddhism, Islam, and Christianity Community social organizations	Traditional health and illness beliefs Use of traditional medicines Traditional practitioners: Chinese doctors and herbalists	Liver cancer Stomach cancer Coccidioidomycosis Hypertension Lactose intolerance
African West Coast (as slaves) Many African countries West Indian Islands Dominican Republic Haiti Jamaica	National languages Dialect, pidgin, creole, Spanish, and French	Close personal space	Present over future	Family, many female, single parents Large, extended family networks Strong church affiliation within community Community social organization	Traditional health and illness beliefs Folk medicine tradition Traditional healer: rootworker	Sickle cell anemia Hypertension Cancer of the esophagus Stomach cancer Coccidioidomycosis Lactose intolerance
Europe Germany England Italy Ireland Other European countries	National languages Many learn English immediately	Noncontact people Aloof Distant Southern countries: closer contact and touch	Future over present	Nuclear families Extended families Judeo-Christian religions Community social organizations	Primary reliance on modern health care system Traditional health and illness beliefs Some remaining folk medicine traditions	Breast cancer Heart disease Diabetes mellitus Thalassemia
Native American 500 Native American tribes Aleuts Eskimos	Tribal languages Use of silence and body language	Space very important and has no boundaries	Present	Extremely family oriented Biological and extended families Children taught to respect traditions Community social organizations	Traditional health and illness beliefs Folk medicine tradition Traditional healer: medicine man	Accidents Heart disease Cirrhosis of the liver Diabetes mellitus
Hispanic countries Spain Cuba Mexico Central and South America	Spanish or Portuguese primary language	Tactile relationships Touch Handshakes Embracing Value physical presence	Present	Nuclear family Extended families *Compadrazzo:* godparents Community social organizations	Traditional health and illness beliefs Folk medicine tradition Traditional healers: *curandero, espiritista, partera, señora*	Diabetes mellitus Parasites Coccidioidomycosis Lactose intolerance

Compiled by Rachel Spector, RN, PhD.

Guidelines for Communicating With Culturally Diverse Clients   Box 16-1

* *Plan care based on the communicated needs and cultural background.* When care is being planned for persons from other cultures, it must be consistent with the lifestyle and unique needs of the client that have been communicated to you and mutually agreed on (Geissler, 1991; Grossman, 1996).
* *Modify communication approaches to meet cultural needs.* A factor that commonly interferes with care delivery to a person from another culture is confusion and fear concerning the treatment process. The fact that a non–English-speaking client is ill and receiving treatment can interfere with the client's normal ability to communicate. You must be attentive to signs of anxiety and respond in a reassuring manner.

    Some cultures are primarily oral and do not rely on a written form of communication. In such cases the spoken word holds greater meaning and power. For example, Hmongs are considered an oral cultural group. For these individuals the formation of and acceptance in a social group is primarily dependent on the spoken word (Shadick, 1993). When interacting with individuals from an oral culture, you must remember that if the teaching-learning process is to be effective, instruction must be oral.
* *Understand that respect for the client and communicated needs is central to the therapeutic relationship.* The need to communicate respect for the client is a nursing concept that crosses all cultural boundaries. Regardless of the language spoken or the cultural orientation, communication is increased and interpersonal distance is reduced when your approach focuses on individuals and their emotional and physical needs. Communication of respect is central to a focus on emotional needs. Respect for clients is communicated by a kind and attentive approach whereby you clearly listen to what the client says. Active listening techniques are used, such as encouraging clients to share thoughts and feelings by reflecting back what has been heard. Be attentive to how listening is communicated in the client's culture. For example, for some persons listening may be indicated by eye contact, whereas for others listening may mean having the listener turn a listening "ear." Predictions about what the client is trying to express may be made to encourage elaboration. At the heart of the task of hearing is the art of listening (Martin, 1995). Listening communicates genuine interest and

caring. The feeling of being heard is powerful, reducing distance and drawing people together into positive interpersonal interactions. An attitude of flexibility, respect, and interest can bridge barriers of distance imposed by culture and role.
* *Communicate in a nonthreatening manner.* The interview should be started in an unhurried manner with adherence to acceptable social and cultural amenities. It is usually wise to start with general social topics. During the information-gathering stage, ask general rather than specific questions. Allow time for the respondent to give what appears to be unrelated information. In some cultures a direct approach appears rude and uncaring. For example, persons of European background and Hispanics often value "small talk" and will not relate optimally to you if you talk only about illness-related matters. Many persons, specifically Asians and Hispanics, respond better to a nondirective approach with open-ended questions than to direct questions and answers (Giger and Davidhizar, 1999).
* *Use validating techniques in communication.* Although validating techniques are always important, they are especially important when the client is from a different culture. Be alert for feedback indicating that the client does not understand and use restating and validating techniques, such as "Did I hear and understand you correctly?" When you have difficulty understanding, it may help to find out precisely what the topic is (e.g., "Are you telling me where you're having pain?"). By determining the topic, the number of words can be decreased. If the message is not understood, it may be helpful to have the client try to convey the message in another way (e.g., through pointing or imitation). Never pretend to understand a message. People usually know when they are understood. By pretending, you convey to the client that the message is not important (Pore, 1995).
* *Adopt special approaches when the client speaks a different language.* A client who enters the health care system without being able to speak the same language as the caregivers is easily frightened and frustrated. Without the availability of words, you must relate to the client on an affective level. A tone and facial expression of caring can reduce the client's fear. Locating an interpreter should be a priority when caring for these clients.

---

thought to be so profound that African-American clients may be unable to use available health care services. These variables may also explain why morbidity and mortality rates are higher for African-Americans than for the rest of the general population. Although underrepresented in the general population, African-Americans remain overrepresented among the health statistics for life-threatening illness.

Life expectancy for African-Americans continues to lag behind that for whites. The life expectancy for African-Americans is 71.0 years, compared with 76.4 years for whites (U.S. Department of Commerce, Bureau of Census, 2000). African-Americans continue to have a higher infant mortality (11.2 per 1000 live births in 1993), compared with white Americans (9.4 per 1000 live births in 1993) (National Center for Health Statistics, 2000). In 1997 the rate of deaths for African-American males was 55% higher for heart disease, 26% higher for cancer, 180% higher for stroke, and 100%

higher for lung disease than for the rest of the general U.S. population (National Center for Health Statistics, 1998).

THE FAMILY SYSTEM.   In 1998, 46.0% of African-American families were matrifocal (female headed with no husband present), compared with 13.0% of white families (National Center for Health Statistics, 1998). Even when there is a male present in the home, African-American families are oriented around women. This has implications for health care because within the African-American family structure the wife and/or mother is often charged with the responsibility for protecting the health of the family members. The African-American woman is expected to assist each family member in maintaining good health and in determining treatment if a family member is ill.

Some African-American families are composed of large networks and tend to be very supportive during times of crisis and illness. Large-network groups can have both positive and negative effects on wellness, illness, and recovery behaviors. Nonetheless, it is important to include all the members of the network in the planning and implementation of health care.

CULTURAL HEALTH PRACTICES.   Some of the African-Americans who were reared in the rural South may have been treated by folk practitioners and may not have encountered a physician until they reached adulthood. They are more likely to turn to a neighborhood folk practitioner when they become ill. Folk medicine is still used within the African-American community, and some African-Americans may go to physicians primarily to get medications that require a prescription.

BIOLOGICAL VARIATIONS.   Several categories of diseases have a higher incidence in the African-American population, including the human immunodeficiency virus (HIV), cardiovascular disease, and alcoholism. Since the first reported case of acquired immunodeficiency syndrome (AIDS) in 1981, HIV/AIDS has become a major cause of morbidity and mortality among African-Americans. In fact Ward and Duchin (1998) noted that the death rate from AIDS was 4 times greater for African-American males than for white males. African-American females fare even worse, with a death rate 9 times greater than that of white females (Ward and Duchin, 1998).

The incidence of hypertension is significantly higher in African-Americans. The onset of hypertension occurs at an earlier age, and the elevation in blood pressure is more severe and associated with a higher mortality, especially in cardiovascular diseases. The Joint National Committee (1999) concluded that the prevalence of hypertension increases with age at a greater rate for African-Americans than for whites. In addition, the prevalence is greater in African-American men in the young adult and middle years. In later years, hypertension is equally distributed among African-American men and women.

Cardiovascular disease remains the leading cause of morbidity and mortality in the United States for all demographic groups. The major causes of death due to cardiovascular disease are myocardial infarction and cerebral vascular accident (National Center for Health Statistics, 1998). The age-adjusted mortality rate for myocardial infarction in black males exceeds that of whites. Data from the 1980-1991 Heart and Stroke Statistics Update indicate that the age-adjusted death rate from myocardial infarction was highest among African-American males and females compared with white males and females (Liao and Cooper, 1995). African-American women tend to develop coronary artery disease much earlier than white women. In addition, the death rate for African-American women under age 55 is twice that for white women. Until age 75 the mortality from coronary artery disease is higher in African-American women compared with women of other racial backgrounds (Woods, 1998).

Sickle cell anemia is the most common genetic disorder in the United States. This illness affects predominantly African-Americans. This is a chronic, incurable disorder that includes symptoms of chronic anemia and fatigue, and in acute crises hospitalization is required to manage joint pain, thrombosis, and fever. One problem frequently associated with this disorder is substance abuse. People with sickle cell anemia are at greater risk for substance abuse to gain control of the joint pain.

Alcoholism is another health problem in the African-American community, contributing to reduced longevity. There are high incidences of acute and chronic alcohol-related diseases among African-Americans, such as alcoholic fatty liver; hepatitis; cirrhosis of the liver, heart disease; cancers of the mouth, larynx, tongue, esophagus, and lung; and unintentional injuries and homicide (Ronan, 1987).

Several causes of alcohol abuse and misuse in African-Americans have been identified in the literature. A primary factor is economics. Many African-American men drink as a result of unemployment, which leads to depression and frustration because of the inability to meet financial commitments.

Hispanic-Americans

Hispanic-Americans are the fastest growing group of people in the United States today and are expected to become the largest ethnic minority group in the United States within the first decade of the twenty-first century. Between 1980 and 1990 the number of Hispanic-Americans residing in the United States grew by 53% (U.S. Department of Commerce, Bureau of Census, 2000). This tremendous growth is related to higher birth rates than the rest of the general population and substantial influx of immigrants from Mexico, Central America, and South America. Projections indicate that the Hispanic-American population will double its current size by the year 2020 and triple its current size by 2050 (U.S. Department of Commerce, Bureau of Census, 2000).

A major issue for some Hispanic-Americans is lack of citizenship. Many Mexican-Americans gain entry into the United States by simply walking across the border. The lack of citizenship is a barrier to gaining education, skills, stable jobs, decent living conditions, and government benefits.

THE FAMILY SYSTEM.   For many Hispanic-Americans extended family relationships have special significance, and the family is perhaps the most significant social organization. The major dominating theme of the traditional Hispanic-American family is the need for collective achievement of the family as a group. Thus the need for family collective achievement and other family needs supersede the needs of individual members. Also, any dishonor or shame that an individual member experiences is considered a reflection on the entire family. The Hispanic-American family takes pride in family endeavors and generally does not seek help from outsiders to solve problems or meet needs. Many Hispanic-American families place a great deal of value on having many relatives living nearby. The local extended family is tightly integrated, its members have frequent face-to-face encounters, and they provide one another with mutual aid.

Within the Hispanic-American family, the father has the dominant role, assuming responsibility for being head of the house and the decision maker. For the male family member, there is a strong sense of machismo that is not compatible with the loss of self-esteem or authority. The wife or mother of the family has a primary role of keeping the family cohesive. Although the mother may influence family decisions, she does not have a dominant role in the family.

CULTURAL HEALTH PRACTICES.   An external locus of control influences the way in which an individual views health. Some individuals may believe that health may be the result of good luck or a reward from God for good behavior. For some Hispanic Americans, health is a state of equilibrium in the universe wherein the forces of "hot," "cold," "wet," and "dry" must be balanced. This concept is thought to have originated with the early Hippocratic theory of health and the four humors. According to the Hippocratic theory, the body humors (e.g., blood, phlegm, black bile, and yellow bile) vary in both temperature and moisture. Persons who subscribe to this theory believe that health exists only when these four humors are in balance. Thus health can be maintained by diet and other practices that keep the four humors in balance. Illness, on the other hand, is believed to be misfortune or bad luck, a punishment from God for evil thoughts or actions, or a result of the imbalance of hot and cold or wet and dry.

The concept of balance dominates much of the Hispanic-American worldview regarding the cause and treatment of illness. Good health implies that one is in proper balance with God, the family, fellow human beings, and the church. Illness is often believed to be a result of an imbalance in the social or spiritual aspects of life.

FOLK MEDICINE.   Operating within the folklore system of beliefs and practices are several levels of healers. The first healer sought out is a member of the family; if the health problem is or becomes more complicated, healers within the community are sought. The family member healer is generally female and is respected for her knowledge of folk medicine. This individual may be a wife/mother, grandmother, or revered elderly relative. The healing practices are passed down in the family from mother to daughter. If the client does not improve, there is usually an intermediary person who directs the client to the *jerbero* or *curandero*.

The *jerbero* is a folk healer who specializes in using herbs and spices for preventive and curative purposes. This person grows and distributes herbs and spices and explains how to use them effectively. The more serious physical and mental/emotional illnesses are brought to the *curandero* (male folk healer) or *curandera* (female folk healer).

BIOLOGICAL VARIATIONS.   Several categories of diseases have a high incidence in Hispanic-Americans. The following section will highlight the impact of diabetes mellitus, heart disease, communicable diseases, obesity, and HIV on this cultural group.

In Mexican-Americans not only is the incidence of diabetes 5 times the national average, but also complications are also more frequent. Hispanic-Americans suffer primarily from type 2 diabetes, with diabetes ranking as the third leading cause of death for Hispanic women between the ages of 45 and 74 (Vasquez, 1997).

Hispanic-Americans in the San Antonio heart study were found to be less knowledgeable about preventing heart attacks and were not engaging in risk-reducing behaviors as often as non-Hispanic whites (Derenowski, 1990). Researchers noted that cardiovascular risk reduction and changes in lifestyle are necessary components of education for some Mexican-Americans. In providing this education, however, you must remember to address cultural differences such as health values, ethnic care practices, family life patterns, and dietary practices. The whole family should be committed to developing and sustaining the lifestyle changes if they are to be successful.

It is essential when you are working with Hispanic-Americans to realize that approximately 85% of the health problems common in Hispanic-Americans involve communicable diseases (National Center for Health Statistics, 1998, 2000). These include respiratory tract infections, diarrhea, skin disorders, and nutritional problems, particularly during the first year of life. In the United States the population that is most at risk for the incidence and transmittal of tuberculosis includes newly arrived immigrants, including Mexicans (Phipps, 1997). Because there is a high prevalence of tuberculosis in Mexico, it is thought that Mexican-Americans may have a higher predisposition for tuberculosis than other Americans.

Hepatitis C has also been found to occur at a higher rate among Hispanic-Americans. It is estimated that more people could die from the complications of hepatitis C than from AIDS (Cronin, 1997). Some 70% of the cases result in liver damage, which leads to death. Lifestyle changes such as avoiding alcohol can prolong length and quality of life for persons with hepatitis C.

There is a growing incidence of childhood obesity noted among Hispanic-Americans and particularly among Mexican-Americans. Alexander and Blank (1988) suggest that the increasing incidence of obesity in Mexican-American children may be a result of mothers believing a fat baby is a healthy baby. The mothers in this study had a greater body mass index than did mothers in a control group. These subjects also had "pushier" feeding practices with their children. To prevent the complications of adult obesity stemming from childhood obesity, you should identify mothers and their children who are at risk for obesity.

Asian-Americans

THE FAMILY SYSTEM.   For most Asian-Americans, the family is the basic institution of society and as such provides lifelong protection and guidance to the individual (Figure 16-2). The roles and structure of the family are generally well defined, with extensive terminology designating kinship relationships. In most Asian-American families, the father is the head of the household but shares the rights and authority with his spouse.

The immediate family includes parents, unmarried children, sometimes the husband's parents, and sons with their wives and children. The extended family may include other

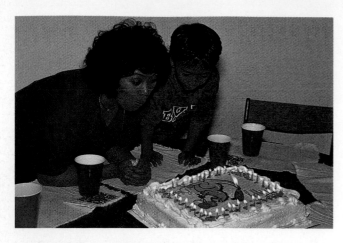

FIGURE 16-2 Blending of Asian culture and American practices at a child's birthday.

close relatives who live in the same community. For some Asian-American families, the eldest son has the responsibility of carrying on the family name, of taking over for the parents when they become elderly, and of following through with religious and ancestral observances.

After arriving in the United States, many Asian-Americans (e.g., Hmongs, Vietnamese, and Laotians) are forced to reverse traditional roles. Persons who are traditionally "providers" become the "recipients." For example, Vietnamese-American women initially upon arriving in this country are more likely to gain employment because "women's jobs" such as maids, sewing machine operators, and food service workers are more plentiful than male-oriented unskilled jobs. Thus the Asian-American male is often forced to reverse roles with his wife, becoming the recipient instead of the provider. Likewise, Asian-American children often assume the role of translator for non-English-speaking parents. Because Vietnamese-American children have assimilated very rapidly into the U.S. society, they are more likely than their parents to find gainful employment. Among some Asian-American families, a role reversal creates intergenerational conflicts (Gold, 1992).

CULTURAL HEALTH PRACTICES.   A naturalistic explanation for illness encourages a search for a natural or obvious cause of symptoms. For example, illness may be associated with rotten food or "poisonous water," in an obvious cause-and-effect relationship. To counteract the effects of these natural elements, an informal body of knowledge has been collected about indigenous medicinal herbs, therapeutic diets, and simple medical and hygienic measures. The information is usually transmitted orally and often treated with secrecy, remaining inside the clan or extended family.

The supernaturalistic explanation for disease lays the blame on supernatural powers, such as gods, demons, or spirits. The illness is considered a punishment for a fault, for a violation of religious or ethical codes, or for an act of omission causing displeasure to a deity.

Metaphysical explanation is built on the theory that nature and the body operate within a delicate balance between two opposite elements: the yin and the yang (e.g., female and male, dark and light, or hard and soft). In medicine the opposites are expressed as "hot" and "cold," and health is the result of a balance between hot and cold elements. This results in harmonious functioning of the organs and harmony with the environment. An excess or shortage in either direction causes discomfort and illness.

BIOLOGICAL VARIATIONS.   Several categories of diseases occur with high incidence in Asian-Americans. The following section will highlight the impact of cancer, diabetes mellitus, and coronary artery disease on this cultural group.

Cancer of the stomach, esophagus, and liver occurs more frequently among Japanese-Americans than among white counterparts (Overfield, 1995). In addition, diets high in salt-cured foods and nitrites and poor in vitamin C intake have been commonly associated with greater incidence of stomach cancer. Also, drinking hot tea may contribute to the development of esophageal cancer.

Pockets of high incidences of diabetes and obesity have been noted among the Japanese in Hawaii. These higher incidences may be a result of a combination of diet and lifestyle.

Longitudinal research noting the incidence of coronary artery disease has been conducted on the Japanese in Japan, in Hawaii, and on the U.S. mainland. The mortality from coronary artery disease (and breast and colon cancer) has been attributed to variations in diets and lifestyles of Asian, Hawaiian, and mainland Japanese.

Native American Indians

According to the recent census, there were 1.9 million Native Americans among 10 different tribes living in the United States. The Cherokee and Navajo tribes had the largest populations. Native American populations were found in Arizona, Oklahoma, New Mexico, Alaska, California, North Carolina, South Dakota, New York, Montana, Washington, and Minnesota (U.S. Department of Commerce, Bureau of Census, 2000). Providing culturally appropriate nursing care is complicated by the fact that each nation or tribe of Native Americans has its own language and religion, and belief-system practices differ significantly among groups and among members of the same tribe.

There is a clear distinction between American Indian (AI) and Alaska Native (AN). Thus when the term Native American Indian is used, it is intended to imply tribes residing in the continental United States. Today, although many Native American Indians remain on reservations and in rural areas, an equal number also reside in cities (U.S. Department of Commerce, Bureau of the Census, 1998).

The Synder Act of 1921 provides the basic authority for health care for Native American Indians and Alaska Natives. The Bureau of Indian Affairs assumed responsibility as a federal branch for providing health care services for the Navajo people until 1954. In 1954 this responsibility was transferred to the Indian Health Service.

THE FAMILY SYSTEM.   Native Americans are extremely family oriented, but the term *family* has a much broader

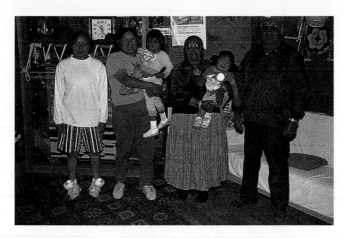

FIGURE **16-3**   Native American Indian family in front of a display at a local festival.

meaning than just the nuclear family (Figure 16-3). The biological family is the center of social organization and includes all members of the extended family. There are some tribes, such as the Navajo, for example, who are traditionally a matriarchal society. This means that when a couple marries, the husband makes his home with his wife's relatives, and his family becomes one of several units that live in a group of adjacent homes or other type of dwellings. The family is considered so important in the Navajo culture that to be without relatives is to be really poor. Children learn from infancy that the family and the tribe are of paramount importance.

Historically, Native American people have been guided by sacred myths and legends that describe the tribe's evolution from inception to the present time. Supernatural beings portrayed in these stories symbolize the culture, in which religion and healing practices are blended with each other. Values and beliefs intrinsic to culture and religion form the Navajo day-to-day living experiences.

CULTURAL HEALTH PRACTICES.   Traditional Native American Indian concepts focus on the need for the individual to be in harmony with the surrounding environment and with the family. Health and religion cannot be separated within the Native American world. The linkage between traditional religion and healing ceremonies found among Native American Indians is obvious.

NATIVE AMERICAN HEALERS.   Native American healers spend many years learning their skills and serving as apprentices. There are a variety of healers within each tribe, including herbalists, diagnosticians, and medicine men. Medicine men and medicine women have *jists,* or medicine bundles, containing symbolic and sacred items, including corn pollen, feathers, stones, arrowheads, and other instruments used for healing and blessing.

Keep in mind that a Navajo client needs to feel in harmony with the environment. Therefore the environment must be structured in such a way that this harmony is promoted. If you were to deny or not allow the client the op-

portuntiy to achieve harmony with other people, animals, plants, nature, weather, and supernatural forces, the client would not be able to obtain a sense of assurance in relation to physical, social, psychological, and spiritual health.

BIOLOGICAL VARIATIONS.   Several categories of diseases have a high incidence in Native American Indians. The following section will highlight the impact of diabetes mellitus, alcoholism, and suicide on this cultural group.

Type 2 diabetes mellitus is a major health problem for Native Americans, occurring as early as the teens or early 20s. The earlier onset leads to an earlier onset of complications and excessive mortality in the early and middle adult years. Age-specific death rates for diabetes appear to be 2.6 times higher for Native Americans between 25 and 54 years of age than those for the rest of the general U.S. population (U.S. Department of Health and Human Services, Indian Health Service, 1992). In addition, the complications from diabetes among Native Americans are appearing with distressing frequency.

In whites, alcohol is metabolized "fairly efficiently" by the liver enzyme dehydrogenase. In contrast, in Native Americans and Asians it is metabolized by aldehyde dehydrogenase (ALDH), which works faster, often causing circulatory and unpleasant effects such as facial flushing and palpitations (Kudzma, 1992).

Approximately 85% to 90% of American Indians have been found to have the high-activity variant of ALDH, which means that the alcohol they consume is rapidly converted to acetaldehyde. However, the next step, conversion of acetaldehyde to acetic acid, is delayed in 35% to 70% of American Indians. It is because of these enzyme differences that a majority of American Indians experience a rapid onset initially and thereafter a slow decrease in blood acetaldehyde levels. Alcoholism exists among Native Americans in very high percentages.

Suicide is another major contributor to death in Native Americans. Men are at higher risk than women for suicide (U.S. Department of Health and Human Services, Indian Health Service, 1992). The mental health of Native Americans is complicated by the pressures created by traditional cultural demands, attempts at assimilation of Western values, and the availability of alcohol. Suicide is associated with alcohol abuse, which in turn is a symptom of a people attempting to assimilate into a rapidly changing society.

IMPLICATIONS FOR NURSING PRACTICE

Each culture has specific practices that you must be sensitive to in order to provide culturally diverse care. Some African-Americans may believe that good health is equated with one's ability to read the signs of nature or being in "God's good graces"; education and spiritual support may be important interventions. You need to educate the client and family on causation of illness within the context of the client's cultural beliefs. In addition, the client's religious community can play an integral role in health promotion and health care.

In addition to cultural differences, English may be a second language for many clients. For some clients their only language may be their language of origin, and it is very frightening to not understand English or to have to rely on others for communication. It is important that you establish methods for communication early in the caregiving situation. These communication interventions must meet the client's and health care provider's needs simultaneously, they must be reliable, and they must be understood by all.

Because some clients may rely on folk and alternative therapies, recognize the importance of folk medicine practices mentioned earlier. Acknowledging the client's reliance on folk health practices and religious beliefs will promote a more individualized plan of care. The family can be of great assistance to you in incorporating some of the folk medicine methods into the plan of care.

Whenever possible you should try to incorporate the client's cultural medical practices into the plan of care. For example, the use of relaxation or acupuncture may be very effective for some Asian clients. These types of alternative therapies are also becoming popular in traditional health care practices, so you do have access to practitioners of alternative therapies (see Chapter 29).

The access to health care for culturally diverse populations may be somewhat limited due to the cultural and language differences, lack of insurance, or unemployment. As a result the use of screening and prevention may often be overlooked. You can begin to educate clients with regard to health maintenance practices, doing so in a manner that complements their own health beliefs.

It is essential to understand differences in individuals as they relate to cultural heritage. It is also important to appreciate that each client and family are culturally unique and bring to the care environment this uniqueness. In addition, you also bring to the client-nurse relationship a personal cultural heritage. It is essential to refrain from imposing personal values and beliefs on the client and to respect the uniqueness and differences each of you brings to the care environment.

Key Terms

culture, p. 410
cultural values, p. 410

ethnicity, p. 410
folk medicine, p. 411
race, p. 410

stereotyping, p. 410
transcultural nursing, p. 410

Key Concepts

- Culture is a patterned behavioral response that develops over time as a result of being imprinted on the mind through social and religious structures and intellectual and artistic manifestations.
- Transcultural nursing is viewed as a culturally sensitive practice that is client centered.
- As the cultural diversity of the United States continues to expand, it is important that you be knowledgeable about a variety of cultures, their health beliefs and practices, their folk medicines, their religious and social practices, and nutritional patterns.
- To provide culturally sensitive care it is important to remember that each individual is culturally unique and as such is a product of past experiences, cultural beliefs, and cultural norms.
- Folk medicine is practiced in a variety of cultures and affects health practices of clients from diverse populations.
- Knowledge of biological variations within cultural groups help you in assessing clients' risk factors for diseases.

Critical Thinking Activities

1. What influence does culture have on cultural beliefs, illness, and wellness behaviors?
2. In what ways does communication present barriers to culturally competent care, even when you and the client speak the same language?
3. Mr. Sanchez is a 60-year-old man seeking care for a cough, fatigue, and weight loss. He is diagnosed with bronchitis and type 2 diabetes. He has lived in the United States for 5 years and is a Spanish-speaking field laborer. His food is Mexican-American, with very few fruits and vegetables. Identify in what ways Mr. Sanchez's time orientation, spatial needs, and health patterns differ from Western culture. How may culture and health practices affect his compliance or adherence to a particular treatment regimen?

Review Questions

1. Culture is described as:
   1. a patterned behavioral response based on generational influences.
   2. a patterned behavioral response based solely on religious practices.
   3. a patterned behavioral response developed over time based on social and religious structures and intellectual and artistic influences.
   4. a patterned behavioral response developed over time based on developmental stages, social and religious structures, and intellectual and artistic influences.
2. Transcultural nursing provides:
   1. competent nursing care that is culturally sensitive to the client's and/or family's individual needs.
   2. competent nursing care that is culturally sensitive to the social needs of the client and/or family.
   3. competent nursing care that is culturally sensitive to the practices of the client's culture of origin.
   4. competent nursing care that is culturally sensitive to the practices of the client's culture of residence.
3. When providing care to clients with varied cultural backgrounds, it is important to recognize that:
   1. cultural considerations must be put aside if basic needs are in jeopardy.
   2. generalizations about behavior of a particular groups may be inaccurate.
   3. current health standards should determine the acceptability of cultural practices.
   4. similar reactions to stress will occur when individuals have the same cultural background.
4. The most important factor in providing culturally sensitive nursing care is:
   1. communication.
   2. time orientation.
   3. biological variations.
   4. environmental controls.
5. To be effective in meeting the client's cultural needs, you must:
   1. treat all client alike.
   2. be aware of client's cultural differences.
   3. act as if you are comfortable with the client's behavior.
   4. avoid asking questions about the client's cultural background.

References

Alexander M, Blank J: Factors related to obesity in Mexican American preschool children, *Image J Nurs Sch* 20(2):79, 1988.

Aruffo J and others: AIDS knowledge in low-income and minority populations, *Public Health Rep* 106(2):115, 1991.

Birchenall J: *Mosby's textbook for the home care aide,* St. Louis, 1997, Mosby.

Bullough VL, Bullough B: *Health care for the other Americans,* East Norwalk, Conn, 1982, Appleton-Century Crofts.

Caudle P: Providing culturally sensitive health care to Hispanic patients, *Nurse Pract* 18(12):40, 1993.

Centers of Disease Control and Prevention: *HIV surveillance report: estimated incidence of AIDS and deaths of persons with AIDS, adjusted for delays in reporting, by quarter-year of diagnosis/death, United States, January 1985 through June 1997,* 1997, Atlanta, 1977 Centers for Disease Control and Prevention.

Cronin M: Billboard campaign spotlights growing hepatitis C epidemic, *Seattle Times,* p. A1, July 30, 1997.

Derenowski J: Coronary heart disease in Hispanics, *J Cardiovasc Nurs* 4(4):13, 1990.

Geissler E: Transcultural nursing and nursing diagnosis, *Nurs Health Care* 12(4):190, 1991.

Giger J, Davidhizar R: *Transcultural nursing: assessment and intervention,* ed 3, St. Louis, 1999, Mosby.

Gold S: Mental health and illness in Vietnamese refugees, *West J Med* 157(3):290, 1992.

Grossman D: Cultural dimensions in home health care nursing, *Am J Nurs* 96(7):33, 1996.

Hilsop TG and others: Participation in the British Columbia cervical cytology screening program by Native Indian Women, *Can J Public Health* 83(5):344, 1992.

Information please almanac, Boston, 1998, Houghton Mifflin.

Joint National Committee: The sixth report of the Joint National Committee on detection, evaluation, and treatment of high blood pressure, Washington, DC, 1999, National Institutes of Health, National Heart, Lung, and Blood Institute.

Kudzma E: Drug responses: all bodies are not created equal, *Am J Nurs* 92:48, 1992.

Liao Y, Cooper R: Continued adverse trends in coronary heart disease mortality among blacks, 1980-1991, *Public Health Rep* 110: 572, 1995.

Martin B: The difficult art of listening, *Gospel Herald* 88(48):1, 1995.

National Center for Health Statistics: *Health, United States, 1996-97 and injury chartbook.* Hyattsville, Md, 1997, Center for Health Statistics.

National Center for Health Statistics: *Healthy people 2010,* Hyattsville, Md, 2000, Public Health Service.

Overfield RT: *Biologic variations in health and illness: race, age and sex differences,* ed 2, Reading, Mass, 1995, Addison-Wesley.

Phipps W: The patient with pulmonary problems. In Long BC and others, editors: *Medical surgical nursing: concepts and clinical practice,* ed 6, St. Louis, 1997, Mosby.

Pore S: I can't understand what my patient is saying. *Adv Nurs Pract,* p. 17, July 1995.

Ronan L: Alcohol-related health risks among black Americans, *Alcohol Health Res World* 12:36, 1987.

Shadick K: Development of a transcultural health education program for the Hmong, *Clin Nurse Spec* 7(2):48, 1993.

Spector R: *Cultural diversity in health and illness,* Stamford, Conn, 1996, Appleton & Lange.

U.S. Department of Commerce, Bureau of the Census: *Top 25 American Indian tribes for the United States: 1990 and 1980,* Internet release, Washington, DC, Aug 1995, US Government Printing Office.

U.S. Department of Commerce, Bureau of Census: Population profiles of the United States, Internet update, Washington, DC, 2000, US Government Printing Office.

U.S. Department of Health and Human Services, Indian Health Service: Prevalence of HIV and AIDS in American Indians and Alaska Natives, *IHS Primary Care Provider* 17(5):66, 1992.

Vasquez S: Diabetes alert: high-fat, genetics make Hispanics prone to the disease, *Rocky Mountain News,* p. 3d, May 20, 1997.

Ward J, Duchin J: U.S. Epidemiology of HIV and AIDS. In Volberding P, Jacobson M: *AIDS clinical review,* New York, 1998, Marcel Dekker.

Woods S: Can aspirin prevent coronary heart disease in women? *Women's Health in Primary Care* 1:210, 1998.

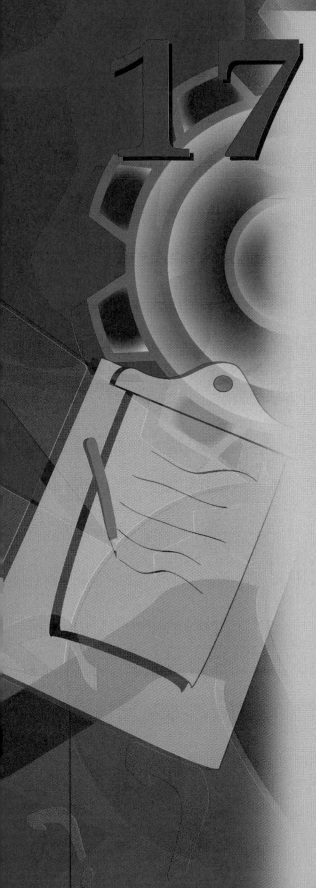

17

Spiritual Health

Objectives

- Define key terms.
- Describe the relationship between faith, hope, and spiritual well-being.
- Compare and contrast the concepts of religion and spirituality.
- Discuss the relationship of spirituality to an individual's total being.
- Perform an initial assessment of a client's spirituality.
- Discuss nursing interventions designed to promote spiritual health.
- Evaluate attainment of spiritual health.

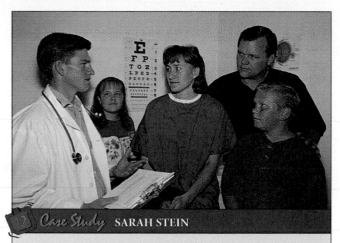

Case Study   SARAH STEIN

Sarah Stein is a 48-year-old college professor, diagnosed 3 months ago with breast cancer. She is married to Joe, an insurance salesman, and is the mother of two children: Valerie, who is 16 years of age, and Peter, who is 12. Surgeons removed Sarah's cancerous tumor and two involved lymph nodes. Lymphatic involvement increases the risk that the cancer might spread. Sarah has completed a course of radiation and now visits the local cancer clinic with her husband 3 times a week for a course of chemotherapy. She has received instruction from one of the clinic nurses about the side effects of chemotherapy. Both Sarah and Joe discuss their concern for their children. Their son is preparing for his bar mitzvah, which is only 6 months away. Sarah hopes to attend the ceremony but worries about how she will feel. Valerie, their daughter, has been showing behavioral outbursts since her mother's illness.

Jeff is a 36-year-old, married student nurse assigned to the oncology clinic. One of the clinic case managers, who serves as Jeff's preceptor, assigns Jeff to follow Sarah during her clinic visits. Jeff is in his last semester at school and hopes to get a position in the clinic after graduation. Sarah's experience is significant for Jeff because he has children in the same age-group and wonders how they might react to their mother being ill.

During one of their clinic visits, Sarah and Joe spent some time discussing ways to manage chemotherapy side effects with Jeff. Jeff has noticed that Sarah and Joe appear very calm and relaxed when discussing cancer therapy. Joe explains, "What happens will happen, but we both have a lot of faith in God." Sarah responds, "Even though I know I have cancer, I hope to be able to attend my son's bar mitzvah next year. Joe is my support, and together I know we will make it."

---

*T*he word *spirituality* derives from the Latin word *spiritus,* which refers to breath or wind. The spirit gives life to a person. It signifies whatever is at the center of all aspects of a person's life (Dombeck, 1995). **Spirituality** is an awareness of one's inner self and a sense of connection to a higher being, nature, or to some purpose greater than oneself (Reed, 1987). A person's health depends on a balance of physical, psychological, sociological, cultural, developmental, and spiritual variables. This **holistic** view of health is the focus and heart of nursing practice. Spiritual care is often an overlooked part of nursing; however, the spiritual dimension does not exist in isolation from our physical and psycholog-

ical being (Humphreys, 2000). Spirituality is an important factor that helps to achieve the balance needed to maintain health and well-being and to cope with illness. Research on clients with chronic illness and survivors of abuse has shown that spirituality can reduce a person's distress and even enhance personal growth and empowerment (O'Neil and Kenny, 1998; Humphreys, 2000).

Too often in nursing, clinicians de-emphasize the spiritual dimension of human nature (Calabria and Macrae, 1994), either because it is not scientific enough or is difficult to measure or because there are health care providers who do not believe in God or an ultimate being. Frequently spirituality and religion are interchanged, but spirituality is a much broader and more unifying concept than religion. Florence Nightingale described spirituality as the sense of a presence higher than human, the divine intelligence that creates and sustains (Calabria and Macrae, 1994). The human spirit is powerful, and it can be integrated into a nurse's approach to care. Nursing care involves helping clients to use their spiritual resources as they identify and explore what is meaningful in their lives and to find ways to cope with illness and life's stressors.

SCIENTIFIC KNOWLEDGE BASE

Recently, health care research has shown the association between spirituality and health. There may be beneficial health outcomes when an individual is able to engage personal beliefs in a higher power and sense a source of strength or support. Turner and Clancy (1986) studied clients with chronic low back pain and found that increased use of praying and hoping was related to decreased pain intensity. Prayer is frequently used as a method of coping and is effective in minimizing physical stressors. Humphreys (2000) found that battered women's experience of distress was reduced by the personal variable of spirituality. Research has also shown that meditation is successful in treating chronic pain, insomnia, anxiety, and depression (Culligan, 1996).

The relationship between spirituality and healing is not completely understood. However, it is the individual's intrinsic spirit that seems to be the factor in healing. When clients are given a placebo (sugar pill) instead of a prescribed medication, often they improve, not because of the sugar pill but because of their belief in the effect of the treatment. The placebo phenomenon shows that healing can take place because of believing.

Research is showing a link between the mind, body, and spirit. An individual's beliefs and expectations can and do have effects on the person's physical well-being (Coe, 1997). Many of these effects may be tied to hormonal and neurological function. Relaxation exercises and guided imagery, for example, have been shown to improve individuals' immune function (Kiecolt-Glaser and others, 1985). Laughter raises pain thresholds, boosts antibodies, reduces stress hormones, relieves tension, and elevates mood (Kellar, 2001). A person's inner beliefs and convictions can become powerful resources for healing. As a nurse you will be more successful in helping clients achieve desirable health outcomes after learning to support clients and families spiritually.

NURSING KNOWLEDGE BASE
Concepts in Spiritual Health

It is important for you to understand the concepts that are at the foundation of spiritual health. The concepts of spirituality, faith, hope, spiritual well-being, and religion give direction in understanding the view each individual has of life and its value.

SPIRITUALITY.   Spirituality is unique for each of us. Our definition of spirituality is influenced by our culture, development, life experiences, beliefs, and values about life. Our spirituality enables us to love, have faith and hope, seek meaning in life, and to nurture relationships with others. Reed (1992) explains that spirituality offers a sense of connectedness intrapersonally (connected with oneself), interpersonally (connected with others and the environment), and transpersonally (connected with God, the unseen, or a higher power). Through connectedness one is able to move beyond the stressors of everyday life and find comfort. Elements of spirituality found in the literature include **spiritual well-being,** spiritual needs, and spiritual awareness. There are two important characteristics of spirituality about which most authors agree: (1) it is a unifying theme in people's lives, and (2) it is a state of being.

There are individuals who either do not believe in the existence of God (**atheist**) or who believe that any ultimate reality is unknown or unknowable (**agnostic**). This does not mean that spirituality is not an important concept for the atheist or agnostic. Atheists search for meaning in life through their work and relationships with others (Burnard, 1988). Because atheists feel they are alone, they sense a strong responsibility for themselves. They also tend to believe in a joint responsibility for others. In acting for themselves, they feel they should also act for all of humankind. It is important for agnostics to discover meaning in what they do or how they live. Burnard (1988) explains that since agnostics find no ultimate meaning for the way things are, they believe that we as people bring meaning to what we do.

Spirituality is an integrating theme in our lives. Farran and others (1989) provide a model to show how spirituality represents the totality of one's being, serving as the overriding perspective that unifies the various aspects of an individual (Figure 17-1). Spirituality spreads throughout the physiological, psychological, and sociological dimensions of a person's life, whether or not the individual acknowledges or develops it (see Figure 17-1).

FAITH.   The concept of **faith** has two uses described in the literature. In the first, faith is defined as a cultural or institutional religion, such as Buddhism, Christianity, or Islam. Second, faith is a relationship with a divinity, higher power, authority, or spirit that incorporates a reasoning faith (belief) and a trusting faith (action) (Benner, 1985). Reasoning faith

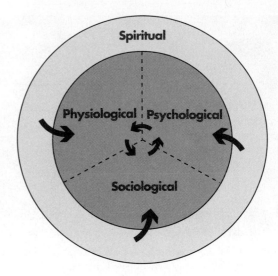

FIGURE **17-1**   The spiritual dimension: the unifying approach. (Modified from Farran CJ and others: Development of a model for spiritual assessment and intervention, *J Religion Health* 28[3]:185, 1989.)

is a person's belief and confidence in something for which there is no proof. It is an acceptance of what our reasoning cannot reach. Sometimes it involves a belief in a higher power, spirit guide, God, or Allah (Fryback, 1993). However, faith also might be the manner in which a person chooses to live life. Faith in this sense enables action. For example, a person might believe that having a positive outlook on life is the best way to achieve life's goals. The belief that comes with faith involves **transcendence,** or an awareness of that which cannot be seen or known in ordinary physical ways (Reed, 1987). It gives purpose and meaning to an individual's life, allowing for action. For example, cancer clients who have faith in a positive outlook on life might pursue more knowledge about their disease and continue to pursue daily activities rather than resign themselves to the disease's symptoms. Fryback (1993) studied clients diagnosed with human immunodeficiency virus (HIV) and found faith to be an inner power that enabled clients to act, to go on with life, and to gain a sense of freedom from their illness.

RELIGION.   Religion is associated with the "state of doing," or a specific system of practices associated with a particular denomination, sect or form of worship. Emblen (1992) defines religion as a system of organized beliefs and worship that a person practices to outwardly express spirituality. Many persons practice a faith or belief in the doctrines of a specific religion or sect, such as the Lutheran church within Christianity or Orthodox Judaism. Religion influences how the person exercises a faith of belief and action. For example, a Buddhist believes in Four Noble Truths: life is suffering, suffering is caused by desire, suffering can be eliminated by eliminating desire, and to eliminate desire, one follows an eightfold path (Giger and Davidhizar, 1995). The path includes right understanding, purpose, speech, conduct, vocation, effort, thinking, and meditation. A Buddhist turns inward, valuing self-control, whereas a Christian looks to the love of God to provide enlightenment and direction in life.

When providing spiritual care to clients you must know the differences between religion and spirituality. Religious care helps clients maintain their faithfulness to their belief systems and worship practices. Spiritual care helps people maintain personal relationships and a relationship to a higher being or life force, to identify meaning and purpose in life.

HOPE.   Spirituality is a key element in hope. When a person has the attitude of something to live for and look forward to, hope is present. **Hope** is a multidimensional concept that provides comfort while enduring life threats and personal challenges (Morse and Doberneck, 1995). It is a concept closely associated with faith. Hope is energizing, giving individuals a motivation to achieve and the resources to use toward that achievement. People express hope in all aspects of their lives as a force that helps them deal with life stressors. Hope is an invaluable personal resource whenever someone is faced with a loss (see Chapter 22) or a challenge that seems difficult to achieve. Morse and Doberneck (1995) conducted research with four different groups of clients: clients undergoing heart transplant, spinal cord injured clients, breast cancer survivors, and breast-feeding mothers intending to continue nursing while employed. Their work identified seven concepts of hope, revealing the complexity of hope and how very unique it can be for each individual (Box 17-1).

Spiritual Health

Individuals gain spiritual health by finding a balance between their life values, goals, and belief systems and their relationships within themselves and with others. Throughout life an individual may grow more spiritual, becoming increasingly aware of the meaning, purpose, and values of life. In times of stress, illness, loss, or recovery a person may turn to previous ways of responding or adjusting to a situation. Often these coping styles lie within the person's spiritual beliefs.

Spirituality begins as children learn about themselves and their relationships with others. Many adults experience spiritual growth by entering into lifelong relationships. An ability to care meaningfully for others and the self is evidence of a healthy spirituality. Older adults often turn to important relationships and the giving of themselves to others as spiritual tasks.

Spiritual Problems

When illness, loss, grief, or a major life change affects a person, spiritual resources help the person move to recovery. Without spiritual resources, concerns and doubts can develop within an individual. **Spiritual distress** is a nursing diagnosis, defined as the disruption in the "life principle" that fills a person's entire being and that integrates and transcends one's biological and psychosocial nature (North

Conceptual Components of Hope   Box 17-1

- A realistic initial assessment of threat or predicament
- The envisioning of options and setting of goals
- Bracing or preparing for negative outcomes
- A realistic assessment of personal resources and external conditions/resources
- The seeking out of mutually supportive relationships
- The continuous evaluation for signs that reinforce the selected goals
- A determination to endure

Modified from Morse JM, Doberneck B: Delineating the concept of hope, *Image J Nurs Sch* 27(4);277, 1995.

American Nursing Diagnosis Association, 2001). A catastrophic illness, for example, can upset a person's spiritual well-being sufficiently to cause doubt and loss of faith. Spiritual distress may cause the person to feel alone or even abandoned by resources that at one time were very nurturing. Individuals may question their spiritual values, raising questions about their whole way of life and purpose for living. Spiritual distress also occurs when there is conflict between a person's beliefs and prescribed health regimens or the inability to practice usual rituals.

ACUTE ILLNESS.   Sudden, unexpected illness that threatens a client's life, health, and/or well-being can create significant spiritual distress. For example, the 50-year-old man who has a heart attack and the 20-year-old who is injured in a motor vehicle accident both face crises that may threaten their spiritual health. The illness or injury creates an unanticipated scramble to integrate and cope with new realities (e.g., disability). People look for ways to remain faithful to their beliefs and value systems through use of spiritual resources. Often conflicts develop around a person's beliefs and the meaning of life. Anger is not uncommon, and clients may express it against God, their families, themselves, or the nurse. The strength of clients' spirituality influences their ability to cope with sudden illness and how quickly recovery can begin. Yim and Vande Creek (1996) have developed a spiritual healing critical pathway for coronary artery bypass clients. Their research has shown that knowledge of a person's spiritual well-being can be used to maximize a client's recovery. Hope and the ability to speak about life values and to gain meaning from illness influence a client's ability to recover from heart surgery. This has important implications for nurses to use appropriate interventions that help clients find purpose and worth to move forward and recover.

CHRONIC ILLNESS.   Persons with chronic illness often suffer debilitating symptoms that change their lifestyles. The uncertain and long-term character of chronic illness, along with the potential for outcomes such as pain, changes in body image, and the need to confront death, can lead to spiritual distress (O'Neill and Kenny, 1998). Clients struggle with questions about the meaning and

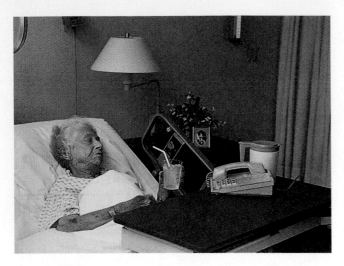

FIGURE 17-2 Dispiritedness can affect a person's adjustment to illness.

purpose of their lives because their independence can be threatened, causing fear, anxiety, and an overall dispiritedness (Figure 17-2). A person's spirituality can be a significant factor in how he or she adapts to the changes resulting from chronic illness. Successfully adapting to those changes can strengthen a person spiritually. A reevaluation of life may occur. Those who are able to use their spiritual resources have a much better chance to reestablish a self-identity and live to their potential.

TERMINAL ILLNESS. Terminal illness commonly causes fear of physical pain, isolation, the unknown, and dying (Turner and others, 1995). Clients may have an uncertainty about what death means and thus be susceptible to spiritual distress. There are also clients who have a spiritual sense of peace that enables them to face death without fear. Individuals experiencing a terminal illness often find themselves reviewing their life and questioning its meaning. Common questions asked include, "Why is this happening to me" or "What have I done?" Family and friends can be affected just as much as the client. Terminal illness causes members of the family to ask important questions about its meaning and how it will affect their relationship with the client (see Chapter 22).

Fryback (1993) learned how people with a terminal illness describe health. Clients identified the following three domains of health: mental-emotional, spiritual, and physical. The spiritual domain was seen as essential for health and included having a relationship with a higher power, recognizing mortality, and striving for self-actualization. Although many of the participants in the study either attended church or stated a desire to do so, others found that spirituality was not dependent on a religion or church. They associated health with belief in a higher power that gave them faith and the ability to love. The study revealed that when terminally ill clients have a perception of being unhealthy, it is not due to the disease but to being unable to live their lives fully and do the things they desire.

NEAR-DEATH EXPERIENCE. You may care for a client or have a family member who has had a near-death experience (NDE). An NDE is a psychological phenomenon of people who have either been close to clinical death or have recovered after being declared dead. It is not associated with a mental disorder (Basford, 1990). Persons who experience an NDE after cardiopulmonary arrest, for example, often tell the same story of feeling themselves rising above their bodies and watching caregivers initiate lifesaving measures. Most individuals describe passing through a tunnel to a bright light, encountering people who preceded them in death, and feeling an inner tranquility and peace. Instead of moving toward the light, they learn it is not time for them to die and they return to life.

Clients who have an NDE are often reluctant to discuss it, thinking family or caregivers will not understand. Isolation and depression can occur. However, individuals experiencing an NDE who can discuss it openly with family or caregivers find acceptance and meaning from this powerful experience. They consistently report positive aftereffects, including a positive attitude and spiritual development (Turner and others, 1995). After a client has survived a cardiopulmonary arrest, it is important for you to remain open and give the client a chance to explore what happened.

CRITICAL THINKING
Synthesis

The helping role is an important domain of nursing practice (Benner, 1984). Clients look to nurses for a different kind of help than that sought from other health care professionals. Expert nurses acquire the ability to anticipate the personal issues affecting clients' abilities to receive and seek help, including their spiritual well-being. Critical thinking knowledge and skills help you to enhance clients' spiritual well-being and health and to assist those in need of help and support in engaging their own spirituality for healing and recovery. While using the nursing process, you will apply knowledge, experience, attitudes, and standards in providing appropriate spiritual care.

KNOWLEDGE. Your knowledge about the concept of spirituality and a client's faith and belief systems helps to provide appropriate spiritual care. A client's faith history may reveal the individual's beliefs toward life, health, and a Supreme Being. Knowledge of a client's culture might provide additional insight into a person's spiritual practices. In addition, good communication principles (see Chapter 8) and caring (see Chapter 15) will help you to establish therapeutic trust with clients. An individual's spiritual beliefs are very personal and relational. When you are able to convey caring and openness to individuals, you will be more successful in promoting honest discussion about their spiritual beliefs.

When caring for clients with terminal illness, knowledge of loss and grief dynamics (see Chapter 22) is important. A person's reaction to loss is in part a function of the grief response, influenced by the person's spirituality. Another area of knowledge to consider while providing spiritual care is that of family dynamics (see Chapter 20). For many individuals, their spiritual health is often integrated with the relationships between family members. Family theory and the principles of family systems are important to consider in planning spiritual care for your client.

Another area of knowledge for you to reflect on is your own spiritual beliefs and values. Differentiate your personal spirituality from that of the client. This becomes important during the delivery of care, when you must be able to engage a client spiritually rather than try to exercise personal spiritual convictions. Your role is not to solve the spiritual problems of clients but to provide an environment where spirituality can be expressed (Humphreys, 2000).

Finally, a sound understanding of ethics and values (see Chapter 4) is also essential to providing spiritual care. A person's values or beliefs about the worth of a given idea, attitude, or custom are linked to the individual's spiritual well-being. Application of ethical principles ensures respect for a client's spiritual and religious convictions.

EXPERIENCE.   Recognizing that spirituality is more than religion, you need to consider personal views and philosophies about life and reflect on whether your own spirituality can be beneficial in assisting clients. If you sense a personal faith and hope regarding life, it is likely that you will be better able to help clients. Previous experiences with dying clients, clients with chronic disease, or clients who have experienced significant losses can provide lessons in how to help clients face difficult challenges and how to offer support to family and friends.

ATTITUDES.   Do not presume to know how a client might react to illness or loss. Humility becomes very important, particularly when caring for clients from diverse cultural and/or religious backgrounds. You must recognize any limitations in knowledge about a client's spiritual beliefs and religious practices and be willing to pursue the knowledge needed to provide appropriate, individualized care. Also exhibit integrity: realize the importance of refraining from expressing your opinions about religion or spirituality when they conflict with that of the client. Finally, show confidence in dealing with spiritual issues as you build a caring relationship with the client. Confidence works to build trust.

STANDARDS.   A good critical thinker must be complete and ensure that information about a client is significant and relevant when making decisions about clients' spiritual needs. The nature of a person's spirituality is complex and highly individualized. It is important to conduct a complete assessment of the client's spiritual beliefs and resources. Assumptions must be avoided regarding the client's religion and beliefs. Significance and relevance are standards of critical thinking that ensure you explore the issues that are most meaningful to clients and most likely to affect their spiritual well-being. Ethical standards of care must also be applied when providing spiritual care.

NURSING PROCESS

Application of the nursing process from the perspective of a client's spiritual needs is not simple. It goes beyond assessing a client's religious practices. Understanding a client's spirituality and then appropriately identifying the level of support and resources needed requires a new, broader perspective. Heliker (1992) describes the importance of shared community and compassion. *Compassion* comes from the Latin words *puti* and *cum,* meaning "to suffer with." *Community* is derived from the Latin word meaning "fellowship." To be compassionate is to "enter into places of pain, to share in brokenness with other human beings" (Heliker, 1992). To practice compassion as a nurse requires awareness of the very human tie between clients and a healing community. Remove any personal biases or misconceptions from your assessment, and be willing to share and discover another person's meaning and purpose in life, sickness, and health. Learn to look beyond a personal view when establishing a client relationship. This means identifying the common values that make us human and respecting the commitments and values that make humans unique.

Another important aspect of spiritual care is recognizing that a client does not have to have a spiritual problem. Clients bring certain spiritual resources for you to use as resources to help them assume healthier lives, recover from illness, or face impending death. Supporting and recognizing the positive side of a client's spirituality goes a long way in delivering effective, individualized nursing care.

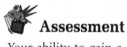 **Assessment**

Your ability to gain a reliable picture of clients' spirituality may be limited if you have only periodic contact with clients (e.g., outpatient settings) or if you fail to build therapeutic relationships with them. But once you establish a trusting relationship with a client, you and the client can reach a point of learning together, and spiritual caring can occur. Learn to consciously integrate an attitude of spiritual care into the nursing process. Your assessment should focus on aspects of spirituality most likely to be influenced by life experiences, events, and questions in the case of illness and hospitalization (Table 17-1). Conducting an assessment can be therapeutic because it conveys a level of caring and support. When you understand the overall approach to spiritual assessment you can enter into thoughtful discussions with the client, gain a greater awareness of the personal resources the client brings to a situation, and then incorporate the resources into an effective plan of care.

The JAREL spiritual well-being scale (Figure 17-3) was developed by nurse researchers to provide nurses and other health care professionals with a simple tool for assessing a client's spiritual well-being (Hungelmann and others, 1996). The tool was developed for clients from Christian, non-Christian, and atheist belief systems. Items on the tool comprise three key dimensions: the faith/belief dimension, life/self-responsibility, and life-satisfaction/self-actualization.

The tool is simple to use, requiring clients to rate their level of agreement with each item along a five-point scale (strongly agree to strongly disagree). For clients with visual or literacy problems, you can read the items and record the client's response. If the client's score on any item, group of items, or a particular dimension is low, it may indicate an area to explore further (Hungelmann and others, 1996). The tool can help you explore any perceptions or concerns a client might have. For example, if a client disagrees about accepting life situations, you need to spend time learning how the client accepts and manages his or her illness. Remember, when using any spiritual assessment tool, do not impose your personal value systems on the client. This is particularly true when the client's values and beliefs are similar to yours because it can then become very easy to make false assumptions.

FAITH/BELIEF. Individuals have some source of authority and guidance in their lives that leads them to choose and act on their beliefs. The authority can be a Supreme Being, a code of conduct, a religious leader, family or friends, oneself,

Example of a Focused Client Assessment		Table 17-1
Factors to Assess	Questions and Approaches	Physical Assessment Strategies
Past experiences with loss	Tell me how your life was affected when you lost your wife? How would you describe the ways you cope spiritually when faced with difficult times?	Observe client's facial expressions and mannerisms during the discussion.
Fear of the unknown resulting from a terminal illness	Describe the people who mean the most to you. In what way do you look to them for support? Do you consider yourself a spiritual person? If so, what gives you comfort? If not, what provides you a sense of peace?	Fear can be associated with anxiety. Be alert for changes in vital signs. Observe the client's mood, willingness to initiate conversation, and interest in surroundings.

DIRECTIONS: PLEASE CIRCLE THE CHOICE THAT **BEST** DESCRIBES HOW MUCH YOU AGREE WITH EACH STATEMENT. CIRCLE ONLY **ONE** ANSWER FOR EACH STATEMENT. THERE IS NO RIGHT OR WRONG ANSWER.

		Strongly Agree	Moderately Agree	Agree	Disagree	Moderately Disagree	Strongly Disagree
1.	Prayer is an important part of my life.	SA	MA	A	D	MD	SD
2.	I believe I have spiritual well-being.	SA	MA	A	D	MD	SD
3.	As I grow older, I find myself more tolerant of others' beliefs.	SA	MA	A	D	MD	SD
4.	I find meaning and purpose in my life.	SA	MA	A	D	MD	SD
5.	I feel there is a close relationship between my spiritual beliefs and what I do.	SA	MA	A	D	MD	SD
6.	I believe in an afterlife.	SA	MA	A	D	MD	SD
7.	When I am sick I have less spiritual well-being.	SA	MA	A	D	MD	SD
8.	I believe in a supreme power.	SA	MA	A	D	MD	SD
9.	I am able to receive and give love to others.	SA	MA	A	D	MD	SD
10.	I am satisfied with my life.	SA	MA	A	D	MD	SD
11.	I set goals for myself.	SA	MA	A	D	MD	SD
12.	God has little meaning in my life.	SA	MA	A	D	MD	SD
13.	I am satisfied with the way I am using my abilities.	SA	MA	A	D	MD	SD
14.	Prayer does not help me in making decisions.	SA	MA	A	D	MD	SD
15.	I am able to appreciate differences in others.	SA	MA	A	D	MD	SD
16.	I am pretty well put together.	SA	MA	A	D	MD	SD
17.	I prefer that others make decisions for me.	SA	MA	A	D	MD	SD
18.	I find it hard to forgive others.	SA	MA	A	D	MD	SD
19.	I accept my life situations.	SA	MA	A	D	MD	SD
20.	Belief in a supreme being has no part in my life.	SA	MA	A	D	MD	SD
21.	I cannot accept change in my life.	SA	MA	A	D	MD	SD

FIGURE **17-3** JAREL spiritual well-being scale. (Copyright 1987 by Hungelmann J, Kenkel-Rossi E, Klassen L, Stollenwerk R, Marquette University College of Nursing, Milwaukee, WI 53201.)

| Religious Beliefs About Health | | Table 17-2 |
Religious/Cultural Group	Health Care Beliefs	Response to Illness
Hinduism	Accepts modern medical science.	Illness is caused by past sins. Prolonging life is discouraged.
Sikhism	Accepts modern medical science.	Females to be examined by females. Removing undergarments causes great distress.
Buddhism	Accepts modern medical science.	May refuse treatment on holy days. Nonhuman spirits invading the body cause illness. May want a Buddhist priest. May permit withdrawal of life support. Does not practice euthanasia.
Islam	Must be able to practice the Five Pillars of Islam. May have a fatalistic view of health.	Uses faith healing. Family members are a comfort. Group prayer is strengthening. May permit withdrawal of life support. Does not practice euthanasia.
Judaism	Believes in the sanctity of life. God and medicine must have a balance. Observance of the Sabbath is important. May refuse treatments on the Sabbath.	Visiting the sick is an obligation. They are obligated to seek care. Euthanasia is forbidden. Life supports are discouraged.
Protestants/Catholics	Accept modern medical science.	Use prayer, faith healing. Appreciate visits from clergy. Some will use laying on of hands. Holy communion is commonly used. Last rites given when individual near death (Catholic).
Navajos	Concepts of health have a fundamental place in their concept of humans and their place in the universe.	Blessingway is a practice that attempts to remove ill health by means of stories, songs, rituals, prayers, symbols, and sand paintings (Sobralske, 1985).
Appalachians	Life and health are controlled by nature. Accept folk healers. Good Christian members of community are called as servants to minister to disabled (Giger and Davidhizar, 1995).	Dislike hospitals. Tend to be noncompliant in following medical regimens but expect to be helped directly when seeking episodic treatment.

or a combination of sources. Faith in an authority provides a sense of confidence that guides a person in exercising beliefs and experiencing growth. You can assess a person's faith in an authority by asking, "To what or whom do you look for guidance in life?" The client's response will likely open the door for a meaningful discussion. Listen carefully, and explore what is meaningful to the client.

Determine if the client has a religious source of guidance that conflicts with medical treatment plans. This can seriously affect the treatment options nurses and other health care providers can offer clients. For example, if a client is a Jehovah's Witness, blood products cannot be accepted as a form of treatment. Christian Scientists often refuse any medical intervention, believing that their faith will heal them.

It is also important to understand a client's philosophy of life. Asking the client, "Describe for me what is most important in your life" or "Tell me what gives your life meaning or purpose" may help to assess what is the basis of the client's spiritual belief system. This information reveals the client's spiritual focus and may help to reflect the impact illness, loss, or disability has on the person's life. Depending on a client's religious practices, views about health and the response to illness may influence how you will provide support (Table 17-2).

LIFE AND SELF-RESPONSIBILITY.   Spiritual well-being includes life and self-responsibility (Hungelmann and others, 1996). Individuals who can accept change in life, make decisions about their lives, and are able to forgive others in times of difficulty have a higher level of spiritual well-being. During illness clients often are unable to accept limitations or know what to do to regain a functional and meaningful life. Their sense of helplessness may reflect spiritual distress. However, if a client is able to adapt to changes and seek solutions for how to deal with any limitations, spiritual well-being reflects an important coping resource. Assess the extent a client understands any limitations or threats posed by an illness and the manner in which the client has chosen to adjust to them. You might ask, "Tell me how you feel about the changes caused by your illness" and "How do these changes affect what you now need to do?"

LIFE SATISFACTION.   Spiritual well-being seems to be tied to a person's satisfaction with life and what he or she has accomplished (Hungelmann and others, 1996). When persons are satisfied with life and the manner in which they are using their abilities, there is more energy available to deal with new difficulties and to resolve problems. Hasse and others (1992) have found satisfaction with someone or something to be associated with acceptance. Acceptance is the process of resolving issues within oneself or dealing with life experiences and is closely tied to hope and spirituality. You can assess a client's satisfaction with life by asking, "How happy or satisfied are you with your life?" or "Tell me to what extent you feel satisfied with what you have accomplished in life."

FELLOWSHIP AND COMMUNITY.   Fellowship is one kind of relationship an individual can have with other persons (Farran and others, 1989), including immediate family, close friends, associates at work or school, fellow members of a church, and neighbors. More specifically, this includes the extent of the community of shared faith between clients and their support networks. Ask the client, "With whom do you have a bond or find the greatest source of support in times of difficulty?" or "When you have faced difficult times in the past, who has been your greatest resource?"

Your assessment should explore the extent and nature of a person's support networks and their relationship with the client. It is unwise to assume that a given network offers the kind of support a client desires. For example, calling the client's clergy to request a visit might be inappropriate if the client finds little fellowship with that individual or the community that the individual represents. Does the client have one significant fellowship or several? What is the level of support received from the community? Do they visit, say prayers, or support the client's immediate family? You need to learn whether openness exists between the client and those persons with whom a fellowship has formed.

RITUAL AND PRACTICE.   The use of rituals and practice is easy to assess and can help you understand a client's spirituality. Rituals include participation in a religious group or private worship, prayer, sacraments such as baptism or communion, fasting, singing, meditating, scripture reading, and making offerings or sacrifices. Different religions have established various rituals for certain life events. For example, Buddhists practice baptism later in life and find burial or cremation acceptable at death. Muslims wash the body of a dead family member and wrap it in white cloth with the head turned toward the right shoulder. Orthodox and Conservative Jews have their newborn sons circumcised 8 days after birth. Determine whether a client's usual rituals or practices have been interrupted as a result of illness or hospitalization. A ritual can provide a client with structure and support during difficult times. If rituals are important to the client, use them as part of your nursing intervention.

VOCATION.   Individuals express their spirituality daily in life routines, work, play, and relationships (Farran and others, 1989). Spirituality can be used in their vocation in life and be part of their identity. Determine if illness or hospitalization has altered the person's ability to express some as-

Case Study   **SYNTHESIS IN PRACTICE**

Jeff has anticipated the next visit by Sarah and Joe Stein to the clinic. He has spent time learning more about Sarah's disease and treatment plan so that he can better explain what to expect as chemotherapy progresses. Jeff recognizes that Joe usually comes to the clinic with Sarah and has been described by her as a strong source of support. However, Jeff does not know enough about the couple's relationship and wants to explore this further. The role of family members in providing support, particularly with regard to decision making, is important for Jeff to understand before a plan of care can be developed. In reviewing information about loss and grieving, Jeff recognizes that Sarah shows acceptance of her disease because she is able to discuss cancer and the plan for treatment. Jeff knows that as clients begin to accept the fact of being diagnosed with a life-threatening disease, it is important to offer opportunities to share feelings and to begin to provide time to discuss future plans.

Jeff's previous experience with clients with cancer has taught him that when clients express hope, they seem to be able to move forward and cope with the challenges of their disease. During the last clinic visit, Sarah expressed an intermediate hope, to be able to attend her son's bar mitzvah. Jeff reflected on that experience and thinks that Sarah and Joe may have a strong sense of spiritual well-being that will help them cope with cancer. Further assessment will be necessary.

Jeff wants to be complete in assessing Sarah and Joe's level of spiritual health. Jeff is Lutheran and is not well informed about the couple's religion, Judaism. However, he knows that the Jewish sense of community is very strong and that it is important to learn more about how members of the Stein's temple or synagogue play a role in offering support to the family. Jeff recognizes that spiritual well-being is more complex than simply religion. He spends time reflecting on his own value and belief systems so that he can remain open and receptive to understanding the spiritual belief systems that Sarah and Joe possess.

pect of spirituality. Expression of spirituality may include showing an appreciation for life in the variety of things people do, living in the moment and not worrying about tomorrow, appreciating nature, expressing love toward others, and being productive. Assess whether the client loses the ability to express a sense of relatedness to something greater than the self (Fryback, 1993). Questions might include, "Has your illness affected the way you live your life spiritually, at home or where you work?" or "Has your illness affected your ability to express what's important in life for you?" If illness or loss prevents an individual from exercising his or her spirituality, you must understand the implications psychologically, socially, and spiritually and find ways to offer guidance and support.

CLIENT EXPECTATIONS.   Before completing your spiritual assessment, learn what the client expects from you and other caregivers. If the client senses your compassion, an expectation might involve maintaining a trusting and open relationship. In addition, it might be important that the client perceive caregivers to be accepting of religious practices or rituals. Asking the client what expectations are held of caregivers can be very beneficial in establishing a strong nurse-client partnership.

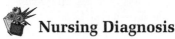 Nursing Diagnosis

When reviewing a spiritual assessment to identify appropriate nursing diagnoses, you will know a great deal about the client's spirituality. Exploring a client's spirituality may reveal responses to health problems that require nursing intervention, or it may reveal a strong set of resources for the client to use in coping (Box 17-2). As you identify nursing diagnoses for a client, it is important to recognize the significance that spirituality has for all types of health problems. Pain, fear, anxiety, and self-care deficit are just some examples of nursing diagnoses that will require you to apply spiritual care principles.

Three nursing diagnoses accepted by the North American Nursing Diagnosis Association (NANDA) pertain specifically to spirituality. *Readiness for enhanced spiritual well-being* is based on defining characteristics that show a pattern of inner strength and interconnectedness that comes from inner faith and hope (NANDA, 2000). Your assessment will reveal that the client has a strong faith; is in harmony with self, others, and a higher power; and has a good sense of the purpose and meaning of life. A client with enhanced spiritual well-being has resources to draw on when faced with other nursing diagnoses. You can help the client explore how to use these resources when facing health problems.

The nursing diagnoses of *spiritual distress* and *risk for spiritual distress* create different clinical pictures. Defining characteristics from your assessment will show patterns that reflect a person's actual or potential dispiritedness (e.g., expressing concern with the meaning of life and beliefs, anger toward God, and verbalizing conflicts about personal beliefs). Clients likely to be at risk for spiritual distress include those who have poor relationships, have experienced a recent loss, or are suffering some form of mental or physical illness. Defining characteristics must be validated and clarified with the client before you can make a diagnosis and develop a plan of care. With spiritual care, the importance of your own spiritual well-being and perceptions cannot be overemphasized. Do not impose your personal beliefs. Be sure any diagnosis has an accurate related factor (e.g., a situational loss or relationship conflict) so that your interventions can be purposeful and goal directed.

Planning

During planning, integrate the knowledge gathered from assessment and knowledge relating to resources and therapies available for spiritual care to develop an individualized plan of care (see care plan). Match the client's needs with those interventions that are supported and recommended in the clinical and research literature. Focus on building a caring relationship with the client so that you might enter into a healing relationship together.

Nursing Diagnoses for Box 17-2
CLIENTS IN NEED OF SPIRITUAL CARE

- Anxiety
- Anxiety, death
- Coping, compromised family
- Coping, ineffective
- Family processes, interrupted
- Fear
- Grieving, anticipatory
- Loneliness, risk for
- Self-esteem, situational low
- Sorrow, chronic
- Spiritual distress
- Spiritual well-being, readiness for enhanced

GOALS AND OUTCOMES.   A spiritual plan of care must include realistic and individualized goals along with relevant outcomes. This will require you to collaborate closely with the client in setting goals and outcomes and ultimately choosing nursing interventions. In cases where spiritual care requires helping clients adjust to loss or stressful situations, goals may be long term (e.g., regaining spiritual comfort or affirming a purpose in life). Short-term goals, such as renewing participation in religious practices, may be helpful to allow a client to move toward a more spiritually healthy situation. Outcomes must relate to what you have learned about the client. For example, if you know a client once practiced regular prayer and meditation, an outcome for the goal of regaining spiritual comfort might be stated, "Client will reinstitute regular prayer and meditation daily."

SETTING PRIORITIES.   Spiritual care is very personalized. You must establish a relationship allowing you to know what the client's priorities are. If you have developed a mutually agreed-on plan with the client, he or she should be able to relate what is most important. Spiritual priorities need not be sacrificed for physical care priorities. In the case of a terminally ill client, for example, spiritual care may be the most important intervention you can provide.

CONTINUITY OF CARE.   To ensure ongoing spiritual care, it may become necessary to involve family members, significant others, and clergy to lend support. This means you learned from the assessment which individuals or groups have formed a fellowship with the client. These individuals can become involved in all levels of your plan. The client's support network may assist in sharing quiet moments of prayer, reading scripture to the client, and even giving physical care. In a hospital setting the pastoral care department can be a valuable resource. These professionals can provide insight about how and when to best support clients and families.

Implementation

If a client is in spiritual distress or has a health problem that requires the client to use spiritual resources, a caring relationship between you and the client is necessary. Both you and the client must feel free to let go and discover together

Case Study Nursing Care Plan   SPIRITUALITY

ASSESSMENT

Sarah has been told her prognosis is promising, although treatment will be needed to prevent spread of her disease. Sarah expresses a **connectedness with her God**, "I do not feel alone; God is with me. I have a better appreciation of each day God gives me, and I believe God will help me see my son's bar mitzvah." Sarah and Joe **attend synagogue regularly and hope to continue** doing so even during the chemotherapy. Jeff learns that Joe encourages Sarah and has been trying to arrange work so that he can take her to the clinic. This means that since their mother's illness, he has less time in the evening to spend with the children. In the past, Joe and Sarah have always had discussions with the children during mealtime, but this has been difficult. **Members of their synagogue have offered support** by taking Sarah to the clinic if Joe is unable.

Sarah worries about her children. During the last month she has spent less time with Valerie and Peter because of her cancer treatment and resultant fatigue. Peter is having some difficulty with studying for the bar mitzvah. He is also doing poorly in school. Valerie has recently expressed concern that her mother might die. Both children reportedly have been acting angrily toward their parents. Before Sarah's illness the children were very **close to their parents and shared their faith in God.**

*Defining characteristics are shown in bold type.

NURSING DIAGNOSIS

Readiness for enhanced spiritual well-being related to renewed appreciation of life after cancer diagnosis.

PLANNING

GOAL	EXPECTED OUTCOMES
Client will restore connectedness with children (within 2 months)	Client, husband, and children will discuss client's beliefs about the future and her hope of having the cancer cured (to be met in 2 weeks). Client will report son and daughter's ability to discuss fears with mother (to be met in 4 weeks).

IMPLEMENTATION

STEPS	RATIONALE
1. Plan a conference late in afternoon at cancer clinic where children can attend to hear discussion of mother's progress. Establish a presence, and express a realistic hope of mother's prognosis.	Ensures children will have accurate perception of mother's clinical condition and course. Offering compassionate presence and support aids clients' spiritual well-being (Peri, 1995).
2. Encourage client to discuss with family the meaning life now has for her after being diagnosed with breast cancer.	Situations seen from the individual's point of view will enhance understanding and sensitivity on the part of the family.
3. Recommend use of storytelling to reminisce with family about experiences that were positive and representative of mutual support.	Storytelling allows a pattern to emerge that describes client's way of life filled with meaning. Helps family understand need for mutual love and support (Heliker, 1992).
4. Encourage client and husband to focus a discussion with children on their fears about mother's well-being.	Gives children opportunity to discuss their primary concerns and to clarify their roles as part of the family.

EVALUATION

- Have client and husband report on outcomes of discussions with children.
- Observe interactions between parents and children.
- Ask client to describe feelings she has when communicating with children about cancer.

---

the meaning illness or loss poses for the client and the impact it has on the meaning and purpose of life. Achieving this level of understanding with a client enables you to deliver care in a sensitive, creative, and appropriate manner.

HEALTH PROMOTION.   Spiritual care should be a central theme in promoting an individual's overall well-being. Spirituality is one personal resource that affects the balance between health and illness. The interventions described here under health promotion can be used at any level of health care.

ESTABLISHING PRESENCE.   Clients have reported that the presence of nurses contributes to a sense of well-being and

provides hope for recovery (Clark and others, 1991). Behaviors that establish your presence include giving attention, answering questions, listening, and having a positive and encouraging (but realistic) attitude. Presence is part of the art of nursing. Benner (1984) explains that presence involves "being with" a client versus "doing for" a client. Presence is being able to offer a closeness with the client: physically, psychologically, and spiritually. Presence can help to prevent emotional and environmental isolation.

When health promotion is the focus of care, your presence becomes important in instilling confidence in clients' abilities to take the steps necessary to remain healthy. You can convey a caring presence by listening to clients' concerns, willingly involving family in discussions about the client's health, and showing self-confidence when providing health instruction.

Trust is fundamental to any relationship. The attitude you convey when first interacting with a client sets the tone for all conversations (see Chapter 8). Listening to the meaning of what a client says is most important. It involves paying attention to the person's words, tone of voice, and entering his or her frame of reference. By observing expressions and body language of the client, you can find cues to help assist the client in exploring ways to achieve inner peace, take action, or do whatever a situation demands (Hungelmann and others, 1996). Peri (1995) concludes that the role of nurses is not to solve the spiritual problems of clients but to provide an environment where spirituality can be expressed.

SUPPORTING A HEALING RELATIONSHIP.   When giving spiritual care, look beyond isolated client problems and recognize the broader picture of a client's holistic needs. For example, do not just look at a client's back pain as a problem to solve with quick remedies but rather how the pain influences the client's ability to function and achieve goals established in life. A holistic view enables you to assume a helping role. Within a helping role, nurses learn to establish healing relationships (Benner, 1984). Three steps are evident when a healing relationship develops between a nurse and client:

1. Mobilizing hope for the nurse and for the client
2. Finding an interpretation or understanding of the illness, pain, anxiety, or other stressful emotion that is acceptable to the client
3. Assisting the client in using social, emotional, or spiritual resources (Benner, 1985)

Central to a healing relationship is mobilizing the client's hope. Hope motivates people to face challenges in life. You can help a client find realistic things to hope for. A client newly diagnosed with diabetes might hope to learn how to manage the disease so as to continue a productive and satisfying way of life. A terminally ill client may hope to attend a daughter's graduation and live each day to the fullest.

Hope has both short- and long-term implications. From a long-term perspective, hope gives individuals a determination to endure and carry on with life's responsibilities. In the short-term view, hope provides an incentive for constructive coping with obstacles and for finding ways to realize the object of hope. Hope is future oriented and helps a client work toward recovery. You can help clients achieve hope by working with them to find explanations for their situations that are mutually acceptable. Then help each client realistically exercise hope. This might include supporting a client's positive attitude toward life or a desire to be informed and to make decisions.

To further support a healing relationship, remain aware of the client's spiritual resources and needs. It is always important for clients to be able to express and exercise their beliefs and to find spiritual comfort. When illness or treatment create confusion or uncertainty for the client, you must recognize the possible effect this can have on a client's well-

being. How can spiritual resources be used and strengthened? Having a clear sense of what illness may hold for an individual helps the person to apply all resources toward recovery.

ACUTE CARE.   Within an acute care setting, support and enhancement of a client's spiritual well-being can be a challenge when the focus of health care seems to be one of treatment and cure rather than care. Display a soothing presence and supportive touch as you administer nursing therapies. The client may be fearful of experiencing an illness that would threaten loss of control and looks for someone to offer competent direction. Your artful use of hands, encouraging words of support, and calm and decisive approach will establish a presence that builds trust. Work closely with clients to maximize resources that support their spirituality.

SUPPORT SYSTEMS.   Use of support systems is of course important in any health care setting. Clark and others (1991) found that support systems provided clients with the greatest sense of well-being during hospitalization. Support systems serve as a human link connecting the client, the nurse, and the client's lifestyle before an illness. Part of the client's caregiving environment is the regular presence of family and friends viewed by the client as supportive. Plan care with the client and the client's support network to promote the interpersonal bonding that is needed for recovery. The support system becomes an important resource in conducting the religious rituals on which a client relies.

When a client depends on family and friends for support, encourage them to visit the client regularly. Provide for privacy, and encourage the family to be themselves during visits to provide the spiritual comfort that they are capable of sharing. Often illness and the hospital environment produce unknowns that intimidate family members and friends. Help the family to feel welcome and use their support and presence to promote the client's healing. Including family members in prayer, for example, is a thoughtful gesture if it is appropriate to the client's religion, and if family members are comfortable participating. Encouraging the family to bring meaningful religious symbols to the client's bedside can offer significant spiritual support.

Other important resources to clients are spiritual advisors and members of the clergy. A hospital's pastoral care department can assist in notifying community clergy of their congregant's admission. When pastoral care is unavailable, ask if clients desire to have their clergy notified of their hospitalization. All clergy should be made welcome on nursing units. When requested by clients or families, keep clergy informed of any physical, psychosocial, or spiritual concerns affecting the client. Show respect for clients' spiritual values and needs by willingly cooperating with others giving spiritual care and by facilitating the administration of sacraments, rites, and rituals.

DIET THERAPIES.   Food and nutrition are important aspects of nursing care. Food is also an important component of some religious observances. For example, some Hindu and

---

Outcome Evaluation for **SARAH STEIN**   Box 17-4

Nursing Action	Client Response/Finding	Achievement of Outcome
Ask Sarah to describe how children reacted to discussion with her and Joe. Did children express concerns? During next clinic visit observe manner in which Sarah and children interact.	Children initially did not speak, only listened. With Joe's encouragement, daughter began to express her fears. Both children come to clinic with Sarah. They spontaneously ask questions of staff. Daughter stands close to mother and asks if chemotherapy infusion is uncomfortable.	Outcome partially met. Recommend an additional session with children. Children showing closeness to mother and interest in her well-being. Recommend a final family conference after last round of chemotherapy.

Gerontological Nursing Practice   Box 17-3

- Religious activities and attitudes are very common among older adults. A large proportion of older adults claim that religion helps them to cope both when asked directly about religion as a source of strength in difficult times and when asked indirectly about how they coped with stressful life events (Koenig, 1987).
- The very old are more likely to be interested in the nonorganizational aspects of religion than in active participation (Courtney and others, 1992).
- Consideration and a belief in the afterlife increases as adults grow older. Visits from clergy, social workers, lawyers, and even financial advisors can be made available so clients feel prepared. Leaving a legacy to loved ones prepares the older adult to leave the world with a sense of meaning (Ebersole and Hess, 1998). Legacies may include oral histories, works of art, publications, photographs, or some other object of significance.

Islamic sects are vegetarians. Muslims are not allowed to eat pork, and fasting is done during the month of Ramadan. Orthodox Jewish clients observe kosher dietary restrictions. Native Americans have food practices influenced by individual tribal beliefs. As with many aspects of a particular culture or religion, food and the rituals surrounding the preparation and serving of food can be important to a client's spirituality. When possible, integrate the client's dietary preferences into daily care. Consult with the health care institution's dietitian. In the event that a hospital or other health care agency cannot prepare food in the preferred way, the family may be asked to bring meals fitting into any dietary restrictions posed by the client's condition.

SUPPORTING RITUALS. You can become active in your clients' spiritual care by supporting clients' participation in spiritual rituals and activities. This is especially important for older adults (Box 17-3). Plan care to allow time for religious readings, spiritual visitations, or even attendance at religious services. Some churches and synagogues offer audiotapes of religious services. Allow family members to plan a prayer session or an organized reading when appropriate. Taped meditations, religious music, and televised religious services provide other effective treatment options. Be respectful of icons, medals, prayer rugs, or crosses that clients bring to a healthcare setting to be sure they are not accidentally lost or misplaced.

RESTORATIVE AND CONTINUING CARE

PRAYER AND MEDITATION. The act of prayer gives an individual the opportunity to renew personal faith and belief in a higher being in a specific, focused way that may be highly ritualized and formal or quite spontaneous and informal. Prayer has been shown to be an effective coping resource for physical and psychological symptoms. Clients may pray in private or pursue opportunities for group prayer with family, friends, or clergy. You can be supportive of prayer by giving the client privacy if desired, learning if the client wishes to have you participate, and by suggesting prayer when it is known to be a coping resource for the client. If prayer is not suitable for a client, an alternative may be to read from a book selected by the client or from poetry or inspirational texts.

Meditation can be effective in creating a relaxation response that reduces daily stress. Meditation exercises can give clients relief from chronic pain, insomnia, anxiety, and depression and can help in coping with the side effects of uncomfortable therapy. Individuals who regularly—twice a day, for 10 or 20 minutes—sit quietly in a comfortable position with their eyes closed and repeat a sound, phrase, or sacred word in rhythm with their breathing, disregarding intrusive thoughts as they do so, experience decreased metabolism and heart rate, easier breathing, and slower brain waves (Culligan, 1996). Chapter 29 addresses relaxation approaches.

Evaluation

CLIENT CARE. Attainment of spiritual health is a lifelong goal. Clients will experience the need to clarify values (see Chapter 4), reshape philosophies, and live those experiences that help to shape purpose in life. As you provide spiritual care, always evaluate whether planned outcomes and goals were achieved (Box 17-4). Compare the client's level of spiritual health with the behaviors and perceptions noted in the nursing assessment (see case study). For example, if your assessment found the client losing hope, the follow-up evaluation involves a discussion to determine if the client has regained an attitude of something to live for. Family and friends

Case Study   EVALUATION

Sarah returns to the clinic the week after establishing the plan with Jeff. A member of the synagogue accompanies Sarah because Joe is out of town on a business trip. Jeff wants to evaluate whether Sarah has begun to spend time with the children to discuss the effect her experience has had on them. Jeff asks, "Tell me, Mrs. Stein, have you had a chance yet to try any of the approaches we talked about last week to give the kids a chance to talk about their feelings? If so, what were the results?" Sarah reports, "Yes, Joe and I spent a couple of hours Saturday evening talking about what all of this means. It was during a time when we have always tried to be together as a family, and the kids seemed to appreciate it. They asked many questions. They are looking forward to coming to the clinic Thursday. I hope this will help them settle down a bit and feel less frightened." Jeff also determines that Sarah has spoken with close friends from her synagogue and they plan to visit her this week. The client also is going to see the physical therapist today.

In an effort to evaluate if Sarah's expectations were met, Jeff asks, "Do you believe we have helped you so far with your concerns about your children? Your faith is strong, and it is my hope you have felt comfortable in talking about your worries." Sarah replies, "The best thing you have done is listen and recognize how important my family is to me. Your suggestions have helped so far; I am encouraged by them."

DOCUMENTATION NOTE
The client visited the clinic for her third week of chemotherapy. She denies nausea but is complaining of some soreness in the mouth and a loss of hair. She asks questions readily and has made an appointment with the physical therapist as recommended. She has expressed hope that her children will feel less frightened over the diagnosis. The children will be attending the next clinic visit.

with whom the client seeks to have fellowship can be a useful source of evaluative information. Successful outcomes should reveal the client developing an increased or restored sense of connectedness with family, maintaining, reviewing, or re-forming a sense of purpose in life and, for some, a confidence and trust in a Supreme Being or higher power.

For clients with a serious or terminal illness, evaluation focuses on the goal of helping the client retain faith and hope or express openly the uncertainties life poses. Evaluate how the client is accepting the illness and whether hope has enabled the client to recognize individual mortality and focus on living for each day. Fryback (1993) found that the terminally ill, regardless of whether they followed a formal religion, held a belief in a higher power, which gave them a sense they were not alone. Do not assume all clients have such faith. However, your support aims to help clients accept their destiny and to be at peace.

CLIENT EXPECTATIONS.   Evaluate whether client expectations were met. Evaluating spiritual care requires determining if the client's spiritual practices were respected and if the quality of the nurse-client relationship was supportive. Both the client and family should be able to relate if opportunities were offered for religious rituals. With respect to the nurse-client relationship, does the client express trust and confidence in you? Is the client able to discuss those things that are important spiritually? Taking time to ask the client to reflect on the quality of the nurse-client relationship is time well spent. Asking the client, "Have I helped you to become comfortable in saying what you feel is important to you spiritually?" will determine whether an effective healing relationship was developed.

Key Terms

agnostic, *p. 422*
atheist, *p. 422*

faith, *p. 422*
holistic, *p. 421*
hope, *p. 423*
spiritual distress, *p. 423*

spirituality, *p. 421*
spiritual well-being, *p. 422*
transcendence, *p. 422*

Key Concepts

- Attending to a client's spirituality ensures a holistic focus to nursing practice.
- Frequently spirituality and religion are interchanged, but spirituality is a much broader and more unifying concept than religion.
- An individual's beliefs and spiritual well-being can influence physical function.
- Faith and hope are closely linked to a person's spiritual well-being, providing an inner strength for dealing with illness and disability.
- Religion is a system of organized beliefs that a person practices to outwardly express his or her spirituality.
- Being an atheist or agnostic does not eliminate spirituality as an important resource for a client.

- Research suggests there may be a link between a client's spirituality and potential for healing.
- Acute and chronic illness, terminal illness, and near-death experiences pose spiritual problems for individuals.
- The provision of appropriate spiritual care requires you to critically apply knowledge from principles related to caring, cultural care, loss and grief, and therapeutic communication.
- Avoid biases when assessing and planning spiritual care.
- Learning to practice caring and compassion helps you to discover a client's life values and meaning.
- Fellowship with other persons can be a source of hope for a client.
- Clients often have spiritual strengths that you as the nurse can use as resources to help them assume healthier lives.

- Interruptions or changes to customary religious practices may affect the support that religion contributes to a person's well-being.
- Common religious rituals include private worship, prayer, singing, use of a rosary, and scripture reading.
- The personal nature of spirituality requires open communication and the establishment of trust between you and the client.

- Establishing presence involves giving attention, answering questions, having an encouraging attitude, and conveying a sense of trust.
- Part of a client's caregiving environment can be the regular presence of family, friends, and spiritual advisors.

Critical Thinking Activities

1. Mr. Bruns is a terminally ill client suffering from acquired immunodeficiency syndrome (AIDS). He has expressed a sense of abandonment by friends and even family as his disease has progressed. The nurse finds him crying, "Oh, I feel that God has left my life." How might the nurse offer him spiritual support?
2. Norma Lee is a 72-year-old woman with advanced glaucoma who had surgery on her right knee 5 days ago. Her close friend and neighbor, who assisted in administering her eye drops, recently died. The friend also regularly drove Mrs. Lee to church and attended services with her. The registered nurse (RN) from the home health agency is visiting to evaluate Ms. Lee for home health aid services. How might the nurse help Ms. Lee continue exercising her religious rituals?
3. Consider a typical clinical situation in which you might enter a client's room and find that the client is experiencing serious symptoms (e.g., pain, nausea, or shortness of breath). You are able to help resolve the client's symptoms, but then the client asks you, "Do you believe in God?" Consider how you might respond.

Review Questions

1. You enter the hospital room to discover that your client is crying quietly in bed. You walk to the bedside, announce your entry, place your hand on the client's shoulder, and softly ask, "Can you tell me what is bothering you?" In this example you are demonstrating:
   1. coaching.
   2. presence
   3. establishing hope.
   4. offering social resource.
2. Health care treatment is discouraged on a holy day by:
   1. Islam.
   2. Hinduism.
   3. Buddhism.
   4. Christianity.
3. During your assessment of a client at a neighborhood health clinic you learn that the client recently lost his job as a store manager. The client has no presenting health problems. He continues to take his medication regularly for high blood pressure. The client's wife is in the waiting room, and when the client walked into the examination room, you observed the two arguing about what to tell the physician. The client may likely be experiencing the nursing diagnosis of:
   1. spiritual distress.
   2. coping, ineffective.
   3. spiritual distress, risk for.
   4. health maintenance, ineffective.
4. You have been caring for a client recently diagnosed with colon cancer. You enter the client's room prepared to assess vital signs and to determine if the client is having any discomfort. The client interrupts you and says, "You know, I really am worried about how my family is going to take all of this." You stop placing the blood pressure cuff around the client's arm and say, "Tell me what concerns you have." You are demonstrating an intellectual standard for critical thinking called:
   1. humility.
   2. completeness.
   3. significance.
   4. risk taking.
5. Hope is a concept related to spirituality that can best be described as:
   1. satisfaction with someone or something.
   2. having a bond with another person for ongoing support.
   3. having confidence in something for which there is no proof.
   4. knowing a threat exists and preparing for any undesired outcomes.
6. For Hindus it is important to consider that:
   1. some sects are vegetarians.
   2. followers must observe fast days.
   3. many individuals avoid meats containing blood.
   4. members abstain from alcohol and caffeine.

References

Basford TK: *Near death experience: an annotated bibliography,* New York, 1990, Garland.

Benner DG: *Baker encyclopedia of psychology,* Grand Rapids, Mich, 1985, Baker Book House.

Benner P: *From novice to expert,* Menlo Park, Calif, 1984, Addison-Wesley.

Burnard P: The spiritual needs of atheists and agnostics, *Prof Nurse* 4(3):130, 1988.

Calabria M, Macrae, J, editors: *Suggestions for thought by Florence Nightingale: selections and commentaries,* Philadelphia, 1994, University of Pennsylvania Press.

Clark CC and others: Spirituality: integral to quality care, *Holist Nurs Pract* 5(3):67, 1991.

Coe RM: The magic of science and the science of magic: an essay on the process of healing, *J Health Soc Behav* 38(3):1, 1997.

Courtey BC and others: Religiosity and adaptation in the oldest old. In Poon LW, editor: *The Gengea centenarian study,* Amityville, NY, 1992, Baywood.

Culligan K: Spirituality and healing in medicine, *America*, p 17, August 31, 1996.

Dombeck MB: Dream-telling: a means of spiritual awareness, *Holist Nurs Pract* 9(2):37, 1995.

Ebersole P, Hess P: *Toward healthy aging*, ed 5, St. Louis, 1998, Mosby.

Emblen JD: Religion and spirituality defined according to current use in nursing literature, *J Prof Nurs* 8(1):41, 1992.

Farran CJ and others: Development of a model for spiritual assessment and intervention, *J Religion Health* 28(3):185, 1989.

Fryback PB: Health for people with a terminal diagnosis, *Nurs Sci Q* 6(3):147, 1993.

Giger JN, Davidhizar RE: *Transcultural nursing: assessment and intervention*, ed 2, St. Louis, 1995, Mosby.

Haase JE and others: Simultaneous concept analysis of spiritual perspective, hope, acceptance, and self-transcendence, *Image J Nurs Sch* 24(2):141, 1992.

Heliker D: Reevaluation of a nursing diagnosis: spiritual distress, *Nurs Forum* 27(4):15, 1992.

Humphreys J: Spirituality and distress in sheltered battered women, *J Nurs Scholarship*, 32(3):273, 2000.

Hungelmann J and others: Focus on spiritual well-being: harmonious interconnectedness of mind-body-spirit—use of the JAREL spiritual well-being scale, *Geriatr Nurs* 17(6):262, 1996.

Kellar P: Mind-body medicine, *Midwest Pain Society Update*, p 3, July 2001.

Kiecolt-Glaser JK and others: Psychosocial enhancement of immunocompetence in a geriatric population, *Health Psychol* 4:25, 1985.

Koenig H: Religion and well-being in later life (abstract), *Proceedings of the Third Congress of the International Psychogeriatric Association*, Chicago, 1987.

Morse JM, Doberneck B: Delineating the concept of hope, *Image J Nurs Sch* 27(4):277, 1995.

North American Nursing Diagnosis Association: *NANDA Nursing diagnoses: definitions and classifications 2001-2002*, Philadelphia, 2001, The Association.

O'Neill DP, Kenny EK: Spirituality and chronic illness, *Image J Nurs Sch* 30(3):275, 1998.

Peri TC: Promoting spirituality in persons with acquired immunodeficiency syndrome: a nursing intervention, *Holist Nurs Pract* 10(1):68, 1995.

Reed PG: Spirituality and well-being in terminally ill hospitalized adults, *Res Nurs Health* 10:335, 1987.

Reed PG: An emerging paradigm for the investigation of spirituality in nursing, *Res Nurs Health* 15:349, 1992.

Sobralske M: Perceptions of health: Navajo Indians, *Top Clin Nurs* 7(3):32, 1985.

Turner JA, Clancy S: Strategies for coping with chronic low back pain: relationship to pain and disability, *Pain* 24:355, 1986.

Turner RP and others: Religious or spiritual problems: a culturally sensitive diagnostic category in the DSM IV, *J Nerv Ment Dis* 183(7):435, 1995.

Yim RJR, Vande Creek L: Unbinding grief and life's losses for thriving recovery after open heart surgery, *Caregiver J* 12(2):8, 1996.

18

Growth and Development

Objectives

- Define key terms.
- Compare the frameworks for growth and development as described by major developmental theorists.
- Describe the growth and development changes that occur in individuals from conception through old age.
- Identify factors that can facilitate or interfere with normal growth and development of individuals at each stage of life.
- Specify the physical and psychosocial health concerns of infants, children, adolescents, and adults.
- Use knowledge of growth and development to enhance use of the nursing process for individuals across the life span.
- Identify specific nursing interventions for the health promotion of clients across the life span.
- Use critical judgment to determine appropriate teaching topics for individual clients across the life span.

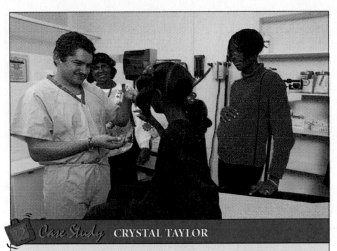

Case Study CRYSTAL TAYLOR

Crystal Taylor, a 25-year-old black young adult, is the single parent of $2^1/_2$-year-old Zachary and $5^1/_2$-year-old Monica and is in the sixth month of a current pregnancy. She lives with her 44-year-old mother and 15-year-old brother. Crystal's 68-year-old maternal grandmother and uncle live next door and often help care for Zachary and Monica. Crystal's family has used the city clinic for years, and she now brings her children to the neighborhood clinic for their health care. Today she has brought Monica to the clinic for her checkup before beginning school.

Louis Ruiz is a 28-year-old student assigned to the clinic, where he is to select a family to follow throughout the semester. Louis, who is married and has a 4-year-old son who attends day care, was a medical technician in the army for 4 years. The clinic is Louis' first clinical experience as a student nurse, and he is eager to become involved in health promotion activities but also anxious about his new role as a professional nurse.

As a nurse, you will care for individuals of all ages. If you look at clients from a developmental perspective, you can provide care that considers the unique needs and level of development of each person.

SCIENTIFIC KNOWLEDGE BASE
Growth and Development Theory

The terms *growth* and *development* used together encompass all of the many changes that take place throughout an individual's lifetime (Wong and others, 1999). **Growth** is the measurable aspect of a person's increase in physical dimensions. Indicators of growth include changes in height, weight, teeth and skeletal structures, and sexual characteristics. **Development** is the behavioral aspect of a person's adaptation to the environment. Behaviors that indicate development are increased ability to function such as learning to walk and talk.

Maturation is the biological plan for growth and development. Physical growth and motor development are a function of maturation. Examples of age-related behaviors that follow a specific sequence are sitting, walking, and reading, which are a result of maturation.

A **critical period of development** refers to a specific period when the environment has its greatest effect on a spe-

cific aspect of development (Papalia and Olds, 1995). An example of a critical period in psychological development is language development before puberty. Young children may learn to speak a foreign language without an accent, whereas those beyond puberty may learn to speak a foreign language quite fluently but retain an accent.

THEORIES OF HUMAN DEVELOPMENT. There are a number of human development theories (Table 18-1). Some theories view development as a continuous process, moving from the simple to the more complex. Others consider it as discontinuous, with alternating periods of relative equilibrium and disequilibrium.

Abraham Maslow (1908-1970) developed a theory of human needs from his study of individuals without physical or mental illness (Figure 18-1). He described an ordering (hierarchy) of needs that motivate human behavior that is often depicted as a pyramid composed of five levels. When the most basic needs for hunger, thirst, and so on have been fulfilled, the person strives to satisfy those needs for safety and security on the next highest level. The highest level, self-actualization, the realization of one's potential, is easily interfered with by disturbances at lower levels. This theory has made a valuable contribution to understanding human development through its positive viewpoint and recognition of needs that motivate all humans. It has also been criticized for not differentiating needs according to ages.

According to Kohlberg (1964, 1969), moral development is one component of psychosocial development. It involves the reasons an individual makes a decision about right and wrong behaviors within the culture. Moral development depends on the child's ability to accept social responsibility and to integrate personal principles of justice and fairness. In addition, the child's knowledge of right and wrong and behavioral expression of this knowledge must be founded on respect and regard for the integrity and rights of others. Cognitive development underlies the progression of a person's morality from level to level.

Adult theorists, such as Robert Peck (1955), identify psychological developments as important to healthful adaptation and successful aging of the adult. For example, critical adjustments for middle age involve a shift from physical prowess to mental and emotional flexibility. Critical adjustments for later life require individuals to move beyond concerns with work, physical well-being, and mere existence to a broader view of one's purpose in life.

Many researchers have been critical of Peck's theory because his studies did not include women. In contrast, Carol Gilligan (1982) compared male and female personality development and highlighted the differences. She identified **attachment** within relationships as the most important factor in successful female development. Females learn to value relationships and become interdependent at an earlier age. According to Gilligan (1982), women struggle with the issues of care and responsibility. As women progress toward adulthood, the moral dilemma changes from how to exercise their rights without interfering in the rights of others to

Comparison of Major Development Theories

Table 18-1

Developmental Stage (Approximate Age)	Freud (Psychosexual Development)	Erikson (Psychosocial Development)	Piaget (Logical and Cognitive Development) / Piaget (Moral Development)	Kohlberg (Development of Moral Reasoning)
Infancy (birth to 18 months)	Oral stage	Trust versus mistrust Ability to trust others/sense of own trustworthiness versus withdrawal and estrangement	Sensorimotor period Stage 1—reflexes cause actions Stage 2—repeats pleasing actions Stage 3—makes interesting action last, finds partially hidden object	
Early childhood/ toddler (18 months to 3 years)	Anal stage	Autonomy versus shame and doubt Self-control without loss of self-esteem Ability to cooperate/express self versus compulsive compliance; defiance	Stage 4—coordinates more than one action, finds hidden object Stage 5—tries new actions to see what happens Stage 6—holds idea for later action Preoperational period Preconceptual—uses symbols (language, play) to recall past, represent present, and anticipate future	Level I—preconventional level Stage I—punishment and obedience orientation—obeys rules to avoid punishment
Preschool (3-5 years)	Phallic stage (Oedipus complex; Electra complex)	Initiative versus guilt Realistic sense of purpose/able to evaluate own behavior versus self-denial/self restriction	Intuitive—increased use of symbols; ability to see simple relationships Egocentric—can see things from only one point of view *Heteronomous morality—follows rules of those in authority*	Level 1—preconventional level Stage 2—instrumental relativist orientation—conforms to obtain rewards or favors
Childhood (6-12 years)	Latent stage	Industry versus inferiority Realization of competence/ perseverance versus feeling one will never be any good, withdrawal from school and peers	Concrete operations period Developing logical thinking related to concrete tasks that are immediate and physically present	Level II—conventional level Stage 3—good boy–nice girl orientation—seeks good relations and approval of family group; orientation to interpersonal relations of mutuality
Early adolescence (12-14 years)	Genital stage	Identity versus identity diffusion Coherent sense of self/plan to actualize abilities versus feelings of confusion/indecisiveness or antisocial behavior	Formal operations period Stage 1 (preconventional)—ability to think in abstract manner develops, scientific reasoning emerges Concern about satisfying own needs *Autonomous morality—moral judgments based on mutual respect for the rules and mutual regard for person*	Level II—conventional level Stage 4—society-maintaining orientation—obedience to law and order in society; maintenance of social order—shows respect for authority
Middle adolescence (14-16 years)	Genital stage	Identity versus identity diffusion	Formal operations period Stage 2 (conventional)—ability to order ideas—and possibilities	Level III—postconventional level Stage 5—social contract orientation—concern with individual rights and legal contract; social contract; utilitarian lawmaking perspective
Late adolescence (17-21 years)	Genital stage	Identity versus identity diffusion	Formal operations period Stage 3—true formal thought: construction of all possible combinations of relations; deductive hypothesis testing	Level III—postconventional level Stage 6—universal ethical principle orientation—higher law and conscience orientation; orientation to internal decisions of conscience but without clear rationale or universal principles

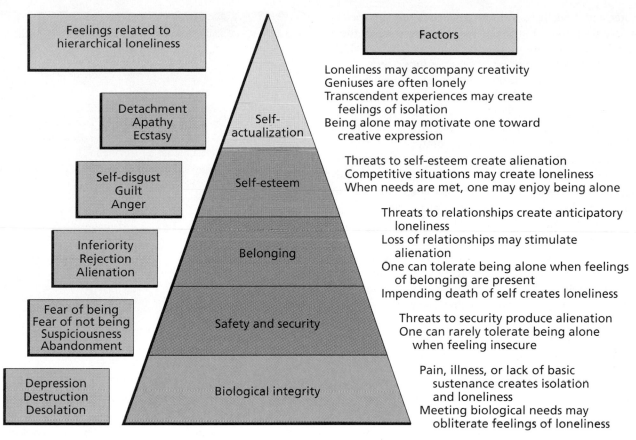

FIGURE **18-1**   Loneliness in relation to Maslow's hierarchy of needs. (Modified from Ebersole P, Hess P: *Toward healthy aging: human needs and nursing responses,* ed 6, St. Louis, 1998, Mosby.)

"how to lead a moral life," which includes obligations to themselves, their families, and people in general.

NURSING KNOWLEDGE BASE

A strong body of knowledge about growth and development gives you good insight regarding how individuals may perceive an event or behave in response to a given situation at a particular age or stage of life. Following is an overview of the stages of life and related health concerns.

Conception and Fetal Development

From the moment of conception, human development proceeds rapidly. The ovum and sperm each carry half the genetic material that guides biochemical processes essential to the developing organism. Abnormalities in the genes or chromosomes can alter health. Other health problems, such as fetal alcohol syndrome, result from environmental factors (e.g., the mother's diet or tobacco use).

Intrauterine life generally lasts 9 calendar or 10 lunar months. The first **trimester** is the first 3 calendar months. After implantation the fetal cells continue to differentiate and develop into essential organ systems. Because several organ systems are developing during the same time, disruption of one system is often associated with disruption of others.

The second trimester is the period from the third to the sixth prenatal months of life. Some organ systems continue basic development during this time, and the functional capabilities of others are refined. By the end of the second trimester most organ systems are complete and can function. The fetus weighs about 0.7 kg (1$^1/_2$ pounds) and is approximately 30 cm (12 inches) long.

During the last 3 months of intrauterine life the fetus grows to approximately 50 cm (20 inches) in length. Weight increases to approximately 3.2 to 3.4 kg (7 to 7$^1/_2$ pounds). The skin thickens, lanugo begins to disappear, and the fetal body becomes rounder and fuller. A tremendous spurt in brain growth begins during this trimester and lasts well into the first few years of life. The central nervous system has established its total number of neurons and connections between neurons, and myelination of nerve fibers progresses rapidly. Damage to the central nervous system during the third trimester can potentially alter higher-level cognitive functions. Exposure to toxic agents and the absence of essential nutrients are the most common causes of damage during this trimester.

HEALTH PROMOTION.   Because the placenta is extremely porous, **teratogens** (agents capable of having adverse effects on the fetus) such as viruses, drugs (prescribed, over-the-counter, and street drugs), alcohol, and environmental pollutants can pass from mother to fetus. The fetal effect of these harmful agents depends on the developmental stage in which exposure takes place. Some teratogens produce defects only if the fetus is exposed to the agent at a critical time when the vulnerable organ is developing. One such teratogen is the rubella or measles virus. This virus can cause spontaneous abortion; stillbirth; or defects of the eyes, ears, and heart, primarily when exposure is in the first trimester.

Many drugs are teratogenic during the period of rapid organ growth in the first trimester. Barbiturates, alcohol, anticonvulsants, and anticoagulants are associated with fetal abnormalities. The benefits of prescribed medications must be weighed against potentially harmful fetal effects. In addition, there is evidence that mothers who smoke deliver infants with lower birth weights than nonsmoking mothers.

You should explore lifestyle changes that can help women abstain from tobacco, alcohol, and drugs not only during pregnancy but also while planning for pregnancy. Preconception counseling is a growing trend in health care. The goal is secure an optimal outcome for mother, fetus, and significant others, which can be achieved with good prenatal care.

Neonate

The neonatal period is the first 28 days of life. The newborn's physical functioning is primarily reflexive, and stabilization of major organ systems is the body's primary task. The average full-term **neonate** weighs 3.4 kg (about $7^1/_2$ pounds), is 50 cm (20 inches) in length, and has a head circumference of 34 cm ($13^1/_2$ inches).

Normal physical characteristics include the continued presence of lanugo on the skin of the back; cyanosis of the hands and feet (acrocyanosis), especially during activity; and a soft, protuberant abdomen. Normal behavioral characteristics of the newborn include periods of sucking, crying, sleeping, and activity. Movements are generally sporadic, but they are symmetrical and involve all extremities. Newborns respond to sensory stimuli, particularly the caregiver's face, voice, and touch.

Early cognitive development begins with innate behaviors, reflexes, and sensory functions. For example, neonates learn to turn to the nipple. Newborns can focus on objects 20 to 25 cm (8 to 10 inches) from their faces and respond to auditory stimuli. Therefore you need to teach parents the importance of talking to their babies and providing appropriate visual stimulation.

HEALTH PROMOTION. Parental concerns during the neonatal period most frequently center on the baby's crying, feeding, eliminating, and sleeping behaviors (Box 18-1). New parents may not be aware of the newborn's immature immune system and may need information about how to protect the baby from infection (e.g., not taking infant to church or grocery story until at least 4 weeks old).

Since 1992 the American Academy of Pediatrics has recommended that for sleeping, infants be placed on their backs or propped on their sides and not placed on thick bedding, sheepskins, waterbeds, or cushions. These measures have been asso-

ciated with a decreased incidence of sudden infant death syndrome (SIDS) (Herda, 1992). Nurses assist parents in attaining the knowledge and skills required to foster the newborn's physical, psychosocial, and cognitive well-being and development. You can help new parents by teaching the phrase "back to sleep" as a reminder to always place children on their backs.

Infant

Growth and development are more rapid during the first 12 months of life than they will ever be again. The infant depends completely on caretakers to provide for basic needs of food and sucking, warmth and comfort, love and security, and sensory stimulation.

Typically infants double their birth weight by 5 months and triple it by 12 months. Their length increases about 1 inch per month during the first 6 months and then $1/_2$ inch per month to the end of their first year. Play provides opportunities for the infant to develop many motor skills. Rattles, plastic stacking rings, and wooden blocks are just a few examples of toys that promote fine motor development of the hands and fingers (Figure 18-2).

HEALTH PROMOTION In addition to those health promotion activities regarding feeding, crying, eliminating, and sleeping for the newborn, new health promotion activities for the 1- to 12-month-old infant are often related to dentition, immunizations, and safety.

The first tooth to erupt is usually one of the lower central incisors at the average age of 7 months. Most babies have six teeth by their first birthday (Behrman and others, 1996). The use of a frozen teething ring and medication to numb the gums is helpful to comfort the irritable infant during teething episodes. Tooth decay can be prevented by providing adequate fluoride through formula or otherwise, cleaning inside the baby's mouth at least once a day with a wet

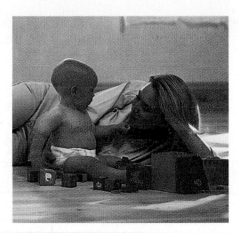

FIGURE **18-2** Playing with blocks helps to develop infant's motor skills. (From Wong DL and others: *Whaley and Wong's nursing care of infants and children,* ed 6, St. Louis, 1999, Mosby.)

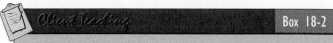

Box 18-2

PARENTS OF INFANTS
- Keeping crib away from radiators, the blast of air ducts, and cords from drapes or blinds
- Expected growth and developmental norms
- Play activities to stimulate gross and fine motor development
- Techniques to encourage development of language
- Readiness for weaning from breast or bottle to cup
- Addition of solid foods and other fluids
- Need for immunizations
- Safety measures related to use of approved car seats, falls, drowning, and use of mouth to explore everything in environment
- Develement of attachment, stranger awareness, and separation anxiety
- Use of voice, eyes, and facial gestures as disciplinary measures
- Signs of illness, measures for assessment (temperature taking), and appropriate action
- Criteria to use when choosing day care

washcloth, and not allowing the baby to take the bottle to bed (VonBurg and others, 1995).

The quality and quantity of nutrition influence the infant's growth and development. Breast-feeding is recommended for infants because human milk contains an appropriate balance of protein, fat, and carbohydrate essential for growth during the first few months and immunoreactive proteins that help protect against infection. Commercially prepared formulas fortified with vitamins and minerals are also acceptable.

The use of immunizations has resulted in a dramatic decline of infectious diseases over the past 50 years. More recently complacency and fears regarding side effects of vaccines have resulted in inadequate immunization of children less than 2 years. Nurses play a major role in assisting community organizations in promoting immunizations and eradicating preventable childhood disease.

Infants' quickly developing motor skills increase their mobility and their ability to place all types of objects in their mouths. Infants need constant supervision when not sleeping. You need to help parents raise their level of awareness regarding potential hazards in their homes. Common accidents during infancy include automobile accidents, aspiration, burns, drowning, falls, poisoning, and suffocation (Box 18-2).

When an infant becomes ill, it is important that you maintain the infant's routine daily care. Whenever this is impossible, limit the number of caregivers who have contact with the infant, and follow the parents' directions for care. If hospitalization is necessary, infants may have difficulty establishing physical boundaries because of repeated bodily intrusions and painful sensations. Limiting these negative experiences and providing pleasurable sensations support early psychosocial development.

Toddler

The toddler period ranges from 12 to 36 months of age. The rapid development of motor skills allows the child to participate in feeding, dressing, and toileting. Toddlers walk in an upright position with a broad-stanced gait, bowed legs, pro-

tuberant abdomen, and arms flung out to the sides for balance. Soon the child begins to navigate stairs, run, jump, stand on one foot for several seconds, and kick a ball.

Because moral development is closely associated with cognitive ability, the moral development of toddlers is only beginning. It is also **egocentric.** Toddlers do not understand concepts of right and wrong. However, they do grasp that some behaviors bring pleasant results and others elicit unpleasant results.

Toddlers are generally able to speak in short sentences, and common questions they ask are, "Who's that?" and "What's that?" By 3 years of age, toddlers have a beginning mastery of speech, are possessive of their toys, and are often heard to say, "That's mine!" They begin to learn that sharing is a desirable behavior when they offer parents toys to hold and the parents express pleasure. Play is frequently solitary in nature. However, toddlers often participate in **parallel play,** playing beside another child with a similar toy or object but not actively interacting through their play. Gradually play begins to include the exchanging or sharing of objects when playing beside another toddler engaged in a similar activity. An example of this **associative play** would be sharing a shovel when playing in a sand pile.

HEALTH PROMOTION.   Slower growth rates are accompanied by a decrease in caloric needs and a smaller food intake. Confirming the child's pattern of growth with standard growth charts can be reassuring to parents concerned about their toddler's decreased appetite (physiological anorexia). Parents are encouraged to offer a variety of nutritious foods, in reasonable servings, for mealtime and snacks. Special dietary considerations must be made for the toddler who is ill, is going to have surgery, or is on a vegetarian diet. Finger foods allow the toddler to be independent and "eat on the run." Toilet training is a major task of toddlerhood. The success of toilet training is based on three primary factors: physical ability to control anal and urethral sphincters (after the child learns to walk), the child's ability to recognize urge and communicate it to the parent, and the desire to please the parent by holding on and letting go at appropriate times. The average age for achieving control is 2 years for daytime and 3 years for nighttime control. Girls usually toilet train earlier than boys (Bloom and others, 1993).

The natural curiosity and the mobility of the toddler, without good reasoning abilities, make him or her an accident waiting to happen. Toddlers seem to want to put everything into their mouths (e.g., bugs, bleach, or electrical cords) or place their hands, feet, or entire bodies into dangerous sites (e.g., electrical outlets, clothes dryers, tubs with very hot water, or pools). They need constant supervision unless they are in a totally child-proofed area such as their bed. Toddlers have little awareness of physical safety, and accidents continue to be the leading cause of death and injury. The most common accidents are burns, drowning, falls, motor vehicle accidents, and poisoning (Behrman and others, 1996). You can often help parents anticipate the safety needs of their toddlers and make appropriate suggestions (Box 18-3).

Whenever toddlers are ill, it is important to provide care consistent with the child's developmental needs. Use the responses of children and their parents to determine children's specific care. Being separated from one's family in an unfamiliar environment when not feeling well is a great stress for a young child to experience. Parents are more likely to remain with their young child when the nurse and members of the health care team create a comfortable environment for them. If a significant caretaker does not remain with the toddler, it is especially important that one nurse assume responsibility for providing the toddler with consistent and appropriate care. Limiting the number of strange caretakers will help establish trust and reduces separation anxiety for the toddler. During times of stress or illness children often return to behaviors of an earlier time that provide them comfort and security. This **regression** of behavior is often disturbing to parents, and they need reassurance that this behavior is normal and that the child will return to more mature behavior patterns when the stressful situation is resolved.

Toddlers cannot clearly identify where pain is felt and often find anything that causes pressure to be intrusive or extremely painful. You can reduce physical discomfort by keeping periods of restraint or immobility to a minimum. A soft voice, physical contact, and a security item can also comfort the child.

Preschool Child

Early childhood is a period between the ages of 3 and 6 years when children refine the mastery of their bodies and eagerly await the beginning of formal education. Many parents find this age-group more enjoyable than toddlerhood because children are more cooperative, can share thoughts with greater accuracy, and can interact and communicate more effectively. Physical development continues to slow, whereas cognitive and psychosocial development accelerates.

Three-year-olds are able to recognize persons, objects, and events by their outward appearance. For example, they prefer having two nickels over a dime because it appears to

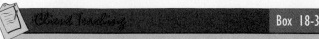

Box 18-3

PARENTS OF TODDLERS

- Expected growth and developmental norms
- Play activities to stimulate gross and fine motor development (e.g., push/pull, nesting toys)
- Physiological anorexia; good nutritional habits and feeding of self
- Techniques to encourage development of language
- Readiness and appropriate methods for toilet training
- Need for autonomy and setting limits on behavior
- Need to set limits and provide firm, gentle discipline to resolve negativism and temper tantrums
- Continued separation anxiety and development of ritualism
- Safety measures including child proofing the home environment (e.g., storage of cleaning products and medication, use of car seats, selection of appropriate safe toys, pool and water precautions, outdoor play, placing plants out of reach and getting rid of poisonous ones)
- Keeping electrical cords out of reach and covering unused electrical outlets
- Blocking stairways and balconies and not leaving infant unsupervised near water
- Not leaving iron on ironing board
- Continued need for immunization and developmental assessments

be more. The continued egocentricity of early thinking makes it difficult to suggest acceptable alternatives to the preschooler. When they are hungry they expect others also to be hungry, and they think they must eat now!

In addition, preschoolers can increasingly solve problems intuitively on the basis of one aspect of a situation. For example, they can classify objects according to size or color but not both, and they can ask questions such as, "Why do they call it the thirty-first day of the month instead of the thirty-last?" They also have a great sense of imagination. Their tall tales may be misinterpreted by adults as lying when they are actually presenting reality from their perspective. Their imagination also contributes to the development of fears, the greatest of which in this age group is the fear of bodily harm. It may be manifested as fear of various animals, the dark, or of procedures such as having their blood pressure measured.

If two events are related to time or space, children link them causally. The hospitalized child, for example, may reason, "I cried last night and that's why the nurse gave me the shot." As children near age 5, they begin to use or can be taught to use rules to understand cause and effect. They then bring to reason from the general to the particular.

HEALTH PROMOTION. Ingestion of large amounts of carbohydrates and fats from junk foods may result in overweight and undernourishment. Encourage parents to role model good eating habits and to offer their children a varied diet that prevents deficiencies and excesses. Children enjoy helping prepare healthy snacks such as

Box 18-4

PARENTS OF PRESCHOOL CHILDREN
- Expected growth parameters and developmental tasks
- Encouraging parents to support their child's sense of initiative and recognizing they will be unable to complete all activities begun
- Nutritional requirements for optimal growth
- Methods to stimulate continued progress in the development of motor skills, language, cognitive skills, and social skills
- Signs of common childhood communicable diseases and measures to reduce their risk and spread
- Criteria to use when evaluating preschool education programs
- Teaching methods used to help preschoolers learn about their health, including nutrition, exercise, and rest
- Safety measures and education related to motor vehicles, tricycles, and fire
- Increased sexual curiosity and need for use of correct anatomical terminology
- Child abuse, including how to protect children, identify signs of abuse, and know community agencies available for assistance
- Great sense of imagination and development of fears, particularly in regard to bodily harm
- Development of conscience

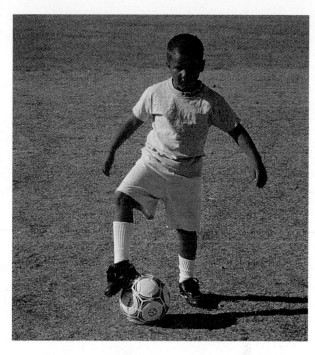

FIGURE 18-3   Coordination improves in school-age children as they gain control over their bodies.

fruit slices, carrot sticks, celery stuffed with peanut butter, and popcorn.

Preschoolers require role modeling and instruction to develop good hygiene measures such as brushing their teeth after meals and sugary snacks, covering their mouth and noses when coughing or sneezing, keeping their fingers out of their noses and eyes, and washing their hands before eating and after using the toilet.

Accidents are the major cause of mortality for this age-group, and motor vehicle accidents (usually as a pedestrian) are the major cause of death. Parents need education to assist in meeting the health promotion needs of their child (Box 18-4). This is a good time for you to teach children to learn what to do in case of fire, safety regulations for crossing the street, the necessity of riding in the back seat of the car, and how to get help when someone is hurt.

When preschoolers become ill, their beginning abilities to reason and understand can make illness less stressful. Although preschoolers have developed object permanence and recognize their parents still exist when out of sight, most tolerate only short absences without becoming distressed. Encourage parents to tell the child when they are leaving and when they will return in terms the child can understand (e.g., after lunch). You should be present when parents leave to provide distraction and support for the child. Strategies for reducing children's fears are allowing the child to sit up for assessments and procedures when possible, demonstrating procedures on another person or doll, allowing the child to see and handle equipment, encouraging parents to be present, allowing the child to assist with a procedure as appropriate, and leaving the room door open at night if the child requests it. Simple and factual information is especially im-

portant to this age-group because of their great sense of imagination.

School-Age Child

The foundation for adult roles in work, recreation, and social interaction is laid during the "middle years" of childhood (ages 6 to 12). Great developmental strides are made in physical, cognitive, and psychosocial skills. Children become "better" at things. For example, they can run faster and farther as proficiency and endurance develop.

Educational experience in school expands the child's world and transitions the child from a life of relatively free play to a life of structured play, learning, and work. The school and home influence growth and development. For optimal development to occur, the child must learn to cope with the rules and expectations of school and peers.

School-age children become more graceful as they gain increasing control over their bodies (Figure 18-3). Strength doubles, and large muscle coordination improves. Participation in the basic gross motor skills of running, jumping, balancing, throwing, and catching refines neuromuscular function and skills. Evidence of fine motor coordination improvement is that most 6-year-old children can easily hold a pencil and print letters and words. By age 12 the child can make detailed drawings and write sentences in script. Assessment of neurological development is often based on fine motor coordination. Teachers often ask school nurses to conduct fine motor assessment of children with questionable ability.

The middle childhood years are often referred to as the "age of the loose tooth," because all of the primary teeth are lost during this period. The secondary teeth are much larger in proportion and are often referred to as "tombstone teeth."

SCHOOL-AGERS AND THEIR PARENTS

- Expected growth parameters and developmental tasks including the middle childhood growth spurt and puberty
- Measures to enhance adjustment to school and reduce school-related stressors
- Promotion of child's sense of industry through opportunities for achievement
- Influence and importance of peers as they learn to follow rules and be competitive
- Development and expression of sexuality, including sex play (e.g., masturbation)
- Parental modeling of safety practices
- Recreational safety including helmets for sports, bicycling, and skateboarding
- Substance abuse (tobacco, alcohol, drugs), including dangers, signs of use, and available community agency support
- Measures to facilitate development of cognitive skills (reading out loud, appropriate use of television, family discussions, regarding school performance and homework) and decision-making skills, including weighing the consequences of actions taken
- Responsibility for health-promoting activities, including nutrition, exercise, and safety

Regular dental visits will validate if children are brushing their teeth with regularity and good technique. As children begin to move away from their family and into the world of school, there are many opportunities for them to gain a sense of competence as they learn reading, writing, and other academic skills; to follow the rules of a new authority person; and to compete and cooperate with peers in play and work. The recognition that a child receives at home for achievements also bolsters the child's developing self-esteem and provides reason to put forth further good efforts. Children's success in work and play leads to an increasing sense of independence and a need to participate in any decisions that involve them. As children move through these middle years of childhood they are confronted with a number of stressors in the school, in their home, and from peers.

The school-age child prefers same-sex peers to opposite-sex peers. In general, girls and boys view the opposite sex negatively. Peer influence becomes diverse during this stage.

HEALTH PROMOTION. Accidents and injuries are major health problems affecting school-age children and are the causative factor in 51% of deaths in this age-group. Motor vehicle accidents, followed by drowning, fires, burns, and firearms are the most frequent fatal accidents. Other major causes of accidents involve recreational activity, most frequently involving bicycles, swings, skateboards, and contact sports. Parents should encourage school-agers to assume some responsibility for their own safety by establishing rules and acting as good role models (Box 18-5).

Blood pressure elevation in childhood is the single best predictor of adult hypertension. This recognition has reinforced the significance of making blood pressure measure-

ment a part of every annual assessment of the child (Purath, 1995). Measure on at least three separate occasions with the appropriate size cuff and in a relaxed situation before concluding that the child's blood pressure is elevated and needs further medical attention. Daily exercise and maintaining normal body weight are important as both interventions and prevention.

ACUTE CARE. During illness, school-agers usually tolerate the absence of their parents better than the younger child because of their reasoning abilities. Although they understand their parents often need to be elsewhere, they want and expect daily visits and intervening phone calls. The items school-agers often bring from home, such as their own pillows and favorite books, give them a sense of security and independence. Honesty, factual information, and interest in their concerns are helpful in establishing a trusting relationship with this age-group.

School-agers can usually pinpoint their pain, describe it with moderate assistance, and may attempt to explain its cause. They may use play to cope with their pain or withdraw in an attempt to deal with their discomfort. They are usually aware that they can receive medication for pain but may not ask for it until the pain is intense. They are quick to learn to use a scale to assess their discomfort. Most school-agers are eager learners who gain much satisfaction from learning to find their various pulses, read a thermometer, or operate the blood pressure machine during hospitalization. Many school-agers can assist in checking their urine for sugar or protein or learn to do their own finger sticks for blood samples. School-agers who become ill are often threatened by a loss of their recently developed independence by needing to use a bedpan, having help with bathing, bed rest, or having someone else select their menus.

Preadolescent

At present, children experience more emotional and social pressures than youngsters 30 years ago. As a result, children 10 to 12 years of age are now having experiences that were once unique to 13- and 14-year-old youths. This transitional period between childhood and adolescence is often referred to as **preadolescence.** Others refer to this period as late childhood, early adolescence, pubescence, and transescence. Physically it refers to the beginning of the second skeletal growth spurt, when the physical changes such as the development of pubic hair and female breasts begin. Children also become more social, and their behavioral patterns become much less predictable.

Adolescent

Adolescence is the transition from childhood to adulthood, usually between 13 and 18 years of age but sometimes extending until graduation from college. The term adolescence refers to the psychological maturation of the individual, whereas *puberty* refers to the point when reproduction is possible. This period is characterized by a steady progression of physical, social, cognitive, psychological, and moral changes. The adaptations required by these changes push adolescents to develop individualized coping mechanisms and styles of behaviors, which they will continue to use or adapt throughout life. Most teenagers successfully meet the challenges of this period.

PHYSICAL DEVELOPMENT.   Although timing varies greatly, physical changes occur rapidly during adolescence. Sexual maturation occurs with the development of primary and secondary sexual characteristics. Primary characteristics are physical and hormonal changes necessary for reproduction. Secondary characteristics externally differentiate males from females.

Height and weight increases accelerate during the prepubertal growth spurt. The growth spurt for girls generally begins between 8 and 14 years of age, with height increases of 2 to 8 inches (5 to 20 cm) and weight increases of 15 to 55 pounds. The male growth spurt usually takes place between 10 and 16 years of age, with height increases of approximately 4 to 12 inches (10 to 30 cm) and weight increases of 15 to 65 pounds.

Girls attain 90% to 95% of their adult height by **menarche** (the onset of menstruation) and reach their full height by 16 to 17 years of age. Boys continue to grow taller until 18 to 20 years of age. Adolescents are sensitive about physical changes that make them different from peers. Thus they are generally interested in the normal pattern of growth, as well as in their personal growth curves.

PUBERTY.   A wide variation exists between the sexes and within the same sex as to when the physical changes of **puberty** begin. Ranges of normal should be used when assessing progress of growth. As with increases in height and weight, the pattern of sexual changes is more significant than their time of onset. Large deviations from normal time frames require attention. Visible and invisible changes take place during puberty as a result of hormonal change.

Language development is fairly complete by adolescence, although vocabulary continues to expand. The primary focus becomes developing diverse communication skills that can be used effectively in many situations and refined later in life. Adolescents need to communicate thoughts, feelings, and facts to peers, parents, teachers, and other persons of authority.

Developing moral judgment depends on cognitive and communication skills and peer interaction. Moral development, begun in early childhood, matures. Adolescents learn to understand that rules are cooperative agreements that can be changed to fit the situation, rather than absolutes. Adolescents learn to apply rules by using their own judgment rather than simply to avoid punishment as in the earlier years. They judge themselves by internalized ideals, which often leads to conflict between personal and group values.

The search for personal identity is the major task of adolescent psychosocial development. Teenagers must establish close peer relationships or remain socially isolated. Erikson (1968) sees identity (or role) confusion as the prime danger of this stage. Teenagers must become emotionally independent

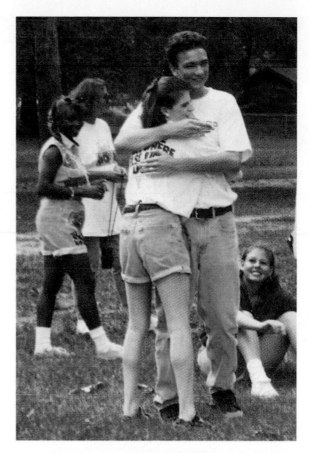

FIGURE **18-4**   Heterosexual relationships are an important part of adolescence. (From Wong DL and others: *Whaley and Wong's nursing care of infants and children,* ed 6, St. Louis, 1999, Mosby.)

from their parents and yet retain family ties. They also need to develop their own ethical systems based on personal values.

Achievement of sexual identity is enhanced by the physical changes of puberty. These changes encourage the development of masculine and feminine behaviors. If these physical changes involve deviations, the person has more difficulty developing a comfortable sexual identity. Adolescents depend on these physical clues because they want assurance of maleness or femaleness and because they do not wish to be different from peers. Sexual identity is also influenced by cultural attitudes, expectations of sex role behavior, and available role models. The masculine and feminine behaviors teenagers see and the expectations they perceive for behaving as a man or woman affect how they express sexuality. Adolescents master age-appropriate sexuality when they feel comfortable with sexual behaviors, choices, and relationships (Figure 18-4).

HEALTH PROMOTION.   A component of personal identity is perception of health. Healthy adolescents evaluate their own health according to feelings of well-being, ability to function normally, and absence of symptoms. Health problems causing severe or long-term alteration of these factors may permanently alter self-identity. Working with parents, you can assist adolescents in taking responsibility for their own health status and practices (Box 18-6).

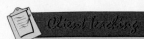

Box 18-6

ADOLESCENTS AND THEIR PARENTS
- Clear, reasonable limits for acceptable behavior and consequences for breaking the rules
- Automobile safety, including driver's education course; use of seat belts; risks to self and others associated with drinking, drugs, and driving; use of helmet by bicyclists and motorcyclists
- Awareness of warning signs of depression and suicide, alternatives to suicide, and methods to deal with a suicidal peer
- Dealing with peer pressure, school-related stressors, anger, and violent feelings through decision-making skills, conflict resolution, and positive coping strategies
- Prevention of unintentional injuries (e.g., classes on use of firearms, danger of swimming alone or under the influence of alcohol or drugs)
- Sexual experimentation and measures to prevent STDs and pregnancy, including abstinence, transmission of infection, symptoms of disease, prophylactic measures, and community organizations that provide assistance
- Allowing increasing independence within limits of safety and well-being
- Providing privacy and unconditional love
- Listening to and respecting the adolescent's viewpoint

The major causes of mortality in the adolescent age period are injuries, homicide, and suicide (Wong and others, 1999). Motor and other vehicular accidents, pregnancy, sexually transmitted diseases (STDs), and substance abuse are major causes of morbidity; mental disorders, chronic illness, eating disorders, and oral health problems are other causes.

Females are more likely to have eating disorders and emotional distress, and males are more often involved in vehicular accidents (Millstein and others, 1993; Bearinger and Blum, 1994). Homicide is the most frequent cause of death among older black adolescents, whereas vehicular accidents are the leading cause of death among white males (U.S. Department of Health and Human Services [USDHHS], 1995).

Health services for adolescents must be readily available, affordable, and approachable if parents and communities expect teens to use them. School-based programs, where instituted, have been well used by adolescents. Health care workers must be skilled in interviewing adolescents and identifying those more at risk. Health promotion activities to be successful must actively involve teenagers at all times. The involvement of teens in organizations that promote responsible behaviors such as Drug Abuse Resistance Education (DARE) and Students Against Drunk Driving (SADD) is a key element. Through your efforts in the school and community, you can make a contribution in meeting the *Healthy People 2010* objectives (USDHHS, 1998a).

Substance abuse is a major concern to those who work with teenagers. All adolescents are at risk for experimental or recreational substance use. You can assess those at risk, educate them to prevent accidents related to substance abuse, and counsel those in rehabilitation.

Suicide is the third leading cause of death in persons between 15 and 24 years of age and the second leading cause of death for white males in this age-group (Centers for Disease Control and Prevention [CDC] 1998b). Depression and social isolation commonly precede a suicide attempt, but suicide most likely results from a combination of several factors. Be alert to the following warning signs, which often occur for at least 1 month before a suicide attempt (Papalia and Olds, 1995):
1. Decrease in school performance
2. Withdrawal from family and friends
3. Drug or alcohol abuse
4. Personality changes such as boredom, anger, apathy, anxiety, panic, and neglect of appearance
5. Appetite and sleep disturbances
6. Talking about death, the hereafter, or suicide
7. Giving away prized possessions

Immediate referrals to mental health professionals should be made when your assessment suggests an adolescent may be considering suicide. Guidance can help focus on the positive aspects of life and strengthen coping abilities.

Sexual experimentation is common among adolescents. Peer pressure, physiological and emotional changes, and societal expectations contribute to heterosexual and homosexual relations. More than 50% of adolescent students have had sexual intercourse during their lifetime, and two thirds of these sexually active teenagers are inconsistent in their use of safe sex. Even after going to a health clinic, only a small percentage use birth control pills correctly all the time (Papalia and Olds, 1995). Consequently STDs and teenage pregnancy are major problems for many adolescents (CDC, 1998a).

The United States has one of the highest rates of teenage pregnancy in the world. Pregnancy rates are higher among older adolescents than they are among younger adolescents (Guttmacher Institute, 1994). Adolescent pregnancy occurs across socioeconomic classes, in public and private schools, among all ethnic and religious backgrounds, and all parts of the country.

ACUTE CARE. Hospitalization imposes rules and separates adolescents from their usual support system, restricts their independence, and threatens their personal identity. Adolescents who are forced into dependency or have their need for privacy ignored may respond with frustration, anger, or self-assertion. Although most hospitals allow peers to visit, some adolescents will isolate themselves until they can compete on an equal basis with peers. The telephone is often the lifeline between adolescents and their friends and helps them maintain their place in their social group. Many adolescents welcome peer visitors, and hospitals often allow the client to go to a lounge or cafeteria with them.

Adolescents who are engaged in emancipating themselves from their parents usually do well with intermittent visiting but expect some type of daily contact. Some will request that their parent remain with them throughout the hospitalization, and others will not object to it, demonstrating that they also experience regression with the stress of illness. It is important that you address the client rather than the parents during the assessment process.

Adolescents can usually describe their pain with minimal assistance, pinpoint its location, and often explain its cause. They are usually aware of the medication they receive for pain and like to be in control of when it is given. Many of them are able to use distraction and relaxation techniques to decrease their discomfort.

Young Adult

Setting the age limits for the young adult period is an even more arbitrary affair than for other age spans. The beginning of this life phase is determined more by the acceptance of adult responsibilities for one's own maintenance than it is by a specific age. Somewhere between the age of 18 and 21, most adults complete the basic education or training they need to enter their chosen occupation, attain employment, set up their own living arrangements, and select a significant other. These changes in their lifestyle are recognized by others as the entrance into adulthood. The completion of this period is usually recognized as 40 years.

Young adults have reached physical maturity, have achieved the highest level of cognitive ability according to Piaget, and are expected to exhibit a high degree of psychosocial maturity. Many young adults recognize that they are continuously in the process of becoming more mature in their behavior.

PHYSICAL DEVELOPMENT.   Young adults usually complete their physical growth by the age of 20. They are usually at their peak of health and less commonly experience severe illnesses compared with other adults. Although physical changes associated with aging have begun, the effects are not great enough to be noticed or require attention (Lewis and others, 2000).

COGNITIVE DEVELOPMENT.   Rational thinking habits and flexibility of thought increase steadily through the adult years. Formal and informal educational experiences, general life experiences, and occupational opportunities dramatically increase conceptual, problem-solving, and motor skills. A rich, stimulating environment for the growing and maturing adult encourages the development of full creative potential.

An understanding of how adults learn will assist you in developing teaching plans for them (see Chapter 9). Adults come to the teaching-learning situation with a background of unique life experiences. Their compliance with regimens such as medications, treatments, or lifestyle changes involves a decision-making process. You should present as much information as the adult needs to make decisions about the prescribed course of treatment.

PSYCHOSOCIAL DEVELOPMENT.   The emotional health of young adults is related to their ability to effectively address personal and social tasks. According to developmental theorists, certain patterns or trends are relatively predictable. Once young adults have begun to work in their chosen area, they have more time and energy to select a mate (if they have

not already done so) and develop a greater sense of intimacy. Many will choose to marry, but an increasing number of young adults are choosing to remain single.

Identifying a preferred occupational area is a major task of young adults. When individuals know their skills, talents, and personality characteristics, occupational choices are easier and they are generally more satisfied with their choices. In the young and middle adult years, job satisfaction has been found to be a major factor in achievement and responsibility.

The developmental tasks of young adults are potentially filled with stressful situations. Most young adults have the physical and emotional resources and support systems to meet the many challenges, tasks, and responsibilities they face. You can often assist young adults in developing time management skills or in mobilizing their resources and support systems, especially when one of their immediate family members is ill or hospitalized.

HEALTH PROMOTION.   Health teaching and health counseling are often directed at assisting clients in improving their health habits. Understanding the dynamics of behavior and habits will assist you in designing interventions that will help the client develop or reinforce health-promoting behaviors. To help clients form positive health habits, you become a teacher and facilitator. You need to remember that you may not be able to change clients' habits but you can raise their level of knowledge regarding the potential impact of behavior on health. Clients have control of and are responsible for their own behaviors. When working with the client you can explain psychological principles of changing habits, offer information about health risks, and provide positive reinforcement of health-directed behaviors and decisions. Barriers to change, such as lack of knowledge or motivation, must be minimized or eliminated to bring about change.

Young adults are generally active and have no major health problems. However, their fast-paced lifestyles may put them at risk for illnesses or disabilities during their middle or older adult years. Violence is the greatest cause of mortality and morbidity among young adults. The U.S. Department of Health and Human Services [USDHHS] (1998b) reported that in 1996 the death rates per 100,000 population for 25- to 34-year-olds were 19.1% for motor vehicle accidents, 13.1% for homicide, and 14.5% for suicide.

Occupational risk factors may be a concern for the young adult. Certain work environments result in exposure to airborne particles, which may cause lung diseases and cancer (see Chapter 27). Cancers resulting from occupational exposures may involve a variety of organs. Young adults need to become aware of the dangers in their environment and take measures to protect themselves.

Poor adherence to routine screening schedules can put the client at risk for severe illnesses because of failed early detection. Clients should be encouraged to perform monthly breast self-examination (BSE), testicular self-examination (TSE), and regular genital self-examination (see Chapter 12). Women should be informed of the benefits and suggested schedule for routine mammography, and men should be informed about the need for regular prostate gland examinations.

Family stressors can occur at any time. Family life has peaks, when everyone in the family works together, and valleys, when everyone appears to pull apart. Situational stressors occur during events such as births, deaths, illnesses, marriages, divorces, and job losses.

The psychosocial assessment allows you to identify areas of particular stress for the young adult. After identifying these stressors, work with the client to modify the stress response. Chapter 21 reviews specific interventions for stress reduction.

Community health programs for young adults are designed to prevent illness, promote health, and detect disease in the early stages. You can contribute to community health by actively planning screening and teaching programs. Family planning, birthing, and parenting skills are program topics in which adults are often interested. Health screening is a good opportunity for you to perform assessment and provide health teaching and health counseling.

ACUTE CARE.   Many young adults do not experience hospitalization, but when they do it is often threatening because it interferes with their employment and fulfillment of family responsibilities. Scheduled hospitalizations allow adults to effectively plan to meet the needs of their families and expectations of their employment. Unanticipated hospitalizations often cause chaos for adults and all those directly involved in their lives. If they do not have a strong support system, they may welcome your help to establish priorities and mobilize their resources. Adults are often impatient with the time and energy requirements that a chronic health problem may require for good management. Support groups can often help clients deal with these challenges.

Middle-Age Adult

Middle adulthood usually refers to those years between 40 and 65 and is often described as that period when one has both grown children and elderly parents (Papalia and Olds, 1995). Personal and career achievements have often already been experienced, along with socioeconomic stability. Using leisure time in satisfying and creative ways is a challenge that, if met satisfactorily, will enable middle adults to prepare for retirement.

PHYSICAL CHANGES.   Accepting and adjusting to the physiological changes of middle age is one of the major developmental tasks of this age period (Havighurst, 1972). Because middle adulthood spans 25 years, many of the physical changes described may not occur until later in the developmental period. Middle-age adults use much energy to adapt self-concept and body image to physiological realities and changes in physical appearance. Table 18-2 summarizes these expected physical changes.

Climacteric is a term used to describe the decline of reproductive capacity and accompanying changes brought about by the decrease in sexual hormones. Men and women are affected differently. Men begin to experience decreased fertility, but they can continue to father children. **Menopause,** when a woman stops ovulating and menstruating, occurs only when 12 months have passed since the last menstrual flow (Lewis and others, 2000). The woman's ability to bear children comes to an end.

COGNITIVE DEVELOPMENT.   Changes in the cognitive function of middle adults are few except during illness or trauma. Performance on intelligence tests indicates increases in some areas, particularly verbal abilities and tasks involving stored knowledge. Although middle-age adults may perform more slowly and not be as adept at solving new or unusual problems, the ability to solve practical problems based on experience peaks at midlife because of the ability to think integratively (Papalia and Olds, 1995).

PSYCHOSOCIAL DEVELOPMENT.   According to Erikson (1968), the primary developmental task of the middle adult years is to achieve generativity, which is the willingness to establish and guide the next generation and care for others. Many find particular joy in assisting their children and other young people to become productive and responsible adults. During this period adult children often begin to help older adult parents. Individuals have the time and interest to become more involved in their church, charitable activities, politics, fund-raising, and other voluntary activities that bring them satisfaction. The opposing developmental trait, stagnation, occurs when people become preoccupied with themselves or self-indulgent or through inactivity become bored, withdrawn, and isolated. Short stagnant periods allow one to gather energy for the next project, but prolonged stagnation may result in destructive behavior toward children and the community.

Expected changes in the middle adult may involved expected events such as children moving away from home or unexpected events such as a marital separation or the death of a spouse or parent. These changes may result in stress that can affect the middle adult's overall level of health.

Career changes may occur by choice or as a result of changes in the workplace or society as a whole. In recent decades, middle adults more often change occupations because they find themselves less satisfied with their present employment. In some cases, technological advances or changes in the direction of industry force middle adults to change work situations. Such changes, especially when unanticipated, may result in stress that affects family relationships, self-concept, and financial security for the later years.

Marital changes that may occur during middle age include death of a spouse, separation, divorce, and the choice of remarrying or remaining single. A widowed, separated, or divorced client goes through a period of loss and grief during which it is necessary to adapt to the change in marital status. If the single middle adult decides to marry, the stressors of marriage are similar to those for the young adult. In

Physiological Changes in the Middle-Age Adult
Table 18-2

Body System	Findings
Integument	Intact condition
	Appropriate distribution of pigmentation
	Slow, progressive decrease in skin turgor
	Graying and loss of hair
Head and neck	Symmetry of scalp, skull, and face
Eyes	Visual acuity by Snellen chart that is less than 20/50
	Loss of accommodation of lens to focus light on near objects
	Pupillary reaction to light and accommodation
	Normal visual fields and extraocular movements
	Normal retinal structures
Ears	Normal auditory structures; acuity of high-pitched sounds may decline
Nose, sinuses, and throat	Patent nares and intact sinuses, mouth, and pharynx
	Location of trachea at midline
	Nonpalpable lateral thyroid lobes
Thorax and lungs	Increased anteroposterior diameter
	Respiratory rate 16-20 breaths per minute and regular
	Normal tactile fremitus, resonance, and breath sounds
Heart and vascular	Normal heart sounds
	Point of maximal impulse: at fifth intercostal space in midclavicular line and 2 cm or less in diameter
	Vital signs
	Temperature: 36.0°-37.6° C (96.8°-99.6° F)
	Pule: 60-100 (conditioned athlete ≈ 50)
	Blood pressure: 95-140/60-90 mm Hg
	All pulses palpable
Breasts	Decreased size resulting from decreased muscle mass
	Normal nipples
Abdomen	No tenderness or organomegaly
	Decreased strength of abdominal muscles
Female reproductive	Change in menstrual cycle and in duration and quality of menstrual flow
	"Hot flashes"
	Change in cervical mucosa
Male reproductive	Normal penis and scrotum
	Prostatic enlargement in some individuals
Musculoskeletal	Decreased muscle mass
	Decreased range of joint motion
Neurological	Appropriate affect, appearance, and behavior
	Lucidity and appropriate level of cognitive ability
	Intact cranial nerves
	Adequate motor and sensory responses

addition, the couple may have to cope with the social expectations and pressures related to middle-age marriage.

The departure of the last child from the home of the middle-age parents may be a stressor. Many parents welcome freedom from child-rearing responsibilities, whereas others feel lonely or without direction. Parents may need to reassess relationships, resolve conflicts, and plan for the future.

The increasing life span in the United States and Canada has led to increased numbers of older adults in the population. Therefore greater numbers of middle-age adults must address the personal and social issues confronting their aging parents. Adult children frequently assume partial or total care-giving responsibilities for their older parents. This means adult children may assist with personal care, decision making, housekeeping, financial, transportation, and medical care management tasks. The burden placed on adult caregivers is increased if they are also employed and continuing to raise children. The middle-age adult and the older adult parent may have conflicting relationship priorities. The older adult may desire to remain independent, while the adult child strives to protect the parent. Negotiations and compromises are useful in defining and resolving such problems.

HEALTH PROMOTION.   Because middle-agers experience physiological changes and face certain health realities, their perceptions of health and health behaviors are often important factors in maintaining health. Middle adults are more prone to stress-related illnesses such as heart attacks, hypertension, migraine headaches, backache, arthritis, cancer, and autoimmune diseases.

The leading causes of death in persons between the ages of 45 and 64 years are heart disease, cancer (primarily lung, breast, and colorectal), stroke, accidental injuries, and chronic obstructive pulmonary diseases. Females' risk for coronary heart disease increases with middle age, particularly after menopause. One in nine women from age 45 to 64 has some form of heart disease or stroke, and one in six men has heart or blood vessel disease.

Middle-age adults should continue the same recommended health practices that were outlined in the young adult section. Additional considerations for the middle-ager include the following:

- Women should have an annual screening mammogram beginning at 40 (American Cancer Society [ACS], 2000).
- Women age 35 with a history of breast cancer should begin annual screening mammograms (ACS, 2000).
- A proctosigmoidoscopic or colonoscopic examination for colorectal cancer should be done at 3- to 5-year intervals after the age of 50, provided that negative examinations have been recorded for 2 consecutive years.
- Annual digital examination of the rectum with stool guaic testing should be performed over the age of 40 (ACS, 2000).
- Women should get between 1000 and 1500 mg of calcium a day and sufficient vitamin D to facilitate calcium absorption to prevent osteoporosis.
- Middle-age adults should recognize that obesity is more of a threat during middle age.

When middle adults seek health care, focus on goals of positive health behaviors and wellness to evaluate health behaviors, lifestyle, and environment. Exercise and fitness clubs, for example, give adults the opportunity to participate in many physical activities.

ACUTE CARE.   Middle-agers hold the same family and occupational concerns regarding hospitalization as do young adults. There may be less stress because of the security of employment or because the children who are still at home are usually old enough to care for themselves. However, those who are underinsured are faced with serious financial threats. Middle-age adults are at risk for a decline in their physical health. The American Cancer Society (2000) reports that most cancer cases affect adults middle-age or older. Chronic health problems such as sickle cell anemia, arthritis, asthma, diabetes, and lung disease require ongoing medical care and may require brief hospitalizations. The middle-age adult is usually interested in his or her health and desires to be informed.

Older Adult

Most older adults are physically active, intelligent, and socially engaging (Figure 18-5). Extended life spans allow many older adults to enjoy their retirement by pursuing interests that they previously had little time for. The percentage of Americans 65 years or older has more than tripled since 1900 and is expected to continue to rise (Lueckenotte, 2000).

Older adulthood traditionally begins after retirement, but the time when people retire varies greatly. Some people re-

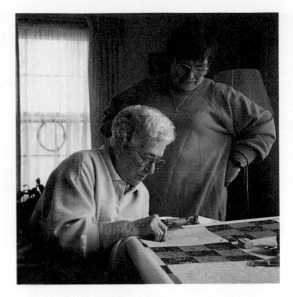

FIGURE **18-5**   Quilting keeps this older adult active.

tire at 50, and others work into their eighties and nineties. It is not unusual for those who write about older adults to divide them into the "young old," who are vital, vigorous, and active, and the "old old," who are frail and infirm. The fastest growing subset is the nearly 3 million people over the age of 85, whose growth rate is nearly 3 times that of the overall older adult population (Lueckenotte, 2000).

Geriatrics is the branch of health care dealing with the physiology and psychology of aging and with the diagnosis and treatment of diseases affecting older adults. **Gerontology** is the study of all aspects of the aging process and its consequences.

Nursing care of older adults poses special challenges because of diversity in clients' physical, cognitive, and psychosocial health. Older adults vary in level of function and productivity. Before making a health assessment, the nurse should be aware of the normal expected findings of physical and psychosocial assessment for an older adult and should consider the normal changes of aging.

PHYSICAL DEVELOPMENT.   The older adult must adjust to the physical changes of aging. These changes are not associated with a disease state but are the normal changes anticipated with aging. The physiological changes that occur with advancing age vary with the client. Table 18-3 describes the general types of physiological changes that can be expected with older adults. Some are visible to the eye, and others are not. They occur in all persons but take place at different rates and depend on accompanying circumstances in an individual's life. As the nurse assessing the older adult client, consider the potential for sensory changes that may influence data gathering.

COGNITIVE DEVELOPMENT.   Older adults often remain alert and highly perceptive until the time of their death. Nevertheless, the misconception that older adults always

Normal Physical Changes of Aging   Table 18-3

System	Normal Findings
Integumentary	
Skin color	Brown age spots and spotty pigmentation in areas exposed to sun; pallor even in absence of anemia
Moisture	Dry, scaly
Temperature	Extremities cooler; perspiration decreased
Texture	Decreased elasticity; wrinkles; folding, sagging.
Fat distribution	Decreased on extremities; increased on abdomen
Hair	Thinning and graying on scalp; axillary and pubic hair and hair on extremities may be decreased; facial hair in men decreased; chin and upper lip hair may be present in women
Nails	Decreased growth rate
Head and neck	
Head	Nasal and facial bones sharp and angular; loss of eyebrow hair in women; men's eyebrows become bushier
Eyes	Decreased visual acuity; decreased accommodation; reduced adaptation to darkness; sensitivity to glare
Ears	Decreased pitch discrimination; diminished light reflex; diminished hearing acuity
Nose and sinuses	Increased nasal hair; decreased sense of smell
Mouth and pharynx	Use of bridges or dentures; decreased sense of taste; atrophy of papillae of lateral edges of tongue; occasionally change in voice pitch
Neck	Thyroid gland nodular; slight tracheal deviation resulting from muscle atrophy
Thorax and lungs	Increased anterior-posterior diameter; increased chest rigidity; increased respiratory rate with decreased lung expansion
Heart and vascular	Significant increase in systolic pressure with slight increase in diastolic pressure; peripheral pulses easily palpated; pedal pulses weaker and lower extremities colder, especially at night; orthostatic hypertension common
Breasts	Diminished breast tissue; pendulous, flabby condition
Gastrointestinal	Decreased salivary secretions, which make swallowing more difficult; decreased peristalsis; decreased production of digestive enzymes; hydrochloric acid, pepsin, and pancreatic enzymes, leading to indigestion and constipation
Reproductive	
Female	Decreased estrogen; decreased uterine size; decreased secretions; atrophy of epithelial lining of the vagina; vaginal dryness
Male	Decreased testosterone; decreased sperm count; decreased testicular size
Urinary	Decreased renal filtration and renal efficiency; subsequent loss of protein from kidney; nocturia
Female	Urgency and stress incontinence from decrease in perineal muscle tone
Male	Frequent urination resulting from prostatic enlargement
Musculoskeletal	Decreased muscle mass and strength; bone demineralization (more pronounced in women); shortening of trunk from intervertebral space narrowing; decreased joint mobility; decreased range of joint motion; kyphosis (usually in women); slowed reaction time
Neurological	Decreased rate of voluntary or automatic reflexes; decreased ability to respond to multiple stimuli; insomnia; shorter sleeping periods

Modified from Ebersole P, Hess P: *Toward healthy aging: human needs and nursing response,* ed 5, St. Louis, 1998, Mosby.

have cognitive impairments and suffer from memory loss and confusion persists. Because cognitive impairment can occur in this age-group, you must be aware of the nature and type of these impairments.

Intelligence testing in late adulthood seems to indicate that fluid intelligence, the ability to solve new problems, declines during late adulthood, but crystallized intelligence, based on learning and experience, may increase or at least is maintained. Practical thinking, specialized knowledge and skills, and wisdom continue to increase, although the mechanics of intelligence often decline. Certain aspects of short-term memory (e.g., numbers) decrease with age, but visual memory, which allows a person to remember how to read, remains strong. Long-term memory for newly learned information decreases significantly with age, but recall for

distant experiences and procedural experiences (e.g., driving) do not seem to be affected in the later years of life. Both intelligence and memory vary greatly among individuals. Most older people who want and need to learn new skills and information can do so when it is presented more slowly over a long period. Continuing mental activity is considered essential to keeping older adults alert, and older people do benefit from memory training (Papalia and Olds, 1995).

Dementia is a broad category of disorders that affect older adults' memory and cognitive function. Vocational and interpersonal functioning is also altered (Lueckenotte, 2000). Clients experience memory impairment, disturbed language (aphasia), impaired motor activity (apraxia), and the inability to recognize objects (agnosia). Certain forms of dementia are acute and treatable. Early recognition is thus important, requiring you to make thorough observations of client behavior, neurological function (see Chapter 12), and laboratory diagnostic studies. Family and friends can be valuable resources in detecting behavioral changes.

Alzheimer's disease is a progressive form of dementia that usually ends in death after a period of 5 to 8 years. The disease progresses in three stages: an early stage involving memory loss; a middle stage involving loss of language skills and motor function; and the final stage involving incontinence, inability to ambulate, and a complete loss of language skills (Brady, 1993).

Long-term abuse of alcohol and drugs can also affect cognitive functioning. The incidence of identified alcohol abuse in older adults is currently less than 10% of that population, but it is expected to rise in the near future as more middle-agers who are accustomed to the use of alcohol enter late adulthood (Thibault and Maly, 1993).

PSYCHOSOCIAL DEVELOPMENT.   The older adult must adapt to many psychosocial changes that occur with aging. Among the more common transitions that occur with aging include retirement, volunteerism, and loss of spousal roles (Ebersole and Hess, 1998). Many older adults also have experienced occupational success and spend their later years forming independent businesses (e.g., consulting, travel agencies, or sales). Despite the changes that occur, the older adult has the potential for developing new and fulfilling life patterns.

Most older adults desire to work as long as they are physically able (Lueckenotte, 2000). The time a person chooses to retire is often based on type of work, status achieved, and length of time employed. When a client describes retirement, it is important to know whether the individual is fully retired, partially retired, or retired from one position to assume another.

Retirement represents a developmental stage that may occupy 30 years of one's life. It may also represent a highly productive and fulfilling period of life. Help clients and their families prepare for retirement by gathering information as to why the client is considering retirement.

Thirty-five percent of the population age 65 and older are engaged in some type of volunteer work. This includes offering assistance for religious and charitable organizations and government and community service programs.

DEATH.   The majority of older adults experience death of spouses, friends, and in some cases children. These losses require individuals to go through a process of grieving (see Chapter 22). Losing a partner that one has lived with for many years in a satisfying relationship is like losing one's self (Lueckenotte, 2000). For many older adults the grief associated with loss of a spouse can last for many years. Experiencing the grieving process requires support from family, nurses, and other health professionals. You can lend support by showing warmth and caring to help the clients feel they are not alone. Helping the client understand the normal process of grief is important (see Chapter 22).

A common misconception is that the death of an older adult is always a blessing and the culmination of a full and rich life. Many dying older adults still have life goals and are not emotionally prepared to die. **Reminiscence,** or life review, is a technique that may facilitate the individual's preparation for the end of life on earth. It is an adaptive function of older adults that allows them to recall the past for the purpose of assigning new meaning to past experiences. Reminiscence is the natural way older adults revive their past in an attempt to establish order and meaning and to reconcile conflicts and disappointments as they prepare for death. You can support reminiscence by sharing some of your own conflicts or ambivalence so as to encourage clients to participate in the process (Ebersole and Hess, 1998). It takes time to help clients truly explore how they feel. The sharing of personal memories requires you and the client to trust one another. You must be patient and recognize it can take several weeks or months for a client to review past hopes and future expectations.

ALONENESS AND LONELINESS.   With advancing age, more people live alone. This is particularly common for older white women. The growing percentage of unmarried individuals, the likelihood of widowhood for women, and the support of families in allowing older adults to maintain their independence all contribute to more individuals living by themselves. However, living alone is not equivalent to the feeling of loneliness. A person can be surrounded by others yet still feel lonely. Ebersole and Hess (1998) define loneliness as an affective state of longing and emptiness, whereas being alone is to be solitary, apart from others, and undisturbed. Many clients choose to be alone or isolated simply because of the desire to gain privacy or an opportunity for self-reflection and creativity. Loneliness on the other hand can be a passive and painful emotion, influenced by psychological, economic, sociological, and physiological factors (see Figure 18-1, p. 439).

It is important to understand the differences between aloneness and loneliness and to be able to recognize which condition is affecting a client. Too often the two concepts are confused. When you see a client spending time alone, if is important to share observations with the client and to determine why the client chooses privacy. The client may desire to be left alone to have time to think about existing concerns or about an illness. It may be necessary to help the client find more time for privacy and to find ways to minimize disturbances (especially for the hospitalized client).

HOUSING AND ENVIRONMENT.   Changes in social roles, family responsibilities, and health status influence the older client's choice of living arrangements. An older adult may need to change living arrangements because of the death of a spouse or a change in health status. A change in an older client's living arrangements may require an extended period of adjustment during which assistance and support will be needed from health care professionals and the client's family.

Housing and the environment as a whole are important because they can have a major impact on the health of the older adult. Nurses are often asked to help clients and their families determine appropriate living arrangements. It is important for you to assess clients' activity level, financial status, access to public transportation and community activities, environmental hazards, and support systems. For example, certain physical problems would make it difficult to live on the second floor or have laundry facilities in the basement. Because falls commonly occur in older adulthood, caregivers should use preventive measures to decrease their incidence. Making changes in the house environment to reduce the client's fear of falling can be helpful. Physical assessment of older adults may reveal risk factors that predispose to falls, such as neuropathy of the feet, severe joint problems, abnormal gait, changes in posture, poor vision, loss of muscle control, and affected memory. Changes that provide a safer environment for older adults are summarized in Chapter 35.

HEALTH PROMOTION.   The possibility of an individual being reasonably healthy and fit in later life often depends on the person's lifestyle. Older adults should continue the same recommended health practices that were introduced in the young adult section. Some older adults will need encouragement to maintain a pattern of physical exercise and activity. It is not too late for an older person to begin an exercise program; however, older adults should have a complete physical examination, which usually includes a stress cardiogram or stress test. Assessment of activity tolerance will help you and the client plan a program that meets physical needs while allowing for physical impairments (Box 18-7).

Most older adults are in good health; however, chronic medical conditions increase dramatically with age. The effect of a particular chronic health problem on mobility and independence depends greatly on the individual. Most older adults are capable of taking charge of their lives and assume responsibility for preventing disability. Coronary artery disease (CAD) remains the leading cause of death in those 65 years of age or older.

Hypertension contributes to both strokes and heart attacks. Blacks are at greater risk than whites, and men are at greater risk than women. The relationship between hypertension and CAD (including myocardial infarction, congestive heart failure, peripheral vascular disease, and stroke) is well documented (Stammer and others, 1993). Lifestyle modifications including weight reduction, adequate physical activity; salt restriction (1 to 2 g/day); limiting alcohol intake; reducing dietary saturated fat and cholesterol; adequate intake of potassium, calcium, and magnesium; and smoking cessation will lower the blood pressure and reduce the incidence of CAD (Lueckenotte, 2000).

Malignant neoplasms are the second most common cause of death among older adults. The organs most commonly affected are the lung, prostate, colon, rectum, pancreas, bladder, skin, breast, and uterus (ACS, 2000). Early detection and treatment are important. Older adults should continue cancer risk reduction practices and screenings recommended for the middle-age adult.

Sensory impairments are common in the older adult (Chapter 35). These changes are frequently the result of the normal aging process. The nurse can aid the other adult in identifying resources to help correct visual and auditory problems. The sense of touch usually remains strong. Older adults who often become victims of social isolation are often deprived of touching and holding, which convey affection and friendliness. The touch of nurses and all caregivers who work with older adults can serve to provide sensory stimulation, reduce anxiety, relieve physiological and emotional pain, orient the person to reality, and provide comfort, particularly during the dying process.

Dental problems are common in older adults. They can lead to changes in taste and a decrease in nutritional intake. Because of missing teeth or poorly fitting dentures, older adults may restrict their diet to soft foods. Help prevent dental and gum disease through health education. In addition to teaching the older adult to maintain routine dental care, teach specific measures to reduce the risk of gum disease.

As a group, adults over 65 years of age are the greatest users of prescription drugs. Many drugs may interact with one another, potentiating or negating the effect of another drug. Some drugs cause confusion; affect balance; cause dizziness, nausea, or vomiting; or promote constipation or urinary frequency. **Polypharmacy,** the prescription, use, or administration of more medications than are indicated clinically, is a common problem of older adults. The combined use of multiple drugs can cause serious untoward effects.

HEALTH CARE SERVICES.   A variety of health care services are available to the population. Chapter 2 outlines a variety of services such as day care centers and respite care used frequently by older adults and their families. Home care services and homemaker services prevent or delay institutionalization for older adults who need assistance with self-care and activities of daily living.

Situations of declining health, decreased physical and human resources, and increased dependence may necessitate the older adult's institutionalization in a long-term care facility. Such a facility provides extended residential, intermediate, or skilled nursing care, medical care, and personal and psychosocial services. The decision for institutional care is not easy to make, and the family requires a great deal of support. In addition, the family may need your help in locating the proper facility to meet the needs of the client. When possible, the facility chosen should be close to the client's and family's home to provide accessibility for visits.

ACUTE CARE.   Hospitalization of older adults is often disturbing to them because the environment and routines are very different from those they are accustomed to. Even those who are able to live independently with some assistance from their families may become temporarily disoriented by the strange surroundings of a hospital. Monitor the client for confusion, and encourage frequent visitation by family members. In addition, use reality orientation techniques to help reorient the older adult who has been disoriented by a change in environment, surgery, illness, or emotional stress.

Reality orientation is a communication modality used for making the client aware of time, place, and person. The major purposes of reality orientation include restoring clients' sense of reality; improving their level of awareness; promoting socialization; elevating clients to a maximal level of independent functioning, and minimizing confusion, disorientation, and physical regression. Environmental changes within a hospital, such as the bright lights and lack of windows in intensive care and the noise from nearby roommates, often lead to disorientation and confusion. The client's environment and the nursing personnel are constantly changing in the hospital, and the immediate environment is unstable, making coping and adaptation difficult. Anticipate disorientation and confusion as a consequence when older adults are hospitalized, and incorporate reality orientation interventions into their care.

When an older adult is hospitalized or has an acute or chronic illness, the related physical dependence makes it difficult for the person to maintain a positive body image. You can have an influence on the older adult client's appearance. Help the client maintain a pleasant appearance and present a socially acceptable image.

CRITICAL THINKING
Synthesis

When caring for an individual client or family, many factors will influence your care. You and your clients bring unique backgrounds and personal experiences to each care setting. Although these individual perspectives may not be openly discussed, they do influence the care. Both you and your clients will have preexisting ideals as to how to best meet developmental needs. You will use your knowledge, experience, attitudes, and standards to best meet the individual needs of each client and his or her family.

KNOWLEDGE.   Before beginning the assessment of an individual, review the developmental theories, outlined earlier, that relate to the client. In addition, recognize that familiarity with physical developmental milestones, psychosocial developmental crises, cognitive development, and health concerns for each age-group is essential if you are going to be effective in assisting clients to attain optimal health.

Another important area of knowledge to consider when caring for a client's development needs is that of cultural diversity. Together with the client, explore the cultural variations in family roles and relationships as they influence an individual's development, to have a clear understanding of client needs.

EXPERIENCE.   You who are parents or have been involved in the teaching of children are aware that the thinking abilities of individuals of different ages differ and it is necessary to change one's approach to gain their cooperation. Your previous experiences with individuals of various ages through family or other relationships will make it easier for you to determine appropriate or inappropriate behaviors and health concerns related to that age-group.

ATTITUDES.   Humility is an important attitude for you to apply when collecting data about a client's developmental history. It is easy to form opinions about clients developmental needs on the basis of developmental theory and related psychosocial principles. However, as is the case in any nursing situation, do not assume you know what the client's needs are without gathering a clear picture of a client's physical and psychosocial health concerns. Often information about the client's health practices will reflect the client's cultural background, which may be very different from yours. Creativity is a valuable critical thinking attitude when you conduct an assessment of an infant or child. Often you must incorporate play or other activities into the assessment to better visualize the child's physical developmental capacities.

STANDARDS.   Critical thinking standards help ensure that the right decisions are made. When developing a plan of care that incorporates growth and development principles and approaches, strive to apply the intellectual standards of relevance and completeness. It is important that you do not employ a developmental approach that does not fit with the client's level of maturation. For example, having a preschooler attempt a motor skill that is not within his or her ability would be irrelevant and inappropriate for promoting developmental enrichment. When selecting a plan of care, you need to be sure the plan uses psychosocial, cognitive, and physical approaches that complement and strengthen the client's developmental abilities.

Also use professional standards when providing care to clients of various age-groups. For example, when supporting parents' health promotion practices it is important to refer to standards for immunizations. These standards help to determine not only the required immunizations for certain age-groups but also the parents' success in ensuring a child is im-

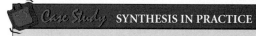

Factors to Assess	Questions and Approaches	Physical Assessment Strategies
Home safety	Ask client about the location of household cleaners, medications.	Observe client's home environment.
		Observe child's play area.
	Ask about history of home-based accidents.	
Health promotion activities	Ask mother about childhood immunization.	Obtain actual immunization history.
	Review child's usual food intake.	Obtain serial weight and height measurements and compare with standards.
	Review child's usual play activities.	Ask child to color, draw, skip, and jump.
Sibling interaction	Ask parent about child's interactions with siblings.	Observe child playing and interacting with sibling.
	Ask parent about any change in child's behavior, independence when sibling was born.	

Example of a Focused Client Assessment   Table 18-4

munized. Similarly, a variety of standards have been established for health screening of adult age-groups, and you should refer to these standards when providing client education.

NURSING PROCESS

Assessment

Nursing assessment of individuals across the life span requires you to be familiar with the physiological, cognitive, and psychosocial changes that occur during each stage of development and the health concerns for each age-group. Table 18-4 is an example of a focused assessment for a school-age child. A number of assessment tools facilitate concise but comprehensive data collection for individuals of various ages. During the health history, physical assessment, and developmental assessment, observe the interactions between the individual and any family member present. Data gathered will provide information regarding the client's lifestyle, level of functioning, family relationships, health concerns, and health promotion activities.

Throughout life, illness and hospitalization are stressful experiences. The ability of individuals to cope is affected by their level of development, their coping skills, their previous experiences with illness and hospitalization, the seriousness of the diagnosis, the degree to which the illness interferes with their activities of daily living and their lifestyle, and the availability of a support system. Your assessment should demonstrate an awareness of specific client concerns at various stages of life.

CLIENT EXPECTATIONS.   During your assessment it is important to determine what clients and/or their families expect from the caregiver. At the beginning of a home visit ask, "What do you think is most important for us to accomplish today?" or when preparing to leave, ask, "Have we met your expectations for this visit?" In the outpatient setting ask what expectation(s) the client and/or family have for the visit. In the hospital setting it is wise to determine if and who family members which to participate in the care of the client and how members of the health team can be most helpful to them. As the client's primary nurse, you should begin each day with a brief assessment to determine any change in condition and the client's perceptions of the care received.

Case Study   **SYNTHESIS IN PRACTICE**

Louis has selected Crystal Taylor and her family to follow throughout this semester of his nursing program. As he prepares to begin an assessment, he focuses on 5½-year-old Monica, who has been brought by Crystal to the clinic for a checkup before beginning school. Louis will recall the physical, psychosocial, and cognitive developmental characteristics that are typical of the older preschool child and prepare to use this information as a basis for his observations. Louis will engage Monica in play activities with dolls to ensure that observations of her physical abilities are relevant and complete. He is also interested in any concerns Crystal has regarding Monica's health. In preparation for doing anticipatory guidance with Monica and her mother he reviews types of accidents common among her age-group and appropriate health promotion activities. He is also interested in observing the quality of the interaction between Monica and her mother and assessing how Crystal copes with being a single parent.

As the parent of a 4-year-old, Louis knows the importance of immunizations in keeping children free of many contagious diseases with serious consequences, and he is aware that children are not admitted to school without the completion of certain immunizations. His own child has made him very conscious of the great fear young children have for bodily harm and the fact that Monica may have difficulty cooperating with an injection. He recalls the approach he has used to help his own son cooperate with and recover from the discomfort of an injection. Louis refers to the standards for immunizations that are updated twice yearly by the American Academy of Pediatricians, the American Academy of Family Physicians, and Centers for Disease Control and Prevention (CDC) to determine Monica's immunization needs. Louis knows that the key to his having a positive effect on the practice of health promotion activities by Crystal Taylor's family members is the development of trust through positive interactions.

Louis's nursing instructors have informed him that he is responsible for encouraging health promotion activities among his clients. Louis recognizes that *Healthy People 2010: National Health Promotion and Disease Prevention Objectives* can be a guide for choosing health promotion activities for Crystal's family (see Chapter 1). Louis knows he must be accepting of Ms. Taylor as a single parent and assess the resources she has to support health promotion in her family. Understanding that Crystal likely has some definite ideas about parenting and health promotion will ensure that Louis is complete in assessing client needs and in offering appropriate suggestions to support Crystal and her family.

Nursing Diagnosis

Your nursing assessment of the client reveals clusters of data from the nursing history, physical examination, and developmental assessment. These data include defining characteristics, which you analyze through critical thinking to select the nursing diagnoses that apply. Accuracy is important because the defining characteristics help to differentiate the nursing diagnosis that applies to the clinical situation. For example, *parental role conflict* and *impaired parenting* are two distinctly different nursing diagnoses. You must carefully review all information before selecting the nursing diagnosis applicable to the client's and family's needs. Defining characteristics for the nursing diagnosis of *ineffective sexuality patterns* would include factors such as difficulties or limitations in sexual functioning, expressions of concern about sexuality, and inappropriate verbal and nonverbal sexual behavior. Box 18-8 contains examples of nursing diagnoses for clients with developmental problems across the lifespan.

The second part of the nursing diagnostic statement states suspected causes or related factors for the client's response to the health problem. Revealed in the assessment data, the related factors allow you to target specific interventions toward the client's diagnosis. For example, the nursing diagnosis of *ineffective sexuality patterns* might be related to the stress of an impaired relationship with a significant other, fear of pregnancy, or lack of a significant other. The related factors are different, and each would require different nursing strategies.

Planning

GOALS AND OUTCOMES.   The plan addresses each identified nursing diagnosis by determining goals, client outcomes, and interventions for the alleviation or resolution of the diagnosis. The goal for each nursing diagnosis identifies a specific and measurable client outcome that is realistic and reflects the client's highest level of wellness and independence in function. An example of a goal is "Client acquires healthy psychosocial behavior within 3 months." An example of an outcome is "Client participates in health promotion activities within 6 weeks." See the care plan on page 457 for detailed examples of goals and outcomes.

Collaboration with clients and their families is essential when determining goals and outcomes. Clients' degree of participation in planning depends on their developmental status, as well as physiological and psychological condition. For example, because young children may be unable to articulate feelings and needs, their parents must become involved in establishing goals. The participation of clients and their families in this process will increase their motivation for achievement of identified goals and outcomes.

SETTING PRIORITIES.   During the planning phase of the nursing process, you formulate a plan of care that is directed toward the identified nursing diagnoses for the client. Chosen nursing diagnoses are addressed in order of priority,

with the most pressing problems receiving immediate attention. Prioritizing of nursing diagnoses is based on such factors as the nature of the problem (e.g., whether it is life threatening, interferes with activities of daily living, or affects level of comfort) and the degree of importance attributed to the problem by the client or family. Maslow's theory of human needs is helpful as a guide when arranging nursing diagnoses in order of priority.

CONTINUITY OF CARE.   Collaboration and consultation with other members of the health care team provide valuable resources for care for clients throughout the life span. Such collaboration can identify community resources to help parents of a child with developmental disabilities or can help a family find adult day care activities for an older adult. In addition, these resources can assist in providing continuity in discharge planning.

Discharge planning should begin at the time of admission to the hospital because the length of stay is usually very brief. Effective planning involves the health care team, the client, and the client's support system. Nursing interventions should be individualized for the client and modified accordingly for home- or hospital-based nursing care. Needed referrals to community agencies should be made to coincide with the client's arrival home.

Implementation

You will provide developmental interventions in collaboration with the client and the family or significant others. It is important that you keep clients and their families as active in this process as possible. Interventions are appropriate for both the client's developmental level and the client's unique needs and thus support and promote normal developmental processes. Collaboration with a variety of health team members facilitates the provision of optimal care for clients.

Earlier in this chapter, nursing strategies for health promotion and acute care were discussed for each age-group.

Case Study Nursing Care Plan   HEALTH-SEEKING BEHAVIORS

ASSESSMENT

Louis's physical assessment reveals that Monica's weight of 45 pounds places her between the 50th and 75th percentiles, and her height of 46 inches places her on the 75th percentile for age $5^1/_2$ years on the growth grid. In comparison with her $2^1/_2$-year-old brother, she appears thinner with longer legs. She has a gap-toothed grin from the loss of a front tooth. Monica is able to do all of the items for a 6-year-old on the Denver II (Denver Developmental Screening Test). This includes the gross motor skill of balancing on each foot for 6 seconds; the language ability to define seven words such as house and banana; the fine motor skill of copying a square; and the reported personal/social skills of brushing teeth and dressing without assistance, preparing her own cereal, and playing a board game. It was also noted that she does not squint or hold the story book at an unusual distance form her eyes. She enjoys showing and telling Louis about the pictures she is coloring and often giggles. **Her mother reports that Monica is very protective of and bossy with her brother, and she always wants to sit on Crystal's lap when she is holding Zachary.** Crystal denies that Monica has ever been involved in any accident that required a visit to the doctor, but **she did say she had found Monica playing with her father's cigarette lighter one day.** Crystal reports that Monica rides a tricycle with ease but has no experience with a bicycle.

When Louis inquires, Crystal tells him that she is feeling tired but well during this pregnancy and that she has been told she is doing well during her prenatal clinic appointments. **Crystal wants to be sure that Zachary and Monica have all their health care up-to-date before the baby comes, because she knows the baby will keep her busy and she wants them to be healthy.** Louis asks Crystal how she plans to prepare Monica and Zachary for the new sibling. She tells him that other than informing them of the event, she has not done anything in particular. Monica did ask her mother why she was getting so fat, and Crystal told her that she has a baby brother or sister growing in a special place inside her tummy. She is expecting that Monica will soon want to know how the baby will get out, but so far she has not asked. **Crystal asks Louis what suggestions he has for preparing her children for the arrival of the new baby.**

*Defining characteristics are shown in bold type.

NURSING DIAGNOSIS

Health-seeking behaviors related to a lack of knowledge regarding age-related health promotion activities.

PLANNING

GOAL	EXPECTED OUTCOMES
Crystal will become more knowledgeable about health concerns related to her children's ages within the next 3 months.	Crystal will begin to discuss the safety needs of her children with all other family members who participate in their care before her next clinic visit. Crystal will talk to other family caregivers and Monica about protecting Monica from the danger of playing with fire before the next clinic visit. Crystal will begin to prepare Monica and Zachary for the birth of a sibling before the next clinic visit. Crystal will make sure her children keep appointments for well-baby or well-child checkups and receive appropriate immunizations.

IMPLEMENTATION

STEPS	RATIONALE
1. Provide Crystal with handouts that describe safety measures according to age of child.	Handouts provide initial information and allow for a quick review of information whenever needed (Wong and others, 1999).
2. Discuss with Crystal measures to decrease Monica's risk for playing with fire.	Adults must remember to keep potentially hazardous items out of reach of children; a lighter, like a match, is an adult tool (Wong and others, 1999).
3. Provide Crystal with a list of books about preparing children for a new sibling.	The list will assist Crystal in finding these books in a bookstore or at the local library.
4. Encourage Crystal to write appointment dates for well-child checkups on a pocket calendar she carries in her purse and to keep a copy of her children's immunization records with the calendar.	Placement of all appointments and records in one central area makes them available for reference whenever needed.

EVALUATION

- Ask Crystal to report on success of holding a discussion about child safety with the family.
- Ask Monica to talk about the arrival of a new baby in the family.
- Observe Monica during the next clinic visit to see if she continues to play with the lighter.

Restorative care measures for older adults were also outlined. You can refer to each of the developmental age-groups for specific interventions regarding age-related health concerns. It is important to remember that a client's developmental needs should be incorporated into any plan of care, regardless of the nature of the client's health problem. Whether the client has serious physiological alterations or merely is seeking health promotion information, developmental care considerations ensure a more individualized and thorough nursing approach.

Outcome Evaluation for **CRYSTAL TAYLOR**   Box 18-9

Nursing Action	Client Response/Finding	Achievement of Outcome
Crystal received handouts describing safety measures.	Crystal locked up medicines and cleaning agents. She was able to get grandmother to move medicines and cleaning agents to a locked cabinet.	Crystal is beginning to modify home and home of grandmother for safety risks.
Crystal received an appointment book for next visit and an up-to-date immunization schedule.	Crystal kept next appointment. Crystal provided child's school with an up-to-date record of immunizations.	Crystal needs to continue to keep appointments for well-baby or well-child checkups and receive appropriate immunizations.
Crystal received list of books and tapes to prepare children for arrival of new sibling.	Children were able to talk about the "almost new baby." "Baby is coming for Halloween."	Preparation for new sibling is progressing, but remains ongoing.

Case Study **EVALUATION**

Louis sees Crystal 1 month later when she returns to the clinic for a scheduled prenatal visit. She has left the children at home with their grandmother. While she waits to see her primary caregiver, Louis takes the opportunity to evaluate the progress she has made in meeting expected outcomes. Louis asks Crystal if she has been able to find any of the list of books he had given her about preparing young children for the birth of a sibling. Crystal reports that the librarian helped her locate two books, one appropriate for her toddler and the other one for Monica. She adds that the children loved the books and want her to read them every night at bedtime. Louis asks her if she thinks the content of the books was the kind of information she wanted to share with her children, and she replies that they explained childbirth so simply it really made it easy for her to talk about the new baby with both children.

During the previous clinic visit, Louis had also given Crystal pamphlets that described important safety measures for infants and young children. He asks her if she has discussed any of this information with any family members. Crystal tells him that her mother and grandmother have looked at the pamphlets and have told her it is a big responsibility to watch those two grandchildren and that they are very hard to keep up with. She also reports that they have all talked to Monica about not playing with candles, matches, or lighters. She tells Louis about the evening news on TV talking about a child who hid in her bedroom playing with a

lighter and caught herself and the mattress on fire and almost died. The story seemed to scare Monica, and they talked about what young children should do if anything caught fire around them. She says Monica has often brought up the situation and asked what happened to the little girl on TV.

Crystal asks Louis if he will be there for her next prenatal appointment, and he tells her that the plans to be. He asks if there is anything in particular that she would like to talk about next time, and Crystal replies, "Just tell me how I can manage a new baby and my other two at the same time!" Before leaving, Crystal again tells Louis she likes having him be with her at each clinic visit and that he has given her helpful information. Louis is satisfied that they are developing a good relationship and that he has assisted her in developing her knowledge base for managing health promotion activities for her children.

DOCUMENTATION NOTE
After the primary caregiver has documented Crystal's prenatal visit, Louis adds the following documentation in Crystal's clinic chart:

"While waiting for primary caregiver, client reports that she has begun to prepare her two children for the birth of a new sibling through reading books and talking about the event. States she has shared safety measures for children, particularly in regard to fire, with family caregivers. Has requested additional information pertaining to child rearing; will assess further during next visit."

Evaluation

CLIENT CARE.   During evaluation measure the client's progress and the degree to which the planned interventions were effective in meeting the expected outcomes and goals of care (see case study). Evaluate the client's behavioral response to the interventions, and thus determine the success or failure of the nursing action. This might include observing family members interact, having the client describe health promotion habits, or visiting the home to see if suggestions for improving child safety were followed. Both you and the client and/or family evaluate if the expected outcomes were met in the manner anticipated. When outcomes are not met, a review must determine if they are realistic, if the interventions are appropriate, or if there is a need to modify an approach.

Ongoing evaluation is necessary to ensure that progress toward defined goals is achieved (Box 18-9).

CLIENT EXPECTATIONS.   Nurse-client relationships are often long-term when a developmental plan of care is implemented. Always remember to determine if the client's expectations of care are continuing to be met. Over time the client's expectations can change. To add to the complexity of evaluation, expectations may be varied when family members are involved. Basic to understanding the client and family members' expectations is trust. When you and the client have established trust, it becomes easier to evaluate on a frequent basis how your relationship with the client is proceeding and whether the client senses his or her health care needs are being adequately and professionally addressed.

Key Terms

adolescence, *p. 444*
Alzheimer's disease, *p. 452*
associative play, *p. 441*
attachment, *p. 437*
climacteric, *p. 448*
critical period of development, *p. 437*
dementia, *p. 451*

development, *p. 437*
egocentric, *p. 441*
geriatrics, *p. 450*
gerontology, *p. 450*
growth, *p. 437*
maturation, *p. 437*
menarche, *p. 445*
menopause, *p. 448*
neonate, *p. 440*

parallel play, *p. 441*
polypharmacy, *p. 453*
preadolescence, *p. 444*
puberty, *p. 445*
reality orientation, *p. 454*
regression, *p. 452*
reminiscence, *p. 452*
teratogens, *p. 439*
trimester, *p. 439*

Key Concepts

- Growth and development are orderly, predictable, interdependent processes that continue throughout the life span.
- Growth is most rapid during the prenatal and infancy stages and continues to slow until the second skeletal growth spurt announces that puberty is approaching.
- People progress through similar stages of growth and development but at an individual pace and with individual behaviors.
- Theories of growth and development provide nurses with a framework for understanding the behavior of individuals.
- Erikson identified psychosocial development crises for each stage of life that must be resolved in a positive manner to achieve optimal emotional health.
- Piaget identified how the individual's cognitive development changes and progresses through the various stages of life.
- Cognitive abilities develop from birth through adolescence and continue to mature during young and middle adulthood.
- Physiological, cognitive, and psychosocial development continue across the life span, and you must be familiar with normal expectations to determine potential problems and promote normal development.
- Accidental injuries are the major cause of death in individuals between 1 and 25 years of age, and their prevention should be a focus of many health promotion activities.
- Immunizations across the life span help individuals develop their protection against infections.
- All adult age-groups need to practice healthy habits regarding nutrition, exercise, medical screening practice, life style, and so on.
- Young adults have few health problems but need to develop positive health habits to avoid many health problems in middle and late adulthood.
- The health concerns of the middle adult commonly involve hormonal changes, stress-related illnesses, screening for health problems, and adoption of positive health habits.
- The health concerns of older adults are commonly related to their ability to continue to care for themselves and any health problems they have.

Critical Thinking Activities

1. Zachary at 2½ years of age is admitted to the hospital with a second-degree burn on the palm of his right hand. This is the second hospitalization day on the burn unit. What measures can the nursing staff take to increase his sense of security and promote his sense of autonomy?
2. Monica, 5½ years old, is having a checkup in preparation for beginning school. The nurse needs to perform a number of procedures, which Monica may perceive as threatening because of their intrusive or invasive nature (e.g., measure her blood pressure, check her throat, and look in her ears). What nursing approaches will be most likely to gain her cooperation?
3. Crystal is concerned that her 15-year-old brother may soon become sexually active and wants to be sure that he knows the risks involved and how to protect himself from STDs (including acquired immunodeficiency syndrome [AIDS]) and from becoming a father before he is ready for the responsibility. As a nurse, how would you advise her?
4. Crystal's 44-year-old mother began having very short, light menstrual periods several months ago and has not had a period for 2 months. She tells you during her checkup that she thinks she is experiencing an early menopause and does not need to use birth control any longer. What information should you give her?
5. Crystal's 40-year-old uncle has felt healthy and has not had a checkup for a number of years. Crystal has convinced him to go to the clinic for a checkup. What should his assessment include?

Review Questions

1. While assessing for a toddler's growth and developmental status, it is important to remember that:
   1. each toddler has the same set of communication skills.
   2. each toddler progresses at the same rate of development.
   3. the toddler may have sufficient motor skills to assist in self-care activities.
   4. the toddler does not have sufficient motor skills to assist in self-care activities.

Continued

Review Questions—cont'd

2. When teaching safety tips to the parents of a preschooler, you need to tell the parents that the major cause of mortality is:
   1. violence.
   2. poisonings.
   3. infectious illness.
   4. motor vehicle accidents.
3. During an assessment, a client indicates that the school performance of her 16-year-old daughter has declined and the girl is withdrawn, appears bored, and no longer takes pride in caring for possessions. You feel that these assessment findings may most likely be related to:
   1. dislike of school.
   2. increased risk for suicide.
   3. normal changes of adolescence.
   4. a breakup with her boyfriend.
4. When assessing young adults, you will find that this population usually has a high level of wellness. However, it is important to direct health care education toward activities related to:
   1. health promotion.
   2. primary prevention.
   3. tertiary prevention.
   4. secondary prevention.

5. When you suspect that your client is a victim of domestic violence, you need to know that clients' risk for violence increases when:
   1. they seek medical treatment.
   2. they experience their first violent attack.
   3. they seek law enforcement intervention.
   4. they initiate a plan to remove themselves from the violent environment.
6. According to the American Cancer Society, women should have an annual screening mammogram beginning at:
   1. 30 years of age.
   2. 35 years of age.
   3. 40 years of age.
   4. 45 years of age.
7. According to the American Cancer Society, people should have stool guiaic testing beginning at:
   1. 30 years of age.
   2. 35 years of age.
   3. 40 years of age.
   4. 45 years of age.
8. Women should increase their daily calcium intake to 1000 to 1500 mg to prevent:
   1. arthritis.
   2. osteoporosis.
   3. hypertension.
   4. coronary artery disease.

References

American Cancer Society: *2000 cancer facts and figures,* New York, 2000, The Society.

Bearinger L, Blum R: Adolescent health care. In Wallace H and others, editors: *Maternal and child health practices,* ed 4, Oakland, Calif, 1994, Third Party Publishing.

Behrman RE and others: *Nelson textbook of pediatrics,* ed 15, Philadelphia, 1996, WB Saunders.

Bloom DA and others: Toilet habits and continence in children: an opportunity sampling in search of normal parameters, *J Urol* 149(5):1087, 1993.

Brady PF: Mental health of the aging. In Johnson B, editor: *Psychiatric-mental health nursing: adaptation and growth,* ed 3, Philadelphia, 1993, JB Lippincott.

Centers for Disease Control and Prevention: 1998 guidelines for the treatment of sexually transmitted disease, *MMWR Morb Mortal Wkly Rep* 47(RR-1):1, 1998a.

Centers for Disease Control and Prevention: Youth risk behavior surveillance—United States, *MMRW Morb Mortal Wkly Rep* 47(55-3):1, 1998b.

Ebersole P, Hess P: *Toward healthy aging: human needs and nursing response,* ed 5, St. Louis, 1998, Mosby.

Erikson E: *Identity: youth and crisis,* New York, 1968, WW Norton.

Freud S: *An outline of psychoanalysis,* New York, 1949, Norton.

Gilligan C: *In a different voice,* Cambridge, Mass, 1982, Harvard University Press.

Guttmacher Institute: *Sex and America's teenagers,* New York, 1994, Alan Guttmacher Institute.

Havighurst RJ: Successful aging. In Williams RH and others, editors: *Process of aging,* vol 1, New York, 1972, Atherton Press.

Herda JA: Nursing interventions aimed at reducing risks of SIDS, *Pediatr Nurs* 18(5):531, 1992.

Kohlberg L: Development of moral character and moral ideology. In Hoffman ML, Hoffman LNW, editors: *Review of child development research,* vol 1, New York, 1964, Russell Sage Foundation.

Kohlberg L: Stages and sequence: the cognitive-developmental approach to socialization. In Goslin DA, editor: *Handbook of socialization theory and research,* Chicago, 1969, Rand McNally.

Lewis SM and others: *Medical/surgical nursing: assessment and management of clinical problems,* ed 5, St. Louis, 2000, Mosby.

Lueckenotte AG: *Gerontologic nursing,* ed 2, St. Louis, 2000, Mosby.

Millstein S and others: Adolescent health promotion: rationale, goals, and objectives. In Millstein S and others, editors: *Promoting the health of adolescents: new directions for 21st century,* New York, 1993, Oxford University Press.

Papalia DE, Olds SW: *Human development,* ed 6, St. Louis, 1995, McGraw-Hill.

Peck RC: Psychological developments in the second half of life. In Anderson JE, editor: *Psychological aspects of aging,* Washington, DC, 1955, American Psychological Association.

Piaget J: *The origins of intelligence in children,* New York, 1952, International Universities Press.

Purath J: Pediatric hypertension: assessment and management, *Pediatr Nurs* 21(2):173, 1995.

Stammer J and others: Blood pressure, systolic and diastolic, and cardiovascular risks, *Arch Intern Med* 153(5):598, 1993.

Thibault JM, Maly RC: Recognition and treatment of substance abuse in the elderly, *Prim Care* 20(1):155, 1993.

U.S. Department of Health and Human Services, Public Health Service: *Healthy people 2010 objectives,* Washington, DC, 1998a, Office of Disease Prevention and Health Promotion.

U.S. Department of Health and Human Services, Public Health Service: *National vital statistics report final data for 1996,* 47(9), Hyattsville, Md, 1998b, Centers for Disease Control and Prevention, National Center for Health Statistics.

U.S. Department of Health and Human Services, Public Health Service: *Monthly vital statistics report: advance report of final mortality statistics, 1992,* 43(6), supplement, Hyattsville, Md, 1995, Centers for Disease Control and Prevention, National Center for Health Statistics.

VonBurg MM and others: Baby bottle tooth decay: a concern for all mothers, *Pediatr Nurs* 21(6):515, 1995.

Wong DL and others: *Whaley and Wong's nursing care of infants and children,* ed 6, St. Louis, 1999, Mosby.

19

Self-Concept and Sexuality

Objectives

- Define key terms.
- Discuss factors that influence the following components of self-concept: body image, self-esteem, roles, and identity.
- Identify stressors that affect each of the four components of self-concept.
- Discuss ways in which your self-concept and nursing activities can affect your client's self-concept.
- Discuss your role in maintaining or enhancing a client's sexual health.
- Define sexuality as a component of personality.
- Describe key concepts of sexual development in the adult and older adult.
- Apply the nursing process to promote a client's self-concept and sexual health.

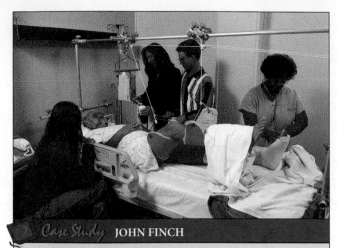

Case Study **JOHN FINCH**

John Finch is a 46-year-old white man who was admitted to the hospital 2 days ago after a motor vehicle accident. He is married and has two teenage children. He was involved in a single-vehicle accident when his car skidded on ice. He sustained crushing injuries to both of his lower legs. He was transferred to the orthopedic unit from a rural hospital near his home. Surgery was performed on admission, and an external fixation device was applied to his right leg. He is scheduled for an open reduction and internal fixation of his left tibia in the morning. This surgery will include performing a skin graft over the injury site. Because of the extent of his injuries, there are questions regarding how functional his lower extremities will be in the future; the surgeon has mentioned the possibility of amputation. The surgeon is worried about performing the surgery because Mr. Finch is a Jehovah's Witness and has refused any blood products. The surgery consent has been signed. A progress note indicates his physicians have talked with him repeatedly about the danger of blood loss and questioned his refusal of blood products. Mr. Finch has remained firm regarding no administration of blood products. He has expressed his religious beliefs and his faith in his beliefs. The unit staff has expressed concern among themselves regarding his decision. Mr. Finch has consistently been polite to the staff. Since admission he has experienced considerable pain and required regular administration of morphine. Repositioning often causes pain. When he is moved during daily care, he has very specific requests regarding how he wants to be turned and positioned. Because of the pain and the extent of his injuries, Mr. Finch is immobile and unable to engage in most of his personal care.

Mia Kendal is a 28-year-old freshman nursing student assigned to care for Mr. Finch. Mia is married and working part-time as a certified nursing assistant (CNA) at a local long-term care facility while in school. She worked as a CNA for 7 months before beginning nursing school. She has had personal experience with orthopedic injuries, because she was in a skiing accident several years ago and understands the experience of having a fractured femur that requires surgery (open reduction and internal fixation). Changes in health status often result in stressors that affect a person's self-concept and sexuality. Such stressors influence a person's ability to interact with others and to function effectively. Mia's knowledge of self-concept and sexuality can aid in identifying stressors that affect the client and promote effective planning to support the client's growth and adaptation to change.

SELF-CONCEPT

▌NURSING KNOWLEDGE BASE

How people see themselves affects how they care for themselves both physically and emotionally. People with poor self-concepts will often have difficulty caring for themselves in a way that supports physical and emotional health.

Self-concept represents how people view themselves. It is a combination of conscious and unconscious feelings, attitudes, and perceptions. Self-concept affects behaviors and relationships with others.

Development of Self-Concept

The development of a self-concept is a complex process involving many variables. Erikson's (1963) psychosocial theory of development is helpful in understanding the key tasks individuals face at various stages of development. Erikson describes eight stages, which end with senescence. Each stage builds on the tasks of the former stage. In each stage of development, an individual faces certain tasks that, if not positively completed, may negatively influence self-concept and lead to difficulty in subsequent stages.

As a nurse you will use Erikson's theory to identify the stage of psychosocial development a client is likely to be experiencing, assess if the client is in that particular stage, and determine how the client is negotiating the task(s) of that particular stage (Box 19-1). Awareness of the client's developmental stage aids in knowing what may be important to the person in that particular stage of development and how to select appropriate nursing interventions.

Components of Self-Concept

There are four components of self-concept: body image, self-esteem, roles, and identity. Each aspect develops from birth onward and reflects the changes that take place throughout life. Although they will be considered as separate aspects, they overlap and are interrelated.

Body image involves experiences and attitudes related to the body, including appearance, perceptions regarding masculinity and femininity, physical abilities, and capabilities (Drench, 1994). Cultural and societal norms influence what each person considers an acceptable body (Figure 19-1). If a person's body deviates markedly from cultural norms, body image and thus self-concept may be negatively affected (Newell and Marks, 2000). Concerns regarding body image are often most pronounced during adolescence and aging.

People generally adapt slowly to physical changes. For example, it may take someone who has lost a great deal of weight a long time to incorporate the thin self into the self-concept. Formerly obese people may tell you there is still a "fat person" inside.

Self-esteem is our emotional evaluation of self-worth. Self-esteem is influenced both by our own evaluation of our worth and the evaluation of others. The love and approval received as an infant and child heavily influences an individ-

Erikson's Developmental Tasks and Key Areas Relating to Self-Concept

Box 19-1

TRUST VERSUS MISTRUST (BIRTH TO 1 YEAR)
Relationship to caregiver

AUTONOMY VERSUS DOUBT AND SHAME (1 TO 3 YEARS)
Success in gaining control of bodily functioning (including dressing, feeding, talking, and walking)
Beginning independence

INITIATIVE VERSUS GUILT (3 TO 6 YEARS)
Trying out new things
Imagination
Using language more effectively to meet needs

INDUSTRY VERSUS INFERIORITY (6 TO 12 YEARS)
Achieving recognition for skills and accomplishments in "the world"
Involved in school and group activities with peers

IDENTITY VERSUS ROLE CONFUSION (PUBERTY TO 18 TO 21 YEARS)
Continued involvement with peers (important to be a part of peer group)
Experiencing body changes associated with puberty
Exploring relationships with those found sexually attractive
Beginning to consider vocation/career

INTIMACY VERSUS ISOLATION (18 TO 21 TO 40 YEARS)
Forming and maintaining intimate relationships with significant other(s) and family
Forming relationships with peers at work

GENERATIVITY VERSUS SELF-ABSORPTION (40 TO 65 YEARS)
Reconsideration of life direction and goals
Consideration of changing appearance and functioning as ages
Broadening circle of concern to include the future of the community and/or world

EGO INTEGRITY VERSUS DESPAIR (65 YEARS TO DEATH)
Examining life and satisfaction with "contributions"
Interest in "nurturing" the next generation

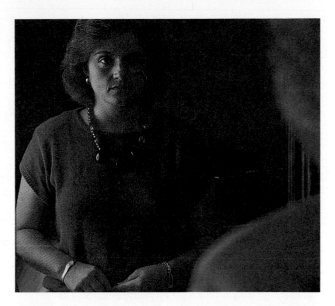

FIGURE **19-1**   A person's appearance influences body image.

time. Another person may identify strongly with a life role, such as a teacher.

Stressors Affecting Self-Concept

A self-concept stressor is any factor or change, whether real or perceived, that threatens body image, self-esteem, performance of roles, or sense of identity (Figure 19-2). The response to various self-concept stressors is as unique as the individual experiencing the stress. A person's perception of the situation is the most important factor determining his or her response. For example, a man who has had a heart attack may perceive that this means he will no longer be able to be the aggressive businessman he has prided himself as being. This perception of what the heart attack will mean to his lifestyle could lead to depression. Another man could see his heart attack as a message to slow down and enjoy his life. This perception could lead to gratitude to have a chance to change his life and make more time for the things he values.

BODY-IMAGE STRESSORS.   When the body changes in appearance or function, the body image may be affected. An individual's perception of the change and the relative importance of body image in the individual's self-concept affect the significance of a loss of function or a change in appearance. For example, if a woman considers her breasts key to her femininity, a mastectomy could negatively affect her body image. To a construction worker, use of his hands may be key to his worth as a person; a traumatic amputation would be devastating.

SELF-ESTEEM STRESSORS.   People with high self-esteem are generally happier, more optimistic, and more able to cope with demands and stressors than those with low self-esteem (Anderson, 2000). People with low self-esteem tend to feel unloved and often experience depression and anxiety. Illness, surgery, or accidents that interrupt or change life pat-

ual's self-esteem. When love and approval are not given, the child frequently has a low self-esteem. A child's developing self-esteem is also related to how the child evaluates himself or herself at school and within the family. Adults are also influenced by the evaluation of significant others. Thus successful experiences in one's world, such as in a particular job or in a group of friends, tend to promote positive self-esteem.

Roles also influence self-concept. A **role** is a set of behaviors that have been approved by the family, community, and culture as appropriate in particular situations. A person's role, such as student, nurse, or parent, influences how the person sees himself or herself. A person's perception of personal performance in a role influences self-esteem.

The fourth component of self-concept is **identity.** Identity involves the persistent individuality and sameness of a person over time and in various circumstances. It implies a consciousness of being oneself, distinct and separate from others. This element of self-concept is what might lead a person to say, "I'm a fighter," because this is the way the person perceives himself or herself facing life circumstances over

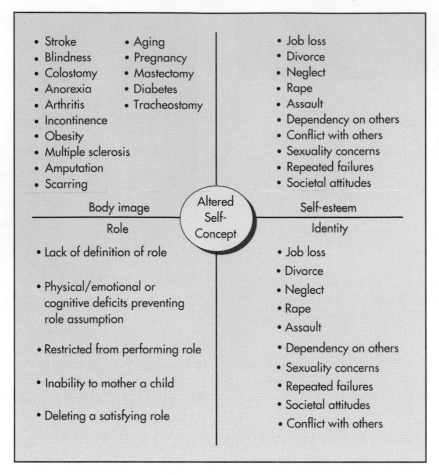

- Stroke
- Blindness
- Colostomy
- Anorexia
- Arthritis
- Incontinence
- Obesity
- Multiple sclerosis
- Amputation
- Scarring

- Aging
- Pregnancy
- Mastectomy
- Diabetes
- Tracheostomy

- Job loss
- Divorce
- Neglect
- Rape
- Assault
- Dependency on others
- Conflict with others
- Sexuality concerns
- Repeated failures
- Societal attitudes

Body image   Altered Self-Concept   Self-esteem

Role   Identity

- Lack of definition of role

- Physical/emotional or cognitive deficits preventing role assumption

- Restricted from performing role

- Inability to mother a child

- Deleting a satisfying role

- Job loss

- Divorce

- Neglect

- Rape

- Assault

- Dependency on others

- Sexuality concerns

- Repeated failures

- Societal attitudes

- Conflict with others

FIGURE 19-2   Examples of stressors that can affect a person's self-concept.

terns may decrease the feeling of self-esteem. Chronic illnesses may require changes in lifestyle and job performance that affect self-esteem.

ROLE STRESSORS.   Throughout life a person undergoes many role changes. For example, when a woman has a child, she becomes a mother. The new role of mother will entail many changes in behavior if the woman is to be successful in her new role. Certain chronic illnesses can alter a person's ability to carry out various roles, which may affect self-esteem and identity.

IDENTITY STRESSORS.   Identity is closely tied to physical appearance and ability. Individuals face significant stress in terms of their identity as physical appearance, level of health, or abilities to carry out life activities change. Although identity is challenged throughout the life span, adolescence is one of the critical periods for identity stress. Adolescence is a time of change, insecurity, and anxiety. The changes in body and emotion, peer pressure, and the unclear role of adolescence in our society cause much anxiety. An adult generally has a more stable identity and a more firmly held image of self. Once a person's identity is stable, the adult can better weather stressors such as marriage, divorce, menopause, aging, and retirement.

How the Nurse Can Influence a Client's Self-Concept

As a nurse you can positively influence a client's self-concept. Often you are the first health care provider to see the client. Your words and actions can convey sincere interest and acceptance and can have a profound impact on the client. In addition, you can favorably influence client outcomes by recognizing and including self-concept issues and problems in planning care. For example, when working with a client who is scheduled for a mastectomy, you can contact Reach to Recovery (a support group for mastectomy clients) to plan to have another woman who has experienced a mastectomy visit the client after surgery. Seeing another woman who has undergone a mastectomy helps the client realize that she can still be an attractive woman who is able to do what she wants to in her life, thus positively influencing her self-concept.

How you respond to clients who have experienced changes in body appearance sets the stage for how they come to see themselves. The client with a change in body functioning or appearance is often extremely sensitive to your verbal and nonverbal responses. Your positive and matter-of-fact approach to care can serve as a model for both the client and family for acceptance of any body changes.

There are general nursing measures, such as building a trusting nurse-client relationship and appropriately including the client in decision making, that can be supportive of most clients' self-concept. There are also measures you can implement that are specific to a particular individual (e.g., supporting clients' use of alternative healing techniques or methods of spiritual expression).

CRITICAL THINKING
Synthesis

As you begin to care for a client, think about the factors that are part of critical thinking. Synthesizing all these factors will help you make good clinical decisions. When a client's self-concept is threatened, you must use your knowledge of self-concept, critical thinking attitudes and intellectual standards, and your own previous experience to provide a quality approach to care. Using a critical thinking approach ensures your care is purposeful and individualized to your client's needs.

KNOWLEDGE.   In addition to considering the various aspects of a client's self-concept, knowledge of how various medications and chronic pain influence functioning and thinking may be helpful. Many medications have actions and side effects that can influence a client's sense of identity. When you care for clients who might have alterations in self-concept, be particularly alert to the client who is experiencing chronic pain. Chronic pain predisposes a person to decreased ability to function, irritability, and decreased sleep. These changes can negatively affect self-concept.

Another area of knowledge to consider is the client's cultural background. The importance persons place on such things as appearance, performance in a role, and acceptance by others can be influenced culturally (see Chapter 16).

EXPERIENCE.   Throughout life, all individuals, including nurses, have experience with self-concept issues. Personal memories of changes in appearance or times when the ability to carry out usual roles was affected by a temporary illness can help you become empathetic with clients who are experiencing stressors to their self-concept. Past experiences with clients who have undergone changes in self-concept or experienced self-concept stressors can also provide useful insight in how to work effectively with a current client.

ATTITUDES.   An attitude to use when caring for clients with threats to self-concept is one of independence. Do not accept other professionals' assessments and conclusions regarding a client without personally considering and thinking through the situation. If you do, you may miss important data and fail to implement interventions that could be useful in helping the client move toward a higher level of functioning. For example, if you hear several health care providers talking about a client's lack of progress and relating it to a lack of motivation, you could fail to explore the resources the client sees as being available. The client may be unaware that there are resources within the community to

provide support. Approaching the client with an attitude of independence helps you to see options that might not otherwise be evident.

STANDARDS.   There are several codes of professional conduct for nurses, but each reflects a commitment to the principle of respect for client autonomy. Autonomy relates to individuals' having the freedom to choose their own life plan and ways of being moral. Supporting clients' autonomy to make choices and live their lives in keeping with their values and beliefs supports the development and maintenance of a strong and positive self-concept.

When a client's self-concept is threatened, you must avoid stereotypical perceptions. For example, you cannot let your personal beliefs affect how you care for a client who has undergone divorce or is a victim of rape. Be aware of the possibility of biases and instead act ethically.

NURSING PROCESS

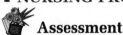

Assessment

The nursing assessment should focus on each component of self-concept, actual and potential self-concept stressors, and coping patterns. Much of the data regarding self-concept is most effectively gathered through observation of clients' nonverbal behavior and paying attention to the content of clients' conversations rather than through direct questioning (Box 19-2). Notice the manner in which individuals talk about the people in their lives. This can provide clues to both stressful and supportive relationships and to key roles. Use knowledge of developmental stages to determine what areas are likely to be important to the client, and inquire about these aspects of the person's life. For example, you might ask a 44-year-old about his or her family and job. Key targeted questions will likely provide data related to role performance, identity, self-esteem, stressors, and coping patterns (Table 19-1).

The nursing assessment should also include consideration of previous coping behaviors; the nature, number, and intensity of the stressors; and the client's internal and external resources. Knowledge of how a client has dealt with stressors in

Factors to Assess	Questions and Approaches	Physical Assessment Strategies
	Example of a Focused Client Assessment	**Table 19-1**
Identity	If I did not know you, how would you describe yourself to me?	Observe client interacting with family, friends. Observe client's appearance. Observe client's nonverbal responses.
Body Image	Is there something about your body you'd change? If so, what is it?	Observe client's nonverbal responses. Observe for answers indicating marked divergence from expected answers (e.g., "I would weigh 150 lb less" or "I would not be [a certain culture].") These responses indicate great discomfort.
Self-esteem	Observe client for marked changes in weight. How do you feel about yourself? Are you accomplishing what you want in your life so far?	Weigh client. Note statements of not liking oneself or poor goal achievement. Observe for verbalization of hopelessness. Observe for signs of hopelessness (e.g., poor physical appearance, inability to attempt to solve problems). Observe for statements of dissatisfaction.
Roles	Do you feel you have been able to be a (mother, daughter, wife, husband, father, son) in your family in the way you wanted to be? Do you feel you have been able to be a (teacher, lawyer, housewife, etc.) in your career the way you wanted to be?	

Case Study SYNTHESIS IN PRACTICE

As Mia prepares to care for Mr. Finch, she recalls what she has learned about self-concept. She recognizes that his accident and resulting injuries are likely to be significant stressors in regard to his self-concept. Being in the hospital and his dependence on the staff for personal care threaten his sense of independence. His inability to work for the next several months and the questions about his returning to preaccident mobility affect his ability to carry out his occupation as a plumber. His role of provider for his family is threatened, as is his role of an "able-bodied man." Recognizing the significance of these changes and their possible influence on his self-concept, Mia plans to assess what it is like for Mr. Finch to be in the hospital and if he is thinking about his future (e.g., finances and work).

Mia remembers that after her own accident, her initial concerns were with her pain and surgery. It was not until several days after surgery that she began to consider the impact her changed mobility would have on her life. This knowledge will guide her in knowing that assessing Mr. Finch's current concerns is important. It may be some time before he begins to consider the impact of his accident on other aspects of his life.

When Mia is reading Mr. Finch's chart before meeting him, she overhears two staff members taking about Mr. Finch and his "pickiness" about positioning. They are expressing their distress at how long it takes to complete his care because of his specific requests in regard to his personal hygiene and positioning. Mia realizes that the staff may not be aware of the extent of Mr. Finch's pain and how his requests for care in movement might be related to his pain or to fear of further injury. Mia hears the comments but recognizes that she will make her own independent assessment of his status and needs. She recognizes that if she allows others' attitudes to influence her view of Mr. Finch, she will be less likely to develop a therapeutic relationship or to be able to effectively support him in coping.

As Mia reads the surgeon's progress notes relating to Mr. Finch's upcoming surgery and his repeated refusals to accept blood products, she recognizes an issue of autonomy. She will be alert to the responses of others to his decision. She will also be alert for an opportunity to explore with him what it has been like to make choices based on his beliefs when others have repeatedly asked him to make different choices.

the past provides insight into the client's style of coping. Not all issues are addressed in the same way by clients, but many times one uses a familiar coping pattern for newly encountered stressors. Exploring resources and strengths, such as helpful significant others, can be important in gathering a thorough assessment. Also determine how the client perceives the situation. What is viewed as a crisis by one client may be seen as less significant by another client. For example, one client might express fear over needing to have a colonoscopy and biopsy, whereas another client may see the need for the diagnostic testing as just a part of growing older.

CULTURAL VARIABLES. When assessing self-concept you need to be attuned to the client's cultural background. Cultural heritage can influence each of the aspects of self-concept. The behaviors expected in various roles can differ from culture to culture. What is viewed as attractive in terms of body appearance varies between cultures (see Chapter 16). Cultural beliefs regarding what is attractive, such as certain makeup or jewelry, will influence a person's body image and self-esteem. Identity will be influenced by characteristics that are valued in a particular culture (Giger and Davidhizar, 1999).

CLIENT EXPECTATIONS. Also important in assessing self-concept are the client's expectations. For example, if you were caring for a client who is experiencing anxiety related to an upcoming diagnostic study you might ask the client if he or she thinks the relaxation exercise you have been practicing together might help. The client's response will provide you with valuable information about the client's beliefs and attitudes regarding the effectiveness and appropriateness of the interventions. Asking the client how he or she believes interventions will make a difference in the problem can provide an opportunity to discuss the client's goals and expectations.

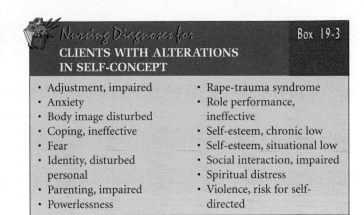

Box 19-3

Nursing Diagnoses for
CLIENTS WITH ALTERATIONS
IN SELF-CONCEPT

- Adjustment, impaired
- Anxiety
- Body image disturbed
- Coping, ineffective
- Fear
- Identity, disturbed personal
- Parenting, impaired
- Powerlessness
- Rape-trauma syndrome
- Role performance, ineffective
- Self-esteem, chronic low
- Self-esteem, situational low
- Social interaction, impaired
- Spiritual distress
- Violence, risk for self-directed

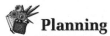

Nursing Diagnosis

In analyzing data regarding a client's self-concept, review the data collected on body image, role, self-esteem, and identity. Alterations to any of these areas may reveal data that result in a nursing diagnosis. Making nursing diagnoses in the realm of self-concept is complex (Box 19-3).

Often, isolated data could be defining characteristics for more than one nursing diagnosis. For example, a client might express feelings of regret and inadequacy. These are defining characteristics for both *anxiety* and *situational low self-esteem*. To make the most appropriate nursing diagnosis, you must be open to seeing the possibilities of both nursing diagnoses. In fact, the awareness that the client is demonstrating defining characteristics of more than one nursing diagnosis can guide you in gathering specific data to differentiate the underlying problem.

To further assess the possibility of anxiety, you might consider the following defining characteristics of anxiety: Is the person experiencing increased muscle tension, shakiness, a sense of being "rattled," or restlessness? These symptoms would suggest *anxiety* as the more appropriate diagnosis. On the other hand, if the person expresses a predominantly negative self-appraisal, evaluation of self as unable to handle situations or events, and difficulty making decisions, these characteristics would suggest the more appropriate nursing diagnosis to be *situational low self-esteem*.

To further aid you in differentiating between these two diagnoses, information regarding recent events in the person's life and how the person has viewed himself or herself in the past would provide insight into the most appropriate nursing diagnosis. In this example, the two nursing diagnoses are closely related. The person might have several defining characteristics from each diagnosis, but as additional data are gathered, usually the most appropriate or predominant nursing diagnosis becomes evident. If this is not the case, you can consider consulting with other nurse colleagues or a mental health professional to help identify the priority problem.

It is also important to have sufficient data to correctly identify the factors contributing to the nursing diagnosis. These factors will be reflected in the "related to" component of the nursing diagnostic statement. If a thorough database is not gathered before formulating the nursing diagnosis, diagnostic errors are likely. For example, a nurse was working with a 62-year-old woman who was admitted because of chronic back pain. The client demonstrated signs of anxiety (inattentiveness and frequent startling) and reported that she did not sleep well and had a loss of appetite. The nurse knew that the client had undergone diagnostic testing to rule out cancer as the cause of the back pain. The nurse made the following nursing diagnosis: *anxiety related to possibility of cancer.* The nurse later learned that the woman was anxious because her grandson had been in a serious car accident and was in intensive care. This example illustrates the danger in making a diagnosis without sufficient data.

Planning

Realistic planning to enhance and support a client's self-concept is based on your assessment data. For interventions to be effective, they must be acceptable to the client and realistic within the context of the client, setting, and community resources.

GOALS AND OUTCOMES. The first step in effective planning is the development of goals and outcome criteria. To formulate a goal, consider a realistic resolution of the nursing diagnosis for this particular person. Consult with your client to develop realistic goals and expected outcome criteria. Consulting with family, other health care providers, and community resources can also provide valuable input and guidance in planning. Once the goal has been formulated, consider how the clues that alerted you to the problem would change if the problem were diminished. These changes should be reflected in the outcome criteria (see care plan). For example, a client is diagnosed with *situational low self-esteem related to recent job loss.* The defining characteristics she demonstrates are saying that she just cannot seem to do anything right these days and expressing shame about losing her job. The goal is that the client's self-esteem will improve within 1 week. Appropriate outcome criteria might be that the client discusses areas of her life where she is functioning well and says she realizes that losing her job does not mean she is a bad person.

SETTING PRIORITIES. In some cases nursing diagnoses relating to the client's self-concept need a greater priority

Case Study Nursing Care Plan **ALTERATIONS IN SELF-CONCEPT**

ASSESSMENT

Mia learns from Mr. Finch's chart that he was transferred from his local hospital 70 miles away to the acute care center. The transfer was made because of the extent of his injuries and the need for specialized orthopedic treatment. He had been in essentially good health up until the time of the accident.

When Mia first goes in to meet Mr. Finch, she finds he makes eye contact and answers her questions, but his **answers are brief** and to the point, without elaboration. As Mia spends more time with Mr. Finch, his eye contact increases but the answers to her questions remain brief. He is **restless** and **shifts frequently in the bed.** Mr. Finch tells Mia that before the accident he had a near ideal life. He describes his family as a source of pleasure and satisfaction. He tells her briefly about a recent trip the family took and the adventures of the two teenagers. He describes his work as OK. He states, "Fixing pipes is not the most exciting thing in the world, but it pays the bills and I know how to do it."

In gathering the nursing history, Mia learns that Mr. Finch has had **trouble sleeping** since admission. He says that in addition to the pain, there is **too much to think about.** Specifically, he says, "You know, they may not be able to save my legs."

In reviewing the flow sheets since administration, Mia notes that Mr. Finch's **appetite has been recorded as poor and he usually only eats one quarter to one half of his meals.**

*Defining characteristics are shown in bold type.

NURSING DIAGNOSIS

Anxiety related to pain, uncertainty of outcome of upcoming surgery, and treatment of injuries.

PLANNING

GOAL

Client's anxiety will be diminished within 1 week.

EXPECTED OUTCOMES

Client will state that his anxiety/worry is less within 3 days.

Client will discuss his concerns openly with a staff person within 3 days.

Client will report having slept for 4 consecutive hours during the night within 1 week.

Client will report an increased appetite and will eat at least three quarters of his meals within 1 week.

IMPLEMENTATION

STEPS

1. Help the client to define his level of anxiety (use the terminology the client is comfortable with; e.g., worried, nervous).
2. Encourage and support client's visual adaptive coping skills used in the past.

3. Encourage the client to express concern verbally.

4. Decrease the number of new stressors (e.g., answer client's call bell promptly, explain procedures, decrease unnecessary noise).

5. Treat pain before it becomes moderate to severe.
6. Teach the client progressive relaxation techniques.

RATIONALE

Anxiety is highly individualized, and different clients manifest anxiety in varying degrees (Read, 1999).

Most clients have developed effective coping skills during their lives. Supporting these coping skills in currently stressful situations can aid adaptation (Newell and Marks, 2000).

Verbalizing a concern can allow the client to be more objective about what is happening.

Reduction in the number and duration of stressors improves the ability to cope and resolve stress and stress-related anxieties (Read, 1999).

Pain is a stressor that can increase anxiety.

Relaxation is psychophysiologically in opposition to anxiety. Relaxation is energy conserving and nurturing (Sundeen and others, 1998).

EVALUATION

- Explore with the client his current level of anxiety.
- Ask the client how he slept the night before.
- Inquire regarding the client's appetite, and monitor the amount of food eaten from meal trays.
- Explore with the client his concerns, and note areas he discusses.
- Observe nonverbal clues regarding eye contact and degree of restlessness during discussion.

---

than those diagnoses of physiological origin. For example, a 20-year-old woman newly diagnosed with type 1 diabetes also has *situational low self-esteem related to the presence of a chronic illness.* This diagnosis must have high priority because as your client's self-esteem improves, so will her ability to manage her diabetes correctly.

CONTINUITY OF CARE. Considering the current health care delivery system, much of your client's care will occur in the home or restorative care settings. It is important that you plan for this aspect of care as well. As you anticipate discharge planning, consult and collaborate with other members of the health care team and community resources. For example, you are caring for a client with a recent medical diagnosis of breast cancer who prefers a neighborhood breast cancer support group instead of the university-based cancer support group. Identifying such a community group will provide continuity of care for your client as she and her family learn to adapt to the illness.

Implementation

Once you develop the goals and outcome criteria for a client, select nursing interventions that help move the client toward the goals of care. Remember to keep the client an active participant in the plan of care. Select interventions based on the client's nursing diagnosis. Developing interventions that influence the etiological factors decrease the problem reflected in the nursing diagnosis.

HEALTH PROMOTION.   You may have the opportunity to work with clients to help them develop healthy lifestyle measures that contribute to a healthy self-concept. These include measures that support adaptation to stress, such as sound nutrition and regular exercise within the client's capabilities. Measures that promote adequate sleep and rest and stress-reducing practices also contribute to a healthy self-concept. As a nurse you are in a unique position to identify specific lifestyle practices that may place your client at risk for an alteration in self-concept. For example, a woman brings her baby to the well-baby clinic. When taking a family history, you note that the woman is very knowledgeable about the needs of her newborn. However, she comments that although she has lost much of her pregnancy weight, her husband refers to her as fat. She says, "No matter what I do, I'll always be fat, even though I only eat once a day." You have an unique opportunity to further assess this problem and determine methods to resolve her body image disturbance.

ACUTE CARE.   In the acute care setting, you will likely meet clients who are experiencing threats to their self-concept. Clients may be faced with the need to adapt to an altered body image as a result of surgery or other physical change. Often a visit by someone who has experienced similar changes and adapted to them is helpful. The timing of such a visit is important. You must be sensitive to the client's level of acceptance of the change. Forcing confrontation with the change before the client is ready could delay the person's acceptance. For example, a man may be admitted to an acute care facility for treatment of a multiple fracture resulting from a motor vehicle accident. In gathering the nursing history, you learn of lifestyle practices such as too little rest, a large number of life changes occurring simultaneously, or excessive use of alcohol. These factors are suggestive of self-concept disturbances or put him at risk for self-concept disturbances. In this situation, you have the opportunity to talk with him to determine how he sees the various lifestyle elements, to help him see the behavior as potentially problematic, and to make appropriate referrals or provide needed health teaching.

In the acute care setting, the client's family can assist in improving or maintaining self-concept. In supporting their family member, it is important that the family not let "good intentions" remove the client from family decisions. Helping the client maintain involvement, roles, and responsibilities, assists in promoting the client's self-concept.

RESTORATIVE AND CONTINUING CARE.   In a long-term nurse-client relationship in a home health or restorative care environment, you often have the opportunity to work with a client to reach the goal of attaining a more positive self-concept. Interventions designed to help a client reach the goal of adapting to changes in self-concept or attaining a positive self-concept are based on the premise that the client first develops insight and self-awareness concerning problems and stressors and then acts to solve the problems and cope with the stressors. This approach, outlined by Stuart and Laraia (2000), involves a number of levels of intervention (e.g., expanded self-awareness, self-exploration, and planning realistic goals) (Table 19-2). Interventions proceed a step at a time to promote increasing awareness and help the client efficiently solve problems.

You can increase the client's self-awareness by establishing a trusting relationship that allows the client to openly explore feelings. Open exploration can make the situation less threatening for the client and encourages behaviors that expand self-awareness.

Accepting the client's feelings and thoughts, helping the client to clarify interactions with others, and being empathetic all encourage the client's self-exploration. Assisting the client in self-evaluation involves helping the client to define problems clearly and identifying positive and negative coping mechanisms. Work closely with the client to help analyze adaptive and maladaptive responses, contrast different alternatives, and discuss outcomes.

Assist the client is committing to decisions and actions to achieve goals by teaching the client to move away from ineffective coping mechanisms and develop successful coping strategies. Supporting client attempts at health promotion is essential, because with each success another attempt can be made. Supporting adaptive, flexible coping is central to promoting a positive self-concept.

Clients who experience threats to or alterations in self-concept often benefit from collaboration with mental health and community resources to promote increased awareness. Knowledge of available community resources, such as counseling and peer support groups, allow you to make appropriate referrals. Social service involvement may also be indicated.

Evaluation

CLIENT CARE.   Evaluate the effectiveness of nursing interventions based on the goals and expected outcome criteria (Box 19-4). If you developed realistic individual goals and outcome criteria, you can reassess the client to see if he or she has attained the changes that were desired. Key indicators of self-concept can be the client's nonverbal behaviors. For example, a client who has had difficulty making eye contact may

Principle	Rationale	Nursing Action
Goal: Expand Client's Self-Awareness		
Work with resources client possesses.	Some resources, such as self-control and self-perception, are needed as foundations for later nursing care.	Confirm identity. Provide support measures to reduce anxiety. Approach client in an undemanding way. Accept and attempt to clarify any verbal or nonverbal communication. Prevent client isolation. Help establish simple routine. Help set limits on inappropriate behavior. Orient client to reality. Reinforce appropriate behavior.
Maximize client's participation in therapeutic relationship.	Mutuality is necessary for client to assume ultimate responsibility for behavior and coping responses.	Gradually increase activities and tasks that provide positive experiences. Assist in personal hygiene and grooming. Encourage client to care for self. Gradually increase client's participation in decisions that affect care. Convey that client is a responsible individual.
Goal: Encourage Client's Self-Exploration		
Show interest in and accept client's feelings and thoughts.	When nurse shows interest in and accepts client's feelings and thoughts, the nurse helps client to do so also.	Attend to and encourage client's expression of emotions, beliefs, behavior, and thoughts—verbally, nonverbally, symbolically, or directly. Use therapeutic communication skills and empathetic responses. Note use of logical and illogical thinking and reported and observed emotional responses.
Help client clarify self-concept and relationships to others through self-disclosure.	Self-disclosure and understanding self-perceptions are prerequisites to bringing about future change; this may, in itself, reduce anxiety.	Elicit client's perceptions of strengths and weaknesses. Help describe ideal self. Identify self-criticisms. Help describe how client perceives relationships to other people and events.
Be aware and have control of your own feelings.	Self-awareness allows nurse to model authentic behavior.	Be open to your own feelings. Accept your positive and negative feelings. Practice therapeutic use of self: share your feelings with client, describe how another might have felt, and mirror your perception of client's feelings.
Respond empathetically, not sympathetically, emphasizing that power to change lies with client.	Sympathy can reinforce client's self-pity; rather, nurse should communicate that client's life situation is subject to one's own control.	Use empathetic responses and monitor yourself for feelings of sympathy or pity. Reaffirm that client is not helpless or powerless when dealing with problems. Convey verbally and behaviorally that client is responsible for behavior, including choice of maladaptive or adaptive coping responses. Discuss your client's scope of choices, areas of strength, and coping resources available.
Goal: Assist Client in Forming Realistic Goals		
Help client identify alternative solutions.	Only when all possible alternatives have been evaluated can change be effected.	Help client understand that one can only change oneself, not others. If client holds inconsistent perceptions, instruct client that changing beliefs or ideals can bring him or her closer to reality. If self-concept is not consistent with behavior, assist client in changing behavior to conform to self-concept and beliefs. Mutually review use of coping resources.
Help client conceptualize realistic goals.	Goal setting that includes clear definition of expected change is necessary.	Encourage client to form personal (not nurse's) goals. Mutually discuss emotional and practical consequences of each goal. Help client define concrete change to be made. Encourage client to enter new experiences for growth potential. Use role modeling and role playing when appropriate.

Modified from Stuart GW, Laraia MT: *Principles and practice of psychiatric nursing,* ed 7, St. Louis, 2000, Mosby.

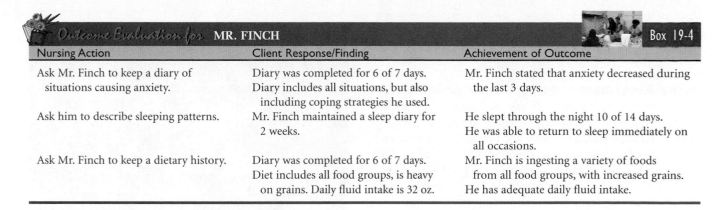

Outcome Evaluation for MR. FINCH   Box 19-4

Nursing Action	Client Response/Finding	Achievement of Outcome
Ask Mr. Finch to keep a diary of situations causing anxiety.	Diary was completed for 6 of 7 days. Diary includes all situations, but also including coping strategies he used.	Mr. Finch stated that anxiety decreased during the last 3 days.
Ask him to describe sleeping patterns.	Mr. Finch maintained a sleep diary for 2 weeks.	He slept through the night 10 of 14 days. He was able to return to sleep immediately on all occasions.
Ask Mr. Finch to keep a dietary history.	Diary was completed for 6 of 7 days. Diet includes all food groups, is heavy on grains. Daily fluid intake is 32 oz.	Mr. Finch is ingesting a variety of foods from all food groups, with increased grains. He has adequate daily fluid intake.

Case Study   EVALUATION

Mia is absent from the acute care hospital for 2 weeks. When she returns, she is again assigned to care for Mr. Finch. Since she last cared for him, he has undergone two surgeries, the surgery that was scheduled for the day after she was there and another surgery to do a second graft when the first did not take. Mr. Finch is glad to see her. He tells her that he is in a "much better place" now than when they first met. The second skin graft is not doing well, and the surgeons have talked with Mr. Finch about further surgery. He is questioning whether further surgery to save his left leg is reasonable. The prognosis for functioning of the leg even if it heals is not good. He tells Mia he thinks that if further surgery is required he will choose an amputation. He says, "You know, I now can see I'll be OK even if they have to amputate my leg. If I had it to do over again, I would have made that choice when they did the second surgery. But it took me awhile to realize that I will not have the same functioning in my legs regardless of what they do. And I can live without my leg." As he relates what had happened over the last 2 weeks and the upcoming plans to transfer him to a hospital near his home, his speech is animated and he makes frequent eye contact. During the course of the day, Mia notices that his restlessness has decreased. He reports that his appetite has returned, and he ate all of both his breakfast and his lunch. He also reports that he has become more accustomed to the hospital and is sleeping most of the night.

Documentation Note

Mia documents Mr. Finch's progress toward the goal as follows:

Client's anxiety has decreased, as evidenced by his statement that he is in a "much better place" now than when he was first admitted. Client reports sleeping most of the night and eating all of his last two meals. He is more open in discussing his condition and prognosis, and he is less restless.

demonstrate a more positive self-concept by making more frequent eye contact during conversation. Patterns of interacting can also reflect changes in self-concept. For example, a client who has been hesitant to express his or her views may more readily offer opinions and ideas as self-esteem increases.

CLIENT EXPECTATIONS. If you have developed a good rapport with the client, the client may well be able to tell you how things are going and whether expectation were met from his or her perspective. You may be able to encourage this by re-

viewing what has happened over time. This offers the opportunity to share perceptions and encourages the client to consider and voice how he or she has experienced any changes.

SEXUALITY

Sexuality involves the whole person. It includes a person's sense of femaleness or maleness. Sexuality involves biological, psychological, sociological, spiritual, and cultural dimensions of the person's being. In addition, sexuality influences values, attitudes, behaviors, and relationships with others, including the need to be emotionally close (MacLaren, 1995).

Because of the all-encompassing nature of sexuality, nurses should consider a client's sexual health. The intimacy of the nurse-client relationship, whether it is involved in providing physical care or discussing the impact of a recent diagnosis, provides a unique opportunity for discussing a person's sexual concerns.

SCIENTIFIC KNOWLEDGE BASE
Sexual Development

As a person grows and develops, so does his or her sexuality. Each stage of development brings changes in sexual functioning, sexual focus, and sexual relationships (see Chapter 18). People who maintain sexual health throughout their life have demonstrated a slower rate of decline in activity as they age (Read, 1999). This chapter focuses primarily on sexual development and changes in the adult and older adult client.

ADULTHOOD. The adult has gained physical maturation but is continuing to explore and define emotional maturation in relationships. Sexual health has been defined as "the integration of the somatic, emotional, intellectual, and social aspects of sexual being, in ways that are positively enriching and that enhance personality, communication, and love" (World Health Organization, 1975). People can be sexually healthy in numerous ways. Sexual activity is often defined as a basic need, but sexual desire can be channeled into other forms of intimacy throughout a lifetime.

All sexually active adults, as they develop intimate relationships, should learn techniques of stimulation and sexual response that are satisfying to themselves and their sexual partners. Some adults may need information or therapy to achieve mutually satisfying sexual relationships.

OLDER ADULTHOOD.   The capacity for sexuality is life-long (Figure 19-3). Theoretically people can engage in sex as far into old age as they choose, and many are active well into their ninth decade (Read, 1999). The best indicator for continued sexual satisfaction with aging is a regularly active sex life during adulthood and into later life (Masters and others, 1992). Older people may face health concerns and societal attitudes that may make it difficult for them to continue sexual activity. Although declining physical abilities may make sex as they knew it painful or impossible, with sympathetic intervention they can experiment with and learn alternative ways of sexual expression. For example, older adults who experience joint dysfunction may find greater comfort in a side-lying position during intercourse. Research has consistently shown that many older adults remain sexually active and value this expression (Johnson, 1996).

Sexual Orientation

Sexual orientation is a clear, persistent sexual preference for persons of one sex. Based on studies by Kinsey and others (1948, 1953), most people are heterosexual; a smaller percentage are homosexual (gay or lesbian) and bisexual. Gays or lesbians may keep their sexual orientation hidden or be more open about their sexual preference. The process of "coming out" involves self-acknowledgment, self-acceptance, and self-disclosure (Alexander and LaRosa, 1994). "Coming out" can be particularly difficult because of **homophobia,** an irrational fear of homosexuality, displayed by some individuals.

Contraception

The decisions that women and men make regarding contraception have far-reaching effects on their lives. Effective contraception involves factors relating to the sexually active couple, the method of contraception, the consistency of use, and the compliance with the requirements of the particular contraceptive method. Personal characteristics that have been identified as positively influencing contraceptive use include motivation to avoid unintended pregnancy, ability to plan, comfort with sexuality, and previous contraceptive use (Beckman and Harvey, 1996).

Numerous contraceptive options are available to sexually active couples. Some methods do not require a prescription, whereas other methods do require intervention by a health care provider. Nonprescription contraceptive methods include abstinence, timing of intercourse in regard to the menstrual cycle, and various barrier methods. Abstinence from sexual intercourse is 100% effective. Barrier methods include over-the-counter spermicidal products that are placed into the vagina before intercourse to create a spermicidal barrier between the uterus and ejaculated sperm. A condom, frequently called a "rubber," is a thin latex sheath that fits over the penis. Condoms provide a barrier against all sexually transmitted diseases (STDs). Vaginal spermicides and condoms are most effective when instructions are carefully fol-

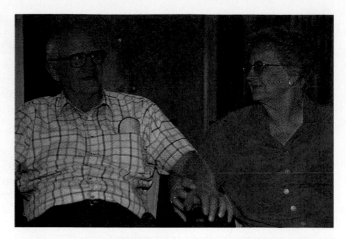

FIGURE **19-3**   Sexuality is important across the life span.

lowed; their combined use has been found to be more effective in preventing pregnancy than the use of either alone. Effectiveness varies with each method and with the consistency of use. The percentage of women experiencing an accidental pregnancy using these nonprescription methods ranges from 3% to 36% (Hatcher and others, 1994).

Contraception methods that require the intervention of a health care provider include hormonal contraception, the intrauterine device (IUD), the diaphragm or cervical cap, and sterilization. Hormonal contraception is available in several forms, including oral contraceptive pills, intramuscular injection, subdermal implant, and IUDs that contain progesterone.

Sterilization is the most effective contraception method other than abstinence. It is considered permanent. Female sterilization, or tubal ligation, involves cutting, tying, or otherwise ligating the fallopian tubes. In male sterilization, or vasectomy, the vas deferens that carries the sperm away from the testicles is cut and tied.

Sexually Transmitted Disease

A **sexually transmitted disease** is an infectious process spread through sexual contact; this includes oral, genital, or anal sexual activity. At present STDs are epidemic, with the highest prevalence being among teens and young adults (McIlhaney, 2000). Acquired immunodeficiency syndrome (AIDS) continues to receive wide public attention; however, often STDs also need to be considered. Prevalent STDs include syphilis, gonorrhea, chlamydia, genital warts, the human papillomavirus (HPV), and herpes simplex virus (HSV) type 2.

▌ NURSING KNOWLEDGE BASE

Sexuality is an important aspect of a person's identity. Clients' perception of their sexuality may affect how they care for themselves both physically and emotionally. A person's sexual beliefs, preferences, and activity can have an effect on issues and decisions affecting sexuality. In addition, altered sexual health can affect a person's self-concept and relationships with others, and physical and emotional health.

Issues and Decisions

Issues relating to sexuality are significant for most people. Nurses encounter clients who are making decisions or working with issues related to sexuality on a regular basis. Understanding some of the decisions and issues clients may be facing can increase your effectiveness in assisting clients to reach their maximum level of health in the area of sexuality.

ABORTION.   Abortion remains an issue that stimulates heated discussions. Reasons for selecting an abortion vary and may include a decision to terminate an untimely pregnancy or a choice to abort a fetus known to have a defect incompatible with life. The woman and her partner who have chosen an abortion may experience a sense of loss, grief, and/or guilt. Guilt may surface immediately or may be more covert and manifest by sexual dysfunction or inappropriate perceptions. Women have reported sensations of loss and psychological problems 2 years after the abortion (Major and others, 2000).

Alterations in Sexual Health

Alterations in sexual health can occur from a variety of situations (e.g., illness, infertility, trauma, and abuse). It is important that the clinician understand the reason for changes in the client's sexual health. Frequently a professional specializing in altered sexual health is needed·to assist the client and partner in resuming a satisfying sexual relationship.

SEXUALITY AND INTIMACY FOLLOWING ILLNESS. The response to changes in sexuality and intimacy following an illness depends on the person's self-concept, family support, support of sexual partner, lifestyle, and self-perceptions regarding sexuality (Hordern, 2000). Most health professionals fail to address sexual needs of their clients (Middleman, 1999). Understanding the impact of a diagnosis, treatment, and medications on your client's perception of sexuality or sexual performance can result in a treatment plan that has minimal effect on your client's sexual health. Your client is more likely to adhere to a treatment plan if medications that alter sexual function are only prescribed when there is no alternative.

INFERTILITY.   Infertility is defined as the inability to conceive after 1 year of unprotected intercourse. If a couple desires to conceive but cannot, the individuals may experience a sense of failure. Couples who are unsuccessful in conceiving or carrying a child to full term must be referred to a fertility specialist to assist in determining the cause and individualized treatment of infertility.

SEXUAL ABUSE.   Sexual abuse is widespread in our society and crosses all socioeconomic and ethnic groups. It is estimated that from one fourth to one half of all females experience some type of sexual abuse by the age of 18 (Guidry, 1995; Bohn and Holz, 1996). Most often this abuse is at the hands of an intimate partner or family member. Abuse may begin, continue, or even intensify during pregnancy. Sexual abuse is also an issue for males. Studies indicate that one in six young boys has experienced at least one sexually abusive incident before reaching adulthood (Guidry, 1995). Sexual abuse has far-ranging effects on physical and psychological functioning. Women who have been sexually abused are disproportionately frequent users of health care resources (Bohn and Holz, 1996).

When abuse is reported or recognized, immediate treatment should be mobilized for the victim and the family. All family members may require therapy to promote healthy interactions and relationships.

SEXUAL DYSFUNCTION.   The causes of **sexual dysfunction** may be physiological or psychological. Sometimes the cause of a dysfunction cannot be identified or is a combination of several factors. Common chronic illnesses that can contribute to sexual dysfunction include diabetes mellitus, kidney disease, alcoholism, neurological disorders, hormone deficiencies, multiple sclerosis, and vascular insufficiency. In addition, side effects of medications can also contribute to sexual dysfunction.

▌CRITICAL THINKING
Synthesis

Sexuality is complex and related to self-concept, as well as to physical and emotional health. Critical thinking involves considering all variables affecting a client's sexuality. Reflect on your personal and professional experiences to provide appropriate interventions for the client's care.

KNOWLEDGE.   When you consider the sexuality of clients, think about knowledge regarding sexual development, sexual orientation, sexual response, STDs, contraception, and alterations in sexual health. Also helpful is knowledge regarding self-concept. Body image will affect how a person interacts with actual and potential sexual partners. Self-esteem influences how people perceive their personal attractiveness. This will affect how they interact with others. People who perceive themselves as attractive will interact more openly and spontaneously, thus inviting a relationship. People with low self-esteem will be less relaxed and less open to relating. Another important knowledge base to consider when caring for clients with sexuality problems is communication (see Chapter 8). Use of therapeutic communication techniques establishes a relationship that encourages your clients to express their concerns.

EXPERIENCE.   Your own sexuality and sexual experience can provide a valuable resource for understanding a client's experiences. In addition, your own sexual experiences can add to understanding about what a first sexual encounter may have been like or what it is like to broach the topic of STDs before intercourse. In addition to personal experience related to sexuality, use what you have learned through working with other clients as you assess and work with current clients.

ATTITUDES.   In approaching clients about their sexuality and sexual functioning, an attitude of risk taking can be helpful. Certainly for novice nurses, it can be unnerving to inquire about another person's sexual functioning. You may worry that the client will not appreciate being asked about sexuality and sexual practices. However, clients want to know how medications, treatments, and surgical procedures influence their sexual relationship. Your willingness to risk asking a client about sexual issues can move you to a place of greater comfort in discussing sexuality. With experience you will come to recognize that many clients welcome the opportunity to talk about their sexuality. When clients are experiencing difficulty in sexual relating, they often appreciate the nurse bringing up the subject. Once the topic is broached, the client can talk about concerns and explore possible ways to resolve the problem.

STANDARDS. Ethical standards may come into play when you are faced with caring for a client whose sexual practices and values differ from your own. The American Nurses Association (ANA) code of ethics (2001) states, "The nurse provides services with respect for human dignity and the uniqueness of the client, unrestricted by considerations of social or economic status, personal attributes, or the nature of health problems."

Ethical standards also come into play in regard to reporting of STDs. An element in both the ANA code of ethics (1985) and the International Council of Nurses code for nurses (2000) is the protection of the public. This involves reporting certain diseases and/or incidents of abuse to the appropriate health officials so that follow-up can be instituted. Most states mandate a report to a social service agency if abuse is suspected.

NURSING PROCESS

 Assessment

Sexuality involves physical, psychological, social, and cultural variables. You must assess all relevant factors to determine a client's sexual well-being. Many nurses find that they are uncomfortable talking about sexuality with clients. To increase comfort in discussing sexuality, build a sound knowledge base, including understanding of healthy sexuality, the most common sexual dysfunctions, and the effects of medical therapies on sexual function. Also important is assessment of your own comfort level when discussing sexuality. Remember that you do not need to have all the answers to a client's questions or problems.

SEXUAL HEALTH HISTORY. Every complete nursing history should include a few questions related to sexual functioning. Start with a general statement such as "Sex is an important part of life and can be affected by our health status" or "To better understand your health, it is useful to know if you have concerns about your sexual function." Other questions for adults may include the following:
1. How do you feel about the sexual aspect of your life?
2. How has your illness, medication, or impending surgery affected your sex life?

3. It is not unusual for people with your condition to experience some sexual problems. What has been your experience.

Explore the client's use of contraception and safe sex practices. Adolescents may best respond to a question such as, "Many teenagers have questions about STDs or whether their bodies are developing at the right rate. Do you have any questions about sex?"

FACTORS INFLUENCING SEXUAL FUNCTION. In gathering a sexual history, consider physical, functional, relationship, lifestyle, and self-esteem factors that may influence sexual functioning. Sexual desire and function may be influenced, positively or negatively, by a variety of physical factors. For example, sexual intercourse may result in pain or discomfort from arthritis, angina, endometriosis, or lack of vaginal lubrication. Sexual performance can be altered by neuropathies, vascular deficiencies, and hormonal alterations. Even anticipation that sex may hurt, such as postpartum or postoperatively, can lessen sexual desire. Learn to what extent these physical factors affect a client's sexual performance.

Medications may affect sexual desire or cause physical changes that affect performance. Drinking alcohol or using drugs may cloud judgment and result in activities that may lead to STDs or pregnancy. Gather a complete history of any medications or illicit drugs the client is taking. You may also need to obtain the same information for the client's partner.

Self-perceptions may lead to personal and emotional conflict involving sexuality. Lower self-esteem can negatively influence sexual functioning. Communication skills play a critical role in the partner's sexual compatibility. Try to learn how clients feel about their sexuality and the ability to perform sexually. Ask clients if they feel comfortable when they are relating to their partner and whether there is an openness in the interaction.

A variety of normal change associated with aging can affect sexual function. Women experience a reduction in vaginal secretions, and the vagina becomes shorter and does not expand as well to accommodate the penis (Lueckenotte, 2000). Orgasmic contractions are fewer and may be accompanied by painful uterine contractions. In men, the penis may not become firm as quickly and may not be as firm as at a younger age. Ejaculation can take longer to achieve and may be shorter in duration, and erection often diminishes more quickly. Nursing assessment includes a history of past sexual experiences, perceptions, and difficulties.

SEXUAL HEALTH PRACTICES. *Safe sex* is a term used to describe responsible sexual behavior aimed at preventing the spread of STDs, including AIDS. Responsible sexual behavior includes knowing one's sexual partner, being able to openly discuss sexual and drug use behaviors with the partner, and using protective devices.

SEXUAL DYSFUNCTION. Be alert for indications of sexual dysfunction. Consider the nature of physical problems, medications, and the factors that can put a client at risk for sexual dysfunction.

Signs and Symptoms That May Indicate Current Sexual Abuse or a History of Sexual Abuse

Box 19-5

Bruises	Premenstrual syndrome
Lacerations	Sleep pattern disturbances
Abrasions	Nightmares
Burns	Repetitive dreams
Frequent visits to health care providers	Insomnia
Vague symptoms	Depression
Headaches	Anxiety
Gastrointestinal problems	Fear
Eating disorders	Decreased self-esteem
Abdominal pain	Difficulty developing trust
Vaginal pain	Difficulties with intimate relationships
Dysmenorrhea	Substance abuse

Modified from Bohn D, Holz K: Sequelae of abuse: health effects of childhood sexual abuse, domestic battering, and rape, *J Nurse Midwifery* 41(6):442, 1996.

SEXUAL ABUSE.   Be alert to clues that may suggest abuse (Box 19-5). In addition, observe the interaction between the client and partner for additional clues. Controlling behaviors such as speaking for the woman or belittling her are suggestive of emotional and perhaps physical or sexual abuse (Bohn and Holz, 1996). If you suspect abuse, interview the client privately. A client will probably not admit to problems of abuse with the sexual partner present. Some of the following questions may be useful: "Are you in a relationship in which someone is hurting you?" or "Have you ever been forced to have sex when you didn't want to?" These questions avoid using the frightening and sometimes confusing terms *abuse* and *rape*. If you ask questions related to abuse, tell the client that the answers will be confidential.

CLIENT EXPECTATIONS.   As in the case of any client assessment, it is important to understand the client's expectations regarding care. Questions such as "What do you expect from us in the way we perform your care?" or "How can we best meet your needs?" give the client the opportunity to express any desires. When nursing care involves consideration of the client's sexuality, the need for sensitivity, confidentiality, and understanding are likely client expectations.

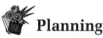 **Nursing Diagnosis**

Possible nursing diagnoses related to sexual functioning are listed in Box 19-6. Clues to help you identify defining characteristics of a possible nursing diagnosis include surgery of reproductive organs or changes in appearance, chronic fatigue or pain, past or current physical abuse, chronic illness, and developmental milestones such as puberty or menopause. Interventions depend on selecting the correct related factors.

Identifying a nursing diagnosis regarding sexuality often requires clarification with the client to establish that

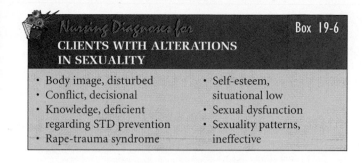

Nursing Diagnoses for   Box 19-6

CLIENTS WITH ALTERATIONS IN SEXUALITY

- Body image, disturbed
- Conflict, decisional
- Knowledge, deficient regarding STD prevention
- Rape-trauma syndrome
- Self-esteem, situational low
- Sexual dysfunction
- Sexuality patterns, ineffective

the nursing diagnosis defining characteristics exist and that the client perceives difficulty with regard to sexuality. Determining the contributing factors is important. Including all relevant contributing factors can help to focus effective planning. For example, the nursing diagnosis *ineffective sexuality patterns related to acceptance of recent mastectomy* might be appropriate for a woman who has recently undergone a mastectomy. Further expanding the "related to" section to include more about how the mastectomy is affecting sexuality would be helpful. Altered sexuality could be related to postoperative pain or fear of pain, fear of diminished attractiveness, and/or difficulty in moving. The approaches to each of these factors would be slightly different.

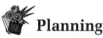 **Planning**

GOALS AND OUTCOMES.   Involve the client when developing a plan of care. If the client agrees, include the sex partner as well. For planning to be effective, the client must be involved in setting goals and outcome criteria. For example, for the nursing diagnosis *ineffective sexuality patterns related to recent mastectomy and fear of pain* you might explore with the client what she envisions as a satisfactory recovery after her mastectomy. This would give the client the opportunity to share, for example, that she would like to return to her presurgical sexual relationship with her partner. She might specify that she wants to feel comfortable having her remaining breast caressed and to engage in intercourse 1 to 2 times per week, without experiencing pain.

SETTING PRIORITIES.   Clients who are undergoing surgeries that alter their body image (e.g., mastectomies or colostomies) also have changes in perceptions of their sexuality (Hordern, 2000). For these clients resuming sexual activities may have priority. It is important that you determine if this is your client's need and plan for this accordingly. For example, you may need to plan for private time for your client and partner to quietly sit in the room and have dinner and watch a movie without any interruptions.

CONTINUITY OF CARE.   Planning in the area of sexuality may include referrals to a clinical psychologist, social worker, or sex therapist. Sexual conflict in marriage or trauma over past sexual assault or incest may require intensive treatment with mental health professionals or a certified sex therapist.

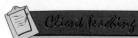

PROMOTING SEXUAL FUNCTION

Box 19-7

- Refrain from drinking alcohol 1 to 2 hours before sexual activity.
- Encourage partners to discuss what types of intimate behavior provide the most sexual stimulation and satisfaction.
- Explain options available for contraception.
- Discuss side effects of medications that commonly alter sexual function and response.
- For a client with cardiac dysfunction, encourage use of the usual position during intercourse and selection of a time of day when the client feels rested.
- Explain that safe sex involves the following practices: avoidance of multiple or anonymous partners, prostitutes, and other people with multiple sex partners; avoidance of sexual contact with a person who has a genital discharge, genital warts, herpes, other suspicious lesions, or a medical diagnosis of HIV or hepatitis B; avoidance of oral/anal sex; avoidance of genital contact with oral sores; and use of latex condoms and diaphragms along with spermicides.

Gerontological Nursing Practice   Box 19-8

- Females may benefit from use of an artificial water-based lubricant during intercourse.
- Alternative positions for intercourse (e.g., side-lying, lying on a bed with legs over the side) may decrease discomfort during intercourse.
- A longer period of foreplay helps the male to achieve penile firmness.
- Conserve strength by not working hard at the beginning of intercourse, so as to avoid tiring before climax.
- Resume foreplay or use time for touching and talking so as to achieve a second orgasm.

From Lueckenotte A: *Gerontologic nursing* ed 2, St. Louis, 2000, Mosby.

 Implementation

Good nursing includes promoting sexual health, as well as caring for clients in acute and restorative settings. Nurses can promote sexual health by helping clients understand their problems and explore methods to deal with them effectively.

HEALTH PROMOTION.   Exploring a person's sexuality and providing useful sex education require good communication skills. The environment and timing should provide privacy, uninterrupted time, and client comfort. For example, discuss contraception methods with a woman in an office rather than in the examination room when she is only partially clothed. Plan the discussion so there are no interruptions, and sit down while showing your interest and readiness to support her needs.

Teaching topics on sexuality vary (Box 19-7). Education may offer explanation of normal developmental changes. For example, you might talk to a school-age child about the appearance of pubic hair. Provide details of physiological changes resulting from illness or treatment effects as a part of general health care. This encourages clients to ask questions or voice concerns about personal functioning. Box 19-8 summarizes special considerations for the older adult.

When discussing sexual health with clients of childbearing age, always consider your client's cultural and religious beliefs regarding contraception. The discussion may include their desire for children, usual sexual practices, and acceptable methods of contraception. When teaching about contraceptives, include scheduling or frequency of sex, comfort with genital touching, and comfort with interruption of sexual acts. Review all methods of contraception to provide necessary information for an informed client choice. The best method is the one the client will use consistently.

Individuals having more than one sex partner or whose partner had other sexual experiences need to learn more about safe sex practices. Provide information on STD transmission and symptoms, use of condoms, and high-risk sexual activities (e.g., anal sex). Safe sex may also consider the client's emotional risks within a relationship. Role play may be a useful teaching tool to help the client learn to say "No" or negotiate with a partner to use a condom.

Nursing interventions that address client alterations in sexual patterns or sexual dysfunction raise awareness, assist clarification of issues or concerns, and provide information. Recognize when clients' needs exceed their expertise. Referral to a sexual counselor may be necessary.

ACUTE CARE.   Illness and surgery can be significant situational stressors. Clients may experience major physical changes, the effects of drugs or treatments, and the emotional stress of prognosis and future limited function. Sexuality, as a component of personality, may be affected by both physical and psychological aspects of illness. Never assume that sexual functioning is not a concern merely because of an individual's age or severity of prognosis. After identifying concerns, address them in the context of the person's value system. When a client experiences physical limitations to sexually performing, you might suggest therapies such as planning sexual activity when the client is rested, experimenting with positions that are more comfortable, encouraging partners to give one another more time to achieve arousal, and encouraging the use of foreplay to increase sexual arousal. For example, a client experiencing joint pain may appreciate a discussion of how the side-lying position can be effective in intercourse. Use of fantasy or a sense of playfulness may add new romance or stimulation to a long-term relationship.

RESTORATIVE AND CONTINUING CARE.   In the home environment it is important to assist clients in creating an environment comfortable for sexual activity. This may involve making recommendations for ways to rearrange the client's bedroom to accommodate any limitations. For example, wheelchair-bound clients may prefer being able to move the chair close up to the side of the bed at an angle that allows the partner to assume a coital position more easily. Clients and partners need to know how to accommodate barriers such as Foley catheters or drainage tubes that may make coital positioning difficult.

In the long-term care setting, facilities should make proper arrangements for privacy during an older client's sexual experience (Lueckenotte, 2000). The ideal situation is to set up a pleasant room that can be used for a variety of activities but may also be reserved by the older adult for private visits with a spouse or partner. This may not be possible. Another option is to use the client's room and make other arrangements for the client's roommate. Although privacy of clients is important, they should not be left alone in a situation in which they may injure themselves (Lueckenotte, 2000).

 ## Evaluation

CLIENT CARE. Review goals and outcome criteria that were developed during the planning process and determine if they have been met. In addition, consider the overall status of the identified problems or nursing diagnoses. This will require a follow-up discussion with the client to determine if the level of satisfaction with sexual performance or sexual function has improved. Sometimes the goal and outcome criteria may have been achieved but sexual functioning is still not ideal. Consider what other steps might be appropriate.

CLIENT EXPECTATIONS.   In evaluating care provided to clients with sexual alterations or those in need of sexual health education, determine if the client's expectations are met. After determining the progress in care, ask if the client thinks that nursing care was effective and supportive. Remain aware of any personal limitations in being able to counsel the client. Referrals to other health care providers may still be necessary.

Key Terms

body image, *p. 462*
homophobia, *p. 472*

identity, *p. 463*
role, *p. 463*
self-concept, *p. 462*
self-esteem, *p. 462*

sexual dysfunction, *p. 473*
sexual orientation, *p. 472*
sexually transmitted disease, *p. 472*
sexuality, *p. 471*

Key Concepts

- The self-concept is an integrated set of conscious and unconscious feelings, attitudes, and perceptions about oneself.
- Components of self-concept are body image, self-esteem, roles, and identity.
- Roles are learned through socialization; they involve the expectations of others about behavior in particular positions (e.g., family member, employee).
- You should be aware of how your self-concept and nursing actions can affect a client's self-concept.
- Sexuality is related to all dimensions of health; therefore sexual concerns or problem should be addressed as a part of nursing care.

- Attitudes toward sexuality vary widely and are influenced by spirituality, society's values, the media, family, and other factors. You should not judge a client's sexual preferences and needs.
- Sexual development involves some kind of sexual behavior or growth in all developmental stages.
- Sexual health involves physical and psychosocial aspects and contributes to an individual's sense of self-worth and positive interpersonal relationships.
- A client's sexuality is affected by development and life changes, ethical decisional issues, fertility, personal and emotional conflicts, illness, and hospitalization; you help the client adapt to situations and maintain healthy sexuality.

Critical Thinking Activities

1. Jack Fisher is a 28-year-old manager of a local food store. He comes to his primary care provider for blood work before his upcoming marriage. The nurse knows Mr. Fisher because he has been coming to the clinic for minor health issues over the past 4 years. In talking with Mr. Fisher, the nurse learns that this is his first marriage, the woman he is marrying has a 3-year-old son, and although he has spent a good deal of time with his fiancée's 3-year-old son he has not lived in a household with young children since his own childhood. The nurse recognizes that Mr. Fisher will be undergoing several role changes related to his upcoming marriage. What new roles will he likely be taking on? How might the nurse explore with Mr. Fisher his readiness to assume new roles and his awareness of the possible stress of taking on new roles?

2. Mrs. Smith, a 48-year-old married woman, is scheduled for a hysterectomy tomorrow. She expresses concern regarding whether this is the right choice. What issues may be influencing Mrs. Smith? How do you proceed with her care?

3. Mr. Jackson is 65 years old and is admitted with postdiabetic ketoacidosis. During his stay you notice great intimacy (hand holding, kissing, massage, affectionate names) expressed between Mr. and Mrs. Jackson. How might you approach the topic of sexuality? What is relevant information to provide regarding age and disease state?

4. Kathy Lane is a 20-year-old college student. She is being seen in the clinic for an STD. What strategies would you use to assess her sexual activity and safe sex practices? What would your teaching priorities be?

Review Questions

1. When you are caring for a client after mastectomy, interventions to promote physiological stability and pain control are necessary. In addition, you also need to design nursing interventions directed toward improving her:
   1. mobility.
   2. self-concept.
   3. activity tolerance.
   4. self-care activities.
2. Adolescents are at risk for body image disturbance. An accurate statement about body image is that:
   1. body image is not influenced by the opinions of others.
   2. body image only refers to the external features of a person.
   3. body image includes actual and perceived perceptions of one's body.
   4. physical changes during adolescence are quickly incorporated into the person's body image.
3. A person's clear, persistent preference for another person of one sex or the other is known as:
   1. sexual response.
   2. sexual behavior.
   3. sexual preference.
   4. sexual orientation.
4. Inability or difficulty in sexual functioning caused by physiological or psychological factors or both is called:
   1. sexual behavior.
   2. sexual response.
   3. sexual orientation.
   4. sexual dysfunction.
5. Gender identity is the individual's:
   1. sexual behavior.
   2. sexual orientation.
   3. sense of being feminine or masculine.
   4. sense of preferring one sex over the other.

References

Alexander LL, LaRosa JH: *New dimensions in women's health,* Boston, 1994, Jones & Bartlett.

American Nurses Association: *Code for nurses with interpretive statements,* Kansas City, MO, 2001, The Association.

Anderson E: Self-esteem and optimism in men and women infected with HIV, *Nurs Res* 49(5):262, 2000.

Beckman LJ, Harvey SM: Factors affecting the consistent use of barrier methods of contraception, *Obstet Gynecol* 88(10):65S, 1996.

Bohn D, Holz K: Sequelae of abuse: health effects of childhood sexual abuse, domestic battering, and rape, *J Nurse Midwifery* 41(6):442, 1996.

Drench M: Changes in body image secondary to disease and injury, *Rehabil Nurs* 19(1):31, 1994.

Erikson EH: *Childhood and society,* ed 2, New York, 1963, WW Norton.

Forrest JD, Frost JJ: The family planning attitudes and experiences of low-income women, *Fam Plan Perspect* 28(11-12):246, 1996.

Giger JN, Davidhizar RE: *Transcultural nursing: assessment and intervention,* ed 3, St. Louis, 1999, Mosby.

Guidry HM: Childhood sexual abuse: role of the family physician, *Am Fam Physician* 51(2):407, 1995.

Hatcher RA and others: *Contraceptive technology,* New York, 1994, Irvington.

Hordern A: Intimacy and sexuality for the woman with breast cancer, *Cancer Nurs* 23(3):230, 2000.

International Council of Nurses: *ICN code of ethics for nurses,* Geneva, 2000, 3 place, Jean-Marteau, CH-1201, The Association.

Johnson B: Older adults and sexuality: a multidimensional perspective, *J Gerontol Nurs* 22(2):6, 1996.

Kinsey AC and others: *Sexual behavior in the human male,* Philadelphia, 1948, WB Saunders.

Kinsey AC and others: *Sexual behavior in the human female,* Philadelphia, 1953, WB Saunders.

Lueckenotte L: *Gerontologic nursing,* ed 2, St. Louis, 2000, Mosby.

MacLaren A: Primary care for women: comprehensive sexual health assessment, *J Nurse Midwifery* 40(2):104, 1995.

Major B and others: Psychological responses of women after first-trimester abortion, *Arch Gen Psychiatry,* 57(8):777, 2000.

Masters W and others: *Human sexuality,* Boston, 1992, Little, Brown.

McIlhaney JS: Sexually transmitted infection and teenage sexuality, *Am J Obstet Gynecol* 183(2):334, 2000.

Middleman AB: Review of sexuality education in the United States for health professionals working with adolescents, *Curr Opin Pediatr* 11(4):283, 1999.

Newell R, Marks I: Phobia nature of social anxiety in patients with facial disfigurement, *Br J Psychiary* 176:177, 2000.

Read J: ABC of sexual health: sexual problems associated with infertility, pregnancy, and aging, *Br Med J* 318(7183):587, 1999.

Stuart GW, Laraia MT: *Principles and practice of psychiatric nursing,* ed 7, St. Louis, 2000, Mosby.

World Health Organization: *Education and treatment in human sexuality: the training of health professionals,* WHO Teach Rep Ser, 572, Geneva, 1975, The Organization.

Family Context in Nursing

Objectives

- Define key terms.
- Examine current trends in the American family.
- Discuss common family forms and their health implications.
- Assess the way family structure and pattern of functioning affect the health of family members and the family as a whole.
- Compare family as context with family as client and explain the way these perspectives influence nursing practice.
- Use the nursing process to provide for the health care needs of the family.
- Interpret both external and internal factors that promote family health.

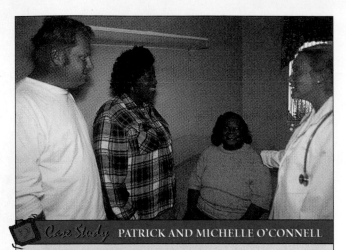

Case Study PATRICK AND MICHELLE O'CONNELL

Patrick and Michelle O'Connell have been married 9 years and live in Auburn, Maine. Patrick is 38 years old, and after being employed by the state in the Department of Public Safety for the past 8 years, he has recently learned that he is in danger of being laid off in the next round of cuts. Patrick has been diagnosed with borderline hypertension and admits his stress level is an 8 on a scale of 1 to 10. He enjoys watching TV, playing war games on the computer, and playing with the family's pet dogs and cats. The family's health insurance is provided through Patrick's job. Michelle is 32 years old, is employed part-time as a receptionist at a building supply company, and attends nursing school. They are a child-free couple by choice. Michelle received a diagnosis of cervical cancer 3 months after their wedding, however, and had a vaginal hysterectomy 2 years ago. Michelle has been very worried about their financial problems and her grandmother's health problems, and she fears needing to work full-time. She describes herself as spiritual and attends church occasionally.

Michelle plays the role of keeping the couple connected to their extended families. Because each of their parents divorced and either have since remarried or are cohabitating, they have four sets of parents and 28 step-, half, and whole brothers and sisters between them. Michelle manages the household duties and finances, works, and goes to school. She is the oldest daughter in her family and is the only one of the siblings to keep in contact with her grandmother, Lois. Michelle has learned from the visiting nurse that Lois's condition is worsened—she is becoming more forgetful and less tolerant of physical activity related to severe heart disease. Michelle worries about what she can do from 2 hours away geographically. Lois needs continuous support, and for Lois to move in with her, Michelle would have to rid the house of pets, which Lois is allergic to, and her home would require major renovations to accommodate her 80-year-old grandmother.

Bethany, age 28, is the nursing student assigned to Lois in her community health rotation. She sees Lois living alone in a clean mobile home in a nice park. She understands that Lois has been widowed 17 years and that she receives Social Security and has Medicare. However, she cannot afford supplemental insurance to pay for her medications. Bethany is concerned about Lois's financial situation, especially in light of the fact the visiting nurse has said Lois may need different living arrangements.

Major changes have occurred in the concept and structure of the family, but it is clear that the family remains the central institution in American society. The current general assumption is that although the family is in transition and may look very different from the family of the 1950s, the concept of family is here to stay. Although contemporary families have their share of problems and challenges, they are characterized by three important attributes: durability, resiliency, and diversity.

Family durability is the term for the intrafamilial system of support and structure that may extend beyond the walls of the household. The players may change, the parents may remarry, the children may or may not leave home as adults, but the "family" transcends long periods and inevitable lifestyle changes.

Family resiliency is the ability to cope with expected and unexpected stressors. The family's ability to adapt to role changes, developmental milestones, and crises shows resilience. The goal of the family is not only to survive "the challenge" but also to thrive and grow as a result of the newly gained knowledge.

Family diversity is the attention to uniqueness. Some families will be experiencing marriage for the first time and having children in later life, whereas others are grandparents at the same age. Every person within a familial unit has specific needs, strengths, and important developmental considerations. As nurses it is our job first to understand the makeup, structure, function, and coping capacity of the family and then to see how to design nursing interventions appropriate to the family's strengths and weakneses.

SCIENTIFIC KNOWLEDGE BASE
Concept of Family

Family evokes a visual image of adults and children living together in a satisfying, harmonious manner. Families are, however, as diverse as the individuals that compose them, and clients have deeply ingrained values about their families that deserve respect. Thus each individual defines the family. In other words, think of the **family** as a set of relationships that the client identifies as family or as a network of individuals who influence each other's lives whether there are actual biological or legal ties.

Family Forms

Family forms are patterns of people who are considered to be family members. Although all families have some things in common, each family form has unique problems and strengths. Keep an open mind about what constitutes a family so that potential resources and concerns are not overlooked. Several family forms are described in Box 20-1.

CURRENT TRENDS AND NEW FAMILY FORMS. Families are smaller today. People are marrying later, women are delaying childbirth, and couples are choosing to have fewer children or none at all. Divorce rates have tripled since the 1950s, and although the rate appears to have stabilized, it is

Family Forms   Box 20-1

NUCLEAR FAMILY

This family consists of husband and wife (and perhaps one or more children).

EXTENDED FAMILY

This family includes relatives (aunts, uncles, grandparents, and cousins) in addition to the nuclear family.

SINGLE-PARENT FAMILY

This family is formed when one parent leaves the nuclear family because of death, divorce, or desertion or when a single person decides to have or adopt a child.

BLENDED FAMILY

This family is formed when parents bring unrelated children from prior or foster parenting relationships into a new joint living situation.

ALTERNATE PATTERNS OF RELATIONSHIPS

These relationships include multiadult households, "skip-generation" families (grandparents caring for grandchildren), communal groups with children, "nonfamilies" (adults living alone), cohabitating partners, and homosexual couples.

estimated that 60% of marriages will end in divorce (U.S. Bureau of the Census, 2001).

Adolescent pregnancy is an ever-increasing concern. The majority of these adolescents continue to live with their families. A teen pregnancy tends to have long-term consequences for the mother and often severely stresses family relationships and resources. Teen fathers have stressors placed on them as well when their partner becomes pregnant. As a result, both of these adolescents are often struggling with the normal tasks of development and identity but now are also forced to accept responsibility that they may not be ready for physically, emotionally, socially, and/or financially.

Although unable to marry by law in many states, homosexual couples define their relationship in family terms. Approximately half of all gay male couples live together, compared with three fourths of lesbian couples. Individuals in same sex relationships have become more open about their sexual preference and more vocal about their legal rights.

The fastest-growing age-group is 65 years and older. For the first time in history the average American has more living parents than children, and children are more likely to have living grandparents and even great-grandparents. This "graying" of America has affected the family life cycle, perhaps most significantly for middle-age adults. As a result there are fewer family members available to take care of and assist older adults (Ganong and others, 1998). This generation is finding that they must balance the needs of their offspring and the needs of their aging parents, sometimes at the expense of their own well-being and resources. Caring for a frail or chronically ill relative is a primary concern for a growing number of families (Marks, 1998).

FACTORS INFLUENCING FAMILY FORMS.   Families face many challenges, including changing structures and roles in

the changing economic status of society. There are family challenges related to divorce and the aging of its older members. There are two additional trends that social scientists identify as threats or concerns facing the family: (1) changing economic status (e.g., declining family income, need for dual incomes, decreased health insurance or lack of access to health care, and growing hunger and homelessness) and (2) family violence (Voydanoff and Donnelly, 1999).

Making ends meet is a daily concern for many people because of the declining economic status of families. Even though two-income families have become the norm, real family income has not increased since 1973. Families at the lower end of the income scale have been particularly affected, and single-parent families are especially vulnerable.

The statistics regarding family violence are disturbing. Clemen-Stone and others (1998) reported that 2.7 million children were reported abused or neglected in 1991, up from 1.1 million in the preceding 11 years, and the need for foster care increased by almost 50%. The inflicting of emotional and physical pain on family members occurs in more than half of all households in the United States; approximately 50 million people are victimized each year. Emotional, physical, and sexual abuse occurs toward spouses, children, older adults, and across all social classes. The cause of family violence is complex and multidimensional. Factors associated with violence include stress, poverty, social isolation, psychopathology, and the cycle of violence—the intergenerational transmission of violence.

STRUCTURE AND FUNCTION.   Each family has a unique structure and way of functioning. **Family structure** is based on organization (i.e., the ongoing membership of the family and the pattern of relationships). Relationships can be numerous and complex. For example, a woman's relationships may include wife-husband, mother-son, and mother-daughter and employee-boss, boss-employee, and work colleague-colleague, each with different demands, roles, and expectations.

Although the definitions of structure vary, ask the following questions: "Who is included in the family?" "Who performs which tasks?" and "Who makes which decisions?" Structure may enhance or detract from the family's ability to respond to the expected and unexpected stressors of daily life. Very rigid or very flexible structures can threaten the functioning of the family. A rigid structure specifically dictates persons permitted to accomplish a task and may also limit the number of persons outside the immediate family allowed to assume these tasks. For example, the mother might be considered the only acceptable person to provide emotional support for the children and/or to perform all of the household chores. The husband may be the only acceptable person to provide financial support, maintain the vehicles, do the yard work, and/or do all of the home repairs. A change in the health status of the person responsible for a task places a burden on the family because no other person is available, willing, or considered acceptable to assume that task (Call and others, 1999). An extremely open structure can also present problems for the family. Stability that oth-

Stages of the Family Life Cycle		Table 20-1
Family Life Cycle Stage	Emotional Process of Transition: Key Principles	Changes in Family Status Required to Proceed Developmentally
Between families: unattached young adult	Accepting parent-offspring separation	Differentiation of self in relation to family of origin Development of intimate peer relationships Establishment of self in work
Joining of families through marriage: newly married couple	Commitment to new system	Formation of marital system Realignment of relationships with extended families and friends to include spouse
Family with young children	Accepting new generation of members into system	Adjusting marital system to make space for children Taking on parenting roles Realignment of relationships with extended family to include parenting and grandparenting roles
Family with adolescents	Increasing flexibility of family boundaries to include children's independence	Shifting of parent-child relationships to permit adolescents to move into and out of system Refocus on midlife marital and career issues Beginning shift toward concerns for older generation
Launching children and moving on	Accepting multitude of exits from and entries into family system	Renegotiation of marital system as dyad Development of adult-to-adult relationships between grown children and their parents Realignment of relationships to include in-laws and grandchildren Dealing with disabilities and death of parents (grandparents)
Family in later life	Accepting shifting of generational roles	Maintaining own or couple functioning and interests in the face of physiological decline; exploration of new familial and social role options Support for more central role for middle generation Making room in system for wisdom and experience of older adults; supporting older generation without overfunctioning for them Retirement; change in role Dealing with loss of spouse, siblings, and other peers, and preparation for own death; life review and integration

Data from Vaughan-Cole B and others: *Family nursing practice*, St. Louis, 1998, Mosby.

erwise leads to automatic action during a crisis or rapid change is often absent.

Vaughan-Cole and others (1998) describe functioning as "what the family does." **Family functioning** involves the processes used by the family to achieve its goals. These processes include communication among family members, goal setting, conflict resolution, nurturing, and use of internal and external resources. The reproductive, sexual, economic, and educational goals once considered central family goals no longer apply to all families. Although many families pursue these goals at various times during their development, the provision of psychological support remains an important goal throughout the life span.

DEVELOPMENTAL STAGES. Families, like individuals, change and grow over time. Although families are far from identical to one another, they have a basic pattern and similarity in experiences resulting in predictable stages. Each of these developmental stages has its own challenges, needs, and resources and includes tasks that need to be completed before the family can successfully move on to the next stage (Table 20-1).

FAMILY AND HEALTH. **Family health** influences family functioning. When the family satisfactorily meets its goals through adequate functioning, its members tend to feel positive about themselves and their family. Conversely, when they do not meet goals, families view themselves as ineffective. Constant stress resulting from inadequate functioning can adversely affect an individual family member's health (Voydanoff and Donnelly, 1999). Constant stress may disrupt cardiovascular function, blood pressure, and circulating neuroendocrine substances, and these disruptions may cause poor health (see Chapter 21). Maladaptive behaviors within the family have a negative impact on the health of members and the overall ability of the family to nurture and meet its goals (Johnson, 1998). Poor communication inhibits the family's ability to identify problems, make decisions, and solve problems. Good health may not be highly valued by the client and by the family, and in fact detrimental practices may be accepted. In some cases a family member may provide mixed messages about health. For example, a parent may continue to smoke while telling children that smoking is bad for them. Family environment is crucial because health behavior reinforced in early life has a strong influence on later health practices.

Although a family can be a source of stress, it can also be a protective resource and during stressful events protect family members from negative stress-related outcomes (Patterson, 1995). Recently health promotion research has started to focused on the stress-moderating effect of "hardiness" as a factor that contributes to long-term health. Vaughan-Cole and others (1998) note that **family hardiness** encompasses the internal strengths and durability of the family unit. It is characterized by a sense of control over the outcome of life events and hardships. A hardy family views a change as beneficial and growth-producing.

NURSING KNOWLEDGE BASE

To begin work with families, you need a scientific knowledge base in family theory and an adequate knowledge base in family nursing. To apply the concepts of family theory in nursing practice, consider how the concepts interact to affect the care that is delivered to the family. Family nursing is practiced in all practice settings and is emphasized in all health care environments.

Family Nursing: Family as Environment and as Client

In caring for a family, your goal is to help the family and its individual members reach and maintain maximum health in any given situation. Bradley (1996) examines the shift of health care focus from the individual to the family. With earlier discharges and technological advances, the informal care delivery system assumes the greatest role in providing care and support to clients (Call and others, 1999). You must be aware that family members affect the client and that clients, in turn, affect their families. A family nursing focus includes both **family as context** and **family as client** (Figure 20-1). Both approaches recognize that a nursing intervention for one member influences all members and affects family functioning. The family is viewed as an irreducible whole that is not understood by knowledge of individual members alone (Newby, 1996). Families are continually changing; therefore it is important for you to understand that the family is more complex than simply a combination of individual members.

FAMILY AS CONTEXT.   With family as context the primary focus is the health and development of an individual member existing within a specific environment. Although the nursing process concentrates on the individual's health status, you assess the extent to which the family provides for the individual's basic needs. Families provide more than just material essentials, so their ability to help the client meet psychological needs and life goals and strive for optimal health must also be considered.

FAMILY AS CLIENT.   With this approach the family is the primary focus of nursing care. Family patterns and processes are studied. The nursing process concentrates on the extent to which these patterns and processes are consistent with reaching and maintaining family and individual health.

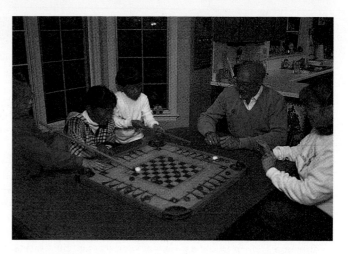

FIGURE **20-1**   Observing family interactions assists in understanding family functioning.

CRITICAL THINKING

Critical thinking is crucial in the care of clients and their families. The elements of critical thinking require synthesis and ongoing evaluation of the family. The care of a family as a client is an ongoing mutually acceptable relationship, not just a product or care plan tool for you to follow like a cookbook recipe. There is ongoing thought, analysis, and reflection required to meet the goals and needs of the clients and their families.

Synthesis

The scientific knowledge and family nursing knowledge bases enable you to identify the needs of both clients and their families. Assess the family as context, family as client, family systems theory, family life-cycle perspective, family structure and functioning, and family health. Combine knowledge about the family and its functioning with nursing knowledge of holistic practice.

KNOWLEDGE.   The health and functioning of each member in the family to some degree depends on the health of the other levels of the family system. Family care draws on knowledge from growth and development, psychology, basic and social sciences, and the family life-cycle. When a family is in a transitional phase of the life-cycle perspective (e.g., birth of a first child) and there is an additional stressor to the family unit (e.g., chronic illness), it creates considerable anxiety within the family system. Knowledge of stress and coping can assist in family care.

EXPERIENCE.   Your past experiences in a related situation often helps you to problem solve. We all draw on life experience even if we are not able to draw on nursing knowledge. Experiences with your own family members can assist in designing family-centered care. Remember how illness may have brought family members closer together because they all shared duties, roles, and responsibilities, or in some cases

Factors to Assess	Questions and Approaches	Physical Assessment Strategies
Family resources	Ask if there are significant relatives and friends not occupying immediate residence.	
	What are the family's strengths and coping skills?	When possible, observe family member interaction.
	How does the family obtain health services?	Review past medical experiences of the family.
Family patterns	Ask who works outside the home, type of work, and hours worked.	Observation of family members as they make decisions (e.g., regarding health care, discharge planning) will help obtain this information. Obtaining family pattern information requires long-term interaction with the family unit.
	Determine how the work of the home (e.g., housekeeping, shopping, repairs) is done.	
	Ask how child-rearing responsibilities are divided.	
	Determine decision-making strategies (e.g., day-to-day decisions, financial decisions, health care decisions).	
Family function	Ask about family's short- and long-term goals regarding a variety of subjects (e.g., childrearing, retirement, health care).	Observe communication patterns with individual family members.
	Ask individual members about their own short-term and long-term goals.	Observe communication and interaction patterns within the family.
	Ask if realization of goals is changed as a result of current health problems.	

how it pulled families apart. Your use of experience-related information needs to be considered carefully because no two families are alike.

ATTITUDES. You can identify the client's needs and begin to solve problems by keeping an open mind and applying creativity, perseverance, and risk taking. Respect for your client's family structure and function, beliefs, values, and expectations enables you to develop a comprehensive, multidisciplinary plan *in partnership with* the client and family.

STANDARDS. As a nurse you must use applicable nursing content area standards (e.g., obstetrical or gerontological) plus delivery area standards (e.g., home care, acute care, or long-term care) and ethical and professional standards when providing care to the family. Because a portion of family-centered nursing may be provided in community-based, clinic, or restorative care settings, as well as in the acute care setting, any information about the family must be kept confidential, and documentation of pertinent information must be accurate, consistent, and accountable.

NURSING PROCESS

The nursing process is the same whether the focus is family as client or family as context. It is also the same as that used with individuals and incorporates the needs of the family and those of the client.

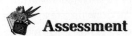 **Assessment**

It is essential for you to assess the family (Table 20-2). Although the family as a whole differs from individual members, the measure of family health must be more than a summation of the health of all members. Areas included in fam-

ily assessment are the form, structure, and function of the family; its developmental stage; and its progress toward or accomplishment of developmental tasks. Cultural background is an important variable when assessing the family because race and ethnicity affect structure and function and influence health beliefs and values. Begin assessment by considering the attitudes of family members and the client toward the family. To determine the family form and membership, ask the client, "Whom do you consider your family?" or "With whom do you share strong emotional feelings?" If the client is unable to express a concept of family, ask with whom the client lives, spends time, and shares confidences, and then ask the client to validate this observation: "Do you consider this person to be family or like family to you?" To further assess the family structure, ask questions that determine the power structure and patterning of roles and tasks, for example, "How are the tasks divided in your family?" "Who does the laundry?" "Who mows the lawn?" and "Who decides on where to go on vacation?"

Assessment of family functions may include the ability to provide emotional support for members, the ability to cope with their current health problem or situation, the appropriateness of their goal setting, and progress toward achievement of tasks of the developmental stage. Because families' goals vary, measures of family health care must be flexible. During assessment, assess whether the family can provide and allocate sufficient economic resources and if the family's social network is extensive enough to provide support.

CLIENT EXPECTATIONS. Families, like individual clients, have certain expectations for care. The family may expect to be consulted as a whole unit when discussing care of their loved one, or the family may wish to have a designated decision maker. The family may expect the health care system to

Case Study SYNTHESIS IN PRACTICE

Bethany assesses Lois's health care demands, and basic physiological needs. She analyzes the role strain on Michelle and how this affects her relationship with Patrick. She operates under the ethical principle of beneficence and tries to do the most good for the most people in this case. She understands that Lois wants to stay in her home, and Michelle wants Lois to do what will make her happiest. Patrick wants Michelle to do whatever will not aggravate Michelle's stress level or force her to quit school, because they may soon have to depend on more income from her.

If the family is viewed as context, Bethany focuses on the client as an individual. Bethany assesses Patrick's knowledge of ways to manage his blood pressure (e.g., strategies for reducing the number of high-sodium foods in the diet, realistic opportunities to reduce the number and extent of perceived stressors in work and family environments, and knowledge and skill in stress management such as relaxation or biofeedback techniques).

If the family is viewed as client, Bethany assesses the family's current dietary patterns and their desire and resources for changing the patterns. She determines the demands placed on the hypertensive client and the family. The family's capabilities to support the hypertensive member's development and use of stress management are also assessed.

---

meet all of their needs, not only those related to health issues. When meeting the family's expectations, be clear whether the family is the client and receiver of care or whether the family member is the client and receiver of care. Determining these expectations early in the assessment can avoid problems resulting from misunderstandings in the future.

Nursing Diagnosis

Nursing assessment results in clustering pertinent data that support nursing diagnoses and identifying areas in which functioning is inadequate or deficient and intervention is needed. The nursing diagnosis selected may include the family's health needs, current and potential health problems, level of wellness, or a combination of these areas. In addition, the diagnostic statement should indicate possible related factors.

The nursing diagnosis often focuses on the family's ability to cope with their current situation, whether it is an acute illness, an anticipated developmental transition, or negative behaviors that threaten short-term or long-term health (Box 20-2). Appropriate use of internal and external resources can allow the family to cope with day-to-day challenges and with unexpected occurrences that threaten health and equilibrium. The nursing diagnosis might also focus on changes in family processes or roles of members. During times of acute illness the family can become extremely distressed and focus solely on the ill member, neglecting the needs of the other family members. The diagnosis of *risk for caregiver role strain,* for example, should always be considered a possibility when long-term care of a family member is necessary.

Nursing diagnosis involves a database about the family and potential stressors that pose a threat to the stability of

Box 20-2 Nursing Diagnoses for CLIENTS WITH FAMILY-CENTERED NEEDS

- Caregiver role strain, risk for
- Coping, compromised family
- Coping, disabled family
- Coping, readiness for enhanced family
- Family processes, interrupted
- Parenting, impaired
- Role performance, ineffective
- Spiritual well-being, readiness for enhanced
- Violence, risk for other directed

---

the family unit (Patterson, 1995; Call and others, 1999). Identifying the correct related factor or factors is essential to choosing the appropriate plan of care.

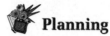 Planning

GOALS AND OUTCOMES.   After you develop nursing diagnoses, the next step is to plan care with the family. Goal setting must be mutual, and the goals must be concrete, realistic, compatible with the family's developmental stage, and acceptable to the family.

Nursing practice may be enhanced by a family-focused approach (St. John and Rolls, 1996). Goals for a care plan that incorporates a family approach may include those that view the family as client or the family as context or a combination of the two. The client situation and availability of family members dictate the type of goals that are feasible. A broad goal could be "The family functions at its optimal level," with the expected outcome being "Communication between family members is appropriate, direct, and clear." Family members are able to confront and resolve conflict in a healthy way. *The broader the goals, however, the less measurable and practical they become.* For specific examples, see the care plan.

SETTING PRIORITIES.   Setting priorities can focus on the client, the client/family unit, or the family alone. It is imperative that the plan of care and priorities be clearly understood and agreed on by the family and the client. The priorities for the client and family may indeed be different. For example, the priority for the client may be to obtain physiological or emotional stability, self-care, or progress to a rehabilitation facility. However, the family priorities may include obtaining temporary housing so they can be near their ill family member, spiritual support, assistance with decision making, or understanding the complexities of the health care delivery system. In some instances the priorities of the family and client are different but require simultaneous interventions.

CONTINUITY OF CARE.   Collaboration with family members is essential during planning. A positive collaborative relationship is based on mutual respect and trust, and it is facili-

Care Study Nursing Care Plan COMPROMISED FAMILY COPING

ASSESSMENT

Patrick and Michelle are **caregivers to Michelle's grandmother,** Lois, who has heart disease. Lois suffers fatigue and forgetfulness and poses numerous caregiving demands. She frequently **complains about how Michelle offers assistance** with household chores. Michelle and Patrick have frequent arguments over how to best help Lois, because they live 2 hours away. Patrick has been experiencing **an increase in his blood pressure.** Michelle is **not eating regularly** and has **difficulty sleeping.** They both share concerns as to what will happen to Lois.

*Defining characteristics are shown in bold type.

NURSING DIAGNOSIS

Caregiver role strain related to increasing needs and unrealistic expectations.

PLANNING

GOAL

Husband and wife will gain improved understanding of stress and adaptive management techniques (5/1).

Husband will accept wife's household role limitations (3/30).

Husband and wife will accept non–family member help if needed (3/30).

EXPECTED OUTCOMES

Husband and wife will be able to identify and perform a share of caregiving activities (4/30).

Husband will not demonstrate impatient behavior (if tasks are not done at home) while wife performs some caregiving activities (3/27).

Husband and wife will be comfortable with help non–family member can give with household roles (3/27).

IMPLEMENTATION

STEPS

1. Discuss with Patrick and Michelle the effects of stress on themselves and the family and techniques to reduce the stressors or the response to stress.

2. Provide a list of support services and groups for Patrick and Michelle.

3. Consult with Patrick and Michelle to establish a list of community resources, housekeeping agencies, friends, and volunteers to assist with caregiver tasks and household activities.

RATIONALE

Identification of specific stressors and the effects of the stress on an individual or group must occur before techniques to reduce the stress can be effective (Patterson, 1995; Vaughan-Cole and others, 1998).

Intergenerational assistance between parent and adult child is complex and at times requires some support. Identification of community-based support groups is one means to provide assistance to the caregiver in adjusting to the increased responsibilities (Voydanoff and Donnelly, 1999).

Provides a potential list of resources. Having a list available provides the family with the security of a backup system.

EVALUATION

- Ask Patrick and Michelle to describe caregiving activities they each will be able to perform.
- Observe husband interacting with wife during home visit for signs of frustration and violent temper that may impede Michelle's functioning and her caregiving activities for Lois.
- Observe effectiveness of combined efforts of husband and wife, and determine if they are sufficient. If not, consider suggesting non–family member assistance.

---

tated by allowing the family to feel as "in control" as possible (Danielson and others, 1993). For example, offering alternative actions and asking family members for their own ideas and suggestions can reduce feelings of powerlessness. Collaboration also extends to other health care professionals. Collaborating with other disciplines and using good delegation skills increases the likelihood of continuity of care throughout the client's stay in a health care facility and return to the community. Using the expertise of other disciplines is particularly important for discharge planning because referrals are often necessary to ensure that long-term goals will be attained.

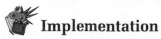
Implementation

Family interventions include nursing actions that increase members' abilities in a certain area, remove barriers to health

care, and do things that the family cannot do for themselves. You may guide family members in problem solving and provide practical service and concrete aid. For example, as a health educator you provide accurate health information about diagnosis and prognosis that helps the family caregiver to understand and anticipate needs and concerns of a care recipient. Caregivers are not born with the knowledge of how to be caregivers, and older adults are not born with the knowledge of how to accept dependency (Box 20-3). A moderately flexible structure is generally most beneficial to the family. Nursing interventions therefore may involve modulating the family patterns away from extremely rigid or flexible structures if either extreme causes problems related to the health of an individual or the family as a whole. You must work within the family structure when providing care and not attempt to change the structure.

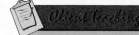

Box 20-3

Gerontological Nursing Practice

- The nurse must consider caregiver strain; caregivers are usually either spouses, who may also be an older adult and may have declining physical stamina, or middle-age children, who often have other responsibilities.
- Later-life families may have a different social network than younger families because friends and same-generation family members may have died or been ill themselves. The nurse may need to look for social support within the community and church's affiliation.
- Greater physical health impairment increases the risk of the older adult's depression.
- As in the other stages of life, members of later-life families need to be working on developmental tasks (see Chapter 18).

Box 20-4

Client Teaching

HEALTH PROMOTION
- Instruct client and family members about medication, treatment, and future appointments.
- Provide specific strategies for modification in family's nutritional, exercise, and coping patterns.
- Provide new parents with immunization schedules and community resources for obtaining necessary immunizations.
- Contact national organizations for resources, publications, and low-cost membership for parents (e.g., Children's Defense Fund, Family Resource Coalition).

HEALTH PROMOTION.   It is important to include health promotional activities as part of your family-centered nursing care. Encourage clients and families to reach their optimum level of wellness. Identifying attributes that contribute to healthy and resilient families has been a focus of ongoing research for at least three decades (Patterson, 1995). "Strong" families that adapt to transitions, crises, and change tend to be characterized by clear communication, problem-solving skills, a commitment to each other and to the family unit, and a sense of cohesiveness and spirituality (Johnson, 1998). Prevention programs aimed at enhancing or developing these attributes are available for families and children in many communities (Thomas, 1994). You need to be aware of family-oriented offerings so that clients can be referred as needed. Often health promotion behaviors that you need to encourage are tied to the developmental stage of the family, for example, effective prenatal care for the child-bearing family and adherence to immunization schedules for the child-rearing family (Box 20-4).

One approach for meeting the family goal of promoting health is the use of family strengths. Families are not accustomed to looking at their own system as one that has positive components. You can help the family become aware of its own unique strengths, thereby increasing its potential and capabilities. Family strengths include clear communication, adaptability, healthy child-rearing practices, support and nurturing among family members, active community participation, and the use of crisis for growth. Individualized interventions can help the family focus on its strengths instead of its problems and weaknesses (see care plan, p. 486).

CHALLENGES FOR FAMILY NURSING.   Multidisciplinary collaboration is essential in family nursing. The needs of individual members and the family as a client can be diverse. Always confer with family members to determine if they are receptive to the use of referral services. Also consider how collaboration with other disciplines can improve family function.

Cultural sensitivity in family nursing requires recognizing the diverse ethnic, cultural, and religious backgrounds of the family and its members, including the differences and similarities that exist within the same family. Different-age family members may have different folk remedies, health care beliefs, and religious influences. Using effective and respectful communication techniques enables you to determine the family's strengths and areas for potential problems.

ACUTE CARE.   The family is becoming more of the focus, and nursing will need to take more of a role in emphasizing family and client needs within the context of health care delivery in a managed care environment. Clients are discharged from acute care settings very quickly. Family members must maintain their jobs while also providing assistance during the client's recovery. It is a challenge to prepare family members to assist with health care or to locate appropriate community resources. When family members assume the role of caregiver, they may lose support from significant others. You must assess the family's willingness and ability to assume care responsibilities.

RESTORATIVE AND CONTINUING CARE.   Family nursing emphasizes maintenance of a clients' functional abilities. This means working closely with the family in making sure the home environment is adaptive to the client's strengths and limitations. Referral to home health nursing is essential. The home health nurse can assist in educating family members in providing ongoing care and making changes in the home so that the client can be self-sufficient.

 Evaluation

CLIENT CARE.   When the client's family functions as context, evaluation focuses on attainment of client needs. Thus evaluation is client centered, although nursing measures may have involved assisting the client in adapting to the family environment. The response of the client is compared with predetermined outcomes (Box 20-5).

When the family is the client, the measure of family health must be more than an evaluation of the health of all family members. For example, the family's attainment of family developmental tasks may be a useful criterion. The nurse evaluates the family's change in functioning and their satisfaction with the new level of functioning.

Evaluation is an ongoing process. Goals and interventions are modified as needed. Evaluation must come not only from your observations, but also from the client's and family's perspectives. This comprehensive evaluation helps to determine that the health care team is meeting the expecta-

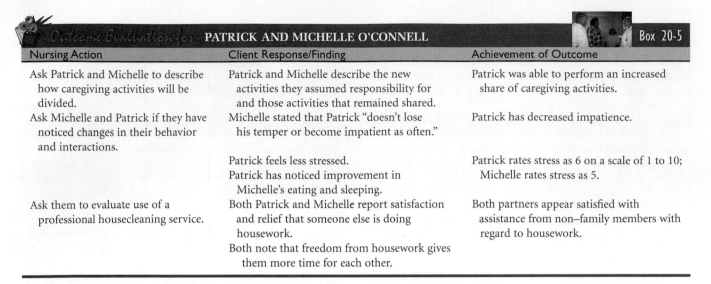

Outcome Evaluation for PATRICK AND MICHELLE O'CONNELL   Box 20-5

Nursing Action	Client Response/Finding	Achievement of Outcome
Ask Patrick and Michelle to describe how caregiving activities will be divided.	Patrick and Michelle describe the new activities they assumed responsibility for and those activities that remained shared.	Patrick was able to perform an increased share of caregiving activities.
Ask Michelle and Patrick if they have noticed changes in their behavior and interactions.	Michelle stated that Patrick "doesn't lose his temper or become impatient as often."	Patrick has decreased impatience.
	Patrick feels less stressed.	Patrick rates stress as 6 on a scale of 1 to 10; Michelle rates stress as 5.
	Patrick has noticed improvement in Michelle's eating and sleeping.	
Ask them to evaluate use of a professional housecleaning service.	Both Patrick and Michelle report satisfaction and relief that someone else is doing housework.	Both partners appear satisfied with assistance from non–family members with regard to housework.
	Both note that freedom from housework gives them more time for each other.	

Case Study EVALUATION

Bethany visits Lois periodically throughout the semester and checks to see how the family's short-term goals are coming along for caregiving and maintaining their own family life. She checks to see how Lois's goals are being fulfilled regarding her care in the home, activity tolerance, and forgetfulness. Bethany assesses Michelle's stress level with school, home, and long-distance planning around her grandmother's needs. To assess Michelle and Patrick, she may request that a family meeting be arranged once a month. This ongoing evaluation requires a multidisciplinary effort from the home health nurse who knows the family best, the family members themselves, their physician who is involved, and the chaplain, social worker, and nutritionist who are involved. The nurse is the true coordinator and evaluator of care provided, and Bethany knows this.

Bethany learns through the course of the semester that Patrick has been able to begin implementing some of the more positive coping strategies he has learned. He is also able to help Michelle around the house with some of the daily chores and finances. He also assists twice a month with cleaning Lois's home. When he realized how important his help has become to everyone in the family, he felt more needed and wanted to help. Michelle has more free time to concentrate on her studies every other night so she can "hurry through school to get a better job to help their financial future plans," as she and Patrick have wanted. One day a week and every other weekend she spends with Lois to observe her grand-mother's condition, help to plan her care, ease Lois's loneliness, and reduce the number of paid nursing care hours per week.

Bethany had discussed the long-term goals of including the community in Lois's care. A registered nurse visits for 1 hour per week, a hospice volunteer takes Lois to the Senior Enrichment Program on Mondays, Lois receives Meals on Wheels a couple of days per week, and a clergyman visits once per week. Lois has regional transportation for those times when Michelle or the volunteer is unavailable, and she receives paid CNAs from a local agency for overnights. In addition, Lois sees the nurse practitioner one month and the physician the next. The CNA overnight service is used during the week, and the cost is divided among all the family members who live too far away to help with Lois's care. Michelle has found family members willing to take turns caring for Lois during the weekends that Michelle stays with Patrick.

Documentation Note
Patrick and Michelle are participating in family meetings; both report that sitting down together helps them deal with the stress of their jobs, school, and the care of Lois. Michelle feels that she and Patrick are partners in the work of the family. The overnight care of Lois by the CNA has helped relieve some of the stress. Both Patrick and Michelle know that Lois will eventually need nursing home care and have begun looking at placements together.

---

tions of family members, as well as family members meeting the expectations of the health care team.

Use critical thinking skills and clinical decision making to evaluate your client's responses to interventions. Often the client and/or family does not know how care could be delivered differently or better. For example, they may think a pain medication does not work at all; however, an adjustment in scheduling may be all that is required. Each client and family is unique. Family nursing requires the use of therapeutic communication skills, scientific and family nursing knowledge, critical thinking skills, knowledge of oneself, and extensive learning about the clients and their families.

CLIENT EXPECTATIONS. It is important to obtain the family's perspective of nursing care: how the care was planned and delivered, whether it was delivered satisfactorily, whether it met the family's goals, and if not, what they think was needed instead. With a truly trusting relationship between you and your client, this information can be obtained to create an even more positive atmosphere. This evaluation is continuous throughout the care planning to modify or adjust care delivery techniques (e.g., how soon the home health nurse was able to make a visit, adequacy of comfort measures, or timeliness of care) or even to adjust care delivery personnel.

Key Terms

family, p. 480
family as client, p. 483

family as context, p. 483
family forms, p. 480
family functioning, p. 482

family hardiness, p. 483
family health, p. 482
family structure, p. 481

Key Concepts

- The family has a significant impact on the lives of its members.
- Family members mutually influence one another's health beliefs, practices, and status.
- Because the concept of family is highly individualized, you should base care on the client's attitude toward family.
- Specific family forms tend to have typical family health problems with which the nurse should be familiar.

- The family's structure and functioning significantly influence its health and ability to respond to health problems.
- The nurse can view the family as an important context for the individual family member, can view the family unit as the client, or both. The approach for any family depends in part on the situation.
- Measures of family health involve more than a summation of all individual members' health.
- Social class, economic stability, and racial and ethnic background influence the family's health.

Critical Thinking Activities

1. Imagine one of your clients is a young child with a contagious illness. List some suggestions you might give the parents to deal with the care of the child and to provide a positive family life for the client's siblings. How would your approach differ if the child were from a single-parent family?
2. Think of the family in which you grew up. Describe the values and attitudes you learned in this environment and the influence they may have on how you view your client's family and health practices.

3. You are caring for an intergenerational family that consists of an 80-year-old grandmother, who is in the last stages of heart and kidney failure, and a married couple in their 40s, Jane and Harry. Both Jane and Harry are teachers and take additional summer jobs. Jane and Harry have three children. Rachael (16 years old), Harry Jr. (13 years old), and Kathy (11 years old). What are the stressors placed on this family? When the grandmother's health status changes, what additional stressors do you anticipate?

Review Questions

1. Family functioning involves:
   1. the process used by the family to achieve its goals.
   2. the patterns of people who are considered to be family members.
   3. the ongoing membership of the family and the pattern of relationships.
   4. the intrafamilial system of support and structure extending beyond the walls of the household.
2. Family structure is:
   1. the process used by the family to achieve its goals.
   2. the patterns of people who are considered to be family members.
   3. the ongoing membership of the family and the pattern of relationships.
   4. the intrafamilial system of support and structure extending beyond the walls of the household.
3. Family assessment includes:
   1. assessing individual family members separately.

   2. assessing only those members living in the household.
   3. assessing only the client's perception of family interaction.
   4. assessing individual family members and their interactions with one another and the client.
4. When planning care for the family as a client, you need to:
   1. consider the developmental stage of the family.
   2. include only the ill family member and the significant other.
   3. understand that the family will always help to achieve the health goals of an ill member of the family.
   4. understand that cultural background is an important variable to consider when developing nursing interventions.
5. When working with a family with a rigid family structure, interventions are designed to:
   1. attempt to change the family structure.
   2. include only the most flexible family member.
   3. create interventions that require minimal change.
   4. provide solutions for problems only when they arise.

References

Bradley SF: Processes in the creation and diffusion of nursing knowledge: an examination of the developing concept of family-centered care, *J Adv Nurs* 23(4):722, 1996.

Call KT and others: Caregiver burden from a social exchange perspective: caring for older people after hospital discharge, *J Marriage Fam* 61:688, 1999.

Centers for Disease Control and Prevention, U.S. Public Health Service: HIV/AIDS surveillance reports, 10(2), 1998.

Clemen-Stone S and others: *Comprehensive approach to community health nursing,* St. Louis, 1998, Mosby.

Danielson DB and others: *Family, health and illness,* St. Louis, 1993, Mosby.

Friedman MM: *Family nursing: theory and assessment,* ed 2, New York, 1992, Appleton-Century-Crofts.

Ganong L and others: Attitudes regarding obligations to assist an older parent or stepparent following later-life remarriage, *J Marriage Fam* 60:595, 1998.

Johnson ED: The effect of family functioning and family sense of competence on people with mental illness, *Fam Relat* 47:443, 1998.

Marks NF: Does it hurt to care? Caregiving, work-family conflict, and midlife well-being, *J Marriage Fam* 60:951, 1998.

Newby NM: Chronic illness and the family life-cycle. *J Adv Nurs* 23(4):786, 1996.

Patterson ED: The effect of family functioning and family sense of competence on people with mental illness, *Fam Relat* 47:443, 1995.

St. John W, Rolls C: Teaching family nursing: strategies and experiences, *J Adv Nurs* 23(1):91, 1996.

Thomas HS: Conceptual underpinnings of the family support movement, *J Pediatr Health Care* 8(2):57, 1994.

U.S. Bureau of the Census: *Statistical abstracts of the United States: 2000,* Washington, DC, 2001, U.S. Government Printing Office.

Vaughan-Cole B and others: *Family nursing practice,* St. Louis, 1998, Mosby.

Voydanoff P, Donnelly BW: Multiple roles and psychological distress: the intersection of the paid worker, spouse, and parent roles with the role of the adult child, *J Marriage Fam* 61:725, 1999.

Ward JW, Duchin JS: The epidemiology of HIV and AIDS in the United States, *AIDS Clin Rev,* p 1, 1997-1998.

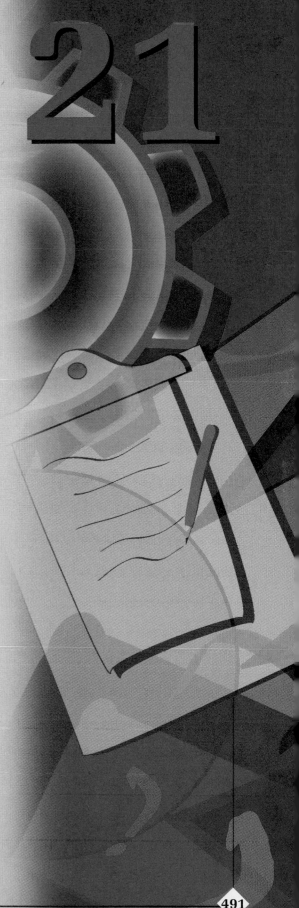

Stress and Coping

21

Objectives

- Define key terms.
- Describe the three stages of the general adaptation syndrome.
- Discuss the integration of stress theory with nursing theories.
- Formulate nursing diagnoses based on assessment data.
- Describe stress management techniques beneficial for coping with stress.
- Discuss the process of crisis intervention.
- Develop a care plan for clients experiencing stress.
- Discuss how stress in the workplace can affect the nurse.

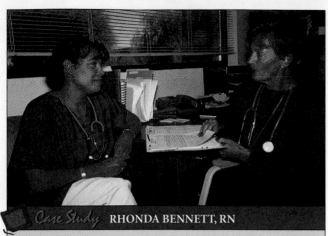

Case Study **RHONDA BENNETT, RN**

Rhonda Bennett is a 35-year-old married mother of three children who has worked as a registered nurse for City Hospital since her graduation from a community college 15 years ago. She began her career on a general medical unit and through the years has earned a reputation as a skilled and compassionate nurse. She presently is the nurse manager in the medical intensive care unit and has always felt very happy with her job.

Rhonda's family life is also of great importance to her. She serves as a Girl Scout leader and a soccer coach. Until last year she also enjoyed playing tennis with her husband, who was self-employed as a contractor. Within the past year, however, he has had several hospitalizations related to chest pain, panic attacks, and, finally, a spontaneous pneumothorax. As a result, he has been much less involved in his work and has a decreased income. He has bouts of depression that result in Rhonda's shouldering responsibility for the family alone. Hoping to help her husband overcome his depression by spending more time with him, Rhonda has reduced her community involvement, but chose to take the manager's job for a year for an increase in salary to help pay the family's accumulated debt. Because of Rhonda's employment, the Bennetts have been able to maintain their home and standard of living.

After a year of declining profitability, City Hospital has announced a "major restructuring" effort. Based on comments that the administration has made, Rhonda knows that she will almost certainly lose her job. She feels overwhelmed by the burden of being breadwinner, mother, wife, and nurse to her family. She is unable to ask for help, but she wishes that someone could take care of *her*. She has tried to "put on a face" of confidence, but every day it is becoming harder to keep going. She feels defeated and hopeless, has no energy, and is having difficulty organizing her thoughts. Her boss has noticed that Rhonda often complains of severe headaches and has become especially concerned since Rhonda tearfully confided that she cannot sleep and therefore has begun drinking at night to help herself "unwind." Because of these behaviors, Rhonda has been referred to the hospital's employee health office. This department has been charged with the duty of helping employees cope with the stresses associated with being laid off.

Becky Howard is the nurse in the employee health office who has been assigned to do preliminary screening and crisis intervention with staff members who will be laid off. She has a bachelor's degree in nursing and extensive experience working both in acute care hospitals and on a crisis intervention telephone hot line. She is a 52-year-old divorced mother of four children and has been hired by City Hospital on a temporary basis to help manage the employee response to restructuring and layoffs.

Stress is a topic of interest to all of us. **Stressors** are disruptive forces operating within or on any system (Neuman, 1995). Knowing about **stress** is important not only so health care professionals can recognize stress in clients and families and intervene effectively, but also because professionals are affected by stressful events that occur in the course of clinical practice. You must be able to recognize in your own life the signs and symptoms of stress and be knowledgeable about stress management techniques to aid personal coping in yourself, as well as with your clients and their families.

You can experience stress as a consequence of daily life events and experiences. Stress can stimulate thinking processes and help you stay alert to your environment. How you react to stress depends on how you view and evaluate the impact of the stressor, its effect on your situation and support at the time of the stress, and your usual coping mechanisms. Stress is a universal part of the human experience and is necessary for survival, affecting every person regardless of age, gender, race, economic condition, or educational level. Stress can provide stimulation and motivation, as well as cause discomfort and retreat. However, when stress overwhelms a person's existing coping mechanisms, a crisis results (Aguilera, 1998).

SCIENTIFIC KNOWLEDGE BASE

Over 60 years ago Walter Cannon proposed the **fight-or flight-response** to stress, which is arousal of the sympathetic nervous system (Aldwin, 2000). This reaction prepares a person for action by increasing heart rate; diverting blood from the intestines to the brain and striated muscles; and increasing blood pressure, heart rate, respiratory rate, and blood sugar levels. In the 1930s, 40s, and 50s Hans Selye enlarged on Cannon's fight-or-flight hypothesis to describe the **general adaptation syndrome (GAS),** a three-stage reaction to stress (Selye, 1991). The GAS describes how the body responds to stressors through the alarm reaction, the resistance stage, and the exhaustion stage. The GAS can be triggered either directly by a physical event or indirectly by a psychological event (Lazarus, 1999).

General Adaptation Syndrome

The GAS is an immediate physiological response of the body to stress and involves several body systems, especially the autonomic nervous system and the endocrine system (Table 21-1). When a physical demand is made on the body, such as an injury, the GAS is initiated by the pituitary gland. In addition, the pituitary gland is closely linked to the hypothalamus, another part of the brain, which secretes **endorphins.** Endorphins are hormones that act on the mind like morphine and opiates, producing a sense of well-being and reducing pain (Lazarus, 1999). In this way the GAS defends us against stress both by activating the neuroendocrine system and by providing endorphins that decrease our awareness of the pain.

During the **alarm reaction** rising hormone levels result in an increased blood volume, blood glucose levels, epinephrine and norepinephrine amounts, heart rate, blood flow to muscles, oxygen intake, and mental alertness (Selye, 1991).

Indicators of Stress

Table 21-1

System	Assessment Findings	System	Assessment Findings
Physical		**Psychological—cont'd**	
Cardiovascular	Tightness of chest	Cognitive—cont'd	Poor concentration
	Increased heart rate		Inattention to detail
	Elevated blood pressure		Orientation to past instead of present
Respiratory	Breathing difficulty		Decreased creativity
	Tachypnea		Slower thinking, reactions
Neuroendocrine	Headaches, migraines		Learning difficulties
	Fatigue, exhaustion		Apathy
	Insomnia, sleep disturbances		Confusion
	Feeling uncoordinated		Lower attention span
	Restlessness, hyperactivity		Calculation difficulties
	Tremors (lips, hands)		Memory problems
	Profuse sweating (palms)		Distressing dreams
	Dry mouth	Emotional	Disruption of logical thinking
Gastrointestinal/	Cold hands and feet		Blaming others
genitourinary	Urinary frequency		Lack of motivation to get up in the morning
	Nausea, diarrhea, vomiting		Crying tendencies
	Weight gain or loss of more than		Lack of interest
	10 lb		Irritability
	Change in appetite		Isolation
	Gastrointestinal bleeding		Diminished initiative
Diagnostic	Blood in stools/vomitus		Negative thinking
	Elevated blood glucose level	Behavior/lifestyle	Worrying
Musculoskeletal	Backaches, muscle aches		Decreased involvement with others
	Bruxism (clenched jaw)		Change in activity level
	Slumped posture		Withdrawal
Reproductive	Amenorrhea		Suspiciousness
	Failure to ovulate		Change in communication
	Impotency in men		Change in interactions with others
	Loss of libido		Increased or decreased food intake
Immunological	Frequent or prolonged colds/flu		Increased smoking or alcohol intake
Psychological			Overvigilance to environment
Cognitive	Forgetfulness/preoccupation		Excessive humor or silence
	Denial		No exercise
	Increased fantasy life		Type A personality

In addition, the pupils of the eyes dilate to produce a greater visual field. This change in body systems prepare an individual for fight or flight and may last from 1 minute to many hours. If the stressor poses an extreme threat to life or remains for a long time, the person progresses to the second stage, resistance.

During the **resistance stage** the body stabilizes and responds in an opposite manner to the alarm reaction. Hormone levels, heart rate, blood pressure, and cardiac output return to normal, and the body repairs any damage that may have occurred. However, if the stressor remains, and there is no adaptation, the person enters the third stage, exhaustion.

The **exhaustion stage** occurs when the body can no longer resist the effects of the stressor and when the energy necessary to maintain adaptation is depleted. The physiological response is intensified, but the person's energy level is compromised, and adaptation to the stressor diminishes. The body is unable to defend itself against the impact of the event, physiological regulation diminishes, and, if the stress continues, death may result.

Physiological responses to stress also include immunological responses. The immune system differentiates between self and nonself, so that under normal conditions one's own cells are not treated as threats, in the way that bacteria, viruses, parasites, or toxins are treated. Problems occur when the immune system makes a too vigorous response and an autoimmune illness develops. The mechanisms through which stress affects the immune system are unclear (Aldwin, 2000).

Selye (1991) noted that a prolonged state of stress can cause disease. Stress can make people ill as a result of (1) increased levels of powerful hormones that change our bodily processes; (2) coping choices that are unhealthy, such as not getting enough rest or a proper diet or use of tobacco, alcohol, or caffeine; and (3) neglect of warning signs of illness or prescribed medicines or treatments (Monat and Lazarus, 1991).

REACTION TO PSYCHOLOGICAL STRESS.   The GAS is activated indirectly for psychological threats, which are different for each person and produce differing reactions (Box 21-1). Lazarus (1999) maintains that a person is under stress

Factors Influencing the Response to Stressors   Box 21-1

INTENSITY

Minimal, severe, or somewhere in between. The greater the perceived magnitude of the stressor, the greater the stress response.

SCOPE

The pervasiveness with which a stressor affects a person's total being. The greater the scope of a stressor, the greater the stress response.

DURATION

The length of time the person is exposed to the stressor. The greater the duration, the greater the stress response.

NUMBER AND NATURE OF OTHER STRESSORS PRESENT

Multiple stressors experienced simultaneously or a succession of single stressors with no opportunity for the person to rest and regroup results in a greater stress response.

PREDICTABILITY

Being able to anticipate the occurrence of an event, even if one cannot control it, generally results in a reduced experience of stress.

LEVEL OF PERSONAL CONTROL

Believing that one has control over an unpleasant experience, even if that control is never exercised or the belief is erroneous, lessens the level of associated stress and anxiety.

FEELINGS OF COMPETENCE

Greater self-confidence in one's ability to manage a stressful event results in less tension and anxiety.

COGNITIVE APPRAISAL

The greater the personal meaning of an event, the greater the stress associated with it. Thus the same event may cause differing levels of stress in different people.

AVAILABILITY OF SOCIAL SUPPORTS

The emotional concern and support of other people reduce the negative effects of stressful events.

---

only if the person evaluates the event or circumstance as personally significant. Evaluating an event for its personal meaning is called **primary appraisal.** If primary appraisal results in the person's identifying the event or circumstance as a harm, loss, threat, or challenge, the person has stress. If stress is present, **secondary appraisal** focuses on possible coping strategies.

Coping is the person's effort to manage psychological stress (Lazarus, 1999). Effectiveness of coping strategies depends on the individual's needs. For this reason no single coping strategy works for everyone or for every stress. The same person may cope differently from one time to another. In stressful situations people may use a combination of problem-focused coping and emotion-focused coping. In other words, when under stress, we obtain information and take action to change the situation, as well as regulating our emotions tied to the stress. In some cases we avoid thinking about the situation or change the way we think about it, without changing the actual situation itself (Lazarus, 1999).

Lazarus (1999) suggests that not only does the type of stress make a difference, but that people's goals, their beliefs about themselves and the world, and personal resources determine how they cope with stress. "Resources include intelligence, money, social skills, supportive family and friends, physical attractiveness, health and energy, and ways of thinking, such as optimism" (Lazarus, 1999).

Types of Stress

Selye identified two types of stress; these are **distress,** or damaging stress, and **eustress,** stress that protects health. However, the idea of healthy stress has become controversial because it is difficult to tell whether a person has benefitted from stress or is coping by denying the stress in some way (Aldwin, 2000). There are several types of stress, including work stress, family stress, chronic stress, acute stress, daily hassles, trauma, and crisis. "Work and family stress interact, family being the background for work stress, and work the background for family stress" (Lazarus, 1999). One person may look at a stimulus and see it as a challenge, leading to mastery and growth. Another sees the same stimulus as a threat, leading to stagnation and loss. Lazarus suggests a spillover of stresses between work and home. The individual with family responsibilities and a full-time job outside the home may experience chronic stress. Chronic stress occurs in stable conditions and from stressful roles. Another example of chronic stress is living with a long-term illness. Conversely, acute stress is provoked by time-limited major or minor events that are threatening for a relatively brief period. Further complicating chronic or acute stress are daily hassles that are recurrent, such as commuting to work, maintaining a house, dealing with difficult people, and managing money.

A **crisis** implies that a person is facing a turning point in life. That is, previous ways of coping are not effective and the person must change. Gerald Caplan, in 1964, described crisis intervention. Caplan distinguished two types of crises, those associated with changing developmental levels, or **developmental crises,** and **situational crises.** A basic assumption of crisis theory is that a person can either advance or regress as a result of a crisis, depending upon how the crisis is managed (Lazarus, 1999).

NURSING KNOWLEDGE BASE

Nurses have proposed theories related to stress and coping. Because stress plays a central role in vulnerability to disease, symptoms of stress often require nursing intervention.

Nursing Theory and the Role of Stress

Neuman's systems model is based on the concepts of stress and reaction to stress. This nursing theory views nursing as being responsible for developing interventions to prevent or reduce stressors on the client or to make them more bearable for the client (Neuman, 1995). Because the Neuman model is a systems model, you may use it to understand your clients' individual responses to stressors and also families' and communities' responses. All systems experience multiple stressors, each of which has a differing potential to disturb the person's, family's, or community's balance. For example, these may be intrapersonal stressors, such as an illness or injury; interpersonal stressors, such as an argument or misunderstanding between two people, or extrapersonal stressors, such as financial concerns, that impinge on the person from life circumstances. Every person has developed a set of responses to stress that constitute the "normal line of defense" (Neuman, 1995). This line of defense helps to maintain health and wellness. However, when "physiological, psychological, sociocultural, developmental, or spiritual influences" are unable to buffer stress, the normal line of defense is broken, and disease can result. In this belief, Neuman's systems model coincides with Selye's general adaptation syndrome.

Neuman's systems model stresses the importance of accuracy in assessment and interventions that promote optimal wellness using primary, secondary, and tertiary prevention strategies. According to Neuman's theory of nursing, the goal of primary prevention is to promote client wellness by stress prevention and reduction of risk factors. Secondary prevention occurs after symptoms appear. You determine the meaning of the illness and stress to the client and the client's needs and resources for meeting them. Tertiary prevention begins when the client system is becoming more stable and recovering. At the tertiary level of prevention you support rehabilitation processes involved in healing, moving the client back to wellness and the primary level of disease prevention. Neuman's model of nursing views the person, family, or community as constantly changing in response to the environment and stressors.

Pender's health promotion model proposes that health promotion is directed toward increasing the level of well-being of an individual or group, but primary, secondary, and tertiary prevention focus on avoiding negative events (Pender, 1996). Pender considers stress reduction strategies important to reduce threats to well-being, to help people fulfill their potential and shape and maintain health behaviors. To change behavior, your client must initiate the change and behave differently in interactions. People want to live in ways that enable them to be as healthy as possible and to be capable of assessing their own abilities and assets. Based on these assumptions of the capability and desire of people to be healthy, Pender suggests strategies for prevention and health promotion related to stress management.

Situational, Maturational, and Sociocultural Factors

Potential stressors and coping mechanisms vary across the life span. For example, adolescence, adulthood, and old age bring different stressors. Appraisal of stressors, amount and type of social support, and coping strategies are balancing factors when assessing stress, and all depends on previous

---

✦ *Gerontological Nursing Practice*   Box 21-2

- Coping ability of older adults is related to their previous lifestyle, adaptation to retirement, adjustments to minor ailments, openness to both feelings and ideas, and maintenance of social activities and contacts (Aguilera, 1998).
- Older adults with multiple losses, including job status, mobility, health, vision, spouse, mental acuity, and home, are more vulnerable to needing institutional support (Aguilera, 1998).
- The most common problem in later adulthood is probably depression (Aguilera, 1998).
- When assessing an older adult for stress, you should be aware of the tendency to stereotype the person's appearance and symptoms as part of the normal aging process (Aguilera, 1998).
- It is critical to differentiate signs of stress and crisis from dementia and from acute confusion, a condition that can be life threatening. Examine the person's current medical history as part of the assessment.

---

life experiences (Aguilera, 1998). Furthermore, environmental and social stressors place people who are vulnerable at higher risk for prolonged stress.

SITUATIONAL FACTORS.   Situational stress can arise from job changes, either one's own or that of a family member, and relocation. Stressful job changes can include promotions, transfers, downsizing, restructuring, changes in supervisors, and additional responsibilities. Adjusting to chronic illness is another situational stress. Common diseases that provoke stress are obesity, hypertension, diabetes, depression, asthma, and coronary artery disease. Furthermore, being a family caregiver for someone with a chronic illness such as Alzheimer's disease is known to cause stress (Aguilera, 1998).

MATURATIONAL FACTORS.   Stressors vary with life stage. Preadolescents experience stress related to self-esteem issues, changing family structure due to divorce or death of a parent, or hospitalizations. As adolescents search for their identity with peer groups and separate from their families, they undergo stress. In addition, they face questions about using mind-altering substances, sexuality, jobs, school, and career choices that cause stress. Stress for adults center around major changes in life circumstances (Aguilera, 1998). These include the many milestones of beginning a family and a career, losing parents, seeing children leave home, and accepting physical aging. In old age, stressors include multiple losses; concerns about income, nutrition, and transportation; the effects of aging and chronic illness; and confronting societal stereotypes about old age (Box 21-2).

SOCIOCULTURAL FACTORS.   Environmental and social stressors can lead to developmental problems. Potential stressors that could affect any age group, but that are especially stressful for young people, include prolonged poverty, physical handicap, and chronic illness. Children are vulnerable when relationships with parents and caregivers are lost through divorce, imprisonment, or death or when parents have mental illness or substance abuse disorders. Furthermore, living under conditions of continuing violence, disintegrated neighborhoods, or homelessness is damaging for people of any age, but especially for young people (Pender, 1996).

Posttraumatic Stress Disorder

Posttraumatic stress disorder (PTSD) affects people who have experienced accidents; violent events, such as rape or domestic abuse; war; and natural disasters such as floods or fires (Aguilera, 1998). PTSD symptoms may appear to be a normal response to a traumatic event; however, if the symptoms persist beyond 3 months, the diagnosis of PTSD can be made. Nevertheless, symptoms may first appear months or years after the traumatic event. People with PTSD may experience a **flashback,** or "a recollection so strong that the individual thinks he is actually experiencing the trauma again or seeing it unfold before his eyes" (Aguilera, 1998).

CRITICAL THINKING

Synthesis

When examining your role with a client experiencing stress, consider your client's perception of the stress and examine your own frame of reference as a nurse. You will be entering into the nurse-client relationship with your own past experiences and your views about your responsibilities related to helping the client cope with his or her stress.

In addition, the client will also have expectations of you. Interacting with a client who is experiencing stress requires you to have confidence in yourself and integrity in dealing with a client who may be temporarily vulnerable. Assess the client's situation accurately, and be especially aware of your ethical responsibility in caring for someone who many have diminished autonomy due to stress.

KNOWLEDGE. Physiological changes occur in the client experiencing the alarm reaction, resistance stage, and exhaustion stage of the general adaptation syndrome. Apply knowledge of those physiologic changes. Your knowledge of communication principles will help you to assess client's behaviors. Determining the ability of the client to cope with the stress is of utmost importance. If the client's usual coping skills are unsuccessful, you will need to use crisis intervention counseling.

EXPERIENCE. Your experience teaches you to understand the client's unique perspective. View every person as an individual, recognizing that no two people are exactly alike. Experience with clients will also help you to recognize responses to stress. In addition, your own personal experiences with stress and coping will increase your ability to empathize with a client who is temporarily immobilized by stress. Understanding the client's position enables you to intervene more effectively.

ATTITUDES. You must be confident in the belief that stress can be effectively managed. Clients who are over-

whelmed and perceive events as being beyond their capacity to cope will rely on you as an expert. Clients will respect your advice and counsel and gain confidence from your belief in their ability to move past the stressful event or illness. Clients overwhelmed by life events are often unable, at least initially, to act on their own behalf and require either direct intervention or guidance. Integrity is an essential attitude through which you are reminded to respect the client's perception of or perspective about the stressor. Effort must be made to have clients explain their unique viewpoint and situation.

STANDARDS. Make accurate assessment of a client's stress, coping mechanisms, and support system before intervening. You must be able to clearly and precisely understand a client's perception of the stress and focus on factors significant to the client's well-being. In addition, select interventions that respect the individuality of the client.

NURSING PROCESS

 Assessment

Assessment of a client's stress level and coping resources requires that you first establish a trusting nurse-client relationship because you will be asking the client to share personal and sensitive information (see Chapter 8). You learn from the client both by asking questions and by making observations of nonverbal behavior and the client's environment. Synthesize the information you obtain, and adopt a critical thinking attitude while observing and analyzing client behaviors. Often the client has difficulty expressing exactly what is most bothersome about the situation until there is an opportunity to discuss it with someone who has time to listen.

Stress can occur to a family or a community, as well as to an individual. Stress to a family might be from a critically ill family member, the sudden loss of a job, a move, or becoming homeless. Stress to a community might be a natural disaster such as a major flood or the sudden, unexpected death of a beloved teacher or teenager. Individuals experience stress and difficulty in coping while others are also experiencing the stress in their own ways.

SUBJECTIVE FINDINGS. When you assess a client's stress level and coping resources, sit with the client in comfortable chairs in a private setting facing each other. Assume a listening posture, establish eye contact, and allow time for the client to talk to you. Gather information about the health status of the client from the client's perspective, and begin the process of developing a trusting relationship with the client. Use the interview to determine the client's view of the stress, coping resources, any possible maladaptive coping, and adherence to prescribed medical recommendations, such as medication or diet (Monat and Lazarus, 1991) (Table 21-2). If the client is using denial as a coping mechanism, be alert to

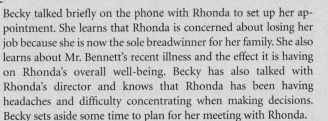

Example of a Focused Client Assessment		Table 21-2
Factors to Assess	**Questions and Approaches**	**Physical Assessment Strategies**
Perception of stressor	Ask the client what is of most concern at this time. Ask the client about problems sleeping, eating, working, and concentrating. Ask whether the client has had accidents in the home, in the car, or on the job.	Observe nonverbal behavior and expressions of feelings that indicate anxiety, fear, anger, irritability, or tension.
Available coping resources	Ask the client about current friendships and contacts with family members. Ask what the client has done in the past to cope with similar problems or stress. Ask how the client spends leisure time.	Observe whether the person is alone or with others. Observe grooming and hygiene. Observe the person's communication skills. Observe if the person is able to ask for help. Observe developmental level and sociocultural circumstances.
Maladaptive coping used	Ask about use of tobacco, alcohol, drugs, medications, and caffeine.	Observe for effects of smoking, alcohol, drugs, and caffeine.
Adherence to healthy practices	Ask if the client sees a physician or nurse practitioner regularly for checkups. Ask about nutritional habits, exercise, use of seat belts, helmets (if applicable), and safe sex.	

Case Study   SYNTHESIS IN PRACTICE

Becky talked briefly on the phone with Rhonda to set up her appointment. She learns that Rhonda is concerned about losing her job because she is now the sole breadwinner for her family. She also learns about Mr. Bennett's recent illness and the effect it is having on Rhonda's overall well-being. Becky has also talked with Rhonda's director and knows that Rhonda has been having headaches and difficulty concentrating when making decisions. Becky sets aside some time to plan for her meeting with Rhonda.

Becky takes time to reflect on other employees she has recently seen in the employee health office. Many of the registered nurses have had physical complaints of stress including headaches, sleep problems, changes in eating habits, and flare-ups of existing medical problems. Becky knows she wants to be thorough in assessing the types of problems Rhonda has been experiencing. Previous experience with other employees also has taught Becky the importance of learning about the employee's family and the type of support they offer, and the person's appraisal of the situation.

After talking with Rhonda on the phone, Becky detects a great deal of anxiety but also some anger. Becky knows it is important

to build trust with Rhonda as quickly as possible. As a single parent, Becky can identify with Rhonda's crisis of being the sole financial support for the family. Yet Becky decides not to tell her life history to Rhonda because it is important to recognize that no two persons have exactly the same experience or use the same coping strategies to get through difficult times. Becky wants to conduct an accurate assessment of Rhonda's problems, and she reminds herself that Rhonda's perspective of life will be unique. Becky plans to allow Rhonda time to fully describe her feelings and to listen carefully to the message being conveyed. Becky wants to be able to work closely with Rhonda and establish priorities that are realistic for her to achieve.

Finally, Becky can identify with Rhonda's job concerns. As a staff member of the employee assistance program, Becky's role is to be the employee's advocate while at the same time trying to help the employee return as a productive member of the workforce. Keeping Rhonda's concerns confidential will be important. It will be Rhonda's choice as to whether she will choose to discuss her visits with her manager.

whether the person is overlooking necessary information. As in all interactions with the client, you must respect the confidentiality and sensitivity of the information shared.

OBJECTIVE FINDINGS.   Obtain objective findings related to stress and coping through your observation of the appearance and nonverbal behavior of the client. Observe grooming and hygiene, gait, characteristics of the client's handshake, actions of the client while sitting, quality of speech, eye contact, and the attitude of the client toward you during the interview (see Chapter 12). Before the interview begins or at the end of the interview, depending upon the

anxiety level of the client, take basic vital signs to assess for physiological signs of stress such as elevated blood pressure, heart rate, or respiratory rate.

CLIENT EXPECTATIONS.   A central point relating to stress is the importance of your understanding the meaning of the precipitating event to the client and the ways in which stress is affecting the client's life. Allow time for the client to express priorities for coping with stress. For example, in the case of a woman who has just been told that a breast mass was identified on a routine mammogram, it would be important for you to know what the client wants and needs most from you. Although some persons in this situation might identify their need for information about biopsy or mastectomy as their personal priority, other women might need guidance and support in discussing how to share the news with family members. Remember also that in some cases, when nothing can be done to change or improve the situation, allowing the client to use denial as a coping mechanism can be helpful. Gaining an understanding of client expectations does not mean that you will exclude certain types of care that are important simply because a client does not identify them as needs. However, by inquiring about client expectations and priorities, you will be better able to ensure that *all* the client's needs will be addressed in some way.

Nursing Diagnosis

Nursing diagnoses for people experiencing stress generally focus on coping (Box 21-3). Specifically, major defining characteristics of *ineffective coping* include verbalization of an inability to cope and an inability to ask for help. You identify defining characteristics when you ask the client what is of most concern at the time of the interview and, importantly, when you allow the client sufficient time to answer. Observe for nonverbal signs of anxiety, fear, anger, irritability, and tension in a client who is experiencing ineffective coping. Other defining characteristics include the presence of life stress, an inability to meet role expectations and basic needs, alteration in societal participation, self-destructive behavior, change in usual communication patterns, high rate of accidents, excessive food intake, drinking, smoking, and sleep disturbances. Identify these behaviors as part of your subjective and objective data collection.

Crisis differs from stress in the degree of severity, although there are also many similarities between stress and crisis (Shontz, 1975). A client whose stress is so severe that the person is unable to cope in any ways that have worked before is experiencing a crisis. A crisis is devastating and requires use of all resources available. Unlike stress, which ends when the stressor is gone, the effects of a crisis can last for years (Shontz, 1975).

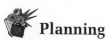

Planning

GOALS AND OUTCOMES. Desirable goals for persons experiencing stress are (1) coping, (2) family coping, (3) caregiver emotional health, and (4) psychosocial adjustment: life change (Johnson and others, 2000). Interventions for stress and improved coping include coping enhancement and **crisis intervention** from the Nursing Interventions Classification (NIC) (McCloskey and Bulechek, 2000). In addition, by synthesizing assessment information about the particular stress and nursing diagnosis for your client, resources available, and goals identified by you and the client together, you are able to select individualized interventions.

Your nursing interventions may be designed within the framework of primary, secondary, and tertiary prevention.

At the primary level of prevention, design nursing activities directed to identifying individuals and populations who may be at risk for stress (Stuart and Wright, 1995). Your nursing interventions at the secondary level include actions directed at symptoms, such as protecting the client from self-harm. Tertiary-level interventions have the purpose of assisting your client in readapting and might include relaxation training and time management training. According to Pender's health promotion model (1996), you and the client assess the level and source of the existing stress and determine the appropriate points for intervention to reduce the stress.

Just as your assessment of the client's stress and coping depends on the client's perception of the problem and coping resources, your interventions develop a partnership with the client and support system, usually the family. In the case of a family or community stressor and impaired family or community coping, your view of the situation and resources would be broader.

SETTING PRIORITIES. Prioritizing needs has special meaning for a person experiencing stress or crisis (see care plan). The first question to be answered is, "Why did you come for help today?" or "What happened in your life that is *different?*" This requires some focusing by the client. Next, learn about the client's perception of the event, available situational supports, and what the person usually does when there is a problem the client cannot solve (Aguilera, 1998). As in all areas of nursing, safety of the client and others in the client's environment is your first priority. You need to learn if the person is suicidal or homicidal by asking directly. For example, you might ask, "Are you thinking of killing yourself or someone else?" If so, you need to determine if the person has a plan and to determine how lethal the means are.

If suicide or homicide is not an issue, examine other potential threats to the safety of vulnerable people who are under the care of the client. Provide for their temporary care or supervision if necessary. Determine the degree of disruption in the person's life with work, school, home, and family. When immediate assessment is completed and safety is assured, begin the problem-solving process (Aguilera, 1998).

CONTINUITY OF CARE. You need to collaborate with occupational therapists, dietitians, or pastoral care profes-

Case Study Nursing Care Plan   STRESS AND INDIVIDUAL COPING

ASSESSMENT

When Becky Howard first meets Rhonda, she is immediately struck by Rhonda's appearance. She observes Rhonda showing signs of being nervous, **frequently licking her lips, picking at her fingernails, and being easily startled.** Rhonda's **vital signs show changes in response to stress:** pulse 120, respirations 24, blood pressure 168/84. Rhonda appears thin and pale and reports that she has **lost 15 lb in the last 3 months.** Her appetite has been poor, and she has stopped cooking meals, instead picking up fast food for her family at night. She also reports **difficulty in falling and remaining asleep at night.** In discussing her situation, including both fear of losing her job and being unable to support her family, Rhonda **uses poor eye contact** and then **bursts into tears and expresses feelings of being overwhelmed.** Rhonda admits to having started **drinking at night to help herself "unwind."** During the discussion, Rhonda also talks about **feelings of shame and embarrassment.** She has always been the one to care for other people, and she is ashamed that she cannot "get a grip" on her own life. She cannot easily accept herself in a "client" role and **thinks of herself as a failure for not coping better.** Rhonda has high expectations of herself as a wife, mother, and nurse.

*Defining characteristics are shown in bold type.

NURSING DIAGNOSIS

Ineffective coping related to threatened job loss and multiple family stresses and responsibilities.

PLANNING

GOAL	EXPECTED OUTCOMES
Client will demonstrate coping strategies in relation to threat of job loss and family security within 1 month.	Client will return to normal sleep pattern, requiring less than 1 hour to fall asleep and staying asleep all night. Client will have three meals a day, joining family during evening meals within 1 week. Client will participate in a support group offered by the counselor at the employee assistance program in 1 week. Client will begin to verbally express feelings of loss and powerlessness in an environment that is both supportive and "safe" in 2 weeks. Client will set time frame to pursue employment opportunities in 2 weeks.

IMPLEMENTATION

STEPS	RATIONALE
1. Set appointment at employee assistance program clinic with client 2 times a week. Provide an atmosphere of acceptance.	In order for treatment goals to be accomplished in a short time, client must see therapist as being likable, reliable, and understanding (Aguilera, 1998).
2. Define the problem from the information given by client. Explore possible alternative solutions, and give specific directions as needed. At the next session evaluate results with client. If none of the solutions has been effective, work together to find others.	Client's primary appraisal of the stressor and her secondary appraisal of her coping strategies define the stressful situation for the person experiencing the stress (Lerman and Glanz, 1997).
3. Encourage client to identify a realistic description of a change in her roles.	Everyone needs a purpose in life and to be able to identify what is personally meaningful (Manning and others, 1999).
4. Explore client's previous achievements of success.	Emphasizing the positive helps a person feel more optimistic, which can lead to positive actions and results (Manning and others, 1999).
5. Encourage client to identify own strengths and abilities.	To manage stress and cope with change people must know their strengths and abilities and what is important to them (Manning and others, 1999).
6. Provide information on cost-free counseling and support groups.	Talking with others can relieve tension for a person, and helping others, as in a support group setting, can reduce self-absorption and reduce stress (McCloskey and Bulechek, 2000).

EVALUATION

- Ask client to report over the course of a week ability to fall asleep and hours slept per night.
- Weigh client regularly, and ask for a report on food intake over a week's time.
- Observe personal hygiene, attitude toward therapy, and expressions of despair.
- Continue to assess for suicide potential or other signs of worsening depression.
- Discuss with client her perceptions of counseling and support group in terms of meeting her needs for support and assistance with problem solving.
- Have client present revised resume for review and job interview selections.

STRESS MANAGEMENT
- Instruct the client to reduce the frequency of stress-inducing situations by
  - Serving on work-site committees to improve working conditions or policies, such as flextime, child-care benefits, reasonable work assignments, and reducing workplace hazards
  - Analyzing new job possibilities if necessary
  - Avoiding excessive change in lifestyle such as moving when other stress is present
  - Using time blocking to schedule personal time to adjust to changes
  - Using time management skills to become more organized and set priorities
- Instruct the client how to increase her resistance to stress by
  - Exercising regularly
  - Enhancing self-esteem by using positive self-talk and by becoming successful in a skill for which the person takes pride
  - Learning to be assertive
  - Developing alternatives to goals that are problematic
  - Building coping resources such as social support, continuing education, a financial reserve, and an improved personal appearance
- Train the client in skills that help reduce the physiological reaction to stress, including biofeedback, relaxation training, and imagery.

Modified from Pender, NJ: *Health promotion in nursing practice*, ed 3, Stamford, Conn, 1996, Appleton & Lange.

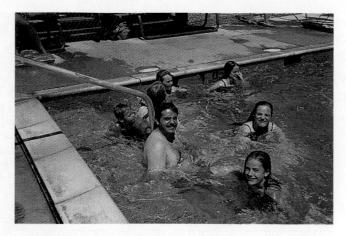

FIGURE **21-1**   A regular exercise program reduces tension and promotes relaxation. (Courtesy Michael S. Clement, MD, Mesa, Ariz.)

sionals. There will be times when the scope of nursing practice is insufficient to meet all of the client's needs. Clients experiencing stress from medical conditions or psychiatric disorders will present needs that will make it necessary for you to consult with advanced practice mental health nurses, psychiatrists, psychologists, or psychiatric social workers. Such a multidisciplinary approach to care is often most effective in addressing the holistic needs of the client. Your role is to recognize the need for collaboration and consultation, inform the client about potential resources, and make arrangements for interventions, such as consultations, group sessions, or therapy as needed.

Implementation

HEALTH PROMOTION.   Three primary modes of intervention for stress are to decrease stress-producing situations, increase resistance to stress, and learn skills that reduce physiological response to stress (Pender, 1996) (Box 21-4). You are in a position to educate clients and families about the importance of health promotion.

REGULAR EXERCISE.   A regular exercise program improves muscle tone and posture, controls weight, reduces tension, and promotes relaxation. In addition, exercise reduces the risk of cardiovascular disease and improves cardiopulmonary functioning (Figure 21-1). Clients who have a his-

tory of a chronic illness, who are at risk for developing an illness, or who are older than 35 years of age should begin a physical exercise program only after discussing the plan with a physician. In general, for a fitness program to have positive physical effects, a person should exercise at least 3 times a week for 30 to 40 minutes.

SUPPORT SYSTEMS.   A support system of family, friends, and colleagues who will listen, offer advice, and provide emotional support benefits a client experiencing stress. There are many support groups available to individuals, such as those sponsored by the American Heart Association, the American Cancer Society, local hospitals and churches, and mental health organizations.

TIME MANAGEMENT.   Time management techniques include developing lists of tasks to be performed in order of priority, for example, those tasks that require immediate attention, those that are important and can be delayed, and those tasks that are routine and can be accomplished when time become available. In many cases setting priorities helps individuals identify tasks that are not necessary or perhaps can even be delegated to someone else.

GUIDED IMAGERY AND VISUALIZATION.   Guided imagery is based on the belief that a person can significantly reduce stress with imagination. Guided imagery is a relaxed state in which a person actively uses imagination in a way that allows visualization of a soothing, peaceful setting. Typically the image created or suggested uses many sensory words to engage the mind and offer distraction and relaxation (see Chapter 29).

PROGRESSIVE MUSCLE RELAXATION.   In the presence of anxiety-provoking thoughts and events, a common physiological symptom is muscle tension. Physiological tension will be diminished through a systematic approach to releasing tension in major muscle groups. Typically a relaxed state is achieved through deep chest breathing, and then the client is directed to alternately tighten and relax muscles in specific groupings (see Chapter 29).

ASSERTIVENESS TRAINING.   Assertiveness is a skill for helping individuals communicate effectively regarding their needs and desires. The ability to resolve conflict with others through assertiveness training is important for reducing stress. When assertiveness is taught in a group setting, benefits of the experience are increased.

JOURNAL WRITING.   For many people, keeping a private, personal journal provides a therapeutic outlet for stress, and it is well within the realm of nursing to suggest journal keeping to clients experiencing difficult situations. In a private journal, clients can express a full range of emotion and vent their honest feelings without hurting anyone's feelings and without concern for how they might appear to others.

STRESS MANAGEMENT IN THE WORKPLACE.   Rapid changes in health care technology, diversity in the workforce, organizational restructuring, and changing work systems can place stress on nurses (Manning and others, 1999). Additional causes of job stress include particular job assignments, difficult schedules, shift work, fear of failure, and inadequate support services, and not knowing where you stand (Manning and others, 1999). Burnout occurs as a result of chronic stress. Burnout is "a syndrome of emotional exhaustion, depersonalization of others, and perceptions of reduced personal accomplishment, resulting from intense involvement with people in a care-giving environment" (Aguilera, 1998).

If you recognize feelings of burnout, you can make changes in your behavior to cope with workplace stress. An important step is identifying the limits and scope of your responsibilities at work (Aguilera, 1998). Recognizing the areas over which you have control and can change and those that you do not have responsibility for is a vital insight. Making a clear separation between work and home life is crucial as well. Strengthening friendships outside of the workplace, arranging for temporary social isolation for personal "recharging" of emotional energy, and spending off-duty hours in interesting activities all help reduce burnout.

ACUTE CARE

CRISIS INTERVENTION.   When stress overwhelms a person's usual coping mechanisms and demands mobilization of all available resources, it becomes a crisis (Shontz, 1975). A crisis creates a turning point in a person's life because it changes the direction of a person's life in some way (Shontz, 1975). According to Aguilera (1998), the precipitating event usually occurs from 1 to 2 weeks before the individual seeks help, but it may have occurred within the past 24 hours. Generally a crisis is resolved in some way within approximately 6 weeks. Crisis intervention aims to return the person to a precrisis level of functioning and to promote growth.

Because an individual's or family's usual coping strategies are ineffective in managing the stress of the precipitating event, the use of new coping mechanisms is required. This experience, which forces the use of unfamiliar strategies, can result either in a heightened awareness of previously unrecognized strengths and resources or in deterioration in functioning. Thus a crisis is often referred to as a situation of both danger and opportunity. Some persons or families will emerge from a crisis state functioning more effectively, whereas others may find themselves weakened, and still others completely dysfunctional.

Crisis intervention is a specific type of brief psychotherapy with prescribed steps (Aguilera, 1998). Crisis intervention is more directive than traditional psychotherapy or counseling and can be used by any member of the interdisciplinary health care team who has been trained in its techniques. The basic approach is problem solving and focuses only on the problem presented by the crisis.

When using a crisis intervention approach, you help the client make the mental connection between the stressful event and the client's reaction to it. You need to do this because the person may be unable to see the whole situation clearly. You also need to help the person become aware of present feelings, such as anger, grief, or guilt, to help the individual reduce feelings of tension. In addition, you need to help the client explore coping mechanisms, perhaps identifying ways of coping the client had not thought of. Finally, you need to help increase the scope of the person's social contacts if the person had been internally focused and isolated (Aguilera, 1998).

RESTORATIVE AND CONTINUING CARE.   A person under stress recovers when the stress is removed or coping strategies are successful; however, a person who has experienced a crisis has changed, and the effects may last for years or for the rest of the person's life (Shontz, 1975). The final stage of adapting to a crisis is acknowledgment of the long-term implications of the crisis (Shontz, 1975). If a person has successfully coped with a crisis and its consequences, he or she becomes a more mature and healthy person. When a person has recovered from a stressful situation, the time is right for introducing stress management skills to reduce the number and intensity of stressful situations in the future.

Evaluation

CLIENT CARE.   By evaluating the goals and expected outcomes of care, you know if your nursing interventions were effective and if the client is coping with the identified stress. Review the behaviorally stated, measurable goals, and assess whether or not the client has met the criteria for success as stated in the outcomes. If the nursing interventions have not been effective in helping the client achieve targeted goals, you must reevaluate the strategies implemented and revise the plan of care in light of the client's current health status.

To evaluate the client experiencing stress, observe client behaviors and talk with the client and family, if appropriate.

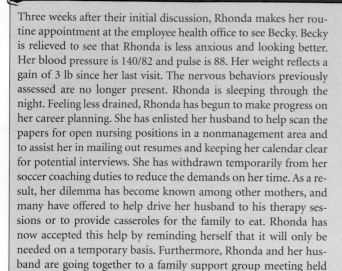

Case Study **EVALUATION**

Three weeks after their initial discussion, Rhonda makes her routine appointment at the employee health office to see Becky. Becky is relieved to see that Rhonda is less anxious and looking better. Her blood pressure is 140/82 and pulse is 88. Her weight reflects a gain of 3 lb since her last visit. The nervous behaviors previously assessed are no longer present. Rhonda is sleeping through the night. Feeling less drained, Rhonda has begun to make progress on her career planning. She has enlisted her husband to help scan the papers for open nursing positions in a nonmanagement area and to assist her in mailing out resumes and keeping her calendar clear for potential interviews. She has withdrawn temporarily from her soccer coaching duties to reduce the demands on her time. As a result, her dilemma has become known among other mothers, and many have offered to help drive her husband to his therapy sessions or to provide casseroles for the family to eat. Rhonda has now accepted this help by reminding herself that it will only be needed on a temporary basis. Furthermore, Rhonda and her husband are going together to a family support group meeting held every week at his rehabilitation facility. She is finding the encouragment of that group to be of benefit to her and an important addition to her individual counseling sessions with her employee assistance program counselor. Although the Bennett family has not yet found full resolution for their stress, they are making progress toward achievable, short-term goals.

Documentation Note
Client reports feelings of increased hopefulness and return to normal sleep and eating patterns. She is taking Zoloft, 100 mg daily, as prescribed by her personal physician, Dr. Smith, and is returning to see him for follow-up in 1 week. She is attending weekly counseling with Dr. Moody and also a rehab support group with husband. Her blood pressure today is 140/82, pulse 88, and she had a weight gain of 3 lb in the last 3 weeks. She has requested instruction in relaxation techniques. We will continue to follow the present plan, and she will return for follow-up in 2 weeks.

Outcome Evaluation for **FOR RHONDA BENNETT**   Box 21-5

Nursing Action	Client Response/Finding	Achievement of Outcome
Ask Rhonda about suicidal thoughts.	Rhonda states that she wants to continue to live and to find solutions for her problems.	Demonstrates coping through ability to discuss feelings openly; she needs further counseling.
Discuss with Rhonda her ability to ask for assistance when she needs it.	Rhonda has set an appointment with a self-help group offered by an employee assistance program.	Willing to call on others for help; may need to feel comfortable seeking help from friends.
Observe Rhonda's personal hygiene, attitude toward therapy, and expressions of loss and powerlessness.	Rhonda will begin to verbally express feelings of loss and powerlessness.	Confidence related to past experience with health behavior (Johnson and others, 2000).
Ask Rhonda to identify areas in her life that she can change to reduce stress.	Rhonda will ask friend to consider being the soccer coach.	Verbalizes sense of control over personal life (Johnson and others, 2000).
Ask Rhonda to identify own strengths and abilities.	Rhonda will establish a career plan.	Modifies lifestyle as needed (Johnson and others, 2000).
Ask Rhonda to report over the course of a week ability to fall asleep and hours slept per night.	Rhonda reports improves appetite; she still takes an hour to fall asleep but only awakens once.	Quality of sleep improving.

Remember that coping with stress can take time. If you are in a setting where contact with a client must end before resolution of goals has been achieved, it is important for you to refer clients to appropriate resources so that progress is not delayed or interrupted.

CLIENT EXPECTATIONS.   It is crucial that you maintain ongoing communication with clients regarding the plan of care. Clients under severe stress, or trauma, often experience feelings of powerlessness, vulnerability, and loss of control. You can help to reduce these feelings by actively involving clients and families in the process of problem identification (assessment), prioritizing, and goal setting and evaluation. Involving clients in these processes gives them an opportunity to direct their energy in a positive way and moves them toward taking greater responsibility for health maintenance and promotion.

Engaging the client as a partner in health care sets the stage for open communication. In such an environment the client can feel more freedom to give important feedback to you about interventions that are successful and can help you better understand why some interventions fail to meet the established goals.

An essential part of the evaluation process is collaborating with clients to determine if their own expectations from nursing have been met (Box 21-5). Any revision in the plan of care must then include steps to address client expectations.

Key Terms

alarm reaction, *p. 492*
coping, *p. 494*
crisis, *p. 494*
crisis intervention, *p. 498*
developmental crises, *p.494*
distress, *p. 494*

endorphins, *p. 492*
eustress, *p. 494*
exhaustion stage, *p. 493*
fight-or-flight response, *p. 492*
flashback, *p. 496*
general adaptation syndrome (GAS),
 p. 492
primary appraisal, *p. 494*

resistance stage, *p. 493*
secondary appraisal, *p. 494*
situational crises, *p. 494*
stress, *p. 492*
stressor, *p. 492*

Key Concepts

- The general adaptation syndrome is an immediate physiological response of the whole body to stress and involves several body systems, especially the autonomic nervous system and the endocrine system. Physiological responses to stress also include immunological changes.
- Stress can make people ill as a result of (1) increased levels of powerful hormones that change our bodily processes; (2) coping choices that are unhealthy, such as not getting enough rest or a proper diet or use of tobacco, alcohol, or caffeine; and (3) neglect of warning signs of illness or prescribed medicines or treatments.
- A person is under psychological stress only if the person evaluates the event or circumstance as personally significant. Such an evaluation of an event for its personal meaning is called primary appraisal.
- There are several types of stress, including work stress, family stress, chronic stress, acute stress, daily hassles, trauma, and crisis. Rapid changes in health care technology, diversity in the workforce, organizational restructuring, and changing work systems can place stress on nurses.

- Potential stressors and coping mechanisms vary across the life span, from childhood through adolescence, adulthood, and old age.
- Coping means making an effort to manage psychological stress. Coping is a process that is constantly changing to manage demands on a person's resources.
- Three primary modes for stress intervention are to decrease stress-producing situations, increase resistance to stress, and learn skills that reduce physiological response to stress.
- Posttraumatic stress disorder affects people who have experienced accidents, violent events, war, and natural disasters.
- A client whose stress is so severe that the person is unable to cope in any ways that have worked before is experiencing a crisis. A crisis is a turning point in life and can be developmental or situational.
- Generally a crisis is resolved in some way within approximately 6 weeks. Crisis intervention aims to return the person to a precrisis level of functioning and to promote growth.

Critical Thinking Activities

1. You are caring for a 30-year-old single mother who has recently received a diagnosis of metastatic breast cancer. She is the sole provider for three young children (all under 7 years of age). Discuss the various stressors that will need to be considered when writing an appropriate discharge plan.
2. A client comes to the emergency department with complaints of dizziness, which are not related to any physical finding on examination. During the health history the client reports that her life is very stressful and she is barely coping. She finalized her divorce 3 months ago, is working 32 hours per week, and is attending college. Her ex-husband recently lost his job and can no longer pay

child support. Finally, she tearfully confesses that she thinks she might be pregnant but does not want her ex-husband to know. Develop nursing diagnoses related to this situation.
3. An older adult woman is admitted to the hospital with a fractured hip. Before her injury she lived with her husband, who suffers from advancing Alzheimer's disease. While she is hospitalized, he is staying with a niece who lives 100 miles away, but this cannot be a permanent situation because her niece is also in frail health. The client has no children who can help her when she returns home. She is concerned not only about who will care for her after she is discharged but also about her husband. What approach would be the best to take in establishing goals for treatment?

Review Questions

1. While assessing a person for effects of the general adaptation syndrome, you should be aware that:
   1. heart rate increases in the resistance stage.
   2. blood volume increases in the exhaustion stage.
   3. vital signs return to normal in the exhaustion stage.
   4. blood glucose level increases during the alarm reaction stage.

2. While teaching a person with hypertension about how stress can cause illness, you explain that:
   1. hypertension causes stress by suppressing immunity.
   2. some antihypertensive medications cause stress and illness.
   3. a person who takes antihypertensive medication has an immunity to stress.
   4. stress may cause a person to forget to take medication and thereby cause illness.

Continued

Review Questions—cont'd

3. A child who has been in a house fire comes to the emergency department with her parents. The child and parents are upset and tearful. In your first assessment for stress you should say:
   1. "Tell me whom I can call to help you."
   2. "Tell me what bothers you the most about this experience."
   3. "I will contact someone who can help get you temporary housing."
   4. "I will sit with you until other family members can come help you get settled."

4. Another nurse is talking with you about the stress she feels on the job. You recognize that:
   1. nurses who feel stress usually pass the stress along to their clients.
   2. a nurse who feels stress is ineffective as a nurse and should not be working.
   3. nurses who talk about feeling stress are unprofessional and should calm down.
   4. nurses frequently experience stress with the rapid changes in health care technology and organizational restructuring.

5. When assessing a child for the effects of stress, you would observe that:
   1. children are resilient and cope with stress better than adults.
   2. children provoke more stress in others than they experience themselves.
   3. stressors and coping methods are different for children than older people.
   4. ways of coping that will be effective for a child are similar to those of the child's parents.

6. You are evaluating the coping success of a client experiencing stress from being newly diagnosed with multiple sclerosis and psychomotor impairment. You realize that the client is coping successfully when the client says:
   1. "I am going to learn to drive a car so I can be more independent."
   2. "My sister says she feels better when she goes shopping, so I will go shopping."
   3. "I have always felt better when I go for a long walk. I will do that when I get home."
   4. "I am going to attend a support group to learn more about multiple sclerosis and what I will be able to do."

7. You know that the client is recovering from the stress of an emergency surgery when the client says:
   1. "I am going to change jobs."
   2. "I am learning progressive relaxation training."
   3. "I plan to have plastic surgery while I am here in the hospital."
   4. "I am planning to sell my house and move within the next 6 weeks."

8. When doing an assessment of a young woman who was in an automobile accident 6 months before, you learn that the woman has vivid images of the crash whenever she hears a loud, sudden noise. You recognize this as:
   1. social phobia.
   2. acute anxiety.
   3. posttraumatic stress disorder.
   4. borderline personality disorder.

9. A family tells the community mental health nurse that their adult mentally retarded son is experiencing hallucinations. This has begun very recently and had not happened before. They are frightened for him and do not know what to do. In addition, they are living below the poverty level on their pensions and have only enough money to last from one month to the next. The nurse helps them set the following goal:
   1. after a psychiatric evaluation, investigate a group home for the son.
   2. with help from the nurse, obtain suitable housing and additional financial resources.
   3. develop a plan to take in a renter so that they can have a better income.
   4. obtain a psychiatric evaluation and stabilization on antipsychotic medication to be covered by Medicaid.

References

Aguilera D: *Crisis intervention: theory and methodology,* St. Louis, 1998, Mosby.

Aldwin C: *Stress, coping, and development,* New York, 2000, Guilford.

Johnson M and others, editors: *Nursing outcomes classification (NOC),* ed 2, St. Louis, 2000, Mosby.

Johnson M and others: *Nursing diagnoses, outcomes, and interventions: NANDA, NOC, and NIC linkages,* St. Louis, 2001, Mosby.

Lazarus R: *Stress and emotion: a new synthesis,* New York, 1999, Springer.

Lerman C, Glanz K: Stress, coping, and health behavior. In Glanz K and others, editors: *Health behavior and health education: theory, research, and practice,* ed 2, San Francisco, 1997, Jossey-Bass.

Manning G and others: *Stress: living and working in a changing world,* Duluth, Minn, 1999, Whole Person Associates.

McCloskey J, Bulechek G, editors: *Nursing Interventions Classification (NIC),* ed 3, St. Louis, 2000, Mosby.

Monat A, Lazarus R: *Stress and coping: an anthology,* New York, 1991, Columbia University Press.

Neuman B: *The Neuman systems model,* ed 3, Stamford, Conn, 1995, Appleton & Lange.

Pender NJ: *Health promotion in nursing practice,* ed 3, Stamford, Conn, 1996, Appleton & Lange.

Selye H: History and present status of the stress concept. In Monat A, Lazarus R, editors: *Stress and coping: an anthology,* New York, 1991, Columbia University Press.

Shontz F: *The psychological aspects of physical illness and disability,* New York, 1975, Macmillan.

Stuart G, Wright L: Applying the Neuman systems model to psychiatric nursing practice. In Neuman B: *The Neuman systems model,* ed 3, Stamford, Conn, 1995, Appleton & Lange.

Loss and Grief

22

Objectives

- Define key terms.
- Identify your role in assisting clients with problems related to loss, death, and grief.
- Describe and compare the phases of grieving from Kübler-Ross, Bowlby, and Worden.
- List and discuss five basic categories of loss.
- Describe the dimensions of hope.
- Describe characteristics of a person experiencing grief.
- Discuss variables that influence a person's response to grief.
- Develop a care plan for a client or family experiencing loss and grief.
- Describe effective nursing interventions for clients experiencing grief.
- Discuss principles of palliative care.
- Describe the procedure for care of the body after death.
- Discuss the nurse's own loss experience when caring for dying clients.

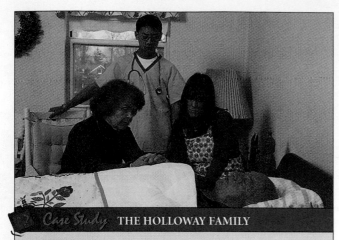

Case Study THE HOLLOWAY FAMILY

Mr. Holloway is a 73-year-old man with a history of colon cancer diagnosed 18 months ago and treated with surgery and chemotherapy. As a result of surgery he has experienced incontinence and chronic diarrhea. Chemotherapy has caused oral ulcers and loss of appetite. He was recently admitted to the hospital for evaluation and treatment of severe anemia and dehydration. When diagnostic studies revealed widespread metastases of the cancer to his liver and lungs, his oncologist decided to stop all chemotherapy. Medical treatment now includes pain management, blood replacement, and rehydration. The discharge plan is for Mr. Holloway to receive hospice care at home and be made comfortable in his remaining days.

Living in the household with Mr. Holloway are his wife of 53 years and their only child, a single daughter who is 38 years old. Mr. Holloway's daughter has taken a leave of absence from her teaching job and moved back home to help care for him during his final illness. His wife, however, is unwilling to accept that he is near death. She continues to insist, "If he would only eat right, take vitamins, and go to a gym, he would regain his strength and recover." Mr. Holloway's wife and daughter argue often about how best to help him. He becomes visibly upset when they argue and often is very withdrawn and tearful. The Holloways have few ties to the community and very limited social support. The health care team is concerned about how they will cope now that Mr. Holloway is ready for discharge.

Peter Wong is a 22-year-old nursing student in his last year of education, completing a rotation in community health. He considers himself fortunate to have never lost a family member to death and has never been assigned to care for a terminally ill client. When he learns that he will be providing home health care for Mr. Holloway and his family, he becomes anxious. He feels unprepared to intervene effectively with the sadness and conflict in the Holloway household. Peter arranges a time to talk with his instructor about his concerns. The instructor assures him that he is competent and that this will be a good opportunity to learn.

L oss and grief are experiences that affect not only clients and their families but the nurses who care for them as well. The intense emotions associated with grief are caused by very real, concrete losses. Death of a client, for example, leaves one feeling powerless. Most nurses enter the profession with the intent of helping clients recover from illness and move toward health promotion. It is frightening to learn that knowledge, skill, and technology cannot always come together to result in cure. As a nurse, you will have the opportunity to help clients and families face devastating losses and accept the reality of impending death. Providing care for clients in crisis and at the end of life requires knowledge and caring to help bring comfort to clients and families even when hope for cure is gone.

SCIENTIFIC KNOWLEDGE BASE
Loss

Loss comes in many forms based on the values and priorities learned within one's sphere of influence, including one's family, friends, society, and culture. A person experiences loss in the absence of an object, person, body part or function, emotion, or idea that was formerly present (Table 22-1). Losses may be actual or perceived. An **actual loss** is any loss of a person or object that can no longer be felt, heard, known, or experienced by the individual. Examples could include the loss of an arm, child, relationship, or role at work. Lost objects that have been valued by a client include any possession that is worn out, misplaced, stolen, or ruined by disaster. For example, a child may grieve over the loss of a favorite toy or pet. A **perceived loss** is any loss that is tangible and uniquely defined by the grieving client. It may be less obvious to others. An example is the loss of confidence or prestige. Perceived losses are easily overlooked or misunderstood, yet the process of grief follows the same sequencing and progression as actual losses. Individual interpretation makes a difference in how the perceived loss is uniquely valued and the response that one will have during grieving.

Losses may also be maturational, situational, or both. A **maturational loss** includes any change in the developmental process that is normally expected during a lifetime. One example would be a mother's feeling of loss as a child goes to school for the first time. Events associated with maturational loss are part of normal life transitions, but the feelings of loss persist as grieving helps a person cope with the change. **Situational loss** includes any sudden, unexpected, external event that is not predictable. Often this type of loss includes multiple losses rather than a single loss, such as an automobile accident that leaves a driver paralyzed, unable to return to work, and grieving over the loss of the passenger in the accident.

The type of loss and the perception of the loss influence the degree of grief a person experiences. Each individual responds to loss differently. It is incorrect to assume that the loss of an object does not generate the same level of stress as loss of a loved one. The value an individual places on the lost object (e.g., a family pet) determines the emotional response to the separation. As a nurse you must assess the special meaning that a loss has for a client and its effect on the client's health and well-being.

Hospitalization and chronic illness or disability are special circumstances that have multiple associated losses. When persons enter a hospital, they lose their privacy, control over body functions and their daily routines, their mod-

Types of Loss

Table 22-1

Definition	Implications of Loss
Loss of external objects (e.g., loss, misplacement, deterioration, theft, destruction by natural causes)	Extent of grieving depends on object's value, sentiment attached to it, and its usefulness.
Loss of a known environment (e.g., moving from a neighborhood, hospitalization, a new job, moving out of intensive care unit)	Loss occurs through maturational or situational events and through injury or illness. Loneliness or newness of unfamiliar setting threatens self-esteem and makes grieving difficult.
Loss of a significant other (e.g., being promoted, moving, or running away; loss of a family member, friend, trusted nurse, acquaintance, or animal companion)	Significant other typically fulfills another person's need for psychological safety, love and belonging, and self-esteem.
Loss of an aspect of self (e.g., body part, psychological or physiological function)	Illness, injury, or developmental changes result in loss of aspect of self that causes grief and permanent changes in body image and self-concept.
Loss of life (e.g., death of family member, friend, or acquaintance; own death)	Loss of life creates grief for those left behind. Person facing death often fears pain, loss of control, and dependency on others.

esty, and any illusions that they may have about their personal indestructibility. A chronic or debilitating illness adds concern over financial security. Furthermore, long-term illness may require a job change, threaten independence, and force alterations in lifestyle. Even a brief illness or hospitalization requires temporary shifts in family role functioning. Chronic or debilitating illness may pose a major threat to the stability of relationships.

Death is the ultimate loss. Although death is part of the continuum of life and a universal and inevitable part of being human, it is also a mystical event that generates anxiety and fear. Death ends the relationship that bind families and individuals together and separates people from the physical presence of persons who influence their lives. Even in the presence of a strong spiritual grounding, facing death is often difficult for the dying person, as well as for the person's family, friends, and caregivers. A person's terminal illness reminds close friends and associates of their own mortality. Death is generally not part of most persons' day-to-day experience. Callahan (1995) suggests that talking about death has been banished from our society, from our everyday lives, from our language, and even our thinking. Feelings of guilt, anger, and fear arise when death must finally be faced. It may cause family members and caregivers to withdraw at a time when the dying person needs their love and support. The way a person approaches dying will be influenced by personal fundamental beliefs and values, culture, spirituality, and the quality of the emotional support available.

Grief

Grief is the emotional and behavioral response to loss. It is manifested in a variety of ways that are unique to an individual and based on personal experiences, cultural expectations, and spiritual beliefs (Farber and others, 1999) (see Chapter 16 and 17). Successful mastery of grief after a loss occurs when one adapts through **mourning** and moves forward in one's life experiences with a minimum of disruptions (Engel, 1964). Mourning is the **grieving process.** It involves working through the grief until an individual accepts and adapts to one's expectations to go on in life without that

which was lost. The mourning or grieving process is not linear. It does not proceed in sequential stages that can be precisely predicted. Rather, an individual will move back and forth across phases of mourning many times, possibly extending over a period of several years, before the process is completed. Three theorists have studied grief and loss and offer explanations for the process of grieving: Kübler-Ross (1969), Bowlby (1980), and Worden (1982) (Table 22-2).

KÜBLER-ROSS'S STAGES OF DYING.   The framework for Kübler-Ross's theory is behavior oriented and includes five stages (see Table 22-2, p. 508). During **denial** an individual acts as though nothing has happened and may refuse to believe or understand that a loss has occurred. In the **anger** stage, the individual resists the loss and may strike out at everyone and everything. During **bargaining,** the individual postpones awareness of the reality of the loss and may try to deal in a subtle or overt way as though the loss can be prevented. A person finally realizes the full impact and significance of the loss during the **depression** stage. During depression the individual may feel overwhelmingly lonely and withdraw from interpersonal interaction. Finally, during the stage of **acceptance,** the individual accepts the loss and begins to look to the future.

BOWLBY'S PHASES OF MOURNING.   Bowlby's attachment theory (1980) is the foundation for his theory on mourning. Attachment is described as an instinctive behavior that leads to the development of affectional bonds between children and their primary caregiver. These bonds are present and active throughout the life cycle. Later the bonds are generalized to other persons with whom individuals form close relationships. Attachment behavior ensures our survival because it keeps us in close contact with persons who can offer us protection and support.

Bowlby describes four phases of mourning (see Table 22-2). As in the case of the other mourning theories, a person can move back and forth between any two of the phases while responding to the loss. The phase of **numbing** may last from a few hours to a week or more and may be interrupted by peri-

The Grief Process		Table 22-2
Kübler-Ross's Five Stages of Dying	Bowlby's Four Phases of Mourning	Worden's Four Tasks of Mourning
Denial	Numbing	Accepting the reality of loss
Anger	Yearning and searching	
Bargaining		
Depression	Disorganization and despair	Working through the pain of grief
	Reorganization	Adjusting to the environment without the deceased
Acceptance		Emotionally relocating the deceased and moving on with life

ods of extremely intense emotion. The grieving person may describe this phase as feeling "stunned" or "unreal." The second phase of **yearning and searching** arouses emotional outbursts of tearful sobbing and acute distress in most persons. A person may also experience less openly an intense yearning for the object or individual who is lost. This phase may last for months or years. During the phase of **disorganization and despair** an individual engages in an endless examination of how and why the loss occurred. It is common for the person to express anger at anyone who might be responsible. Gradually this examination gives way to an acceptance that the loss is permanent. During the final phase of **reorganization,** which may require a year or so, the person begins to accept unaccustomed roles, acquire new skills, and build new relationships.

WORDEN'S FOUR TASKS OF MOURNING. Worden's four tasks of mourning (1982) imply that persons who mourn can be actively involved in helping themselves and can be assisted by outside intervention. The tasks typically require a minimum of a full year to work through.

- Task I: *To accept the reality of the loss.* Even when a death has been expected, there is always some period of disbelief and surprise that the event has really happened. This task involves the processes required to accept that the person or object is gone and will not return.
- Task II: *To work through the pain of grief.* Even though people respond to loss differently, it is not possible to experience a loss and work through grief without emotional pain. Individuals who deny or shut off the pain prolong their grief.
- Task III: *To adjust to the environment in which the deceased is missing.* A person does not realize the full impact of the loss for at least 3 months. At this point many visitors and friends stop calling and the person is left to ponder the full impact of loneliness. People completing this task must take on roles formerly filled by the deceased, including some tasks that they never fully appreciated.

- Task IV: *To emotionally relocate the deceased and move on with life.* The goal of this task is not to forget the deceased or give up the relationship with the deceased but to have the deceased take a new, less prominent place in a person's emotional life. This is often the most difficult task to complete because people fear that if they make other attachments they will forget their loved one or become disloyal. A person completes this stage after realizing that it is possible to love other people without loving the deceased person less.

ANTICIPATORY GRIEF. The process of disengaging or "letting go" that occurs before an actual loss or death has occurred is called **anticipatory grief.** For example, once a person or family receives a terminal diagnosis, they begin the process of saying good-bye and completing life affairs. The process becomes more stressful when the client is unable to make decisions due to a deterioration in health. Unless guided by a client's explicit decisions regarding end-of-life care, the family shoulders the responsibility of deciding whether to continue life-sustaining measures. The family must weigh factors such as the client's values and choices, the medical facts and probabilities, the burden of treatment, the expected future quality of life for the client, and the limitations of their own emotional resources (Tilden and others, 2001).

When the actual process of dying is extended for a long time, persons in the client's family may have few symptoms of grief once the death occurs. This seeming absence of grief symptoms may result because the family has engaged in a slow grief process over time. By the time the actual moment of death arrives, much of the shock, denial, and tearfulness have already been experienced.

There are risks in anticipatory grieving. Family members may withdraw emotionally from the client too soon, leaving the client with no emotional support as death approaches. There may also be complications if a person who was thought to be near death survives. Family members may then have difficulty reconnecting and may even be resentful that the person has lived past life expectancy.

COMPLICATED BEREAVEMENT. **Bereavement** is the state of thought, feeling, and activity that follows loss. A person may have difficulty progressing through the normal phases or stages of grieving, and bereavement then becomes complicated. In these cases bereavement appears to "go wrong" and loss never resolves. This can threaten a person's relationships with others. Complicated bereavement can take on any of the following forms:

- Chronic grief: active acute mourning that never resolves, but extends for many years without remission. Persons verbalize an inability to "get past" the grief.
- Delayed grief: active grieving is held back, only to resurface later, usually in response to a trivial loss or upset. For example, a wife may only grieve a few weeks after the death of her spouse, only to become hysterical and sad a year later when she loses her car keys. The extreme sadness is a delayed response to the death of her husband.

- Exaggerated grief: persons become overwhelmed by grief, and they cannot function. This may be reflected in the form of severe phobias or alcoholism and substance abuse.
- Masked grief: persons develop symptoms (e.g., alteration in sleeping or eating) that are not recognized as grief related.

APPLICATION OF GRIEF THEORY TO OTHER TYPES OF LOSS.   Although grief theories apply mainly to the way individuals cope with the death of a loved one, each also applies to other losses. The theories are also relevant when describing the way persons respond to the loss of body function, as in the case of organ transplantation or heart attack, and disability such as amputation of a limb or a stroke. Grief theory also applies to individuals who progress through stages of mourning for lost independence, body integrity, and a change in body image. These individuals experience emotional pain that is very real as they progress through the stages of grieving.

▌ NURSING KNOWLEDGE BASE
Factors Influencing Loss and Grief

The way an individual perceives a loss and responds to it with grief and mourning will be heavily influenced by many factors.

HUMAN DEVELOPMENT.   Persons of differing ages and stages of development will display different and unique symptoms of grief. For example, toddlers are unable to understand loss or death but they feel great anxiety over loss of objects and separation from parents. School-age children experience grief over the loss of a body part or function. They often associate misdeeds with causing death. Middle-age adults usually begin to reexamine life and are sensitive to their own physical changes. Older adults often experience anticipatory grief because of aging and the possible loss of self-care abilities (Box 22-1). The loss of others poses a significant threat to the older adult's lifestyle. A person's level of growth and development helps to explain the individual's ability to understand loss and what it may mean in life (see Chapter 18). It also influences how an individual chooses to react.

SOCIOECONOMIC STATUS.   Socioeconomic status influences a person's ability to obtain options and use support mechanisms when coping with loss. Generally an individual feels greater burden from a loss when there is a lack of financial, educational, or occupational resources. For example, a client with limited financial resources may not be able to replace a home lost in a fire or may not be able to purchase necessary medications to manage a newly diagnosed disease. These clients require referral to community agencies that can provide needed resources.

PERSONAL RELATIONSHIPS.   When loss involves a loved one, the quality and meaning of the relationship severed are

Gerontological Nursing Practice   **Box 22-1**

FACTORS INFLUENCING GRIEF IN OLDER ADULTS
- Physical changes accompanying aging
- Loss of employment
- Loss of social respect
- Loss of relationships
- Loss of self-care capabilities
- Fear of loss of control
- Sense of fulfillment and contributions made
- Personality traits
- Feelings of self-worth
- Functional ability retained

critical in understanding a person's grief experience. It has been said that to lose your parents is to lose your past, to lose your spouse is to lose your present, and to lose your child is to lose your future. When a relationship between two individuals has been very close and well connected, it can be very difficult for the one left behind to cope. The support that clients receive from family and friends is based in part on their relationships with members of their social network and the manner and circumstances of their loss. When clients do not receive supportive understanding and compassion from others, they become unable to handle grief and look to the future.

NATURE OF THE LOSS.   The ability to resolve grief depends on the meaning of the loss and the situation surrounding the loss. The ability to accept help from others influences whether the bereaved will be able to cope effectively. The visibility of the loss influences the support a person receives. For example, the total loss of one's home from a tornado will bring support from the community, whereas a private loss of an important possession may bring less support. The suddenness of a loss can often cause slower resolution from grief. For example, a sudden and unexpected death is generally more difficult for a family to accept that one following a long-term chronic disease.

CULTURE AND ETHNICITY.   Interpretation of a loss varies greatly with a person's cultural and ethnic background. The expression of grief generally arises from cultural background and family practices. Culture affects how a support system or family is to behave (see Chapter 16). For example, in the Western hemisphere the grieving process is usually personal and private, with individuals showing restrained emotion. However, the ceremonies surrounding a person's death offer time for grief resolution and reminiscing. In Eastern nations, respect for the dead is shown by loud wailing and physical demonstration of grief for a specified period of time. Despite these trends, members of the same ethnocultural background often respond to loss and death to differing degrees. Research has shown that ethnicity is strongly related to attitudes toward life-sustaining treatments during terminal illness (Blackhall and others, 1999).

SPIRITUAL BELIEFS. Individuals' spirituality significantly influences their ability to cope with loss (see Chapter 17). A person's faith in a higher power or influence, the community of fellowship with friends, and the use of religious rituals and practices are just some of the spiritual resources a client may depend upon during loss. Loss can sometimes cause internal conflicts about spiritual values and the meaning of life.

Coping With Grief and Loss

In order for you, as a nurse, to provide the necessary support clients and families require during loss, it is necessary to understand how people normally cope with grief and loss. Your nursing interventions will involve reinforcement of these coping strategies or introduction of approaches that help clients learn new strategies (see Chapter 21).

HOPE. **Hope** is the anticipation of a continued good, an improvement, or lessening of something unpleasant. It is a multidimensional concept that is energizing (Miller and Powers, 1988; Nowotny, 1991; Bierman and others, 1998). Hope enhances coping skills and even influences a person's survival (Doka, 1993). A person often reveals hope through an expression of expectations for life, the present, and the future. Often in terminal illness a client focuses hope on milestones (e.g., a child's high school graduation or the completion of an important project at work), significant events (e.g., an upcoming anniversary), or for the relief of pain or other disabling symptoms (Weissman and others, 1999). A person's spiritual distress is often based on their definition of hope or lack of hope (Stepnick and Perry, 1992). Persons may view hope as encouragement to work toward recovery. Others may view hope more negatively by not being able to see any future favorable outcomes.

   Hope can be found in all aspects of life as a force that helps persons cope with life stressors. It has purpose and direction and gives reason for being (Post-White and others, 1996). The existence and maintenance of hope depend on a person having strong relationships and a sense of emotional connectedness to others. Nurses and other health professionals may provide that personal connectedness essential to hope. In studies with cancer clients, hope has been found to help individuals find meaning in their illness (Fryback, 1993). When clients with cancer face uncomfortable symptoms or increasing disability, hope enables them to face the discomforts of their disease and continue to value living as fully as possible. Chapter 17 discusses hope and its relationship to spirituality.

▌CRITICAL THINKING
Synthesis

When you care for a client who has experienced a loss, successful critical thinking requires a synthesis of knowledge, experiences with loss and grief, and information gathered from clients and families. In addition, you must apply critical thinking attitudes and intellectual and professional standards to provide appropriate and responsive nursing care. Each client enters the health care setting at a different developmental, spiritual, and cultural place and with different expectations. You will learn to consider all of these factors when providing a comprehensive plan of care.

KNOWLEDGE. Knowledge of the grief process will help you understand the responses and needs of your client and family. You must also have a clear understanding of the nature of the loss, how the client and family perceive the loss, and how the loss affects their lives. Applying knowledge of therapeutic communication principles (see Chapter 8) enables you to explore the loss thoroughly with a client to understand all influential factors. Knowledge of the pathophysiology of the related illness that is threatening loss will help you offer clients and families a realistic explanation of what they can expect about the course of the illness. Understanding the cultural meanings loss and death pose for a specific family will allow you to individualize your approach. Finally, principles of caring (see Chapter 15) and an understanding of family dynamics (see Chapter 20) will enable you to provide compassionate care.

EXPERIENCE. Most of us have experienced some type of loss: loss of a friend, a family pet, a beloved family member. Personal experience with loss prepares you to understand what loss means and to anticipate the emotional experience a client is feeling. When you have previously cared for clients experiencing loss or those who have died, the lessons are invaluable. Reflect upon those experiences and consider how you might apply what you have learned to care for your next client.

ATTITUDES. Risk taking, self-confidence, and humility are key attitudes that will help you to make accurate judgments and decisions about your clients. Many nurses become anxious when caring for clients who grieve. Being with a client or family who is mourning requires a personal risk. One must learn to accept clients' discomfort in the interest of being supportive.

   Self-confidence goes hand in hand with risk taking. Confidence helps you to understand that in the absence of something to do or say, what a client needs most is the personal connection with someone who cares. By silently sharing a moment of sadness with a client or family, you communicate caring and send the message that the client's feelings and emotions are respected and accepted.

   You cannot know everything there is to know about a client's loss. Humility helps you to put aside personal assumptions about how loss might be interpreted by the client and to remain open to hearing and understanding the client's beliefs, thoughts, and concerns.

STANDARDS. You are ethically bound to provide the best quality care to clients at all times. You must be diligent and sensitive in maintaining the client's physical integrity, preserving modesty and dignity, administering comfort measures and guarding confidentiality.

Clients facing death have the right to some self-determination in their final days. Living wills are legal documents that state individuals' wishes regarding life support, organ donation, and other considerations regarding their death (see Chapter 3). Other documents such as *A Patient's Bill or Rights* and *The Dying Person's Bill of Rights* (Box 22-2) are honored at hospitals and often posted in prominent areas. You also have the moral responsibility to support clients in the expression of their personal faith or spirituality as death approaches.

The intellectual standards of significance and relevance are important when caring for clients suffering loss. These standards guide your assessment in revealing what is most important and relevant to the client's situation and experience. Your assessment may take more time, but you will be able to acquire information that provides for a sensitive and thorough approach to your care.

NURSING PROCESS

Assessment

Begin with an open mind and accepting attitude as you assess a client who has experienced a loss. Do not assume to know how or if the client and family experience grief. Also do not assume a particular behavior indicates grief. Allow clients to share what is happening in their own way so that you can determine how the client is actually reacting (Table 22-3). This will allow you to determine what phase of grief the client is experiencing. Help clients and families find a time and place to express their grief and describe their experience (Figure 22-1). It is recommended that you interview clients and families separately unless a client requests having family members present.

First assess the meaning of the loss to the individuals involved. Examples of topics to explore are summarized in Table 22-4. Many variables affect grief, so consider each of them in your assessment in order to have a broad database.

Interview the client and family using honest and open communication. Listen carefully, and observe the client's responses and behaviors. Assume a neutral perspective and be alert for nonverbal cues. Summarize and validate any impressions you form with the client and family so that appropriate nursing diagnoses can be made. Other health care workers will contribute to your database, including physicians, social workers, and members from pastoral care.

COPING RESOURCES.   Determine what behaviors and outside resources typically help clients cope with difficulties. Ask open-ended questions or statements to enable the client to provide details: "Tell me how you find ways to adjust when times get difficult" or "Tell me whom you go to when you are experiencing difficult times." Use of direct questions

---

The Dying Person's Bill of Rights	Box 22-2

I have the right to be treated as a living human being until I die.

I have the right to maintain a sense of hopefulness, however changing its focus may be.

I have the right to be cared for by those who can maintain a sense of hopefulness, however changing this might be.

I have the right to express my feelings and emotions about my approaching death in my own way.

I have the right to participate in decisions concerning my care.

I have the right to expect continuing medical and nursing attention even though "cure" goals must be changed to "comfort" goals.

I have the right not to die alone.

I have the right to be free from pain.

I have the right to have my questions answered honestly.

I have the right not to be deceived.

I have the right to have help from and for my family in accepting my death.

I have the right to die in peace and dignity.

I have the right to retain my individuality and not be judged for my decisions that may be contrary to beliefs of others.

I have the right to discuss and enlarge my religious and/or spiritual experiences, whatever these may mean to others.

I have the right to expect that the sanctity of the human body will be respected after death.

I have the right to be cared for by caring, sensitive, knowledgeable people who will attempt to understand my needs and will be able to gain some satisfaction in helping me face my death.

From Barbus AJ: The dying person's bill of rights, *Am J Nurs* 75:99, 1975.

Example of a Focused Client Assessment   Table 22-3

Factors to Assess	Questions and Approaches	Physical Assessment Strategies
Phase of grief	Tell me how you are feeling now. Validate client's feelings: 　　You seem angry, tell me more about that . . . 　　You seem very sad, tell me more . . .	Observe client's behaviors: 　Presence of crying 　Frequent sighing 　Poor eye contact
Survivor's response to sudden loss	It is so difficult to lose someone so quickly: What has your (wife, child, spouse) meant to you in your life? What are your feelings right now? Are you feeling guilty because . . . ? Could you really have prevented this?	Observe nonverbal behaviors as members of family interact together 　Tone of conversation 　Detaches or walks away from members of family 　Seeks physical closeness from member of family

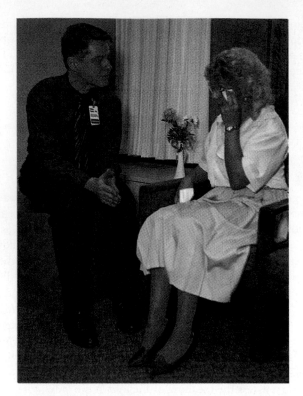

FIGURE 22-1 Nurses assist family members in finding resources to help with the grieving process.

As Peter Wong prepares to meet the Holloway family for the first time, he mentally reviews all of the information that will be essential in making an accurate assessment. He has read extensively about colon cancer and has tried to anticipate key symptoms to look for in a client who has metastases to the lungs and liver. He will attempt to be sensitive to any embarrassment Mr. Holloway might feel about his incontinence. He has read that family members experience grief in their own way, with roles and responsibilities shifting. Mr. Holloway is facing his own death and has become very dependent. Regardless of Mrs. Holloway's seeming denial, she is being forced to assume new responsibilities as her husband's health deteriorates. Mr. Holloway's daughter has already given up her home and job to care for her father. The stress of Mr. Holloway's condition may be exaggerated by the conflict between these two women as the needs of the family change.

Peter has no past experience with death, but he has cared for critically ill clients. Humility and the willingness to take risks will be key attitudes to have in working with this family. If they ask him what he knows about death, he can honestly tell them that he thinks it must be very difficult to live through so many stresses. He will ask them to discuss their perceptions and feelings with him, and he will try to understand their feelings and accept them. If family members express emotions, Peter will try to show confidence that he knows he does not need to "fix" things. He just needs to be there to share their sadness. If they ask questions he cannot answer, he will have the humility to admit that he does not know and will try to obtain the information for them or put them in contact with someone who can help.

Peter will be especially careful to attend to Mr. Holloway's complaints of pain and discomfort and teach family members how to position him and medicate him when no nurses are in the home. He will respect Mr. Holloway's privacy, modesty, and need for dignity, especially in the face of medical problems such as incontinence. At school and at hospice, he will take care to protect confidentiality. He will help the family discuss important subjects such as preparation for death and will be sensitive to Mr. Holloway's need and desire to discuss his wishes regarding his death.

may help you determine if activities such as relaxation exercises, meditation, reading, or exercise help clients deal with stressors. These coping resources may become invaluable in your plan of care.

GRIEF BEHAVIORS.   Assessment of the client and family includes consideration of the stages of grief and the type of behaviors they exhibit. While you observe the client's behavior, you can assess the effects of the loss. No two people grieve exactly the same way. However, most persons who grieve have at least some outward signs and symptoms that are associated with grief. These signs fall into several categories, including feelings, physical sensations, cognitions or thought patterns, and behaviors (Box 22-3). The purpose in observing and noting these signs and symptoms of grief is not to document a stage or phase of mourning but rather to guide interventions and evaluate outcomes.

A loss takes place in a social context. In the case of a family experiencing a death, the family begins to reorganize itself as soon as the client is no longer able to fulfill the same number and types of roles. When a person is disabled, both the client and family undergo a similar reorganization, realigning roles and responsibilities to meet the new demands. Assess the entire family's response to loss, recognizing that family members may be dealing with different aspects of grief than the client.

END-OF-LIFE DECISIONS.   When a client is experiencing a terminal illness, family members must face end-of-life deci-

sions. The stress that families experience when deciding whether to withdraw life-sustaining treatments is very high (Tilden and others, 2001). Although more and more clients have living wills, it is important for family members to know a client's wishes in regard to life-sustaining measures. The Study to Understand Prognoses and Preferences for Outcomes and Risks of Treatments (SUPPORT Principal Investigators, 1995) found that a larger proportion of clients received prolonged aggressive treatments even when clients and families had indicated preference for palliative care rather than life extension. As a nurse you must assess the client's and family's wishes for the type of treatment desired as a terminal illness progresses. Family members often face complex decisions with unresolved burdens and guilt, limited knowledge, and an inability to conceptualize the dying trajectory or how a person's final days or weeks will be experienced (Forbes and others, 2000). Determine the client's or family's preferences and goals for end-of-life care. Does the client want to try all avail-

Assessment Factors for Grieving		Table 22-4
Factors	**Areas/Suggested Questions to Explore**	

Hope	Goals, worth, adaptations to future changes
	Examples:
	    What do you expect now that . . . ?
	    How do you feel about yourself?
	    Tell me what you will do now that . . . ?
	    What do you expect to help you through this . . . ?	

Nature of relationships	Functions of family, community, society
	Examples:
	    How long have you known the dying client?
	    What role did the dying client play in your family?
	    What is your relationship? Will it change?
	    What contributions have been made by the client?
	    How do you interpret the potential loss? By the client? By the significant other?
	    How will family relationships change as a result of the loss?	

Social support system	Availability of health care workers, timing, family needs
	Examples:
	    Who is present? Absent? Supportive? Nonsupportive?
	    Are they always actually available or do they just say, "Call me if you need me"?
	    Are they helpful, or do they avoid the issues offered for discussion by the client?
	    Do they use a listening ear approach rather than a judgmental approach?
	    Is the client's self-esteem built up and supported?	

Nature of loss	Death issues: personal, family, or community; private or group; actual versus perceived; functional
	    versus dysfunctional or disenfranchised; recognized or not by society
	Examples:
	    What is your belief about death?
	    How do you define death?
	    Define the loss in your own terms.
	    What factors will help you grieve?
	    What factors will interfere with grieving?
	    What support does the grieving significant other have? Are these persons available when needed?
	    What past experiences have you had? Outcomes?
	    What has helped you cope in the past? What has not? Can you identify coping behaviors?	

Cultural and spiritual beliefs	Values, practices, customs, attitudes, clergy, spiritualist
	Examples:
	    How is this person valued based on spiritual and cultural expectations?
	    How does the loss of a limb change this valuing?
	    How does the client or significant other perceive physical death? Meaning of life?
	    How should the body (or part) be treated when removed?
	    What traditions are required to show value of all life?
	    Can religious practices interfere with medical treatment?
	    Who has the right to say "yes" or "no"? Legally? Ethically? Can the court interfere?	

Loss of personal life goals	Actual or perceived individual losses affecting future decisions and options
	Examples:
	    What is your goal in life for . . . ?
	    How was this changed with this diagnosis? Surgery?
	    How have things changed since the accident (e.g., an automobile accident causing permanent
	        quadriplegia)?
	    How will your role change your personal goals?
	    What planning has occurred for your own life?
	    How does your perception of the problem differ from the client's view?	

able treatments? Does the family insist on use of a feeding tube for continued nutritional support? When life support requires use of a mechanical ventilator, is this something the client refuses? If you feel uncomfortable in assessing a client's wishes, find a health care provider who is experienced with discussing end-of-life care issues.

NURSE'S EXPERIENCE WITH GRIEF.   When caring for clients experiencing grief, it is important for you to assess your own emotional well-being. Self-reflection, which is a part of critical thinking, becomes a valuable tool in asking whether your personal sadness is related to caring for the client or to unresolved personal experiences from the past. It is not wrong

Symptoms of Normal Grief Box 22-3

FEELINGS
Sadness
Anger
Guilt or self-reproach
Anxiety
Loneliness
Fatigue
Helplessness
Shock/numbness (lack of
feeling)
Yearning
Emancipation/relief

**COGNITIONS
(THOUGHT PATTERNS)**
Disbelief
Confusion
Preoccupation about the
deceased
Sense of the presence of the
deceased
Hallucinations
Hopelessness ("I'll never be
OK again")

PHYSICAL SENSATIONS
Hollowness in the stomach
Tightness in the chest
Tightness in the throat
Oversensitivity to noise
Sense of depersonalization
("Nothing seems real")
Feeling short of breath
Muscle weakness
Lack of energy
Dry mouth

BEHAVIORS
Sleep disturbances
Appetite disturbances
Absentminded behavior
Dreams of the deceased
Sighing
Crying
Carrying objects that be-
longed to the deceased

Nursing Diagnoses for
**CLIENTS/FAMILIES EXPERIENCING
LOSS AND GRIEF** Box 22-4

- Anxiety
- Caregiver role strain
- Coping, compromised
family
- Coping, ineffective
- Denial, ineffective
- Grieving, anticipatory
- Grieving, dysfunctional
- Hopelessness
- Powerlessness
- Social Isolation
- Spiritual distress
- Spiritual well-being,
readiness for enhanced

to have personal feelings and emotions. However, it is inappropriate to put your personal family situation before the client. Part of being a professional is knowing when to get away from a situation and take care of oneself.

CLIENT EXPECTATIONS. Take time to assess the client's and family's expectations for nursing care. The client's perceptions and expectations will influence how you prioritize nursing diagnoses. For example, if clients perceive that their level of pain and discomfort is severe, they will be less attentive to any attempts you make to discuss the significance of their loss. It will become a priority for you to make a client comfortable before you can institute any meaningful discussion or counseling. Be sure to assess the client's expectations within the context of the loss by asking questions such as, "How can we help you cope with your loss?" and "What do you feel is necessary from us for you to be able to resolve the grief you feel?"

It is important for you to give family members the chance to explain how they perceive your role and what their goals are for the health care team. This part of the assessment helps you to clarify any misunderstanding that might exist. For example, the family may have very unrealistic expectations regarding the type of treatment available to the client and the anticipated effects. Taking time to assess what clients and families expect and desire from nursing care helps to ensure an individualized and comprehensive plan of care.

Nursing Diagnosis

After thorough and thoughtful data collection, identify nursing diagnoses applicable to the client's clinical situation.

Clustering of client or family behaviors, actual or potential losses, the client's attempts at coping, and data involving the nature and meaning of the loss lead to individualized nursing diagnoses (Box 22-4).

The presence of one or two defining characteristics is usually insufficient to make an accurate diagnosis. Be vigilant and carefully review the data you have and consider competing diagnoses. For example, if a client who is dying manifests crying or tearfulness, displays anger, and reports nightmares, this could signal several possible nursing diagnoses because these characteristics are common to more than one diagnosis. Possibilities include *pain, ineffective coping,* and *spiritual distress.* You must examine all available data and inquire about the presence of other behaviors and symptoms until you feel comfortable in selecting an accurate diagnosis.

Identify the appropriate related factor for each diagnosis. For example, *dysfunctional grieving related to loss of the ability to walk from paralysis* will require different interventions than *dysfunctional grieving related to the loss of a job.* Clarification of the related factor will ensure that appropriate interventions are elected for the client's care.

When a client is seriously ill, as in the case of a terminal illness, several nursing diagnoses will likely apply. In addition to diagnoses pertinent to grieving, you will likely diagnose problems reflecting the client's physical and psychological condition. Some of these diagnoses are common to grieving, such as *anxiety* or *imbalanced nutrition.* In these situations your interventions must focus on supporting or resolving grief before the other diagnoses can be resolved.

Planning

Grieving is the natural response to loss and has a therapeutic value. Plan your nursing care to meet the physical, emotional, developmental, and spiritual needs of your client and family (see care plan). Support the client's self-esteem and right to autonomy by including the client in decisions about the plan of care. Encourage ongoing involvement of the family when appropriate.

GOALS AND OUTCOMES. Establish realistic goals and expected outcomes based on the client's nursing diagnoses. Consider the client's available resources, such as physical

Case Study Nursing Care Plan   **LOSS AND GRIEF**

Assessment

During Peter's home visit, he finds Mr. Holloway appearing to be in reasonably good physical condition 1 week after discharge. His appetite has improved, and his mouth ulcers have disappeared. He continues to have bowel incontinence, however, and he has become very unsteady while walking. One night he fell while attempting to get out of bed and badly bruised his face. Peter finds Mr. Holloway easy to talk with and very receptive to Peter's questions. Mr. Holloway is easily moved to tears when talking about his situation, yet he becomes more relaxed when talking with Peter about memories of his younger years. He confides that his wife **disappears for hours every day** and **does not seem to realize how ill her husband really is.** Mr. Holloway states, "I know this is very **hard for her to accept,** but I also know I need her help." When asked about his daughter, Mr. Holloway reports that she appears tired and has not been sleeping well. "I think she feels as though she doesn't know what to do."

During Peter's visit, Mrs. Holloway comes into the room. She begins to **describe plans for their summer vacation, still 9 months away.** She avoids Peter's question about what she and her daughter have done to deal with Mr. Holloway's symptoms. Instead she suggests that her husband might benefit from "getting some exercise and eating a more balanced diet." Peter asks to talk with Mrs. Holloway alone for a few minutes. During this time, Mrs. Holloway begins to cry and voices her **fear of being unable to support her husband** appropriately. Mrs. Holloway states, **"I still can't believe this is happening to us."** She collects her thoughts and asks Peter what the family should do; both she and her daughter want to be more helpful.

*Defining characteristics are shown in bold type.

Nursing Diagnosis

Compromised family coping related to stress of impending death of father/husband.

Planning

Goal

Client and family understand client's terminal condition and its implications within 1 month.
Family assumes caregiving tasks within 1 week.

Expected Outcomes

Wife and daughter participate in home visits with home health nurse within 3 days.
Client and family set short-term goals together for Mr. Holloway within 1 week.
Wife and daughter will assist with husband's hygiene and safety care within 1 week.
Wife and daughter will identify support resources to use within 1 week.
Mr. Holloway will begin the process of life review, sharing his thoughts with his family within 2 days.

Implementation

Steps

1. Involve Mrs. Holloway and daughter in discussion between home health nurse and Mr. Holloway, focusing instruction on symptom management.

2. Offer time for Mrs. Holloway and daughter to ask questions and discuss course of cancer, the expected trajectory of the disease, and desires for life-sustaining treatment.

3. Explain to family that setting easily achievable goals helps foster hope. Enlist their help to establish goals for the next week.

4. Provide family with names and phone numbers of support groups such as those provided by the hospice and the cancer society.

5. Discuss with Mrs. Holloway and daughter the value of reminiscence as part of looking back and evaluating life and its meaning.

Rationale

Even with a poor prognosis, quality of life can be improved through discussion and planning for possible problems (Poncar, 1994).

Clarifying expectations better prepares individuals to face changes that will develop as cancer progresses (Talle and others, 2000).

Restructuring goals to be more short-term and achievable is a means of supporting and sustaining hope in terminally ill clients (Nowotny, 1991).
Accessing social support helps to facilitate grief and reduce anxiety and feelings of loneliness (Worden, 1982).

Life review is a normal developmental task that needs to be supported as life nears its end (Erikson, 1982). Engaging in this process will help move the family along the process of anticipatory grieving (Worden, 1982).

Evaluation

- During home visit, observe Mrs. Holloway's and daughter's behavior and level of involvement in care.
- Review with family the goals they have established.
- Two weeks after family instruction, ask family to discuss if any problems exist in providing care to Mr. Holloway.
- Ask family about their progress in locating a support group and about their plans to attend.
- Discuss the family's degree of participation in the life review and reminiscence with Mr. Holloway. Evaluate if he becomes less dependent on the nurse to fulfill this role as his family becomes more involved in sharing.

energy, supportive family members, and methods for coping, and integrate them into the goals of care. For example, if a terminally ill client has the diagnosis of *powerlessness,* a goal of "Client will be able to discuss expected course of disease" will be realistic if the client is able to remain attentive and participate in educational discussions without becoming fatigued. An expected outcome of "Client will participate in series of short planned teaching discussions about disease" accounts for the client's need to have short teaching sessions so as to avoid exhaustion.

Goals of care for a client dealing with loss might be long or short term, depending on the nature of the loss and the client's phase of grieving. Because a client may move back and forth between phases of grief, it may become necessary for you to revise goals and outcomes to ensure they are still relevant. While you develop individualized goals of care, remember that ultimately you are assisting clients to adjust to their grief, accept the reality of a loss, regain self-esteem, and renew normal personal relationships as much as possible.

SETTING PRIORITIES. When a client has multiple nursing diagnoses, it is not possible to address all of the problems simultaneously. On any given day or time when you care for a client, two or three problem areas will demand your attention. Always consider what are the client's most urgent physical or psychological needs requiring immediate attention. Then consider the client's expectations and preferences in regard to the priorities of care. If the client is progressing as desired, you may refocus priorities to address unmet needs. For example, a client has experienced the loss of a spouse and has been experiencing imbalanced nutrition and disturbed sleep pattern. If the client reports an improved appetite and has shown a weight gain since the last clinic visit, you can focus more attention of the sleep pattern disturbance. Remember, the client's expectations and preferences should influence how you set priorities. If a terminally ill client places more emphasis on comfort or spiritual support versus other priorities such as mobility or learning about planned treatments, attend to the client's priorities first. Meeting the client's priorities first may then allow you to meet other needs more effectively with less effort.

CONTINUITY OF CARE. Interdisciplinary teams help to identify and meet the needs of those who experience losses. Dietitians, pastoral care professionals, physicians, social workers, psychologists, and other health care providers can assist a client and family in their grief. A coordinated group approach ensures that little is left to chance and that the client's plan of care will be managed well. Often, terminally ill clients will return home and require continued intense nursing care. In that situation, home health nurses will collaborate closely with family members to ensure the client's ongoing needs are met.

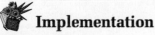

Implementation

HEALTH PROMOTION. Although a return to full function will not be an expected outcome for a terminally ill client or even a person who experiences significant disability or other loss of function, there is always the goal of enabling the client to return to optimal physical and emotional functioning. This does not mean the client and family will not experience sadness or other disturbing emotions, but that they will cope with the stressors in their life. You will assist clients in learning to deal with their loss, to make effective decisions about their health care, and to adjust to any disappointment, frustration, and anxiety created by their loss.

THERAPEUTIC COMMUNICATION. Nursing care of the grieving client and family begins with establishing the significance of their loss. This is difficult if the client is unwilling or unable to express feelings or is experiencing shock or denial. It is important for you to use therapeutic communication strategies that enable the client to discuss the loss and work with you in findings ways to resolve it. Use open-ended questions that allow clients to freely share their thoughts and concerns. Too often the use of closed questions result in the client discussing only what you presume is the problem. Acknowledge the client's grief and show support by use of touch, remaining attentive, and demonstrating other caring behaviors. You will gain the client's trust by showing a desire to become involved with the client at a level that fosters open communication. Listening to the client's story can be very therapeutic and will generally reveal details that enable you to provide very effective interventions.

If a client chooses not to share feelings or concerns, you should convey a willingness to be available when needed. If you are reassuring and respectful of the client's needs and expressed preferences for privacy, a therapeutic relationship will likely develop. Sometimes clients need to begin resolving their grief before they can discuss their loss.

It is important to recognize that some clients will not discuss feelings about their loss. Be observant for expressions of anger, denial, depression, or guilt. Remember, it is important to know your own feelings before encouraging clients to express their anger. Individuals may retaliate against family, staff, or physicians. They can also become demanding and accusing. Remain supportive by letting clients and family members know that feelings such as anger are normal. For example, you might say, "You are obviously upset, I just want you to know I am available to talk if you want." Always be sure to avoid barriers to communication (see Chapter 8) by denying the client's grief, providing false reassurance, or avoiding discussion of sensitive issues.

No topic that a dying client wishes to discuss should be avoided. When you sense that clients desire to begin a discussion, it is important to find time to let them discuss their concerns. This can be very challenging in a busy acute care setting. Respond to questions openly and honestly. Provide information that helps them and their families to understand their condition, the trajectory or future course of their disease, the benefits and burdens of treatment, and clarification of values and goals (Forbes and others, 2000).

PROMOTING HOPE.   Hope can be an energizing resource for clients experiencing loss. For each dimension of hope, there are nursing strategies that promote a client's hope:
- **Affective dimension.** Show empathic understanding of the client's strengths. Reinforce expressions of courage, positive thinking, and realistic goal setting.
- **Cognitive dimension.** Offer information about the illness and correct any misinformation. Clarify or modify client's perceptions.
- **Behavioral dimension.** Assist the client in using personal resources and making use of external supports to balance need for independence with healthy interdependence and dependence.
- **Affiliative dimension.** Encourage clients to foster supportive relationships.
- **Temporal dimension.** Focus on short-term goals as life expectancy diminishes.
- **Contextual dimension.** Encourage development of achievable goals. Reminisce about achievements or positive moments in time so client can derive meaning from suffering.

FACILITATING MOURNING.   There are strategies you can use to help clients move through uncomplicated grief (Worden, 1982). These guidelines are equally helpful for persons who are mourning a death, facing death, and grieving over an actual situational loss.
- **Help the client accept that the loss is real.** Discuss how the loss or illness occurred or was discovered, when, under what circumstances, who told them about it, and other similar topics to help make the event more real and place it in perspective.
- **Support efforts to live without the deceased person or in the face of disability.** Using a problem-solving approach is often helpful. Have clients or family make a list of their problems, help them prioritize them, and then lead them step-by-step through a discussion of how they might tackle each one. Encourage them to make use of family members, community resources, or others who can help.
- **Encourage establishment of new relationships.** Many people will fear that in doing so they will be disloyal. They will need reassurance that new relationships do not mean that they are replacing the person who has died.
- **Allow time to grieve.** It is common to have "anniversary reactions" around the time of the loss in subsequent years. Some people worry that they are going crazy when sadness or other signs of grief recur after a period of relative calm.
- **Interpret "normal" behavior.** Being distractible, having difficulty sleeping or eating, and thinking they have heard the deceased's voice are common behaviors following loss. These symptoms do not mean an individual has an emotional problem or is becoming ill in some way. Reinforce that these behaviors are normal and will resolve over time.
- **Provide continuing support.** Clients and their families may need to talk and may look to you for support for

many months or years following a loss. If you have occasion to see the client or family after an extended time, it is appropriate to inquire about how they are coping. This gives them the opportunity to talk if needed.
- **Be alert for signs of ineffective coping.** Be aware of coping mechanisms that may be harmful, such as alcohol or substance abuse, which can include excessive use of over-the-counter pain killers and sleep aids.

ACUTE CARE
PALLIATIVE CARE.   People facing life-threatening illnesses have many medical and technological advances available to prolong their lives. However, you will care for clients who make the decision to forego high-tech life-sustaining treatment in exchange for a peaceful death. According to the World Health Organization (WHO), when health care providers deliver **palliative care,** they do the following:
- Affirm life and regard dying as a normal process
- Neither hasten nor postpone death
- Provide relief from pain and other distressing symptoms
- Integrate psychological and spiritual aspects of client care
- Offer a support system to help clients live as actively as possible until death
- Offer a support system to help families cope during the client's illness and their own bereavement (Rousseau, 1998)
Palliative care is a philosophy of total care during a client's end of life (EOL). The approach to care usually involves an interdisciplinary team of physicians, nurses, social workers, pastoral care professionals, and pharmacists. A palliative care approach ensures that a client experiences a "good death," free of avoidable pain and suffering, in accord with the client's and family's wishes, and reasonably consistent with clinical, cultural, and ethical standards (Tolle and others, 2000).

As a nurse one of the most important skills in providing palliative care is establishing a caring relationship with both client and family so that you can engage in meaningful communication with them. Next, it becomes very important for you to provide appropriate symptom-control measures to maintain the client's dignity and self-esteem, to prevent abandonment or isolation, and to provide a comfortable and peaceful environment.

Symptom Control.   Comfort for a dying client includes pain control and management of symptoms of disease and therapies. Fear of pain is common in many clients and may heighten perception of discomfort. Assess the character of the client's pain carefully, and individualize therapies. Chapter 29 reviews in detail appropriate principles and options for pain management.

The terminally ill also frequently experience dyspnea, or air hunger. Air hunger can cause great panic in the client and significant stress in the caregiver (Tarzian, 2000). As the client panics, unable to get a breath, the air hunger simply worsens. Tarzian (2000) interviewed nurses who cared for the terminally ill and found that surrendering and sharing control help reduce panic and anxiety in these clients. For example, a client may choose to switch oxygen devices, even though they deliver the same concentration of oxygen. However, if the

Promoting Comfort in the Terminally Ill Client
Table 22-5

Symptoms	Characteristics or Causes	Nursing Implications
Discomfort	Any source of physical irritation may worsen pain.	Provide thorough skin care including daily baths, lubrication of skin, and dry, clean bed linens to reduce irritants.
	As client approaches death, mouth remains open, tongue becomes dry and edematous, and lips become dry and cracked.	Provide oral care at least every 2 to 4 hours. Use soft toothbrushes or foam swabs for frequent mouth care. Apply a light film of petroleum jelly to lips and tongue (see Chapter 26).
	Blinking reflexes diminish near death, causing drying of cornea.	Eye care removes crusts from eyelid margins. Artificial tears reduce corneal drying.
Fatigue	Metabolic demands of a cancerous tumor cause weakness and fatigue.	Help client to identify valued or desired tasks; then help client to conserve energy for only those tasks. Promote frequent rest periods in a quiet environment.
	Exhaustion phase of the general adaptation syndrome causes energy depletion.	Time and pace nursing care activities.
Constipation	Narcotic medications and immobility slow peristalsis.	Give preventive care, which is most effective: increase fluid intake; include bran, whole grain products, and fresh vegetables in diet; encourage exercise.
	Lack of bulk in diet or reduced fluid intake may occur with appetite changes.	
	Constipation can add to discomfort.	Administer prophylactic stool softeners.
Diarrhea	Diarrhea results from disease process (e.g., colon cancer) and complications of treatment or medications.	Assess for fecal impaction. Confer with physician to change medication if possible. Provide low-residue diet.
Urinary incontinence	Incontinence results from progressive disease (e.g., involvement of spinal cord, reduced level of consciousness).	Protect skin from irritation or breakdown. Indwelling urinary catheter or condom catheters may be used.
Inadequate nutrition	Nausea and vomiting can decrease appetite.	Serve smaller portions and bland foods, which may be more palatable.
	Depression from grieving may cause anorexia.	Allow home-cooked meals, which may be preferred by client and gives the family a chance to participate.
Dehydration	As disease progresses, client is less willing or able to maintain oral fluid intake.	Remove factors causing decreased intake; give antiemetics, apply topical analgesics to oral lesions. Reduce discomfort from dehydration; give mouth care minimum of every 4 hours; offer ice chips or moist cloth to lips.

client believes there is a difference, it might be enough to relieve the dyspnea at least briefly. When there are options in respiratory therapy, give the client a choice. Management of air hunger also involves the judicious administration of morphine and **anxiolytics** for relief of respiratory distress.

Clients may also experience nausea as a side effect of medications such as chemotherapy and as a result of severe pain. Nausea can be managed through the administration of antiemetics such as Compazine, provision of frequent mouth care, and individualized diet therapy. Administration of a clear liquid diet may allow a client to maintain fluid intake. Sometimes a client enjoys ice chips. Liquids that increase stomach acidity such as coffee, milk, and citric acid juices, should be avoided. Table 22-5 summarizes nursing care measures for additional symptoms of terminal disease.

Maintaining Dignity and Self-Esteem. You can promote a client's self-esteem and dignity by attending to the client's appearance. Cleanliness, absence of body odors, attractive clothing, and personal grooming all contribute to a sense of worth. When caring for a client's bodily functions, always show an attitude of respect, even when the client becomes dependent. Keep the client's immediate surroundings pleasant by opening curtains and letting the light change from the bright of day to the dark of night. Remove any unpleasant odors from liquid stool or vomitus as soon as possible.

Disabilities experienced by the client may threaten dignity, especially when caregivers take control of the client's life. Allow the client to make nursing care decisions (e.g., how to administer personal hygiene, diet preferences, and timing of nursing care activities). Keep the client well informed about planned therapies and anticipated effects. Provide the client privacy during nursing care procedures and when the client and family need time together.

Preventing Abandonment and Isolation. A terminally ill client is often fearful of dying alone. Therefore it is important to answer the call light quickly and to explain when staff will be giving care and performing assessments throughout the day and night. Avoid placing the client in a private room unless family members do visit and plan to stay around the clock. Clients feel a sense of involvement when sharing a room and interacting with staff. Clients can share conversation and companionship with roommates and visitors.

If family members have difficulty accepting the client's impending death, they may avoid visitation. When family members do visit, it is important to talk with them. It may be useful to give family members helpful hints about what to discuss with clients. For example, you can role model attentive listening and offering reassurance to improve their communication skills. Encourage family to discuss activities other family members are involved in, to reminisce about enjoyable times, and to inquire about the client's concerns. Also help them find simple and appropriate tasks to perform when they visit in the hospital such as feeding the client, washing the client's face, combing hair, and filling out the client's menu. Older adults often become particularly lonely at night and may feel more secure if a family member stays at the bedside during the night. Allow visitors to remain with dying clients at any time if the client wants them. Also know how to contact family members at any time if the client requests a visit or if the client's condition worsens.

Providing a Comfortable and Peaceful Environment. Keep a client comfortable through frequent repositioning, keeping bed linens dry, and controlling extraneous environmental noise. Pictures, cherished objects, cards or letters from family members, and plants and flowers create an environment that is more familiar and comforting. Offer the client frequent back massage, and allow the client to listen to preferred types of music. A comfortable, pleasant environment helps clients to relax, which promotes their ability to sleep and minimizes severity of symptoms.

Providing a client spiritual comfort means that you give clients the opportunity to exercise their faith and spiritual beliefs. As death approaches, clients often seek comfort by discussing their values and beliefs related to life and death. Dying clients seek to find purpose and meaning in life before surrendering to death. They might also feel guilty if they perceive their life to be unfulfilled. Chapter 17 discusses some of the spiritual practices and religious rituals that can support persons who are very sick or dying.

SUPPORT FOR THE GRIEVING FAMILY.   The family may be the primary caregivers when the client chooses to be at home during the last days of life. Family members will require your support and benefit from your teaching them ways to care for their loved one (Box 22-5). This can be emotionally stressful and physically exhausting for the family caregiver. In the home setting provide the opportunity for the family to be temporarily relieved of their duties so they can acquire needed rest and support. Respite care is a resource available through hospice programs. Keep the family informed so that they can anticipate the type of symptoms the client will likely experience and the implications for care. Encourage family members to express their grief with the client and to give the client the opportunity to discuss any remaining concerns or requests.

In the hospital setting, assist in planning a visitation schedule for family members to prevent the client and family from excessive fatigue. Allow young children to visit a dy-

| Box 22-5 |

THE DYING CLIENT'S FAMILY
- Describe and demonstrate feeding techniques and selection of foods to facilitate ease of chewing and swallowing.
- Demonstrate bathing, mouth care, and other hygiene measures, and allow family to perform return demonstration.
- Show video on simple transfer techniques to prevent injury to themselves and the client; help family to practice.
- Describe ways the family can promote the client's comfort, such as frequent rest periods and repositioning.
- Teach family to recognize signs and symptoms to expect as the client approaches death and information on whom to call in an emergency.
- Discuss ways to support the dying person and listen to needs and fears.
- Solicit questions from family, and provide information as needed.

ing parent when the client is able to communicate. At the time of death, help the family to stay in communication with the client through frequent visits, caring silence, touch, and telling the client of their love. After death, assist the family with decision making such as notification of a mortician, transportation of family members, and collection of the client's belongings.

HOSPICE CARE.   **Hospice** care is an alternative for the terminally ill. Generally clients accepted into a hospice program have less than 6 months to live. Hospice is not a facility but a concept for family-centered care designed to assist the client in being comfortable and maintaining a satisfactory lifestyle until death. A nurse's role in hospice is to meet the primary wishes of the dying client and to be open to individual desires of each client (Hospice Care, 1997). The nurse maintains the client's comfort and dignity through choice. A hospice program emphasizes palliative care with the client and family as active participants.

A client in hospice may become hospitalized, but the health care team will coordinate care between the home and inpatient setting. There is always the effort to keep clients at home for as long as possible. The family becomes the caregiver, but if the family cannot meet the client's basic needs, a home health aide or nurse becomes available to assist. The interdisciplinary hospice team provides psychological and physical resources needed for family support.

CARE AFTER DEATH.   If you care for a client at the time of death, you are the best person to provide **postmortem care.** It is important to care for the client's body with dignity and sensitivity. After death the body undergoes many physical changes. Therefore you should provide postmortem care as soon as possible to prevent tissue damage or disfigurement of body parts.

Federal and state legislation require hospitals to formulate policies and procedures based on current laws to validate death, identify potential organ or tissue donors, and to provide postmortem care. For transplantation of organs, remember that the need for ventilatory and circulatory support is necessary until vital organs can be harvested. The family must clearly understand that the equipment (i.e., ventilator) is not keeping the client alive but keeping the physical body in a state so that the organs will not be damaged prior to harvesting. Provide a private area to discuss all of the issues with the family. Offer the family clarification of what defines brain death because support systems must remain in place even after the client is pronounced "dead." Reinforce your explanations throughout the organ retrieval process. Nonvital tissues such as corneas, skin, long bones, and middle ear bones can be harvested when the client is proclaimed dead without maintaining vital functions. Each agency has a staff member designated for organ and tissue request. Organ and tissue donation must be agreed on by the family if no specific documented requests were made by the client before death. Review your state's organ retrieval laws regarding the formal consent process.

If a client dies while in a semiprivate room, temporarily transfer the roommate out of the room if possible to prevent that individual from having to listen to the activities surrounding postmortem care. Prepare the body for postmortem care by making it look as natural and comfortable as possible. A mortician can better prepare a body for interment when it is placed in a supine position with arms at the sides, palms down or across the abdomen. Place a small pillow or folded towel under the head to prevent discoloration from blood pooling. The eyelids usually remain closed if gently held down for a few seconds. Insert the client's dentures to maintain normal facial features. Wash soiled body parts, dress the body in a clean gown, comb or brush the hair, and cover the body to the shoulders with clean linen. Hospital policy will dictate whether tubes such as urinary catheters, intravenous lines, and endotracheal tubes are removed or tied off.

After cleaning the body and removing extraneous equipment, dirty linens, and extra supplies from the room, offer the family the opportunity to view the body. Provide a few private moments for the family to spend with the deceased. It may help to suggest that this is an opportunity to say "goodbye," especially if the family was not present at the time of death. If the family seems hesitant or anxious, give them time to think about it. If the family chooses not to view the body, accept their decision nonjudgmentally. If the family decides to view the body, accompany them into the room so that they are not alone. If the family wishes to have a representative from pastoral care present, arrange for the visit. Remove the client's jewelry and present it and other valuables the family, or allow the family to remove the jewelry themselves. Spend time with the grieving family to answer any questions or respond to any requests. At this time the family is your client.

After the family leave the room, place tags containing the client's name and other identifying information on the client's ankle, wrist, or toe. A rolled-up towel placed under the chin helps to keep the mouth closed. Remove the gown and wrap the body completely in either a shroud or body bag. Most

shroud or body bag kits contain absorbent pads that are placed under the perineal and rectal areas to collect oozing feces or urine from relaxed sphincter muscles. After wrapping the body, place another identification tag on the outside of the shroud or bag. If the client had a known transmissible infection, it may be necessary to use special labeling to alert those who move and store the remains. If family members are not present at the time of death, be sure the client's valuables and belongings are transported with the deceased. At this time either transporters deliver the body to the hospital morgue or the mortician will pick up the body from the client's room. Hospital policies are usually in place to ensure that transport of the body through hallways is as unobtrusive as possible.

Documentation of all of the events surrounding death is important to avoid misunderstandings and to clarify final event's in a client's life. Your notes should reflect time of death (pronounced by a physician), the name of the person who pronounced death, preparation of the body, stipulation of what equipment was left in place, and what valuables or possessions were either given to the family or left with the client. Also document the funeral home that is notified and time the body is removed to the morgue. Complete and accurate documentation offers a summary of activities that can become the focus for risk management or legal investigations.

THE GRIEVING NURSE.   When you have cared for a client for a period of time, it is possible to have deep personal feelings of loss and sadness for the family when the client dies. In these instances you may choose to cope with your own grief by attending the viewing at the mortuary or the funeral. It can be natural for you to go through the grieving process. If you work in an area where you experience multiple losses and fail to process them, you can experience bereavement overload. You might feel frustration, anger, guilt, sadness, anxiety, or other feelings of being overwhelmed. It is important to develop your own support systems that allow time away from the care setting and opportunities for you to share your feelings. Stress management techniques can help to restore your energy and continued enjoyment in your work.

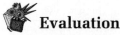 **Evaluation**

CLIENT CARE.   You will care for clients and families at every phase of the grief response. This requires you to remain aware of signs and symptoms of grief, even when clients are not specifically seeking care directly related to a loss. These same signs and symptoms offer criteria to evaluate whether a client is able to deal with a loss and progress through the grief process.

To determine the effectiveness of your nursing interventions, use evaluative measures to identify actual behavioral outcomes (Box 22-6). Compare actual behaviors with expected outcomes to determine the client's health status and the need to revise the plan of care. The goal for a terminally ill client and family is participation in the process of life review.

Outcome Evaluation for FOR THE HOLLOWAY FAMILY		Box 22-6
Nursing Action	Client Response/Finding	Achievement of Outcome
During home visit ask Mrs. Holloway to describe her involvement in care of her husband.	Wife continues to have difficulty helping Mr. Holloway with incontinence but reports that she is regularly assisting daughter during bathing.	Outcome partially met. Provide further encouragement to wife, discuss her continued concerns about providing incontinence care.
Observe Mr. Holloway's daughter provide a bath for her father.	Daughter is able to keep her father involved in conversation during the bath. She bathes him effectively; skin is clean and intact. There are no safety risks observed in her approach.	Outcome met. Reinforce daughter's success in bathing her father. Remain available to answer questions or clarify how to perform any bathing techniques.

Case Study EVALUATION

One week after discussing his proposed interventions with the Holloway family, Peter is pleased to observe on his next visit that Mrs. Holloway is helping Mr. Holloway with his bath. She explains that her daughter is "out taking a break, reading a book in the park." Mrs. Holloway has obtained a walker from the hospital supply store, and Mr. Holloway states that he feels much more secure when he uses it and is less fearful of walking. Mr. Holloway explains that he and his daughter have enjoyed looking through old photo albums together, and in the last day or two Mrs. Holloway has "wanted to join in the fun, too." They are enjoying their time as a family. Mrs. Holloway tells Peter that although Mr. Holloway's incontinence appears to be less, she remains uncomfortable with cleaning up after an accident. She also tells Peter that she and her daughter have inquired about a support group sponsored by the cancer society.

Documentation Note

Peter enters the following note on the client's chart at the home health agency: "Client reports that he is now using walker to ambulate in the home. States he feels more secure. Observed use of walker. Grip strong, posture erect, and gait steady with support. Wife more involved in bathing and interpersonal interaction with client. Wife and daughter working together to provide care. Daughter out of the home during visit, but mood of both client and his wife very positive, cheerful. Bath in progress at time of visit. Client's skin observed to be clear, without redness, tenderness, or evidence of tissue breakdown. Reportedly continues to have incontinent episodes daily. Client complains of recurrent right side pain every 3 to 4 hours, rapidly relieved with current pain medication. Is sleeping at night, waking only once for pain meds. Vital signs: T 98.0, pulse 68, resp. 18, BP 110/60. Family has contacted cancer society regarding support group. Plan is to continue supportive care and current medication management."

Evaluate outcomes of care by asking the client to describe the activities used to review important events in his or her life.

CLIENT EXPECTATIONS.   Maintain open communication with clients to allow them to evaluate their nursing care. Clients who have developed a good relationship with a nurse will feel comfortable in discussing their perceptions of "how things are going." When caring for a terminally ill client, take the time to frequently ask the family about their level of satisfaction. When a client offers feedback or suggestions, you should consider this a sign of a satisfactory relationship. Such suggestions indicate that the client and family perceive that they can approach you with their concerns. Once the client identifies new approaches or problems to be addressed, revise the plan of care to meet these emerging needs. Similarly, you should be encouraged when the client's feedback reflects that progress is being made toward achieving the goals of care.

Key Terms

acceptance, p. 507
actual loss, p. 506
anger, p. 507
anticipatory grief, p. 508
anxiolytics, p. 518
bargaining, p. 507
bereavement, p. 508

denial, p. 507
depression, p. 507
disorganization and despair, p. 508
grief, p. 507
grieving process, p. 507
hope, p. 510
hospice, p. 519
maturational loss, p. 506

mourning, p. 507
numbing, p. 507
palliative care, p. 517
perceived loss, p. 506
postmortem care, p. 519
reorganization, p. 508
situational loss, p. 506
yearning and searching, p. 508

Key Concepts

- The grieving process involves emotional, cognitive, and behavioral responses to an actual or perceived loss.
- Individuals experience different aspects of the grieving process at different times.
- Dying may lead to a grief response similar to that with other kinds of losses.
- Your support of a client's hope can help promote an effective grieving process associated with a loss.
- The individual's reaction to loss is influenced by many factors, including developmental stage, beliefs, roles, culture, relationships, and socioeconomic status.
- The process of mourning is often considered to be composed of "stages" or "phases," yet in reality these phases are not sequential, and the client may move back and forth along a continuum of grief.
- Assessment of the grieving client considers behavioral characteristics that suggest the client's stage of grieving.
- Grief resolution is a process that should be expected to take a year or more, with "anniversary reactions" common for several years following the loss.
- Nursing diagnoses focus on the type of grief experienced by clients or health-related problems common to grieving clients.
- Therapeutic communication is an important nursing intervention to assist the grieving and dying client in coping with loss.
- Nursing care of the grieving and dying client should promote the client's sense of identity, dignity, and self-esteem.
- Nursing care of the terminally ill focuses on promoting comfort and improving the quality of remaining life.
- As death approaches, a client should review and analyze values and beliefs pertinent to the meaning of life and death.
- Assess whether family members are willing to be involved in a dying client's care before using them as resources.
- Evaluation must also include the client's appraisal of the effectiveness of intervention. Clients and families are partners in care planning and delivery.
- Care after death involves caring for the body with dignity and sensitivity.
- The evaluation of nursing care for the grieving and dying client is ongoing and is based on identifiable behavioral changes through the grieving process.
- Your own loss history influences responses to client losses.
- Nurses who work with critically or terminally ill clients experience loss and grief.

Critical Thinking Activities

1. Mr. Vina has just been told that diagnostic tests reveal that his left leg cannot be saved. Surgical amputation is to be scheduled for tomorrow morning. You know that Mr. Vina is a construction worker who relies on the use of his legs. When you enter the client's room you overhear a nurse colleague say to Mr. Vina, "You need to think about the future; there are many options available for artificial legs." Is the nurse's comment appropriate at this time? Give a rationale for your answer.

2. Mrs. Sponszer is undergoing chemotherapy 3 times a week for invasive breast cancer. She is a strong woman who expresses faith that God will help her through this difficult time. Mrs. Sponszer has been active in her church in the past and she and her husband enjoy visiting her grandchildren. She was a full-time English teacher at a local middle school until just a year ago. Describe how you as the nurse might instill hope for Mrs. Sponszer across the following three dimensions: affective, behavioral, and affiliative.

3. Ms. Sarah has the terminal diagnosis of pancreatic cancer. Her mother is her closest relative but only visits for short periods. The client comments that she enjoys her mother's visits very much. Ms. Sarah is very weak and her principal symptoms at this time are nausea and abdominal pain. She enjoys reading and quilting when she feels able to participate in activities. Describe the priorities you would establish for Ms. Sarah's palliative care and how you would provide nursing care.

Review Questions

1. A middle-age man comes to your community clinic for his annual flu examination. In your discussion you learn that he still works at a local law firm; however, he has recently lost two important cases, and his boss has been applying pressure on him "to turn it around." The client may be experiencing:
   1. an actual loss.
   2. a perceived loss.
   3. a situational loss.
   4. a maturational loss.

2. Your client has been diagnosed with terminal brain cancer. When you visit him during rounds, he asks you whether the cancer could have been caused by something he ate or perhaps following exposure to some chemical toxin. Your client is likely experiencing.
   1. Bowlby's phase of numbing.
   2. Kübler-Ross's stage of acceptance.
   3. Worden's task of emotionally relocating.
   4. Bowlby's phase of disorganization and despair.

3. As a community health nurse your job is to provide grief counseling for the citizens of your town, where a major flood has occurred. The loss associated with flooding is best described as:
   1. an actual loss.
   2. a perceived loss.
   3. a situational loss.
   4. a maturational loss.

4. Since the death of his wife, your client has assumed full responsibility for the care of his children. He has noticed over the last few weeks that friends are calling less often. He is most likely in the following phase of mourning:
   1. anticipatory grieving.
   2. Worden's task III of mourning.
   3. Kübler Ross's phase of bargaining.
   4. Bowlby's disorganization and despair.
5. A factor that uniquely influences an older adult's grief response is:
   1. cultural background.
   2. socioeconomic resources.
   3. sense of contributions in life.
   4. support available from family members.

6. A 16-year-old has been admitted to the intensive care unit after suffering a closed head injury in a head-on car collision. The physician and nurse are preparing to approach the family to consider donation of heart and lungs. When working with families in this situation, it is important to explain that:
   1. the ventilator is being used to prevent brain death.
   2. the ventilator maintains organ perfusion until time for harvesting.
   3. tissues such as corneas can be harvested only if the client remains ventilated.
   4. organ donation can occur only if the client has made a request to donate organs in the past.

References

Barbus AJ: The dying person's bill of rights, *Am J Nurs* 75:99, 1975.

Bierman E and others: Assessing access as a first step towards improving the quality of care for very old adults, *J Ambul Care Manage* 21(3):17, 1998.

Blackhall LJ and others: Ethnicity and attitudes towards life-sustaining technology. *Social Science in Medicine* 48:1779, 1999.

Bowlby J: *Attachment and loss,* vol 3, Loss, sadness, and depression, New York, 1980, Basic Books.

Callahan D: Terminating life-sustaining treatment of the demented, *Hastings Cent Rep* 25:25, 1995.

Doka KJ: *Living with life-threatening illness: a guide for patients, their families, and caregivers,* New York, 1993, Lexington.

Engel GL: Grief and grieving, *Am J Nurs* 64:93, 1964.

Erickson E: *Childhood and society,* New York, 1982, Norton.

Farber SJ and others: Issues in end-of-life care: family practice faculty perceptions, *J Fam Pract* 48(7):525, 1999.

Forbes and others

Fryback PB: Health for people with a terminal diagnosis, *Nurs Sci Q* 6(3):147, 1993.

Hospice care, *Mayo Clin Health Lett* 15(7):4, 1997.

Kübler Ross E: *On death and dying,* New York, 1969, Macmillan.

Miller JF, Powers MJ: Development of an instrument to measure hope, *Nurs Res* 37(1):6, 1988.

Nowotny M: Every tomorrow a vision of hope, *J Psychosoc Oncol* 9(3):117, 1991.

Poncar PJ: Inspiring hope in the oncology patient, *J Psychosoc Nurs Mental Health Serv* 32(1):33, 1994.

Post-White J and others: Hope, spirituality, sense of coherence, and quality of life in patients with cancer, *Oncology Nurs Forum* 23(10):1571, 1996.

Rousseau P: Palliative care in managed Medicare—reasons for hope—and for concern, *Geriatrics* 53(11):59, 1998.

Stepnick A, Perry T: Preventing spiritual distress in the dying client, *J Psychosoc Nurs* 30(1):17, 1992.

SUPPORT Principal Investigators: A controlled trial to improve care for seriously ill hospitalized patients, *JAMA* 274:1591, 1995.

Tarzian AJ: Caring for dying patients who have air hunger, *Image J Nurs Sch* 32:137, 2000.

Tilden VP and others: Family decision-making to withdraw life-sustaining treatments from hospitalized patients, *Nurs Res* 50:105, 2001.

Tolle SW and others: Family reports of barriers to optimal care of the dying, *Nurs Res* 49:310, 2000.

Weissman DE and others: Pain assessment and management in the long-term care setting, *Theor Med Bioeth* 20(1):31, 1999.

Worden JW: *Grief counseling and grief therapy,* New York, 1982, Springer.

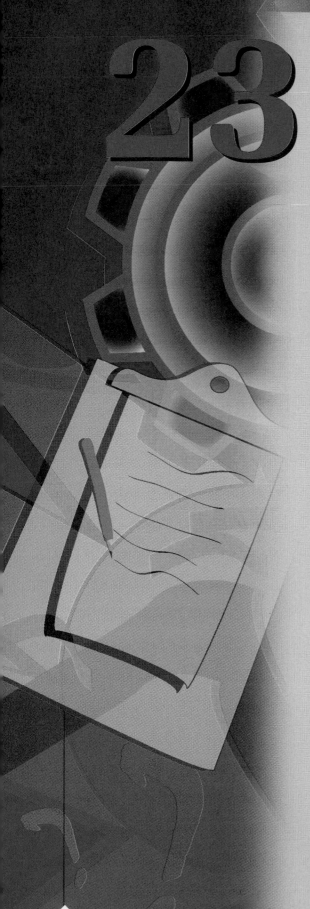

23

Managing Client Care

Objectives

- Define the key terms listed.
- Discuss the importance of education in professional nursing practice.
- Describe the purpose for professional standards of nursing practice.
- Differentiate among the types of nursing care delivery models.
- Describe the elements of decentralized decision making.
- Discuss the ways in which a nurse manager can support staff involvement in a decentralized decision-making model.
- Discuss ways to apply clinical care coordination skills in nursing practice.
- Discuss principles to follow in the appropriate delegation of client care activities.
- Differentiate among structure, process, and quality outcomes.
- Describe an example of a quality improvement project on a nursing unit.

As a student nurse, it is important for you to acquire the necessary knowledge and competencies that ultimately allow you to practice as an entry-level staff nurse (Box 23-1). Regardless of the type of setting you eventually choose to work in as a staff nurse, you will be responsible for practicing professional standards of care, using organizational resources, participating in organizational routines while providing direct client care, using time productively, collaborating with all members of the health care team, and using certain leadership characteristics to manage others on the nursing team (Wywialowski, 1997). The delivery of nursing care within the health care system is a challenge because of the changes that are influencing health professionals, clients, and health care organizations (see Chapter 2). However, change offers opportunities. As you develop the knowledge and skills to become a staff nurse you will learn what it takes to effectively manage the clients you care for and to take the initiative in becoming a leader among your professional colleagues.

Entry-Level Staff Nurse Competencies	Box 23-1

Identify organizational resources (people, equipment, services), and determine when they are needed.
Work within various nursing care delivery models.
Use position descriptions to establish the scope and limitations of one's own and other nursing team members' practices.
Manage time purposefully and productively.
Prioritize client needs and related care.
Exhibit flexibility in providing care within available time constraints.
Show initiative and creativity as leadership qualities.
Use decision-making skills.
Defend one's own decisions.
Work with other health team members.
Resolve conflicts within the health team.
Delegate care activities appropriately.

Modified from Wywialowski EF: *Managing client care*, ed 2, St. Louis, 1997, Mosby.

PROFESSIONALISM

Nursing is a profession. A person who acts professionally is conscientious in actions, knowledgeable in the subject, and responsible to self and others. Professions possess the following characteristics.

- An extended education of members and a basic liberal education foundation
- A theoretical body of knowledge leading to defined skills, abilities, and norms
- Provision of a specific service
- Autonomy in decision making and practice
- A code of ethics for practice

Nursing shares each of these characteristics, offering an opportunity for the growth and enrichment of all its members.

Professional Registered Nurse Education

As a profession, nursing requires that its members possess a significant amount of education. There are various educational routes for becoming a **professional registered nurse (RN)**. Currently in the United States an individual can become an RN by completion of an associate degree, diploma, or baccalaureate degree program. In Canada there are currently only diploma and baccalaureate degrees. Nursing education provides the solid foundation for practice, and it must respond to changes in health care created by scientific and technological advances.

After completion of the professional education program, RN candidates in the United States must pass the National Council Licensure Examination for Registered Nurses (NCLEX-RN), which is administered by the individual state boards of nursing. Regardless of candidates' educational preparation, the examination for RN licensure is the same in every state, ensuring a standardized minimum knowledge base for the client population nurses serve. In Canada the CNA Testing Service (CNATS) administers an examination to qualified candidates in each province. Whether nurses can practice in a state or province other than their own depends on the agreement between the states or provinces involved.

The opportunities in the nursing profession are limitless, but often they require a professional nurse to pursue additional education. A nurse may choose to work toward certification in a specific area of nursing practice. Minimum practice requirements are set based on the certification the nurse is seeking, such as in critical care, oncology, or gerontology. National nursing organizations, such as the American Nurses Association (ANA), have many types of certification that nurses can work toward. After passing the initial examination, the nurse maintains certification by ongoing continuing education and clinical practice.

Advanced Education

There are roles in nursing that require advanced educational degrees. A master's degree in nursing (e.g., master of arts in nursing, [MA], master in nursing [MN], master of science in nursing [MSN]) is generally required for nurses seeking roles as nurse educator, clinical nurse specialist, nurse administrator, or nurse practitioner. The degree provides the advanced clinician with strong skills in nursing science and theory with emphasis in the basic sciences and research-based clinical practice. There are also roles within nursing that require doctoral degrees. Expanding clinical and research roles, new areas of nursing, such as nursing informatics, and the influential presence of nursing in public policy and health care planning are just a few reasons for increasing the number of doctorally prepared nurses. Doctorally prepared nurses are needed to educate beginning nurses and those seeking advanced academic and clinical preparation.

Licensed Practical Nurse Education

A licensed practical or vocational nurse is trained in basic nursing techniques and direct client care. The **licensed practical** nurse **(LPN)** or **licensed vocational nurse (LVN)** practices under the supervision of a registered nurse in a hospital or community health practice setting. An LPN, or in Canada a registered nurse's assistant (RNA), generally receives 1 year of education and training in a community college or other agency. The LPN or LVN is licensed by a board after completing the educational program and passing the licensure examination.

Theory

The practice of professional nursing and nursing knowledge has been developed through nursing theories, global perspectives that help to describe, predict, or prescribe activities for the practice of nursing. Theoretical models provide frameworks for how nurses practice. Typically a theoretical model is integrated through a nursing school's curriculum. Examples include Orem's self-care deficit theory, Benner's primacy of caring, and Roy's adaptation theory. There are also nursing organizations that adopt a nursing theory to serve as the foundation for the organization's standards of nursing care. The ongoing development of nursing theory or nursing science involves generating knowledge to advance and support nursing practice and health care (Chinn and Kramer, 1999).

Service

Nursing is a service profession and a vital and indispensable component of the health care delivery system. Nurses today require a consumer-focused and service-based practice. Clients are more aware and knowledgable about their health care problems, their options, and their rights. As a nurse you must work with the client and family, individualizing care while incorporating their preferences and expectations. Show respect for clients by providing care on time, displaying a caring attitude, considering clients' cultural and social differences, and collaborating with necessary health care providers to ensure a smooth continuation of care from one setting to the next.

Autonomy

Autonomy is an essential element of professional nursing. Autonomy means that a person is reasonably independent and self-governing in decision making and practice. Autonomy is attained through experience, advanced education, and the support of an organization that values the independent role of the nurse. With increased autonomy comes greater responsibility and accountability for the performance of nursing care activities.

Code of Ethics

Nursing has a **code of ethics** that defines the principles by which nurses function (see Chapter 4). In addition, nurses incorporate their own values and ethics into practice. The ANA's *Code of Ethics for Nurses With Interpretive Statements* provides a guide for carrying out nursing responsibilities to ensure quality nursing care and to provide for the ethical obligations of the profession (American Nurses Association, 2001).

STANDARDS OF NURSING PRACTICE

Nursing is a helping, independent profession that provides services that contribute to the health of people. Three essential components of professional nursing are care, cure, and coordination. The care aspect is more than "to take care of"; it is also "caring about." Caring is relational and requires the nurse to understand the client's needs at a level that permits individualization of nursing therapies (see Chapter 15). The promotion of health and healing is the cure aspect of professional nursing. To cure is to assist clients in understanding their health problems and helping them to cope. The cure aspect involves the administration of treatments, and the use of clinical nursing judgment in determining, on the basis of client outcomes, whether the plan of care is effective. Coordination of care involves organizing and timing medical and other professional and technical services to meet the needs of a client. Often a client requires many services simultaneously in order to be well cared for. A professional nurse also supervises, teaches, and directs all of those who are involved in nursing care.

As an independent profession, nursing has increasingly set its own standards for practice. Standards of nursing practice offer guidelines for how nurses are to perform professionally and how they are to exercise the care, cure, and coordination aspects of nursing. Clinical, academic, and administrative nurse experts have developed standards of nursing practice. The ANA has published *Standards of Professional Performance* (Table 23-1).

Standards of Care

In the practice setting it is important to have objective guidelines for providing and evaluating nursing care. Standards of nursing care are developed and established on the basis of strong scientific research and the work of clinical nurse experts. An organization may adopt a general set of standards for nursing care, such as those established by the ANA (American Nurses Association, 1998) (Table 23-2). Individual nursing units or work groups can also establish standards of care to address the unique needs of clients for whom they care. For example, an oncology nursing unit might develop standards of care for pain management and palliative care. Standards of care are important if a legal dispute arises over whether a nurse practiced appropriately in a particular case (see Chapter 3). More importantly standards of care establish the guideline for nursing excellence within an organization.

BUILDING A NURSING TEAM

As educated professionals, nurses want to enjoy their work and achieve success in delivering the best care to their clients (Trofino, 1996). Your education and the commitment you make in practicing within established standards and guidelines will ensure a rewarding professional career. It is also important to work as a member of a cohesive and strong nursing

ANA Standards of Professional Performance

Table 23-1

Standard	Definition	Measurement Criteria
I: Quality of care	The nurse systematically evaluates the quality and effectiveness of nursing practice.	Participates in quality-of-care activities Practice changes are a result of quality-of-care activities Quality-of-care activities are used to initiate changes throughout the health care delivery system
II: Performance appraisal	The nurse evaluates one's own nursing practice in relation to professional practice standards and relevant statutes and regulations.	Engages in performance appraisal on a regular basis Seeks constructive feedback regarding one's own practice Takes action to achieve goals identified during performance appraisal Participates in peer review as appropriate Practice reflects knowledge of current professional practice standards, laws, and regulations
III: Education	The nurse acquires and maintains current knowledge and competency in nursing practice.	Participates in ongoing educational activities related to clinical knowledge and professional issues Seeks experiences to maintain clinical skills Seeks knowledge and skills appropriate to the practice setting
IV: Collegiality	The nurse interacts with, and contributes to the professional development of, peers and other health care providers as colleagues.	Shares knowledge and skills with colleagues Provides peers with constructive feedback regarding their practice Interacts with colleagues to enhance one's own professional nursing practice Contributes to an environment that is conducive to clinical education of nursing students as appropriate Contributes to a supportive and healthy work environment
V: Ethics	The nurse's decisions and actions on behalf of patients are determined in an ethical manner.	Practice is guided by the *Code for Nurses* Maintains patient confidentiality Acts as a patient advocate Delivers care in a nonjudgmental and nondiscriminatory manner that is sensitive to patient diversity Delivers care in a manner that preserves patient autonomy, dignity, and rights Seeks available resources in formulating ethical decisions
VI: Collaboration	The nurse collaborates with the patient, family, and other health care providers in providing patient care.	Communicates with the patient, significant others, and health care providers regarding patient care and nursing's role in the provision of care Collaborates with the patient, family, and other health care providers in the formulation of overall goals and the plan of care and in the decisions related to care and delivery of services Consults with health care providers for patient care as needed Makes referrals, including provisions for continuity of care, as needed

VII: Research	The nurse uses research findings in practice.	Utilizes best available evidence, preferably research data, to develop the plan of care and interventions
		Participates in research activities as appropriate to the nurse's education and position, such as the following:
		    Identifying clinical problems suitable for nursing research
		    Participating in data collection
		    Participating in a unit, organization, or community research committee
		    Sharing research activities with others
		    Conducting research
		    Critiquing research for application to practice
		Uses research findings in the development of policies, procedures, and practice guidelines for patient care

VIII: Resource utilization	The nurse considers factors related to safety, effectiveness, and cost in planning and delivering patient care.	Evaluates factors related to safety, effectiveness, availability, and cost when practice options would result in the same expected patient outcome Assists the patient and family in identifying and securing appropriate and available services to address health-related needs Assigns or delegates tasks as defined by the state nurse practice acts and according to the knowledge and skills of the designated caregiver Assigns or delegates tasks based on the needs and condition of the patient, the potential for harm, the stability of the patient's condition, the complexity of the task, and the predictability of the outcome Assists the patient and family in becoming informed consumers about the cost, risks, and benefits of treatment and care

Reprinted with permission from American Nurses Association: *Standards of clinical practice*, 2nd edition, © 1998 American Nursing Publishing, American Nurses Foundation/American Nurses Association, Washington, DC.

team. An empowering work environment is one that brings out the best in a professional, concentrating on effective client care systems (e.g., client assessment, referral mechanisms, physician-nurse collaboration), supporting risk taking and innovation, focusing on results and rewards, and offering professional opportunities for growth and advancement.

It takes an excellent nurse manager and an excellent nursing staff to achieve an enriching work environment. Together a manager and the nursing staff must share a philosophy of care for their work unit. A philosophy of care incorporates the professional nursing staff's values and concerns for the way in which clients should be viewed and cared for. For example, a philosophy should address the nursing unit's purpose, how staff will work with clients and families, and the standards of care for the work unit. A philosophy is a vision for how nursing is to be practiced. It should inspire the soul and be something about which all staff members can be proud (Hansten and Washburn, 1999). Integral to the philosophy of care is the selection of a nursing care delivery model and management structure that support professional nursing practice.

Nursing Care Delivery Models

A nursing care delivery model should be designed to help nurses achieve desirable outcomes for their clients. Key factors contributing to this success are decision-making authority for nurses giving direct care and effective methods of communicating with their colleagues, with physicians, and with other health care providers (Duchene, 1992). There are a variety of nursing care delivery models.

FUNCTIONAL NURSING.   Functional nursing is a model of care that is task-focused, not client-focused. In this model, tasks are divided, with one nurse assuming responsibility for specific tasks, for example, hygiene and dressing changes, whereas another nurse may assume responsibility for medication administration. Typically a lead nurse responsible for a specific shift assigns available nursing staff members according to their qualifications, their particular abilities, and tasks to be completed. Nurses become highly competent with the tasks that are repeatedly assigned to them. The major disadvantages of functional nursing are problems with continuity of care, absence of a holistic view of clients, and the possibility that care will become mechanical (Duchene, 1992). In other words, a task-focused approach does not ensure that patient care needs are met shift to shift. Communication is not always clear, because a single nurse is not responsible for the overall care of the client.

TEAM NURSING.   In team nursing an RN leads a team that is composed of other RNs, LPNs or LVNs, and nurse assistants or technicians. The team members provide direct client care to groups of clients, under the direction of the RN team leader. In this model, nurse assistants are given client assignments rather than being assigned particular nursing tasks.

The team leader develops client care plans, coordinates care delivered by the nursing team, provides care requiring complex nursing skills, problem solves with physicians and members of other disciplines, and assists the team in evaluating the effectiveness of their care (Wywialowski, 1997). Limitations to the model include the lack of time the team leader spends with clients. Depending on the mix of staff members, this may mean that clients see an RN infrequently. Risks exist if an RN is unable to make necessary client assessments and be involved in important clinical decision making. Nurses may not be assigned to the same clients each day, which potentially may cause lack of continuity of care. An advantage of team nursing is the collaborative style that encourages each member of the team to help the other members.

TOTAL PATIENT CARE.   Total patient care delivery was the original care delivery model developed during Florence Nightingale's time. A registered nurse (RN) is responsible for all aspects of care for one or more clients. The RN may delegate aspects of care to an LPN or unlicensed staff, but retains accountability for care of all assigned clients. The nurse works directly with the client, family, physician, and health care team members. The model typically has a shift-based focus. The same nurse does not necessarily care for the same client over time. Continuity of care from shift to shift or day to day can be a problem if staff members do not clearly communicate client needs to one another.

PRIMARY NURSING.   The primary nursing model of care delivery was developed with the aim of placing RNs at the bedside and improving the professional relationships among staff members (Manthey, 1980). The model became more popular in the 1970s and early 1980s as hospitals began to employ more RNs. Primary nursing supports a philosophy regarding nurse and client relationships. Primary nursing is a model of care delivery whereby an RN assumes responsibility for a caseload of clients over time. Typically the RN selects the clients for his or her caseload and cares for the same clients during their hospitalization or stay in the health care setting. The RN assesses client needs, develops a care plan, and ensures that appropriate nursing interventions are delivered to the client.

Primary nursing maintains continuity of care across shifts, days, or visits. It can be applied in any health care setting. When a primary nurse is off-duty, associate nurses, including LPNs or other RNs follow through with the developed plan of care. If there are differences in opinion as to client needs, associates and primary nurses collaborate to redefine the plan as needed.

Although primary nursing may require the presence of more professional staff members, this does not mean that the model is more costly. Care consistently managed by a single professional can minimize delays in therapies, improve collaboration with other professionals, and enhance the client-nurse relationship.

CASE MANAGEMENT.   Case management is a delivery of care approach that coordinates and links health care services to

ANA Standards of Care	Table 23-2

Standard	Measurement Criteria
Assessment The nurse collects patient health data.	Data collection involves the patient, significant others, and health-care providers when appropriate. The priority of data collection is determined by the patient's immediate condition or needs. Pertinent data are collected using appropriate assessment techniques. Relevant data are documented in a retrievable form. The data collection process is systematic and ongoing.
Nursing Diagnosis The nurse analyzes the assessment data in determining diagnoses.	Diagnoses are derived from the assessment data. Diagnoses are validated with the patient, significant others, and health care providers, when possible. Diagnoses are documented in a manner that facilitates the determination of expected outcomes and plan of care.
The nurse identifies expected outcomes individualized to the patient.	Outcomes are derived from the diagnoses. Outcomes are mutually formulated with the patient and health care providers, when possible. Outcomes are culturally appropriate and realistic in relation to the patient's present and potential capabilities. Outcomes are attainable in relation to resources available to the patient. Outcomes include a time estimate for attainment. Outcomes provide direction for continuity of care. Outcomes are documented as measurable goals.
Planning The nurse develops a plan of care that prescribes interventions to attain expected outcomes.	The plan is individualized to the patient and patient's condition or needs. The plan is developed with the patient, significant others, and health care providers, when appropriate. The plan reflects current nursing practice. The plan provides for continuity of care. Priorities for care are established. The plan is documented.
Implementation The nurse implements the interventions identified in the plan of care.	Interventions are consistent with the established plan of care. Interventions are implemented in a safe and appropriate manner. Interventions are documented.
Evaluation The nurse evaluates the patient's progress toward attainment of outcomes.	Evaluation is systematic, ongoing, and criterion-based. The patient, significant others, and health care providers are involved in the evaluation process, when appropriate. Ongoing assessment data are used to revise diagnoses, outcomes, and the plan of care as needed. Revisions in diagnoses, outcomes, and the plan of care are documented. The effectiveness of interventions is evaluated in relation to outcomes. The patient's responses to interventions are documented.

Reprinted with permission from American Nurses Association: *Standards of clinical practice,* 2nd edition, © 1998 American Nurses Publishing, American Nurses Foundation/American Nurses Association, Washington, DC.

clients and their families (see Chapter 2). Case management involves a professional nurse maintaining responsibility for client care from admission to after discharge (Duchene, 1992). What is unique about case management is that clinicians, either as individuals or as part of a collaborative group, oversee the management of clients with specific case types (e.g., clients with specific diagnoses presenting complex nursing and medical problems) and are usually held accountable for some standard of cost management and quality. A case manager coordinates a client's acute care in the hospital, for example, and then follows the client after discharge home. Case managers may not provide direct care but instead they collaborate with and supervise the care delivered by other staff members and actively coordinate client discharge planning. Many organizations use critical pathways, which are multidisciplinary treatment plans, in a case management delivery system (see Chapter 2).

Box 23-2

Responsibilities of the Nurse Manager

Assist staff in establishing annual goals for the unit and the systems needed to accomplish goals.

Monitor professional nursing standards of practice on the unit.

Develop an ongoing staff development plan, including one for new employees.

Recruit new employees (interview and hire).

Conduct routine staff evaluations.

Establish self as a role model for positive customer service (customers include clients, families, and other health care team members).

Serve as an advocate for the nursing staff to the administration of the institution.

Submit staffing schedules for the unit.

Conduct regular client rounds and help to solve client or family complaints.

Establish and implement a quality improvement (QI) plan for the unit.

Review and recommend new equipment needs for the unit.

Conduct regular staff meetings.

Conduct rounds with physicians.

Establish and support necessary staff and interdisciplinary committees.

Decentralized Decision Making

Decentralized management, in which decision making is moved down to the level of staff, is very common within health care organizations. It is clear that progressive organizations achieve more when employees at all levels are actively involved. As a result the role of a nurse manager has become critical in the management of effective nursing unit or groups. The diverse responsibilities assumed by nursing managers are highlighted in Box 23-2. To make decentralized decision making work, managers must know how to move decision making down to the lowest level possible. On a nursing unit, it is important for all staff members (RNs, LPNs, LVNs), nurse assistants, and unit secretaries to feel involved. Key elements to the decision-making process are responsibility, authority, and accountability (Cox, 1995).

Responsibility refers to the duties and activities that an individual is employed to perform. A professional nurse's responsibilities in a given role are outlined in a position description describing the nurse's duties in client care and in participating as a member of the nursing unit. Responsibility reflects ownership; it must be given by the individual who oversees the employee, and it must be accepted by the employee. For example, a primary nurse is responsible for completing a nursing assessment of all assigned clients and for developing a plan of care that addresses each of the client's nursing diagnoses. As the plan of care is delivered, the primary nurse is responsible for evaluating whether the plan is successful. This responsibility becomes a work ethic for the nurse in delivering excellent client care.

Authority refers to the right to act in areas where an individual has been given and accepts responsibility (Cox,

1995). For example, a primary nurse, managing a caseload of clients, may discover that members of the nursing team did not follow through on a discharge teaching plan for an assigned client. The primary nurse has the authority to consult other nurses to learn why recommendations on the plan of care were not followed and to choose appropriate teaching strategies for the client that all members of the team will follow. The primary nurse has the final authority in selecting the best course of action for the client's care.

Accountability refers to individuals being answerable for their actions. It involves follow-up and a reflective analysis of one's decisions to evaluate their effectiveness (Cox, 1995). A primary nurse is accountable for his or her clients' outcomes. In the example above, the primary nurse is accountable for ensuring that the client learns the information necessary to improve self-care. By using authority in bringing the nursing team together, the primary nurse determines if collaboration was successful, if continuity in teaching occurred, and if the client and family were able to relate the information taught.

A successful decentralized nursing unit exercises the three elements of decision making on an ongoing basis. An effective manager sets the same expectations for the staff in how decisions are made. Staff members must feel comfortable in expressing differences of opinion and in challenging ways in which the team functions, while recognizing their own responsibility, authority, and accountability. Ultimately, decentralized decision making is the vehicle for realizing the unit's vision of what professional nursing care should be.

STAFF INVOLVEMENT. When decentralized decision making exists on a nursing unit all staff members actively participate in unit activities (Figure 23-1). Because the work environment promotes participation, all staff members benefit from the knowledge and skills of the entire work group. If the staff learns to value knowledge and the contributions of colleagues, better client care becomes an outcome. The nursing manager supports staff involvement through a variety of ways:

1. *Establishment of nursing practice or problem-solving committees.* Staff committees establish and maintain professional nursing practice on a unit. It becomes important for the committees to focus on client outcomes rather than only work issues (e.g., work schedules, supply issues) in order to ensure quality care is delivered on the unit (Hansten and Washburn, 1999). Practice committees become involved in activities such as the review and revision of standards of care, development of policy and procedure, and resolution of repeated client satisfaction issues. A senior staff member usually chairs a committee. Managers might not sit on the committee, but they receive regular reports of committee progress. The nature of work on the nursing unit determines committee membership. At times, members of other disciplines, for example, pharmacy, respiratory therapy, or clinical nutrition, might participate on practice committees.

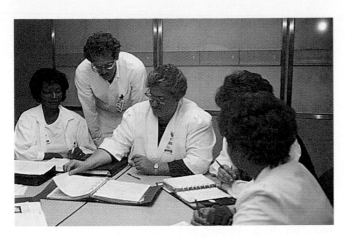

FIGURE **23-1** Nursing staff collaborating on practice issues.

2. *Nurse/physician collaborative practice.* The unit's delivery of care model influences how nurse and physician collaboration can best be fostered. If the unit practices team nursing, it is important for team leaders to regularly participate in physician rounds. If the unit practices primary nursing, the physician should communicate either with each primary nurse or the associate nurse who is assuming care for the client on that day. The manager avoids taking care of problems for the staff. Instead, staff members learn to keep physicians informed on important information about their clients. Open communication is critical.

3. *Interdisciplinary collaboration.* The emphasis on efficiency in health care delivery brings all members of the health care team together. The staff must recognize the importance of prompt referrals and timely communication. Interdisciplinary collaboration involves bringing representatives of the various disciplines together in practice projects, in-services, conferences, and staff meetings.

4. *Staff communication.* In the present health care environment, it is difficult for a manager to get a clear, accurate, and timely message to all members of a nursing staff. Staff members can quickly become uneasy and distrusting if they fail to hear about planned changes on their unit. However, a manager cannot assume total responsibility for all communication. Instead, the manager establishes a variety of approaches to ensure information is communicated quickly and accurately to all staff members. For example, many managers distribute biweekly or monthly newsletters of ongoing unit or health care agency activities. Minutes of staff and practice committee meetings should be posted in an accessible location for all staff members to read. When vital issues regarding the operations of the unit or the organization are to be discussed, the manager should conduct staff meetings. When the unit has practice or quality improvement committees, each member should be assigned responsibility to communicate directly to a select number of staff members. In that way all staff members are contacted and given the opportunity to comment.

5. *Staff education.* A professional nursing staff always grows in knowledge. It is impossible to remain knowledgeable of current medical and nursing practice trends without ongoing education. The nurse manager is responsible for giving staff members the necessary opportunities to remain competent in their practice. This involves planning in-services, sending staff members to professional conferences, and having members present case studies or practice issues during staff meetings.

Leadership Skills for Nursing Students

As you begin to assume clinical assignments, it is important for you not only to learn how to care for clients but also to become a responsible and productive team member. Start by always taking responsibility and accountability for the care you provide your clients. Learn to become a leader by making good clinical decisions, learning from mistakes and seeking guidance, collaborating closely with professional nurses, and striving to improve your performance during each client interaction. Use the following skills to become a competent professional.

CLINICAL CARE COORDINATION. Learn to acquire the skills necessary to deliver client care competently and in a timely and effective manner. In the beginning this might involve only one client, but eventually it will involve groups of clients. Clinical care coordination includes clinical decision making, priority setting, organizational skills, use of resources, time management, and evaluation.

CLINICAL DECISIONS. When you begin a client assignment always conduct a focused but complete assessment of the client's condition and ask what outcomes the client expects in his or her care. This will allow you to know the client so that you can get a grasp of the client's situation, enabling you to recognize the client's responses and patterns during care. Your assessment will also direct you in making accurate clinical decisions as to your client's needs (see Chapter 5). Failing to make accurate clinical judgments about a client can have undesirable outcomes. The client's condition might worsen or remain the same when the potential for improvement has been lost. An important lesson in clinical care is to be thorough. Always attend to the client, look for any cues (obvious or subtle) that point to a pattern of findings, and direct your assessment to explore the pattern further. Accurate clinical decision making keeps you focused on the proper course of action. Never hesitate to ask for assistance when a client's assessment reveals a changing clinical condition.

PRIORITY SETTING. As you begin to make clinical judgments (including nursing diagnoses), a picture of the client's total needs begins to form. While planning care, you must then decide what client needs or problems must be addressed first (see Chapter 6). Wywialowski (1997) describes categories of priority nursing needs of individual clients:

• First-order priority needs—an immediate threat to a client's survival or safety, such as a physiologic episode of obstructed airway, loss of consciousness, or a psychological episode of an anxiety attack

- Second-order priority needs—actual problems for which the client or family has requested immediate help, such as comfort measures, nausea, or a full bladder or bowel
- Third-order priority needs—relatively urgent actual or potential problems that the client or family does not recognize, such as monitoring for postoperative complications, or anticipating teaching needs of a client who may be unaware of side effects of a drug
- Fourth-order priority needs—actual or potential problems with which the client or family may need help in the future, such as teaching for self-care in the home

Many clients can have all four types of priorities, requiring you to make careful judgments in choosing your course of action. Obviously first-order priority needs demand your immediate attention. When a client has diverse priority needs, sometimes it helps to focus on the client's basic needs. For example, a client who is immobilized in traction might report being uncomfortable from being in the same position. The dietary assistant arrives in the room to deliver a meal tray. Instead of immediately assisting the client with the meal, you reposition the client and offer basic hygiene measures. The client will likely become more interested in eating after being made to feel comfortable. The client will also then be more receptive to any instruction you wish to provide.

Over time you will also be required to meet the priority needs of a group of clients. This requires you to know the priority needs of each client within the group: you must assess each client's needs as soon as possible while addressing first- and second-priority needs in a timely manner (Wywialowski, 1997). To identify which clients require assessment first, you rely on information from the change-of-shift report, the agency's classification system that identifies client acuity, and information from the medical record. Over time you will learn to spontaneously rank clients' needs by priority or urgency. Remember to think about the resources you have available, be flexible in recognizing that priority needs can change, and consider how you can use your time wisely.

Priorities must also be made on the basis of client expectations. You might have an excellent plan of care established, but if the client is resistant to certain therapies or disagrees with your approach, little success will be gained. Working closely with the client is important. Share the priorities you define with the client to establish a level of agreement and cooperation.

ORGANIZATIONAL SKILLS.　Implementing a plan of care requires you to be effective and efficient. Effective use of time entails doing the right things, whereas efficient use of time entails doing things right (Wywialowski, 1997). As you address your client's priorities, certain organizational skills will ensure that you become more efficient. Efficient care conserves effort and minimizes interruptions. One way to be efficient is by combining various nursing activities, in other words, doing more than one thing at a time. This of course

takes practice. For example, during medication administration or while obtaining a specimen, combine therapeutic communication skills, teaching interventions, and assessment and evaluation. Always try to establish and strengthen relationships with clients and use any client contact as an opportunity to convey important information. You must always attend to the client's behaviors and responses to therapies to assess if any new problems are developing and to evaluate responses to interventions.

A nursing procedure is easier to perform if you are well-organized. Prepare in advance by having all necessary equipment and supplies available and making sure the client is prepared. Be sure the client is comfortable, positioned correctly for the procedure, and well-informed to increase the likelihood the procedure will go smoothly. Sometimes you may require the assistance of colleagues to perform or complete a procedure (e.g., helping to turn a client for an enema, handing supplies during a dressing change). It is always wise to have the work area organized and preliminary steps completed before asking colleagues for assistance.

When you try to deliver care based on established priorities, events may occur that can interfere with your plans. For example, just as you begin to provide a client's bath, the x-ray technician enters to do a portable chest film. Once the x-ray film is completed, the phlebotomist arrives to draw a sample of blood. Your priorities seem to conflict with the priorities of other health care personnel. It is important to always keep the client's needs as the center of attention. The client may have been experiencing symptoms earlier that required a chest film and laboratory work. In such a case it is important to be sure the diagnostic tests are completed. In another example, the client might be waiting to visit family and the chest film was a routine order from 2 days ago. The client's condition has since stabilized, and the x-ray technician is willing to return later to shoot the film. Attending to the client's hygiene and comfort so that family can visit is more of a priority at this time.

USE OF RESOURCES.　Another important aspect of clinical care coordination is appropriate use of resources. Resources in this case include members of the health care team. In any setting the administration of client care occurs more smoothly when staff members work together. As a student you should always look for opportunities to help other staff members, for example, answer a call light, help a staff member make a bed, or offer to sit and talk with another nurse's client. Also, never hesitate to ask staff members to assist you, especially when there is the opportunity to make a procedure or activity more comfortable and safer for the client. For example, assistance in turning, positioning, and ambulating clients is frequently necessary when clients experience impaired mobility. Having a staff member assist with handling equipment and supplies during more complicated procedures, such as catheter insertion or a dressing change, can help make procedures more efficient. This is an excellent way for you to learn how to delegate aspects of care activities and to work with assistive personnel.

There are also times you must recognize personal limitations and use professional resources for assistance. For example, you may assess a client and find relevant clinical signs and symptoms but be unfamiliar with the client's underlying physical condition. Consulting an RN leads to confirmation of findings and assurance that the proper course of action is taken for the client. Throughout your professional career there are always new experiences. A leader knows his or her limitations and seeks professional colleagues for guidance and support.

TIME MANAGEMENT.   Much of the stress experienced by nurses results from the perception that client needs must be met all at once (Gustafson and others, 1992). This is of course impossible, especially when you are caring for more than one client. One way to manage this stress is through the use of time management skills. These skills involve learning how, where, and when to use your time. Because you have a limited amount of time with clients, it is essential to remain goal-oriented and focused on your clients' priorities. Priorities of care help you in determining, for example, what procedures to perform first, client assessments that must be conducted on an ongoing basis, and the anticipated response of your client to care activities.

One useful time management skill involves keeping a to-do list. When you first begin working with a client or clients, make a list that sequences the nursing activities you must perform. The change-of-shift report may help you sequence activities based on what you learn about your client's condition and the care provided before your arrival to the unit. Consider activities that have specific time limits in terms of addressing client needs, such as administering a pain medication before a scheduled procedure or instructing clients before their discharge home. Also, analyze the items on your list that are scheduled by agency policies or routines. Note which activities need to be done on time and which activities can be done at your discretion (Wywialowski, 1997). The administration of medications must be performed within a specific schedule, but you can also perform other activities while you are in the client's room. Finally, estimate the amount of time needed to complete the various activities. Activities requiring the assistance of other staff members usually take longer since you must plan around their schedule.

Good time management also involves completing one task before starting another. Complete the activities you begin with one client before moving on to the next if possible. Your care will then become less fragmented, and you can better focus on what you are doing for each client. As a result it is less likely that you will make errors in your care.

EVALUATION.   One of the most important aspects of clinical care coordination is evaluation (see Chapter 6). It is a mistake to think that evaluation occurs at the end of an activity. Evaluation is an ongoing process. Once you assess a client's needs and begin therapies directed at a specific problem area, you should immediately evaluate if therapies are effective and the client's response. The process of evaluation compares actual client outcomes with those that are ex-

pected. When expected outcomes are not being met, evaluation reveals the need to continue current therapies for a longer period, revise approaches to care, or introduce new therapies. Throughout the day as you care for a client anticipate when you need to return to the bedside to evaluate your care, for example, 30 minutes after a medication was administered, 15 minutes after an intravenous (IV) line has begun infusing, or 60 minutes after discussing discharge instructions with the client and family.

Keeping a focus on evaluation of the client's progress lessens the chance of becoming distracted by the tasks of care. It is common to assume that staying focused on planned activities ensures that care is performed appropriately. However, task orientation does not ensure good client outcomes. The competent nurse learns that at the heart of good organizational skills is the constant inquiry into the client's condition and progress toward an improved level of health.

TEAM COMMUNICATION.   As a part of a nursing team, each nurse is responsible for open, professional communication. Regardless of the setting, nurses learn that an enriching, professional environment is one in which staff members respect one another's ideas, share information, and keep one another informed. On a busy hospital unit this means keeping colleagues informed about clients with emerging problems, physicians who have been called for consultation, and unique approaches that solved a complex nursing problem. In a clinic setting it may mean sharing unusual diagnostic findings or conveying important information regarding a client's source of family support. One way of fostering good team communication is by setting expectations of one another. Always treat colleagues with respect, listen to the ideas of other staff members without interruption, be honest and direct in what you say, and be responsible for your actions without displacing anger or frustration on co-workers (Kreitzer and others, 1997). An efficient team knows it can count on all members when needs arise. Sharing expectations of what, when, and how to communicate is a step toward establishing a strong work team.

DELEGATION.   The art of effective delegation is a skill nursing students need to observe and practice to improve their own management skills. Delegation is the process of assigning part of one person's responsibility to another qualified person with his or her consent (Bernard and Walsh, 1995). One purpose of delegation is to improve efficiency. Asking a staff member to obtain an ordered specimen while the nurse attends to a client's pain medication request effectively prevents a delay in the client gaining pain relief. Delegation can also provide job enrichment. A nurse shows trust in colleagues by delegating tasks to them and showing staff members that they are important players in the delivery of care. Never delegate a task that you dislike doing or would not do yourself because this can create negative feelings and poor working relationships. Remember that even though the delegation of a task transfers the responsibility and authority to another person, the delegator retains accountability for the delegated tasks.

Professional nurses are finding themselves in situations where more support is needed to do the daily, repetitive tasks of care, such as basic hygiene, specimen collection, and feeding clients. The RN's time is needed to coordinate care delivery for groups of clients, to conduct individual assessments and make professional judgments about a client's health and therapeutic needs, to deliver complex therapies, and to provide client counseling and education. An LPN in acute care can benefit from acquiring support to deliver care to a group of clients whose needs are complex. In long-term care settings the LPN directs care and relies on assistive personnel to provide basic care measures. A nurse simply cannot do all the work necessary to care for groups of clients.

To be able to perform your professional responsibilities as a nurse you must learn how to work effectively with other staff members. Each health care member has a set of job responsibilities that contribute to the overall care of clients. As a nurse, your job will be to help the care team work efficiently. Because you will oversee the care of groups of clients, it will become necessary at times for you to delegate work to others.

The American Nurses Association (1995) defines **delegation** as transferring responsibility for the performance of an activity or task while retaining accountability for the outcome. For example, you may delegate catheter care to a patient care technician whom you know is trained and competent to perform the skill after you have assessed the condition of the client's catheter and perineal tissues. However, you are ultimately accountable for having the client receive catheter care. When delegating responsibilities to a competent individual, you as the RN still remain accountable for the overall nursing care of the client (Parkman, 1996). Thus you must exercise good judgment at all times in deciding what tasks to delegate and in what situations. The National Council of State Boards of Nursing offers guidelines for delegation of tasks in accordance with an RN's legal scope of practice (Box 23-3).

It is important to recognize that in regard to delegation to assistive personnel, tasks are delegated, not clients. Further, a task is not automatically delegated because it is a task but because it is appropriate for the task to be performed by someone else. For example, as the nurse you are always responsible for the assessment of a client's ongoing status, but if a client is stable, you may delegate vital sign monitoring to assistive personnel. Leah Curtin (1994), a well-known nurse administrator, wrote that assistive personnel should not be at the bedside but at the nurse's side. It is important for you to have assistive personnel work as your assistants or partners and take on tasks that you determine are safe and appropriate for them to provide. A nurse must know how to give clear instructions, effectively prioritize client needs and therapies, and be able to give staff members timely and meaningful feedback.

Here are a few tips on appropriate delegation (Keeling and others, 2000):

- *Assess the knowledge and skills of the delegate:* Determine what assistive personnel know and what they can do by asking open-ended questions that will elicit conversation and details on what the person knows; for example, "How

The Five Rights of Delegation   Box 23-3

RIGHT TASK
The task is delegable for a specific client, such as tasks that are repetitive, require little supervision, and are relatively noninvasive.

RIGHT CIRCUMSTANCES
Appropriate client setting, available resources, and other relevant factors are considered.

RIGHT PERSON
The right person is delegating the right tasks to the right person to be performed on the right person.

RIGHT DIRECTION/COMMUNICATION
A clear, concise description of the task, including its objective, limits, and expectations, is given.

RIGHT SUPERVISION
Appropriate monitoring, evaluation, intervention as needed, and feedback are provided.

Modified and reprinted with permission from National Council of State Boards of Nursing, Inc: *Delegation: concepts and decision-making process,* Chicago, 1995, The Council.

do you usually put the cuff on when you measure a blood pressure?" or "Tell me how you prepare the tubing before you give an enema."
- *Match tasks to the delegate's skills:* Know what skills are included in the training program for assistive personnel at your facility. Determine if personnel have learned critical thinking skills, such as knowing when a client may be in harm or knowing what changes to report.
- *Communicate clearly:* Always provide unambiguous and clear directions by describing a task, the desired outcome, and the time period within which the task should be completed. Never give instructions through another staff member. Make the person feel as though he or she is part of the team. For example, "I'd like you to help me by getting Mr. Floyd up to ambulate before lunch. Be sure to check his blood pressure before he stands and write your finding on the graphic sheet. OK?"
- *Listen attentively:* Listen to the response of assistive personnel after you provide directions. Do they feel comfortable in asking questions or requesting clarification? If you encourage a response, listen to what the person has to say. Be especially attentive if the staff member has been given a deadline to meet by another nurse. Help sort out priorities.
- *Provide feedback:* Always give assistive personnel feedback regarding performance, regardless of outcome. Let them know of a job well-done. If an outcome is undesirable, find a private place to discuss what occurred, any miscommunication, and how to achieve a better outcome in the future.

Quality Improvement

Managing client care involves your active participation not only in clinical care management activities but also in quality improvement (QI). The Joint Commission on Accreditation of Healthcare Organizations (JCAHO) (2000) defines **quality**

improvement as an approach to the continuous study and improvement of the processes of providing health care services to meet the needs of clients and others. Among the processes that most directly influence clients are those that make up nursing practice. Typically in health care, however, many individuals are involved in a single process of care. For example, medication delivery involves the nurse who prepares and administers the drug, the physician who prescribes the medication, the pharmacy that prepares the dosage, the secretary who communicates orders and changes, and the transporter who may deliver medications. With so many individuals involved, it is important for you as a professional to become involved in finding ways to make processes more efficient and effective for better quality client care.

The focus of quality care is outcomes. Outcomes are the conditions to be achieved as a result of care delivery. An **outcome** tells whether interventions are effective, whether clients progress, how well standards are being met, and whether changes are necessary. When nursing staff members think in terms of outcomes, their actions become much more purposeful and focused on improving the condition of their client's health. Two types of outcomes are important to differentiate (Peters, 1995):

Professional outcomes: Measures of the professional caregiver's performance. For example, the RN is responsible for the ongoing assessment of clients' status and will communicate changes in a client's condition to appropriate health team members.

Client outcomes: Measures of the client's status after receiving care. For example, following use of guided imagery and relaxation a client will report a reduction in the severity of hip pain.

A well-organized QI program focuses on processes or systems that significantly contribute to outcomes. A systematic approach is needed organizationally to ensure that everyone supports a continuous QI philosophy. This begins with the organizational culture, where all staff members understand their responsibility toward maintaining and improving quality. On a unit level the nursing manager is responsible for supporting a unit-based QI program. As a member of the nursing team you will participate in recognizing trends in nursing practice, identifying when recurrent problems develop, and initiating opportunities to improve the quality of care. For example, after reviewing clients who have undergone hip surgery, a nursing staff member might ask, "Are our clients regaining functional mobility without severe pain?", "Is the proper analgesic being administered?", "Is rehabilitation delayed?" The QI process begins at the staff level, where problems are defined. This requires staff members to know the standards or guidelines that define quality. In order to judge if clients with hip surgery have functional mobility impaired by poor pain management, there must be an agreement as to how functional clients should be after surgery and how pain is to be managed. Figure 23-2 outlines an organization's framework for quality by showing the relationship of the mission, vision, and values of a nursing organization to its professional standards and standard of care guidelines. The mission, vision, and values serve as the

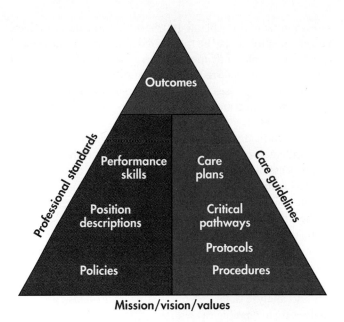

FIGURE **23-2**   Framework for quality. (Data from Peters DA: Outcomes: the mainstay of a framework for quality care, *J Nurs Care Qual* 10[1]:61, 1995.)

framework for defining professional standards and nursing care guidelines, which are found in the workplace in the form of policies, protocols, and procedures, for example. Ultimately a nursing organization with a strong foundation of practice is able to provide quality care and achieve excellent client outcomes.

Unit practice committees review activities or services considered most important in providing quality care to clients. To identify the greatest opportunity for improving quality, the committees consider those activities that are high-volume (greater than 50% of a unit's activity), high-risk (potential for trauma or death), and problem areas (potential problem for client, staff, or institution). For example, on the orthopedic unit, hip surgery is high volume, older adults over age 80 years have more postoperative complications, and a recurrent problem has been family dissatisfaction with clients' pain control. Staff members will review all available information and then select a **quality indicator** as the focus of their QI project. The three types of indicators are structure, process, and outcome. Structure indicators evaluate the structure or systems for delivering care: an example is whether patient-controlled analgesic pumps are delivered in a timely manner. Process indicators evaluate the manner in which care is delivered: an example is the process of pain assessment. Outcome indicators, as described earlier, evaluate the end result of care: an example is a client's report of pain severity and use of analgesics.

After selecting a quality indicator, staff members determine ways to quantitatively measure the indicator. The occurrence of an indicator or the percentage of times the indicator is observed (e.g., the number of clients who have their pain assessed on return from the operating room) is a common measure. A threshold is a standard set by staff members for determining if a problem exists. In the example of pain assessment, anything below 100% would indicate a problem. Lower thresholds may be tolerated depending on the indicator; for example, staff members may set an 80% threshold for clients being referred to a community resource after discharge. In many cases variations in quality indicators are to be expected. Staff members must decide what level of variation is tolerated.

Once indicators are chosen, staff members will collect data and analyze their findings. Depending on the indicator, this process might include client observations or interviews, medical record review, or staff interviews. What is important in data collection is to collect data on the right criteria and to then have adequate data from which to make decisions. Many organizations have made QI so important that formal research studies are conducted. In this case the process of data collection and analysis can be very formal. When simple evaluation studies are conducted, staff members will collect and analyze data, determine if problems exist, and then analyze their possible causes.

Monitoring of quality indicators evaluates whether a specifically defined process reaches desired outcomes. If results exceed or meet a threshold no problem has been identified and the process is performing well. When thresholds for satisfactory care are not met staff members must try to find the cause of problems. For example, if there is a proven delay in patient-controlled analgesic pumps arriving on the nursing unit, thus preventing proper orientation of clients to the use of the pump before surgery, the unit practice committee must recommend solutions. When a process is not working well, one of the models for QI (e.g., Focus-PDCA) may be used. This allows staff members to structure problem analysis and resolution in order to improve the process of care. It is often appropriate to organize an expert team who knows the process well. For example, the committee working on patient-controlled analgesia might include staff nurses, colleagues from pharmacy, and staff members from the equipment supply area. Focus-PDCA is an acronym for the following: find the process to improve, organize a team that knows the process, clarify current knowledge of the process, understand causes of process variation, and select a process improvement. Once the improvement is selected the committee will then Plan, Do, Check, Act.

It often takes several meetings before a group can agree on the proper actions to take. After reviewing all options the committee eventually selects the best approach for improving the process and achieving desired outcomes. It is important to establish actions likely to be successful. For example, the orthopedic unit decides that since they have a large number of clients receiving patient-controlled analgesia, the nearby satellite pharmacy will begin to prepare the pumps instead of the central pharmacy. Nursing staff members will be able to order the pumps directly through the satellite center, reducing delivery time significantly.

After implementing an action plan, staff members must reevaluate its success. The change may be positive or negative. For example, the new pump delivery process reduces waiting time by 50%. However, if the problem remains, a new plan of action is necessary. The QI process is similar to the nursing process (see Chapter 6) in that when desired outcomes are not met, the staff reinstitutes the QI process.

The results of QI activities must be communicated to staff members in all appropriate organizational departments. If findings and results are not communicated, practice changes will likely not occur. Revision of policies and procedures, modification of standards of care, and implementation of system changes are examples of ways that an organization may respond. Over time, incorporation of a QI program benefits the client, the professional staff, and the organization.

Key Terms

Key Concepts

- A profession possesses the characteristics of extended education, theory, service, autonomy, and a code of ethics.
- The essential components of professional nursing are care, cure, and coordination.
- Standards of care offer objective guidelines for nurses to provide care and to evaluate care.
- A manager must set a philosophy for a work unit, ensure appropriate staffing, mobilize staff and institutional resources to achieve objectives, motivate staff members to carry out their work, set standards of performance, and make the right decisions to achieve objectives.
- Consideration conveys mutual trust, respect, and rapport between the manager and staff members.
- Empowering staff members brings out the best in a manager and allows him or her concentrate on effective client care systems, to support risk taking and innovation, and to focus on results and rewards.
- Nursing care delivery models vary by the responsibility of the RN in coordinating care delivery and the roles other staff members play in assisting with care.

- Critical to the success of decentralized decision making is making staff members aware that they have the responsibility, authority, and accountability for the care they give and the decisions they make.
- A nurse manager can foster decentralized decision making by establishing nursing practice committees, supporting nurse-physician and interdisciplinary collaboration, setting and implementing quality improvement (QI) plans, and maintaining timely staff communication.
- Clinical care coordination involves accurate clinical decision making, establishing priorities, efficient organizational skills, appropriate use of resources and time management skills, and an ongoing evaluation of care activities.

- Each member of a nursing work team is responsible for open, professional communication.
- When done correctly delegation can improve job efficiency and job enrichment.
- You must exercise good judgment at all times in deciding what tasks to delegate and in what situations.
- QI initiatives are designed to maintain or improve the outcomes of nursing practice.
- After a nursing staff evaluates a quality problem, an action plan must be developed to improve the process and outcomes.
- The results of QI activities must be communicated to staff members in all appropriate organizational departments.

Critical Thinking Activities

1. Mr. Tanaka is scheduled for surgery at 1 PM to repair torn ligaments in his knee. It is the first time he has had surgery. It is now 11:30 AM and the operating room (OR) has notified nursing that they will pick up Mr. Tanaka in 30 minutes. Mr. Lines enters the room to complete the preoperative checklist for Mr. Tanaka and to make final preparations for surgery. He finds the client moving about restlessly in bed and reluctant to talk. What should be Mr. Lines's priority in this situation: continue preparation for surgery, perform an assessment of the client, or call the OR to delay pickup?

2. Lisa is a student nurse assigned to two clients. She begins her afternoon by checking first on Mrs. Rhodes, a 49-year-old married schoolteacher who is being discharged in approximately 2 hours after a right lumpectomy that morning for cancer of the breast. She examines the surgical site and begins to take Mrs. Rhodes's blood pressure. The call light system at the bedside comes on, and the unit secretary lets Lisa know that her second client, Mr. Sawyer, has finished lunch and wants to ambulate down the hall. Mr. Sawyer had surgery 2 days ago for acute appendicitis. Lisa tells Mrs. Rhodes that she will return in just a moment and leaves to check on Mr. Sawyer. When Lisa arrives in Mr. Sawyer's room, he tells her that he wants a pain medication. While preparing the medication, Lisa notices that Mrs. Rhodes's blood pressure should have been checked again 10 minutes ago. How might Lisa have managed her time more wisely?

3. Don, the evening RN, is preparing to assess Mr. Sequera, who experienced a myocardial infarction 4 days ago and who will ambulate down the hall for the first time this evening, and Mrs. Lennox, a client newly admitted with gastrointestinal bleeding. Don finds that Mr. Sequera is resting comfortably and visiting with his daughter. He is eager to start walking. Mrs. Lennox is very restless and experiencing discomfort from her nasogastric tube. The physician has ordered stool specimens to be collected. Which of these two clients should Don delegate to the nurse technician, Linda?

Review Questions

1. While administering medications, June realizes she has given the wrong dose of a medication to a client. June acts by completing an incident report and notifying the client's physician. This is an example of June exercising:
   1. authority.
   2. responsibility.
   3. accountability.
   4. decision making.

2. During morning rounds, Rhea assesses Mr. Nile's condition. The client had major heart surgery 2 days ago. His vital signs are stable. Rhea finds that Mr. Nile's incision is clean and healing well. Mr. Niles complains of pain in his lower leg where the vein graft was removed. Rhea finds that the IV infusion is running on time but only 100 ml remains before the infusion runs out. An order exists for the IV infusion to continue. The client is likely to be discharged in 2 days if he continues to progress. A second order of priority is:
   1. the need to replace the IV bag with a new one.
   2. Mr. Niles's need to have an analgesic administered for his leg pain.

   3. Mr. Niles's need to receive instruction on complications of wound healing.
   4. the need for Rhea to determine if the pharmacy has delivered IV solutions ordered for the day.

3. During the change-of-shift report you receive the following information on four different clients:
   - Mr. Tighe had trouble during the night. His blood pressure dropped to 70/50, and the physician ordered an increase in his IV fluids to raise the pressure. The physicians believe he might be bleeding from his surgery. His last blood pressure was 90/60. He might go back to the operating room if he does not stabilize.
   - Mrs. Adams is a difficult client. She called out for assistance all through the night. I think she is afraid of returning home. She has no one to help her once she is discharged.
   - Ms. Dye was admitted last evening from the emergency department following an auto accident. They took her to the operating room for an open reduction of her right femur, which was fractured. She rested well after returning, but she just called out for a pain medication when I came to give report.

Continued

- Mr. Spagnoli is due to be discharged this morning. He is anxious to get all his medications so he can leave as soon as his family arrives.

The first client you should visit during your morning rounds is:
1. Ms. Dye.
2. Mr. Tighe.
3. Mrs. Adams.
4. Mr. Spagnoli.

4. Sharon checks her client, Mr. Rawls, a 62-year-old man who was admitted to the hospital with pneumonia. Mr. Rawls has been coughing profusely and has required nasotracheal suctioning. He also has an IV infusion of antibiotics. Mr. Rawls is febrile with a temperature of 101° F (38.3° C). Mr. Rawls asks Sharon if he can perhaps have a bed bath since he has been perspiring profusely. The task for Sharon to delegate to the nurse assistant working with her today is:
1. vital signs.
2. changing IV dressing.
3. nasotracheal suctioning.
4. administering a bed bath.

5. Jennifer, an RN, is working with Ken, a nurse assistant. Jennifer has completed morning rounds on her assigned clients and is giving Ken directions for what he needs to do for the next hour.

An appropriate way to provide directions when delegating nursing care is:
1. "Ken, why don't you go to room 20A and see what Mr. Wilson needs."
2. "Ken, I would like you to take all the vital signs for rooms 12 and 13 and let me know if there are any problems."
3. "Ken, would you start Mrs. McNamara's bath while I check on the IV line in room 14. I will help you with turning her so I can assess her skin and decide on the turning schedule we will need to follow."
4. "Ken, I want you to help Mr. Nelson off the bedpan and while you are at it get a specimen if he passed any stool. I don't think I can go in his room one more time, so I would appreciate your help."

6. An example of a quality improvement (QI) outcome indicator is the:
1. rate of postoperative wound infection.
2. percentage of time remaining narcotics are counted by nursing staff every shift.
3. number of patients receiving postoperative education on possible surgical complications.
4. time it takes for a client to be transported from the emergency department to an inpatient nursing unit.

References

American Nurses Association: Position statement on registered nurse utilization of assistive personnel, *Am Nurse* 25(2):7, 1995.

American Nurses Association: *Standards of clinical practice,* ed 2, Washington, DC, 1998, The Association.

American Nurses Association: *Code of ethics for nurses with interpretive statements,* Washington, DC, 20001, The Association.

Bernard L, Walsh M: *Leadership: the key to professionalization in nursing,* ed 2, St. Louis, 1995, Mosby.

Canadian Nurses Association: *A definition of nursing practice: standards for nursing practice.* Ottawa, 1986, The Association.

Chinn PL, Kramer MK: *Theory and nursing: integrated knowledge development,* ed 2, St. Louis, 1999, Mosby.

Cox S: Managing the workplace 2000. Seminar conducted at Barnes-Jewish Hospital, St. Louis, 1995. Curtin L: The heart of patient care, *Nurs Manage* 25(5):7, 1994.

Duchene P: Organizing care. In Sullivan EJ, Decker PJ: *Effective management in nursing,* ed 3, Redwood City, Calif, 1992, Addison-Wesley.

Gustafson D and others: Stress and time management. In Sullivan EJ, Decker PJ: *Effective management in nursing,* ed 3, Redwood City, Calif, 1992, Addison-Wesley.

Hansten R, Washburn M: Seven steps to shift from tasks to outcomes, *Nurs Manage* 30(7):25, 1999.

Joint Commission on Accreditation of Healthcare Organizations: *An introduction to quality improvement in health care,* Chicago, 2000, The Commission.

Keeling B and others: Appropriate delegation, *Am J Nurs* 100(12):24, 2000.

Kreitzer MJ and others: Creating a healthy work environment in the midst of organizational change and transition, *JONA* 27(6):35, 1997.

Manthey M: *The practice of primary nursing,* St. Louis, 1980, Mosby.

National Council of State Boards of Nursing: *Delegation: concepts and decision-making process,* Chicago, 1995, The Council.

Parkman CA: Delegation: are you doing it right? *Am J Nurs* 96(9):43, 1996.

Peters DA: Outcomes: the mainstay of a framework for quality care, *J Nurs Care Qual* 10(1):61, 1995.

Trofino J: Vision: a professional model for nursing practice, *Nurs Manage* 27(3):43, 1996.

Wywialowski E: *Managing client care,* ed 2, St. Louis, 1997, Mosby.

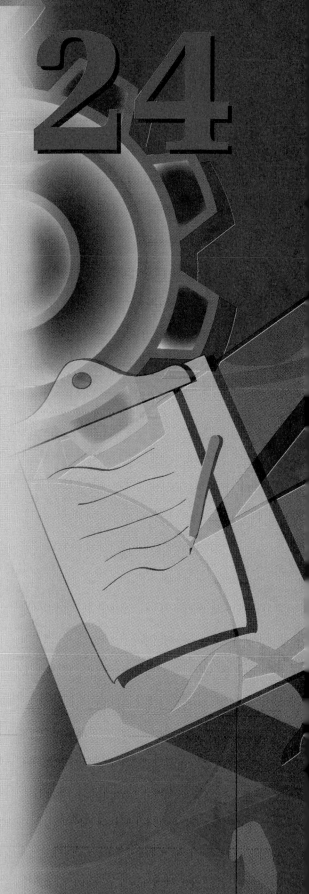

Exercise and Activity

Objectives

- Define key terms.
- Describe the role of the skeleton, skeletal muscles, and nervous system in the regulation of movement.
- Discuss physiological and pathological influences on body alignment and joint mobility.
- Assess clients for impaired body alignment, exercise, and activity.
- Formulate nursing diagnoses for clients experiencing problems with exercise and activity.
- Write a nursing care plan for a client with impaired body alignment and activity.
- Describe the interventions for maintaining proper alignment, assisting a client in moving up in bed, repositioning a client needing assistance, and transferring a client from a bed to a chair.
- Evaluate the nursing care plan for maintaining body alignment and activity.

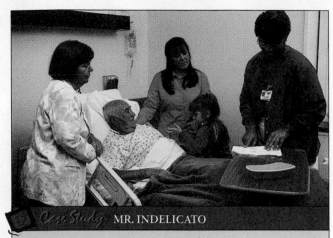

Case Study   MR. INDELICATO

Mr. Indelicato is a 72-year-old man who is going to be hospitalized for surgery on his right knee. His general level of health is good in that he does not have any underlying illnesses, such as cardiovascular illness, diabetes mellitus, or other musculoskeletal illnesses. He relates the problem with his knees to previous sports injuries. He repeatedly "twisted the knee" while playing racquetball. He knows that he hurt his knee at least 6 times over the last 30 years while playing the sport. He first sought medical advice and treatment about 6 years ago. His last injury to his knee was approximately "5 or 6 years ago, and it hasn't worked the same since." He has tried various treatments, including physical therapy, rest, and pain medication. His only preoperative medication is Motrin 600 mg every 6 to 8 hours. He chooses to have surgery so he can get back to being active. He and his wife are very active and do enjoy golf, tennis, and bike riding. In addition, they have an active social life of attending the theater, dinner with friends, and visiting their children and grandchildren. Mr. Indelicato's wife is in good health as well. He feels they are very fortunate in that neither one has any illnesses or takes any prescribed medication.

Marilyn Sweeney is a 40-year-old nursing student completing her second clinical semester. She has just finished rotating through a general surgical unit and is spending the remaining 6 weeks in the orthopedic/rehabilitation division of the agency. Her assignment is to follow this patient through his surgery and rehabilitation.

The actions of walking, turning, lifting, or carrying are all common in the provision of nursing care. Such activities require muscle exertion. To reduce the risk of injury to the client or yourself, you must know and practice proper **body mechanics.** This includes knowledge of the actions of various muscle groups, understanding of the factors involved in the coordination of body movement, and familiarity with the integrated functioning of the skeletal, muscular, and nervous systems.

SCIENTIFIC KNOWLEDGE BASE

The coordinated efforts of the musculoskeletal and nervous systems to maintain balance, posture, and body alignment during lifting, bending, moving, and performing activities of daily living provide the foundation for body mechanics. If you properly implement these activities, the risk of injury to the musculoskeletal system is reduced and body movements are facilitated, allowing physical mobility without muscle strain and excessive use of muscle energy.

Body Alignment

Body alignment refers to the relationship of one body part to another body part along a horizontal or vertical line. Correct alignment reduces strain on musculoskeletal structures, maintains adequate **muscle tone,** and contributes to balance.

Body Balance

Body balance is achieved when a relatively low **center of gravity** is balanced over a wide, stable base of support, and a vertical line falls from the center of gravity through the base of support. The base of support is the foundation. When the vertical line from the center of gravity does not fall through the base of support, the body loses balance.

Body balance is also enhanced by posture. The term **posture** means maintaining optimal body position. It means a position that most favors function, requires the least muscular work to maintain, and places the least strain on muscles, ligaments, and bones (Thibodeau and Patton, 1999).

You maintain proper body alignment and posture by using two simple techniques. First, widen the base of support by separating your feet to a comfortable distance. Second, bring the center of gravity closer to the base of support to increase balance. This is achieved by bending the knees and flexing the hips until you are squatting and still maintaining proper back alignment by keeping the trunk erect.

Coordinated Body Movement

Weight is the force exerted on a body by gravity. When an object is lifted, the lifter must overcome the object's weight and be aware of its center of gravity. In symmetrical objects, the center of gravity is located at the exact center of the object. The force of weight is always directed downward. An object that is unbalanced has its center of gravity away from the midline and falls without support. Like unbalanced objects, clients who fail to maintain a balance with their center of gravity are unsteady, placing them at risk for falling. You must be able to identify such clients and intervene with them in such a way that safety is maintained.

Friction

Friction is the effect of rubbing or the resistance that a moving body meets from the surface on which it moves. As you turn, transfer, or move a client up in bed, you need to overcome friction. Friction is reduced by following some basic principles. The greater the surface area of the object to be moved, the greater the friction.

A passive or immobilized client produces greater friction to movement. Thus, when possible, use some of the client's strength and mobility when lifting, transferring, or moving the client up in bed. This can be done by explaining the procedure and telling the client when to move. For instance, friction is decreased if the client can bend his or her knees as you assist him or her to move up in the bed. Friction is also reduced by lifting rather than pushing a client. Lifting has an upward component and decreases the pressure between the client and the bed or the chair. The use of a lift sheet reduces friction because the client is more easily moved along the bed's surface.

Regulation of Movement

Coordinated body movement involves the integrated functioning of the skeletal, muscular, and nervous systems. Because these three systems cooperate so closely in mechanical support of the body, they are often considered as a single functional unit.

SKELETAL SYSTEM. Bones perform five functions in the body: support, protection, movement, mineral storage, and hematopoiesis (blood cell formation). Two of these functions, support and movement, are most important. In support, bones serve as the framework and contribute to the shape, alignment, and positioning of the body parts. In movement, bones with their **joints** constitute levers for muscle attachment. When muscles contract and shorten, they pull on bones, producing joint movement (Thibodeau and Patton, 1999).

JOINTS. An articulation, or joint, is the connection between bones. Each joint is classified according to its structure and degree of mobility. On the basis of connective structures, joints are classified as fibrous, cartilaginous, and synovial (Huether and McCance, 2000). Fibrous joints fit closely together and are fixed, permitting little if any movement. The cartilaginous joint has little movement but is elastic and uses cartilage to unite separate body surfaces.

The synovial or true joint is a freely moveable joint and the body's most mobile, numerous, and anatomically complex joint. There are seven structural characteristics of synovial joints: joint capsule, synovial membrane, articular cartilage, joint cavity, menisci, ligaments, and bursae (Thibodeau and Patton, 1999).

LIGAMENTS. Ligaments are white, shiny, flexible bands of fibrous tissue that bind joints and connect bones and cartilages. Ligaments are elastic and aid joint flexibility and support. In some areas of the body, ligaments also have a protective function. For example, ligaments between vertebral bodies prevent damage to the spinal cord during back movement.

TENDONS. Tendons are white, glistening, fibrous bands of tissue that connect muscle to bone. Tendons are strong, flexible, and inelastic and occur in various lengths and thicknesses.

CARTILAGE. Cartilage is nonvascular, supporting connective tissue with the flexibility of a firm, plastic material. The gristlelike nature of cartilage permits it to sustain weight and serve as a shock-absorber pad between articulating bones. It is located chiefly in the joints and in the thorax, trachea, larynx, nose, and ear (Thibodeau and Patton, 1999).

SKELETAL MUSCLE. In addition to facilitating movement, muscles determine body form and contour. Muscles span at least one joint and attach to both articulating bones. When contraction occurs, one bone is fixed while the other moves. The origin is the point of attachment that remains still; the insertion is the point that moves when the muscle contracts (Thibodeau and Patton, 1999).

MUSCLES CONCERNED WITH MOVEMENT. The muscles of movement are located near the skeletal region, where movement is caused by a lever system (Thibodeau and Patton, 1999). The lever system makes the work of moving a weight or load easier. It occurs when specific bones, such as the humerus, ulna, and radius, and the associated joints, such as the elbow, act as a lever. Thus the force applied to one end of the bone to lift a weight at another point tends to rotate the bone in the direction opposite that of the applied force. Muscles that attach to bones of leverage provide the necessary strength to move the object.

MUSCLES CONCERNED WITH POSTURE. Gravity pulls on parts of the body all the time; the only way the body can be held in position is for muscles to exert pull on bones in the opposite direction. Muscles accomplish this counterforce by maintaining a low level of sustained contraction. Poor posture places more work on muscles to counteract the force of gravity. This leads to fatigue and can eventually interfere with bodily functions and cause deformities.

MUSCLE GROUPS. The antagonistic, synergistic, and antigravity muscle groups are coordinated by the nervous system and maintain posture and initiate movement. Antagonistic muscles bring about movement at the joint. During movement the active mover muscle contracts while its antagonist relaxes. For example, during **extension** of the arm, the active mover, the triceps brachii, contracts, and the antagonist, the biceps brachii, relaxes.

Synergistic muscles contract to accomplish the same movement. When the arm is flexed, the strength of the contraction of the biceps brachii is increased by contraction of the synergistic muscle, the brachialis.

Antigravity muscles are involved with joint stabilization. These muscles continuously oppose the effect of gravity on the body and permit a person to maintain an upright or sitting posture. In an adult the antigravity muscles are the extensors of the leg, the gluteus maximus, the quadriceps femoris, the soleus muscles, and the muscles of the back.

Skeletal muscles support posture and carry out voluntary movement. The muscles are attached to the skeleton by tendons, which provide strength and permit motion.

NERVOUS SYSTEM. Movement and posture are regulated by the nervous system. The major voluntary motor area, located in the cerebral cortex, is the motor strip (precentral gyrus). A majority of motor fibers descend from the motor strip and cross at the level of the medulla. The motor fibers from the right motor strip initiate voluntary movement for the left side of the body, and motor fibers from the left motor strip initiate voluntary movement for the right side of the body. Transmission of the impulse from the nervous system to the musculoskeletal system is an electrochemical event that requires a neurotransmitter, chemicals that transfer the electric impulse from the nerve to the muscle.

PROPRIOCEPTION. Posture is also regulated by the nervous system and requires coordination of proprioception and balance. Proprioception is the awareness of the position of the body and its parts (Huether and McCance, 2000). Proprioception is monitored by proprioceptors located on nerve endings in muscles, tendons, and joints. While a person carries out activities of daily living, proprioceptors monitor muscle activity and body position. When a person walks, the proprioceptors on the bottom of the feet monitor pressure changes. Thus when the bottom of the moving foot comes in contact with the walking surface, the individual automatically moves the stationary foot forward.

BALANCE. **Balance** is assisted through control by the nervous system, specifically by the cerebellum and the inner ear. The major function of the cerebellum is to coordinate all voluntary movement. Within the inner ear are the fluid-filled semicircular canals. When the head is suddenly rotated in one direction, the fluid remains stationary for a moment, whereas the canal turns with the head. This allows a person to change position suddenly without losing balance.

Principles of Body Mechanics

Using principles of body mechanics during routine activities also prevents injury. Teach colleagues and clients' families to lift, transfer, or position clients properly. For example, teaching a client's family how to transfer the client from bed to chair increases and reinforces the family's knowledge and provides opportunity to consistently demonstrate proper body mechanics (Box 24-1).

Pathological Influences on Body Alignment, Exercise, and Activity

Many pathological conditions affect body alignment, exercise, and activity. A few of these conditions include congenital defects; disorders of bones, joints, and muscles; central nervous system damage; and musculoskeletal trauma.

CONGENITAL DEFECTS. Congenital abnormalities affect the efficiency of the musculoskeletal system in regard to alignment, balance, and appearance. Osteogenesis imperfecta is an inherited disorder that affects bone. Bones are porous, short, bowed, and deformed; as a result, children experience curvature of the spine and shortness of stature. Scoliosis is a structural curvature of the spine associated

---

Principles of Body Mechanics	Box 24-1

The wider the base of support, the greater the stability of the nurse.
The lower the center of gravity, the greater the stability of the nurse.
The equilibrium of an object is maintained as long as the line of gravity passes through its base of support.
Facing the direction of movement prevents abnormal twisting of the spine.
Dividing balanced activity between arms and legs reduces the risk of back injury.
Leverage, rolling, turning, or pivoting requires less work than lifting.
When friction is reduced between the object to be moved and the surface on which it is moved, less force is required to move it.
Reducing the force of work reduces the risk of injury.
Maintaining good body mechanics reduces fatigue of the muscle groups.
Alternating periods of rest and activity helps to reduce fatigue.

---

with vertebral rotation. Muscles, ligaments, and other soft tissues become shortened. Balance and mobility are affected in proportion to the severity of abnormal spinal curvatures (Huether and McCance, 2000).

DISORDERS OF BONES, JOINTS, AND MUSCLES. Osteoporosis is a well-known and well-publicized disorder of aging in which the density or mass of bone is reduced. The bone remains biochemically normal but has difficulty maintaining integrity and support. The cause is uncertain, and theories vary from hormonal imbalances to insufficient intake of nutrients (Huether and McCance, 2000).

Joint mobility can be altered by inflammatory and noninflammatory joint diseases and by articular disruption. Inflammatory joint disease (e.g., arthritis) is characterized by inflammation or destruction of the synovial membrane and articular cartilage and systemic signs of inflammation. Noninflammatory diseases have none of these characteristics, and the synovial fluid is normal (Huether and McCance, 2000).

CENTRAL NERVOUS SYSTEM DAMAGE. Damage to any component of the central nervous system that regulates voluntary movement results in impaired body alignment and mobility. For example, the motor strip in the cerebrum can be damaged by trauma from a head injury. The amount of voluntary motor impairment is directly related to the amount of destruction of the motor strip. A client with a right-sided cerebral hemorrhage and damage to the right motor strip may have left-sided hemiplegia.

MUSCULOSKELETAL TRAUMA. Musculoskeletal trauma can result in bruises, contusions, sprains, and fractures. A fracture is a disruption of bone tissue continuity. Fractures most commonly result from direct external trauma. They can also occur because of some deformity of the bone, as with pathological fractures of osteoporosis.

NURSING KNOWLEDGE BASE

Knowledge from areas of nursing practice enables you to meet the activity and exercise needs of the client. Growth and development changes, behavioral aspects, and cultural and ethnic origin are a few areas of knowledge that must be incorporated into the plan of care.

Growth and Development

Throughout the life span the body's appearance and functioning undergo change. Knowledge of growth and development (see Chapter 18) enables you to anticipate types of activities clients can perform. The newborn infant's spine is flexed and lacks the anteroposterior curves of the adult. As growth and stability increase, the thoracic spine straightens, and the lumbar spinal curve appears, which allows sitting and standing. As the baby grows, musculoskeletal development permits support of weight for standing and walking. The toddler's posture is awkward because of the slight swayback and protruding abdomen (Wong and others, 1999). From the third year through the beginning of adolescence, the musculoskeletal system continues to grow and develop. Greater coordination enables the child to perform tasks that require fine motor skills. With aging changes in musculoskeletal function may limit client activity.

Behavioral Aspects

You should take into consideration the client's knowledge of exercise and activity, barriers to a program of exercise and physical activity, and current exercise behavior or habits. Clients are more open to developing an exercise program if they are at the stage of readiness to change their behavior (Prochaska and others, 1994). Clients' decisions to change behavior and include a daily exercise routine in their lives may occur gradually with repeated information that is individualized to their needs and lifestyle (Box 24-2).

Cultural and Ethnic Origin

Exercise and physical fitness is beneficial to all people. When developing a physical fitness program for culturally diverse populations, you must consider what motivates individuals to exercise and what activities are deemed appropriate and enjoyable.

CRITICAL THINKING
Synthesis

It is important that you synthesize knowledge, experience, attitudes and standards when developing care for a client with activity intolerance or improper body mechanics. Doing so will help you prevent complications, promote rehabilitation, and promote a timely return of clients to their home.

KNOWLEDGE. When you begin the process of problem solving for client care, a variety of concepts must be considered and woven together to provide the best outcome for the

---

General Guidelines for Initiating and Maintaining an Exercise Program   Box 24-2

The client will most likely initiate and maintain an exercise program if the individual:
  Perceives a net benefit
  Chooses an enjoyable activity
  Feels competent doing the activity
  Feels safe doing the activity
  Can easily access the activity on a regular basis
  Can fit the activity into the daily schedule
  Feels that the activity does not generate financial or social costs that he or she is unwilling to bear
  Experiences a minimum of negative consequences such as injury, loss of time, negative peer pressure, and problems with self-identity
  Is able to successfully address issues of competing time demands
  Recognizes the need to balance the use of labor-saving devices and sedentary activities with activities that involve a higher level of physical exertion.

From National Institutes of Health Consensus Development Panel on Physical Activity and Cardiovascular Health: Physical activity and cardiovascular health, *JAMA* 276(3):241, 1996.

---

client. Knowledge of the musculoskeletal system exercise physiology and health alterations that create problems for the client in the area of exercise and activity lay the foundation for decision making and planning care.

EXPERIENCE. You may have taken care of other clients with problems associated with improper body mechanics or lack of exercise and activity. These experiences help you to anticipate client needs such as pain control, positioning, transferring, and support of activities of daily living. Visits to a physical or occupational therapy unit in a hospital or community setting can increase your experiential base. In addition, you can use experience from a personal exercise plan to help your client develop an individualized exercise program.

ATTITUDES. Creativity is an attitude you must possess because problems with activity and exercise are often prolonged. The more creative your approach for improving activity tolerance and mobility skills, the greater chance for success. This is especially important with children. When a child makes strides toward greater mobility, you can make it a game by giving the child stickers in pretty colors to symbolize success (Wong and others, 1999).

STANDARDS. At all times promote the client's independence while adhering to the prescribed rehabilitation plan and maintaining client safety. The use of professional standards such as those from the National Institutes of Health Consensus Development Panel on Physical Activity and Cardiovascular Health (1996) provides valuable guidelines for exercise and physical fitness.

NURSING PROCESS

Assessment

The assessment includes the client's present activity tolerance and information about preillness functioning. Assessment of body alignment and posture can be carried out with the client standing, sitting, or lying down. Table 24-1 presents focused examples of factors to assess related to activity intolerance, questions and approaches, and physical assessment strategies.

Through assessment you will be able to determine normal physiological changes in growth and development; deviations related to poor posture, trauma, muscle damage, or nerve dysfunction; and any learning needs of clients. In addition, assessment can provide opportunities for clients to observe their posture and obtain important information about other factors that contribute to poor alignment, such as fatigue, malnutrition, and psychological problems.

BODY ALIGNMENT. The first step in assessing body alignment is to put your client at ease, so unnatural or rigid positions are not assumed. When you assess body alignment of an immobilized or unconscious client, pillows and positioning supports should be removed from the bed if not contraindicated and the client placed in the **supine** position.

STANDING. Assessment for your client includes the following: the head is erect and midline; body parts are symmetrical; the spine should be straight with normal curvatures (cervical concave, thoracic convex, and lumbar concave); the abdomen is comfortably tucked; the knees should be in a straight line between the hips and ankles and slightly flexed; the feet should be flat on the floor and pointed directly forward and slightly apart to maintain a wide base of support; and the arms should hang comfortably at the sides (Figure 24-1). The client's center of gravity is in the midline, and the line of gravity is from the middle of the forehead to a midpoint between the feet. Laterally the line of gravity runs vertically from the middle of the skull to the posterior third of the foot (Wilson and Giddens, 2000).

SITTING. Assessment of your client includes the following: the head is erect, and the neck and vertebral column are in straight alignment; the body weight is distributed on the buttocks and thighs; the thighs are parallel and in a horizontal plane (be careful to avoid pressure on the popliteal nerve and blood supply); the feet are supported on the floor; and the forearms are supported on the armrest, in the lap, or on a table in front of the chair.

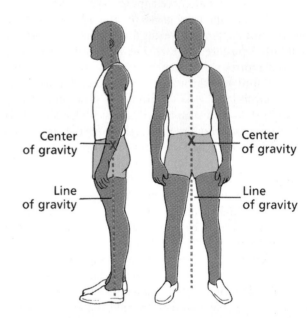

FIGURE **24-1**   Correct body alignment with standing.

Factors to Assess	Questions and Approaches	Physical Assessment Strategies
Range of motion (ROM)	Ask if client has limited movement in joints. Ask if client has a history of connective tissue disorders, fractures, and/or damage to ligaments or tendons.	Observe client's gait and ability to carry out activities of daily living (ADLs). Inspect joints for deformity. Measure ROM of affected joints.
Pain	Ask if client experiences pain or discomfort upon movement. Ask if client needs pain medication before ambulating (with assistance), particularly after surgical procedure. Ask client to rate pain on a scale of 1 to 10.	Inspect joints for redness or swelling indicating potential inflammatory process. Observe for objective signs of pain such as grimacing, moaning, increasing respiratory rate, pulse, and blood pressure. (NOTE: These objective signs may not always be present, and it is best to ask client if pain is present.)
Activity tolerance	Ask if client feels fatigued. Ask if client is experiencing difficulty with ADLs because of muscle weakness. Ask if client feels short of breath, palpitations, light-headed, or dizzy.	Observe for signs of fatigue. Observe client's performance of ADLs. Observe client for paleness, obtain vital signs, and compare to baseline measures.

Example of a Focused Client Assessment   Table 24-1

Your assessment of alignment in the sitting position is particularly important for the client with neuromuscular disorders, muscle weakness, muscle paralysis, or nerve damage. A client with these alterations has diminished sensation in affected areas and is unable to perceive pressure or decreased circulation. Proper sitting alignment reduces the risk of musculoskeletal system damage in such a client.

RECUMBENT. Assessment of your client requires that the client be placed in the lateral position with all but one pillow and all positioning supports removed from the bed. The vertebrae should be in straight alignment without observable curves. This assessment provides baseline data concerning the client's body alignment.

Conditions that create a risk of damage to the musculoskeletal system when lying down include impaired mobility (e.g., traction), decreased sensation (e.g., hemiparesis from a stroke), impaired circulation (e.g., diabetes), and lack of voluntary muscle control (e.g., spinal cord injuries).

When a client is unable to change position voluntarily, you assess the position of body parts while the client is lying down. The vertebrae should be in straight alignment without any observable curves. The extremities should be in alignment and not crossed over one another. The head and neck should be aligned without excessive flexion or extension.

MOBILITY. Your assessment of client mobility determines the client's coordination and balance while walking, the ability to carry out activities of daily living, and the ability to participate in an exercise program. The assessment of mobility has three components: range of joint motion, gait, and exercise.

RANGE OF MOTION. Assessing **range of motion (ROM)** is one of the first assessment techniques used to determine the degree of limitation or injury to a joint. Assess ROM to collect data to answer questions about joint stiffness, swelling, pain, limited movement, and unequal movement (see Chapter 12). Limited range of motion may indicate inflammation such as arthritis, fluid in the joint, altered nerve supply, or contractures. Increased mobility (beyond normal) of a joint may indicate connective tissue disorders, ligament tears, and possible joint fractures.

GAIT. **Gait** is the manner or style of walking, including rhythm, cadence, and speed. Assessing gait allows you to draw conclusions about balance, posture, and the ability to walk without assistance (see Chapter 12). You should note conformity, a regular smooth rhythm, symmetry in the length of leg swing, smooth swaying related to the gait phase, and a smooth, symmetrical arm swing (Wilson and Giddens, 2000).

EXERCISE. Exercise is physical activity for conditioning the body, improving health, maintaining fitness, or providing therapy for correcting a deformity or restoring the overall body to a maximal state of health. When a person exercises, physiological changes occur in body systems (Box 24-3).

During exercise, muscle tone, size, and strength increase, and cardiopulmonary conditioning is improved. As a result, the person is able to exercise longer with each strengthening of the muscles. Joint mobility is also enhanced because the exercise itself requires movement of body parts.

ACTIVITY TOLERANCE. **Activity tolerance** is the kind and amount of exercise or work a person is able to perform (Box 24-4). Assessment of activity tolerance is necessary when planning physical activity for clients with acute or chronic illness and provides you with baseline data (Ackley and Ladwig, 2001).

CLIENT EXPECTATIONS. In assessing the client's expectations concerning body alignment and joint mobility, you first need insight into your client's perception of what is normal or acceptable in regard to mobility. For example, one of the factors affecting posture, alignment, and mobility is freedom from pain. If exercising is painful or tiresome to the client, compliance and commitment to desired interventions may be lacking. Clients may be content with their present range of motion or

---

Effects of Exercise   Box 24-3

CARDIOVASCULAR SYSTEM
Increased cardiac output
Improved myocardial contraction, thereby strengthening cardiac muscle
Decreased resting heart rate
Improved venous return

PULMONARY SYSTEM
Increased respiratory rate and depth followed by a quicker return to resting state
Improved alveolar ventilation
Decreased work of breathing
Improved diaphragmatic excursion

METABOLIC SYSTEM
Increased basal metabolic rate
Increased use of glucose and fatty acids
Increased triglyceride breakdown
Increased gastric motility
Increased production of body heat

MUSCULOSKELETAL SYSTEM
Improved muscle tone
Increased joint mobility
Improved muscle tolerance to physical exercise
Possible increase in muscle mass
Reduced bone loss

ACTIVITY TOLERANCE
Improved tolerance
Decreased fatigue

PSYCHOSOCIAL FACTORS
Improved tolerance to stress
Reports of "feeling better"
Reports of decrease in illness (e.g., colds, influenza)

Data from Huether SE, McCance KL: *Understanding pathophysiology,* ed 2, St. Louis, 2000, Mosby; Hoeman SP: *Rehabilitation nursing: process, application, and outcomes,* ed 3, St. Louis, 2001, Mosby.

Case Study   SYNTHESIS IN PRACTICE

As Marilyn prepares to assess Mr. Indelicato, she reviews anatomy and physiology related to the musculoskeletal system and exercise physiology. She gathers information about the expected surgery, anticipated recovery, and physical therapy. During her previous rotation she cared for postoperative clients and knows relevant postoperative care, measures to promote client comfort, and the implications of inactivity on postoperative recovery.

Marilyn knows that it is important to assist Mr. Indelicato in a prompt immediate postoperative recovery and to engage him in a steady, progressive physical therapy program. Although she has cared for clients who have required physical therapy, Marilyn has never cared for a client requiring continuous passive motion equipment. She has acquired and read literature about this equipment, and she consulted with the physical therapist who will be assigned to Mr. Indelicato.

Marilyn approaches this clinical experience with energy and creativity. She plans to collaborate and implement individualized care to promote Mr. Indelicato's comfort, to increase activity, and to improve range of joint motion.

mobility and may not perceive a need for improvement. Unless there is a real threat to health maintenance, forcing the client to accept your perspective is a breach of standards of care.

Nursing Diagnosis

Assessment of the client's body alignment and joint mobility provides related clusters of data or defining characteristics that lead to the identification of nursing diagnoses (Box 24-5).

Alterations in body alignment and joint mobility can result from developmental changes, postural abnormalities, abnormalities in bone formation, impaired muscle development, damage to the central nervous system, or direct trauma to the musculoskeletal system. In some instances alterations in joint mobility or alignment may be one of the defining characteristics of a separate nursing diagnosis and not the actual nursing diagnosis. Nursing diagnoses often focus on the individual's ability to move. The diagnostic label should direct nursing interventions. For example, in the nursing care plan the diagnostic label *impaired physical mobility* is supported by the characteristics: difficulty in moving his knee and reduced range of joint motion. The related factor is supported by the assessment of pain.

Planning

During planning you will use data gathered during assessment and critical thinking to develop an individualized plan of care. Identifying client needs and, in collaboration with the client and family, integrating these needs with the goals and outcomes of care, care priorities, and restorative and continuing care needs enable you to develop a plan of care to optimize the client's exercise and activity levels.

GOALS AND OUTCOMES.   Once the nursing diagnoses have been defined, you and the client set goals and expected

Factors Influencing Activity Tolerance   Box 24-4

PHYSIOLOGICAL FACTORS
Skeletal abnormalities
Muscular impairments
Endocrine or metabolic illnesses (e.g., diabetes mellitus, thyroid disease)
Hypoxemia
Decreased cardiac function
Decreased endurance
Impaired physical stability
Pain
Sleep pattern disturbance
Prior exercise patterns
Infectious processes and fever

EMOTIONAL FACTORS
Anxiety
Depression
Chemical addictions
Motivation

DEVELOPMENTAL FACTORS
Age
Sex

PREGNANCY
Physical growth and development of muscle and skeletal support

Modified from Phipps WJ and others: *Medical surgical nursing,* ed 6, St. Louis, 1999, Mosby.

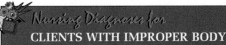

Nursing Diagnoses for   Box 24-5
CLIENTS WITH IMPROPER BODY MECHANICS AND IMPAIRED JOINT MOBILITY

- Activity intolerance
- Body image, disturbed
- Injury, risk for
- Mobility, impaired physical
- Pain, acute
- Pain, chronic
- Skin integrity, impaired

outcomes to direct interventions. The plan should include consideration of any risks for injury to the client and preexisting health concerns. It is especially important to have knowledge of the client's previous functional status and home environment. Your client's family or significant others should be included in the care plan.

SETTING PRIORITIES.   Care planning is individualized to the client, taking into consideration the client's most immediate needs. The immediacy of any problem is determined by the effect the problem has on the client's mental and physical health. For example, if a client is in acute pain, relief of pain is a priority that must be met before exercise can be initiated. Because of the many skills associated with the care of clients with activity intolerance, improper body mechanics, and/or impaired mobility, such as turning, transferring, and positioning, it may be easy to overlook the complications associated with these nursing and medical diagnoses.

Case Study Nursing Care Plan IMPAIRED PHYSICAL MOBILITY

ASSESSMENT

Joseph Indelicato is a 72-year-old man hospitalized for surgery on his right knee. Over the past 5 years, he has continued to experience pain and decreased mobility. He is now *2 days postoperative* following right total knee replacement. His incision is healing, and there is no edema or erythema. He rates his **pain as 6 to 7 on a 10-point scale** and is using a **patient-controlled analgesia pump.** He uses a **continuous passive motion (CPM) machine 4 times a day.** His degree of **knee flexion is now 60 degrees.** He is able to **ambulate to the bathroom with the aid of a walker.**

*Defining characteristics are shown in bold type.

NURSING DIAGNOSIS

Impaired physical mobility related to pain and limited joint motion.

PLANNING

GOAL

Client will gain optimal range of motion (ROM) of right knee.

Client will maintain optimum level of comfort.

EXPECTED OUTCOMES

Client will gain a minimum of 90 degrees flexion in right knee.
Client will ambulate full length of hall by discharge.
Client's pain will be 3 to 4 on a 10-point scale by discharge.
Client's will verbally report pain controlled by oral analgesics.

IMPLEMENTATION

STEPS

1. Provide analgesics 30 minutes before ROM exercises or use of CPM machine.
2. Teach client and family muscle-strengthening exercises.

3. Teach client and family proper use of walker.

RATIONAL

Peak actions of analgesic will occur as client begins exercise (Gahart and Nazareno, 2002).
Exercise improves circulation to the area and strengthens extremity for ambulation.
Prevents injury and loss of function.

EVALUATION

- Measure degree of knee flexion.
- Observe client's ROM or use of CPM machine.
- Observe client ambulate.
- Ask client to rate level of pain on a 10-point scale.

Therefore you must be vigilant in monitoring the client and supervising assistive personnel in carrying out activities to prevent complications and potential injury.

CONTINUITY OF CARE.   Planning also involves an understanding of the client's need to maintain motor function and independence. Collaboration with other members of the health care team, for example, physical or occupational therapists, will be especially important for these clients. Long-term rehabilitation may be necessary, and discharge planning is begun when a client enters the health care system. In addition, always individualize a plan of care directed at meeting the actual or potential needs of the client (see care plan).

Implementation

HEALTH PROMOTION.   In recent years the rate of injuries in occupational settings has increased dramatically. Half of all back pain is associated with manual lifting tasks (Gassett and others, 1996). The most common back injury is strain on the lumbar muscle group, which includes the muscles around the lumbar vertebrae. Injury to these areas affects the ability to bend forward, backward, and side to side. The ability to rotate the hips and lower back is also decreased. To protect the client and yourself, proper body mechanics must be learned and mastered (Box 24-6).

Client Teaching   **Box 24-6**

BODY MECHANICS
- People are more likely to do something if they believe they will be able to perform successfully. They also have to believe that a skill or action will make a positive difference.
- Clients should exercise joints only as ordered by the physician. Increases in discomfort should be reported immediately and not attributed to the exercise activity.
- Family members should be taught the safe use of adaptive aids (e.g., transfer belts, lifts) to assist with transfers and activities in the home.
- Mobility aids are valuable in promoting energy conservation and decreasing fatigue, further promoting compliance with activity.
- Clients and caregivers should assess and stabilize their centers of gravity to promote safety in lifting and positioning.

LIFTING TECHNIQUES.   Before lifting, assess the weight to be lifted and what assistance, if any, is needed. If help is needed, you should assess if a second person is adequate or if mechanical assistance is needed. Once the amount of needed assistance is determined, these steps are followed:

1. Tighten stomach muscles and tuck pelvis. *Provides balance and protects the back.*

2. Bend at the knees. *Maintains your center of gravity and lets the strong muscles of the legs do the lifting (Figure 24-2).*
3. Keep the weight to be lifted as close to the body as possible. *Places the weight in the same plane as the lifter and close to the center of gravity for balance.*
4. Maintain the trunk erect and the knees bent. *Multiple muscle groups work together in a synchronized manner (Gassett and others, 1996).*
5. Avoid twisting. *Twisting can overload your spine and lead to serious injury.*
6. The best height for lifting vertically is approximately 2 feet off the ground and close to the lifter's center of gravity (Gassett and others, 1996). *Maintains center of gravity and improves balance.*

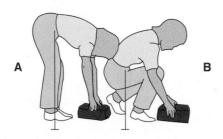

FIGURE **24-2**   Incorrect (**A**) and correct (**B**) body position for lifting.

To reach an object overhead you should do the following:
1. Use a safe, stable step stool or stepladder for elevation. Avoid standing on tiptoe with the feet together. *Maintains base of support, elevates the center of gravity, and improves balance.*
2. Stand as close to the shelf as possible. *Decreases the amount of time you must support the weight of the object with the arms.*
3. Transfer the weight of the object from the shelf to the arms and over the base of support. *Maintains your base of support and aligns the weight of the object close to your center of gravity.*

ACUTE CARE

POSITIONING TECHNIQUES.   Clients with impaired nervous or musculoskeletal system functioning, clients with increased weakness, or those restricted to bed rest benefit from therapeutic positioning (Hoeman, 2001). During client positioning determine areas of bony prominences where pressure, friction, and shear cause the most wear and tear. Through the use of proper positioning and pressure-relief methods, these areas can be protected (see Chapter 34).

In general, clients should be repositioned as needed and at least every 2 hours if they are in bed and every 20 to 30 minutes if they are sitting in a chair. Those clients with contractures or who are at greater risk for skin breakdown over

Devices Used for Proper Positioning	Table 24-2
Devices	Uses and Descriptions
Pillows	Pillows should be of appropriate size for the body part to be positioned. They provide support, elevate body parts, and splint incisional areas.
Foot boots	**Foot boots** maintain feet in dorsiflexion. Boots should be removed at least 2 to 3 times per day to assess skin integrity and joint mobility.
Trochanter rolls	**Trochanter rolls** prevent external rotation of legs when clients are in the supine position. To form a trochanter roll, a cotton bath blanket or a sheet is folded lengthwise to a width extending from the greater trochanter of the femur to the lower border of the popliteal space (Figure 24-3). The roll is placed under the buttocks and then rolled away from the client until the thigh is in a neutral position or an inward position with the patella facing upward.
Sandbags	**Sandbags** provide support and shape to body contours; they immobilize extremities and maintain specific body alignment. They can be used in place of or in addition to the trochanter roll.
Hand rolls	**Hand rolls** maintain the thumb slightly adducted and in opposition to the fingers; they maintain fingers in a lightly flexed position (Figure 24-4). Hand rolls can be made by folding a washcloth in half, rolling it lengthwise, and securing the roll with tape. The roll is placed against the palmar surface of the hand. Evaluate the position of the hand to make certain the hand is in a functional position.
Hand-wrist splints	**Hand-wrist splints** are individually molded for the client to maintain proper alignment of the thumb in slight **adduction** and the wrist in slight dorsiflexion. These splints should be used only for the client for whom they were made.
Trapeze bar	The **trapeze bar** descends from a securely fastened overhead bar attached to the bed frame (Figure 24-5). The trapeze allows the client to use upper extremities to raise the trunk off the bed, to assist in transfer from bed to wheelchair, or to perform upper arm–strengthening exercises.
Side rails	**Side rails** are bars positioned along the sides of the length of the bed. They are designed to increase client's ability to move and turn in bed, for example, rolling from side to side or sitting up in bed.
Bed boards	**Bed boards** are plywood boards placed under the entire surface of the mattress. They are useful for increasing back support and alignment, especially with a soft mattress.
Wedge pillow	A wedge or abductor pillow is a triangular-shaped pillow made of heavy foam. It is used to maintain the legs in **abduction** following total hip replacement surgery.

bony prominences need repositioning more frequently. Additional variables influencing frequency of position changes include level of comfort, amount of spontaneous movement, presence of edema, loss of sensation, and overall physical and mental status (Hoeman, 2001).

Several devices are available for the nurse to use in maintaining good body alignment for clients while clients are being positioned (Table 24-2). Various positions are described in the following paragraphs. The methods of positioning clients are described in Skill 24-1.

Fowler's Position. The head of the client's bed is elevated 45 to 60 degrees, and the client's knees are slightly elevated, avoiding pressure on the popliteal vessels. The head rests against the mattress or a small pillow for support. Pillows can be used to maintain natural alignment of the hands, wrists, and forearms. Supports must permit flexion of the hips and proper alignment of the normal curves in the cervical, thoracic, and lumbar vertebrae (Metzler, 1996).

Supine Position. The supine position is when the client rests on the back. A small, flat pillow supports the head, neck, and upper shoulders (Hoeman, 2001). Pillows, trochanter rolls (see Table 24-2), and hand rolls or arm splints are used to increase comfort and reduce injury to the skin or musculoskeletal system. (Metzler, 1996). The risk of aspiration is greater with this position; thus the supine position should be avoided when your client is confused, agitated, experiencing a decreased level of consciousness, or at risk for aspiration.

The mattress should be firm enough to support the cervical, thoracic, and lumbar vertebrae. Pressure on the back of the legs should be avoided. A foot support is used to prevent **footdrop,** maintain proper alignment, and provide freedom of movement for the feet.

Prone Position. Prone is when the client is in the face-down position. Before placing a client in the **prone** position, assess the client's medical record for any possible complications such as increasing intracranial pressure or cardiopulmonary disease (Hoeman, 2001). Assist the client in lying on the abdomen. The head is turned to the side. This facilitates respiration and drainage of oral secretions. A pillow is placed under the head for comfort and relief from pressure. As an alternative, a wedge can be placed under the client's chest, or arms flexed over the head, if it is more comfortable. Place a pillow under the lower leg; this promotes relaxation. If a pillow is unavailable, the client's ankles should be in **dorsiflexion** over the end of the mattress. Body alignment is poor when the ankles are continuously in **plantar flexion** and the lumbar spine remains in **hyperextension.** Lung expansion may be compromised in this position, especially in the obese.

Lateral Position. In the lateral (or side-lying) position, the client is supported on the right or left side with the opposite arm, thigh, and knee flexed and resting on the bed. A pillow is placed under your client's head to keep the head, neck, and spine in alignment. The upper arm is flexed and supported with a pillow (Metzler, 1996). The upper leg is flexed at the hip and knee and positioned on a small pillow (Hoeman, 2001). Clients who are obese or older may not be able to tolerate this position for any length of time.

Text continued on p. 558

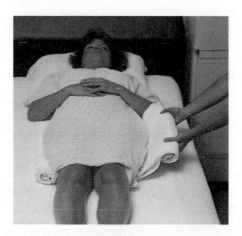

FIGURE **24-3** Trochanter roll.

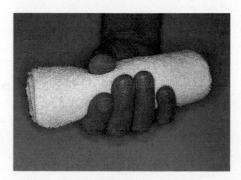

FIGURE **24-4** Hand roll.

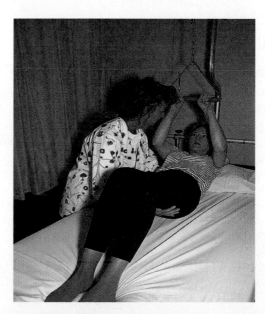

FIGURE **24-5** Client using a trapeze bar.

Skill 24-1
MOVING AND POSITIONING CLIENTS IN BED

DELEGATION CONSIDERATIONS

The skills of moving and positioning clients in bed can be delegated to assistive personnel.

- Instruct caregiver on any limitations affecting movement and positioning of client in bed.
- Evaluate caregiver's transfer and positioning skills.

EQUIPMENT

- Pillows
- Footboard (optional)
- High-top sneakers
- Trochanter roll
- Sandbag
- Hand rolls
- Side rails

STEPS	RATIONALE
1. Assess client's body alignment and comfort level while client is lying down.	Provides baseline data for later comparisons. Determines ways to improve position and alignment.
2. Assess for risk factors that may contribute to complications of immobility:	Increased risk factors require client to be repositioned more frequently.
a. Paralysis: hemiparesis resulting from cerebrovascular accident (CVA); decreased sensation.	Paralysis impairs movement; muscle tone changes; sensation can be affected. Because of difficulty in moving and poor awareness of involved body part, client is unable to protect and position body part for self.
b. Impaired mobility: traction or arthritis or other contributing disease processes.	Traction or arthritic changes of affected extremity result in decreased ROM.
c. Impaired circulation	Decreased circulation predisposes client to pressure sores.
d. Age: very young, aged	Premature and young infants require frequent turning because their skin is fragile. Normal physiological changes associated with aging predispose older adults to greater risks for developing complications of immobility.
e. Level of consciousness and mental status	Comatose or semicomatose clients are unable to verbalize areas of skin pressure, increasing the risk for skin breakdown.
3. Assess client's physical ability to help with moving and positioning:	Use client's mobility and strength. Determines need for additional help. Ensures client's and your safety.
a. Age	Elderly client will move more slowly with less strength.
b. Level of consciousness and mental status	Determines need for special aids or devices.
	Clients with altered levels of consciousness may not understand instructions and may be unable to help.
c. Disease process	Cardiopulmonary disease may require client to have head of bed elevated.
d. Strength, coordination	Determines amount of assistance provided by client during position change.
e. ROM	Limited ROM may contraindicate certain positions.
4. Assess physician's orders. Clarify whether any positions are contraindicated because of client's condition (e.g., spinal cord injury; respiratory difficulties; certain neurological conditions; presence of incisions, drain, or tubing).	Placing client in an inappropriate position could cause injury.
5. Assess for tubes, incisions, and equipment (e.g., traction).	Will alter positioning procedure and may affect client's ability to independently change positions.
6. Assess ability and motivation of client, family members, and primary caregiver to participate in moving and positioning client in bed in anticipation of discharge to home.	Determines ability of client and caregivers to assist with positioning.
7. Raise level of bed to comfortable working height, and get extra help if needed.	Raises level of work to your center of gravity and provides for client's and your safety.
8. Explain procedure to client.	Decreases anxiety and increases client cooperation.

STEPS	RATIONALE
9. Position client flat in bed if tolerated.	Repositioning from a flat position decreases friction and possible shear on client's skin.
10. Keep client aligned.	

• *Critical Decision Point*
Before flattening bed, account for all tubing, drains, and equipment to prevent dislodgment or tipping if caught in mattress or bed frame as bed is lowered.

STEPS	RATIONALE
A. **Move Immobile Client up in Bed (One Nurse)**	
(1) Place client on back with head of bed flat. Stand on one side of bed.	Enables you to assess body alignment. Reduces gravity's pull on client's upper body.
(2) Remove pillow from under head and shoulders, and place pillow at head of bed.	Prevents striking client's head against head of bed.
(3) Begin at client's feet. Face foot of bed at 45-degree angle. Place feet apart with foot nearest head of bed behind other foot (forward-backward stance). Flex knees and hips as needed to bring arms level with client's legs. Shift weight from front to back leg, and slide client's legs diagonally toward head of bed.	Positioning is begun at client's legs because they are lighter and easier to move. Facing direction of movement ensures proper balance. Shifting weight reduces force needed to move load. Diagonal motion permits pull in direction of force. Flexing knees lowers your center of gravity and uses thigh muscles rather than back muscles.
(4) Move parallel to client's hips. Flex knees and hips as needed to bring arms level with client's hips.	Maintains correct body alignment. Brings you closest to object to be moved and lowers center of gravity. Uses thigh muscles rather than back muscles.
(5) Slide client's hips diagonally toward head of bed.	Aligns client's hips and feet.
(6) Move parallel to client's head and shoulders. Flex knees and hips as needed to bring arms level with client's body.	Maintains proper body alignment. Brings you closer to object to be moved. Lowers center of gravity. Uses thigh muscles rather than back muscles.
(7) Slide arm closest to head of bed under clients' neck, with hand reaching under and supporting client's opposite shoulder.	Supports clients' head and neck, maintaining alignment and preventing injury during movement.
(8) Place other arm under client's upper back.	Supports client's body weight and reduces friction during movement.
(9) Slide client's trunk, shoulders, head, and neck diagonally toward head of bed.	Realigns client's body on one side of bed.
(10) Elevate side rail. Move to other side of bed, and lower side rail.	Protects client from falling out of bed.
(11) Repeat procedure, switching sides until client reaches desired position in bed.	
(12) Center client in middle of bed, moving body in same three sections.	Maintains proper body alignment. Provides ample room for turning, positioning, and other nursing activities.
B. **Assist Client in Moving up in Bed (One or Two Nurses)**	
(1) Remove pillow from under head and shoulders, and place pillow at head of bed.	Prevents striking client's head against head of bed.
(2) Face head of bed.	Facing direction of movement prevents twisting of your body while moving client.
(a) Each nurse should have one arm under client's shoulders and one arm under client's thighs.	

STEPS	RATIONALE
(b) Alternative position: position one nurse at clients' upper body. Nurse's arm nearest head of bed should be under client's head and opposite shoulder; other arm should be under client's closest arm and shoulder. Position other nurse at clients' lower torso. The nurse's arms should be under client's lower back and torso.	Prevents trauma to client's musculoskeletal system by supporting shoulder and hip joints and evenly distributing weight.
(3) Place feet apart, with foot nearest head of bed behind other foot (forward-backward stance).	Wide base of support increases balance. Stance enables you to shift body weight as client is moved up in bed, thereby reducing force needed to move load.
(4) When possible, ask client to flex knees with feet flat on bed.	Decreases friction and enables client to use leg muscles during movement.
(5) Instruct client to flex neck, tilting chin toward chest.	Prevents hyperextension of neck when moving client up in bed.
(6) Instruct client to assist moving by pushing with feet on bed surface.	Reduces friction. Increases client mobility. Decreases workload.
(7) Flex knees and hips, bringing forearms closer to level of bed.	Increases balance and strength by bringing your center of gravity closer to client. Uses thighs instead of back muscles.
(8) Instruct client to push with heels and elevate trunk while breathing out, thus moving toward head of bed on count of three.	Prepares client for move. Reinforces assistance in moving up in bed. Increases client cooperation. Breathing out avoids Valsalva maneuver.
(9) On count of three, rock and shift weight from front to back leg. At the same time client pushes with heels and elevates trunk.	Rocking enables you to improve balance and overcome inertia. Shifting your weight counteracts client's weight and reduces force needed to move load. Client's assistance reduces friction and workload.

C. Move Immobile Client up in Bed With Drawsheet or Pull Sheet (Two Nurses)

STEPS	RATIONALE
(1) Place drawsheet or pull sheet under client, extending from shoulders to thighs; return to supine position.	Supports client's body weight and reduces friction during movement.
(2) Position one nurse at each side of client.	Distributes weight equally between nurses.
(3) Grasp drawsheet or pull sheet firmly near the client.	
(4) Place feet apart with forward-backward stance. Flex knees and hips. Shift weight from front to back leg, and move client and drawsheet or pull sheet to desired position in bed.	Facing direction of movement ensures proper balance. Shifting weight reduces force needed to move load. Flexing knees lowers center of gravity and thighs instead of back muscles.
(5) Realign client in correct body alignment.	Prevents injury to musculoskeletal system.

D. Position Client in Supported Fowler's Position (See Illustration)

STEPS	RATIONALE
(1) Elevate head of bed 45 to 60 degrees.	Increases comfort, improves ventilation, and increases client's opportunity to socialize or relax.
(2) Rest head against mattress or on small pillow.	Prevents flexion contractures of cervical vertebrae.

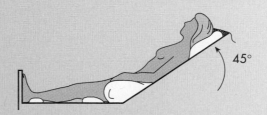

45°

STEP 8D   Fowler's position with footboard in place.

STEPS	RATIONALE
(3) Use pillows to support arms and hands if client does not have voluntary control or use of hands and arms.	Prevents shoulder dislocation from effect of downward pull of unsupported arms, promotes circulation by preventing venous pooling, and prevents flexion contractures of arms and wrists.
(4) Position pillow at lower back.	Supports lumbar vertebrae and decreases flexion of vertebrae.
(5) Place small pillow or roll under thigh.	Prevents hyperextension of knee and occlusion of popliteal artery from pressure from body weight.
(6) Place small pillow or roll under ankles.	Prevents prolonged pressure of mattress on heels.

- *Critical Decision Point*

*To keep feet in proper alignment and prevent footdrop, place **footboard** at bottom of client's feet.*

E. Position Hemiplegic Client in Supported Fowler's Position

STEPS	RATIONALE
(1) Elevate head of bed 45 to 60 degrees.	Increases comfort, improves ventilation, and increases client's opportunity to relax.
(2) Position client in sitting position as straight as possible.	Counteracts tendency to slump toward affected side. Improves ventilation and cardiac output; decreases intracranial pressure. Improves client's ability to swallow and helps to prevent aspiration of food, liquids, and gastric secretions.
(3) Position head on small pillow with chin slightly forward. If client is totally unable to control head movement, hyperextension of the neck must be avoided.	Prevents hyperextension of neck. Too many pillows under head may cause or worsen neck flexion contracture.

- *Critical Decision Point*

If the client has a paralyzed extremity, provide support for involved arm and hand on over-bed table in front of client. Place arm away from client's side and support elbow with pillow.

- *Critical Decision Point*

Position flaccid *hand in normal resting position with wrist slightly extended, arches of hand maintained, and fingers partially flexed; may use section of rubber ball cut in half; clasp client's hands together.*

- *Critical Decision Point*

Position spastic *hand with wrist in neutral position or slightly extended; fingers should be extended with palm down or may be left in relaxed position with palm up. At times it may be difficult to position spastic hands without the use of specially made splints for the client.*

STEPS	RATIONALE
(4) Flex knees and hips by using pillow or folded blanket under knees.	Ensures proper alignment. Flexion prevents prolonged hyperextension, which could impair joint mobility.
(5) Support feet in dorsiflexion with firm pillow or footboard.	Prevents footdrop. Stimulation of ball of foot by hard surface has tendency to increase muscle tone in client with extensor spasticity of lower extremity.

F. Position Client in Supine Position

STEPS	RATIONALE
(1) Be sure client is comfortable on back with head of bed flat.	Some clients' physical conditions will not tolerate supine position.
(2) Place small rolled towel under lumbar area of back.	Provides support for lumbar spine.
(3) Place pillow under upper shoulders, neck, or head.	Maintains correct alignment and prevents flexion contractures of cervical vertebrae.
(4) Place trochanter rolls or sandbags parallel to lateral surface of client's thighs.	Reduces external rotation of hip.
(5) Place small pillow or roll under ankle to elevate heels (see illustration for Step 8 D).	Reduces pressure on heels, helping to prevent pressure sores.
(6) Place footboard or firm pillows against bottom of client's feet.	Maintains dorsiflexion and prevents footdrop.
(7) Place foot splints on client's feet.	Maintains feet in dorsiflexion. Prevents footdrop.

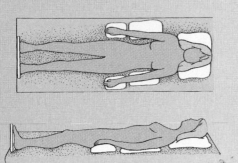

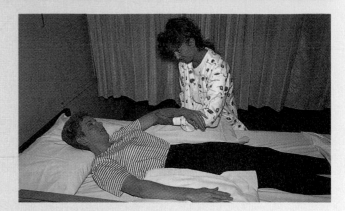

STEP 8 F(8)   Supine position with pillows in place.

STEPS	RATIONALE
(8) Place pillows under pronated forearms, keeping upper arms parallel to client's body (see illustrations).	Reduces internal rotation of shoulder and prevents extension of elbows. Maintains correct body alignment.
(9) Place hand rolls in client's hands. Consider physical therapy referral for use of hand splints.	Reduces extension of fingers and abduction of thumb. Maintains thumb slightly adducted and in opposition to fingers.

G. Position Hemiplegic Client in Supine Position

STEPS	RATIONALE
(1) Place head of bed flat.	Necessary for positioning in supine position.
(2) Place folded towel or small pillow under shoulder or affected side.	Decreases possibility of pain, joint contracture, and subluxation. Maintains mobility in muscles around shoulder to permit normal movement patterns.
(3) Keep affected arm away from body with elbow extended and palm up. (Alternative is to place arm out to side, with elbow bent and hand toward head of bed.)	Maintains mobility in arm, joints, and shoulder to permit normal movement patterns. (Alternative position counteracts limitation of ability of arm to rotate outward at shoulder [external rotation]. External rotation must be present to raise arm overhead without pain.)

• *Critical Decision Point*
Position affected hand in one of the recommended positions for flaccid or spastic hand (see p. 553).

STEPS	RATIONALE
(4) Place folded towel under hip of involved side.	Diminishes effect of spasticity in entire leg by controlling hip position.
(5) Flex affected knee 30 degrees by supporting it on pillow or folded blanket.	Slight flexion breaks up abnormal extension pattern of leg. Extensor spasticity is most severe when client is supine.
(6) Support feet with soft pillows at right angle to leg.	Maintains foot in dorsiflexion and prevents footdrop. Pillows prevent stimulation to ball of foot by hard surface, which has tendency to increase muscle tone in client with extensor spasticity of lower extremity.

H. Position Client in Prone Position

STEPS	RATIONALE
(1) Roll client over arm positioned close to body, with elbow straight and hand under hip. Position on abdomen in center of bed.	Positions client correctly so alignment can be maintained.
(2) Turn client's head to one side and support head with small pillow (see illustration).	Reduces flexion or hyperextension of cervical vertebrae.
(3) Place small pillow under client's abdomen below level of diaphragm (see illustration).	Reduces pressure on breasts of some female clients and decreases hyperextension of lumbar vertebrae and strain on lower back.
(4) Support arms in flexed position level at shoulders.	Maintains proper body alignment. Support reduces risk of joint dislocation.

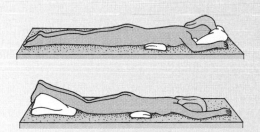

STEP 8 H(2-3)   Prone position with pillows in place.

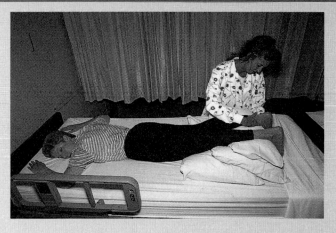

STEP 8 H(5)   Prone position with pillows supporting lower legs.

(5) Support lower legs with pillow to elevate toes (see illustration).	Prevents footdrop. Reduces external rotation of hips. Reduces mattress pressure on toes.

I. Position Hemiplegic Client in Prone Position

• *Critical Decision Point*
Increase frequency of positioning if pressure areas begin to appear, joint mobility becomes impaired or worsened, or client complains of discomfort. Consult with physical and occupational therapists as needed.

(1) Move client toward unaffected side.	Creates room for proper client alignment in center of bed when client is rolled onto abdomen.
(2) Roll client onto side.	
(3) Place pillow on client's abdomen.	Prevents sagging of abdomen when client is rolled over; decreases hyperextension of lumbar vertebrae and strain on lower back.
(4) Roll client onto abdomen by positioning involved arm close to client's body, with elbow straight and hand under hip. Roll client carefully over arm.	Prevents injury to affected side.
(5) Turn head toward involved side.	Promotes development of neck and trunk extension, which is necessary for standing and walking.
(6) Position involved arm out to side, with elbow bent, hand toward head of bed, and fingers extended (if possible).	Counteracts limitation of arm's ability to rotate outward at shoulder (external rotation). External rotation must be present to raise arm over head without pain.
(7) Flex knees slightly by placing pillow under legs from knees to ankles.	Flexion prevents prolonged hyperextension, which could impair joint mobility.
(8) Keep feet at right angle to legs by using pillow high enough to keep toes off mattress.	Maintains feet in dorsiflexion.

J. Position Client in Lateral (Side-Lying) Position

(1) Lower head of bed completely or as low as client can tolerate.	Provides position of comfort for client and removes pressure from bony prominences on back and buttocks.
(2) Position client to side of bed.	Provides room for client to turn to side.
(3) Prepare to turn client onto side. Flex client's knee that will not be next to mattress. Place one hand on client's hip and one hand on client's shoulder.	Positioning will set up leverage for easy turning.

• *Critical Decision Point*
Clients at risk for pressure ulcer development require the 30-degree lateral position (see Chapter 34).

(4) Roll client onto side toward you.

Rolling client toward you decreases trauma to tissues. In addition, client is positioned so leverage on hip makes turning easy.

(5) Place pillow under client's head and neck.

Maintains alignment. Reduces lateral neck flexion. Decreases strain on sternocleidomastoid muscle.

(6) Bring shoulder blade forward.

Prevents client's weight from resting directly on shoulder joint.

(7) Position both arms in slightly flexed position. Upper arm is supported by pillow level with shoulder; other arm, by mattress.

Decreases internal rotation and adduction of shoulder. Supporting both arms in slightly flexed position protects joints. Ventilation is improved because chest is able to expand more easily.

(8) Place tuck-back pillow behind client's back. (Make by folding pillow lengthwise. Smooth area is slightly tucked under client's back.)

Provides support to maintain client on side.

(9) Place pillow under semiflexed upper leg level at hip from groin to foot (see illustrations).

Maintains leg in correct alignment. Prevents pressure on bony prominence.

(10) Place sandbag parallel to plantar surface of dependent foot.

Maintains dorsiflexion of foot. Prevents footdrop.

K. Position Client in Sims' (Semiprone) Position

(1) Lower head of bed completely.

(2) Be sure client is comfortable in supine position.

Provides for proper body alignment while client is lying down.

(3) Position client in lateral position, lying partially on abdomen.

Prepares client for position.
Client is rolled only partially on abdomen.

(4) Place small pillow under client's head.

(5) Place pillow under flexed upper arm, supporting arm level with shoulder.

Maintains proper alignment and prevents lateral neck flexion.
Prevents internal rotation of shoulder. Maintains alignment.

(6) Place pillow under flexed upper legs, supporting leg level with hip.

Prevents internal rotation of hip and adduction of leg. Flexion prevents hyperextension of leg. Reduces mattress pressure on knees and ankles.

(7) Place sandbags parallel to plantar surface of foot (see illustration).

Maintains foot in dorsiflexion. Prevents footdrop.

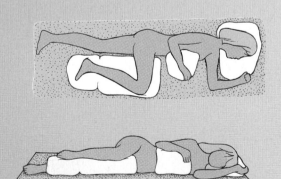
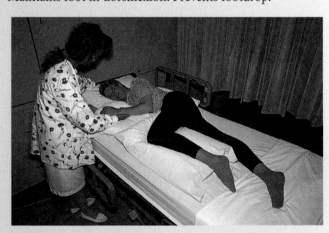

STEP 8 J(9)   Lateral position with pillows in place.

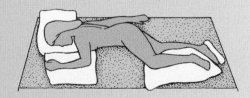

STEP 8 K(7)   Sandbag supporting foot in dorsiflexion.

L. Logrolling the Client (Three Nurses)

- *Critical Decision Point*

Supervise and aid assistive personnel when there is a physician's order to **logroll** *a client. Clients who have suffered from a spinal cord injury or are recovering from neck, back, or spinal surgery often need to keep the spinal column in straight alignment to prevent further injury.*

STEPS	RATIONALE
(1) Place pillow between client's knees.	Prevents tension on the spinal column and adduction of the hip.
(2) Cross client's arms on chest.	Prevents injury to arms.
(3) Position two nurses on side of bed to which the client will be turned. Position third nurse on the other side of bed (see illustration).	Distributes weight equally between nurses.
(4) Fanfold or roll the drawsheet or pull sheet.	Provides strong handles in order to grip the drawsheet or pull sheet without slipping.
(5) Move the client as one unit in a smooth, continuous motion on the count of three (see illustration).	This maintains proper alignment by moving all body parts at the same time, preventing tension or twisting of the spinal column.
(6) Nurse on the opposite side of the bed places pillows along the length of the client (see illustration).	Pillows keep client aligned.
(7) Gently lean the client as a unit back towards the pillows for support (see illustration).	Ensures continued straight alignment of spinal column, preventing injury.

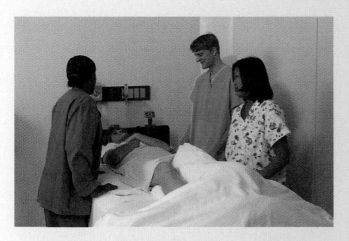

STEP 8 L(3)   Position nurses on each side of client.

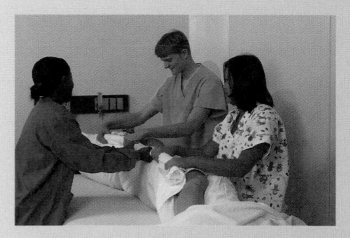

STEP 8 L(5)   Move client as a unit, maintaining proper alignment.

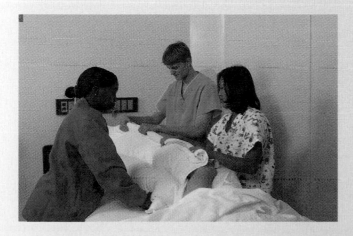

STEP 8 L(6)   Place pillows along client's back for support.

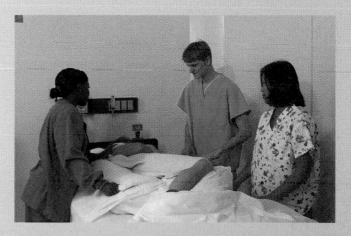

STEP 8 L(7)   Gently lean client as a unit against pillows.

STEPS	RATIONALE

UNEXPECTED OUTCOMES AND RELATED INTERVENTIONS
■ Joint contractures develop or worsen.
  • Improper positioning results in shortening of muscles.
■ Skin shows areas of erythema and breakdown.
  • Frequency of repositioning is inadequate.
  • Place turning schedule above client's bed.
■ Client avoids moving.
  • Indicates fear of pain.
	• Medicate as ordered by a physician to ensure client's comfort before moving.
	• Allow pain medication to take effect before proceeding.
	
	RECORDING AND REPORTING
	■ Record procedure and observations (e.g., condition of skin, joint movement, client's ability to assist with positioning).
	■ Report observations at change of shift and document in nurses' notes.

Sims' Position. In the Sims' position the client is semi-prone on the right or left side with the opposite arm, thigh, and knee flexed and resting on the bed. The Sims' position differs from the side-lying position in the distribution of the client's weight. In this position the client's weight is placed on the anterior ilium, humerus, and clavicle.

Improper positioning can cause unnecessary harm to clients, such as skin breakdown and joint contractures, especially if they have certain preexisting conditions such as peripheral vascular disease or diabetes. Positions that compromise peripheral blood flow may damage nerves as well (Metzler, 1996). Every time your client is repositioned, make certain to check total body alignment, placement of extremities, skin breakdown, and joint contractures.

TRANSFER TECHNIQUES. You often provide care for immobilized clients whose position must be changed, who must be moved up in bed, or who must be transferred from a bed to a chair or a bed to a stretcher. Proper use of body mechanics enables you to move, lift, or transfer clients safely and also protects you from injury to the musculoskeletal system (Skill 24-2).

The following general guidelines should be followed in any transfer procedure:

1. Mentally review the transfer steps before beginning to ensure both the client's safety and yours.
2. Assess the client's mobility and strength to determine the assistance he or she can offer during transfer.
3. Determine the amount and type of assistance you require.
4. Explain the procedure and describe what is expected of the client.
5. Raise the side rail on the side of the bed opposite of where you are standing to prevent the client from falling out of bed on that side.
6. Position the level of the bed to a comfortable and safe height.
7. Arrange equipment (e.g., intravenous [IV] lines, feeding tube, Foley catheter) so it will not interfere with the transfer.
8. Evaluate client for correct body alignment and pressure areas after the transfer.

Transferring is a skill that helps your dependent client attain positions to regain optimal independence as quickly as possible. Physical activity maintains and improves joint motion, increases strength, promotes circulation, relieves pressure on skin, and improves urinary and respiratory functions. It also benefits the client psychologically by increasing social activity and mental stimulation and providing a change in environment. Thus mobilization plays a crucial role in the client's rehabilitation.

One of the major concerns during transfer is the safety of the client and yourself. You prevent self-injury by using correct posture, minimal muscle strength, and effective body mechanics and lifting techniques. Always be aware of the client's motor deficits, ability to aid in transfer, and body weight. As a rule of thumb, if in doubt GET HELP to transfer a client.

Many special problems must be considered in transfer. A client who has been immobile for several days or longer may be weak or dizzy or may develop **orthostatic hypotension** (a drop in blood pressure) when transferred (Phipps and others, 1999). A client with neurological deficits may have paresis (muscle weakness) or paralysis unilaterally or bilaterally, which complicates safe transfer. A flaccid arm may sustain injury during transfer if unsupported. As a general rule, use a transfer belt and obtain assistance for mobilization of such clients.

JOINT MOBILITY AND AMBULATION

Range-of-Motion Exercises. The easiest intervention to maintain or improve joint mobility for clients and one that can be coordinated with other activities is the use of range-of-motion exercises. In **active range-of-motion exercises,** the client is able to move his or her joints. In contrast, as the nurse, you move the client's joints in **passive range-of-motion exercises.** The use of these exercises enables you to systematically assess and improve the client's joint mobility (Table 24-3).

Joints that are not moved periodically can develop contractures, a permanent shortening of a muscle followed by the eventual shortening of associated ligaments and tendons. Over time the joint may become fixed in one position, and the client loses normal use of the joint. For the client who does not have voluntary motor control, passive range-of-motion exercises are the exercises of choice.

The older adult has a decline in physical activity and changes in joints that may predispose the client to problems with mobility, and joint flexibility may be limited. You can

Text continued on p. 565

Skill 24-2

Using Safe and Effective T

DELEGATION CONSIDERATIONS

The skills of effective transfer techniques can be delegated to assistive personnel. Clients who are transferred for the first time after prolonged bed rest, extensive surgery, critical illness, or spinal cord trauma usually require supervision by professional nurses.

- Instruct caregiver to seek assistance when moving or lifting heavy client.
- Instruct caregiver on any client limitations that may affect safe transfer techniques.
- Evaluate caregiver's transfer and positioning skills.

EQUIPMENT

- Transfer belt, sling or lapboard (as needed), nonskid shoes, bath blankets, pillows
- Wheelchair: position chair at 45-degree angle to bed, lock brakes, remove footrests, lock bed brakes
- Stretcher: position at right angle (90 degrees) to bed, lock brakes on stretcher, lock brakes on bed
- Mechanical/hydraulic lift: use frame, canvas strips or chains, and hammock or canvas strips

STEPS	RATIONALE
1. Assess the client for the following:	Provides information relative to the client's abilities, physical status, ability to comprehend, and the number of individuals needed to provide safe transferring.
a. Muscle strength (legs and upper arms)	Immobile clients have decreased muscle strength, tone, and mass. Affects ability to bear weight or raise body.
b. Joint mobility and contracture formation	Immobility or inflammatory processes (e.g., arthritis) may lead to contracture formation and impaired joint mobility.
c. Paralysis or paresis (spastic or flaccid)	Client with central nervous system damage may have bilateral paralysis (requiring transfer by swivel bar, sliding bar, or Hoyer lift or unilateral paralysis, which requires belt transfer to "best" side. Weakness (paresis) requires stabilization of knee while transferring. Flaccid arm must be supported with sling during transfer.
d. Orthostatic hypotension	Determines risk of fainting or falling during transfer. Immobile clients may have decreased ability for autonomic nervous system to equalize blood supply, resulting in drop of 15 mm Hg or more in blood pressure when rising from sitting position.
e. Activity tolerance	Determines ability of client to assist with transfer.
f. Level of comfort	Pain may reduce client's motivation and ability to be mobile. Pain relief before transfer enhances client participation.
g. Vital signs	Vital sign changes such as increased pulse and respiration may indicate activity intolerance (see Chapter 11).
2. Assess client's sensory status: a. Adequacy of central and peripheral vision b. Adequacy of hearing c. Loss of peripheral sensation	Determines influence of sensory loss on ability to make transfer. Visual field loss decreases client's ability to see in direction of transfer. Peripheral sensation loss decreases proprioception. Clients with visual and hearing losses need transfer techniques adapted to deficits. Clients with cerebrovascular accident (CVA) may lose area of visual field, which profoundly affects vision and perception.

- *Critical Decision Point*
Clients with hemiplegia also may "neglect" one side of the body (inattention to or unawareness of one side of body or environment), which distorts perception of the visual field.

3. Assess client's cognitive status:	Determines client's ability to follow directions and learn transfer techniques.

- *Critical Decision Point*
Clients with head trauma or CVA may have perceptual cognitive deficits that create safety risks. If client has difficulty in comprehension, simplify instructions and maintain consistency.

STEPS	RATIONALE

4. Assess client's level of motivation:
  a. Client's eagerness versus unwillingness to be mobile
  b. Whether client avoids activity and offers excuses
	Altered psychological states reduce client's desire to engage in activity.

5. Assess previous mode of transfer (if applicable).	Determines mode of transfer and assistance required to provide continuity. Transfer belts should be used with all clients being transferred for the first time and thereafter as deemed necessary.
6. Assess client's specific risk of falling when transferred.	Certain conditions increase client's risk of falling or potential for injury. Neuromuscular deficits, motor weakness, calcium loss from long bones, cognitive and visual dysfunction, and altered balance increase risk of injury.
7. Assess special transfer equipment needed for home setting. Assess home environment for hazards.	Transfer ability at home is greatly enhanced by prior teaching of family and support persons, assessment of home for safety risks and functionality, and provision of applicable aids.
8. Explain procedure to client.	Increases client participation.
9. Transfer client.	
A. Assist Client to Sitting Position (Bed at Waist Level)	
(1) Place client in supine position.	Enables you to assess client's body alignment continually and to administer additional care, such as suctioning or hygiene needs.
(2) Face head of bed at a 45-degree angle, and remove pillows.	Proper positioning reduces twisting of your body when moving the client. Pillows may cause interference when the client is sitting up in bed.
(3) Place feet apart with foot nearer bed behind other foot, continuing at a 45-degree angle to the head of the bed.	Improves balance and allows transfer of body weight as client is moved to sitting position.
(4) Place hand farther from client under shoulders, supporting client's head and cervical vertebrae.	Maintains alignment of head and cervical vertebrae and allows for even lifting of client's upper trunk.
(5) Place other hand on bed surface.	Provides support and balance.
(6) Raise client to sitting position by shifting weight from front to back leg.	Improves balance, overcomes inertia, and transfers weight in direction in which client is moved.
(7) Push against bed using arm that is placed on bed surface.	Divides activity between arms and legs and protects back from strain. By bracing one hand against mattress and pushing against it as client is lifted, part of weight that would be lifted by your back muscles is transferred through your arm onto mattress.
B. Assist Client to Sitting Position on Side of Bed With Bed in Low Position	
(1) Turn client to side, facing you on side of bed on which client will be sitting (see illustration).	Decreases amount of work needed by client and you to raise client to sitting position.
(2) With client in supine position, raise head of bed 30 degrees.	Prepares client to move to side of bed and protects from falling.
(3) Stand opposite client's hips. Turn diagonally so you face client and far corner of foot of bed.	Places your center of gravity nearer client. Reduces twisting of your body because you are facing direction of movement.

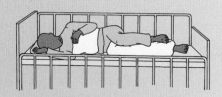

STEP B(1) Side-lying position.

STEPS	RATIONALE
(4) Place feet apart with foot closer to head of bed in front of other foot.	Increases balance and allows you to transfer weight as client is brought to sitting position on side of bed.
(5) Place arm nearer head of bed under client's shoulders, supporting head and neck.	Maintains alignment of head and neck as you bring client to sitting position.
(6) Place other arm over client's thighs (see illustration).	Supports hip and prevents client from falling backward during procedure.
(7) Move client's lower legs and feet over side of bed. Pivot toward rear leg, allowing client's upper legs to swing downward.	Decreases friction and resistance. Weight of client's legs when off bed allows gravity to lower legs, and weight of legs assists in pulling upper body in sitting position.
(8) At same time, shift weight to rear leg and elevate client (see illustration).	Allows you to transfer weight in direction of motion.
(a) Remain in front until client regains balance, and continue to provide physical support to weak or cognitively impaired client.	Reduces client risk for falling. Immobilized clients may experience lightheadedness or dizziness when assuming a sitting position.

C. Transferring Client From Bed to Chair With Bed in Low Position

(1) Assist client to sitting position on side of bed. Have chair in position at 45-degree angle to bed.	Positions chair within easy access for transfer.
(2) Apply transfer belt or other transfer aids.	Transfer belt maintains stability of client during transfer and reduces risk of falling (Owens and others, 1999). Client's arm should be in sling if flaccid paralysis is present.
(3) Ensure that client has stable nonskid shoes. Weight-bearing or strong leg is placed forward, with weak foot back.	Nonskid soles decrease risk of slipping during transfer. Always have client wear shoes during transfer; bare feet increase risk of falls. Client will stand on stronger, or weight-bearing, leg.
(4) Spread feet apart.	Ensures balance with wide base of support.
(5) Flex hips and knees, aligning knees with client's knees (see illustration).	Flexion of knees and hips lowers the center of gravity to object to be raised; aligning knees with client's allows for stabilization of knees when client stands.

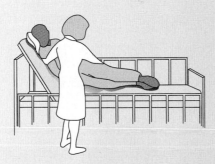

STEP B(6)   Nurse places arm over client's thighs.

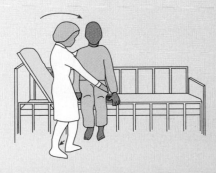

STEP B(8)   Nurse shifts weight to rear leg and elevates client.

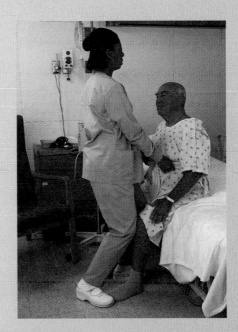

STEP C(5)   Nurse flexes hips and knees, aligning knees with client's knees.

STEPS	RATIONALE

(6) Grasp transfer belt from underneath.

Transfer belt is grasped at client's side to provide movement of client at center of gravity. Clients with upper extremity paralysis or paresis should never be lifted by or under arms.

• *Critical Decision Point*
A transfer belt or walking belt with handles should be used in place of the under-axilla technique. The under-axilla technique has been found to be physically stressful for nurses and uncomfortable for patients (Owens and others, 1999).

(7) Rock client up to standing position on count of three while straightening hips and legs and keeping knees slightly flexed (see illustration). Unless contraindicated, client may be instructed to use hands to push up if applicable.

Rocking motion gives client's body momentum and requires less muscular effort to lift client.

(8) Maintain stability of client's weak or paralyzed leg with knee.

Ability to stand can often be maintained in paralyzed or weak limb with support of knee to stabilize.

(9) Pivot on foot farther from chair.

Maintains support of client while allowing adequate space for client to move.

(10) Instruct client to use armrests on chair for support and ease into chair (see illustration).

Increases client stability.

(11) Flex hips and knees while lowering client into chair (see illustration).

Prevents injury to you from poor body mechanics.

(12) Assess client for proper alignment for sitting position. Provide support for paralyzed extremities. Lapboard or sling will support flaccid arm. Stabilize leg with bath blanket or pillow.

Prevents injury to client from poor body alignment.

(13) Praise client's progress, effort, or performance.

Continued support and encouragement provide incentive for client perseverance.

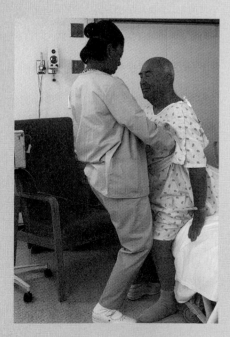 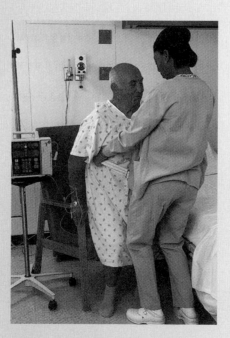 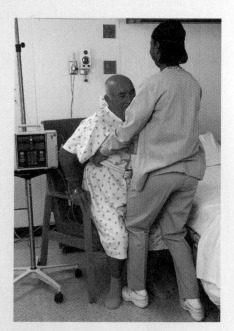

STEP C(7) Nurse rocks client to standing position.

STEP C(10) Client uses armrests for support.

STEP C(11) Nurse eases client into chair.

STEPS	RATIONALE

D. Perform Three-Person Carry From Bed to Stretcher (Bed at Stretcher Level)

(1) Three nurses stand side by side facing side of client's bed.

Prevents twisting of nurses' bodies. Client's alignment is maintained.

(2) Each person assumes responsibility for one of three areas: head and shoulders, hips and thighs, and ankles.

Distributes client's body weight evenly.

(3) Each person assumes wide base of support with foot closer to stretcher in front and knees slightly flexed.

Increases balance and lowers center of gravity of person lifting.

(4) Arms of lifters are placed under client's head and shoulders, hips and thighs, and ankles, with fingers securely around other side of client's body (see illustration).

Distributes client's weight over forearms of lifters.

• ***Critical Decision Point***
Verify that clients with spinal cord injuries are stabilized before transfer. The inexperienced care provider should not attempt to move the spinal cord–injured client.

(5) Lifters roll client toward their chests. On count of three, client is lifted and held against nurses' chests.

Moves workload over lifters' base of support. Enables lifters to work together and safely lift client.

(6) On second count of three, nurses step back and pivot toward stretcher, moving forward if needed.

Transfers weight toward stretcher.

(7) Gently lower client onto center of stretcher by flexing knees and hips until elbows are level with edge of stretcher.

Maintains nurses' alignment during transfer.

(8) Assess client's body alignment, place safety straps across body, and raise side rails.

Reduces risk of injury from poor alignment or falling.

E. Use Hoyer (Mechanical/Hydraulic) Lift to Transfer Client From Bed to Chair

(1) Bring lift to bedside.

Ensures safe elevation of client off bed. (Before using lift, be thoroughly familiar with its operation.)

(2) Position chair near bed, and allow adequate space to maneuver lift.

Prepares environment for safe use of lift and subsequent transfer.

(3) Raise bed to high position with mattress flat. Lower side rail.

Maintains center of gravity.

(4) Keep bed side rail up on side opposite you.

Maintains client safety.

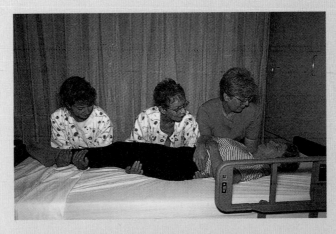

STEP D(4)   Proper positioning of lifters during three-person transfer.

STEPS	RATIONALE
(5) Roll client away from you.	Positions client for use of lift sling.
(6) Place hammock or canvas strips under client to form sling (see illustration). With two canvas pieces, lower edge fits under client's knees (wide piece), and upper edge fits under client's shoulders (narrow piece).	Two types of seat are supplied with mechanical/hydraulic lift: hammock style is better for clients who are flaccid, weak, and need support; canvas strips can be used for clients with normal muscle tone. Hooks should face away from client's skin. Place sling under client's center of gravity and greatest portion of body weight.
(7) Raise bed rail.	Maintains client safety.
(8) Go to opposite side of bed and lower side rail.	
(9) Roll client to opposite side and pull hammock (strips) through.	Completes positioning of client on mechanical/hydraulic sling.
(10) Roll client supine onto canvas seat.	Sling should extend from shoulders to knees (hammock) to support client's body weight equally.
(11) Remove client's glasses, if appropriate.	Swivel bar is close to client's head and could break eyeglasses.
(12) Place lift's horseshoe bar under side of bed (on side with chair).	Positions lift efficiently and promotes smooth transfer.
(13) Lower horizontal bar to sling level by releasing hydraulic valve. Lock valve.	Positions hydraulic lift close to client. Locking valve prevents injury to client.
(14) Attach hooks on strap (chain) to holes in sling. Short chains or straps hook to top holes of sling; longer chains hook to bottom of sling.	Secures hydraulic lift to sling.
(15) Elevate head of bed.	Positions client in sitting position.
(16) Fold client's arms over chest.	Prevents injury to paralyzed arms.
(17) Pump hydraulic handle using long, slow, even strokes until client is raised off bed.	Ensures safe support of client during elevation.
(18) Use steering handle to pull lift from bed and maneuver to chair.	Moves client from bed to chair.
(19) Roll base around chair.	Positions lift in front of the chair in which client is to be transferred.
(20) Release check valve slowly (turn to left) and lower client into chair (see illustration).	Safely guides client into back of chair as seat descends.

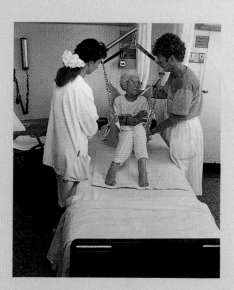

STEP E(6)   Proper placement of sling under client.

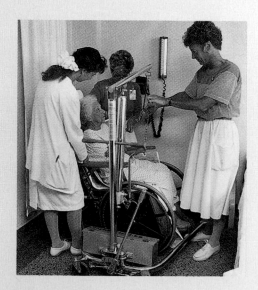

STEP E(20)   Use of hydraulic lift to lower client into chair.

STEPS	RATIONALE
(21) Close check valve as soon as client is down and straps can be released.	If valve is left open, boom may continue to lower and injure client.
(22) Remove straps and mechanical/hydraulic lift.	Prevents damage to skin and underlying tissues from canvas or hooks.
(23) Check client's sitting alignment and correct if necessary.	Prevents injury from poor posture.
(24) Wash hands.	Reduces transmission of microorganisms.

UNEXPECTED OUTCOMES AND RELATED INTERVENTIONS

- Client unable to comprehend and follow directions for transfer.
  - Cognitive impairment affects learning and retention.
  - Reassess continuity and simplicity of instruction.
- Client sustains injury on transfer.
  - Indicates improper transfer technique was used.
  - Evaluate incident that caused injury (e.g., assessment inadequate, change in client status, improper use of equipment).
  - Complete incident report according to institution policy.
- Client's level of weakness does not permit active transfer.
  - Physical impairments require increased assistance from nursing personnel.
  - Increase bed activity and exercise to heighten tolerance.
- Client continues to bear weight on non–weight-bearing limb.
  - Certain conditions (e.g., hip fractures) need to be non–weight bearing through healing process.
  - Reassess client's understanding of weight-bearing status.
- Client transfers well on some occasions, poorly on others.
  - Transfers may be difficult when client is fatigued or in pain; assess before transfer (allow for a rest period before transferring, or medicate for pain if indicated).
  - Periodic confusion may also alter performance.
- Client is unable to stand for time required in transfer.
  - Results from increased fatigue, orthostatic hypotension, or pain.
  - Provide for adequate assistance during transfer.
- Localized areas of erythema develop that do not disappear quickly.
  - Early signs of pressure sores (see Chapter 34).

RECORDING AND REPORTING

- Record procedure, including pertinent observations: weakness, ability to follow directions, weight-bearing ability, balance, ability to pivot, number of personnel needed to assist, and amount of assistance (muscle strength) required.
- Report any unusual occurrence to nurse in charge. Report transfer ability and assistance needed to next shift or other caregivers. Report progress or remission to rehabilitation staff (physical therapist or occupational therapist).

recommend approaches that help older adults to use proper body mechanics and prevent injury (Box 24-7).

Mechanical devices are available for specific joints, which place these joints through continuous passive motion (CPM). These CPM machines are used postoperatively to place joints through a selective repetitive range of motion. The machine can be set to certain degrees of joint mobility with increasing joint mobility or flexion as the goal. The most common clients who use the CPM machine are those who have undergone some form of total joint replacement surgery.

Unless contraindicated, the nursing care plan should include exercising each joint through as nearly a full range of motion as possible. Passive range-of-motion exercises should be initiated as soon as the client loses the ability to move the extremity or joint. The following guidelines apply to the use of range-of-motion exercises:

1. Provide explanation to the client; this elicits cooperation and assistance.
2. Start slowly; movements should be smooth and easy.
3. Flexion of the joint can continue until slight resistance is felt; do not move a joint to the point of pain; avoid hyperextending the joint.
4. Work from distal joints to proximal joints on one extremity at a time.
5. Provide support for joints distal to the joint being manipulated.
6. Assess client closely for signs of generalized fatigue.
7. When exercises are completed, make certain to leave joints in correct alignment position.

Walking. Joint mobility is also increased by walking. In the normal walking posture the head is erect; the cervical, thoracic, and lumbar vertebrae are aligned; the hips and knees have appropriate flexion; and the arms swing freely in alternation with the legs. Illness or trauma can reduce activity tolerance, necessitating a need for assistance with walking or the use of mechanical devices such as crutches, canes, or walkers.

Text continued on p. 569

Range-of-Motion Exercises

Table 24-3

Body Part	Type of Joint	Type of Movement	Range (degrees)	Primary Muscles
Neck, cervical spine	Pivotal	Flexion: bring chin to rest on chest	45	Sternocleidomastoid
		Extension: return head to erect position	45	Trapezius
		Hyperextension: bend head back as far as possible	10	Trapezius
		Lateral flexion: tilt head as far as possible toward each shoulder	40-45	Sternocleidomastoid
		Rotation: turn head as far as possible in circular movement	180	Sternocleidomastoid, trapezius
Shoulder	Ball and socket	Flexion: raise arm from side position forward to position above head	180	Coracobrachialis, biceps brachii, deltoid, pectoralis major
		Extension: return arm to position at side of body	180	Latissimus dorsi, teres major, triceps brachii
		Hyperextension: move arm behind body, keeping elbow straight	45-60	Latissimus dorsi, teres major, deltoid
		Abduction: raise arm to side to position above head with palm away from head	180	Deltoid, supraspinatus
		Adduction: lower arm sideways and across body as far as possible	320	Pectoralis major
		Internal rotation: with elbow flexed, rotate shoulder by moving arm until thumb is turned inward and toward back	90	Pectoralis major, latissimus dorsi, teres major, subscapularis
		External rotation: with elbow flexed, move arm until thumb is upward and lateral to head	90	Infraspinatus, teres major, deltoid

Range-of-Motion Exercises—cont'd

Table 24-3

Body Part	Type of Joint	Type of Movement	Range (degrees)	Primary Muscles
Shoulder —cont'd	Ball and socket— cont'd	Circumduction: move arm in full circle (**Circumduction** is combination of all movements of ball-and-socket joint.)	360	Deltoid, coracobrachialis, latissimus dorsi, teres major
Elbow	Hinge	Flexion: bend elbow so that lower arm moves toward its shoulder joint and hand is level with shoulder	150	Biceps brachii, brachialis, brachioradialis
		Extension: straighten elbow by lowering hand	150	Triceps brachii
Forearm	Pivotal	Supination: turn lower arm and hand so that palm is up	70-90	Supinator, biceps brachii
		Pronation: turn lower arm so that palm is down	70-90	Pronator teres, pronator quadratus
Wrist	Condyloid	Flexion: move palm toward inner aspect of forearm	80-90	Flexor carpi ulnaris, flexor carpi radialis
		Extension: move fingers so that fingers, hands, and forearm are in same plane	80-90	Extensor carpi ulnaris, extensor carpi radialis brevis, extensor carpi radialis longus
		Hyperextension: bring dorsal surface of hand back as far as possible	89-90	Extensor carpi radialis brevis, extensor carpi radialis longus, extensor carpi ulnaris
		Abduction (radial flexion): bend wrist medially toward thumb	Up to 30	Flexor carpi radialis, extensor carpi radialis brevis, extensor carpi radialis longus
		Adduction (ulnar flexion): bend wrist laterally toward fifth finger	30-50	Flexor carpi ulnaris, extensor carpi ulnaris
Fingers	Condyloid hinge	Flexion: make fist	90	Lumbricales, interossesus volaris, interosseus dorsalis
		Extension: straighten fingers	90	Extensor digiti quinti proprius, extensor digitorum communis, extensor indicis proprius
		Hyperextension: bend fingers back as far as possible	30-60	

Continued

Range-of-Motion Exercises—cont'd

Table 24-3

Body Part	Type of Joint	Type of Movement	Range (degrees)	Primary Muscles
Fingers—cont'd	Condyloid hinge	Abduction: spread fingers apart	30	Interosseus dorsalis
		Adduction: bring fingers together	30	Interosseus volaris
Thumb	Saddle	Flexion: move thumb across palmar surface of hand	90	Flexor pollicis brevis
		Extension: move thumb straight away from hand	90	Extensor pollicis longus, extensor pollicis brevis
		Abduction: extend thumb laterally (usually done when placing fingers in abduction and adduction)	30	Abductor pollicis brevis
		Adduction: move thumb back toward hand	30	Adductor pollicis obliquus, adductor pollicis transversus
		Opposition: touch thumb to each finger of same hand		Opponeus pollicis, opponeus digiti minimi
Hip	Ball and socket	Flexion: move leg forward and up	90-120	Psoas major, iliacus, iliopsoas, sartorius
		Extension: move back beside other leg	90-120	Gluteus maximus, semitendinosus, semimembranosus
		Hyperextension: move leg behind body	30-50	Gluteus maximus, semitendinosus, semimembranosus
		Abduction: move leg laterally away from body	30-50	Gluteus medius, gluteus minimus
		Adduction: move leg back toward medial position and beyond if possible	30-50	Adductor longus, adductor brevis, adductor magnus
		Internal rotation: turn foot and leg toward other leg	90	Gluteus medius, gluteus minimus, tensor fasciae latae
		External rotation: turn foot and leg away from other leg	90	Obturatorius internus, obturatorius externus

Range-of-Motion Exercises—cont'd

Table 24-3

Body Part	Type of Joint	Type of Movement	Range (degrees)	Primary Muscles
Hip—cont'd	Ball and socket	Circumduction: move leg in circle		Psoas major, gluteus maximus, gluteus medius, adductor magnus
Knee	Hinge	Flexion: bring heel back toward back of thigh	120-130	Biceps femoris, semitendinosus, semimembranosus, sartorius
		Extension: return leg to the floor	120-130	Rectus femoris, vastus lateralis, vastus medialis, vastus intermedius
Ankle	Hinge	Dorsal flexion: move foot so that toes are pointed upward	20-30	Tibialis anterior
		Plantar flexion: move foot so that toes are pointed downward	45-50	Gastrocnemius, soleus
Foot	Gliding	Inversion: turn sole of foot medially	10 or less	Tibialis anterior, tibialis posterior
		Eversion: turn sole of foot laterally	10 or less	Peroneus longus, peroneus brevis
Toes	Condyloid	Flexion: curl toes downward	30-60	Flexor digitorum, lumbricales pedis, flexor hallucis brevis
		Extension: straighten toes	30-60	Extensor digitorum longus, extensor digitorum brevis, extensor hallucis longus
		Abduction: spread toes apart	15 or less	Abductor hallucis, interosseus dorsalis
		Adduction: bring toes together	15 or less	Adductor hallucis, interosseus plantaris

Assisting a Client in Walking. Assisting the client in walking requires preparation. Assess the client's activity tolerance, strength, coordination, and balance to determine the type of assistance needed. Also assess the client's orientation, and determine if there are any signs of distress. This would preclude attempts at ambulation.

Evaluate the environment for safety before ambulation; this includes the removal of obstacles, a clean and dry floor, and the establishment of rest points should the client's activity tolerance become less than expected. The client should also wear supportive, nonslipping shoes. Resting points should be established in the event the client's activity tolerance is less than was estimated or the client becomes dizzy.

When preparing a client for ambulation, dangling is an important technique. The client should be assisted to a position of sitting at the side of the bed and should rest for 1 to 2 minutes before standing. The longer the period of immobility, the greater the physiological changes. This is especially true regarding changes in circulation. When the client has been flat for extended periods, blood pressure may drop

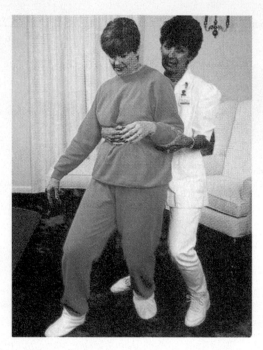

FIGURE 24-6   Ease the client down to the floor by bending your knees, keeping your back straight. (From Birchenall JM, Streight ME: *Mosby's textbook for the home care aide,* St. Louis, 1997, Mosby.)

when the client stands. Dangling helps to prevent this. After standing, the client should remain stationary for a minute or two before moving. If the client becomes dizzy, the bed is still nearby and you can quickly ease him or her back to bed.

Several methods are used for assisting a client with ambulation. Provide support at the waist by using a gait belt so the client's center of gravity remains midline. Clients should not lean to one side because then their center of gravity is no longer midline, which distorts their balance, and their risk of falling is increased.

The client who appears unsteady or complains of dizziness should be returned to the closest bed or a chair. If the client has a syncopal episode or begins to fall, you should assume a wide base of support with one foot in front of the other, thus supporting the client's body weight. Gently lower the client to the floor, protecting the client's head. Although lowering a client to the floor is not difficult, practice this technique with a friend or classmate before attempting it in a clinical setting (Figure 24-6).

Clients with hemiplegia (one-sided paralysis) or hemiparesis (one-sided weakness) need assistance in ambulating. Stand by the client's affected side and support the client by holding onto the gait belt around the client's waist and placing the other arm around the inferior aspect of the client's upper arm so that your hand is supporting the client's axilla. The client's unaffected arm is left free to enable the client to assist. Providing support by holding the client's arm is incorrect because, if the client should experience syncope or fall, you cannot easily support the weight and lower the client to the floor. In addition, if the client falls with you holding the arm, the shoulder joint may be dislocated.

The two-nurse method helps to distribute the client's weight evenly. The two nurses stand on either side of the client. Each nurse holds onto the gait belt, and the other arm is around the inferior aspect of the client's arm so that the hands of both nurses are supporting the client's axillae.

RESTORATIVE AND CONTINUING CARE.   Restorative and continuing care involving activity and exercise involves imple-

menting strategies to assist the client in ADLs after the client's need for acute care is no longer warranted. In collaboration with other health care professionals such as physical therapists, you promote activity and exercise by teaching the use of canes, walkers, or crutches, depending on the assistive device most appropriate for the client's condition. Restorative and continuing care includes activities and exercises that restore and improve optimal functioning in the client with chronic musculoskeletal illnesses, such as arthritis, trauma, and other chronic illnesses, such as coronary artery disease (CAD).

ASSISTIVE DEVICES FOR WALKING.   Walkers are extremely light, moveable devices, about waist high and made of metal tubing (Figure 24-7). They have four widely placed, sturdy legs. The client holds the handgrips on the upper bars, takes a step, moves the walker forward, and takes another step.

Canes.   Canes are lightweight, easily moveable devices about waist high, made of wood or metal. Two common types of canes are the single straight-legged cane and the quad cane. The single straight-legged cane is more common and is used to support and balance a client with decreased leg strength. This cane should be kept on the stronger side of the body. For maximum support when walking, the client places the cane forward 15 to 25 cm (6 to 10 inches), keeping body weight on both legs. The weaker leg is moved forward to the cane so that body weight is divided between the

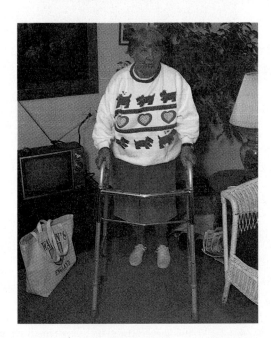

FIGURE **24-7** Client using a walker.

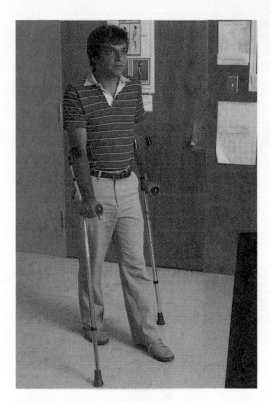

FIGURE **24-9** Double adjustable Lofstrand or forearm crutch.

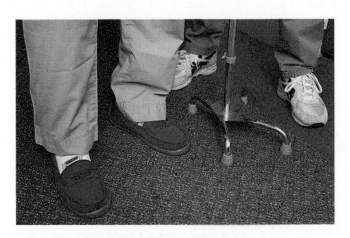

FIGURE **24-8** Quad cane.

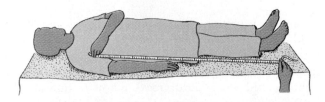

FIGURE **24-10** Measuring crutch length.

cane and the stronger leg. The stronger leg is then advanced past the cane so the weaker leg and the body weight are supported by the cane and weaker leg. During walking, the client continually repeats these three steps. The client must be taught that two points of support, such as both feet or one foot and the cane, are present at all times.

The quad cane provides the most support and is used when there is partial or complete leg paralysis or some hemiplegia (Figure 24-8). The same three steps used with the straight-legged cane are taught to the client.

Crutches. The use of crutches may be temporary, such as after ligament damage to the knee. However, crutches may be needed permanently by a client with paralysis of the lower ex-

tremities. A crutch is a wooden or metal staff. The two types of crutches are the double adjustable Lofstrand or forearm crutch (Figure 24-9) and the axillary wooden or metal crutch. The forearm crutch has a handgrip and a metal band that fits around the client's forearm. The metal band and the handgrip are adjusted to fit the client's height. The axillary crutch has a padded curved surface at the top, which fits under the axilla. A handgrip in the form of a crossbar is held at the level of the palms to support the body. It is important that crutches be measured for the appropriate length and that clients be taught to use their crutches safely, to achieve a stable gait, to ascend and descend stairs, and to rise from a sitting position.

Measuring for Crutches. The axillary crutch is the more common crutch used. Measurements include the client's height, the angle of elbow flexion, and the distance between the crutch pad and the axilla. When crutches are fitted, the length of the crutch should be from three to four finger-widths from the axilla to a point 15 cm (6 inches) lateral to the client's heel (Hoeman, 2001) (Figure 24-10).

The handgrips should be positioned so the client's body weight is not supported by the axillae. Pressure on

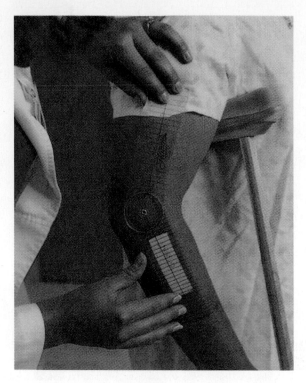

FIGURE **24-11**   Using the goniometer to verify correct degree of elbow flexion for crutch use.

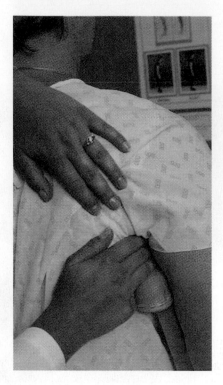

FIGURE **24-12**   Verifying correct distance between crutch pad and axilla.

the axillae increases risk to underlying nerves, which could result in partial paralysis of the arm. Correct position of the handgrips is determined with the client upright, supporting weight by the handgrips with the elbows slightly flexed (20 to 25 degrees). Elbow flexion may be verified with a goniometer (Figure 24-11). When the height and placement of the handgrips have been determined, you should again verify that the distance between the crutch pad and the client's axilla is three to four fingerwidths (Figure 24-12).

Crutch Safety.   Before being allowed to walk independently with crutches, the client should be taught the following safety guidelines:

1. Clients with axillary crutches must be aware of the dangers of pressure on the axilla. Therefore they must not use crutches that fit improperly or lean on their crutches to support body weight.
2. Crutch-dependent clients should be taught to inspect the crutch tips routinely. The rubber tips should be securely attached to the crutches. When the tips are worn, they should be replaced immediately. Rubber crutch tips increase surface friction and prevent the crutches from slipping.
3. Crutch tips should remain dry. If the tips become wet, the client should dry them. Water decreases surface friction and increases the risk that the crutches will slip.
4. The structure of the crutches should also be routinely inspected. Cracks in a wooden crutch decrease the crutch's ability to support weight. Bends in aluminum crutches can alter body alignment, increasing the risk of further damage to the musculoskeletal system.

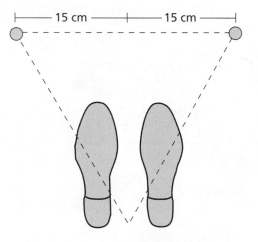

FIGURE **24-13**   Tripod position, basic crutch stance.

5. Clients should be given a list of medical suppliers in their community. This allows the clients to obtain repairs, new rubber tips, handgrips, and crutch pads.
6. Crutch-dependent clients should always have spare crutches and tips on hand.

Crutch Gait.   The **crutch gait** is assumed by alternatively bearing weight on one or both legs and on the crutches. The gait selected by the physician is determined by assessing the client's physical and functional abilities and the disease or injury that resulted in the need for crutches. This section summarizes the basic crutch stance and the four standard gaits: four-point alternating gait, three-point alternating gait, two-point gait, and swing-through gait.

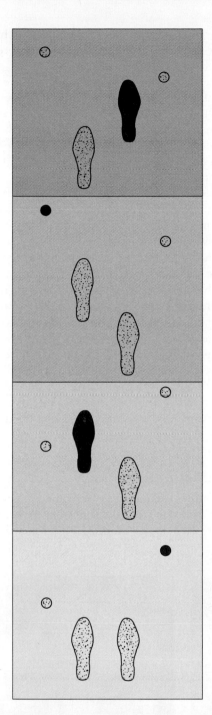

FIGURE **24-14** Four-point alternating gait. Solid feet and crutch tips show foot and crutch tip moved in each of the four phases.

The basic crutch stance is the tripod position, formed when the crutches are placed 15 cm (6 inches) in front of and 15 cm to the side of each foot (Figure 24-13). This position improves the client's balance by providing a wider base of support. The body alignment of the client in the tripod position includes erect head and neck, straight vertebrae, and extended hips and knees. No weight should be borne by the axillae. The tripod position is used before crutch walking.

Four-point alternating or four-point gait gives stability to the client but requires weight bearing on both legs. Each leg

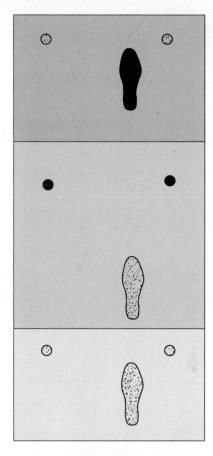

FIGURE **24-15** Three-point gait with weight borne on unaffected leg. Solid foot and crutch tips show weight bearing in each phase.

is moved alternately with each opposing crutch so that three points of support are on the floor at all times (Figure 24-14).

Three-point alternating or three-point gait requires the client to bear all of the weight on one foot. In a three-point gait, weight is borne on both crutches and then on the uninvolved leg, and the sequence is repeated (Figure 24-15). The affected leg does not touch the ground during the early phase of the three-point gait. Gradually the client progresses to touchdown and full weight bearing on the affected leg.

The two-point gait requires at least partial weight bearing on each foot (Figure 24-16). The client moves a crutch at the same time as the opposite leg, so the crutch movements are similar to arm motion during normal walking.

The swing-through gait is frequently used by paraplegics who wear weight-supporting braces on their legs. With weight placed on the supported legs, the client places the crutches one stride in front and then swings to or through the crutches while they support the client's weight.

Crutch Walking on Stairs.   When ascending stairs on crutches, the client usually uses a modified three-point gait (Figure 24-17). The client stands at the bottom of the stairs and transfers body weight to the crutches. The unaffected leg is advanced between the crutches to the stairs. The client then shifts weight from the crutches to the unaf-

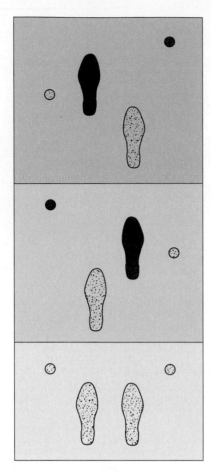

FIGURE **24-16** Two-point gait with weight borne partially on each foot and each crutch advancing with opposing leg. Solid areas indicate leg and crutch tips bearing weight.

fected leg. Finally, the client aligns both crutches on the stairs. This sequence is repeated until the client reaches the top of the stairs.

To descend the stairs (Figure 24-18), a three-phase sequence is also used. The client transfers body weight to the unaffected leg. The crutches are placed on the stair, and the client begins to transfer body weight to the crutches, moving the affected leg forward. Finally, the unaffected leg is moved to the stairs with the crutches. Again, the client repeats the sequence until reaching the bottom of the stairs.

Sitting in a Chair With Crutches.   As with crutch walking and crutch walking up and down stairs, the procedure for sitting in a chair involves phases and requires the client to transfer weight (Figure 24-19). First, the client gets positioned at the center front of the chair with the posterior aspect of the legs touching the chair. Then the client holds both crutches in the hand opposite the affected leg. If both legs are affected, as with a paraplegic who wears weight-supporting braces, the crutches are held in the hand on the client's stronger side. With both crutches in one hand, the client supports body weight on the unaffected leg and crutches. While still holding the crutches, the client grasps the arm of the chair with the remaining hand and lowers the body into the chair. To stand, the procedure is reversed, and the client, when fully erect, should assume the tripod position before beginning to walk.

 Evaluation

CLIENT CARE.   All nursing interventions are evaluated by comparing the client's actual response to the expected outcomes for each goal (Box 24-8). You will evaluate

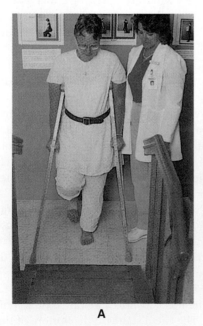 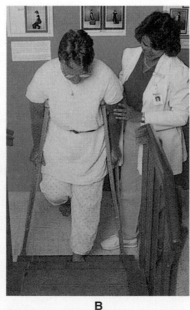 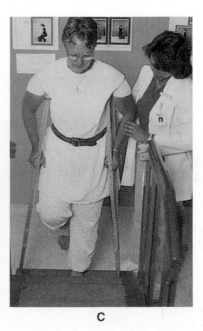

| A | B | C |

FIGURE **24-17** Ascending stairs. **A,** Weight is placed on crutches. **B,** Weight is transferred from crutches to unaffected leg on stairs. **C,** Crutches are aligned with unaffected leg on stairs.

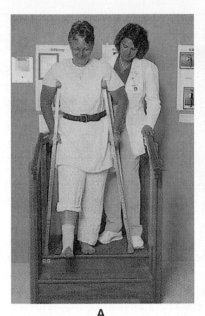
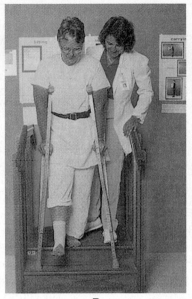
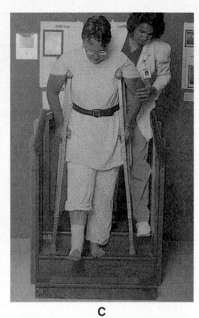

A **B** **C**

FIGURE **24-18** Descending stairs. **A,** Body weight on unaffected leg. **B,** Body weight transferred to crutches. **C,** Unaffected leg aligned on stairs with crutches.

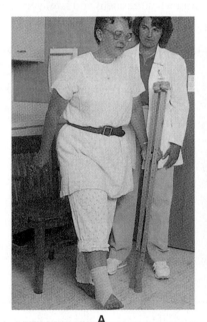
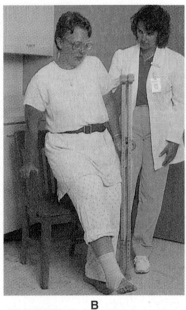
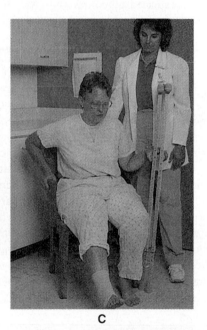

A **B** **C**

FIGURE **24-19** Sitting on chair. **A,** Both crutches are held by one hand. Client transfers weight to crutches and unaffected leg. **B,** Client grasps arm of chair with free hand and begins to lower herself into chair. **C,** Client completely lowers herself into chair.

Outcome Evaluation for **MR. INDELICATO** Box 24-8

Nursing Action	Client Response/Finding	Achievement of Outcome
Measure degree of knee flexion.	Able to flex knee to a 60-degree angle. Complains of pain at 70 degrees flexion.	Outcome partially met. Determine need for analgesic before flexion exercises.
Observe Mr. Indelicato's ROM or use of CPM machine.	Able to perform ROM and using CPM machine.	Outcome met. Mr. Indelicato expresses understanding of need for ROM and CPM machine.
Observe Mr. Indelicato's ambulation.	Steady gait with aid of walker.	Outcome met. Demonstrates correct use of walker.
Ask Mr. Indelicato to rate level of pain on a 10-point scale.	Mr. Indelicato reports a 7 on the pain scale during use of CPM machine.	Outcome not met. Need to provide analgesic before use of CPM machine.

Case Study EVALUATION

It has been 5 weeks since Marilyn began to care for Mr. Indelicato. For the last 4 weeks she has followed him in the outpatient rehabilitation setting. Mr. Indelicato has progressed steadily to increase both weight bearing and range of joint motion on the affected knee. His pain was more difficult to manage. Mr. Indelicato expected pain to be completely resolved on hospital discharge and did not expect pain to follow his physical therapy. Marilyn and the physical therapist worked with Mr. Indelicato and his orthopedic surgeon to identify pain-control measures following physical therapy. Currently Mr. Indelicato takes 600 mg of Motrin 45 minutes before physical therapy and every 8 to 12 hours thereafter. Mr. Indelicato reports that his pain is now almost totally gone. He is now working on increasing strength so he can return to golf and bike riding. He says he will probably give up racquetball and tennis.

specific outcomes designed to demonstrate improved activity and exercise. If expected outcomes are not achieved, you will need to revise the care plan. The success in meeting each outcome is based on the use of evaluative measures such as ROM, ability of client to ambulate, and activity/exercise tolerance.

CLIENT EXPECTATIONS.   For the client with alterations in body mechanics or joint mobility, the effectiveness of nursing interventions is measured by the success of meeting the client's expected outcomes and goals of care. For some clients with altered body mechanics or joint mobility, maintenance of joint mobility will be easily accomplished and will not be a priority goal. For others, return of joint mobility and maintenance of body alignment will be the most important outcome and all interventions will be directed toward its accomplishment.

For you to evaluate the client's perception of the interventions, you must first have knowledge of the client's expectations concerning joint mobility, posture, or body alignment. What is acceptable or anticipated on your part may be vastly different from what the client and family members anticipate or can accept.

Key Terms

abduction, *p. 548*

active range-of-motion exercises, *p. 558*

activity tolerance, *p. 545*

adduction, *p. 548*

balance, *p. 542*

bed boards, *p. 548*

body mechanics, *p.540*

center of gravity, *p. 540*

circumduction, *p. 567*

crutch gait, *p. 572*

dorsiflexion, *p. 549*

extension, *p. 541*

foot boots, *p. 548*

footdrop, *p. 549*

friction, *p. 540*

gait, *p. 545*

hand rolls, *p. 548*

hand-wrist splints, *p. 548*

hyperextension, *p. 549*

Hoyer lift, *p. 563*

joints, *p. 541*

logroll, *p. 557*

muscle tone, *p. 540*

passive range-of-motion exercises, *p. 558*

plantar flexion, *p. 549*

orthostatic hypotension, *p. 558*

posture, *p. 540*

prone, *p. 549*

range of motion (ROM), *p. 545*

sandbags, *p. 548*

side rails, *p. 548*

supine, *p. 544*

trapeze bar, *p. 548*

trochanter rolls, *p. 548*

Key Concepts

- The term *body mechanics* describes the coordinated efforts of the musculoskeletal and nervous systems as a person moves, lifts or bends.
- Muscles primarily associated with movement are located near the skeletal region, where movement results from leverage.
- Muscles primarily associated with posture are located in the lower extremities, trunk, neck, and back.
- Balance is controlled by the cerebellum and inner ear.
- Body alignment is the positioning of joints, tendons, ligaments, and muscles in various body positions.
- Body balance is achieved when there is a wide base of support, the center of gravity falls within the base of support, and vertical line falls from the center of gravity through the base of support.
- Developmental stages influence body alignment and mobility.
- Conditions that affect body alignment and mobility include postural abnormalities, altered bone formation or joint mobility, impaired muscle development, central nervous system damage, and musculoskeletal system trauma.
- Assessment of a client's mobility enables you to determine the client's coordination, balance, and ability to complete activities of daily living and makes it possible to evaluate or plan an exercise program.
- Assessing gait allows you to draw some conclusions about the client's balance, posture, and ability to walk without assistance.

- Clients with impaired body alignment require nursing interventions to maintain them in the supported Fowler's, supine, prone, side-lying, and Sims' positions.
- Transfer techniques require the use of correct body mechanics.

- Mechanical devices, such as canes and walkers, require specific nursing interventions to promote walking.

Critical Thinking Activities

1. Mrs. Smith is a 42-year-old woman who suffered a spinal cord injury. She is admitted on your shift. What do you think would be the safest technique for moving Mrs. Smith from side to side? In addition, what information concerning body alignment, positioning, and transfer should be included in the report to the oncoming nurse?

2. A client has a trapeze bar across the bed, trochanter rolls, and a footboard. Explain the rationale for each of these devices in maintaining proper body alignment.

3. Mr. Brown has just undergone extensive abdominal surgery. What assessment parameters need to be considered before moving and positioning him in bed? What precautions should you take before transferring Mr. Brown to the chair for the first time?

Review Questions

1. A client begins to fall during ambulation. To prevent the client from injury you should:
   1. call for assistance.
   2. slide her down your body to the floor.
   3. instruct the client to sit in the nearest chair.
   4. contact the physician and document the fall.
2. A principle of good body mechanics includes:
   1. keeping knees in locked position.
   2. maintaining a wide base of support.
   3. bending at the waist to maintain center of gravity.
   4. holding objects away from the body for better leverage.
3. Passive range-of-motion exercises prevent:
   1. contractures.
   2. osteoporosis.
   3. muscle atrophy.
   4. renal calculi formation.
4. A necessary safety precaution when ambulating a client is to:
   1. have family members present.
   2. have client wear well-fitting rubber-soled shoes or slippers.
   3. have at least two people present to assist the client.
   4. be sure no pain medication was given for at least 3 hours before ambulation.

5. The piece of equipment that would work best to help ambulate an unsteady client is:
   1. a walker.
   2. crutches.
   3. a wheelchair.
   4. a mechanical lift device.
6. A device that helps prevent footdrop is the:
   1. foot roll.
   2. footboard.
   3. trochanter roll.
   4. ankle-foot splints.
7. Two nurses are standing on opposite sides of the bed to move a client up in bed with a drawsheet. In relation to the client, the nurses should be standing even with the:
   1. hips.
   2. chest.
   3. knees.
   4. shoulders.
8. A physician orders partial weight bearing on the left foot of a client with a broken ankle and full weight bearing on the right foot. The gait that the client would use is the:
   1. two-point.
   2. four-point.
   3. three-point.
   4. swing-through.

References

Ackley BJ, Ladwig GB: *Nursing diagnosis handbook: a guide to planning care,* ed 5, St. Louis, 2001, Mosby.

Birchenall JM, Streight ME: *Mosby's textbook for the home care aide,* St. Louis, 1997, Mosby.

Dawe D, Moore-Orr R: Low-intensity, range of motion exercise: invaluable nursing care for elderly patients, *J Adv Nurs* 21(4):675, 1995.

Gahart BL, Nazareno AR: *2002 intravenous medications: a handbook for nurses and allied health professionals,* St. Louis, 2002, Mosby.

Gassett RS and others: Ergonomics and body mechanics in the work place, *Nurs Clin North Am* 27-4(10):861, 1996.

Hoeman SP: *Rehabilitation nursing: process, application and outcomes,* ed 3, St. Louis, 2001, Mosby.

Huether SE, McCance KL: *Understanding pathophysiology,* ed 2, St. Louis, 2000, Mosby.

Metzler DJ: Positioning your patient properly, *Am J Nurs* 96(3):33, 1996.

National Institutes of Health Consensus Development Panel on Physical Activity and Cardiovascular Health: Physical activity and cardiovascular health, *JAMA* 276(3):241, 1996.

Owens B and others: What are we teaching about lifting and transferring patients? *Res Nurs Health* 22:3, 1999.

Prochaska JO and others: *Changing for good,* New York, 1994, William Morrow.

Phipps WJ and others: *Medical surgical nursing,* ed 6, St. Louis, 1999, Mosby.

Thibodeau GA, Patton KT: *Anatomy and physiology,* ed 4, St. Louis, 1999, Mosby.

Wilson SF, Giddens JF: *Health assessment for nursing practice,* ed 2, St. Louis, 2000, Mosby.

Wong DL and others: *Whaley & Wong's nursing care of infants and children,* ed 6, St. Louis, 1999, Mosby.

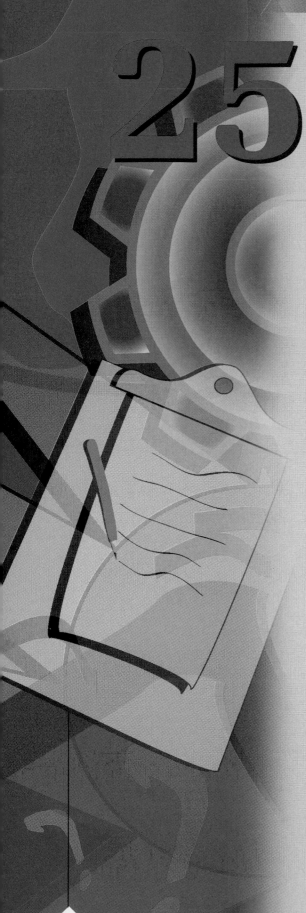

25

Safety

Objectives

- Define key terms.
- Describe how unmet basic physiological needs of oxygen, nutrition, temperature, and humidity can threaten safety.
- Discuss methods to reduce physical hazards and the transmission of pathogens.
- Discuss the specific risks to safety as they pertain to developmental age.
- Identify factors to assess when it becomes necessary to physically restrain a client.
- Describe four categories of safety risks in a health care agency.
- Describe assessment activities designed to identify a client's physical, psychological, and cognitive status as it relates to safety.
- State nursing diagnoses associated with risks to safety.
- Develop a nursing care plan for clients whose safety is threatened.
- Describe nursing interventions specific to the client's age for reducing risk of falls, fires, poisonings, and electrical hazards.
- Describe methods to evaluate interventions designed to maintain or promote safety.

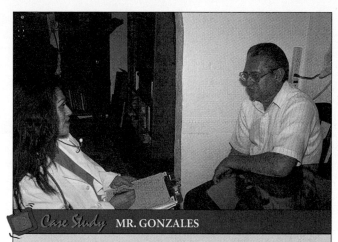

Case Study MR. GONZALES

Mr. Gonzales is a 68-year-old man who has lived alone in a senior apartment building since his wife died 6 months ago. He and his wife were born in Mexico but came to live in the United States shortly after they were married. He is retired from a produce warehouse where he worked for 37 years. He and his wife raised three sons, who are all married and have families of their own. The closest son is 45 minutes away by car. Mr. Gonzales is generally healthy but has some hearing loss from the noisy warehouse job and some "arthritis." He expects to live at least as long as his father, who lived to be 92 years old. Since his wife's death, Mr. Gonzales has attended Catholic mass every day at his parish church, where his wife had attended daily.

Joani Green, a 25-year-old married mother of two, is currently a senior nursing student at the local college. As part of the clinical requirements for the home care course, she and her partner are conducting health screenings and providing health promotion education for the residents of the apartment building where Mr. Gonzales lives. Part of her screening will include Mr. Gonzales's home environment.

Safety, the freedom from psychological and physical injury, is a basic human need. Health care, provided in a safe manner, and a safe community environment are essential for a client's well-being. One of your primary responsibilities as a nurse is to protect clients from harm. You can increase a client's safety by including interventions for a safe environment in your plan of care.

SCIENTIFIC KNOWLEDGE BASE

Vulnerable groups that often require help in achieving a safe environment include infants, children, older adults, the ill, the physically and mentally disabled, the illiterate, and the poor. To be effective, you need to understand factors that contribute to a safe environment in the home or health care agency and thoroughly assess the environment for threats to safety. You also need to understand how a client's safety is affected by alterations in mobility, sensory function, and cognitive function (see Chapters 33 and 35). A safe environment includes meeting basic human needs, reducing physical hazards, and reducing transmission of pathogens.

Basic Human Needs

Basic human needs that may be at risk from a variety of environmental hazards include the physiological needs of adequate oxygen, nutrition, and optimum temperature and humidity.

OXYGEN.   A common environmental hazard in the home is an improperly functioning heating system. A furnace that is not properly vented may introduce carbon monoxide into the environment. **Carbon monoxide** is a colorless, odorless, poisonous gas produced by the combustion of carbon or organic fuels. This gas binds strongly with hemoglobin, preventing the formation of oxyhemoglobin and thus reducing the supply of oxygen delivered to the tissues (see Chapter 27). Low concentrations can cause nausea, dizziness, headache, and fatigue. Higher concentrations can be fatal (Air Pollution Fact Sheet, 1998).

NUTRITION.   In the home, clients need to properly refrigerate, store, and prepare food. The client needs a refrigerator with a freezer compartment to keep perishable foods fresh. An adequate, clean water supply is needed for drinking and to wash fresh produce and dishes. Foods must be adequately cooked to kill any residing organisms. Foods that are inadequately prepared or stored increase the client's risk for infections and **food poisoning.** Although most food-borne diseases are bacterial, the hepatitis A virus is spread by fecal contamination of food, water, or milk (Williams, 2000).

TEMPERATURE.   A person's comfort zone is usually between 18.3° and 23.9° C (65° and 75° F). Temperature extremes, which often occur during the winter and summer, affect comfort, productivity, and safety. Exposure to severe cold for prolonged periods causes frostbite and accidental **hypothermia** (see Chapter 11). Older adults, the young, clients with cardiovascular conditions, clients who have ingested drugs or excess alcohol, and the homeless are at high risk for hypothermia. Exposure to extreme heat can change the body's electrolyte balance and raise the core body temperature, resulting in **heatstroke** or **heat exhaustion.** People at risk from high environmental temperatures should avoid extremely hot, humid environments or heat exhaustion may result.

HUMIDITY.   The relative humidity of the air may affect a client's health and safety. Relative humidity is the amount of water vapor in the air compared with the maximum amount of water vapor that the air could contain at the same temperature. Increasing the environmental humidity can have therapeutic benefits for clients with upper respiratory infections because humidity helps to liquefy pulmonary secretions and improves breathing.

Physical Hazards

Physical hazards in the environment can threaten a person's safety and result in physical or psychological injury or death. Motor vehicle accidents are the leading cause of unintentional death, followed by falls, poisonings, drownings, fires, and burns (Accident Facts, 1998). As a nurse you can play an important role by anticipating potential hazards in the health care setting and client's home and then implementing appropriate nursing interventions.

Common hazards in the home include inadequate lighting, barriers along normal walking paths and stairways, and lack of safety devices. Inadequate lighting can cause eyestrain while the client carries out daily activities. Poorly illuminated stairs or walkways can increase the risk of injury from falls. Injuries frequently result from accidental contact with objects on stairs, floors, bedside tables, closet shelves, refrigerator tops, and bookshelves. Older adults, clients with impaired vision, and clients with impaired mobility are at greater risk of injury due to falls. Assess the client's home for clutter and observe the condition of stairways, bathrooms, and limited-access areas to be sure safety devices are in place, such as handrails around toilets and grab bars in showers.

A **poison** is any substance that impairs health or destroys life when ingested, inhaled, or absorbed by the body. Poisons can impair the function of every major organ system. In the home accidental poisonings are a greater risk for the toddler, preschooler, and young school-age child, who often ingest household cleaning solutions, medications, or personal hygiene products. Poisoning is also a risk for health care providers who daily work around chemicals such as mercury and toxic cleaning agents. Mercury is commonly found in glass thermometers and mercury sphygmomanometers. Health care workers and clients can be exposed to mercury when there is equipment breakage. When a person has ingested a poisonous substance or come in contact with a chemical that is absorbed through the skin, emergency treatment is required. Specific antidotes or treatments are available for only some types of poisons.

Home fires are a major cause of death and injury. The leading cause of fire deaths is careless smoking, with most fire deaths occurring between the hours of 11 PM and 8 AM. Many fatal fires are the result of individuals smoking in bed and accidentally falling asleep. Another problem related to fatal fires is a failure to keep fresh batteries in home smoke detectors.

Pathogen Transmission

Pathogens and parasites pose a threat to client safety. A **pathogen** is any microorganism capable of producing an illness (see Chapter 10). Probably the most common means of transmission of pathogens is by the hands. For example, if an individual infected with hepatitis A does not wash hands thoroughly after having a bowel movement, the risk of transmitting the disease during food preparation is great. One of the most effective ways to limit the transmission of pathogens is the medical aseptic practice of hand washing.

Insects and rodents are carriers of pathogens. For example, some mosquitoes are carriers of malaria, and the rat or mouse can transmit rat-bite fever. Uncontrolled mosquito and rodent populations increase the risk of these diseases. Clients living at the poverty level may reside in homes that are not maintained by the landlords. Rat and roach infestation are common problems.

The transmission of pathogens and parasites is also controlled by adequate disposal of human waste. Without a satisfactory sewer and waste system, the population is at risk for illnesses such as typhoid fever and hepatitis.

The transmission of disease from person to person can be reduced, and often prevented, by immunization. Immunization is the process by which resistance to an infectious disease is produced or augmented. Active immunity is acquired by injecting a small amount of weakened or dead organisms and modified toxins from the organism (toxoids) into the body. Passive immunity occurs when antibodies produced by other persons or animals can be introduced into a person's bloodstream for protection against a pathogen. All adult clients should be encouraged to have their children immunized and to receive regular immunizations for influenza and tetanus.

Health care agencies are concerned with the processing of biohazardous wastes. It is important that you properly dispose of needles, surgical dressings, and syringes to prevent the risk of exposure to the general population and employees. Bed linens and client gowns contaminated by body fluids must also be properly cleansed or disposed of to reduce threats to safety.

▌NURSING KNOWLEDGE BASE

Threats to safety are influenced by a person's developmental stage, lifestyle habits, mobility status, sensory and cognitive impairments, and safety awareness. In the United States accidents are the leading cause of death in people between 1 and 34 years of age and the fifth leading cause overall (Fact Book for the Year 2000, 2001). It is important to be aware of the threats to safety and to teach clients, parents, and other caregivers how to lessen the dangers.

Developmental Level

INFANT, TODDLER, AND PRESCHOOLER.   Injuries are the leading cause of death in children over age 1 (Wong and others, 1999). The nature of an injury is closely related to normal growth and development. For example, the incidence of lead poisoning is highest in late infancy and toddlerhood because of the increase in oral activity and the ability to explore the environment. Accidents involving children are largely preventable, but parents need to be aware of specific dangers at each stage of growth and development. Accident prevention requires health education for parents and the removal of dangers whenever possible.

SCHOOL-AGE CHILD.   When children enter school, their environment expands to include the school, the means of transportation to and from school, and after-school activities. School-agers are learning how to perform more complicated motor activities and oftentimes are uncoordinated. Instruct parents and teachers about safe practices to follow at school and during play. Teach school-age children involved in team and contact sports rules for playing safely and how to use protective safety equipment. Head injuries are a major cause of death with bicycle accidents being one of the major causes of such injuries (Pillitteri, 1999). Playground safety is especially important during the summer months. Teach children about safe distances for jumping and climbing, to avoid unsafe and isolated areas, and to keep away from strange dogs.

ADOLESCENT.   As children enter adolescence, they develop greater independence and a sense of identity. The adolescent begins to separate emotionally from the family, and the peer group begins to have a stronger influence. Adolescent behavior is characterized by wide variations that swing from childlike to mature behavior (Wong and others, 2000). To relieve the tensions associated with the physical and psychosocial changes of this developmental stage, adolescents may begin smoking and using drugs. This increases the risk of accidents such as drowning and motor vehicle accidents. To assess for possible substance abuse, have parents look for environmental and psychosocial clues. Environmental clues include the presence of drug-oriented magazines, beer and liquor bottles, drug paraphernalia, blood spots on clothing, and the continual wearing of long-sleeved shirts in hot weather and dark glasses indoors. Psychosocial clues include failing grades, change in dress, increased absenteeism from school, isolation, increased aggressiveness, and changes in interpersonal relationships.

When adolescents learn to drive, they must be taught to comply with rules and regulations regarding use of a car. Most schools have driver's education programs. The regular use of a seat belt should be strongly encouraged.

ADULT.   Threats to an adult client's safety are often related to lifestyle habits. The client who excessively uses alcohol or drugs, for example, is at greater risk for motor vehicle accidents. The adult experiencing a high level of stress is at greater risk for accidents and certain stress-related illnesses such as headaches, gastrointestinal disorders, and infections.

OLDER ADULT.   The physiological changes associated with aging, effects of multiple medications, psychologic factors, and acute or chronic disease increase the older adult's risk for falls and other types of accidents such as burns and car accidents (Ebersole and Hess, 2001). Adults over age 75 are particularly subject to falls. Most falls occur within the home, specifically in the bedroom, bathroom, and kitchen. Fifty percent of accidents are caused by environmental factors such as broken stairs, icy sidewalks, inadequate lighting, throw rugs, and exposed electrical cords (Edelman and Mandle, 1998). Older adults typically fall while transferring from beds, chairs, and toilets; getting into or out of bathtubs; tripping over carpet edges or doorway thresholds; and slipping on wet surfaces or descending stairs.

Other Risk Factors
LIFESTYLE.   Lifestyle can increase safety risks. People who drive or operate machinery while under the influence of chemical substances or work at jobs that are inherently more dangerous are at greater risk of injury. People who are preoccupied by stress or anxiety are more accident-prone because they fail to recognize the source of potential accidents, such as a cluttered stair or a stop sign.

IMPAIRED MOBILITY.   A client with impaired mobility has many kinds of safety risks. Immobilization can predispose a client to physiological and emotional hazards, which in turn can further restrict mobility and independence (see Chapter 33). Physically challenged clients are at greater risk for injury when entering motor vehicles and buildings not equipped for the handicapped.

SENSORY IMPAIRMENTS.   Clients with visual, hearing, or communication impairments are at greater risk for injury. Such clients may not be able to perceive a potential danger or express need for assistance (see Chapter 35).

COGNITIVE IMPAIRMENTS.   Cognitive impairments associated with delirium, dementia, and depression, place clients at greater risk for injury. These conditions contribute to altered concentration and attention span, impaired memory, and orientation changes. Clients can become easily confused about their surroundings and are prone to falls and burns.

SAFETY AWARENESS.   Some clients are unaware of safety precautions, such as keeping medicine, poisonous plants, or other poisons away from children or reading the expiration date on food products. Your nursing assessment will identify the client's level of knowledge regarding home safety so that deficiencies can be corrected with an individualized care plan.

Risks in the Health Care Agency
Clients in health care settings are at risk for falls, client-inherent accidents, procedure-related accidents, and equipment-related accidents. Learn to recognize factors associated with these risks, and take steps to prevent or minimize accidents.

FALLS.   Among older adults, most falls occur in the home; however, 10% of the falls occur in health care facilities (Fact Book for the Year 2000, 2001). Falls account for up to 90% of all reported incidences in hospitals. In addition, hip fractures result in more hospital admissions than any other injury. Confusion, multiple medical problems, generalized weakness, postural instability, and an unfamiliar environment are major contributors to falling when an older client is hospitalized (Ebersole and Hess, 2001). A risk assessment tool, such as the one developed by Brians and others (1991), can help you assess potential risks before accidents and injuries result (Box 25-1).

CLIENT-INHERENT ACCIDENTS.   Client-inherent accidents are accidents other than falls in which the client is the primary factor causing the accident. Examples are self-inflicted cuts, injuries, and burns; ingestion or injection of

Risk for Falls Assessment Tool

Box 25-1

TOOL 1: RISK ASSESSMENT TOOL FOR FALLS
Directions: Place a check mark in front of elements that apply to your client. The decision of whether a client is at risk for falls is based on your nursing judgment. *Guideline:* A client who has a check mark in front of an element with an asterisk (*) or four or more of the other elements would be identified as at risk for falls.

General Data
___ Age over 60
___ History of falls before admission*
___ Postoperative or admitted for operation
___ Smoker

Physical Condition
___ Dizziness or imbalance
___ Unsteady gait
___ Disease or other problems affecting weight-bearing joints
___ Weakness
___ Paresis
___ Seizure disorder
___ Impairment of vision
___ Impairment of hearing
___ Diarrhea
___ Urinary frequency

Mental Status
___ Confusion or disorientation*
___ Impaired memory or judgment
___ Inability to understand or follow directions

Medications
___ Diuretics or diuretic effects
___ Hypotensive or central nervous system suppressants (e.g., narcotic, sedative, psychotropic, hypnotic, tranquilizer, antihypertensive, antidepressant)
___ Medication that increases gastrointestinal motility (e.g., laxative)

Ambulatory Devices Used
___ Cane
___ Crutches
___ Walker
___ Wheelchair
___ Geriatric (geri) chair
___ Braces

TOOL 2: REASSESSMENT IS SAFE "KARE" (RISK) TOOL
Directions: Place a check mark in front of any element that applies to your client. A client who has a check mark in front of any of the first four elements would be identified as at risk for falls. In addition, when a high-risk client has a check mark in front of the element "Use of a wheelchair," the client is considered to be at greater risk for falls.
___ Unsteady gait, dizziness, or imbalance
___ Impaired memory or judgment
___ Weakness
___ History of falls
___ Use of a wheelchair

Data from Brians LK and others: The development of the RISK tool for fall prevention, *Rehabil Nurs* 16(2):67, 1991.

foreign substances; self-mutilation or setting fires; and pinching fingers in drawers or doors. One of the more common precipitating factors for a client-inherent accident is a seizure. A seizure leads to sudden, violent, and involuntary muscle contractions that may be paroxysmal and episodic, causing loss of consciousness, falling, tonicity (rigidity of muscles), and clonicity (jerking of muscles). Clients with a seizure disorder must be placed under seizure precautions, which are designed to protect clients when seizures occur.

PROCEDURE-RELATED ACCIDENTS. Procedure-related accidents are caused by health care providers and include medication and fluid administration errors, improper application of external devices, and improper performance of procedures such as dressing changes. You can prevent many procedure-related accidents by following your organization's policies and procedures and standards of nursing practice. For example, correct use of body mechanics and transfer techniques reduces the risk of injuries when moving and lifting clients (Chapter 24).

EQUIPMENT-RELATED ACCIDENTS. Accidents that are equipment related result from the malfunction, disrepair, or misuse of equipment or from an electrical hazard caused by a frayed or damaged electrical cord. To avoid injury, make sure you understand how to operate all monitoring or therapy equipment. If you discover faulty equipment, make sure you tag it to prevent it from being used on another client, and promptly report any malfunctions.

CRITICAL THINKING
Synthesis
The synthesis of knowledge, experience, and other elements of critical thinking help you to make clinical decisions. To provide for client safety, you will collect, analyze, and synthesize data to make well-reasoned clinical decisions.

KNOWLEDGE. A complete picture of a client's situation, including physical, psychological, and environmental information, is needed to protect the client from injury. Consider a wide variety of factors (e.g., the client's risk for injury, medications being taken, and the environment where most activities of daily living occur) before you develop a plan of care. Because every client is different, with various strengths and weaknesses, prioritize factors that are threats to safety, and concentrate on those that are probable threats. After considering a client's specific strengths and weaknesses, the client's environment, and the developmental stage, work with the client and family to determine creative interventions.

Example of a Focused Client Assessment		Table 25-1
Factors to Assess	Questions and Approaches	Physical Assessment Strategies
Environment	Ask client about recent or past injuries such as falls or burns; when did injury occur, what precipitated it, where did it occur, was this a recurrence?	Inspect the home environment both inside and outside for potential hazards: focus on the kitchen and bath.
Sensory	Ask client to read label of medication bottle with glasses on.	Observe client's ability to read printed material accurately.
Physical mobility	Ask client about activity or exercise patterns: type of exercise, location where performed, type of footwear.	Observe client's posture, gait, and balance during activities of daily living.

EXPERIENCE. Use clinical and personal experience to recall incidents that occurred with another client or family member and the specific circumstances that led to the situation. For example, your grandmother may have fallen because her slipper became entangled in a throw rug at the top of the stairs. You can use the experience of the grandmother's fall and apply the knowledge gained when you assess a client's home for safety hazards during a home visit.

ATTITUDES. Use of critical thinking attitudes ensures your plan of care for a client's safety is comprehensive. For example, show perseverance in identifying all potential safety risks and threats. Be responsible for collecting unbiased, accurate data that pertain to the client's safety. It is important to show discipline in conducting a thorough review of a client's home environment. View all situations as opportunities to protect the client. Once they occur, injuries may cause pain, immobility, loss of income, or even death.

STANDARDS. The American Nurses Association (ANA) *Standards of Clinical Practice* (1998) includes the concept of safety, stating that nursing interventions are to be implemented competently in a safe and appropriate manner. Safety issues are included in the ANA code of ethics (see Chapter 4) in the statement of the nurse's responsibility to safeguard the client and the public when the incompetent, unethical, or illegal practice of any person affects health care and safety. Regulatory agencies, such as the Joint Commission on Accreditation of Healthcare Organizations (JCAHO) and the Occupational Safety and Health Administration (OSHA) define standards and guidelines related to safety in health care settings.

NURSING PROCESS

Assessment

To conduct a thorough client assessment, consider possible threats to the client's safety, including the client's immediate environment and any individual risk factors. Table 25-1 offers an example of focused assessment questions and assessment strategies. When caring for a client in the home, a home hazard assessment is necessary (Box 25-2). A thor-

Home Hazard Assessment	Box 25-2

Proper lighting inside and outside
Storage areas within easy reach
Appliances in good working order
Extension cords placed along walls
Presence of smoke detectors and a fire extinguisher
Flammable objects away from stove or heaters
Gas pilot lights lit
Hot water thermostat set to 120° F or less
Hand rails or grip bars installed
Nonskid surfaces in the bathroom, tub, or shower
Floor coverings secured and floors free of clutter
Furniture promotes ease of mobility
Medications stored properly and not outdated
Telephone accessible and includes emergency phone numbers

ough hazard assessment covers topics such as adequacy of lighting, presence of safety devices, placement of furniture or other items that may create barriers, condition of flooring, and safety of the kitchen and bathrooms. When you assess the home, walk through the rooms with the client and discuss how the client normally conducts daily activities and whether the environment poses problems. For example, when assessing adequacy of lighting, inspect areas where the client moves and works, particularly outside walkways, steps, interior halls, and doorways. Getting a sense of the client's routines helps you to recognize safety hazards.

In a health care facility, determine if any hazards exist in the immediate care environment. Does the placement of equipment pose barriers when the client attempts to ambulate? Does positioning of the client's bed allow the client to safely reach items on a bedside table? Are self-care items in a bathroom arranged for accessibility? Be sure to collaborate with the hospital's clinical engineering staff to ensure equipment functions properly.

Your nursing history will include data about the client's level of wellness to determine if any underlying conditions pose a threat to safety. For example, assess the client's activity tolerance, gait, muscle strength and coordination, balance, and vision. Consider the client's developmental level when you analyze your data. Also review if the client is taking any medications or undergoing any procedures that pose risks. For example, use of a diuretic increases the frequency of voiding and may result in the client using toilet facilities more often. Falls often occur when clients must get out of bed quickly because of urinary urgency. When you assess an older adult, recognize the types of physical changes that increase the risk of injury (Box 25-3).

CLIENT EXPECTATIONS.   When you care for clients with safety needs, ask what they expect from your care. For example, "How can I provide care that will make you feel safe?" or "After we walk through your home, tell me what is im-

portant that we do to help you feel safe." In some cases a client's and family's expectations of what is safe may not be appropriate. When this happens, you must intervene and educate both the client and family regarding safe practices concerning everyday decisions, use of medications and medical equipment, and the environment. When clients are uninformed or inexperienced, threats to their safety can occur.

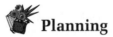 **Nursing Diagnosis**

Gather data from your nursing assessment and analyze clusters of defining characteristics to identify relevant nursing diagnoses. Include specific related or contributing factors to individualize your nursing care. For example, the nursing diagnosis *risk for injury* could be related to altered mobility, or it could be related to sensory alteration (e.g., visual). Altered mobility would lead you to select such nursing interventions as range-of-motion (ROM) exercises or teaching the proper use of safety devices such as side rails, canes, or crutches. Visual impairment as the related factor would lead you to select different interventions such as keeping the area well lighted; orienting the client to the surroundings; or keeping eyeglasses clean, handy, and well protected. When you do not identify the correct related factor, the use of inappropriate interventions can increase a client's risk of injury. For example, not evaluating the home environment for hazards could result in sending a hospitalized client back home only to return with an additional injury (Box 25-4).

Planning

Clients with actual or potential risks to safety require a nursing care plan with interventions that will prevent and minimize threats to safety. Your interventions must be designed to help a client feel safe to interact freely within the environment. The total plan of care will address all aspects of client needs and use resources of the health care team and the community when appropriate.

GOALS AND OUTCOMES.   Planning and goal setting need to be done in collaboration with the client, family, and other members of the health care team. Remember to keep goals realistic, within the resources available to the client. When you involve the client and family in planning, they will be more alert to safety risks and potential hazards. For example, you may develop a goal "Reduce the number of falls" in a client with Parkinson's disease who falls frequently at home. An expected outcome would include "Client reduces barriers to reaching the bathroom." You may then suggest the intervention that the client sleep in a bedroom closest to the bathroom. After collaborating with the family, however, the alternative of a bedside commode is selected.

SETTING PRIORITIES.   Prioritize client nursing diagnoses and interventions that are most important in terms of risk to safety and health promotion. You may need to select more than one nursing diagnosis that best represents a

---

Physical Assessment Findings in the Older Adult That Increase the Risk of Accidents   Box 25-3

MUSCULOSKELETAL CHANGES
Muscle strength decreases
Joints become less mobile
Brittle bones due to osteoporosis
Posture changes; some kyphosis is common
Range of motion (ROM) is limited

NERVOUS SYSTEM CHANGES
All voluntary or autonomic reflexes are slower
Decreased ability to respond to multiple stimuli
Decreased sensitivity of touch

SENSORY CHANGES
Peripheral vision and lens accommodation decrease
Lens may develop opacity
Stimuli threshold for light touch and pain increases
Hearing is impaired because high-frequency tones are less perceptible

GENITOURINARY CHANGES
Increased nocturia
Increased occurrence of incontinence

Modified from Ebersole P, Hess P: *Geriatric nursing and healthy aging,* St. Louis, 2001, Mosby.

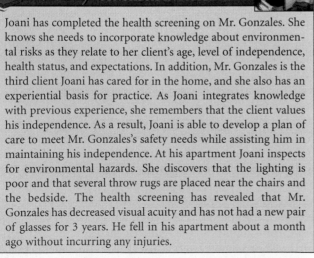

Case Study   **SYNTHESIS IN PRACTICE**

Joani has completed the health screening on Mr. Gonzales. She knows she needs to incorporate knowledge about environmental risks as they relate to her client's age, level of independence, health status, and expectations. In addition, Mr. Gonzales is the third client Joani has cared for in the home, and she also has an experiential basis for practice. As Joani integrates knowledge with previous experience, she remembers that the client values his independence. As a result, Joani is able to develop a plan of care to meet Mr. Gonzales's safety needs while assisting him in maintaining his independence. At his apartment Joani inspects for environmental hazards. She discovers that the lighting is poor and that several throw rugs are placed near the chairs and the bedside. The health screening has revealed that Mr. Gonzales has decreased visual acuity and has not had a new pair of glasses for 3 years. He fell in his apartment about a month ago without incurring any injuries.

client's particular needs. For example, the nursing diagnoses *risk for poisoning* and *deficient knowledge* may be important for an older client who takes several medications and has an impaired memory. Priority nursing interventions would include ways to reduce accidental poisoning (e.g., large labels on medication containers, use of dose dispensers, and having a family member prepare medications) and teaching safe

methods of taking medications, within a client's learning capabilities (see care plan).

CONTINUITY OF CARE.   It is important for you to help clients with safety needs develop a link within their community that helps to maintain a safe environment. Hospitalized clients need to learn how to identify and select resources within their community that will enhance safety once they return home. For example, an older adult may need to go to an adult day care center during weekdays when family members are working and unable to provide regular assistance.

Implementation

Your nursing interventions will be directed toward maintaining the client's safety in all types of settings. Providing a safe environment includes health promotion, developmental interventions, and environmental protection. Each of these

---

Nursing Diagnoses for Box 25-4
CLIENTS WITH SAFETY RISKS

- Body temperature, risk for imbalanced
- Home maintenance, impaired
- Injury, risk for
- Knowledge, deficient
- Poisoning, risk for

- Sensory perception, disturbed
- Suffocation, risk for
- Thought processes, disturbed
- Trauma, risk for

Case Study Nursing Care Plan   **RISK FOR INJURY**

ASSESSMENT

Mr. Gonzales is a 68-year-old man **with diminished visual acuity** who lives in an apartment with **throw rugs on the floors and poor lighting.** He states that he **cannot read the labels on his medication bottles** very well and sometimes takes his medication from memory. When observed walking, he **does not pick his feet very high up off the floor, and his movements appear stiff.**

*Defining characteristics are shown in bold type.

NURSING DIAGNOSIS

Risk for injury related to altered mobility and decreased visual acuity.

PLANNING

GOAL	EXPECTED OUTCOMES
Client's environment will be adapted to motor, sensory, and cognitive developmental needs (within 2 months).	Client will list hazards within 1 week. Modifiable hazards will be reduced 100% within 1 month.

IMPLEMENTATION

STEPS	RATIONALE
1. Review with client the potential risks for accidents observed in the home.	An accurate home assessment will identify threats to a client's safety.
a. Remove throw rugs.	Throw rugs can roll up or bunch to create an uneven walking surface.
b. Increase lighting to a minimum of 75 watts per light.	Adequate lighting reduces the likelihood of falling over objects or bumping into them.
c. Label medication bottles clearly in bold, large print.	Clearly labeled medication bottles reduce the risk of a medication error.
2. Stress the importance of making safety modifications in the home, and give specific instructions for prevention of burns, falls, and poisoning.	Advance guidance is important in preventing potential injuries (Edelman and Mandle, 1998).
3. Arrange for client to visit ophthalmologist and have a new prescription written for eyeglasses.	Reduced visual acuity can be corrected. Routine eye examinations are recommended annually for clients with identified risk factors (Ebersole and Hess, 2001).
4. Encourage client to take 20-minute walks in the neighborhood at least 3 times per week.	Maintenance of a physically active lifestyle can delay age changes associated with cardiovascular, respiratory, and musculoskeletal function (Ebersole and Hess, 2001).

EVALUATION

- Observe environment for elimination of threats to safety.
- Reassess client's motor, sensory, and cognitive status for appropriate environmental modifications.
- Revisit client in 2 weeks to determine if visit to ophthalmologist was made and if regular walks are being taken.

areas of implementation is appropriate in acute and restorative care settings.

HEALTH PROMOTION. The emphasis in health care today is on health promotion. Edelman and Mandle (1998) describe passive and active strategies aimed at health promotion. Passive strategies are implemented through government legislation (e.g., sanitation and clean water laws). Active strategies involve the individual and include changes in lifestyle and participation in wellness programs.

You can participate in health promotion activities by supporting legislation, by acting as a positive role model, and by recommending safety measures in the home, school, neighborhood, and workplace.

DEVELOPMENTAL INTERVENTIONS

INFANT, TODDLER, AND PRESCHOOLER. Growing, curious children depend on adults to protect them from injury. Educate young parents or guardians about reducing risks of injuries to children and teach ways to promote safety in the home (e.g., preventing access to poisonous substances, correct use of safety seats, use of safe toys, and placement of safety covers on electrical outlets (see Chapter 18). For example, as a pediatric nurse you can teach new parents about removal of poisonous substances from easy-to-reach storage areas and the importance of supervised play.

SCHOOL-AGE CHILD. School-age children increasingly explore their environment. They have friends outside their immediate neighborhood; and they become more active in school, church, and the community. Teach children to wear seat belts whenever riding in a car, to wear a helmet when riding a bicycle, skateboard, or scooter, and to keep adults informed of where they are. Also teach children how to cross the street safely and to refrain from talking to or accepting rides or gifts from strangers.

ADOLESCENT. Risks to the adolescent's safety involve many factors outside the home because much of their time is spent away from home and with their peer group. However, adults serve as role models for adolescents and, through providing examples, setting expectations, and providing education, can help adolescents minimize safety risks. Box 25-5 lists measures that will help you and parents prevent accidents during adolescence.

ADULT. Risks to young and middle-age adults frequently result from lifestyle factors such as child rearing, high-stress states, inadequate nutrition, and abuse of drugs or alcohol. You can help adults understand their safety risks and guide them in making lifestyle modifications by referring them to resources such as smoking cessation and stress management classes. Also encourage adults to exercise regularly, to practice relaxation techniques, and to acquire adequate sleep (see Chapter 28).

OLDER ADULT. Elimination of threats to the safety of the older adult focuses primarily on accidents. Advancing age and concurrent physiological changes predispose older adults to falls (Box 25-6) (see Chapter 18). Certain disease states common to older adults, such as arthritis or cerebrovascular accidents, and the effects of many medications such as sedatives, diuretics, and laxatives increase chances of injury. Nursing interventions designed to prevent falls and compensate for the physiological changes of aging are listed in Table 25-2.

Gerontological Nursing Practice | Box 25-6

- Because of visual impairments, teach clients to keep living areas well lighted and free of clutter, to keep eyeglasses in good condition, and to avoid night driving.
- Older adults have musculoskeletal changes that make movement difficult and increase the risk of falling. Teach clients to use assistive devices in proper working order (canes, rails in tub and bathroom, and elevated seats).
- Advise older adults to avoid smoking in bed, to lower thermostats on water heaters, to avoid overloading electrical outlets, and to install and maintain smoke detectors in the house.
- Older adults may have slowed reaction time. Teach clients safety tips for avoiding automobile accidents.
- Older adults frequently have some impairment of memory. Teach clients about the proper handling and storage of food and safe methods of scheduling and taking medications.
- Older adults have physiological changes that result in slower metabolism of drugs. Teach clients about drug interactions and signs and symptoms of drug toxicity to report to their health care provider.
- Older adults may suffer from an irreversible dementia. Assist family caregivers in understanding the nature of dementia. Teach them ways to match expectations with the client's capabilities, how to incorporate earlier life skills and interests, and to provide a calm, caring, and structured environment.

Client Teaching | Box 25-5

ACCIDENT PREVENTION FOR ADOLESCENTS
- Enroll teenagers in a driver's education course. Practice drives with them in good and bad weather. Teach them to handle a motor vehicle in a skid.
- Teach them to wear seat belts while driving or as passengers.
- Instruct them not to drive after using a psychoactive substance or enter an automobile when the driver has been using such substances.
- Form a contract with teenagers: if they drink at a party, they will call home for a ride with no questions asked.
- Help them to develop safe eating, sleeping, and relaxation habits.
- Inform them of the dangers of psychoactive substances.
- Recognize changes in adolescents' behavior and mood. Listen to them.
- Do not try to be a buddy; remain a parent.
- Teach them safe use of the Internet.

Measures to Prevent Falls in Older Adults

Table 25-2

Measure	Rationale
Home or Health Care Facility	
Stairs	
Install treads with uniform depth of 9 inches (22.5 cm) and 9-inch risers (vertical face of steps).	If stairs are of uniform size, older adult does not have to continually adjust vision.
Install uniform-textured or plain-colored surfaces on each tread, and mark edge of tread with contrasting color.	Uniform textures or color help to decrease vertigo. Marking edge of tread provides obvious visual clue to end of stair.
Ensure proper lighting of each tread. Block sun or lightbulb glare with translucent shades or screen, or use lower-wattage bulbs.	Older adults' vision is unable to adjust quickly to changes in lighting.
Ensure adequate head room so that users do not have to duck to negotiate stairs.	Sudden changes in head position may result in dizziness.
Remove protruding objects from staircase walls.	Decreased peripheral vision may prevent client from seeing object; moving to avoid protruding objects may disrupt balance.
Maintain outdoor walkways and stairs in good condition and free of holes, cracks, and splinters.	Decreased visual acuity can prevent client from seeing any structural defect.
Handrails	
Install smooth but slip-resistant handrail at least 2 inches (5 cm) from wall.	Two-inch distance allows client to grasp handrail firmly for support.
Secure handrail firmly so that user's weight is supported, especially at bottom and top of stairway.	Older adult has greatest risk of falling at top and bottom of stairs because center of gravity is being shifted and balance is unstable.
Install grab rails in bathroom near toilet and tub.	This enables client to have support while rising from sitting to standing position.
Floors	
Ensure clients wear properly fitting shoes or slippers with nonskid surface.	Reduces chances of slipping.
Secure all carpeting, mats, and tile; place nonskid backing under small rugs.	Sudden slip may cause dizziness and inability to regain balance.
Place bath mats or nonskid strips on bathtub or shower stall floors.	Wet surfaces increase the risk of falling.
Secure electrical cords against baseboards.	Prevents tripping.
Maintain proper illumination in areas both inside and outside where the client moves and walks.	Reduces the risk of falling due to eyestrain.
Health Care Facility	
Orientation	
Place disoriented clients in room near nurses' station.	Provides for more frequent observation by nursing staff.
Maintain close supervision of confused clients.	Confused client often attempts to wander out of bed or room.
Show the client how to use the call light at the beside and in bathroom, and place within easy reach.	Location and use of the call light is essential to client safety.
Place bedside tables and over-bed tables close to the client.	Prevents client from searching or overreaching for items such as eyeglasses, dentures, hearing aid, or telephone.
Remove clutter from bedside tables, hallways, bathrooms, and grooming areas.	Eliminates potential hazards and promotes client independence.
Have the client rise from the bed or chair slowly.	Prevents dizziness resulting from postural hypotension
Leave one side rail up and one down on the side where the oriented and ambulatory client gets out of bed.	Client can use the side rail for support when getting in and out of bed and to position self once in bed.
Transport	
Lock beds and wheelchairs when transferring a client from a bed to a wheelchair or back to bed.	Provides stability and support during transfer.
Place side rails in the up position and secure safety straps around the client on a stetcher.	Prevents the client from rolling off the stretcher.

Provide information about neighborhood resources to help the older adult maintain an independent lifestyle. Older adults frequently relocate to new neighborhoods and must get acquainted with new resources such as modes of transportation, church schedules, and food resources (e.g., Meals on Wheels). Although retired from their jobs, older adults have a wealth of past experiences to aid volunteer organizations. Some retirees may even enjoy reentering the work force in a new capacity. Information about assistance resources, such as daily "hello" programs, emergency services, and elder abuse hot lines, is also helpful.

ENVIRONMENTAL INTERVENTIONS.   To eliminate environmental threats, your nursing interventions should include general preventive measures and specific measures to reduce the risk of accidental injuries.

GENERAL PREVENTIVE MEASURES.   Your nursing interventions can contribute to a safer environment by helping clients meet their basic physiological needs. To ensure that oxygen availability is not threatened, encourage clients to have their furnaces inspected each season for proper functioning. Carbon monoxide detectors are available for installation in the home. To achieve a comfortable level of humidity in the home, the client might attach a humidifier to the furnace or, in the case of clients who have upper respiratory tract infections, use a room humidifier while sleeping. You can teach basic techniques for food handling and preparation so that nutritional needs are met safely (e.g., wash hands before and after food preparation, clean cutting surfaces thoroughly with soap and water, cook food thoroughly, and refrigerate food after preparation). To prevent injury from exposure to temperature extremes, educate older adults or clients who enjoy outdoor activities about signs and symptoms of frostbite, hypothermia, heatstroke, and heat exhaustion and how to avoid these conditions.

Adequate lighting and security measures in and around the home, including the use of night-lights, exterior lighting, and locks on doors and windows, enable clients to reduce the risk of injury from falls or crime. The local police department and community organizations often have safety classes available on how not to become a victim of crime. If clients have a history of falling and live alone, you may recommend they obtain an electronic safety alert device to wear. This device, when activated by the wearer, alerts a monitoring site to call emergency services for assistance.

Within the health care setting, you can eliminate physical hazards by removing clutter, extra equipment, and furniture from traffic areas. Always be sure an ambulatory client has a clear path to the bathroom. Keeping the bathroom light on also helps clients ambulate safely.

To control pathogen transmission, teach clients how and when to wash hands (e.g., following toileting, before food preparation, and before wound care). Clients should also know how to dispose of infected material such as wound dressings and used needles in the home. For example, heavy plastic containers such as 1-L soda bottles are excellent for needle disposal. Encourage clients to contact neighborhood community governments for guidelines on waste disposal methods.

SPECIFIC SAFETY CONCERNS.   There are specific interventions that you as a nurse can implement to ensure client safety.

Falls.   By modifying a client's environment you can reduce risk for falls. For example, a heavy client may need a bed, wheelchair, or commode specifically designed to support the additional weight. A client with impaired mobility would benefit from having the home organized so it becomes unnecessary to walk up or down stairs. In a health care facility, explain to clients how to use the call light or intercom system and be sure the call device is always placed close to the client. For clients needing assistance to ambulate, respond as quickly as you can when call lights are turned on so that the client does not attempt to get out of bed without help. Keep the immediate environment safe by removing excess furniture and equipment and providing clients with rubber-soled shoes or slippers for walking or transferring. Inspect canes, walkers, and crutches to be sure rubber tips are intact and all connections are tightened.

You can further minimize the risk of falls by implementing certain safeguards and by teaching the family ways to reduce the risk of falls (see Table 25-2, p. 587). Confused and disoriented clients or clients who repeatedly fall or try to remove medical devices (e.g., oxygen equipment, IV lines, dressings) may require the temporary use of restraints or side rails to keep them from falling out of bed. Restraints are not a solution to a client problem, but rather a temporary means to maintain client safety.

Physical Restraint.   A physical **restraint** is a physical or mechanical device that cannot be removed by the client, restricts the client's physical activity or normal access to the body, and is not a usual part of treatment indicated by the client's condition or symptoms (Zusman, 2001). The use of restraints is associated with serious complications due to immobilization, such as pressure ulcers, constipation, and incontinence. In some cases death has resulted because of restricted breathing and circulation. There have been cases where clients have hung themselves in a restraint while trying to get out of bed while restrained. Loss of self-esteem, humiliation, and agitation are also serious concerns. Because of these risks, current legislation emphasizes reducing the use of restraints. Regulatory agencies such as JCAHO and the Health Care Financing Administration (HCFA) enforce standards for the safe use of restraint devices. A restraint-free environment should be your first goal for all clients. Always try alternatives such as more frequent observation, involvement of family during visitation, frequent reorientation, and the introduction of familiar stimuli (e.g., knitting or crocheting, looking at family photos) within the environment to reduce behaviors that often lead to restraint use.

Alternatives to Restraints   Box 25-7

Involve clients and families in planning care; explain all procedures and treatments to them.

Encourage family and friends to stay, or utilize sitters for clients who need continuous supervision.

Use a wedge cushion in a chair or wheelchair to position the client back in the chair, hindering unassisted ambulation.

Assign confused or disoriented clients to rooms near the nurses' station. Observe these clients frequently.

Provide appropriate visual and auditory stimuli (e.g., family pictures, clock, radio).

Eliminate bothersome treatments as soon as possible. For example, discontinue tube feedings and begin oral feedings as quickly as the client's condition allows.

Use relaxation techniques (e.g., music, massage).

Institute exercise and ambulation schedules as the client's condition allows.

Provide scheduled toileting, especially during peak fall times, such as 6-8 AM and 4-6 PM.

Consult with physical and occupational therapists to enhance clients' abilities to carry out activities of daily living.

Evaluate all medications clients are receiving to determine if the medication is having the desired therapeutic effect.

Conduct ongoing assessment and evaluation of clients' care and their ongoing response to care.

Modified from Quinn CA: The advanced practice nurse and changing perspectives on physical restraint, *Clin Nurs Spec* 10(5):223, 1996.

In keeping with current trends toward health promotion, your assessment techniques and modifications of the environment are effective alternatives to restraints (Box 25-7). You might use the **AMBULARM** device for the client who climbs out of bed unassisted and is in danger of falling. This device is worn on the leg and signals when the leg is in a dependent position such as over the side rail. A weight-sensitive bed and chair alarm are designed to warn nursing staff when a client attempts to leave the bed or chair unassisted. A Sensormat, placed under the client's hips, signals an audible alarm when the client tries to get up. These devices may avoid physical restraints and prevent a client fall.

When restraints are required to protect the client or others, involve the client and family in the decision to use restraints. Assist them in adapting to this change by explaining the purpose of the restraint, expected care while the client is in restraints, and that the restraint is temporary and protective. Nursing homes are required to obtain informed consent from family members before using restraints. As with other procedures, you must follow specific guidelines when using physical restraints (Skill 25-1). The overall objectives for restraint use include the following:

1. Reduce the risk of client injury from falls
2. Prevent interruption of therapy such as traction, intravenous (IV) infusions, nasogastric tube feeding, or Foley catheter
3. Prevent the confused or combative client from removing life support equipment
4. Reduce the risk of injury to self or others

For legal purposes you must know agency-specific policies for appropriate use and monitoring of a restrained client. The use of a restraint must be clinically justified and be a part of the client's prescribed medical treatment and plan of care. A physician's order is required and must be based on a face-to-face assessment of the client. The order must be current and specify the duration and circumstances under which restraints are to be used. Your nursing interventions will focus on preventing complications of restraints, such as hazards of immobility, a decreased sense of self-esteem, and increased agitation. You should collaborate with other members of the health care team to design fall prevention programs and a restraint-free environment for the client. The goal is to discontinue the use of restraints as soon as possible.

Side Rails. A side rail can be used to increase a clients' mobility and stability in bed or when moving from bed to chair. Side rails also help to prevent the unconscious or sedated client from rolling out of bed. Always check agency policy about the use of side rails; they can be considered a restraint when used to prevent an ambulatory client from voluntarily getting out of bed. The use of side rails alone for a disoriented client may cause only more confusion and further injury. Frequently a confused client or one determined to get out of bed because of pain, toileting needs, or anxiety attempts to climb over the side rail or out at the foot of the bed. Either attempt usually results in a fall. Your interventions to reduce a client's confusion should first focus on the cause. Confusion is frequently mistaken for a client's attempt to explore the environment or to self-toilet. If all efforts to reduce confusion or restlessness fail and the client is at risk for injury to self or others, a restraint may be necessary. However, remember the goal is to remove the restraint at the earliest possible time. When side rails are raised, be sure the bed is in the lowest position possible.

Fires. A fire is always possible in the home or health care setting. Accidental home fires typically result from smoking in bed, careless extinguishing of cigarette butts in trash cans, grease fires, use of space heaters, or electrical fires resulting from faulty wiring or appliances. Institutional fires typically result from a client smoking in bed or from an electrical or anesthetic-related fire. Regardless of where the fire occurs, it is important to have an evacuation plan in place. Know where fire extinguishers and gas shut-off valves are located, and know how to activate a fire alarm.

To reduce the risk of fires in the home, have clients inspect the condition of cooking equipment and appliances, particularly irons and stoves. For clients with visual deficits, it helps to have dials installed with large numbers or symbols on temperature controls. Smoke detectors should be placed strategically throughout the home (e.g., in a kitchen and near a bedroom) so that occupants in a home can be alerted when a fire breaks out.

Text continued on p. 595

Skill 25-1
USE OF RESTRAINTS

DELEGATION CONSIDERATIONS

Assessment of client's behavior, level of orientation, selection of appropriate restraint alternative, need for restraints, appropriate type to use, and specific assessments related to oxygenation, skin integrity, and neurovascular status should not be delegated to assistive personnel. However, the following aspects of the skill may be delegated to assistive person-nel: correct placement of the restraint; observing for constriction of circulation, skin integrity, adequate breathing; when and how to change client's position; providing ROM and skin care, toileting, and opportunities for socialization.

EQUIPMENT
- Proper restraint: jacket, belt, extremity, or mitten
- Padding

STEPS	RATIONALE
1. Assess if a client needs a restraint. Does the client continually try to interrupt needed therapy? Is the client repeatedly trying to ambulate independently, creating a serious risk of injury?	Restraints are used only when other measures fail to prevent interruption of therapies such as traction, endotracheal intubation, IV infusions, or nasogastric tube feedings; to prevent a confused or combative client from self-injury by getting out of bed or falling out of bed; to prevent client from removing urinary catheters, surgical drains, or life support equipment; and to reduce risk of injury to others by client.
2. Assess client's behavior, such as confusion, disorientation, agitation, restlessness, combativeness, or inability to follow directions.	If client's behavior continues despite attempts to eliminate cause of behavior, use of physical restraint may be needed.
3. Review agency policies regarding restraints. Check physician's order for purpose and type of restraint, location, and duration of restraint. Determine if signed consent for use of restraint is needed.	Physician's order is necessary to apply restraints. The least restrictive type of restraint should be ordered. Because restraints limit client's ability to move freely, nurse must make clinical judgments appropriate to client's condition and agency policy. If nurse restrains client in emergency situation because of violent or aggressive behavior that presents an immediate danger, a face-to-face physician assessment within 1 hour is needed (HCFA, 2000).
4. Review manufacturer's instructions for restraint application before entering client's room.	Nurse should be familiar with all devices used for client care and protection. Incorrect application of restraint device may result in client injury or death.
5. Introduce self to client and family and assess their feelings about restraint use. Explain that restraint is temporary and designed to protect client from injury.	Client and family must be informed about use of restraint. In nursing homes, informed consent must be obtained.
6. Inspect area where restraint is to be placed. Assess condition of skin underlying area on which restraint is to be applied.	Restraints may compress and interfere with functioning of devices or tubes. Assessment provides baseline to monitor client's skin integrity.

- **Critical Decision Point**
Restraints should not interfere with equipment such as IV tubes. They should not be placed over access devices, such as an arteriovenous (AV) dialysis shunt.

STEPS	RATIONALE
7. Approach client in a calm, confident manner. Explain what you plan to do.	Reduces client anxiety and promotes cooperation.
8. Gather equipment and wash hands.	Promotes organization and reduces transmission of microorganisms.
9. Provide privacy. Position and drape client as needed.	Prevents lowering of client's self-esteem.
10. Adjust bed to proper height and lower side rail on side of client contact.	Allows nurse to utilize proper body mechanics and prevent injury.
11. Be sure client is comfortable and in correct anatomical position.	Prevents contractures and neurovascular impairment.
12. Pad skin and bony prominences (if necessary) that will be under the restraint.	Reduces friction and pressure from restraint to skin and underlying tissue.

STEPS	RATIONALE

13. Apply proper-size selected restraint: **Always refer to manufacturer's directions.**

   a. **Jacket (vest or Posey) restraint:** Apply jacket or vest over gown, pajamas, or clothes. Place client's hands through armholes. Jacket restraints have sleeves. They close in back with zippers or hook and loop.

       Vest restraints should have front and back of garment labeled as such. Secure vest according to manufacturer's directions. Some vests secure in the front of the client, and others secure in the back. Adjust to client's level of comfort (see illustration).

Restrains client while lying or reclining in bed and while sitting in chair or wheelchair. Criss-crossing in back can cause risk of death from strangulation. Clothing or gown prevents friction against skin.

   b. **Belt restraint:** Have client in a sitting position. Apply over clothes, gown, or pajamas. Remove wrinkles or creases from front and back of restraint while placing it around client's waist. Bring ties through slots in belt. Help client lie down if in bed. Avoid placing belt too tightly across client's chest or abdomen (see illustrations).

Restrains center of gravity and prevents client from rolling off stretcher or sitting up while on stretcher or from falling out of bed. Tight application may interfere with ventilation.

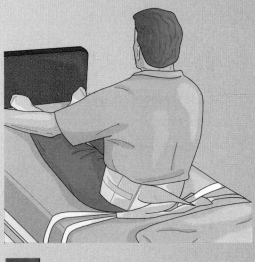

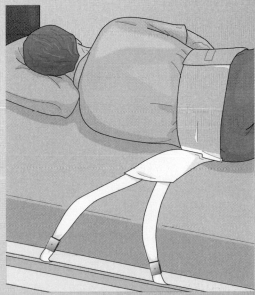

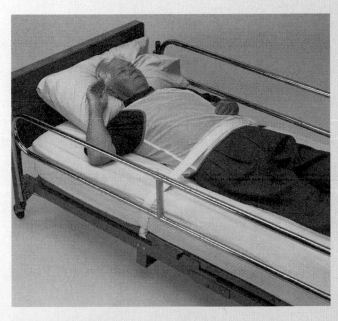

STEP 13A   Vest restraint securely attached to bed frame. (Courtesy JT Posey Co, Arcadia, Calif.)

STEP 13B   Roll belt restraint tied to the bed frame and to an area that does not cause the restraint to tighten when the side rail is raised or lowered. (From Sorrentino SA: *Mosby's textbook for nursing assistants,* ed 5, St. Louis, 2000, Mosby.)

STEPS	RATIONALE

c. **Extremity (ankle or wrist) restraint:** restraint designed to immobilize one or all extremities. Commercially available limb restraints are composed of sheepskin with foam padding (see illustration). Limb restraint is wrapped around wrist or ankle with soft part toward skin and secured snugly in place by Velcro straps.

Maintains immobilization of extremity to protect client from injury from fall or accidental removal of therapeutic device (e.g., IV tube, Foley catheter). Tight application may interfere with circulation.

- *Critical Decision Point*
  Client with wrist and ankle restraints is at risk for aspiration if placed in supine position. Place client in lateral position rather than supine.

d. **Mitten restraint:** thumbless mitten device that restrains client's hands (see illustration). Place hand in mitten, being sure end is brought all the way up over the wrist.

Prevents clients from dislodging invasive equipment, removing dressings, or scratching, yet allows greater movement than a wrist restraint.

14. Attach restraint straps to portion of bed frame that moves when head of bed is raised or lowered (see illustration). **Do not attach to side rails.** Restraint may also be attached with client in chair or wheelchair to chair frame.

Client may be injured if restraint is secured to side rail and it is lowered.

15. When client is in a wheelchair, jacket restraint should be secured by placing ties under armrests and securing at back of chair (see illustration).

Prevents client from sliding and being choked by restraint.

- *Critical Decision Point*
  If ties are not under armrests, clients may be able to slide ties up the back of the chair and free themselves.

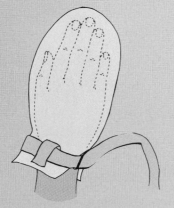

STEP 13C   Placement of wrist restraint.

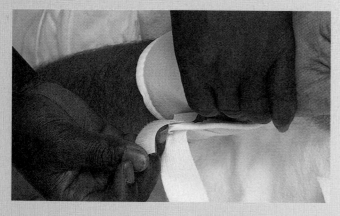

STEP 13D   Mitten restraint.

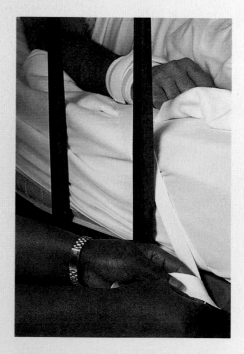

STEP 14   Tie restraint strap to bed frame.

STEPS	RATIONALE
16. Secure restraints with a quick-release tie (see illustrations).	Allows for quick release in an emergency.
17. Insert two fingers under secured restraint (see illustration).	Checking for constriction prevents neurovascular injury.

• *Critical Decision Point*
A tight restraint may cause constriction and impede circulation.

18. Proper placement of restraint, skin integrity, pulses, temperature, color, and sensation of the restrained body part should be assessed **at least every hour** or according to agency policy.	Frequent assessments prevent complications, such as suffocation, skin breakdown, and impaired circulation.

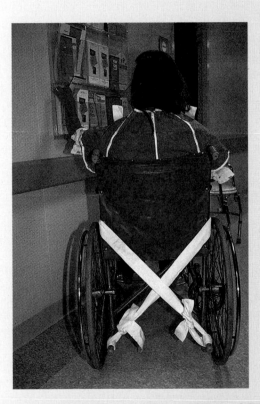

STEP 15   Straps of vest restraint secured at back of chair.

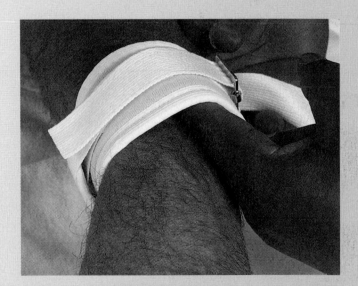

STEP 17   Place two fingers under restraint to check tightness.

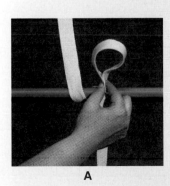 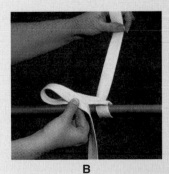 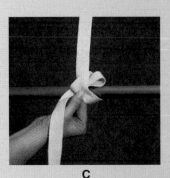 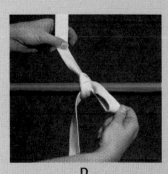

A   B   C   D

STEP 16   The Posey quick-release tie. (Courtesy JT Posey Co, Arcadia, Calif.)

STEPS	RATIONALE
19. Restraints should be removed at least every 2 hours (JCAHO, 2001). If client is violent or noncompliant, remove one restraint at a time and/or have staff assistance while removing restraints.	Provides opportunity to change client's position, perform full ROM, toileting, and exercise and to provide food or fluids.

- *Critical Decision Point*
  Client should not be left unattended while restraints are off.

20. Secure call light or intercom system within reach.	Allows client, family, or caregiver to obtain assistance quickly.

- *Critical Decision Point*
  Restraints restrict movement, making clients unable to perform their activities of daily living without assistance. Providing food and/or fluids and assisting with toileting and other activities is essential.

21. Leave bed or chair with wheels locked. Bed should be in the lowest position.	Locked wheels prevent bed or chair from moving if client attempts to get out. If client falls when bed is in lowest position, chances of injury are reduced.
22. Wash hands.	Reduces transmission of microorganisms.
23. Inspect client for any injury, including all hazards of immobility, while restraints are in use.	Client should be free of injury and not exhibit any signs of immobility complications.
24. Observe IV catheters, urinary catheters, and drainage tubes to determine that they are positioned correctly.	Reinsertion can be uncomfortable and can increase risk of infection or interrupt therapy.
25. Reassess client's need for continued use of restraint at least every 24 hours with the intent of discontinuing restraint at the earliest possible time (JCAHO, 2001). (See agency policy.)	Face-to-face reassessment by physician is required and new order obtained if restraint is to be continued.

UNEXPECTED OUTCOMES AND RELATED INTERVENTIONS

- Skin integrity becomes impaired.
  - Reassess the continued need for the restraint; use a different type of restraint.
  - If restraint is needed, make sure restraint is applied correctly and provide adequate padding.
  - Assess skin, provide appropriate therapy, or remove restraints more frequently.
  - Change wet or soiled restraints.
- Client becomes more confused and agitated after restraints are applied.
  - Determine the cause of the behavior and eliminate the cause if possible.
  - Determine the need for more or less sensory stimulation.
  - Reorient as needed and/or attempt other restraint alternatives.
- Neurovascular status of an extremity is altered, manifested by cyanosis, pallor, edema, or coldness of skin, or client complains of tingling, pain, numbness, or loss of ROM.
  - Remove the restraint immediately and notify the physician.

- Client releases the restraint and suffers a fall or other injury.
  - Attend to the client's immediate physical needs.
  - Notify the physician.
  - Assess the type of restraint and if it was correctly applied.

RECORDING AND REPORTING

- Record client behaviors before you applied restraints.
- Record restraint alternatives you attempted and the client's response.
- Record client's and/or family's understanding of and consent to restraint application.
- Record type and location of the restraint and time applied.
- Record times that you performed assessments and releases while client in restraints.
- Record findings from your assessments related to orientation, oxygenation, skin integrity, circulation, and positioning.
- Record client's behavior and expected or unexpected outcomes after you applied the restraint.
- Record client's response when you removed restraints.
- Also see behavioral restraint flow sheet (Figure 25-1).

Holy Family Hospital and Medical Center
70 East Street, Methuen, MA 01844

BEHAVIORAL RESTRAINT FLOW SHEET
Start new form for each successive renewal.

Page 1 of 2

☐ New Order ☐ Renewal Order	☐ Obtained Physician s Time Limited Order ☐ Face-to-face evaluation by Physician within 1 hour ☐ In-person re-evaluation by the time order expires	Date/Time Restraint Started _____ Date/Time Restraint Ended _____ Total Restraint Time _____

Categorize Emergency Situation:
☐ Substantial risk of serious physical assault
☐ Occurrences of serious physical assault
☐ Substantial risk of self-destructive behavior
☐ Occurrence of serious risk of self-destructive behavior.

Describe Behavior That Requires Use/Continuance Of Restraint:

Alternatives Used Before Restraint:
☐ Verbal de-escalation
☐ Redirecting patient s focus
☐ Activity substitute
☐ Clear, firm limit-setting
☐ Decrease stimuli
☐ Staff-family companionship 1:1
☐ Administer medication
☐ Other (describe):

Type of Restraint Used (check all that apply):
☐ Seclusion
☐ Physical Restraint
☐ Mechanical Restraint
☐ Chemical Restraint

Chemical Restraint

Time	Medication	Dosage	Route

☐ Procedure explained to patient.

☐ Family notified (if appropriate):
Date/Time: _____

☐ Primary physician notified:
Date/Time: _____

Physician Assessment - 1) Clinical justification reviewed; 2) Alternatives/Prevention strategies reviewed; 3) Assessment Summary:

Physician Signature/Date and Time:

BEHAVIORAL RESTRAINT FLOW SHEET
Start new form for each successive renewal.

Page 2 of 2

The patient must be observed 1:1. The RN must assess patient at initiation of restraint and q 15 minutes thereafter.

Key: NN = Nurses Notes; √ = Nursing Assessment/Safety Check Done.	Order Time limits: 4 hours/adult age 18 or older; 2 hours/child and adolescent age 9-17; 1 hour for child under age 9											
Safety Checks and Assessment q 15 minutes Refer to policy for restraint release and removal times.	Date:											
	Time:											
1. Vital Signs: Blood Pressure, Pulse, Respiration												
2. Skin Integrity/Sensation/Joint Mobility												
3. Hydration/Nutrition (T = taken; R = refused)												
4. Elimination (V = voided; R = refused)												
5. Safety Check: comfort, body alignment, circulation												
6. Readiness for Discontinuation of Restraint												
7. Mental Status: 1) maintaining self control, 2) suicidal; 3) homicidal; 4) self-abusive; 5) assaultive; 6) restless; 7) thrashing; 8) calm; 9) sleeping; 10) dissociative; 11) withdrawn; 12) disorganized; 13) organized; 14) crying; 15) threatening; 16) other												
8. Restraint Release/ROM/Reposition per policy												
	RN Initials:											

Signs of injury associated w/application of restraint:

Description of behavior and skin assessment when restraints dicontinued:

RN Signature/Initials:	RN Signature/Initials:	RN Signature/Initials:

Written 6/01

FIGURE 25-1   Behavioral restraint flow sheet. (Courtesy Holy Family Hospital and Medical Center, Methuen, Mass.)

If a fire occurs in a health care agency, you must first protect any clients in immediate danger. All personnel should help to evacuate clients from the area, especially those clients who are closest to the fire. If a client requires oxygen but not life support, discontinue the oxygen, which is combustible and can fuel an existing fire. If the client is on life support, maintain the client's respiratory status manually with an Ambu-bag (see Chapter 27) until the client is moved away from the fire. Direct ambulatory clients to walk by themselves to a safe area or have them as-

Procedural Guidelines for	Box 25-8
INTERVENING IN ACCIDENTAL POISONING	

1. Assess for signs or symptoms of accidental ingestion of harmful substances, such as nausea, vomiting, drooling, lethargy.
2. Identify the type and amount of substance ingested to help determine the correct type and amount of antidote needed.
3. Call the poison control center before attempting any intervention. Poison control centers have information needed to treat poisoned clients or to offer referral to treatment centers.
4. If instructed to induce vomiting:
   a. Infants up to 12 months: 5 to 10 ml of ipecac
   b. Children (1 to 12 years): 1 tablespoon (15 ml) of ipecac
   c. Adults: 2 tablespoons (30 ml) of ipecac
5. Give oral fluids to assist vomiting (if directed):
   a. Children (1 to 12 years): 5 to 15 ml/kg; up to 8 oz of water
   b. Adults: 16 oz of water
6. If requested to do so, save vomitus and deliver to poison control center. Laboratory analysis can determine further treatment.
7. Position victim with head turned to side to reduce risk of aspiration.
8. Vomiting is never induced with the following substances: lye, household cleaners, hair care products, grease or petroleum products, or furniture polish.
9. Vomiting is never induced in an unconscious victim because vomiting increases risk of aspiration.
10. If instructed by poison control center to take person to emergency department, call ambulance. Ambulance personnel will be able to provide emergency measures if needed. In addition, parent or guardian may be too upset to drive safely.

Mercury Spill Cleanup Procedure	Box 25-9

In the event of a mercury spill, follow these steps:
1. Evacuate the room except for a housekeeping crew (if available).
2. Cleanup personnel should wear rubber (latex or vinyl) gloves while handling the mercury.
3. Spray the spill area with a mist of water. This diminishes vaporization of mercury.
4. Ventilate the area. Close interior doors and open any outside windows.
5. Use a suction device such as a syringe without a needle to extract as much of the mercury as possible from the spill site. Put recovered mercury in a leakproof glass or plastic container with a nonmetallic cap or lid. DO NOT VACUUM THE SPILL.
6. Mop the floor with a mercury cleaner (see agency policy).
7. Dispose of collected mercury according to local environmental safety regulations.

sist in moving clients in wheelchairs. Move bedridden clients from the scene by a stretcher, their bed, or a wheelchair, or they may need to be carried. If a client must be carried, be careful not to overextend your physical limits for lifting because an injury to you can result in further injury to the client. If fire department personnel are on the scene, they can also help to evacuate clients.

After a fire has been reported and clients are out of danger, you and other personnel must take measures to contain or put out the fire, such as closing doors and windows, turning off oxygen and electrical equipment, and using a fire extinguisher. The three basic types of fires for which extinguishers are used are paper and rubbish (type A), grease and anesthetic gas (type B), and electrical (type C). Use the appropriate extinguisher for each type.

Your best intervention to prevent fires is to comply with the agency's smoking policies and keep combustible materials away from heat sources. Some agencies have fire doors that are held open by magnets and close automatically when a fire alarm sounds. Make sure that you keep equipment away from these doors.

Poisoning. You can help parents reduce the risk of accidental poisoning by teaching them to keep hazardous sub-

stances out of the reach of children. With adolescents and adults, poisonings are often caused by insect or snake bites. Drug and other substance poisonings in these age-groups are commonly related to suicide attempts or drug experimentation. Teach parents that calling a **poison control center** for information before attempting home remedies can save their child's life. There are guidelines for accepted interventions for accidental poisonings that you can teach a parent or guardian (Box 25-8). In addition, instruct the parent to give milk to neutralize an acid substance or lemon juice or vinegar to neutralize an alkaline substance. Older adults are also at risk for poisoning because diminished eyesight may cause an accidental ingestion of a toxic substance. In addition, the impaired memory of some older adult clients may result in an accidental overdose of prescribed medications. Be sure medications are labeled in large print. Have clients keep poisonous substances out of the bathroom.

In the health care setting it is important for nurses to know how to respond when exposure to a poisonous substance occurs. Mercury is considered a hazardous chemical by OSHA. Common exposures in a hospital include broken thermometers or sphygmomanometers. Mercury enters the body through inhalation and absorption through the skin. Exposures that occur in a hospital setting are usually short term, which may affect the brain or kidney. However, full recovery is likely to occur once the body cleans itself of the contamination. Box 25-9 summarizes steps to take in the event of a mercury spill.

Electrical Hazards. Much of the equipment used in health care settings is electrical and must be well maintained. You can decrease the risk of electrical injury and fire by using properly **grounded** and functional electrical equipment. Teach clients and family how to reduce their risk of electrical injury in the home (e.g., discuss prevention of electrical shock avoidance of use of electrical appliances near water

Outcome Evaluation for **MR. GONZALES**   Box 25-10

Nursing Action	Client Response/Finding	Achievement of Outcome
Observe environment for elimination of threats to safety.	Throw rugs have been removed or replaced with rubber-backed rugs. Lighting has increased to 75 watts except in bathroom and bedroom. Mr. Gonzales is able to identify potential hazards.	Hazards have been reduced. Mr. Gonzales verbalizes adaptation to environmental modifications.
Reassess motor, sensory, and cognitive status for appropriate environmental modifications.	New glasses have been obtained. Mr. Gonzales is able to read medication bottle labels. Mr. Gonzales reports difficulty getting into bathtub due to stiffness. Bathtub floor are without nonskid strips.	Outcome of reducing hazards 100% has not been fully achieved. Mr. Gonzales will purchase nonskid strips for tub floor.

source, methods of grounding appliances, avoidance of operating unfamiliar equipment).

Evaluation

CLIENT CARE.   Evaluate your nursing interventions for reducing threats to safety by comparing the client's response to the expected outcomes for each goal of care. When expected outcomes are not met, your interventions must be revised. It may also be possible that new nursing diagnoses have developed. Apply evaluative measures to determine a client's progress toward outcomes and goals. An example of a goal, outcome, and evaluative measure includes the goal "Client's environment is adapted to motor, sensory, and cognitive developmental needs." An outcome for this goal could be "Modifiable hazards in the home are reduced by 100% within 2 weeks." Your evaluative measures could include "Observe environment for elimination of threats to safety" and "Reassess motor, sensory, and cognitive status for appropriate environmental modifications" (Box 25-10).

Evaluate the client's outcome by comparing what was planned with what resulted, and evaluate how well the plan was implemented. Examine the planned interventions for appropriateness and effectiveness in each situation. By accomplishing goals and outcomes you validate effective care.

CLIENT EXPECTATIONS.   The client has come to expect the highest quality care from you and the health care system.

Case Study   EVALUATION

It has been 2 weeks since the plan of care was implemented for Mr. Gonzales. The hazards have been identified and modifications made. With regular exercise Mr. Gonzales has found that his walking has improved, and now he feels safer about leaving the apartment. The new medication labels have made it easier for Mr. Gonzales to tell his several medications apart. His new glasses will arrive within a few days. The client is currently injury free and now feels better about living to a "ripe old age" like his father. He understands that he can make changes in his environment that will keep him safe. In the last 2 weeks he has not suffered a fall. Joani Green, the student nurse, has a sense of accomplishment in a job well done.

DOCUMENTATION NOTE
Mr. Gonzales's home has improved lighting, and the throw rugs are removed. During good weather and during daylight hours he takes walks in his neighborhood. He is able to list all medications by name, dose, when taken, and significant side effects. No reports of injury.

Expectations as a result of care may include restoration of health, reduction in risks for falling, a safer home environment, and improved recognition of safety risks. Clients are often unaware of the dangers to be found in their homes and workplaces, and many will make the necessary adjustments to keep themselves and loved ones safe and injury free once the dangers have been identified.

Key Terms

AMBULARM, p. 589
carbon monoxide, p. 579

food poisoning, p. 579
grounded, p. 596
heat exhaustion, p. 579
hypothermia, p. 579

pathogen, p. 580
poison, p. 580
poison control center, p. 596
restraint, p. 588

Key Concepts

- A safe environment in a health care agency is comfortable; maintains the client's privacy; and reduces the risks of injury, infection, and untoward effects of treatment or medications.
- In the community a safe environment is one in which basic needs are achievable, physical hazards are reduced, transmission of pathogens and parasites is reduced, pollution is controlled, and sanitation is maintained.
- The transmission of pathogens and parasites is reduced through medical and surgical asepsis, food sanitation, insect and rodent control, and disposal of human wastes.
- Every developmental stage involves assessment of specific safety risks.
- The school-age child is at risk for injury at home, at school, and traveling to and from school.
- Adolescents are at risk for injury from the effects of drug and alcohol abuse.
- Threats to an adult's safety are frequently associated with lifestyle habits.
- Risks of injury for older adults are directly related to the physiological changes of the aging process.
- Risks to client safety within a health care agency include falls and client-inherent, procedure-related, and equipment-related accidents.
- Nursing interventions for promoting safety are individualized for developmental stage, lifestyle, and the environment.
- The nursing care plan to promote safety is continually evaluated to identify new or continued risks to the client.
- Physical restraints should be used only as a last resort, when clients' behavior places them or others at risk for injury.

Critical Thinking Activities

1. While assessing your client who is in a vest restraint, you determine that he is more restless and agitated. What actions will you take?
2. A family member comes to you and reports that the heating pad they brought in for your client caught fire, but they were able to put out the small fire on the mattress. What would you do?
3. You have been assigned to care for an older adult woman who was recently admitted to your unit. Your admission assessment reveals that she is at fall risk due to urinary frequency, an unsteady gait, and recent mental status changes. What fall prevention measures can you take to ensure your client's safety?

Review Questions

1. A confused client is pulling at an IV line during hospitalization. The best nursing intervention for the client's safety would be to:
   1. use an armboard.
   2. apply wrist restraints.
   3. place the client in a vest restraint.
   4. provide closer observation of the client.
2. You discover an electrical fire in a client's room. Your first action would be to:
   1. activate the fire alarm.
   2. evacuate any clients in immediate danger.
   3. confine the fire by closing all doors and windows.
   4. extinguish the fire by using the nearest appropriate fire extinguisher.
3. During the night shift, your client was found wandering in the hall looking for the bathroom. Your initial intervention would be to:
   1. insert a urinary catheter.
   2. assign a staff member to stay with the client.
   3. ask the physician to order a vest restraint.
   4. provide scheduled toileting during the night shift.
4. Your older adult client keeps trying to climb over the bed's side rails. In planning care for this client, you know that:
   1. older adults tolerate restraints well.
   2. older adults must be restrained to protect them from injury.
   3. you are legally liable if you fail to restrain a confused older adult.
   4. older adults are prone to confusion because of a heightened sensitivity to medication.
5. The restraint device that is most restrictive (provides the least movement) for the client is:
   1. the mitten.
   2. the vest.
   3. bilateral wrist restraint.
   4. four bed side rails in the up position.
6. Your medical/surgical unit decides to institute a fall prevention program. You know that:
   1. falls are difficult to prevent.
   2. all clients are at high risk for falling.
   3. a fractured hip is the most common injury after a fall.
   4. older adults are more likely to fall because of the physiological changes of aging.
7. When teaching parents about accidental poisoning in children, you would instruct them to:
   1. give oral fluids.
   2. induce vomiting.
   3. call the poison control center.
   4. drive the child to the emergency department.
8. When providing discharge teaching about home safety to your older client, you know that:
   1. a safe environment promotes client independence.
   2. most accidents in the older adult are related to lifestyle factors.
   3. older clients are reluctant to make necessary environmental changes.
   4. environmental hazards are costly for the older adult on a fixed income.

9. Key elements that place a client at a greater risk for falls include:
   1. history of falls, urinary frequency, smoker.
   2. history of falls, confusion, impaired mobility.
   3. history of falls, age over 60, seizure disorder.
   4. history of falls, sensory impairment, age over 60.

10. In planning discharge teaching aimed at reducing safety risks in the home, you recognize that:
    1. safety risks change in each developmental level.
    2. clients are able to identify what their safety risks are.
    3. your assessment should focus on environmental factors only.
    4. teaching the client and family about home safety is difficult to do in a hospital setting.

References

Accident facts, Itasca, Ill, 1998, National Safety Council.

Air pollution fact sheet, Washington, DC, 1998, Environmental Health Center, National Safety Council.

American Nurses Association: *Standards of clinical practice,* ed 2, Washington, DC, 1998, The Association.

Brians L and others: The development of the RISK tool for fall prevention, *Rehabil Nurs* 16(2):67, 1991.

Ebersole P, Hess P: *Geriatric nursing and healthy aging,* St. Louis, 2001, Mosby.

Edelman CL, Mandle CL: *Health promotion throughout the life span,* ed 4, St. Louis, 1998, Mosby.

Fact book for the year 2000, National Center for Injury Prevention and Control, Centers for Disease Control and Prevention, 2000.

Health Care Financing Administration: *Conditions of participation: interpretive guidelines,* Rockville, Md, 2000. Available at HFCA.gov/quality/462.htm.

Joint Commission on Accreditation of Healthcare Organization: *Comprehensive accreditation manual for hospitals,* Chicago, January 2001, The Commission.

Pillitteri A, *Child health nursing: care of the child and family,* Philadelphia, 1999, Lippincott.

Quinn CA: The advanced practice nurse and changing perspectives on physical restraint, *Clin Nurs Spec* 10(5):223, 1996.

Sorrentino SA: *Mosby's textbook for nursing assistants,* ed 5, St. Louis, 2000, Mosby.

Williams SR: *Basic nutrition and diet therapy,* ed 11, St. Louis, 2000, Mosby.

Wong DL and others: *Whaley and Wong's nursing care of infants and children,* ed 6, St. Louis, 1999, Mosby.

Wong DL and others: *Wong's essentials of pediatric nursing,* ed 6, St. Louis, 2000, Mosby.

Zusman J: *Restraint and seclusion: understanding the JCAHO standards and federal regulations,* ed 3, Marblehead, Mass, 2001, Opus Communications.

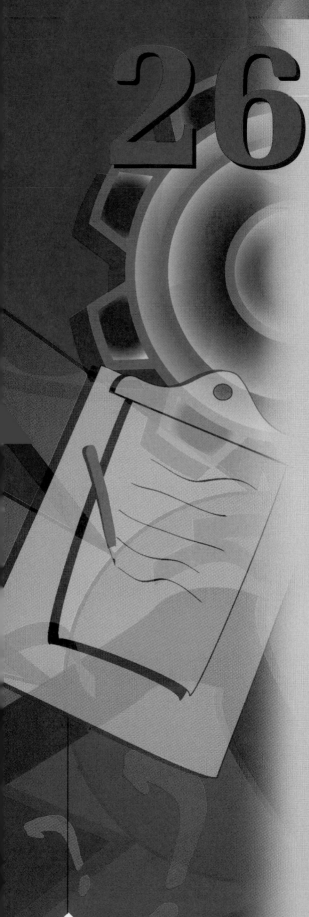

Hygiene

Objectives

- Define key terms.
- Identify common skin problems and related interventions.
- Describe factors that influence personal hygiene practices.
- Discuss conditions that may put a client at risk for impaired skin integrity.
- Describe the types of bathing techniques used for various physical conditions and for clients of various age-groups.
- Perform a complete bed bath and back rub.
- Discuss factors that influence the condition of the nails and feet.
- Explain the importance of foot care for the diabetic client.
- Describe the methods used for cleaning and cutting the nails.
- Discuss conditions that may put a client at risk for impaired oral mucous membranes.
- Discuss measures used to provide special oral hygiene.
- Assist with or provide oral hygiene.
- List common hair and scalp problems and their related interventions.
- Offer hygiene to meet the needs of clients requiring eye, ear, and nose care.
- Describe how hygiene for the older adult may differ from that for the younger client.
- Make an occupied and unoccupied hospital bed.

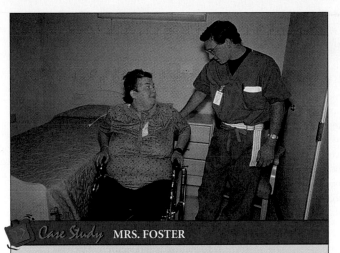

Case Study **MRS. FOSTER**

Mrs. Foster is a 55-year-old woman who has been a resident in a skilled nursing facility for the past 3 years. She has a medical history of multiple sclerosis. Recently she had increased dental problems and had three root canal procedures. Mrs. Foster is married and has three daughters. Her family lives approximately 2 hours from the facility. Today she related the "need to feel better about herself."

James Joseph is a freshman nursing student assigned to the skilled nursing facility. James is 20 years old and single. James has had some experience working with clients who have been in a skilled nursing facility. James has a part-time job in a facility near his home. He knows how important it is for clients to feel comfortable and have their basic needs met.

To provide basic hygiene, James needs to learn about what is important to Mrs. Foster's comfort. When hygiene needs are not fulfilled, clients experience low self-esteem and have difficulties dealing with individuals in their environment. Clients should be given opportunities to maintain self-care needs. At an optimal level of functioning with assistance, this client is at risk for potential self-care deficits, impaired skin integrity, and altered health maintenance. During hygiene you interact with the client to assess the client's readiness to learn and to teach health promotion practices. Preserve as much of the client's independence as possible, ensure privacy, and foster physical well-being.

SCIENTIFIC KNOWLEDGE BASE

Good physical hygiene is necessary for comfort, safety, and well-being. People are usually capable of meeting their own hygiene needs; however, when ill, people may require assistance. Several factors influence hygiene practice. First determine a client's ability to perform self-care, and then provide hygiene care according to your client's needs and preferred practices.

The skin and mucosa cells exchange oxygen, nutrients, and fluids with underlying blood vessels. The cells require adequate nutrition, hydration, and circulation to resist injury and disease. The skin often reflects a change in physical condition by alterations in color, thickness, texture, turgor, temperature, and hydration.

Skin

The skin is an active organ. The skin protects, secretes, excretes, regulates temperature, and is a sense organ (Table 26-1). The three primary layers of the skin are the **epidermis, dermis,** and **subcutaneous** tissue. The epidermis shields underlying tissue against water loss and injury and prevents entry of microorganisms. The dermis contains nerve fibers, blood vessels, sebaceous and sweat glands, and hair follicles. Subcutaneous tissue insulates and cushions the skin. Cleanliness of skin is basic for client comfort.

Feet and Nails

The feet and nails often require special attention to prevent infection, odor, and injury. Problems result from abuse or poor care. The feet are important to physical and emotional health. Foot pain can often change a walking gait, causing strain on different muscle groups. Discomfort while standing or walking can lead to physical and emotional stress.

The nails are epithelial tissues that grow from the root of the nail bed, located in the skin at the nail groove. A normal healthy nail is transparent, smooth, and convex, with a pink nail bed and translucent white tip. Disease can cause changes in the shape, thickness, and curvature of the nail (see Chapter 12).

Oral Cavity and Teeth

The oral cavity is lined with mucous membranes continuous with the skin. The oral or **buccal cavity** consists of the lips surrounding the opening of the mouth, the cheeks running along the side walls of the cavity, the tongue and its muscles, and the hard and soft palate. The oral mucosa is normally light pink and moist.

Hair

Hair growth, distribution, and pattern can indicate general health status (see Chapter 12). Hormonal changes, emotional and physical stress, aging, infection, and certain illnesses can affect hair characteristics. The hair shaft is an inert structure. Changes in its color or condition are caused by hormonal and nutrient deficiencies to the hair follicle.

Care of the Eyes, Ears, and Nose

When you provide hygiene, the client's eyes, ears, and nose also require careful attention. Chapter 39 describes the structure and function of these organs. Cleansing of these sensitive sensory tissues should be done in a way that prevents injury and discomfort to the client. For example, when washing your client's face you are going to be careful not to get soap into the eyes. In addition, the time you spend with your client during hygiene provides an excellent opportunity to ask if there has been any changes in vision, hearing, or sense of smell.

NURSING KNOWLEDGE BASE

Personal preferences for hygiene can be influenced by a number of factors. No two individuals perform hygiene in

Functions of the Skin and Implications for Care		Table 26-1
Function/Description	Implications for Care	

Protection

Epidermis is the relatively impermeable skin layer that prevents entrance of microorganisms. Although microorganisms reside on skin surface and in hair follicles, relative dryness of surface inhibits bacterial growth. Sebum removes bacteria from hair follicles. Acidic pH of skin further slows bacterial growth.

Weakening of epidermis occurs by scraping or stripping its surface as by use of dry razors, tape removal, or improper turning or positioning techniques. Excessive dryness causes cracks and breaks in skin and mucosa that allow bacteria to enter. Emollients soften and prevent moisture loss, soaking improves moisture retention, and hydration of mucosa prevents dryness. However, constant exposure to moisture causes maceration or softening, which interrupts dermal integrity and promotes ulcers and bacterial growth. Keep bed linen and clothing dry. Misuse of soap, detergents, cosmetics, deodorant, and depilatories can cause chemical irritation. Alkaline soaps neutralize protective acid condition of skin. Cleansing removes excess oil, sweat, dead skin cells, and dirt that can promote bacterial growth.

Sensation

Skin contains sensory organs for touch, pain, heat, cold, and pressure.

Minimize friction to avoid loss of stratum corneum, which can increase risk of pressure ulcers. Smoothing linen removes sources of mechanical irritation. Remove rings during bathing to prevent injuring client's skin. Bath water should not be too hot or cold.

Temperature Regulation

Body temperature is controlled by radiation, evaporation, conduction, and convection.

Factors that interfere with heat loss can alter temperature control.
Wet bed linen or gowns increase heat loss.
Excess blankets or bed coverings can interfere with heat loss through radiation and conduction. Coverings can conserve heat.

Excretion and Secretion

Sweat promotes heat loss by evaporation.
Sebum lubricates skin and hair.

Perspiration and oil can harbor microorganism growth. Bathing removes excess body secretions, although excessive bathing can cause dry skin.

the same way, and you provide individualized care only after knowing about the client's unique practices.

Hygiene care is never routine. Because hygiene care often requires intimate contact with the client, use communication skills to promote the therapeutic relationship and to learn about a client's emotional needs. Also use this time to convey caring and respect.

During hygiene care you can also assess your client's readiness to learn about health promotion practices. As you bathe your client, consider the clients' specific physical limitations, beliefs, values, and habits. Individual hygiene preferences do not significantly affect health and can usually be included in the plan of care. Preserve as much of the client's independence as possible, ensure privacy, and foster physical well-being.

Body Image

A client's general appearance may reflect the importance hygiene holds for that person. Body image is a subjective concept of a person's physical appearance. Body image can change frequently and can affect the way in which personal hygiene is maintained. The client's body image may change as the result of surgery, illness, or a change in functional status. Because of these factors you must make an extra effort to promote hygiene.

Social Practices

Social groups also influence hygiene preferences and practices. During childhood, hygiene is influenced by family customs. As children enter adolescence, dating and peer groups influence hygiene practices. Later in life, friends and work groups shape the expectations people have about their personal appearance.

Socioeconomic Status

Economic resources influence the type and extent of hygiene practices used. You should determine whether clients can afford supplies such as deodorant, shampoo, toothpaste, and so on. In the home there may be a need to modify the home environment with safety devices, such as safety bars, nonskid surfaces in the bath, or the addition of a tub chair in order for a client to perform hygienic self-care.

Cultural Variables

A client's cultural beliefs and personal values influence hygiene care. People from diverse cultural backgrounds follow different self-care practices (see Chapter 16). In North America it is common to bathe or shower daily, whereas in some other cultures it is customary to completely bathe only once a week.

Personal Preferences

Each client has individual desires and preferences about when to bathe, shave, and perform hair care. Clients select different products according to personal preferences and needs. These desires should assist you in delivering individualized care for the client. In addition, you should assist the client in developing new hygiene practices or adapting existing ones when indicated by an illness or condition.

Knowledge

Knowledge about the importance of hygiene and its implications for well-being influences hygiene practices. However, knowledge alone is not enough. The client also must be motivated and recognize the benefit to maintain self-care. Often learning about an illness or condition and its influence on the individual encourages the client to improve hygiene. For example, the client with diabetes is aware of the effect of the illness on circulation and the long-term potential for injury. As a result the client is motivated to learn about proper foot hygiene and nail care.

Physical Condition

People with certain illnesses, trauma, or those who have undergone surgery may lack the physical energy and dexterity to perform hygienic care. A client whose arm is in a cast or traction requires assistance with hygiene. Chronic illnesses, such as cardiac disease, cancer, or neurological disorders, may exhaust or incapacitate the client and require you to perform total hygiene.

CRITICAL THINKING

Synthesis

You must synthesize knowledge, draw from experience, use critical thinking attitudes and standards and be knowledgeable about standards of practice. Use practical experience and knowledge from scientific and nursing domains to provide individualized nursing care for clients requiring assistance with hygiene. The client's hygiene needs and practices may differ from your own; therefore you must accept and respect these differences.

KNOWLEDGE. It is important that you understand the implications of proper hygiene for the client's total health status. Proper hygiene promotes skin integrity, a sense of well-being, and improved body image. Knowledge about hygiene practices, which may include cultural, developmental, and pathophysiological factors, provides a scientific basis for identifying and meeting clients' hygiene needs. For example, the diabetic client has specialized needs for nail and foot care. The pathophysiology of diabetes and the impact of the illness on the client's circulation provide you with the scientific knowledge base needed to implement proper foot care practices.

Use knowledge from basic sciences to determine how changes in mobility, aging, exposure to the environment, and disease affect the skin. To effectively identify the hygiene needs of individual clients, use specific knowledge and communication techniques and knowledge of cultural influence with regard to hygiene. These principles assist you in establishing a trusting relationship and basic understanding of the principles of self-concept in identifying and meeting your client's hygiene needs.

Also apply knowledge of physical assessment skills (see Chapter 12) when providing hygiene. A thorough examination of the skin, oral cavity, and peripheral circulation will provide a database to identify hygiene problems and monitor a client's progress over time.

EXPERIENCE. You have your own experiences in meeting specific hygiene needs. In addition, you may have assisted family members with their hygiene. Usually an early clinical experience involves providing hygiene to a client. As your experience increases, your comfort and expertise in meeting the individualized hygiene needs of your clients increase as well.

ATTITUDES. There are multiple critical thinking attitudes that apply to hygiene care. For example, you use creativity to collaborate with the client to determine the best way to meet hygiene needs. You are nonjudgmental and confident when providing care. Because clients' individual physical strength and hygiene practices may differ, it is important that you establish flexibility in the client's schedule to identify needs for periods of rest to lessen the chance of exhaustion during hygiene.

STANDARDS. The use of critical thinking standards ensures that assessment of hygiene needs is comprehensive and accurate. Standards of care are also applied as you advocate for the client. During hygiene care you promote your client's independence while maintaining safety. You must also be mindful of the client's limitations. These concerns for the client establish and maintain self-concept, independence, and mutual respect through advocacy.

NURSING PROCESS

Assessment

Nursing assessment is an ongoing process. You do not assess all body regions before providing hygiene; however, you do routinely observe the client whenever care is given. You must also determine whether the client can tolerate hygiene procedures, which can often be exhausting.

Most assessment occurs while you care for the client's hygiene needs. For example, during oral care the condition of the teeth and mucosa can be observed. Hygiene care allows you to assess for a variety of health care problems and thus helps to set health care priorities (Table 26-2).

ASSESSMENT OF THE SKIN. While assisting a client with personal hygiene, thoroughly assess all external body surfaces. Using inspection and palpation (see Chapter 12), look for alterations, determine the need for hygiene, and note skin changes in response to therapies. Be sure to inspect anterior and posterior surfaces of all body structures.

Observe the skin's color, texture, thickness, turgor, temperature, and hydration, giving special attention to the characteristics most influenced by hygiene measures. Is the skin dry from too much bathing? Are there calluses of the feet that may benefit from soaking?

Example of a Focused Client Assessment
Table 26-2

Factors to Assess	Questions and Approaches	Physical Assessment Strategies
Skin care	Ask client about hygiene practices, frequency, use of soaps, lotions. Ask if client needs assistance to perform hygiene.	Observe client during hygiene activities. Inspect condition of skin and bony prominences.
Mouth	Ask if client has difficulty chewing, change in appetite. Ask if client has dentures. Ask if client has any mouth sores.	Inspect condition of teeth, gums, and mouth. Observe client during mouth care or eating to determine presence of oral pain or discomfort that could impair hygiene practices. Observe fit of dentures. Inspect gums for sores or pressure areas.
Feet	Determine if client is at risk for foot problems (e.g., peripheral vascular disease, callus formation). Obtain information about client's usual practices for foot and nail care.	Watch client walk; observe for limping, uneven gait. Inspect feet for pressure areas. Inspect client's shoes for unequal wear. Inspect nail beds for open sores, trauma, proper nail care.

Common Skin Problems
Table 26-3

Problem	Characteristics	Implications	Interventions
Dry skin	Flaky, rough texture on exposed areas such as hands, arms, legs, or face	Skin may become infected if epidermal layer is allowed to crack.	Bathe less frequently. Use superfatted soap (e.g., Dove) for cleansing. Rinse body of all soap well because residue left can cause irritation and breakdown. Add moisture to air through use of humidifier. Increase fluid intake when skin is dry. Use moisturizing lotion to aid healing process; lotion forms protective barrier and helps maintain fluid within skin. Use creams to clean skin that is dry or irritated by soaps and detergents.
Acne	Inflammatory, papulopustular skin eruption, usually involving bacterial breakdown of sebum; appears on face, neck, shoulders, and back	Infected material within pustule can spread if area is squeezed or picked. Permanent scarring can result.	Wash hair and skin each day with hot water and soap to remove oil. Use cosmetics sparingly because oily cosmetics or creams accumulate in pores and tend to make conditions worse. Dietary restrictions may need to be implemented. Foods found to aggravate condition should be eliminated from diet. Use prescribed topical antibiotics for severe acne.
Skin rashes	Skin eruption that may result from overexposure to sun or moisture or from allergic reaction; may be flat or raised, localized or systemic, pruritic or nonpruritic	If skin is continually scratched, inflammation and infection may occur. Rashes can also cause discomfort.	Wash area thoroughly, and apply antiseptic spray or lotion to prevent further itching and aid healing process. Warm soaks may relieve inflammation.
Contact dermatitis	Inflammation of skin characterized by abrupt onset with erythema, pruritus, pain, and appearance of scaly oozing lesions; seen on face, neck, hands, forearms, and genitalia	Dermatitis is often difficult to eliminate because person is usually in continual contact with substance causing skin reaction. Substance may be hard to identify.	Condition usually disappears when exposure to causative agents (e.g., cleansers, soaps) is avoided.
Abrasion	Scraping or rubbing away of epidermis; may result in localized bleeding and later weeping of serous fluid	Infection occurs easily as result of loss of protective skin layer.	Nurses should always be careful not to scratch clients with their jewelry or fingernails. Wash abrasions with mild soap and water. Dressing or bandage could increase risk of infection because of retained moisture.

Certain conditions place clients at risk for impaired skin integrity (see Chapter 34). You must be particularly alert when assessing clients with reduced sensation, vascular insufficiency, and immobility. The development of pressure ulcers is a common complication that extends hospital stays.

While inspecting the skin, note the presence and condition of lesions. Certain common skin problems affect how hygiene is administered (Table 26-3). Special care is also given to assess less obvious surfaces, such as under the female client's breasts or around perineal tissues. When you

Skin Assessment for the Client With Darkly Pigmented Intact Skin   Box 26-2

Assess localized skin color changes
Any of the following may appear:
- Color darker than surrounding skin, purplish, bluish, eggplant
- Taut
- Shiny
- Induration

Assess for edema (nonpitting swelling)
Importance of lighting for skin assessment:
- Use natural or halogen light
- Avoid fluorescent lamps, which can give the skin a bluish tone

Assess skin temperature:
- Initially may feel warmer than surrounding skin
- Subsequently may feel cooler than surrounding skin
- Use the back of your hand and fingers and, if client's condition permits, no gloves when doing this assessment

Data from Bennett MA: Report of the task force on the implications for darkly pigmented intact skin in the prediction and prevention of pressure ulcers, *Adv Wound Care* 8(6):34, 1995.

observe skin problems, explain proper skin care to the client. You may also educate the client about avoiding irritants, which can worsen the skin condition.

DEVELOPMENTAL CHANGES. Age influences the normal condition of the skin and the type of hygiene required. The neonate's skin is relatively immature and thin. The epidermis and dermis are loosely bound together. You must handle the neonate carefully during bathing to avoid friction, which can result in bruising. A break in the skin can easily cause infection.

The toddler's skin layers are more tightly bound together and thus have a greater resistance to infection and skin irritation. However, because the child is more active and does not have regular hygiene habits, caregivers must be attentive.

During adolescence, growth and maturation of the skin are increased. Sebaceous glands become more active, resulting in **acne.** Eccrine and apocrine sweat glands become fully functional during puberty. More frequent bathing and use of antiperspirants become necessary to reduce body odors.

The condition of an adult's skin depends on hygiene practices and exposure to environmental irritants. Normally the skin is elastic, well hydrated, firm, and smooth. With age the skin loses its resiliency and moisture, and sebaceous and sweat glands become less active. This encourages dry, cracked skin. Daily bathing, inadequate fluid and nutrition, and the use of some soap products may cause the skin of an older adult client to become too dry (Box 26-1). The epithelium thins and elastic collagen fibers shrink, making the skin fragile and subject to bruising and breaking. Use caution when turning and repositioning an older adult client.

CULTURAL CONSIDERATIONS. A client's cultural heritage influences hygiene practices. For example, clients may wear certain garments following their bath. When caring for clients from different cultures, you need to be sensitive to the client's normal practices, such as when and how often bathing is per-

formed, the extent of bathing, and the use of personal care practices. Most of these preferences can be incorporated into the client's hygiene.

When caring for clients with dark skin pigmentation, be aware of unique assessment techniques and skin characteristics unique to highly pigmented skin (see Chapter 34). It is important to provide meticulous skin assessment in clients who are at risk for pressure ulcers (see Chapter 34). Understanding of normal skin assessment characteristics in clients with darkly pigmented skin can assist in early identification of impaired skin integrity (Box 26-2).

ASSESSMENT OF SELF-CARE ABILITY. When a client is unable to bathe or perform personal skin care, you need to provide assistance. To determine whether a client requires a bed bath instead of a tub bath or shower, assess your client's balance, activity tolerance, and muscle strength and coordination. The degree of assistance needed by a client during bathing also depends on the client's vision, the ability to sit without support, hand grasp, and range of motion (ROM) of extremities. If your client has some impairment in cognitive function, you may need to consult with therapists and specialists from other disciplines.

ASSESSMENT OF FEET AND NAILS. Foot care can be incorporated into the client's daily hygiene routine. Often people are unaware of foot or nail problems until pain or discomfort occurs. Problems can result from abuse or poor care of the feet and hands, such as nail biting or trimming nail improperly, exposure to harsh chemicals, and wearing poorly fitting shoes. Assess your clients for nail and foot problems by reviewing developmental factors contributing to alterations, determining the client's type of footwear, and assessing hygiene care practices. Inspect the condition of the nails, and look for lesions, dryness, inflammation, or cracking (Table 26-4).

Common Foot and Nail Problems

Table 26-4

Condition	Characteristics	Implications	Interventions
Callus	Thickened portion of epidermis, consisting of mass of horny, keratotic cells; usually flat, painless, and found on undersurface of foot or on palm of hand; caused by local friction or pressure.	Foot calluses may cause discomfort when wearing tight-fitting shoes.	Wear gloves when using tools or objects that may create friction on palms. Wear comfortable shoes. Soak callus in warm water and Epsom salts to soften cell layers (soaking of feet is contraindicated with diabetic clients). Use pumice stone to remove callus after it softens. Be careful not to use stone on noncallused skin. Applications of creams or lotions can reduce re-formation. Use of orthotic devices (e.g., foam insoles, metatarsal pads, various cushioning devices) redistributes weight and pressure away from callus area.
Corns	Keratosis caused by friction and pressure from shoes; mainly on toes, over bony prominence; usually cone shaped, round, and raised; calluses with painful core.	Conical shape compresses underlying dermis, making it thin and tender. Pain is aggravated by tight-fitting shoes. Tissue can become attached to bone if allowed to grow. Client may suffer alteration in gait because of pain.	Surgical removal may be necessary, depending on location and severity of pain and size of corn. Use oval corn pads carefully, because they increase pressure on toes and reduce circulation.
Plantar warts	Fungating lesion that appears on sole of foot; caused by papillomavirus.	Warts may be contagious, are painful, and make walking difficult.	Treatment ordered by physician may include topical applications of acids, electrodesiccation (burning with electric spark), cryotherapy (freezing) with carbon dioxide or liquid nitrogen, or laser therapy (Osterman and Stuck, 1990).
Athlete's foot (tinea pedis)	Fungal infection of foot; scaliness and cracking of skin between toes and on soles of feet; small blisters containing fluid may appear, apparently induced by constricting footwear (e.g., sneakers).	Athlete's foot can spread to other body parts, especially hands. It is contagious and frequently recurs.	Feet should be well ventilated. Drying feet well after bathing and applying powder help prevent infection. Wearing clean socks or stockings reduces incidence. Physician may order application of griseofulvin, miconazole nitrate, or tolnaftate.
Ingrown nails	Toenail or fingernail growing inward into soft tissue around nail; results from improper nail trimming, poor shoe fit, or heredity.	Ingrown nails can cause localized pain when pressure is applied.	Treatment is frequent hot soaks in antiseptic solution and removal of portion of nail that has grown into skin. Instruct client on proper nail trimming techniques. Professional podiatry may be needed.
Ram's horn nails	Unusually long curved nails.	Attempt by nurse to cut nails may damage nail bed and/or cause infection.	Refer client to podiatrist.
Paronychia	Inflammation of tissue surrounding nail after hangnail or other injury; occurs in people who frequently have their hands in water; common in diabetic clients.	Area can become infected.	Treatment is hot compresses or soaks and local application of antibiotic ointments. Paronychia can be prevented by careful manicuring.
Foot odors	Result of excess perspiration promoting microorganism growth. Faulty foot hygiene or improper footwear may also contribute.		Frequent washing, use of foot deodorants and powders, and clean footwear will prevent or reduce this problem.
Nail fungal infection	Results from excess moisture.	Infection requires treatment with a fungicide.	Wear clean, dry footwear (see athlete's foot).

Risk Factors for Hygiene Problems

Table 26-5

Risks	Hygiene Implications
Oral Problems	
Clients who are unable to use upper extremities due to paralysis, weakness, or restriction (e.g., cast or dressing)	Client lacks upper extremity strength or dexterity needed to brush teeth.
Dehydration, inability to take fluids or food by mouth (NPO)	Causes excess drying and fragility of mucosa; increases accumulation of secretions on tongue and gums.
Presence of nasogastric or oxygen tubes; mouth breathers	Causes drying of mucosa.
Chemotherapeutic drugs	Drugs kill rapidly multiplying cells, including normal cells lining oral cavity. Ulcers and inflammation can develop.
Lozenges, cough drops, antacids, and chewable vitamins over-the-counter (OTC)	Medications contain large amounts of sugar. Repeated use increases sugar or acid content in mouth.
Radiation therapy to head and neck	Reduces salivary flow and lowers pH of saliva; can lead to stomatitis and tooth decay (Danielson, 1988).
Oral surgery, trauma to mouth, placement of oral airway	Cause trauma to oral cavity with swelling, ulcerations, inflammation, and bleeding.
Immunosuppression; alters blood clotting	Predisposes to inflammation and bleeding gums.
Diabetes mellitus	Prone to dryness of mouth, gingivitis, periodontal disease, and loss of teeth.
Poorly fitting dentures	Food may be trapped under denture, causing mouth odor.
Skin Problems	
Immobilization	Dependent body parts are exposed to pressure from underlying surfaces. The inability to turn or change position increases risk for pressure ulcers.
Reduced sensation due to stroke, spinal cord injury, diabetes, local nerve damage	Client does not receive normal transmission of nerve impulses when excessive heat or cold, pressure, friction, or chemical irritants are applied to skin.
Limited protein or caloric intake and reduced hydration (e.g., fever, burns, gastrointestinal alterations, poorly fitting dentures)	Limited caloric and protein intake predispose to impaired tissue synthesis. Skin becomes thinner, less elastic, and smoother with a loss of subcutaneous tissue. Poor wound healing may result. Reduced hydration impairs skin turgor.
Excessive secretions or excretions on the skin from perspiration, urine, watery fecal material, and wound drainage	Moisture is a medium for bacterial growth and can cause local skin irritation, softening of epidermal cells, and skin maceration.
Presence of external devices (e.g., casts, restraint, bandage, dressing)	Device can exert pressure or friction against skin's surface.
Vascular insufficiency	Arterial blood supply to tissues is inadequate, or venous return is impaired, causing decreased circulation to extremities. Tissue ischemia and breakdown may occur. Risk for infection is high.
Foot Problems	
Client unable to bend over or has reduced visual acuity	Client is unable to fully visualize entire surface of each foot, impairing ability to adequately assess condition of skin and nails.
Decreased sensation	Client requires education or foot care or needs referral to podiatrist.
Eye Care Problems	
Reduced dexterity and hand coordination	Physical limitations create inability to safely insert or remove contact lenses.

Chronic foot problems are common with older adults, who may often have dry feet because of a decrease in sebaceous gland secretion, dehydration, or poor condition of footwear. Fissures result in severe itching. One of the more common problems in the older adult population is foot pain (Lueckenotte, 2000).

ASSESSMENT OF THE MOUTH. Oral hygiene helps to maintain the healthy state of the mouth, teeth, gums, and lips. Brushing cleans the teeth of food particles, plaque, and bacteria. It also massages the gums and relieves discomfort resulting from unpleasant odors and tastes. Complete oral hygiene enhances well-being and stimulates the appetite. Your responsibilities in oral hygiene are maintenance and prevention. Help clients to maintain good oral hygiene by teaching correct techniques or by performing hygiene for weakened or disabled clients.

A thorough assessment for problems related to oral hygiene should be included in every client's care (Table 26-5). During the assessment you can inform the client about good oral hygiene habits. You may also refer the client to a specialist if common oral problems are found (Box 26-3). Early identification of poor oral hygiene practices and common oral problems can reduce the risk of gum disease and **dental caries** or cavities.

ASSESSMENT OF HAIR. A person's appearance and feeling of well-being often depend on the way the hair looks and feels. Illness or disability may prevent a client from maintaining daily hair care. An immobilized client's hair soon becomes tangled. Dressings may leave sticky blood or antiseptic solutions on the hair. Proper hair care is important to the client's body image. Brushing, combing, and shampooing are basic hygiene measures for all clients.

Before performing hair care, you must assess the condition of the hair and scalp (Table 26-6). Findings will reveal the frequency and extent of care needed. A client's self-care ability can be altered by conditions such as arthritis, fatigue, and the presence of physical encumbrances (e.g., cast or intravenous [IV] access). Assess your client's physical ability to perform hair care. It is also essential to consider a client's personal hair care practices so every effort can be made to maintain the client's preferred appearance (Box 26-4).

CULTURAL PRACTICES. When caring for clients from different cultures, learn as much as possible about and be sensitive to the clients' customs, beliefs, and practices. Ask the client about preferred hair care methods or any cultural restrictions. For example, African-Americans usually have dry hair. Special lanolin conditioners may be used to maintain conditioning.

ASSESSMENT OF EYES, EARS, AND NOSE. Special attention is given to cleansing the eyes, ears, and nose during the client's bath. Care focuses on preventing infection and maintaining normal organ function. Carefully inspect all external eye structures. Normally the conjunctivae are clear and not inflamed. The eyelid margins are in close approxi-

---

Common Oral Problems — Box 26-3

DENTAL CARIES (CAVITIES)
Caries are most common among young people.
Buildup of plaque causes acid destruction of tooth enamel. Initially appears as chalky, white discoloration of the tooth.

PERIODONTAL DISEASE (PYORRHEA)
Periodontal disease is most common after age 35.
It involves destruction of gingiva (gums) and other supporting structures with bleeding gums, inflammation, and receding gum lines.

OTHER PROBLEMS
Stomatitis (inflammation of the mouth)
Glossitis (inflammation of the tongue)
Gingivitis (inflammation of the gums)
Halitosis (bad breath)
Cheilosis (cracked lips)
Oral malignancy (mouth lumps or ulcers)

Hair and Scalp Problems — Table 26-6

Problem	Characteristics	Implications	Interventions
Dandruff	Scaling of the scalp accompanied by itching; in severe cases, dandruff on eyebrows.	Dandruff causes embarrassment; if dandruff enters eyes, conjunctivitis may develop.	Shampoo regularly with medicated shampoo; in severe cases seek physician's advice.
Ticks	Small gray-brown parasites that burrow into skin and suck blood.	Ticks transmit Rocky Mountain spotted fever, Lyme disease, and tularemia.	Do not pull ticks from skin; sucking apparatus remains and may become infected; place drop of oil or ether on tick, or cover it with petrolatum to ease removal.
Pediculosis capitis (head lice)	Tiny grayish white parasitic insects that attach to hair strands; eggs look like oval particles, resemble dandruff; bites or pustules may be observed behind ears and at hairline.	Head lice are difficult to remove and if not treated may spread to furniture and other people.	Use medicated shampoo for eliminating lice; repeat 12 to 24 hours later, then 10 days after; change bed linens, using isolation precautions required by agency.
Pediculosis corporis (body lice)	Tend to cling to clothing so may not be easily seen; body lice suck blood and lay eggs on clothing and furniture.	Client itches constantly; scratches on skin may become infected; hemorrhagic spots may appear on skin where lice are sucking blood.	Client should bathe or shower thoroughly; after skin is dried, apply lotion for eliminating lice; after 12 to 24 hours another bath or shower should be taken; bag infested clothing or linen until laundered.
Pediculosis pubis (crab lice)	Found in pubic hair; crab lice are grayish white with red legs.	Lice may spread through bed linen, clothing, or furniture or sexual contact.	Shave hair off affected areas; cleanse as for body lice; if lice were sexually transmitted, partner must be notified.
Alopecia	Balding patches in periphery of hair line; hair becomes brittle and broken; caused by improper use of hair curlers and picks, tight braiding, hot styling tools, certain diseases.	Patches of uneven hair growth and loss alter client's appearance. Alopecia is very distressing for all clients, especially women. Male pattern baldness is not caused or accelerated by hair care practices.	Stop hair care practices that damage hair (e.g., teasing hair, hair dyes, excessive heat when blow-drying).

mation with the eyeball, and the lashes are turned outward. The lid margins are normally without inflammation, drainage, or lesions. Flaking skin around the eyebrows may indicate dandruff.

Assessment of the external ear structures includes inspecting the auricle, external ear canal, and tympanic membrane. When performing hygiene, you are most concerned with presence of accumulated cerumen or drainage in the ear canal, local inflammation, or pain.

Assessment of Hair Care — Box 26-4

PHYSICAL CHANGES
Assess condition of hair and scalp (see Chapter 12). Consider age-appropriate changes.
Consider racial or ethnic differences.
Determine reasons for change in distribution or loss of hair.
Check oiliness and texture of hair.
Inspect scalp for lesions, inflammation, infection, or parasites.

SELF-CARE ABILITY
Assess client's ability to grasp comb or brush.
Determine client's ability to physically care for hair.
Does client become easily fatigued?

HAIR-CARE PRACTICES
Assess client's preferences in hair styling.
Identify client's preferences for hair care and shaving products.
Assess adequacy of client's hygiene practices.
Determine client's perceptions of own appearance.
Assess client's socioeconomic background.

Case Study SYNTHESIS IN PRACTICE

Before entering Mrs. Foster's room, James reviews and synthesizes knowledge about the impact of chronic illness on body image and independence, reviews principles of communication, and reviews the pathophysiology for pressure ulcers.

When James arrives in Mrs. Foster's room, he finds her in bed facing the wall. Mrs. Foster does not want to talk; in fact, she is having a difficult time trying not to cry. Initially James begins to straighten up the environment, giving Mrs. Foster some private time.

Previous clinical experience has taught James that clients need to have an opportunity to determine how nursing care is implemented. James engages Mrs. Foster into some discussion regarding how she would like her morning care. James learns that Mrs. Foster was incontinent of stool during the night, and although the nurses did provide perineal care, Mrs. Foster still feels "dirty" and would like a shower. The night nurses told her she would have to wait until her routine shower day, which is 2 days away. At this point in time James feels that assisting Mrs. Foster with a shower is his first priority.

James continues to synthesize knowledge and use previous clinical experience to appropriately analyze assessment data and make his nursing diagnoses. He maintains accurate information and incorporates good communication skills, which will ensure meeting standards for quality care.

Inspect the nares for signs of inflammation, discharge, lesions, edema, and deformity. The nasal mucosa is normally pink, clear, and without discharge. For clients with any form of tubing exiting the nose, you should observe for tissue sloughing, localized tenderness, inflammation, and even bleeding.

USE OF SENSORY AIDS.   For clients who wear eyeglasses, contact lenses, artificial eyes, or hearing aids, you must assess the client's knowledge and methods used to care for the aids, as well as any problems caused by them. Have the client describe the typical approach used in routine care. Compare information gathered with what you know is the proper care technique. Any findings may indicate a need for client education.

SELF-CARE ABILITY.   Assess your client's physical ability to perform eye, ear, and nose care and care of any sensory aids. Clients who are unable to grasp small objects, have limited upper extremity mobility, have reduced vision, or are seriously fatigued require assistance.

CLIENTS AT RISK FOR HYGIENE PROBLEMS.   There are clients who present risks that require more attentive and rigorous hygiene care (see Table 26-5). These risks result from side effects of medications, lack of knowledge, an inability to perform hygiene, or a physical condition that potentially injures the skin, integument, or other structure. For example, an immobilized client with a fever requires more frequent bathing, turning, and positioning to reduce the risk for skin breakdown.

Your assessment must include risks for hygiene problems. Timely identification of these risks results in nursing interventions designed to prevent injury to the skin, feet and nails, and oral mucosa.

CLIENT EXPECTATIONS.   With all nursing care it is important to know the client's expectations. Hygiene is a very personal aspect of care, and clients may indeed have varying expectations. When providing skin care, determine the client's preferences for soaps, lotions, showers, or tub bath. How much privacy does the client wish? Is it important to have hygiene completed before family members visit, or does the client wish the family to assist with hygiene practices? The client has certain expectations in all aspects of hygienic care. Whenever possible, try to incorporate the client's routine practices into hygiene care. Sometimes extra time is needed to offer the client a shampoo. However, hygiene may be one aspect of care where flexibility is easier to achieve.

Nursing Diagnosis

Assessment reveals the condition of the skin, hair, nails, eyes, ears, and nose and the client's need for and ability to maintain personal hygiene. Review all data gathered (e.g., the client's risk for physical immobilization, presence of secretions, or altered circulation and sensation). Clustering defining characteristics reveals the nursing diagnoses related to hygiene. Accurate selection of a diagnosis ensures the client's needs are met (Box 26-5). A nursing diagnosis is accurate only if the appropriate related factors are selected because the diagnosis influences the nursing therapies chosen.

For the diagnosis *bathing/hygiene self-care deficit related to decreased mobility,* you must incorporate principles that will increase mobility to enhance self-care and independence.

Frequent turning or repositioning, using a proper support surface, and removing underlying tubing are good measures. In contrast, the diagnosis *impaired skin integrity related to exposure to body excretions* requires you to choose different therapies. Frequent skin cleansing, controlling sources of wound drainage or incontinence, and timely bed linen changes would be good measures to control the irritation of excretions. Selecting an incorrect related factor for a diagnosis can result in inappropriate and ineffective nursing care.

If your client has foot or nail problems, you may identify a diagnosis *impaired skin integrity related to friction of shoes,* which requires you to make recommendations about footwear to reduce any source of friction. You may also recommend more frequent foot care. Effective nursing care and appropriate nursing interventions result from selecting the correct related factors for a nursing diagnosis.

Planning

During planning use critical thinking to ensure that the plan of care is individualized to meet the client's needs according to the nursing diagnoses identified (see care plan).

Nursing Diagnoses for CLIENTS WITH HYGIENE PROBLEMS
Box 26-5

- Dentition, impaired
- Fatigue
- Health maintenance, ineffective
- Infection, risk for
- Knowledge, deficient
- Mobility, impaired physical
- Oral mucous membrane, impaired
- Powerlessness
- Self-care deficit, bathing/hygiene
- Self-care deficit, dressing/grooming
- Self-esteem disturbance, situational low
- Skin integrity, impaired
- Skin integrity, risk for impaired
- Tissue integrity, impaired
- Tissue perfusion, ineffective peripheral

Case Study Nursing Care Plan 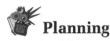 SKIN CARE

ASSESSMENT

Mrs. Foster is very concerned about her physical appearance. She wants to "look her best." She is **in a wheelchair** and **does not have the coordination or muscle strength to independently transfer or stand.** Her skin is intact, but there is **prolonged erythema over ischial pressure areas bilaterally.** Her **skin is dry, her fingernails and toenails are very brittle,** and **she is frequently incontinent of stool and urine.**

*Defining characteristics are shown in bold type.

NURSING DIAGNOSIS

Risk for impaired skin integrity related to impaired mobility and incontinence.

PLANNING

GOAL	EXPECTED OUTCOMES
Client's skin remains intact.	Client's skin is without increased erythema.
	Client's skin remains dry.
	Client's skin is odor free.
	Client feels clean and dry.

IMPLEMENTATION

STEPS	RATIONALE
1. Provide perineal care after each diarrheal episode.	Minimizing skin exposure to moisture decreases irritation and susceptibility to injury (PPPUA, 1993).
2. Change linen after diaphoresis or diarrheal episode.	Changing soiled linen keeps skin free of moisture, which promotes bacterial growth (NPUAP, 1989).
3. Apply lotion to areas that can easily become dried and chapped.	Lotion reduces drying and chapping of skin. Dry, chapped skin impairs skin integrity and is port of entry for bacteria.
4. Monitor length of time any area of redness persists. Determine turning and positioning interval. Turning interval − hypoxia time = suggest interval (e.g., 2 hours − 30 minutes = $1\frac{1}{2}$ hours).	Repositioning reduces pressure and allows for normal hyperemic response (Bennett, 1995).
5. Do **not** massage reddened area.	Massage increases breaks in capillaries in underlying tissues, causing skin breakdown (Maklebust, 1991; USDHHS, 1994).

EVALUATION

- Observe skin for pressure and moisture after each position change, according to turning interval, every $1\frac{1}{2}$ hours.
- Inspect skin for breakdown.
- Ask client how her skin feels after skin care.

In planning care it is important that you identify client goals and outcomes, set priorities for care, and plan for continuity of care.

GOALS AND OUTCOMES.   After you identify and individualize nursing diagnoses, you and the client set goals and expected outcomes to direct nursing interventions. The plan for providing hygienic care should focus on maintaining or improving the condition of the skin and mucosa. Many of your interventions will be performed when the client bathes. You can also set goals for improving client knowledge, providing emotional support, and assisting with ROM exercises.

Considering a client's hygiene preferences before planning is important. The type of hygiene the client desires or requires will determine the supplies and equipment you must prepare. The client's normal lifestyle before admission and hygiene preferences will be incorporated into the care plan.

SETTING PRIORITIES.   The client's condition influences your priorities for delivering hygiene. For example, a seriously ill client usually needs a daily bath because body secretions accumulate, and the client is unable to maintain cleanliness. An older adult client who is awaiting discharge may only need to complete a partial bath before leaving the hospital. Set priorities based on the necessary assistance required by clients who are weakened or have poor muscle strength.

Timing is also important in planning hygiene care. Being interrupted in the middle of the bath for an x-ray procedure can frustrate and embarrass the client. Following extensive diagnostic tests (e.g., stress test), rest may be an important client priority. It may be best to delay hygiene and allow the client to rest.

CONTINUITY OF CARE.   It is important to plan for care throughout the client's hospital visit, discharge to a rehabilitation facility, and home in order to achieve a restored level of wellness. It may be necessary for you to assist the family in developing a plan for providing hygiene care in which the client gradually takes over some self-care responsibility. Be mindful of the equipment and procedures used in the agency so that the client and family are knowledgeable about the care, have the skill needed to provide the care, and have access to necessary equipment. You may also need to collaborate with other health care providers such as physical or occupational therapists. Various community resources may be needed as well.

Implementation

HEALTH PROMOTION, ACUTE CARE, AND RESTORATIVE AND CONTINUING CARE.   The nursing knowledge and skills needed for performing hygiene care are used consistently in all health care settings where health promotion, acute care, and restorative and continuing care are provided.

BATHING AND SKIN CARE.   Instruct clients to follow a few general rules to promote skin health and restore optimal function. Clients should bathe daily unless contraindicated. In hospital settings this is usually done in the morning when more staff are available. Clients should use lotions to moisturize dry skin and bathe in a warm environment, avoiding cold drafts. Clients should routinely inspect their skin for any changes in skin color and texture, and report abnormalities to their primary care provider. The client should handle the skin gently, avoiding excessive rubbing. Finally, clients should be encouraged to eat nutritious foods rich in vitamins and minerals.

Bathing may be done for cleanliness or for a specific therapy, depending on the type of bath. The extent of the bath and the methods used for bathing depend on the client's physical abilities, health problems, and the degree of hygiene required. A **complete bed bath** is for clients who are dependent and require total hygienic care (Skill 26-1).

A **partial bed bath** involves bathing only body parts that would cause discomfort or odor if left unbathed. Aging or dependent clients in need of only partial hygiene or self-sufficient bedridden clients unable to reach all body parts receive partial bed baths.

The tub bath or shower can be used to give a more thorough bath than a bed bath. Washing and rinsing all body parts are easier. Safety is of primary concern because the surface of a tub or shower stall is slippery. Clients vary in how much help they will need. Regardless of the type of bath the client receives, use the following guidelines:

1. Provide privacy. Close the door, or pull room curtains around the bathing area. While bathing the client, expose only the areas being bathed.
2. Maintain safety. When side rails are appropriate to the client's condition, keep them raised while away from the client's bedside. (This is particularly important for dependent or unconscious clients.) Remember clients cannot be restrained from getting out of bed by raising side rails unless there is a physician's order (see Chapter 25). Place the call light in the client's reach if leaving the room.
3. Maintain warmth. The room should be kept warm because the client is partially uncovered and may easily be chilled. Control drafts, and keep windows closed. Keep the client covered by exposing only the body part being washed during the bath.
4. Promote the client's independence as much as possible during bathing activities. Offer assistance as needed.
5. Anticipate needs. Bring a new set of clothing and hygiene products to the bedside or bathroom.

PERINEAL CARE.   **Perineal care** is usually part of the complete bed bath (Skill 26-2). Clients most in need of perineal care are those with perineal secretions (e.g., clients who have indwelling urinary catheters or who are recovering from rectal or genital surgery or childbirth). Excretions allowed to accumulate along the urinary meatus or a suture line can lead to infection. A client able to perform self-care should be allowed to do so. Many nurses are embarrassed about providing perineal care, particularly to clients of the opposite sex. This should not cause you to overlook the client's hygiene needs. A professional, dignified attitude can reduce embarrassment and put the client and you at ease.

Text continued on p. 622

Skill 26-1
BATHING A CLIENT

DELEGATION CONSIDERATIONS

Skills of bathing can be delegated to assistive personnel. It is important to provide caregivers information about the importance of not massaging reddened skin areas, early signs of impaired skin integrity, and when to report changes in the skin to the nurse.

EQUIPMENT

- Two washcloths
- Two bath towels
- Bath blanket
- Soap and soap dish
- Toiletry items (deodorant, powder, lotion, cologne)
- Warm water
- Clean hospital gown or client's own pajamas or gown
- Laundry bag
- Disposable gloves (when risk for contacting body fluids)
- Washbasin

STEPS	RATIONALE
1. Assess client's tolerance for activity, discomfort level, cognitive ability, musculoskeletal function, and the presence of equipment (e.g., intravenous [IV] or oxygen tubing) that may interfere with bathing-hygiene.	Determines client's ability to perform bathing and level of assistance required from you. Also determines type of bath to administer (e.g., tub bath, partial bed bath).

• **Critical Decision Point**

Clients whose levels of independence and mobility change frequently may require more or less assistance during bathing.

STEPS	RATIONALE
2. Assess client's bathing preferences: frequency of and time of day bathing preferred, type of hygiene products used, and other factors related to cultural diversity.	Client participates in plan of care. Promotes client's comfort and willingness to cooperate.
3. Ask if client has noticed any problems related to condition of skin.	Provides you with information to direct physical assessment of skin during bathing.
4. Check physician's therapeutic bath order for type of solution, length of time for bath, body part to be attended.	Therapeutic baths are ordered for specific physical effect, which may include promotion of healing or soothing effect.
5. Review orders for specific precautions concerning client's movement or positioning.	Prevents accidental injury to client during bathing activities. Determines level of assistance required by client.
6. Explain procedure and ask client for suggestions on how to prepare supplies. If partial bath, ask how much of bath client wishes to complete.	Promotes client's cooperation and participation.
7. Adjust room temperature and ventilation, close room doors and windows, and draw room divider curtain.	Warm room that is free of drafts prevents rapid loss of body heat during bathing. Privacy ensures client's mental and physical comfort.
8. Prepare equipment and supplies.	Avoids interrupting procedure or leaving client unattended to retrieve missing equipment.
9. Complete or partial bed bath	
(1) Offer client bedpan or urinal. Provide towel and washcloth.	Client will feel more comfortable after voiding. Prevents interruption of bath.
(2) Wash hands.	Reduces transmission of microorganisms.

• **Critical Decision Point**

Apply gloves if there is an actual or a risk for drainage or secretions on client's skin.

STEPS	RATIONALE
(3) Lower side rail closest to you, and assist client in assuming comfortable supine position, maintaining body alignment. Bring client toward side closest to you. Place hospital bed in high position.	Aids your access to client. Maintains client's comfort throughout procedure. You do not have to reach across bed, thus minimizing strain on back muscles.
(4) Loosen top covers at foot of bed. Place bath blanket over top sheet. Fold and remove top sheet from under blanket. If possible, have client hold bath blanket while withdrawing sheet.	Removal of top linens prevents them from becoming soiled or moist during bath. Blanket provides warmth and privacy.

STEPS	RATIONALE
(5) If top sheet is to be reused, fold it for replacement later. If not, dispose in laundry bag, taking care not to allow linen to contact uniform.	Proper disposal prevents transmission of microorganisms.
(6) Remove client's gown or pajamas. If an extremity is injured or has reduced mobility, begin removal from *unaffected* side. If client has IV access, remove gown from arm *without* IV first. Then remove gown from arm with IV. Remove IV from pole, and slide IV tubing and bag through the arm of client's gown. Rehang IV container and check flow rate (see illustration).	Provides full exposure of body parts during bathing. Undressing unaffected side first allows easier manipulation of gown over body part with reduced range of motion (ROM).
(7) Pull side rail up. Fill washbasin two-thirds full with warm water. Check water temperature, and also have client place fingers in water to test temperature tolerance. Place plastic container of bath lotion in bathwater to warm if desired.	Raising side rail maintains client's safety while you leave bedside. Warm water promotes comfort, relaxes muscles, and prevents unnecessary chilling. Testing temperature prevents accidental burns. Bathwater warms lotion for application to client's skin.
(8) Lower side rail, remove pillow, and raise head of bed 30 to 45 degrees if allowed. Place bath towel under client's head. Place second bath towel over client's chest.	Removal of pillow makes it easier to wash client's ears and neck. Placement of towels prevents soiling of bed linen and bath blanket.

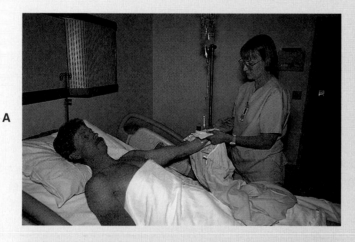
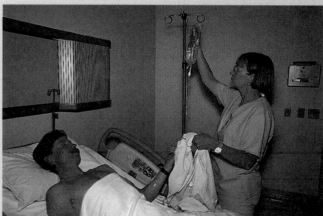
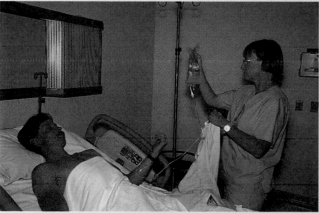
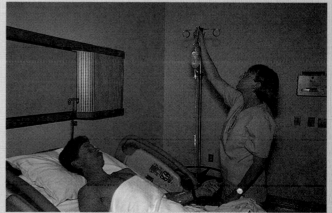

STEP 8A(6) **A,** Remove client's gown. **B,** Remove IV from pole. **C,** Slide IV tubing and bag through arm of client's gown. **D,** Rehang IV bag.

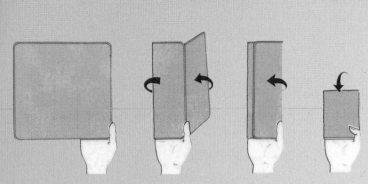

STEP 8A(9)   Steps for folding washcloth to form a mitt.

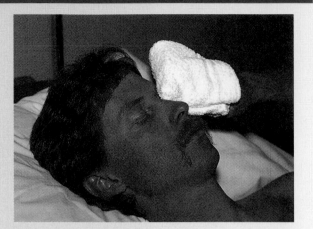

STEP 8A(10)   Wash eye from inner to outer canthus.

STEPS	RATIONALE
(9) Fold washcloth around fingers of your hand to form a mitt (see illustration). Immerse mitt in water and wring thoroughly.	Mitt retains water and heat better than loosely held washcloth; keeps cold edges from brushing against client, and prevents splashing.
(10) Inquire if client is wearing contact lenses. Wash client's eyes with plain warm water. Use different section of mitt for each eye. Move mitt from inner to outer canthus (see illustration). Soak any crusts on eyelid for 2 to 3 minutes with damp cloth before attempting removal. Dry eye thoroughly but gently.	Soap irritates eyes. Use of separate sections of mitt reduces infection transmission. Bathing eye from inner to outer canthus prevents secretions from entering nasolacrimal duct. Pressure can cause internal injury.
(11) Ask if client prefers to use soap on face. Wash, rinse, and dry well forehead, cheeks, nose, neck, and ears. (Men may wish to shave at this point or after bath.)	Soap tends to dry face, which is exposed to air more than other body parts.
(12) Remove bath blanket from client's arm closest to you. Place bath towel lengthwise under arm.	Prevents soiling of linen.
(13) Bathe arm with soap and water using long, firm strokes from distal to proximal areas (fingers to axilla). Raise and support arm above head (if possible) while thoroughly washing axilla.	Soap lowers surface tension and facilitates removal of debris and bacteria when friction is applied during washing. Long, firm strokes stimulate circulation. Movement of arm exposes axilla and exercises joint's normal ROM.
(14) Rinse and dry arm and axilla thoroughly. If client uses deodorant, apply it.	Alkaline residue from soap discourages growth of normal skin bacteria. Excess moisture causes skin maceration, or softening. Deodorant controls body odor.
(15) Fold bath towel in half and lay it on bed beside client. Place basin on towel. Immerse client's hand in water. Allow hand to soak for 3 to 5 minutes before washing hand and fingernails (see Skill 26-3, p. 623). Remove basin and dry hand well.	Soaking softens cuticles and calluses of hand, loosens debris beneath nails, and enhances feeling of cleanliness. Thorough drying removes moisture from between fingers.
(16) Raise side rail and move to other side of bed. Lower side rail and repeat Steps 12 through 15 for other arm.	
(17) Check temperature of bathwater, and change water if necessary.	Warm water maintains client's comfort.

STEPS	RATIONALE

- *Critical Decision Point*

If client is at risk for falling, be sure two side rails are up before obtaining fresh water. Remember, side rails cannot be used as a restraint.

(18) Cover client's chest with bath towel and fold bath blanket down to umbilicus. With one hand, lift edge of towel away from chest. With mitted hand, bathe chest using long, firm strokes. Take special care to wash skinfolds under female client's breasts. It may be necessary to lift breast upward while bathing underneath it. Keep client's chest covered between wash and rinse periods. Dry well.	Draping prevents unnecessary exposure of body parts. Towel maintains warmth and privacy. Secretions and dirt collect easily in areas of tight skinfolds. Skinfolds are susceptible to excoriation if breasts are pendulous.
(19) Place bath towel lengthwise over chest and abdomen. (Two towels may be needed.) Fold blanket down to just above pubic region.	Prevents chilling and exposure of body parts.
(20) With one hand, lift bath towel. With mitted hand, bathe abdomen, giving special attention to bathing umbilicus and abdominal folds. Stroke from side to side. Keep abdomen covered between washing and rinsing. Dry well.	Moisture and sediment that collect in skinfolds predispose skin to **maceration** and irritation.
(21) Apply clean gown or pajama top.	Maintains client's warmth and comfort.

- *Critical Decision Point*

*If one extremity is injured or immobilized, always dress affected side first for easier manipulation of gown over body.**

(22) Cover chest and abdomen with top of bath blanket. Expose near leg by folding blanket toward midline. Be sure perineum is draped.	Prevents unnecessary exposure.
(23) Bend client's leg at knee by positioning nurse's arm under leg. While grasping client's heel, elevate leg from mattress slightly and slide bath towel lengthwise under leg. Ask client to hold foot still. Place bath basin on towel on bed and secure its position next to foot to be washed.	Towel prevents soiling of bed linen. Support of joint and extremity during lifting prevents strain on musculoskeletal structures. Sudden movement by client could spill bath water. (Omit this step if client is unable to hold leg in basin.)
(24) With one hand supporting lower leg, raise it and slide basin under lifted foot. Make sure foot is firmly placed on bottom of basin. Allow foot to soak while washing leg. If client is unable to hold leg, do not immerse; simply wash with washcloth (see illustration).	Proper positioning of foot prevents pressure being applied from edge of basin against calf. Soaking softens calluses and rough skin.

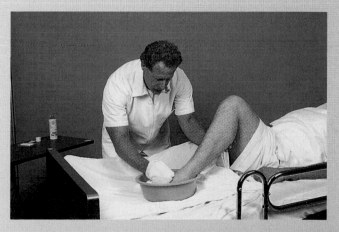

STEP 24

*This step may be omitted until completion of bath; gown should not become soiled during remainder of bath.

STEPS	RATIONALE
(25) Unless contraindicated, use long, firm strokes in washing from ankle to knee and from knee to thigh. Dry well.	Promotes venous return.

• *Critical Decision Point*
Clients with history of deep vein thromboses or blood-clotting disorders should not have their lower extremities washed with long, firm strokes. Use short, light strokes.

STEPS	RATIONALE
(26) Cleanse foot, making sure to bathe between toes. Clean and clip nails as needed (see Skill 26-3, p. 623). Dry well. If skin is dry, apply lotion.	Secretions and moisture may be present between toes. Lotion helps retain moisture and soften skin.

• *Critical Decision Point*
Do not massage any reddened area on client's skin.

STEPS	RATIONALE
(27) Raise side rail and move to other side of the bed. Lower side rail and repeat Steps 22 through 26 for other leg and foot.	
(28) Cover client with bath blanket, raise side rail for client's safety, and change bathwater.	Decreased bathwater temperature can cause chilling. Clean water reduces microorganism transmission.
(29) Lower side rail. Assist client in assuming prone or side-lying position (as applicable). Place towel lengthwise along client's side.	Exposes back and buttocks for bathing.
(30) Keep client draped by sliding both blanket over shoulders and thighs. Wash, rinse, and dry back from neck to buttocks using long, firm strokes. Pay special attention to folds of buttocks and anus. Give a back rub, and change the bathwater.	Maintains warmth and prevents unnecessary exposure. Skinfolds near buttocks and anus may contain fecal secretions that harbor microorganisms. Clean water reduces microorganism transmission.
(31) Apply disposable gloves if not done previously.	Prevents contact with microorganisms in body secretions.
(32) Assist client in assuming side-lying or supine position. Cover chest and upper extremities with towel and lower extremities with bath blanket. Expose only genitalia. (If client can wash, covering entire body with bath blanket may be preferable.) Wash, rinse, and dry perineum (see Skill 26-2, p. 619). Pay special attention to skinfolds. Apply water-repellent ointment to area exposed to moisture.	Maintains client's privacy. Clients capable of performing partial bath usually prefer to wash their own genitalia. Water-repellant ointments (e.g., A and D, Pericare) protect skin from moisture.
(33) Dispose of gloves in receptacle.	Prevents transmission of infection.
(34) Apply additional body lotion or oil as desired.	Moisturizing lotion prevents dry, chapped skin.
(35) Assist client in dressing. Comb client's hair. Women may want to apply makeup.	Promotes client's body image.
(36) Make client's bed (see Skill 26-6, p. 639, and Procedural Guidelines Box 26-10, p. 638).	Provides clean environment.
(37) Remove soiled linen and place in dirty-linen bag. Clean and replace bathing equipment. Replace call light and personal possessions. Leave room as clean and comfortable as possible.	Prevents transmission of infection. Clean environment promotes client's comfort. Keeping call light and articles of care within reach promotes client's safety.
(38) Wash hands.	Reduces transmission of microorganisms.

STEPS	RATIONALE
10. Tub bath or shower	
(1) Consider client's condition, and review orders for precautions concerning client's movement or positioning.	Prevents accidental injury to client during bathing.
(2) Schedule use of shower or tub.	Prevents unnecessary waiting that can cause fatigue.
(3) Check tub or shower for cleanliness. Use cleaning techniques outlined in agency policy. Place rubber mat on tub or shower bottom. Place disposable bath mat or towel on floor in front of tub or shower.	Cleaning prevents transmission of microorganisms. Mats prevent slipping and falling.
(4) Collect all hygienic aids, toiletry items, and linens requested by client. Place within easy reach of tub or shower.	Placing items close at hand prevents possible falls when client reaches for equipment.
(5) Assist client to bathroom if necessary. Have client wear robe and slippers to bathroom.	Assistance prevents accidental falls. Wearing robe and slippers prevents chilling.
(6) Demonstrate how to use call signal for assistance.	Bathrooms are equipped with signaling devices in case client feels faint or weak or needs immediate assistance. Clients prefer privacy during bath if safety is not jeopardized.
(7) Place "occupied" sign on bathroom door.	Maintains client's privacy.
(8) Fill bathtub halfway with warm water. Check temperature of bath water, then have client test water, and adjust temperature if water is too warm. Explain which faucet controls hot water. If client is taking shower, turn shower on and adjust water temperature before client enters shower stall. Use shower seat or tub chair and provide if needed (see illustration).	Adjusting water temperature prevents accidental burns. Older adults and clients with neurological alterations (e.g., spinal cord injury) are at high risk for burn as a result of reduced sensation. Use of assistive devices facilitates bathing and minimizes physical exertion.
(9) Instruct client to use safety bars when getting in and out of tub or shower. Caution client against use of bath oil in tub water.	Prevents slipping and falling. Oil causes tub surfaces to become slippery.
(10) Instruct client not to remain in tub longer than 20 minutes. Check on client every 5 minutes.	Prolonged exposure to warm water may cause vasodilation and pooling of blood, leading to light-headedness or dizziness.

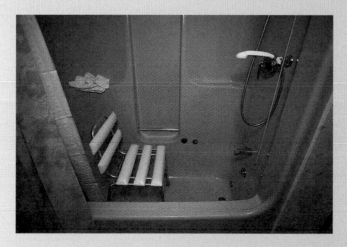

STEP 8B(8)   Shower seat for client safety.

STEPS	RATIONALE
(11) Return to bathroom when client signals, and knock before entering.	Provides privacy.
(12) For client who is unsteady, drain tub of water before client attempts to get out of it. Place bath towel over client's shoulders. Assist client in getting out of tub as needed and assist with drying.	Prevents accidental falls. Client may become chilled as water drains.

• *Critical Decision Point*
Weak or unstable clients need extra assistance in getting out of a tub. Planning for additional personnel is essential before attempting to assist the client from the tub.

STEPS	RATIONALE
(13) Assist client as needed in donning clean gown or pajamas, slippers, and robe. (In home setting client may put on regular clothing.)	Maintains warmth to prevent chilling.
(14) Assist client to room and comfortable position in bed or chair.	Maintains relaxation gained from bathing.
(15) Clean tub or shower according to agency policy. Remove soiled linen and place in dirty-linen bag. Discard disposable equipment in proper receptacle. Place "unoccupied" sign on bathroom door. Return supplies to storage area.	Prevents transmission of infection through soiled linen and moisture.
(16) Wash hands.	
11. Observe skin, paying particular attention to areas that were previously soiled, reddened, or showed early signs of breakdown.	Reduces transfer of microorganisms. Techniques used during bathing should leave skin clean and clear.
12. Observe ROM during bath.	
13. Ask client to rate level of comfort.	Measures joint mobility.

UNEXPECTED OUTCOMES AND RELATED INTERVENTIONS

- Areas of excessive dryness, rashes, or pressure ulcers appear on skin.
  - Review agency skin care policy regarding moisturizing lotions.
  - Limit frequency of complete baths.
  - Complete pressure ulcer assessment (see Chapter 34).
  - Obtain special bed surface if client is at risk for skin breakdown.
- Client becomes excessively fatigued and unable to cooperate or participate in bathing.
  - Reschedule bathing to a time when client is more rested.
  - Clients with breathing difficulties require pillow or elevated head of bed during bath.
  - Notify physician if this is a change in client's fatigue level.

- Client seems unusually restless or complains of discomfort.
  - Schedule client rest periods.
  - Consider analgesia if client complains of pain or discomfort before the bath.

RECORDING AND REPORTING

- Record bath on flow sheet. Note level of assistance required.
- Record condition of skin and any significant findings (e.g., reddened areas, bruises, nevi, or joint or muscle pain).
- Report evidence of alterations in skin integrity to nurse in charge or physician.

Skill 26-2
PROVIDING PERINEAL CARE

DELEGATION CONSIDERATIONS

Skills of perineal care can be delegated to assistive personnel.

- Inform and assist care provider in proper way to position male and female clients.
- Inform care provider about proper positioning of indwelling catheter during perineal care.
- Instruct care provider to inform you if any perineal drainage, excoriation, or rash is observed.

EQUIPMENT

- Washbasin
- Soap dish with soap
- Two or three washcloths
- Bath towel
- Bath blanket
- Waterproof pad or bedpan
- Toilet tissue or diaper wipes
- Disposable gloves

Additional supplies are needed when pericare is given other than during a bath:

- Cotton balls or swabs
- A solution bottle or container filled with warm water or prescribed rinsing solution
- Waterproof bag

STEPS	RATIONALE
1. Identify clients at risk for developing infection of genitalia, urinary tract, or reproductive tract (e.g., presence of indwelling catheter, fecal incontinence).	Secretions that accumulate on surface of skin surrounding female and male genitalia act as reservoir for infection. Tissues traumatized by surgery or by presence of foreign object provide route for introduction of infectious organisms.
2. Assess client's cognitive and musculoskeletal function.	Determines client's ability to perform self-care and determines level of assistance required from you.
3. Apply disposable gloves and assess genitalia for signs of inflammation, skin breakdown, or infection (see Chapter 12). Discard gloves (option: examine genitalia as care is administered).	Determines extent of perineal care required by client.
4. Assess client's knowledge of importance of perineal hygiene.	Clients at risk for infection in perineal area may be unaware of importance of cleanliness. Reflects client's need for education.
5. Explain procedure and its purpose to client.	Helps minimize anxiety during procedure that is often embarrassing to you and client.
6. Prepare necessary equipment and supplies.	Used when administering a bed bath.
7. Pull curtain around client's bed, or close room door. Assemble supplies at bedside.	Maintains client's privacy and ensures orderly procedure.
8. Raise bed to comfortable working position. Lower side rail, and assist client in assuming side-lying position, placing towel lengthwise along client's side and keeping client covered with bath blanket.	Facilitates good body mechanics. Provides easy access to genitalia.
9. Apply disposable gloves.	Eliminates transmission of microorganisms.
10. If fecal material is present, enclose in a fold of underpad or toilet tissue, and remove with disposable wipes. Cleanse buttocks and anus, washing front to back (see illustration). Cleanse, rinse, and dry area thoroughly. If needed, place an absorbent pad under client's buttocks. Remove and discard underpad, and replace with clean one.	Cleansing reduces transmission of microorganisms from anus to urethra or genitalia.

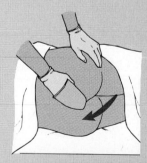

STEP 10   Cleanse buttocks from front to back.

11. Change gloves when they are soiled.

STEPS	RATIONALE
12. Fold top bed linen down toward foot of bed, and raise client's gown above genital area.	Exposes perineal area for easy accessibility.
a. "Diamond" drape female client by placing bath blanket with one corner between client's legs, one corner pointing toward each side of bed, and one corner over client's chest. Tuck side corners around client's legs and under hips. For male client, expose only genital area, using towels or bath blankets to cover client's chest and upper legs.	Prevents unnecessary exposure of body parts and maintains client's warmth and comfort during procedure.
b. Raise side rail. Fill washbasin with warm water.	Prevents client from falling. Proper water temperature prevents burns to perineum.
c. Place washbasin and toilet tissue on over-bed table. Place washcloths in basin.	Equipment placed within nurse's reach prevents accidental spills.
13. Provide perineal care.	
A. Female Perineal Care	
(1) Assist client to dorsal recumbent position.	Provides easy access to genitalia.
(2) Lower side rail, and help client flex knees and spread legs. Note restrictions or limitations in client's positioning.	Provides full exposure of female genitalia. Minimizes degree of abduction in female if position causes pain because of arthritis or reduced joint mobility.
(3) Fold lower corner of bath blanket up between client's legs onto abdomen. Wash and dry client's upper thighs.	Minimizes transmission of microorganisms. Keeping client draped until procedure begins minimizes anxiety. Buildup of perineal secretions can soil surrounding skin surfaces.
(4) Wash labia majora. Use nondominant hand to gently retract labia from thigh; with dominant hand, wash carefully in skinfolds. Wipe in direction from perineum to rectum (front to back). Repeat on opposite side using separate section of washcloth. Rinse and dry area thoroughly.	Skinfolds may contain body secretions that harbor microorganisms. Wiping from perineum to rectum (front to back) reduces chance of transmitting fecal organisms to urinary meatus.
(5) Separate labia with nondominant hand to expose urethral meatus and vaginal orifice. With dominant hand, wash downward from pubic area toward rectum in one smooth stroke (see illustration). Use separate section of cloth for each stroke. Cleanse thoroughly around labia minora, clitoris, and vaginal orifice.	Cleansing method reduces transfer of microorganisms to urinary meatus. (For menstruating women or clients with indwelling urinary catheters, cleanse with cotton balls.)
(6) If client uses bedpan, pour warm water over perineal area. Dry perineal area thoroughly, using front-to-back method.	Rinsing removes soap and microorganisms more effectively than wiping. Retained moisture harbors microorganisms.
(7) Fold lower corner of bath blanket back between client's legs and over perineum. Ask client to lower legs and assume comfortable position.	

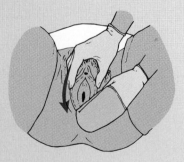

STEP 13A(5)   Cleanse from perineum to rectum (front to back).

STEPS	RATIONALE
B. Male Perineal Care	
(1) Lower side rails, and assist client to supine position. Note restriction in mobility.	Provides full exposure of male genitalia.
(2) Fold lower corner of bath blanket up between client's legs and onto abdomen. Wash and dry client's upper thighs.	Minimizes transmission of microorganisms. Keeping client draped until procedure begins minimizes anxiety. Buildup of perineal secretions can soil surrounding skin surfaces.
(3) Gently raise penis, and place bath towel underneath. Gently grasp shaft of penis. If client is uncircumcised, retract foreskin. If client has an erection, defer procedure until later.	Towel prevents moisture from collecting in inguinal area. Gentle but firm handling reduces chance of client having an erection. Secretions capable of harboring microorganisms collect underneath foreskin.
(4) Wash tip of penis at urethral meatus first. Using circular motion, cleanse from meatus outward (see illustration). Discard washcloth, and repeat with clean cloth until penis is clean. Rinse and dry gently.	Direction of cleansing moves from area of least contamination to area of most contamination, preventing microorganisms from entering urethra.
(5) Return foreskin to its natural position.	Tightening of foreskin around shaft of penis can cause local edema and discomfort.

- **Critical Decision Point**

After administering perineal care, make sure the foreskin is in its natural position. This is extremely important in those clients with decreased sensation in their lower extremities.

(6) Wash shaft of penis with gentle but firm downward strokes. Pay special attention to underlying surface of penis. Rinse and dry penis thoroughly. Instruct client to spread legs apart slightly.	Vigorous massage of penis can lead to erection, which can embarrass client and nurse. Underlying surface of penis may have greater accumulation of secretions. Abduction of legs provides easier access to scrotal tissues.
(7) Gently cleanse scrotum. Lift it carefully, and wash underlying skinfolds. Rinse and dry.	Pressure on scrotal tissues can be painful to client. Secretions collect between skinfolds.
(8) Fold bath blanket back over client's perineum, and assist client in turning to side-lying position.	Draping promotes comfort and minimizes client's anxiety. Side-lying position provides access to anal area.
14. If client has had urinary or bowel incontinence, apply thin layer of skin barrier containing petrolatum or zinc oxide over anal and perineal skin.	Protects skin from excess moisture and toxins from urine or stool (Maklebust, 1991).
15. Remove disposable gloves, and dispose in proper receptacle.	Moisture and body secretions on gloves can harbor microorganisms.
16. Assist client in assuming a comfortable position, and cover with sheet.	Client's comfort helps to minimize stress of procedure.
17. Remove bath blanket, and dispose of all soiled bed linen. Return unused equipment to storage area.	Reduces transmission of microorganisms.
18. Inspect surface of external genitalia and surrounding skin after cleansing.	Thick secretions may cover underlying skin lesions or areas of breakdown. Evaluation determines need for additional hygiene.

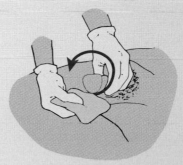

STEP 13B(4)   Use circular motion to cleanse tip of penis.

STEPS	RATIONALE
19. Ask if client feels sense of cleanliness.	Evaluates client's comfort level.
20. Observe for abnormal drainage or discharge from genitalia.	Evaluates presence of infection.

UNEXPECTED OUTCOMES AND RELATED INTERVENTIONS

- Skin and genitalia may be inflamed, with localized tenderness, swelling, and presence of foul-smelling discharge.
  - Bathe area frequently to keep clean and dry.
  - Obtain an order for a sitz bath.
  - Apply protective barrier.
  - Indicates infection or maceration of skin layers. Physician may need to order specific antibaterial, antifungal ointment.
- Client expresses discomfort.
  - Perineal area is not fully cleansed; perform perineal hygiene again.

- Client is unable to describe or perform perineal hygiene.
  - Further instruction is required at a later time.

RECORDING AND REPORTING

- Record procedure and presence of any abnormal findings (e.g., character and amount of discharge, condition of genitalia).
- Record appearance of suture line, if present.
- Report any break in suture line or presence of abnormalities to nurse in charge or physician.

If a client performs self-care, various problems such as vaginal or urethral discharge, skin irritation, and unpleasant odors may go unnoticed. Stress the importance of perineal care in preventing skin breakdown and infection. You must be alert for complaints of burning during urination, localized soreness or excoriation, or perineal pain. Also inspect vaginal and perineal areas and bed linen for signs of discharge.

BACK RUB. A back rub usually follows the bath (see Chapter 29). It promotes relaxation, relieves muscular tension, stimulates skin circulation, and is generally well tolerated by even critically ill clients (Labyak and Metzger, 1997). During the back rub you can assess skin condition.

An effective back rub takes 3 to 5 minutes. You should first ask whether the client would like a back rub because some clients dislike physical contact. You should also consult the client's record for contraindications, such as spinal cord injury, rib fractures, or other painful conditions.

NAIL AND FOOT CARE. For proper foot and nail care, clients should be instructed to protect the feet from injury, keep the feet clean and dry, and wear footwear that fits properly. You can also help the client learn the proper way to inspect the feet for lesions, dryness, or signs of infection. The client, family, or delegated assistive personnel should report any of these conditions to you. Finally, to maintain and promote foot and nail health, clients should visit a podiatrist when necessary.

Foot and nail care involves soaking to soften cuticles and layers of horny cells, through cleansing, drying, and proper nail trimming. You may provide the care in bed for an immobilized client or have the client sit in a chair (Skill 26-3). Take time during the procedure to teach the client proper techniques for cleaning and nail trimming. Measures to prevent infection and promote good circulation should be stressed.

A client with diabetes or peripheral vascular disease is at risk for foot and nail problems because of impaired circulation (Christensen and others, 1991). The American Diabetes Association (ADA) (1999) identifies the following risk conditions associated with an increased risk of amputation: peripheral neuropathy, evidence of increased pressure for callus, erythema, hemorrhage under callus, limited joint mobility, bone deformity, nail pathologic conditions, and peripheral vascular diseases. Although ongoing good foot care can help prevent toe amputation, studies have shown that many clients have not learned proper care. Instruct diabetic clients or clients with peripheral vascular diseases in the following precautions during foot and nail care.

1. Wash the feet daily using lukewarm water; **do not soak.** Thoroughly pat the feet dry, and dry well between the toes.
2. Do not cut corns or calluses or use commercial removers. Consult a physician or podiatrist.
3. If the feet perspire, apply a bland foot powder.
4. If dryness is noted along the feet or between the toes, apply lanolin, baby oil, or even corn oil, and rub gently into the skin.
5. File the toenails straight across and square; do not use scissors or clippers. Consult a podiatrist as needed.
6. Do not use over-the-counter preparations to treat athlete's foot or ingrown toenails. Consult a physician or podiatrist.
7. Avoid wearing elastic stockings, knee-high hose, or constricting garters. Do not cross the legs. Both impair circulation to the lower extremities.
8. Inspect the feet daily, including tops and soles of the feet, heels, and the area between the toes. Use a mirror to inspect all surfaces.
9. Wear clean socks or stockings daily. Socks should be dry and free of holes or darns that might cause pressure.
10. Do not walk barefoot.

Skill 26-3

PERFORMING NAIL AND FOOT CARE

DELEGATION CONSIDERATIONS

The skill of nail and foot care of the nondiabetic client can be delegated to assistive personnel. Inform and assist care provider in proper way to use nail clippers, and caution the care provider to use warm water.

EQUIPMENT

- Washbasin
- Emesis basin
- Washcloth

- Bath or face towel
- Nail clippers
- Orange stick (optional)
- Emery board or nail file
- Body lotion
- Disposable bath mat
- Paper towels
- Disposable gloves

STEPS	RATIONALE
1. Inspect all surfaces of fingers, toes, feet, and nails. Pay particular attention to areas of dryness, inflammation, or cracking. Also inspect areas between toes, heels, and soles of feet.	Integrity of feet and nails determines frequency and level of hygiene required. Heels, soles, and sides of feet are prone to irritation from ill-fitting shoes. Proper footwear is essential in reducing the risk of injury and subsequent ulcer formation (Armstrong and Lavery, 1998).

• **Critical Decision Point**

Clients with peripheral vascular diseases, diabetes mellitus, older adults, and clients whose immune system is suppressed may require nail care from a specialist to reduce the risk for infection.

STEPS	RATIONALE
2. Assess color and temperature of toes, feet, and fingers. Assess capillary refill of nails. Palpate radial and ulnar pulse of each hand and dorsalis pedis pulse of foot; note character of pulses.	Assess adequacy of blood flow to extremities. Circulatory alterations may change integrity of nails and increase client's chance of localized infection when break in skin integrity occurs (Strauss and others, 1998).
3. Observe client's walking gait. Have client walk down hall or walk straight line (if able).	Painful disorders of feet can cause limping or unnatural gait (Armstrong and Lavery, 1998).
4. Ask female clients about whether they use nail polish and polish remover frequently.	Chemicals in these products can cause excessive dryness.
5. Assess type of footwear worn by clients: Are socks worn? Are shoes tight or ill fitting? Are garters or knee-high nylons worn? Is footwear clean?	Types of shoes and footwear may predispose client to foot and nail problems (e.g., infection, areas of friction, ulcerations).
6. Identify client's risk for foot or nail problems:	Certain conditions increase likelihood of foot or nail problems.
a. Older adult	Poor vision, lack of coordination, or inability to bend over contribute to difficulty among older adults in performing foot and nail care. Normal physiological changes of aging also result in nail and foot problems.
b. Diabetes	Vascular changes associated with diabetes reduce blood flow to peripheral tissues. Break in skin integrity places diabetic at high risk for skin infection. Lower-extremity complications of diabetes can involve nerves, muscles, bone, and vasculature, therefore making assessment of and management of foot problems complex (Cooppan and Habershaw, 1995).
c. Heart failure, renal disease	Both conditions can increase tissue edema, particularly in dependent areas (e.g., feet). Edema reduces blood flow to neighboring tissues.
d. Cerebrovascular accident, stroke	Presence of residual foot or leg weakness or paralysis results in altered walking patterns. Altered gait pattern causes increased friction and pressure on feet.
7. Assess type of home remedies clients use for existing foot problems:	Certain preparations or applications may cause more injury to soft tissue then initial foot problem.
a. Over-the-counter liquid preparations to remove corns	Liquid preparations can cause burns and ulcerations.
b. Cutting of corns or calluses with razor blade or scissors	Cutting of corns or calluses may result in infection caused by break in skin integrity.

STEPS	RATIONALE
c. Use of oval corn pads	Oval pads may exert pressure on toes, thereby decreasing circulation to surrounding tissues.
d. Application of adhesive tape	Skin of older adult is thin and delicate and prone to tearing when adhesive tape is removed.
8. Assess client's ability to care for nails or feet: visual alterations, fatigue, musculoskeletal weakness.	Extent of client's ability to perform self-care determines degree of assistance required from you.
9. Assess client's knowledge of foot and nail care practices.	Level of client's knowledge determines client's need for health teaching.
10. Explain procedure to client, including fact that proper soaking requires several minutes.	Client must be willing to place fingers and feet in basins for 10 to 20 minutes. Client may become anxious or fatigued.
11. Obtain physician's order for cutting nails if agency policy requires it.	Client's skin may be accidentally cut. Certain clients are more at risk for infection, depending on their medical condition.
12. Wash hands. Arrange equipment on over-bed table.	Easy access to equipment prevents delays.
13. Pull curtain around bed, or close room door (if desired).	Maintaining client's privacy, reduces anxiety.
14. Assist ambulatory client to sit in bedside chair. Help bed-bound client to supine position with head of bed elevated. Place disposable bath mat on floor under client's feet or place towel on mattress.	Sitting in chair facilitates immersing feet in basin. Bath mat protects feet from exposure to soil or debris.
15. Fill washbasin with warm water. Test water temperature.	Warm water softens nails and thickened epidermal cells, reduces inflammation of skin, and promotes local circulation. Proper water temperature prevents burns.
16. Place basin on bath mat or towel, and help client place feet in basin. Place call light within client's reach.	Clients with muscular weakness or tremors may have difficulty positioning feet. Client's safety is maintained.
17. Adjust over-bed table to low position, and place it over client's lap. (Client may sit in chair or lie in bed.)	Easy access prevents accidental spills.
18. Fill emesis basin with warm water, and place basin on paper towels on over-bed table.	Warm water softens nails and thickened epidermal cells.
19. Instruct client to place fingers in emesis basin and place arms in comfortable position.	Prolonged positioning can cause discomfort unless normal anatomical alignment is maintained.
20. Allow client's feet and fingernails to soak for 10 to 20 minutes. Rewarm after 10 minutes.	Softening of corns, calluses, and cuticles ensures easy removal of dead cells and easy manipulation of cuticle.

• *Critical Decision Point*
Diabetic clients should never soak hands or feet because of increased risk of infection.

21. Clean gently under fingernails with orange stick while fingers are immersed (see illustration). Remove emesis basin and dry fingers thoroughly.	Orange stick removes debris under nails that harbors microorganisms. Thorough drying impedes fungal growth and prevents maceration of tissues.
22. With nail clippers, clip fingernails straight across and even with tops of fingers (see illustration). Shape nails with emery board or file. If client has circulatory problems, do not cut nail; file the nail only.	Cutting straight across prevents splitting of nail margins and formation of sharp nail spikes that can irritate lateral nail margins. Filing prevents cutting nail too close to nail bed (Strauss and others, 1999).

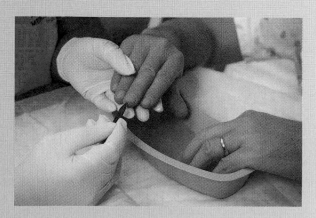

STEP 21   Clean under fingernails with orange stick.

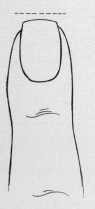

STEP 22   Nails are trimmed straight across.

STEPS	RATIONALE
23. Push cuticle back gently with orange stick.	Reduces incidence of inflamed cuticles.
24. Move over-bed table away from client.	Provides easier access to feet.
25. Put on disposable gloves, and scrub callused areas of feet with washcloth.	Gloves prevent transmission of fungal infection. Friction removes dead skin layers.
26. Clean gently under nails with orange stick. Remove feet from basin, and dry thoroughly.	Removal of debris and excess moisture reduces chances of infection.
27. Clean and trim toenails using procedures in Steps 21 and 22. Do not file corners of toenails.	Shaping corners of toenails may damage tissues.
28. Apply lotion to feet and hands, and assist client back to bed and into comfortable position.	Lotion lubricates dry skin by helping to retain moisture (Strauss and others, 1988).
29. Remove disposable gloves, and place in receptacle. Clean and return equipment and supplies to proper place. Dispose of soiled linen in hamper. Wash hands.	Reduces transmission of infection.
30. Inspect nails and surrounding skin surfaces after soaking and nail trimming.	Evaluates condition of skin and nails. Allows you to note any remaining rough nail edges.
31. Ask client to explain or demonstrate nail care.	Evaluates client's level of learning techniques.
32. Observe client's walk after toenail care.	Evaluates level of comfort and mobility achieved.

UNEXPECTED OUTCOMES AND RELATED INTERVENTIONS

- Nails discolored, rough, and concave or irregular in shape.
  - Increase frequency of nail hygiene because one intervention will not correct long-term problems.
- Cuticles and surrounding tissues may be inflamed and tender to touch.
  - Repeated soakings are necessary to help relieve inflammation and remove layers of cells from calluses or corns.
  - Diabetic clients may require referal to a podiatrist.
- Localized areas of tenderness may occur on feet with calluses or corns at point of friction.
  - Change in footwear or corrective foot surgery may be needed for permanent improvement in corns or calluses.
  - Refer client to podiatrist.

- Ulcer appears between toes.
  - Notify physician.
  - Refer to podiatrist.
  - Provide frequent foot hygiene.

RECORDING AND REPORTING

- Record procedure and observations (e.g., breaks in skin, inflammation, ulcerations).
- Report any breaks in skin or ulcerations to nurse in charge or physician. These are serious in client with peripheral vascular illnesses and illnesses in which client's circlation is impaired. Special foot care treatments may be needed.

11. Wear shoes that fit properly. Soles of shoes should be flexible and should not slip. Lamb's wool can be used between toes that rub or overlap. Shoes should be sturdy, closed in, and not restrictive. Clients with increased plantar pressure (e.g., callus, or erythema) should use footwear that cushions and redistributes pressure (ADA, 1999).

12. Exercise regularly to improve circulation to the lower extremities. Walk slowly, elevate, rotate, flex, and extend the feet at the ankle. Dangle the feet over the side of the bed 1 minute, then extend both legs and hold them parallel to the bed while lying supine for 1 minute, and finally rest 1 minute.

13. Avoid applying hot-water bottles or heating pads to the feet; use extra covers instead.

14. Minor cuts should be washed immediately and dried thoroughly. Only mild antiseptics (e.g., Neosporin ointment) should be applied to the skin. Avoid iodine or Mercurochrome. Contact a physician to treat cuts or lacerations.

ORAL HYGIENE. Good oral hygiene involves cleanliness, comfort, and the moisturizing of mouth structures. Proper care will prevent oral disease. Unfortunately, clients in hospitals or long-term care facilities often do not receive the aggressive care they need. Oral care must be provided on a regular basis. To encourage health promotion and restoration, instruct clients to brush their teeth after each meal and before bedtime and to floss once daily. Acidic fruits in the client's diet can reduce plaque formation. All clients should visit a dentist regularly every 6 months for checkups. To prevent tooth decay, clients may have to change eating habits (e.g., reducing intake of carbohydrates, especially sweet snacks between meals). A well-balanced diet ensures the integrity of oral tissues.

BRUSHING. Thorough toothbrushing at least 4 times a day (after meals and at bedtime) is basic to an effective oral hygiene program. A toothbrush should have a straight handle and brush small enough to reach all areas of the mouth.

Older adult clients with reduced dexterity and grip may require an enlarged handle with an easier grip.

All tooth surfaces should be brushed thoroughly. Commercially made foam rubber toothbrushes are useful for clients with sensitive gums. Electric toothbrushes can be used, but check for electrical hazards. Lemon-glycerin sponges should be avoided because they dry mucous membranes and erode tooth enamel. Moi-Stin is a salivary supplement that improves moisture and texture of the tongue and mucosa.

Clients who receive cancer chemotherapy, radiation, or immunosuppression agents may develop stomatitis and may require certain modifications to oral care. These modifications reduce the discomfort of stomatitis.

When teaching clients about mouth care, recommend that they not share toothbrushes with family members or drink directly from a bottle of mouthwash. Cross-contamination occurs easily. The amount of assistance needed by the client when brushing the teeth may vary (Skill 26-4).

ORAL HYGIENE FOR THE UNCONSCIOUS CLIENT.   Unconscious clients need special attention. While providing hygiene to an unconscious client, you must protect the client from choking and aspirating. The safest technique is to have two nurses provide the care. One does the actual cleaning, and the other removes secretions with suction equipment. While cleansing the oral cavity, never use fingers to hold the mouth open. A human bite is highly contaminated. It may be necessary to perform mouth care at least every 2 hours. Explain the steps of mouth care and the sensations the client will feel. Also tell the client when the procedure is completed (Skill 26-5).

FLOSSING.   Dental flossing is necessary to remove plaque and tartar between teeth. Flossing involves inserting waxed or unwaxed dental floss between all tooth surfaces, one at a time. The seesaw motion used to pull floss between teeth removes plaque and tartar from tooth enamel. If toothpaste is applied to the teeth before flossing, fluoride can come in

Text continued on p. 631

Skill 26-4
PROVIDING ORAL HYGIENE

DELEGATION CONSIDERATIONS
Skills of brushing teeth can be delegated to assistive personnel. Explain how to adapt proceudre to client if at risk for aspiration.
- Inform and assist care provider in proper way to provide toothbrushing.
- Instruct care provider on how to recognize impaired integrity of oral mucosa and the alterations to report.

EQUIPMENT
- Soft-bristled toothbrush
- Nonabrasive fluoride toothpaste or dentifrice
- Dental floss
- Water glass with cool water
- Normal saline or fluoride mouthwash (optional; follow client's preference)
- Emesis basin
- Face towel
- Paper towels
- Disposable gloves

STEPS	RATIONALE
1. Wash hands, and apply disposable gloves.	Reduces transmission of microorganisms. Gloves prevent contact with microorganisms in blood or saliva.
2. Inspect integrity of lips, teeth, buccal mucosa, gums, palate, and tongue (see Chapter 12).	Determines status of client's oral cavity and extent of need for oral hygiene.
3. Identify presence of common oral problems:	Helps determine type of hygiene client requires and information client requires for self-care.
a. Dental caries—chalky white discoloration of tooth or presence of brown or black discoloration	
b. Gingivitis—inflammation of gums	
c. Periodontitis—receding gum lines, inflammation, gaps between teeth	
d. Halitosis—bad breath	
e. Cheilosis—cracking of lips	
f. Stomatitis—inflammation of the mouth	
4. Remove gloves, and wash hands.	Prevents spread of microorganisms.
5. Assess risk for oral hygiene problems:	Certain conditions increase likelihood of impaired oral cavity integrity and need for preventive care.
a. Dehydration, inability to take fluids or food by mouth (NPO)	Causes excess drying and fragility of mucous membranes; increases accumulation of secretions on tongue and gums.
b. Presence of nasogastric or oxygen tubes; mouth breathers	Causes drying of mucosa (Harrell and Damon, 1989).
c. Chemotherapeutic drugs	These drugs kill rapidly multiplying cells, including cancerous tumors and cells lining oral cavity and gastrointestinal tract. Drug effects can lead to stomatitis (Dudjak, 1987).

STEPS	RATIONALE
d. Calcium channel blockers, phenytoin, some amphetamines used to treat hyperactivity in children, and cyclosporine used by organ transplant recipients.	Produces gum overgrowth.
e. Over-the-counter lozenges, cough drops, antacids, and chewable vitamins.	Medications contain large amounts of sugar. Repeated daily use increases sugar or acid content in mouth.
f. Radiation therapy to head and neck	Reduces salivary flow and lowers pH of saliva; can lead to stomatitis and tooth decay (Danielson, 1988).
g. Presence of artificial airway	Increases irritation to gums and mucosa. Excess secretions accumulate on teeth and tongue.
h. Blood-clotting disorders (e.g., leukemia, aplastic anemia)	Predisposes to inflammation and bleeding of gums.
i. Oral surgery, trauma to mouth	Break in mucosa increases risk of infection. Vigorous brushing can disrupt suture lines.
j. Aging	Results in drying and thinning of mucosa.
k. Diabetes mellitus	Prone to dryness of mouth, gingivitis, periodontal disease, and loss of teeth.
6. Determine client's oral hygiene practices:	Allows nurse to identify errors in technique, deficiencies in preventive oral hygiene, and client's level of knowledge regarding dental care.
a. Frequency of toothbrushing and flossing	
b. Type of toothpaste or dentifrice used	
c. Last dental visit	
d. Frequency of dental visits	
e. Type of mouthwash or moistening preparation	Lemon-glycerin preparations can be detrimental. Glycerin is an astringent that dries and shrinks mucous membranes and gums. Lemon exhausts salivary reflex and can erode tooth enamel (Poland, 1987). Mouthwash provides pleasant aftertaste but can dry mucosa after extended use if it has an alcohol base (Blaney, 1986).
7. Assesses client's ability to grasp and manipulate toothbrush. Assessment determines level of assistance required from you.	Older adult clients or persons with musculoskeletal or nervous system alterations may be unable to hold toothbrush with firm grip or manipulate brush.
8. Prepare equipment at bedside.	
9. Explain procedure to client and discuss preferences regarding use of hygiene aids.	Some clients feel uncomfortable about having you care for their basic needs. Client involvement with procedure minimizes anxiety.
10. Place paper towels on over-bed table, and arrange other equipment within easy reach.	Provides accessible work area.
11. Raise bed to comfortable working position. Raise head of bed (if allowed) and lower side rail. Move client, or help client move closer. Side-lying position can be used.	Raising bed and positioning client prevent you from straining muscles. Semi-Fowler's position helps prevent client from choking or aspirating.
12. Place towel over client's chest.	
13. Apply gloves.	Prevents contact with microorganisms or blood in saliva.
14. Apply toothpaste to brush, holding brush over emesis basin. Pour small amount of water over toothpaste.	Moisture aids in distribution of toothpaste over tooth surfaces.
15. Client may assist by brushing. Hold toothbrush bristles at 45-degree angle to gum line (see illustration). Be sure tips of bristles rest against and penetrate under gum line. Brush inner and outer surfaces of upper and lower teeth by brushing from gum to crown of each tooth. Clean biting surfaces of teeth by holding top of bristles parallel with teeth and brushing gently back and forth (see illustration). Brush sides of teeth by moving bristles back and forth (see illustration).	Angle allows brush to reach all tooth surfaces and to clean under gum line, where plaque and tartar accumulate. Back-and-forth motion dislodges food particles caught between teeth and along chewing surfaces.

STEPS	RATIONALE

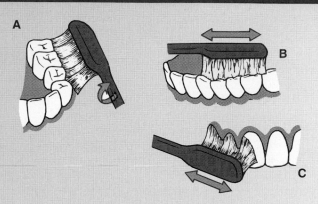

STEP 15   Direction for toothbrush placement. **A,** Forty-five-degree angle brushes gumline. **B,** Parallel position brushes biting surfaces. **C,** Lateral position brushes sides of teeth.

STEPS	RATIONALE
16. Have client hold brush at 45-degree angle and lightly brush over surface and sides of tongue. Avoid initiating gag reflex.	Microorganisms collect and grow on tongue's surface and contribute to bad breath. Gagging may cause aspiration of toothpaste.
17. Allow client to rinse mouth thoroughly by taking several sips of water, swishing water across all tooth surfaces, and spitting into emesis basin.	Irrigation removes food particles.
18. Allow client to gargle to rinse mouth with mouthwash as desired.	Mouthwash leaves pleasant taste in mouth.
19. Assist in wiping client's mouth.	Promotes sense of comfort.
20. Allow client to floss.	Reduces tartar on tooth surfaces.
21. Allow client to rinse mouth thoroughly with cool water and spit into emesis basin. Assist in wiping client's mouth.	Irrigation removes plaque and tartar from oral cavity.
22. Assist client to comfortable position, remove emesis basin and bedside table, raise side rail, and lower bed to original position.	Provides for client comfort and safety.
23. Wipe off over-bed table, discard soiled linen and paper towels in appropriate containers, remove soiled gloves, and return equipment to proper place.	Proper disposal of soiled equipment prevents spread of infection.
24. Wash hands.	Reduces transmission of microorganisms.
25. Ask client if any area of oral cavity feels uncomfortable or irritated.	Pain indicates more chronic problem.
26. Apply gloves, and inspect condition of oral cavity.	Determines effectiveness of hygiene and rinsing.
27. Ask client to describe proper hygiene techniques.	Evaluates client's learning.
28. Observe client brushing.	Evaluates client's ability to use correct technique.

UNEXPECTED OUTCOMES AND RELATED INTERVENTIONS

- Mucosa is dry and inflamed.
  - Increase client's hydration.
  - Apply protectant to client's lips.
- Gum margins are retracted from teeth, with localized areas of inflammation. Bleeding occurs around gum margins.
  - Report findings because client may have an underlying bleeding tendency.
  - Switch to a soft-bristled toothbrush.
  - Avoid too vigorous brushing and flossing.
  - A swab stick containing an aqueous solution of sorbitol, sodium, carboxymethylcellulose, and electrolytes may be used.
- Teeth show signs of dental caries.
  - Refer client to dentist.

RECORDING AND REPORTING

- Record procedure on flow sheet. Note condition of oral cavity in nurses' notes.
- Report bleeding or presence of lesions to nurse in charge or physician.

Skill 26-5
PERFORMING MOUTH CARE FOR AN UNCONSCIOUS OR DEBILITATED CLIENT

DELEGATION CONSIDERATIONS

Skills of brushing teeth of an unconscious or debilitated client can be delegated to assistive personnel. However, you must first assess the client's gag reflex and then inform the assistive personnel of the proper way to position clients for mouth care. For this skill, assistive personnel must be able to safely use the oral suction catheter for clearing oral secretions (see Chapter 27, Skill 27-1). As with all mouth care, care providers must know how to recognize impaired integrity of oral mucosa.

EQUIPMENT

- Antiinfective solution (e.g., diluted hydrogen peroxide) that loosens crusts
- Small soft-bristled toothbrush
- Sponge toothette or tongue blade wrapped in single layer of gauze
- Padded tongue blade
- Face towel
- Paper towels
- Emesis basin
- Water glass with cool water
- Water-soluble lip lubricant
- Small-bulb syringe (optional)
- Suction machine equipment (optional)
- Disposable gloves

STEPS	RATIONALE
1. Wash hands. Apply disposable gloves.	Reduces transmission of microorganisms. Gloves prevent contact with microorganisms in blood or saliva.
2. Test for presence of gag reflex by placing blade on back half of tongue.	Reveals whether client is at risk for aspiration.

- **Critical Decision Point**
  Clients with impaired gag reflex require oral care as well. You must determine the type of suction apparatus needed at the bedside to protect the client's airway against aspiration.

STEPS	RATIONALE
3. Inspect condition of oral cavity (see Chapter 12).	Determines condition of oral cavity and need for hygiene.
4. Remove gloves. Wash hands.	Prevents spread of infection.
5. Assess client's risk for oral hygiene problems (see Skill 26-4, p. 626).	Certain conditions increase likelihood of alterations in integrity of oral cavity structures and may require more frequent care.
6. Position client on side (Sims' position) with head turned well toward dependent side and head of bed lowered. Raise side rail.	Allows secretions to drain from mouth instead of collecting in back of pharynx. Prevents aspiration.
7. Explain procedure to client.	Allows debilitated client to anticipate procedure without anxiety. Unconscious client may retain ability to hear.
8. Wash hands, and apply disposable gloves.	Reduces transfer of microorganisms.
9. Place paper towels on over-bed table and arrange equipment. If needed, turn on suction machine, and connect tubing to suction catheter.	Prevents soiling of table top. Equipment prepared in advance ensures smooth, safe procedure.
10. Pull curtain around bed, or close room door.	Provides privacy.
11. Raise bed to its highest horizontal level; lower side rail.	Use of good body mechanics with bed in high position prevents injury.
12. Position client close to side of bed; turn client's head toward mattress.	Proper positioning of head prevents aspiration.
13. Place towel under client's head and emesis basin under chin.	Prevents soiling of bed linen.
14. Carefully separate upper and lower teeth with padded tongue blade by inserting blade, quickly but gently, between back molars. Insert when client is relaxed, if possible. Do not use force (see illustration).	Prevents client from biting down on your fingers and provides access to oral cavity.

- **Critical Decision Point**
  Never use fingers to separate client's teeth.

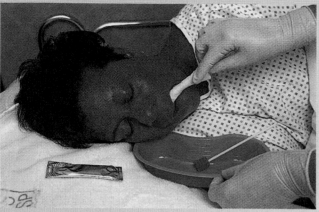

STEP 14   Separate upper and lower teeth with padded tongue blade.

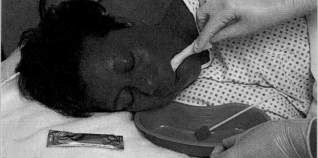

STEP 17   Application of water-soluble moisturizer to lips.

Steps	Rationale
15. Clean mouth using brush or sponge toothettes moistened with peroxide and water. Clean chewing and inner tooth surfaces first. Clean outer tooth surfaces. Swab roof of mouth, gums, and inside cheeks. Gently swab or brush tongue but avoid stimulating gag reflex (if present). Moisten clean swab or toothette with water to rinse. (Bulb syringe may also be used to rinse.) Repeat rinse several times.	Brushing action removes food particles between teeth and along chewing surfaces. Swabbing helps remove secretions and crusts from mucosa and moistens mucosa. Repeated rinsing removes peroxide, which can be irritating to mucosa.
16. Suction secretions as they accumulate, if necessary.	Suction removes secretions and fluid that can collect in posterior pharynx.
17. Apply thin layer of water-soluble jelly to lips (see illustration).	Lubricates lips to prevent drying and cracking.
18. Inform client that procedure is completed.	Provides meaningful stimulation to unconscious or less responsive client.
19. Raise side rails as appropriate or ordered.	Review agency policy and procedures. Raising of all four side rails may be considered a restraint, and a physician's order is needed.
20. Remove gloves, and dispose in proper receptacle.	Prevents transmission of microorganisms.
21. Reposition client comfortably, raise side rail, and return bed to original position.	Maintains client's comfort and safety.
22. Clean equipment and return to its proper place. Place soiled linen in proper receptacle.	Proper disposal of soiled equipment prevents spread of infection.
23. Wash hands.	Reduces transmission of microorganisms.
24. Apply gloves, and inspect oral cavity.	Determines efficacy of cleansing. Once thick secretions are removed, underlying inflammation or lesions may be revealed.
25. Ask debilitated client if mouth feels clean.	Evaluates level of comfort.
26. Assess client's respirations on an ongoing basis.	Ensures early recognition of aspiration.

STEPS	RATIONALE

UNEXPECTED OUTCOMES AND RELATED INTERVENTIONS

- Secretions or crusts remain on mucosa, tongue, or gums.
  - More frequent oral hygiene is needed.
  - A pediatric-size toothbrush may provide better hygiene (Fitch and others, 1999).
- Localized inflammation of gums or mucosa is present.
  - More frequent oral hygiene with soft-bristled toothbrush is needed.
  - Apply OralBalance moisturizing gel to mucosa and massage (Fitch and others, 1999).
  - Chemotherapy and radiation can cause stomatitis. Clients should rinse mouth before and after meals and at bedtime using normal saline or solution of $\frac{1}{2}$ to 1 teaspoon of salt or baking soda to 1 pint of tepid water. To loosen and remove thick mucus, use one part of hydrogen peroxide to four parts of normal saline followed by warm water or saline rinse (Greifzu and others, 1990).

- Lips are cracked or inflamed.
  - Apply OralBalance moisturizing gel to lips or water soluble lubricant.
- Client aspirates secretions.
  - If present, suction oral airways as secretions accumulate to maintain patent airway (see Chapter 27).

RECORDING AND REPORTING

- Record procedure, including pertinent observations (e.g., presence of bleeding gums, dry mucosa, ulcerations, crusts on tongue).
- Report any unusual findings to nurse in charge or physician.

---

direct contact with tooth surfaces, aiding in cavity prevention. Flossing once a day is sufficient. Because it is important to clean all teeth surfaces thoroughly, you should not rush to complete flossing. Placing a mirror in front of the client will help you to demonstrate the proper methods for holding the floss and cleaning between the teeth.

DENTURE CARE.   Clients should be encouraged to clean their dentures on a regular basis to avoid gingival infection and irritation. When clients become disabled, you or the caregiver must assume responsibility for denture care (Box 26-6). Dentures are the client's personal property and need to be handled with care because they can be easily broken. Dentures must be removed at night to give the gums a rest and prevent bacterial buildup. To prevent warping, dentures should be kept covered in water when they are not worn, and they should always be stored in an enclosed, labeled cup with the cup placed in the client's bedside stand. Discourage clients from removing their dentures and placing them on a napkin or tissue because they could be easily thrown away.

HAIR CARE

BRUSHING AND COMBING.   Frequent brushing helps to keep hair clean and distributes oil evenly along hair shafts. Combing prevents hair from tangling. Encourage clients to maintain routine hair care. However, clients with limited mobility and poor coordination and those who are confused or seriously weakened by illness require help. Clients in a hospital or extended care facility appreciate the opportunity to have their hair brushed and combed before being seen by others.

Long hair can easily become matted after a client is confined to bed, even for a short period. When lacerations or incisions involve the scalp, blood and topical medications can also cause tangling. Frequent brushing and combing keep long hair neatly groomed. Braiding can help to avoid repeated tangles. You must ask permission before braiding a client's hair.

To brush hair, part the hair into two sections and separate each into two more sections. It is easier to brush smaller sections of hair. Brushing from the scalp toward the hair ends minimizes pulling. Moistening the hair with water or an alcohol free detangle product makes the hair easier to comb. Never cut a client's hair without written consent.

SHAMPOOING.   Frequency of shampooing depends on a client's daily routines. Remind hospitalized clients that staying in bed, excess perspiration, or treatments that leave blood or solutions in the hair may require more frequent shampooing. For clients at home, the greatest challenge may be to find ways the client can shampoo the hair without injury.

If the client is able to take a shower or bath, the hair can usually be shampooed without difficulty. A shower chair may be used for the ambulatory client who becomes tired or faint. Handheld shower nozzles allow clients to wash the hair during a tub bath or shower. Clients allowed to sit in a chair can usually be shampooed in front of a sink. If the client is forced to sit at the bedside, the hair can be shampooed as the client leans forward over a washbasin.

If a client is unable to sit but can be moved, you may transfer the client to a stretcher for transportation to a sink or shower equipped with a handheld nozzle. Place a towel or small pillow under the client's head and neck, allowing the head to hang slightly over the stretcher's edge. Caution and specific physician's order for shampooing are needed with

Equipment: Soft-bristled toothbrush, denture toothbrush, emesis basin or sink, denture dentifrice or toothpaste, water glass, 4 × 4 inch gauze, washcloth, denture cup, disposable gloves

1. Clean dentures for client during routine mouth care. Dentures need to be cleansed as often as natural teeth.
2. Fill emesis basin with tepid water. (If using sink, place washcloth in bottom of sink, and fill sink with approximately 1 inch of water.)
3. Remove dentures: If client is unable to do this independently, don gloves, grasp upper plate at front with thumb and index finger wrapped in gauze, and pull downward. Gently lift lower denture from jaw, and rotate one side downward to remove from client's mouth. Place dentures in emesis basin or sink.
4. Apply dentifrice or toothpaste to denture, and brush surfaces of dentures (see illustration). Hold dentures close to water. Hold brush horizontally, and use back-and-forth motion to cleanse biting surfaces. Use short strokes from top of denture to biting surfaces of teeth to clean outer tooth surface. Hold brush vertically, and use short strokes to clean inner tooth surfaces. Hold brush horizontally, and use back-and-forth motion to clean undersurface of dentures.

5. Rinse dentures thoroughly in tepid water.
6. Return dentures to client, or store in tepid water in denture cup.

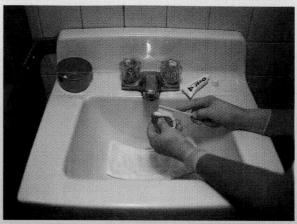

STEP 4

clients with neck injuries because hyperextension of the neck could cause further injury.

When clients are unable to move, sit in a chair, be transferred to a stretcher, or tolerate a wet hair-washing procedure, there a various "dry" shampoo products available. It is important to read manufacturer's guidelines carefully. In general these products are massaged into the client's hair and scalp. Some products may instruct you to apply a towel to remove excess oil and dirt, whereas other products may instruct you to brush product through client's hair.

A final option is to wash the client's hair in the bed. Many institutions require a physician's order for the procedure (Box 26-7).

SHAVING. Shaving facial hair can be done after the bath or shampoo. Women may prefer to shave their legs or axillae while bathing. When assisting a client, take care to avoid cutting the client with razor blades. Clients prone to bleeding (e.g., those receiving anticoagulants or high doses of aspirin) should use an electric razor. Before using an electric razor, check for electrical hazards. Electric razors should be used on only one client because of the risk of infection transmission.

When a razor blade is used for shaving, the skin must be softened to prevent pulling, scraping, or cuts. For example, placing a warm washcloth over the male client's face for a few seconds, followed by application of shaving cream or a lathering of mild soap, softens the skin. If the client is unable to shave, you may perform the shave. To avoid causing discomfort or razor cuts, gently pull the skin taut and use short, firm razor strokes in the direction the hair grows. Short downward strokes work best to remove hair over the upper lip. A client usually can explain to you the best way to move the razor across the skin.

Mustache and Beard Care. Clients with mustaches or beards require daily grooming. Keeping these areas clean is important because food particles and mucus can easily collect in the hair. If the client is unable to carry out self-care, you should do so at the client's request. Never shave off a mustache or beard without the client's consent.

Hair and Scalp Care. To best promote and restore hair and scalp health, clients should be instructed to keep hair clean, combed, and brushed regularly. Clients may also need to know how to check for and remove parasites (see Table 26-6, p. 608). Tell clients to notify their primary health care provider of changes in the texture and distribution of hair.

CARE OF EYES, EARS, NOSE. To maintain optimal health, clients should be instructed in the proper methods of caring for the eyes, ears, and nose. Clients with specific health concerns involving these sensory organs should see the appropriate specialist regularly for checkups and ongoing care. When active, clients should know the best ways of protecting these sensitive organs (e.g., eye protective devices). Older adults experience a variety of changes in sensory function (see Chapter 35). Adapt practice approaches to consider their special needs (Box 26-8).

BASIC EYE CARE. Cleansing the eyes simply involves washing with a clean washcloth moistened in water. Soap may cause burning and irritation (see Skill 26-1, p. 612). Direct pressure should never be applied over the eyeball because it may cause serious injury.

The unconscious client may require more frequent eye care. Secretions may collect along the lid margins and inner canthus when the blink reflex is absent or when the eye does

Equipment: Bath towels, washcloths, shampoo and hair conditioner (optional), water pitcher, plastic shampoo trough, washbasin, bath blanket, waterproof pad, clean comb and brush, hair dryer (optional).

1. Before washing client's hair, determine that there are no contraindications to this procedure. Certain medical conditions, such as head and neck injuries, spinal cord injuries, and arthritis, could place the client at risk for injury during shampooing because of positioning and manipulation of client's head and neck.

2. Inspect the hair and scalp prior to initiating the procedure. This determines the presence of any conditions that may require the use of special shampoos or treatments (e.g., for the removal of dried blood, dandruff).

3. Place waterproof pad under client's shoulders, neck, and head. Position client supine, with head and shoulders at top edge of bed. Place plastic trough under client's head and washbasin at end of trough spout (see illustration). Be sure trough spout or tubing extends beyond edge of mattress.

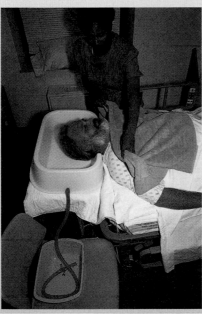

STEP 3

4. Place rolled towel under client's neck and bath towel over client's shoulders.

5. Brush and comb client's hair.

6. Obtain warm water.

7. Ask client to hold face towel or washcloth over eyes.

8. Slowly pour water from water pitcher over hair until it is completely wet (see illustration). If hair contains matted blood, don gloves, apply peroxide to dissolve clots, and then rinse hair with saline. Apply small amount of shampoo.

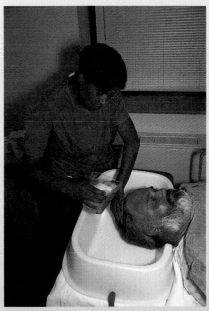

STEP 8

9. Work up lather with both hands. Start at hairline, and work toward back of neck. Lift head slightly with one hand to wash back of head. Shampoo sides of head. Massage scalp by applying pressure with fingertips.

10. Rinse hair with water. Make sure water drains into basin. Repeat rinsing until hair is free of soap.

11. Apply conditioner or cream rinse if requested, and rinse hair thoroughly.

12. Wrap client's head in bath towel. Dry client's face with cloth used to protect eyes. Dry off any moisture along neck or shoulders.

13. Dry client's hair and scalp. Use second towel if first becomes saturated.

14. Comb hair to remove tangles, and dry with dryer if desired.

15. Apply oil preparation or conditioning product to hair, if desired by client.

16. Assist client to comfortable position, and complete styling of hair.

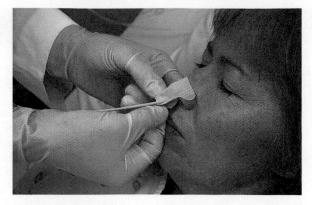

FIGURE **26-1**   Applying new tape over feeding tube.

not totally close. It may be necessary to place an eye patch over the involved eye to prevent corneal drying and irritation. Lubricating eye drops may be given according to the physician's orders.

Eyeglasses.   Eyeglasses are made of hardened glass or plastic that is impact resistant to prevent shattering. Nevertheless, because of the cost, be careful when cleaning glasses and protect them from breakage or other damage when they are not worn. Eyeglasses should be put in a case and in a drawer of the bedside table when not in use.

Warm water is sufficient for cleaning glass lenses. A soft cloth is best for drying to prevent scratching the lens. Plastic lenses in particular are scratched easily, and special cleansing solutions and drying tissues are available.

Contact Lenses.   A contact lens is a thin, transparent, circular disk that fits directly over the cornea of the eye. Contact lenses are designed specifically to correct refractive errors of the eye or abnormalities in the shape of the cornea. They are easy to apply and remove.

Care of contact lenses includes proper cleaning, insertion and removal, and storage. Clients who wear contact lenses usually wear them all day and take care of their own lenses. However, when clients are admitted to hospitals or agencies in unresponsive or confused states it is important to determine if the client is a contact lens wearer and if the lenses are in place. If a seriously ill client is wearing contact lenses and this fact goes undetected, severe corneal injury can result. If you determine that your client has contact lenses in place and the client cannot remove them, seek assistance in removing these lenses from the client's eyes. Once the lenses are removed be sure to document removal of lenses, condition of the client's eyes following lenses removal, and if the lenses were given to a relative or placed with the client's valuables.

Ear Care.   Routine ear care involves cleansing the ear with the end of a moistened washcloth, rotated gently into the ear canal. When cerumen is visible, gentle, downward retraction at the entrance of the ear canal may cause the wax to loosen and slip out. Instruct your client never to use sharp objects such as bobby pins or paper clips to remove cerumen. These objects can cause trauma to the ear canal or rupture the tympanic membrane. In addition the use of cotton-tipped applicators should be avoided because they may cause cerumen wax to become impacted within the ear canal.

When cerumen is impacted it can usually be removed by irrigation. This is done only after verification that your client's tympanic membrane is intact; a perforated tympanic membrane is a contraindication to irrigation.

Before irrigation, instill 2 to 3 drops of glycerin at bedtime; this assists in softening the wax. Two to three drops of hydrogen peroxide are instilled twice a day to assist in loosening the wax. To irrigate the ear, have client sit or lie with the affected ear up. Place a curved emesis basin under the affected ear. Using a bulb irrigating syringe, gently wash the ear canal with 250 ml of warm water. Cold water can cause dizziness and vomiting; hot water increases the risk to the ear canal. Initiate the flow of solution at the top of the canal, which will assist in loosening the wax from the sides of the canal. After the canal is clear, remove any moisture from the ear and inspect the canal for remaning cerumen.

Nose Care.   The client can usually remove secretions from the nose by gently blowing into a soft tissue. Caution the client against harsh blowing that creates pressure capable of injuring the eardrum, nasal mucosa, and even sensitive eye structures. Bleeding from the nares is a key sign of harsh blowing.

If the client is unable to remove nasal secretions, assist by using a wet washcloth or a cotton-tipped applicator moistened in water or saline. The applicator should never be inserted beyond the length of the cotton tip. Excessive nasal secretions can also be removed by gentle suctioning.

When clients have tubes inserted through the nose, change the tape anchoring the tube at least once a day. When tape becomes moist from nasal secretions, the skin and mucosa can easily become macerated. Friction causes tissue sloughing. You should know how to tape tubing correctly to minimize tension or friction on the nares (Figure 26-1). When sloughing occurs, it may be necessary for you to remove the tube and insert one through the other naris.

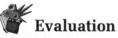

Outcome Evaluation for   MRS. FOSTER

Box 26-9

Nursing Action	Client Response/Finding	Achievement of Outcome
Mrs. Foster is turned every 90 minutes.	Mrs. Foster did not report sensations of pressure, burning, or tingling over bony areas or other areas of the skin. Mrs. Foster was able to assist with position change.	Mrs. Foster's skin remains intact without erythema.
Hygiene and perineal care is following each episode of incontinence.	Mrs. Foster stated that skin felt clean. Mrs. Foster did not report sensations of wetness, burning, pain, or tingling in perineal region.	Mrs. Foster's skin remains dry and intact. Perineal skin is free of odor, redness, or swelling.

Evaluation

The evaluation of hygiene activities includes not only actual client care but also how the client's expectations were met. Combining both of these aspects of evaluation is important in determining the success of hygiene care.

CLIENT CARE.   During and after hygiene, evaluate the success of interventions. The process is dynamic because the client's condition may change (Box 26-9). Always be prepared to revise the care plan based on the evaluation. For example, if a clients' skin continues to be reddened over the sacrum, more frequent turning may be necessary. Systematic evaluation requires you to determine if expected outcomes have been met.

CLIENT EXPECTATIONS.   During assessment you collected data on the client's expectations of care. After hygiene care you need to determine if the client's expectations were met. For example, ask the client if hygiene preferences were met or if family members were able to assist as desired. In addition, ask the client about the care provided, thus determining if the client's expectations were met or whether the client had additional needs.

CLIENT'S ROOM ENVIRONMENT

Attempting to make a client's room as comfortable as the home is one of your priorities. The client's room should be comfortable, safe, and large enough to allow the client and visitors to move about freely. You can control room temperature, ventilation, noise, and odors to create a more comfortable environment. Keeping the room neat and orderly also contributes to the client's sense of well-being.

Maintaining Comfort

The nature of what constitutes a comfortable environment depends on the client's age, severity of illness, and level of normal daily activity. Depending on the client's age and physical condition, the room temperature should be maintained between 20° and 23° C (68° and 74° F). Infants, older adults, and the acutely ill may need a warmer room. However, certain critically ill clients benefit from cooler room temperatures to lower the body's metabolic demands.

Case Study   EVALUATION

James is able to provide Mrs. Foster with a shower and modifies her plan of care to include a shower every other day. Mrs. Foster tells James that she really appreciates having more frequent showers and that they really help her feel and do her best. Although Mrs. Foster is very tired and needs a rest period after the shower, she feels it is worth it. Mrs. Foster knows that James provides the extra effort to her care and the subsequent modification of the care plan, and she is happy and feels somewhat in control of her care.

Documentation Note
Assisted Mrs. Foster in a shower. Nursing care plan was modified to include shower every other day followed by a 30-minute rest period. Physical and occupational therapy times were moved to accommodate shower and rest periods. Mrs. Foster went to the dining room for lunch.

A good ventilation system keeps stale air and odors from lingering in the room. You must protect the acutely ill, infants, and older adults from drafts by ensuring they are adequately dressed and covered with a lightweight blanket.

Good ventilation also reduces lingering odors caused by draining wounds, vomitus, bowel movements, and unemptied bedpans and urinals. Room deodorizers can help remove many unpleasant odors. Always empty and rinse bedpans or urinals promptly. Thorough hygiene measures are the best way to control body or breath odors. Most health care institutions now prohibit smoking. Before using room deodorizers you should determine that the client is not allergic to or sensitive to the deodorizer itself.

Ill clients seem to be more sensitive to common hospital noises. Until the client is familiar with hospital noises, try to control the noise level. You also need to explain the source of any unfamiliar noises.

Proper lighting is necessary for everyone's safety and comfort. A brightly lit room is usually stimulating, but a darkened room is best for rest and sleep. Room lighting can be adjusted by closing or opening drapes, regulating overbed and floor lights, and closing or opening room doors.

Room Equipment

A typical hospital room contains certain basic pieces of furniture. The over-bed table rolls on wheels and can be ad-

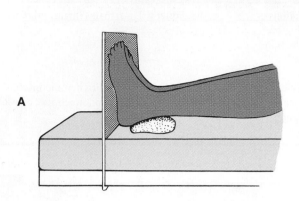
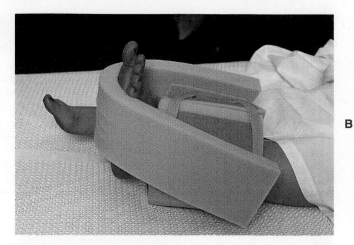
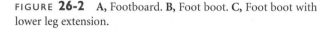
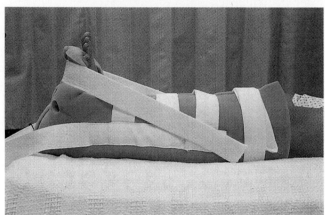

FIGURE **26-2** **A,** Footboard. **B,** Foot boot. **C,** Foot boot with lower leg extension.

justed to various heights over the bed or a chair. Usually two storage areas are under the tabletop. The table provides ideal working space for performing procedures. It also provides a surface on which to place meal trays, toiletry items, and objects frequently used by the client. The bedpan and urinal should not be placed on the over-bed table. The bedside stand is used to store the client's personal possessions and hygiene equipment. The telephone, water pitcher, and drinking cup are commonly found on a bedside stand.

Most hospital rooms contain an armless straight-backed chair and an upholstered lounge chair with arms. The lounge chair is used by the client and visitors and is usually placed at the foot of the bed or beside it. Straight-backed chairs are convenient when temporarily transferring the client from the bed, such as during bed making.

Each room usually has an over-bed light and a floor or table lamp. Moveable lights that extend over the bed from the wall should be positioned for easy reach but moved aside when not in use. Gooseneck or special examination lights are portable standing lights used to provide extra light during bedside procedures.

Other equipment usually found in a client's room includes a call light, a television set or radio, a blood pressure gauge, oxygen and vacuum wall outlets, and personal care items. Special equipment designed for comfort or position-

ing clients include footboards and foot boots (Figure 26-2), special mattresses, and bed boards.

BEDS. Seriously ill clients may remain in bed for a long time. Because a bed is the piece of equipment used most by a client, it should be designed for comfort, safety, and adaptability for changing positions.

The typical hospital bed has a firm mattress on a metal frame that can be raised and lowered horizontally. Different bed positions are used to promote lung expansion, postural drainage, and other interventions (Table 26-7).

The position of a bed is usually changed by electrical controls on the side or foot of the bed or on a bedside table. Clients can thus raise or lower sections of the bed without expending much energy. Instruct clients in the proper use of controls, and caution them against raising the bed to a position that might cause harm. It is generally recommended to keep a bed at a height that is appropriate for easy client transfer.

Beds contain safety features such as locks on the wheels or casters. Wheels should be locked when the bed is stationary to prevent accidental movement. Side rails allow clients to move more efficiently in bed and prevent accidents. Side rails should not be used to restrict a client from moving in bed. When side rails are used as a restraint, a physician's or-

Common Bed Positions

Table 26-7

Position	Description	Uses
Fowler's	Head of bed raised to angle of 45 degrees or more; semisitting position.	Preferred while client eats; used during nasogastric tube insertion and nasotracheal suction; promotes lung expansion.
Semi-Fowler's	Head of bed raised approximately 30 degrees; incline less than Fowler's position.	Promotes lung expansion.
Trendelenburg's	Entire bed tilted downward with head of bed down.	For postural drainage; facilitates venous return in clients with poor peripheral perfusion.
Reverse Trendelenburg's	Entire bed frame tilted downward with foot of bed down.	Used infrequently; promotes gastric emptying and prevents esophageal reflux.
Flat	Entire bed frame parallel with floor.	For clients with vertebral injuries and in cervical traction; used by hypotensive clients; generally preferred by clients for sleeping.

der is required (Chapter 25). The headboard can be removed from most beds. This is important when the medical team must have easy access to the head such as during cardiopulmonary resuscitation.

BED MAKING.   A client's bed should be kept as clean and comfortable as possible. This requires frequent inspections to be sure linen is clean, dry, and free of wrinkles.

Usually make a bed in the morning after the clients' bath or while the client is bathing, in a shower, sitting in a chair eating, or out of the room for procedures or tests. Throughout the day straighten linen that becomes loose or wrinkled. The bed linen should also be checked for food particles after meals and for wetness or soiling. Linen that become soiled or wet should be changed.

When changing the bed linen, follow basic principles of asepsis by keeping soiled linen away from the uniform. Soiled linen is placed in special linen containers before discarding it in the linen hamper. To avoid air currents, which can spread microorganisms, you never fan linen. To avoid transmitting infection, you should not place soiled linen on the floor. If clean linen touches the floor, it is immediately discarded.

During bed making, use proper body mechanics. The bed should always be raised to its highest position before changing linen so you do not have to bend or stretch over the mattress. When making an occupied bed you should also use principles of body mechanics (see Chapter 24).

The clients' privacy, comfort, and safety are important when making a bed. Using side rails, keeping call lights within the client's reach, and maintaining the proper bed position help promote comfort and safety. After making a bed you always return it to the lowest horizontal position to prevent accidental falls.

When possible make the bed while it is unoccupied (Box 26-10). If the client is confined to bed, organize bed-making activities to conserve time and energy (Skill 26-6). When making an unoccupied bed follow the same basic principles as for bed making. The surgical, recovery, or postoperative bed is a modified version of the unoccupied bed. The top covers of a surgical bed are folded to one side or fanfolded to the bottom third of the bed. This allows for easy transfer of client into the bed. After a client is discharged, all bed linen is sent to the laundry, housekeeping personnel clean the mattress and bed, and new bed linen is applied.

LINENS.   Before bed making, it is important to collect not only bed linens but also the client's personal linens. Linens are pressed and folded to prevent the spread of microorganisms and to make bed making easier. Bed linens have a center crease that you place in the center of the bed from the head to the foot. The linens unfold easily to the sides, with creases often fitting over the mattress edge. New linens are applied whenever there is soiling.

Equipment: Linen bag, mattress pad (change only when soiled), bottom sheet (flat or fitted), drawsheet (optional), top sheet, blanket, bedspread, waterproof pads (optional), pillowcases, bedside chair or table, disposable gloves (if linen is soiled), washcloth, and antiseptic cleanser.

1. Determine if client has been incontinent or if excess drainage is on linen. Gloves will be necessary.
2. Assess activity orders or restrictions in mobility in planning if client can get out of bed for procedure. Assist to bedside chair or recliner.
3. Lower side rails on both sides of bed and raise bed to comfortable working position.
4. Remove soiled linen and place in laundry bag. Avoid shaking or fanning linen.
5. Reposition mattress and wipe off any moisture using a washcloth moistened in antiseptic solution. Dry thoroughly.
6. Apply all bottom linen on one side of bed before moving to opposite side. Apply bottom sheet, flat or fitted.
7. Be sure fitted sheet is placed smoothly over mattress. To apply a flat unfitted sheet, allow about 25 cm (10 in) to hang over mattress edge. Lower hem of sheet should lie seam down, even with bottom edge of mattress. Pull remaining top portion of sheet over top edge of mattress.
8. While standing at head of bed, miter top corner of bottom flat sheet (see Skill 26-6, Step 17, p. 640).
9. Tuck remaining portion of unfitted sheet under mattress.
10. Optional: Apply drawsheet, laying center fold along middle of bed lengthwise. Smooth drawsheet over mattress and tuck excess edge under mattress, keeping palms down.
11. Move to opposite side of bed and spread bottom sheet smoothly over edge of mattress from head to foot of bed.
12. Apply fitted sheet smoothly over each mattress corner. For an unfitted sheet, miter top corner of bottom sheet (see Step 8), making sure corner is taut.
13. Grasp remaining edge of unfitted bottom sheet and tuck tightly under mattress while moving from head to foot of bed. Smooth folded drawsheet over bottom sheet and tuck under mattress, first at middle, then at top, and then at bottom.
14. If needed, apply waterproof pad over bottom sheet or drawsheet.

15. Place top sheet over bed with vertical center fold lengthwise down middle of bed. Open sheet out from head to foot, being sure top edge of sheet is even with top edge of mattress.
16. Make horizontal toe pleat: stand at foot of bed and fan fold top sheet 5 to 10 cm (2 to 4 in) across bed. Pull sheet up from bottom to make fold approximately 15 cm (6 in) from bottom edge of mattress.
17. Tuck in remaining portion of sheet under foot of mattress. Then place blanket over bed with top edge parallel to top edge of sheet and 15 to 20 cm (6 to 8 in) down from edge of sheet. (Optional: Apply additional spread over bed.)
18. Make cuff by turning edge of top sheet down over top edge of blanket and spread.
19. Standing on one side at foot of bed, lift mattress corner slightly with one hand, and with other hand tuck top sheet, blanket, and spread under mattress. Be sure toe pleats are not pulled out.
20. Make modified mitered corner with top sheet, blanket, and spread. After triangular fold is made, do not tuck tip of triangle (see illustration).

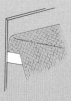

STEP 20

21. Go to other side of bed. Spread sheet, blanket, and spread out evenly. Make cuff with top sheet and blanket. Make modified corner at foot of bed.
22. Apply clean pillowcase.
23. Place call light within client's reach on bed rail or pillow and return bed to height allowing for client transfer. Assist client to bed.
24. Arrange client's room. Remove and discard supplies. Wash hands.

FIGURE **26-3** Equipment for making occupied bed.

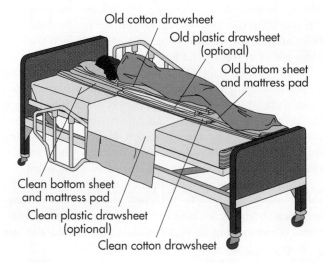

Old cotton drawsheet

Old plastic drawsheet (optional)

Old bottom sheet and mattress pad

Clean bottom sheet and mattress pad

Clean plastic drawsheet (optional)

Clean cotton drawsheet

Skill 26-6
MAKING AN OCCUPIED BED

DELEGATION CONSIDERATIONS

The skill of making an occupied bed can be delegated to assistive personnel. Before delegating this skill, review any precautions or activity restrictions for the client. Be sure assistive personnel know what to do if wound drainage, dressing material, drainage tubes, or IV tubing becomes dislodged or is found in the linens. Instruct the care provider in what to do if client becomes fatigued.

EQUIPMENT (FIGURE 26-3)
- Linen bag(s)
- Mattress pad (needs to be changed only when soiled)
- Bottom sheet (flat or fitted)
- Drawsheet
- Top sheet
- Blanket
- Bedspread
- Waterproof pads and/or bath blankets (optional)
- Pillowcases
- Bedside chair or table
- Disposable gloves (optional)
- Towel
- Disinfectant

STEPS	RATIONALE
1. Assess potential for client incontinence or for excess drainage on bed linen.	Determines need for protective waterproof pads or extra bath blankets on bed.
2. Check chart for orders or specific precautions concerning movement and positioning.	Ensures client safety and use of proper body mechanics.
3. Explain procedure to the client, noting that the client will be asked to turn on side and roll over linen.	Minimizes anxiety and promotes cooperation.
4. Wash hands, and apply gloves (gloves are worn only if linen is soiled or there is risk for contact with body secretions).	Reduces transmission of microorganisms.
5. Assemble equipment, and arrange on bedside chair or table. Remove unnecessary equipment such as a dietary tray or items used for hygiene.	Assembling all equipment provides for smooth procedure and assists in increasing client's comfort. Placing linen on clean surface minimizes spread of infection.
6. Draw room curtain around bed or close door.	Maintains client's privacy.
7. Adjust bed height to comfortable working position. Lower any raised side rail on one side of bed. Remove call light.	Minimizes strain on back. It is easier to remove and apply linen evenly to bed in flat position. Provides easy access to bed and linen.
8. Loosen top linen at foot of bed.	Makes linen easier to remove.
9. Remove bedspread and blanket separately. If spread and blanket are soiled, place them in linen bag. Keep soiled linen away from uniform.	Reduces transmission of microorganisms.
10. If blanket and spread are to be reused, fold them by bringing the top and bottom edges together. Fold farthest side over onto nearer bottom edge. Bring top and bottom edges together again. Place folded linen over back of chair.	Folding method facilitates replacement and prevents wrinkles.
11. Cover client with bath blanket in the following manner: unfold bath blanket over top sheet. Ask client to hold top edge of bath blanket. If client is unable to help, tuck top of bath blanket under shoulder. Grasp top sheet under bath blanket at client's shoulders and bring sheet down to foot of bed. Remove sheet and discard in linen bag.	Bath blanket provides warmth and keeps body parts covered during linen removal.
12. With assistance from another nurse, slide mattress toward head of bed.	If mattress slides toward foot of bed when head of bed is raised, it is difficult to tuck in linen. In addition, it is uncomfortable for the client because the client's feet may be pressed against or hang over the foot of the bed.
13. Position client on the far side of the bed, turned onto side and facing away from you. Be sure side rail in front of client is up. Adjust pillow under client's head.	Turning client onto side provides space for placement of clean linen. Side rail ensures client's safety from forward falls from the bed surface and helps client in moving.

STEPS	RATIONALE
14. Loosen bottom linens, moving from head to foot. With seam side down (facing the mattress), fanfold bottom sheet and drawsheet toward client—first drawsheet, then bottom sheet. Tuck edges of linen just under buttocks, back, and shoulders. Do not fanfold mattress pad if it is to be reused (see illustration).	Prepares for removal of all bottom linen simultaneously. Provides maximum work space for placing clean linen. Later, when client turns to other side, soiled linen can be removed easily.
15. Wipe off any moisture on exposed mattress with towel and appropriate disinfectant.	Reduces transmission of microorganisms.
16. Apply clean linen to exposed half of bed:	
a. Place clean mattress pad on bed by folding it lengthwise with center crease in middle of bed. Fanfold top layer over mattress. (If pad is reused, simply smooth out any wrinkles.)	Applying linen over bed in successive layers minimizes energy and time used in bed making.
b. Unfold bottom sheet lengthwise so that center crease is situated lengthwise along center of bed. Fanfold sheet's top layer toward center of bed alongside the client. Smooth bottom layer of sheet over mattress, and bring edge over closest side of mattress. Pull fitted sheet smoothly over mattress ends. Allow edge of flat unfitted sheet to hang about 25 cm (10 in) over mattress edge. Lower hem of bottom flat sheet should lie seam down and even with bottom edge of mattress (see illustration).	Proper positioning of linen on one side ensures that adequate linen will be available to cover opposite side of bed. Keeping seam edges down eliminates irritation to client's skin.
17. Miter bottom flat sheet at head of bed:	Ensures secure flat sheet will not loosen easily.
a. Face head of bed diagonally. Place hand away from head of bed under top corner of mattress, near mattress edge, and lift.	
b. With other hand, tuck top edge of bottom sheet smoothly under mattress so that side edges of sheet above and below mattress would meet if brought together.	
c. Face side of bed and pick up top edge of sheet at approximately 45 cm (18 in) from top of mattress (see illustration).	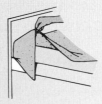
d. Lift sheet, and lay it on top of mattress to form a neat triangular fold, with lower base of triangle even with mattress side edge (see illustration).	STEP 17C Top edge of sheet picked up.

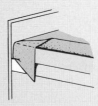

STEP 17D   Sheet on top of mattress in a triangular fold.

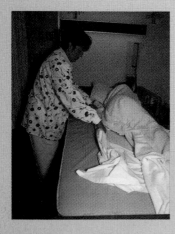

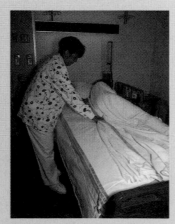

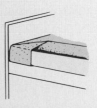

STEP 14   Old linen tucked under client.

STEP 16B   Clean linen applied to bed.

STEP 17E   Lower edge of sheet tucked under mattress

STEPS	RATIONALE

e. Tuck lower edge of sheet, which is hanging free below the mattress, under mattress. Tuck with palms down, without pulling triangular fold (see illustration).

f. Hold portion of sheet covering side of mattress in place with one hand. With the other hand, pick up top of triangular linen fold and bring it down over side of mattress (see illustration). Tuck this portion under mattress (see illustrations).

Mitered corner cannot be loosened easily even if client moves frequently in bed.

18. Tuck remaining portion of sheet under mattress, moving toward foot of bed. Keep linen smooth.

Folds of linen are source of irritation.

19. (Optional) Open drawsheet so that it unfolds in half. Lay centerfold along middle of bed lengthwise, and position sheet so that it will be under the client's buttocks and torso (see illustration). Fanfold top layer toward client, with edge along client's back. Smooth bottom layer out over mattress, and tuck excess edge under mattress (keep palms down).

Drawsheet is used to lift and reposition client. Placement under client's torso distributes most of client's body weight over sheet.

20. Place waterproof pad over drawsheet, with centerfold against client's side. Fanfold top layer toward client.

Protects bed linen from being soiled.

21. Have client roll slowly toward you, over the layers of linen. Raise side rail on working side, and go to other side.

Positions client for removal and placement of linens. Maintains client's safety and body alignment during turning.

22. Lower side rail. Assist client in positioning on other side, over folds of linen. Loosen edges of soiled linen from under mattress (see illustration).

Exposes opposite side of bed for removal of soiled linen and placement of clean linen. Makes linen easier to remove.

23. Remove soiled linen by folding it into a bundle or square, with soiled side turned in. Discard in linen bag. If necessary, wipe mattress with antiseptic solution, and dry mattress surface before applying new linen.

Reduces transmission of microorganisms.

24. Pull clean, fanfold linen smoothly over edge of mattress from head to foot of bed.

Smooth linen will not irritate client's skin.

25. Assist client in rolling back into supine position. Reposition pillow.

Maintains client's comfort.

26. Pull fitted sheet smoothly over mattress ends. Miter top corner of bottom sheet (see Step 17). When tucking corner, be sure that sheet is smooth and free of wrinkles.

Wrinkles and folds can cause irritation to skin.

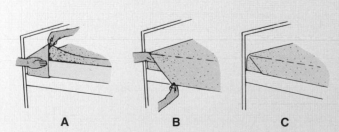

STEP 17F   **A** and **B**, Triangular fold placed over side of mattress. **C**, Linen tucked under mattress.

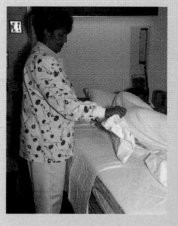

STEP 19   Optional drawsheet.

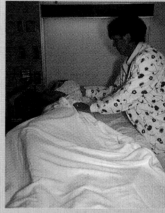

STEP 22   Assisting client to roll over folds of linen.

STEPS	RATIONALE
27. Facing side of bed, grasp remaining edge of bottom flat sheet. Lean back; keep back straight; and pull while tucking excess linen under mattress. Proceed from head to foot of bed. (Avoid lifting mattress during tucking to ensure fit.)	Proper use of body mechanics while tucking linen prevents injury.
28. Smooth fanfolded drawsheet out over bottom sheet. Grasp edge of sheet with palms down; lean back; and tuck sheet under mattress. Tuck from middle to top and then to bottom.	Tucking first at top or bottom may pull sheet sideways, causing poor fit.
29. Place top sheet over client with centerfold lengthwise down middle of bed. Open sheet from head to foot, and unfold over client.	Sheet should be equally distributed over bed by correctly positioning centerfold.
30. Ask client to hold clean top sheet, or tuck sheet around client's shoulders. Remove bath blanket and discard in linen bag.	Sheet prevents exposure of body parts. Having client hold sheet encourages client participation in care.
31. Place blanket on bed, unfolding it so that crease runs lengthwise along middle of bed. Unfold blanket to cover client. Top edge should be parallel with edge of top sheet and 15 to 20 cm (6 to 8 in) from top sheet's edge.	Blanket should be placed to cover client completely and provide adequate warmth.
32. Place spread over bed according to Step 31. Be sure that top edge of spread extends about 2.5 cm (1 in) above blanket's edge. Tuck top edge of spread over and under top edge of blanket.	Gives bed neat appearance and provides extra warmth.
33. Make cuff by turning edge of top sheet down over top edge of blanket and spread.	Protect client's face from rubbing against blanket or spread.
34. Standing on one side at foot of bed, lift mattress corner slightly with one hand and tuck linens under mattress. Top sheet and blanket are tucked under together. Be sure that linens are loose enough to allow movement of client's feet. Making a horizontal toe pleat is an option.	Makes neat-appearing bed. Pressure ulcers can develop on client's toes and heels from feet rubbing against tight-fitting bed sheets.
35. Make modified mitered corner with top sheet, blanket, and spread (see illustration in Box 26-10, p. 638):	Ensures top covers will not loosen easily.
a. Pick up side edge of top sheet, blanket, and spread approximately 45 cm (18 in) from foot of mattress. Lift linen to form triangular fold, and lay it on bed.	
b. Tuck lower edge of sheet, which is hanging free below mattress, under mattress. Do not pull triangular fold.	
c. Pick up triangular fold, and bring it down over mattress while holding linen in place along side of mattress. Do not tuck tip of triangle.	Secures top linen but keeps even edge of blanket and top sheet draped over mattress.
36. Raise side rail. Make other side of bed; spread sheet, blanket, and bedspread out evenly. Fold top edge of spread over blanket and make cuff with top sheet (see Step 33); make modified mitered corner at foot of bed (see Step 35).	Side rail protects client from accidental falls.
37. Change pillowcase:	
a. Have client raise head. While supporting neck with one hand, remove pillow. Allow client to lower head.	Support of neck muscles prevents injury during flexion and extension of neck.
b. Remove soiled case by grasping pillow at open end with one hand and pulling case back over pillow with the other hand. Discard case in linen bag.	Pillows slide out easily, thus minimizing contact with soiled linen.
c. Grasp clean pillowcase at center of closed end. Gather case, turning it inside out over the hand holding it. With the same hand, pick up middle of one end of the pillow. Pull pillowcase down over pillow with the other hand.	Eases sliding of pillowcase over pillow.

STEPS	RATIONALE
d. Be sure pillow corners fit evenly into corners of pillowcase. Place pillow under client's head.	Poorly fitting case constricts fluffing and expansion of pillow and interferes with client comfort.
38. Place call light within client's reach, and return bed to comfortable position.	Ensures client safety and comfort.
39. Open room curtains, and rearrange furniture. Place personal items within easy reach on over-bed table or bedside stand. Return bed to a comfortable height.	Promotes sense of well-being.
40. Discard dirty linen in hamper or chute and wash hands.	Prevents transmission of microorganisms.
41. Ask if client feels comfortable.	Ensures bed linens are clean and smooth.
42. Inspect skin for areas of irritation.	Folds in linen can cause pressure on skin.
43. Observe client for signs of fatigue, dyspnea, pain, or discomfort.	Provides you with data about client's level of activity tolerance and ability to participate in other procedures.

UNEXPECTED OUTCOMES AND RELATED INTERVENTIONS

- Client feels discomfort from linen fold.
  - Tighten sheets.
  - Change client's position frequently.
- Client's skin shows signs of breakdown.
  - Institute skin care measures to reduce risk of pressure ulcer (see Chapter 34).
  - Change client's position frequently.

RECORDING AND REPORTING

- Making an occupied bed need not be recorded.

Key Terms

acne, p. 605
buccal cavity, p. 601
complete bed bath, p. 611

dental caries, p. 607
dermis, p. 601
epidermis, p. 601
maceration, p. 615
oral hygiene, p. 607

partial bed bath, p. 611
perineal care, p. 611
subcutaneous, p. 601

Key Concepts

- Provide clients' daily hygiene needs if they are unable to care for themselves adequately.
- Providing hygiene care gives you the chance to assess external body surfaces and the client's emotional state.
- While providing daily hygiene needs, use teaching and communication skills to develop a relationship with the client.
- The client's personal preferences must always be considered when you plan daily hygiene care.
- You must maintain privacy and comfort when providing the client's daily care.
- During assessment of the skin and oral mucosa, observe characteristics influenced by hygiene.
- Clients who are immobilized and poorly nourished and who have reduced sensation or peripheral circulation are at risk for altered skin integrity.
- Wear gloves during hygiene care when the risk of contacting body fluids is high, and always wear gloves during perineal care.
- Clients with diabetes need special nail and foot care.
- When administering oral care to unconscious clients, take measures to prevent aspiration.
- Evaluation of hygiene care is based on the client's sense of comfort, relaxation, well-being, and understanding of hygiene techniques.

Critical Thinking Activities

1. Mr. Roberts, an 80-year-old widower who lives alone, is admitted to the intensive care unit. He is obese and has poor hygiene. His skin is rough and dry with some areas of excoriation. What are the most important assessments to be made in the situation? What appropriate interventions may be used?

2. Mrs. John, a 30-year-old woman, is admitted to the neurological unit following a spinal cord injury. She is now a quadriplegic. In terms of hygiene needs, what are the priorities in taking care of Mrs. John?

3. Mr. Green, a 52-year-old man, has been on long-term therapy for peripheral vascular disease. He has been on coumarin therapy. Coumarin is an anticoagulant (blood thinner) that is frequently prescribed for clients with circulatory disorders, as is the case with Mr. Green's peripheral vascular disease. What home care instructions are essential in his discharge planning in regard to hygiene?

Review Questions

1. During the first postoperative day following abdominal surgery, your client will probably require a:
   1. shower.
   2. tub bath.
   3. partial bath.
   4. complete bed bath.

2. In addition to bathing, the following intervention may best assist in promoting client comfort:
   1. back rub.
   2. books on tape.
   3. nighttime snack.
   4. postural drainage.

3. The most important priority when providing oral hygiene to the unconscious client is to:
   1. prevent aspiration.
   2. prevent mouth odor.
   3. prevent dental caries.
   4. prevent mouth ulcerations.

4. The goal of meticulous foot care for clients is to:
   1. prevent injury to the toes and feet.
   2. provide routine cleaning of the feet and nails.
   3. to monitor the healing process of foot ulcers.
   4. to determine if the client's shoes are the proper size.

5. The method for trimming nails is:
   1. cut the nail in a curve.
   2. cut the nail straight across.
   3. cut the nail toward the cuticles.
   4. cut the nail to meet the shape of the finger.

6. When providing hygiene to the older adult is important to remember that the older adult's skin is:
   1. fragile with decreased elasticity.
   2. fragile with increased elasticity.
   3. fragile with increased circulation.
   4. fragile with increased muscle mass.

References

American Diabetes Association: Position statement on preventive foot care in people with diabetes: clinical practice recommendations 1999, *Diabetes Care* 22(suppl 1):1, 1999.

Armstrong DG, Lavery LA: Diabetic foot ulcers: prevention, diagnosis and classification, *Am Fam Physician* 57(6):1325, 1998.

Bennett MA: Report of the task force on the implications for darkly pigmented intact skin in the prediction and prevention of pressure ulcers, *Adv Wound Care* 8(6):34, 1995.

Blaney GM: Mouthcare—basic and essential, *Geriatr Nurs* 7:242, 1986.

Christensen MH and others: How to care for the diabetic foot, *Am J Nurs* 91(3):50, 1991.

Cooppan R, Habershaw G: Preventing leg and foot complications, *Patient Care* 29(3):35, 1995.

Danielson LH: Oral care and older adults, *J Gerontol Nurs* 7:242, 1988.

Dudjak LA: Mouthcare for mucositis due to radiation therapy, *Cancer Nurs* 10:131, 1987.

Fitch JA and others: Oral care in the adult intensive care unit, *Am J Crit Care* 8(2):314, 1999.

Greifzu S and others: Oral care is part of cancer care, *RN* 53:43, 1990.

Harrell JS, Damon JF: Prediction of patients' need for mouth care, *West J Nurs Res* 11:748, 1989.

Labyak SE, Metzger BL: The effects of effleurage backrub on the physiological components of relaxation: a meta analysis, *Nurs Res* 46:59, 1997.

Lueckenotte AG: *Gerontologic nursing,* ed 2, St. Louis, 2000, Mosby.

Mahoney DF: Cerumen impaction: prevalence and detection in nursing homes, *J Gerontol Nurs* 54(12):56, 1993.

Maklebust J: Pressure ulcer update, *RN* 41(12):56, 1991.

National Pressure Ulcer Advisory Panel (NPUAP): Pressure ulcer incidence, economics, risk assessment: consensus development conference statement, *Decubitus* 2(2):24, 1989.

Ney DF: Cerumen impaction, ear hygiene practices, and hearing acuity, *Geriatr Nurs* 14(2):70, 1993.

Osterman HM, Struck KM: The aging foot, *Orthop Nurs* 9:43, 1990.

Panel for the Prediction and Prevention for Pressure Ulcers in Adults (PPUA): Assessing risk and preventing pressure ulcers, *Patient Care* 27(7):36, 1993.

Poland JM: Comparing Moi-Stir to lemon glycerin swabs, *Am J Nurs* 87:422, 1987.

Skewes SM: No more bed baths! *RN* 57:34, 1994.

Strauss MB and others: Preventive foot care: a user friendly system for patients and physicians. *Postgrad Med* 103(5):233, 1998.

U.S. Department of Health and Human Services (USDHHS): *Prediction and prevention,* Pub No. 92-0047, 92-0050, Rockville, Md, 1994, PHS, Agency for Health Care Policy and Research.

Oxygenation

27

Objectives

- Define the key terms listed.
- Identify physiological processes in maintaining cardiac output, myocardial blood flow, coronary artery blood flow, ventilation, perfusion, and respiratory gas exchange.
- Explain the relationship between myocardial electrical conduction and pump function.
- Explain how health status, age, lifestyle, and environmental factors can affect oxygenation.
- Identify causes and effects of disturbances in conduction, altered cardiac output, impaired valvular function, myocardial ischemia, and impaired tissue perfusion.
- Identify clinical signs and symptoms of a client with altered oxygenation.
- Perform a nursing assessment of the cardiopulmonary system.
- Develop nursing diagnoses for altered oxygenation.
- Describe nursing interventions to promote, maintain, or restore cardiopulmonary function.
- Develop evaluation criteria for a care plan for the client with altered oxygenation.

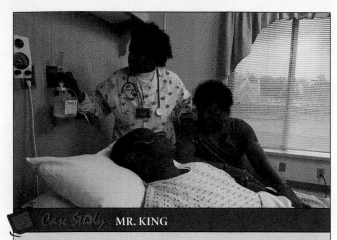

Case Study MR. KING

Mr. King, 74 years old, came to the hospital 2 days ago with complaints of chest pain, weakness, and a high temperature. Mr. King is a retired bookbinder who resides in a mobile home with his wife. Both have preexisting health conditions that put them at risk for pneumonia. Mrs. King is diabetic and takes insulin twice daily. Mr. King has a history of alcohol abuse but at present is not drinking. Both individuals are heavy smokers and have been for more than 50 years. Currently they are not using any external support systems outside the home. Mrs. King performs most of the household duties and grocery shops once each week with the help of her daughter. Mr. King used to help out with the housework, and he loves to tinker in the garden; however, lately he has been unable to do either. His wife states, "All he seems to be able to do is sit in his chair and watch TV."

Mary Brown is a junior nursing student assigned to her first hospital-based clinical experience. Mary has had some experience in health assessment and client teaching related to health promotion activities from her recent clinical rotation in a clinic. In the previous clinical experience, clients were motivated to adjust their at-risk health behaviors, such as smoking or poor diet. Mary feels confident when she arrives in the clinical area this morning because Mr. King has similar health needs to the clinical experiences she has had. However, when Mary goes to meet Mr. King and performs her morning assessment, she is overwhelmed. This client is in a great deal of respiratory distress. It seems that every breath is a struggle for him. Everything that Mary has planned to do seems less important. The client is extremely anxious. His wife is at his side anticipating Mary's every move, and demanding some action.

SCIENTIFIC KNOWLEDGE BASE

Oxygen is a basic human need and is required for life. You will frequently encounter clients who are unable to meet their oxygenation needs, which may be the result of an ineffective pump (heart disease) or ineffective gas exchange (lung disease).

Cardiopulmonary Physiology

The function of the cardiopulmonary system is to provide oxygen to the tissues and remove carbon dioxide and waste products from the body.

STRUCTURE AND FUNCTION. The heart provides the mechanism by which oxygenated blood is sent from the lungs to the body. Once oxygenated blood is delivered, the tissues of the body are able to carry out selected metabolic activities. The cardiovascular system then delivers carbon dioxide and other waste products to the lung for elimination. The pumping action of the heart is essential to maintain oxygen delivery. The four heart valves (tricuspid, pulmonic, mitral, aortic) ensure the one-way flow of blood through the heart.

REGULATION OF BLOOD FLOW. There are multiple regulators of blood flow (Table 27-1). Heart rate affects blood flow because of the interaction between rate and diastolic filling time. With a sustained heart rate greater than 160 beats/min, diastolic filling time decreases, causing **stroke volume** (SV) and **cardiac output** (CO) to decrease. In some situations you will also care for clients with long-term cardiovascular disease whose SV and CO will decrease with heart rates greater than 120 beats per minute. Clients with decreased myocardial reserve may experience decreased SV and CO with a heart rate less than 160 beats per minute. The heart rate of the older adult is slow to increase under stress. To compensate for this, the SV may increase in order to increase the CO and blood pressure (Lueckenotte, 2000).

CONDUCTION SYSTEM. The rhythmic relaxation and contraction of the atria and ventricles depend on continuous, organized transmission of electrical impulses to the muscle. These impulses are generated and transmitted by the conduction system.

The heart's conduction system generates the necessary impulses required to initiate the electrical mechanical chain of events. The autonomic nervous system influences the rate of impulse generation, the transmission speed through the conductive pathway, and the strength of contractions through sympathetic and parasympathetic nerve fibers in the atria and ventricles (the vagus nerve fibers in the atria and ventricles). The vagus nerve (parasympathetic) also innervates sinoatrial and atrioventricular nodes and can reduce the rate of impulse generation.

The conduction system originates with the **sinoatrial (SA) node,** the "pacemaker" of the heart. The SA node is in the right atrium next to the entrance of the superior vena cava. Impulses are initiated at the SA node at an intrinsic rate of 60 to 100 beats per minute. The resting adult rate ranges from 60 to 80 beats per minute. The older adult may have a wide range from the 40s to more than 100 beats per minute (Seidel and others, 1999).

The electrical impulses are then transmitted along intraatrial pathways to the **atrioventricular (AV) node.** The AV node mediates impulse transmission between the atria and the ventricles. Atrial emptying is assisted by delaying the impulse at the AV node before transmitting it through the **bundle of His** and ventricular **Purkinje network.**

The electrical activity of the conduction system is recorded on an **electrocardiogram (ECG)** as waves and

Regulation of Blood Flow
Table 27-1

Regulator	Definition
Cardiac output	Amount of blood ejected from the left ventricle per minute
	Normal range (adult): 4-6 L/min
Cardiac index	Measure of adequacy of the cardiac output; cardiac index equals cardiac output divided by the client's body surface area
	Normal range (adult): 2.5-4 L/min/m^3
Stroke volume	Amount of blood ejected from the ventricle with each contraction
	Normal range (adult): 50-75 ml/contraction
Preload	Amount of blood in the ventricles at end diastole
Afterload	Resistance of the ejection of blood from the left ventricle
Myocardial contractility	Ability of the heart to squeeze blood from the ventricles and prepare for the next contraction

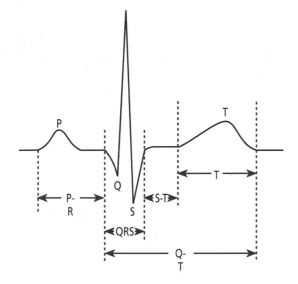

FIGURE **27-1**   Normal ECG waveform. (From Canobbio MM: *Cardiovascular disorders*, St. Louis, 1990, Mosby.)

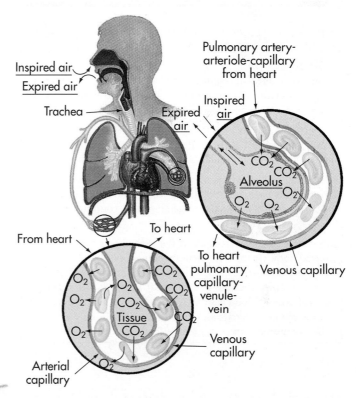

FIGURE **27-2**   Structures of the pulmonary system. The circle denotes the alveoli. (Modified from Wilson SF, Thompson JM: *Mosby's clinical nursing series: respiratory disorders*, St. Louis, 1990, Mosby.)

complexes. An ECG monitors the regularity and path of the electrical impulse through the conduction system; however, it does not reflect the muscular work of the heart. The normal sequence on the ECG is called **normal sinus rhythm (NSR)** (Figure 27-1).

Gas Exchange

For the exchange of respiratory gases to occur, the organs, nerves, and muscles of respiration must be intact and the central nervous system must be able to regulate the respiratory cycle (Figure 27-2).

REGULATION OF RESPIRATION.   Respiratory regulation provides for adequate oxygen to meet the metabolic demand, such as during exercise, infection, or pregnancy (Table 27-2). Respiratory regulation promotes exhalation of metabolically produced carbon dioxide, which is a determinant of acid-base status (see Chapter 14).

Neural and chemical regulators control respiration (Box 27-1). Neural regulation includes the central nervous system control of respiratory rate, depth, and rhythm. Chemical regulation involves the influence of chemicals, such as carbon dioxide and hydrogen ions, on the rate and depth of respiration.

OXYGEN TRANSPORT.   The delivery of oxygen depends on the amount of oxygen entering the lungs (oxygenation), blood flow to the lungs and tissues (perfusion), the oxygen-carrying capacity of the blood (rate of **diffusion**) and the amount of carbon dioxide excreted by the lungs (**ventilation**). The capacity of the blood to carry oxygen is influenced by the amount of dissolved oxygen in the plasma, amount of hemoglobin, and a tendency of hemoglobin to bind with oxygen. Only a relatively small amount

Regulation of Respiration
Table 27-2

Regulator	Definition
Work of breathing	Effort required expanding and contracting the lungs
	Determined by the degree of lung compliance, airway resistance, presence of active expiration, and use of accessory muscles of respiration
Compliance	Degree of elasticity or expandability of the lungs and thorax
Airway resistance	Impedance of airflow through the anatomical airways
Elastic recoil	Tendency of the thoracic cage to contract (relax) after a normal inspiration, resulting in passive expiration

Neural and Chemical Regulation of Respiration
Box 27-1

NEURAL REGULATION
Neural regulation maintains rhythm and depth of respiration, as well as the balance between inspiration and expiration.

CEREBRAL CORTEX
Voluntary control of respiration delivers impulses to the respiratory motor neurons by way of the spinal cord. Voluntary control of respiration accommodates speaking, eating, and swimming.

MEDULLA OBLONGATA
Automatic control of respiration occurs continuously.

CHEMICAL REGULATION
Chemical regulation maintains appropriate rate and depth of respirations based on changes in the blood's carbon dioxide (CO_2), oxygen (O_2), and hydrogen ion (H^+) concentration.

CHEMORECEPTORS
Chemoreceptors are located in the medulla, aortic body, and carotid body. Changes in chemical content of O_2, CO_2, and H^+ stimulate chemoreceptors, which in turn stimulate neural regulators to adjust the rate and depth of ventilation to maintain normal arterial blood gas levels. Chemical regulation can occur during physical exercise and in some illnesses. It is a short-term adaptive mechanism.

of oxygen, about 3%, is dissolved in the plasma. Most oxygen is transported by hemoglobin, which serves as a carrier for oxygen and carbon dioxide. The hemoglobin molecule combines with oxygen to form oxyhemoglobin. The formation of oxyhemoglobin is easily reversible, allowing hemoglobin and oxygen to dissociate, which frees oxygen to enter tissues.

CARBON DIOXIDE TRANSPORT. Carbon dioxide diffuses into red blood cells and is rapidly hydrated into carbonic acid (H_2CO_3). The carbonic acid then dissociates (breaks apart) into hydrogen (H^+) and bicarbonate (HCO_3^-) ions. The hydrogen ion is buffered by hemoglobin and the HCO_3^- diffuses into the plasma (see Chapter 14). Reduced hemoglobin (deoxyhemoglobin) can combine with carbon dioxide more easily than can oxyhemoglobin, and therefore venous blood transports most of the carbon dioxide back to the lungs for excretion in expired air.

Factors Affecting Oxygenation
Any condition that affects cardiopulmonary functioning directly affects the body's ability to meet oxygen demands. The general classifications of cardiac disorders include disturbances in conduction, impaired valvular function, myocardial ischemia, cardiomyopathic conditions, and peripheral tissue hypoxia. Respiratory disorders include hyperventilation, hypoventilation, and hypoxia.

Other pathophysiological processes affecting a client's oxygenation include alterations that affect the oxygen-carrying capacity of blood (e.g., anemia), increases in the body's metabolic demands (e.g., fever, infection), and alterations that affect the client's chest wall movement or the central nervous system.

DECREASED OXYGEN-CARRYING CAPACITY. Hemoglobin carries 97% of oxygen to tissues. Any process that decreases or alters hemoglobin, such as anemia or inhalation of toxic substances, decreases the oxygen-carrying capacity of blood. Carbon monoxide is the most common toxic inhalant decreasing the oxygen-carrying capacity of blood. Hemoglobin tends to bind with carbon monoxide 210 times more readily than with oxygen, creating a functional hypoxemia. Because of the bond's strength, carbon monoxide is not easily dissociated from hemoglobin, making the hemoglobin unavailable for oxygen transport.

DECREASED INSPIRED OXYGEN CONCENTRATION. When the concentration of inspired oxygen declines, the oxygen-carrying capacity of the blood is decreased. Decreases in the fraction of inspired oxygen (F_IO_2) concentration can be caused by an upper or lower airway obstruction limiting delivery of inspired oxygen to alveoli. Decreased environmental oxygen (as occurs at high altitudes) or decreased delivery of inspired oxygen, as the result of an incorrect oxygen concentration setting on respiratory therapy equipment, may also result in a decreased F_IO_2.

HYPOVOLEMIA. Hypovolemia is a reduced circulating blood volume resulting from extracellular fluid losses that occurs in conditions such as shock and severe dehydration. If the fluid loss is significant, the body tries to adapt by increasing the heart rate and constricting peripheral vessels to increase the volume of blood returned to the heart and increase the cardiac output.

Signs and Symptoms of Hypoxemia

Box 27-2

ACUTE
Restlessness
Apprehension
Anxiety
Decreased ability to concentrate
Increased fatigue
Dizziness
Behavioral changes
Increased heart rate
Increased rate and depth of respiration
Increased blood pressure
Pallor
Shortness of breath
Cardiac dysrhythmias, such as premature ventriculare contractions (PVCs), premature atrial contractions (PACs), sinus tachycardia (ST)

LATE
Decreased level of consciousness
Decreased respiratory rate
Decreased blood pressure
Cardiac dysrhythmias, such as ventricular tachycardia (V-tach), ventricular fibrillation (V-fib), asystole
Central cyanosis

CHRONIC
Clubbing of fingers
Cardiac dysrhythmias, such as PVCs, PACs
Increased fatigue
Shortness of breath

INCREASED METABOLIC RATE. Increases in metabolic activity of the body result in an increased oxygen demand. When the body is unable to meet this increased demand, the level of oxygenation falls. An increased metabolic rate is a normal response of the body to pregnancy, wound healing, and exercise because the body is building tissue. Most people can meet the increased oxygen demand and do not display signs of oxygen deprivation.

Fever increases the tissues' need for oxygen. As a result, carbon dioxide production also increases. If the febrile state persists, the metabolic rate remains high and the body begins to break down protein stores, resulting in muscle wasting and decreased muscle mass. Respiratory muscles, such as the diaphragm and intercostals, are also wasted. The body attempts to adapt to the increased carbon dioxide (**hypercapnia**) levels by increasing the rate and depth of respiration to eliminate the excess carbon dioxide. The client's work of breathing increases, and the client will eventually display signs and symptoms of **hypoxemia,** a decreased arterial oxygen level in the blood (Box 27-2). Clients with pulmonary diseases are at greater risk for hypoxemia and hypercapnia, an elevated arterial carbon dioxide level. Client assessment reveals increased rate and depth of respiration, use of the accessory muscles of respiration, use of pursed-lip breathing, and decreased activity tolerance.

CONDITIONS AFFECTING CHEST WALL MOVEMENT. Any condition that reduces chest wall movement can result in decreased ventilation. If the diaphragm cannot fully descend with breathing, the volume of inspired air decreases and less oxygen is delivered to the alveoli and subsequently to tissues.

MUSCULOSKELETAL ABNORMALITIES. Abnormalities in the thoracic region may contribute to decreased oxygenation and ventilation. These can result from abnormal structural configurations, trauma, muscle diseases, or diseases of the nervous system. Abnormal structural configurations impairing oxygenation include those that affect the rib cage, such as pectus excavatum, and those that affect the spinal column, such as kyphosis. The angle of curvature in kyphosis can progress with time, resulting in severe hypoventilation and hypoxemia.

Muscle diseases, such as muscular dystrophy, affect oxygenation of tissues by decreasing the client's ability to expand and contract the chest. Ventilation is impaired, and **atelectasis,** hypercapnia, and hypoxemia can occur.

NERVOUS SYSTEM DISEASES. Myasthenia gravis, Guillain-Barré syndrome, and poliomyelitis are examples of nervous system diseases that affect respiratory functioning and result in hypoventilation. These diseases impair nervous and muscular control. When the nerves and muscles of the respiratory system are affected, impaired ventilation (hypoventilation) occurs.

Disease or trauma involving the medulla oblongata and spinal cord of the central nervous system may impair respiration. When the medulla oblongata is affected, neural regulation of respiration is damaged and abnormal breathing patterns may develop. Damage to the spinal cord can affect respiration in two ways. If the phrenic nerve is damaged, the diaphragm may not descend, thus reducing inspiratory lung volumes and causing hypoxemia. Cervical trauma at C3 to C5 can result in paralysis of the phrenic nerve. Spinal cord trauma below the fifth cervical vertebra usually leaves the phrenic nerve intact but damages nerves that innervate the intercostal muscles, preventing anteroposterior chest expansion.

TRAUMA. Trauma to the chest wall also impairs inspiration. The person with multiple rib fractures can develop a flail chest, a condition in which fractures cause instability in part of the chest wall. This can cause paradoxical breathing in which the lung underlying the injured area contracts on inspiration and expands on expiration.

Chest wall or upper abdominal incisions also decrease chest wall movement because the client exhibits shallow respirations to decrease chest wall movement and reduce incisional pain.

PAIN MANAGEMENT. Excessive or high doses of narcotic analgesics may depress the respiratory center, thus decreasing respiratory rate, depth, and chest wall expansion.

CHRONIC DISEASE. Oxygenation is decreased as a direct consequence of chronic disease and is decreased as a secondary effect, as with anemia. The physiological response to chronic hypoxemia is the development of a secondary polycythemia, which is an increase in red blood cells. This adaptive response is the body's attempt to increase the amount of circulating hemoglobin to increase the available oxygen-binding sites and to improve oxygen transport; as a result the client's oxygenation improves.

Alterations in Cardiac Functioning

Illnesses and conditions that affect cardiac rate, rhythm, strength of contraction, blood flow through the chambers, myocardial blood flow, and peripheral circulation can cause altered cardiac functioning.

DISTURBANCES IN CONDUCTION. Some disturbances in conduction are the result of electrical impulses that do not originate from the SA node. These rhythm disturbances are called **dysrhythmias,** meaning a deviation from the normal sinus rhythm (Table 27-3). Dysrhythmias can occur as a primary conduction disturbances; as a response to ischemia, valvular abnormality, anxiety, and drug toxicity; as a result of caffeine, alcohol, or tobacco use; or as a complication of acid-base or electrolyte imbalance (see Chapter 14).

In addition to the site of impluse origin, cardiac response is used to classify dysrhythmias. The response can be an increase in heart rate or tachycardia (a rate greater than 100 beats per minute), a decrease in rate, or bradycardia (a rate less than 60 beats per minute), premature (early beat) atrial or ventricular beats, or blocked (delayed or absent beat) atrial or ventricular beats.

ALTERED CARDIAC OUTPUT. Failure of the myocardium to eject sufficient blood volume to the systemic and pulmonary circulations can result in heart failure. Failure of the myocardial pump results from primary CAD, cardiomyopathic conditions, valvular disorders, and pulmonary disease.

MYOCARDIAL ISCHEMIA. **Myocardial ischemia** results when the coronary artery does not supply sufficient blood to the myocardium. Decreased perfusion to the myocardium results in chest pain, especially with activity, and your client may have angina or angina pectoris. Angina is the result of decreased blood flow to the myocardium from spasms of the coronary arteries or temporary constriction. When the decreased perfusion is extensive or completely blocked, the tissue becomes necrotic and a **myocardial infarction** occurs. Myocardial infarction presents clinically as severe chest pain, breathlessness, diaphoresis, and usually a fall in blood pressure.

LEFT-SIDED HEART FAILURE. **Left-sided heart failure** is an abnormal condition characterized by impaired functioning of the left ventricle, usually caused by chronically elevated arterial pressures and pulmonary congestion. If left ventricular failure is significant, the amount of blood ejected from the left ventricle drops greatly, resulting in decreased cardiac output.

RIGHT-SIDED HEART FAILURE. **Right-sided heart failure** results from impaired functioning of the right ventricle. This is characterized by venous congestion in the systemic circulation. On assessment your client's jugular veins may be distended and peripheral edema may be present. Right-sided heart failure more commonly results from pulmonary diseases or as an outcome of left-sided or right-sided heart failure.

IMPAIRED VALVULAR FUNCTION. **Valvular heart disease** is an acquired or congenital disorder of a cardiac valve characterized by stenosis and obstructed blood flow or valvular degeneration and regurgitation (backflow) of blood. When stenosis occurs in the semilunar valves (aortic and pulmonic valves), the adjacent ventricles must work harder to move the ventricular volume beyond the stenotic valve. When regurgitation occurs, there is a backflow of blood into an adjacent chamber.

Alterations in Respiratory Functioning

Illnesses and conditions that affect ventilation or oxygen transport cause alterations in respiratory functioning. The three primary alterations are hyperventilation, hypoventilation, and hypoxia.

HYPERVENTILATION. Hyperventilation is an increase in respiratory rate resulting in excess amounts of carbon dioxide elimination. Anxiety, infections, drugs, or an acid-base imbalance can cause hyperventilation. Hypoxia associated with pulmonary embolus or shock may result in hyperventilation. Acute anxiety and an increased respiratory rate may cause loss of consciousness from excess carbon dioxide exhalation.

Fever also causes hyperventilation. For each increase of 1° F, there is a 7% increase in the metabolic rate, thereby increasing carbon dioxide production. The clinical response is increased rate and depth of respiration.

Hyperventilation is also chemically induced. Salicylate (aspirin) poisoning causes excessive stimulation of the respiratory center as the body attempts to compensate for excessive carbon dioxide. Amphetamines also increase ventilation by raising carbon dioxide production. Hyperventilation occurs as the body tries to compensate for metabolic acidosis by producing a respiratory alkalosis. Ventilation increases to reduce the amount of carbon dioxide available to form carbonic acid (see Chapter 14).

Hyperventilation produces many signs and symptoms (Box 27-3).

HYPOVENTILATION. Hypoventilation occurs when ventilation is inadequate to meet the body's oxygen demand or to eliminate carbon dioxide (Box 27-4). As ventilation decreases, arterial carbon dioxide ($PaCO_2$) is elevated. Severe

Common Basic Cardiac Dysrhythmias

Table 27-3

Rhythm Characteristics	Etiology	Clinical Significance	Management
Sinus Tachycardia Regular rhythm, rate 100-180 beats/min (higher in infants), normal P wave, normal QRS complex	Rate increase may be normal response to exercise, emotion, or stressors, such as pain, fever, pump failure, hyperthyroidism, and certain drugs (e.g., caffeine, nitrates, atropine, epinephrine, isoproterenol, nicotine)	May have hemodynamic consequence in client with damaged heart that is unable to sustain increased workloads (increased myocardial oxygen consumption) brought on by persistent increases in heart rate	Correct underlying factors; remove offending drugs

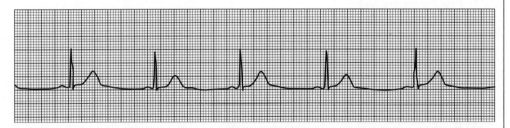

Sinus Bradycardia Regular rhythm, rate <60 beats/min, normal P wave, normal PR interval, normal QRS complex	Rate decrease may be normal response to sleep or in well-conditioned athlete; abnormal drops in rate may be caused by diminished blood flow to SA node, vagal stimulation, hypothyroidism, increased intracranial pressure, or pharmacological agents (e.g., digoxin, propranolol, quinidine, procainamide)	No clinical significance unless associated with signs of impaired cardiac output and symptoms of dizziness, syncope, chest pain	Correct underlying causes; administer atropine, 0.5-1.0 mg IV; may need to implant transvenous pacemaker

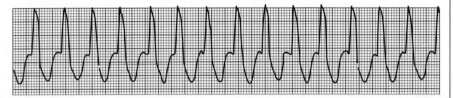

Sinus Dysrhythmia Irregular rhythm; possibly phasic with respiration, slowing during inspiration and increasing with expiration; rate of 60-100 beats/min; normal P wave; normal PR interval; normal QRS complex	Sinus rhythm with cyclical variation caused by vagal impulses that influence rhythm during respiration; occurs commonly in children, young adults, and older adults; usually disappears as heart rate increases	No clinical significance unless heart rate decreases and symptoms of dizziness occur with decreased rate	None indicated unless heart rate decreases and symptoms occur

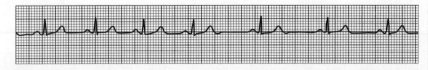

Modified from Canobbio MM: *Cardiovascular disorders,* St. Louis, 1990, Mosby.

Continued

Common Basic Cardiac Dysrhythmias—cont'd

Table 27-3

Rhythm Characteristics	Etiology	Clinical Significance	Management

Supraventricular Tachycardia (SVT)

Sudden, rapid onset of tachycardia with stimulus originating above AV node; regular rhythm; rate 150-250 beats/min; P wave uniform, possibly buried in preceding T wave; PR interval variable, often difficult to measure; normal QRS complex	May begin and end spontaneously or be precipitated by excitement, fatigue, or caffeine, smoking, or alcohol use	Usually no significant impairment; client complains of palpitations and shortness of breath; if persistent or occurring in client with preexisting organic heart disease, may cause decrease in cardiac output and/or blood pressure, resulting in pump failure or shock	Have experienced clinician perform vagal stimulation with carotid sinus massage. Physician may order drugs to decrease ventricular response with medication to block AV conduction: verapamil, 5-10 mg IV push; propranolol slowly IV in 1-mg increments up to 4 mg (contraindicated in clients with heart failure); edrophonium, test dose 1 mg followed by 10 mg IV. Perform cardioversion if resistant to preceding measures

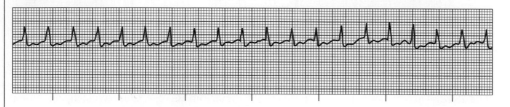

Premature Ventricular Contractions (PVCs)

Irregular rhythm with ectopic beats followed by full compensatory pause; rate normal or increased depending on number of ectopic beats; P wave absent in ectopic beat; PR interval absent; QRS complex widened and distorted; T wave in opposition to R wave	Caused by irritable focus within ventricle, commonly associated with myocardial infarction; other causes include hypoxia, hypocalcemia, acidosis	PVCs occurring frequently (>6/min) or in pairs, indicating increased ventricular irritability	Try to suppress PVCs; if PVCs frequent, administer IV bolus of lidocaine (50-100 mg) followed by continuous IV infusion; administer additional antidysrhythmic agents as needed

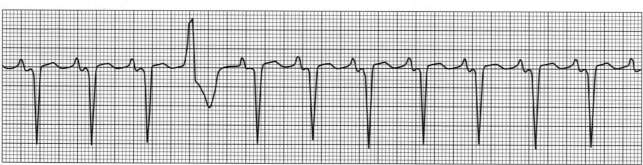

Ventricular Tachycardia

Rhythm slightly irregular, rate 100-200 beats/min, P wave absent, PR interval absent, QRS complex wide and bizarre, >0.12 sec	Caused by irritable ventricular foci firing repetitively, commonly caused by myocardial infarction	Often a forerunner of ventricular fibrillation; if condition persistent and rapid, causes decreased cardiac output because of decreased ventricular filling time	Most episodes terminate abruptly without treatment; administer IV bolus of lidocaine (75-100 mg) followed by continuous IV drip; perform cardioversion

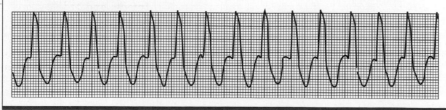

<table>
<tr><td colspan="2">

Signs and Symptoms of Hyperventilation   Box 27-3

</td></tr>
<tr><td>

Tachycardia
Shortness of breath
Chest pain
Dizziness
Light-headedness
Decreased concentration
Paresthesia

</td><td>

Numbness (extremities, circumoral)
Tinnitus
Blurred vision
Disorientation
Tetany (carpopedal spasm)

</td></tr>
</table>

Signs and Symptoms of Hypoventilation   Box 27-4

Dizziness	Cardiac dysrhythmias
Headache (may be occipital only on awakening)	Electrolyte imbalances
	Convulsions
Lethargy	Coma
Disorientation	Cardiac arrest
Decreased ability to follow instructions	

Classification of Hypoxia and Related Causes   Box 27-5

Lowered oxygen-carrying capacity
  Decreased hemoglobin level (e.g., anemia)
  Carbon monoxide poisoning
A diminished concentration of inspired oxygen
  High altitudes
  Obstructed airway
Inability of the tissues to extract oxygen from the blood
  Cyanide poisoning
  Septic shock
Decreased diffusion of oxygen from the alveoli to the blood
  Pneumonia
  Atelectasis
Poor tissue perfusion with oxygenated blood
  Hypovolemic shock
  Cardiogenic shock
  Cardiomyopathy
Impaired ventilation
  Multiple rib fractures or chest trauma
  Spinal cord trauma
  Head trauma

atelectasis, a collapse of the alveoli, can produce hypoventilation. As alveoli collapse, less of the lung can be ventilated and hypoventilation occurs.

When caring for clients with chronic obstructive pulmonary disease (COPD) and chronically elevated $PaCO_2$ levels, remember that inappropriate administration of excessive oxygen can result in hypoventilation. Be aware clients with COPD have adapted to a high carbon dioxide level. Their carbon dioxide–sensitive chemoreceptors are essentially not functioning, and the stimulus to breathe is a decreased PaO_2.

If excessive oxygen is administered, the oxygen requirement is satisfied and the stimulus to breathe is negated. High concentrations of oxygen (e.g., greater than 24% to 28% [1 to 3 L/min]) prevent the PaO_2 from falling and obliterate the stimulus to breathe, resulting in hypoventilation. The excessive retention of carbon dioxide may lead to respiratory arrest. If untreated, your client's status can rapidly decline. Convulsions, unconsciousness, and death can result.

Treatment for hyperventilation and hypoventilation begins by treating the underlying cause, then improving tissue oxygenation, restoring ventilatory function, and achieving acid-base balance.

HYPOXIA. Hypoxia is inadequate tissue oxygenation at the cellular level. Hypoxia results from a deficiency in oxygen delivery or oxygen utilization at the cellular level (Box 27-5). When the PaO_2 level is low (hypoxemia; less than 60 mm Hg), your client is at risk for developing hypoxia. Your client will begin to display signs and symptoms of hypoxemia (see Box 27-2, p. 649).

Hypoxia is a life-threatening condition and if left untreated, can produce cardiac dysrhythmias and death.

Treatment for hypoxia includes administration of oxygen and treatment of the underlying cause.

▮ NURSING KNOWLEDGE BASE

Your nursing knowledge base prepares you to anticipate a client's oxygenation needs. For example, knowledge of a client's developmental status reveals risks for respiratory disorders, as well as client behaviors that may predispose to poor respiratory health. A client's lifestyle patterns can also significantly affect a client's respiratory status. Your knowledge base is critical to accurate problem identification.

Developmental Factors

The developmental stage of the client and the normal aging process can affect tissue oxygenation.

PREMATURE INFANTS. Premature infants are at risk for hyaline membrane disease. **Surfactant** deficiency involves the chemical in the lung that prevents alveolar collapse and is believed to be the cause of hyaline membrane disease. The surfactant-synthesizing ability of the lung develops about the seventh month and may be lacking in preterm infants born before or during the seventh month.

INFANTS AND TODDLERS. Infants and toddlers are at risk for upper respiratory tract infections as a result of frequent exposure to other children and exposure to second-hand smoke. During the teething process some infants develop nasal congestion, which can encourage bacterial growth and increase the potential for respiratory tract infection. Upper respiratory tract infections are usually not dangerous, and infants and toddlers recover with little difficulty. They are also at risk for airway obstruction because of a foreign object (Wong and others, 1999).

SCHOOL-AGE CHILDREN AND ADOLESCENTS. School-age children and adolescents are exposed to respiratory infections and respiratory risk factors, such as secondhand smoke and the increased risk to begin cigarette smoking. A healthy child usually does not have adverse pulmonary effects from respiratory infections. A person who starts smoking in adolescence and continues to smoke into middle age, however, has an increased risk for cardiopulmonary disease and lung cancer.

YOUNG AND MIDDLE-AGE ADULTS. Young and middle-age adults are exposed to many cardiopulmonary risk factors: an unhealthy diet, lack of exercise, stress, and cigarette smoking. Reducing these modifiable factors may decrease the client's risk for cardiac or pulmonary diseases.

Pregnancy causes changes in ventilation. As the fetus grows during pregnancy, the greater size of the uterus pushes abdominal contents up against the diaphragm. During the last trimester of pregnancy the inspiratory capacity declines, resulting in **dyspnea** on exertion and increased fatigue.

OLDER ADULTS. The cardiac and respiratory systems change throughout the aging process. The arterial system develops atherosclerotic plaques, and the systemic blood pressure may rise. The heart rate decreases; the left ventricular wall thickens; and there is decreased myocardial muscle contraction, decreased cardiac output, and thicker, stiffer heart valves (Lueckenotte, 2000).

Many changes in the lung result in decreased effectiveness of the cough mechanism. This puts the older adult at increased risk for respiratory infections (Lueckenotte, 2000). Ventilation and transfer of respiratory gases decline with age. Osteoporotic changes of the thoracic cage prevent the lung from expanding fully, leading to lower oxygen levels (Table 27-4).

Lifestyle Factors

Lifestyle factors that influence respiratory function include nutrition, exercise, cigarette smoking, substance abuse, and anxiety and stress.

NUTRITION. Nutrition affects cardiopulmonary function in several ways. Severe obesity decreases lung expansion, and the increased body weight increases oxygen demands to meet metabolic needs. The malnourished client may experience respiratory muscle wasting, resulting in decreased muscle strength and respiratory excursion. Cough efficiency is reduced secondary to respiratory muscle weakness, putting the client at risk for retention of pulmonary secretions. A client with chronic lung disease requires a diet high in calories.

Diets high in fat increase cholesterol and atherogenesis in the coronary arteries, thus putting your client at risk for

Changes in the Aging Lung

Table 27-4

Function	Pathophysiological Change	Key Clinical Findings
Breathing mechanics	Decreased chest wall compliance	Decreased vital capacity
	Loss of elastic recoil	Increased reserve volume
	Decreased respiratory muscle mass and strength	Decreased expiratory flow rates
Oxygenation	Increased ventilation/perfusion mismatch	
	Decreased cardiac output	Decreased PaO_2
	Decreased mixed venous oxygen	Increased alveolar-arterial oxygen gradient
	Increased physiological dead space	Decreased cardiac output
	Decreased alveolar surface area	
	Decreased carbon dioxide diffusion capacity	
Ventilation control and breathing pattern	Decreased responsiveness of central and peripheral chemoreceptors to hypoxemia and hypercapnia	Decreased tidal volume
		Increased respiratory rate
		Increased minute ventilation
Lung defense mechanisms	Decreased number of cilia and effectiveness of the mucociliary clearance	Decreased airway clearance
	Diminished cough reflex	Increased risk for infection
	Decreased humoral and cellular immunity	Increased risk of aspiration
	Decreased immunoglobulin A (IgA) production	
Sleep and breathing	Decreased ventilatory drive	Increased risk of apnea, hypopnea, and arterial oxygen desaturation during sleep
	Decreased tone of upper airway muscles	
	Decreased arousal	Increased risk of aspiration
		Snoring
		Obstructive sleep apnea
Exercise capacity	Muscle deconditioning and efficiency	Decreased maximum oxygen consumption
	Decreased muscle mass	Breathlessness at low exercise levels
	Decreased reserves	

Data from Pierson DJ: Effects of aging on the respiratory system. In Pierson DJ, Kacmarek RM, editors: *Foundations of respiratory care*, New York, 1992, Churchill Livingstone.

coronary artery disease (CAD). Clients who are obese or malnourished are also at risk for anemia.

EXERCISE. Exercise increases the body's metabolic activity and oxygen demand. The rate and depth of respiration increase, enabling the person to inhale more oxygen and exhale excess carbon dioxide.

A physical exercise program has many benefits (see Chapter 24). People who exercise 3 or 4 times per week for 20 to 40 minutes have a lower heart rate, lower blood pressure, decreased cholesterol, increased blood flow, and greater oxygen extraction by working muscles. The addition of weight training has also shown benefit in decreasing the work of the heart by increasing the efficiency of the other muscles of the body. Fully conditioned people can increase oxygen consumption by 10% to 20% because of increased cardiac output and increased efficiency of the myocardium.

CIGARETTE SMOKING. Cigarette smoking is associated with a number of diseases, including heart disease, chronic obstructive lung disease, and lung cancer. Cigarette smoking can worsen peripheral vascular and coronary artery diseases. The risk of lung cancer is 10 times greater for a person who smokes than for a nonsmoker. Exposure to side-stream smoke increases the risk of lung cancer in the nonsmoker (Centers for Disease Control and Prevention, 2000b).

SUBSTANCE ABUSE. Excessive use of alcohol and other drugs can impair tissue oxygenation in two ways. First, the person who has chronic substance abuse usually has a poor nutritional intake. With the resultant decrease in intake of iron-rich foods, hemoglobin production declines. Second, excessive use of alcohol and certain other drugs can depress the respiratory center, reducing the rate and depth of respiration and the amount of inhaled oxygen. Substance abuse by either smoking or inhaling causes direct injury to lung tissue that can lead to permanent lung damage and impaired oxygenation.

ANXIETY AND STRESS. A continuous state of severe anxiety increases the body's metabolic rate and the oxygen demand. The body responds to anxiety and stress by an increased rate and depth of respiration. Most people can adapt, but some, particularly those with chronic illnesses or acute life-threatening illnesses such as a myocardial infarction, cannot tolerate the oxygen demands associated with anxiety.

CRITICAL THINKING
Synthesis
The care of clients with impaired oxygenation requires you to synthesize knowledge from basic and other sciences, integrate previous learning experiences, apply critical thinking attitudes when caring for clients who may have unhealthy lifestyles, and provide care according to standards of practice.

KNOWLEDGE. When caring for clients with cardiopulmonary problems, you need to incorporate and apply knowledge from physiology and pathophysiology; nutrition; and fluid, electrolyte, and acid-base balance. Your knowledge about health promotion prevents or helps to reduce at-risk behaviors in your clients who are at risk for or have cardiopulmonary problems. During acute care and restorative or continuing care your knowledge assists clients to attain and maintain optimal cardiopulmonary function.

EXPERIENCE. In the acute care setting you will be caring for the client with an acute exacerbation of disease. When your clients require nursing management in the community setting they are usually stable, productive members of the community with little or no change in lifestyle. You may know someone with a cardiac or respiratory illness, perhaps a family member or friend with asthma or COPD. Experience in the care of clients with respiratory disease prepares you to recognize clinical changes and select effective interventions.

ATTITUDES. The critical thinking attitudes of accountability and perseverance will be used as you provide nursing care for clients with cardiopulmonary alterations. You are accountable for the health care information you provide to your clients. In deciding on the approach for a client that has respiratory disease and still smokes, you may choose a matter-of-fact approach, taking into account the client is aware of his or her risk factors. It is unlikely that an older adult with end-stage disease will be willing or able to stop smoking. Acknowledging that your clients already know the risks of smoking and know why they should stop will be received more openly than bombarding them with literature and a lecture.

As a client advocate you may encounter difficult client problems. Perseverance is important to find effective client-centered solutions. For example, when a client has severe cardiac or pulmonary disease and has a limited income, your solutions for promoting health and maintaining client independence are complex. You may need to continue to provide the same information at each visit. Often clients with chronic hypoxemia have a decreased short-term memory, and you will need to reinforce information previously provided.

STANDARDS. The American Heart Association and American Lung Association have specific guidelines for cardiopulmonary nursing care and cardiopulmonary rehabilitation. The American Nurses Association also has guidelines and standards for the care of clients with cardiopulmonary disease.

NURSING PROCESS

Assessment
The nursing assessment of your client's cardiopulmonary functioning should include data collected from the following areas:
- History of the client's baseline and present cardiopulmonary function, past cardiopulmonary illnesses, and

measures the client uses to improve breathing or heart function (e.g., medications, treatments, exercises)
- Physical examination of the client's cardiopulmonary status (see Chapter 12)
- Review of laboratory and diagnostic test results.

NURSING HISTORY.   The nursing history focuses on your client's ability to meet oxygen needs and control symptoms. Ask questions that assist the client in describing symptoms.

RISK FACTORS.   Investigate familial and environmental risk factors, such as a family history of cardiovascular or lung disease or outdoor air quality. Record which blood relatives have the disease and their present level of health or age at time of death. You can obtain information regarding other risk factors by doing the following:
- Determine your client's exercise pattern by asking, "Do you exercise? How often and what type?"
- Obtain a 24-hour diet recall.
- Determine stress and anxiety patterns by asking, "How would you describe your personality? How do you relax?"
- Ask your client if he or she has ever been diagnosed with high blood pressure.
- Ask if there is any family history of diabetes, heart disease, elevated cholesterol, or high blood pressure.
- Determine information on tobacco use by asking, "Do you smoke cigarettes? Number of years? Packs per day? Are you exposed to secondhand smoke?"
- Ask your client his or her usual weight and about any recent weight gains or losses.

Other family risk factors include the presence of infectious diseases, particularly tuberculosis. Determine who in the client's household has been infected and the status of the treatment.

Environmental exposure to many inhaled substances, such as smog, cotton fibers, silicon, second-hand smoke, and asbestos, is closely linked to respiratory disease. Investigate exposures in the client's home and workplace.

An employment history assesses your client's exposure to inhalants. It is particularly important with middle-aged and older adults, who may have worked in places before the onset of regulations to protect workers from carcinogens.

Ask the following:
- Are there environmental conditions that may affect your breathing where you work?
- Have you recently traveled to countries or areas of the United States where you may have been exposed to uncommon respiratory diseases?

FATIGUE.   Fatigue is a subjective sensation reported as a loss of endurance. Fatigue is often an early sign of worsening of the chronic underlying cardiopulmonary disease. To provide a mechanism to objectively measure fatigue, use a visual analog scale with a rating from 0 to 10, with 10 being the worst level of fatigue and 0 representing no fatigue. In addition, ask your clients questions about their perception of fatigue:
- When did you first notice the fatigue? What makes it get better or worse?

- Was the onset sudden or gradual? Is it related to any time of the day or constant throughout the day?
- Does it prevent you from doing what you want to do?

PAIN.   Cardiac pain does not occur with respiratory variations. It is most often substernal and radiates to the left arm and jaw in males. Women may present with epigastric pain, complaints of indigestion, or a choking feeling and dyspnea. Pericardial pain resulting from an inflammation of the pericardial sac is usually nonradiating and may occur with inspiration. Use a visual analog scale to assist the client in describing the pain (see Chapter 29).

Pleuritic chest pain is peripheral and may radiate to the scapular regions. It is worsened by inspiratory maneuvers, such as coughing, yawning, and sighing. Pleuritic pain is caused by an inflammation or infection in the pleural space and is described as knifelike, lasting from 1 minute to hours, and increasing with inspiration.

Musculoskeletal pain may be present following exercise, rib trauma, and prolonged coughing episodes. The pain is also aggravated by inspiratory movements and may easily be confused with pleuritic chest pain.

When assessing pain in clients with cardiopulmonary disease, obtain information specific to cardiac or inspiratory pain. For example, ask your client the following:
- Have you ever had pain in your chest? Explain.
- Where and when do you feel the pain? Does it radiate? Does it change with inspiration?
- What does the pain feel like? Sharp, dull, stabbing?
- Does it occur at rest or with activity?
- How long does it last?
- What makes it better?

BREATHING PATTERNS.   Dyspnea is a clinical sign of hypoxia and manifests as breathlessness. Dyspnea can be associated with clinical signs, such as exaggerated respiratory effort, use of the accessory muscles of respiration, nasal flaring, and marked increases in the rate and depth of respirations. McCarley (1999) found that chronic dyspnea is distress with varying levels of intensity that include long-term physical, psychological, and sociocultural consequences. Use a visual analog scale to help clients objectively assess their dyspnea, with 0 equated with no dyspnea and 10 equated with the worst dyspnea the client has experienced. Measurement of dyspnea on the analog scale helps to show change in the clients' perception of dyspnea.

Orthopnea is an abnormal condition in which the person must use multiple pillows when lying down or must sit to breathe. The number of pillows required for sleep, such as two or three pillows, quantifies the presence and severity of orthopnea.

Wheezing is characterized by a high-pitched musical sound caused by high-velocity movement of air through a narrowed airway. Wheezing may be assessed in asthma, acute bronchitis, or pneumonia. Wheezing can occur on inspiration, expiration, or both. Determine any precipitating factors, such as respiratory infection, allergens, exercise, or stress.

COUGH.   **Cough** is a sudden, audible expulsion of air from the lungs. Coughing is a protective reflex to clear the trachea, bronchi, and lungs of irritants and secretions. Clients with chronic sinusitis may cough only in the early morning, while trying to sleep, or immediately after rising from sleep. This clears the airway of sputum resulting from sinus drainage. Clients with chronic bronchitis generally produce sputum all day, although greater amounts are produced after rising from a semirecumbent or flat position. A **productive cough** results in sputum production that may be swallowed or expectorated. Carefully collect data about the type, amount, color, and quantity of sputum.

If **hemoptysis** (bloody sputum) is reported, determine if it is associated with coughing and bleeding from the upper respiratory tract, from sinus drainage, or from the gastrointestinal tract (hematemesis). Describe the hemoptysis, including amount, color, duration of bleeding, and presence of sputum.

RESPIRATORY INFECTIONS.   Determine if your client has had a Pneumovax or flu vaccine in the past (Centers for Disease Control and Prevention, 2000a). Also ask about any known exposure to tuberculosis and the results of the tuberculin skin test, including type of test and date. Determine the client's risk for human immunodeficiency virus (HIV) infection. Clients with a history of intravenous drug use, blood transfusions, multiple unprotected sexual partners, or a homosexual lifestyle are at risk of developing HIV infection. Clients may not display any symptoms of HIV infection until they present with an opportunistic infection or vague complaints of fatigue and malaise.

MEDICATION USE.   Assess your client's knowledge and ability to correctly take medication (see Chapter 13). Review the client's understanding of medication side effects and what to report to the health care provider. Common drugs monitored by measuring blood levels include theophylline and digitalis preparations. Illicit drugs, particularly parenterally administered narcotics, which are often diluted with talcum powder, can cause pulmonary disorders resulting from the irritant effect of talcum powder on lung tissues.

Many herbals and over-the-counter (OTC) medications can affect the heart rate and blood pressure and promote blood thinning. Ma huang, a naturally occurring ephedrine, increases blood pressure and heart rate and should not be used by clients with cardiopulmonary disease. Clients with asthma should not use ephedrine-containing products as bronchodilators, because they can cause increased bronchospasm and respiratory arrest. Ginseng, garlic capsules, and ginko biloba have properties similar to aspirin and decrease platelet aggregation.

CLIENT EXPECTATIONS.   Knowing what the client expects regarding his or her health and its maintenance assists in determining goals of care, interventions, and use of client education and home care resources.

The client's unwillingness to adhere to a treatment schedule must be assessed. In addition, determine what your client ex-

Case Study **SYNTHESIS IN PRACTICE**

Mr. King's history reveals risk factors accompanying a 40-year history of smoking two packs per day, and he continues to smoke. He has had multiple respiratory infections in the past 5 years, and he complains of chronic cough, especially in the early mornings. Mary's knowledge of physiology and pathophysiology enables her to realize that the shortness of breath is because the infection is obstructing his alveolocapillary membrane, preventing oxygenation of blood in some parts of his lung. She also is aware of his preexisting chronic obstructive pulmonary disease (COPD) and the effects of his smoking. Mary realizes how bad smoking is for this individual, and knowledge from the area of health promotion and restoration can assist her in promoting smoking cessation for Mr. King. From clinical experiences Mary knows the impact of support systems in assisting clients to cope with chronic illnesses. Mary can use creativity and independent thinking to incorporate community and family resources into the plan of care for Mr. King. Mary will need to inquire about his social supports and the availability of smoking cessation programs in his community.

pects from the caregiver. Does the client expect health to improve or expect supportive care? Does your client want to be an active participant in care or for family members to make decisions and provide care?

PHYSICAL EXAMINATION.   The physical examination includes evaluation of the entire cardiopulmonary system (see Chapter 12) (Tables 27-5 to 27-7).

Be mindful of the client's limitations, such as breathlessness or fatigue. You may have to complete your assessment in short sections to allow the client to rest and recover. In addition, it may be necessary to have your initial assessment focus on your client's immediate problems. Table 27-8 gives an example of a focused assessment.

DIAGNOSTIC TESTS.   Diagnostic tests are conducted to determine adequacy of the cardiac conduction system, myocardial contraction, and blood flow; to measure the adequacy of ventilation and oxygenation; and to visualize structures of the respiratory system. Your client may need an ECG, chest x-ray, pulse oximetry, laboratory tests (e.g., arterial blood gases, complete blood count, sputum analysis, cardiac enzymes), cardiac stress test, pulmonary function test, and cardiac catheterization.

Nursing Diagnosis

Your client with an altered level of oxygenation may have nursing diagnoses that are primarily of cardiovascular or pulmonary origin (Box 27-6). Each nursing diagnosis is based on specific defining characteristics and must include the related etiology. The defining characteristics or signs and symptoms identified during your assessment validate the diagnostic label.

During the assessment process, you collected data that accurately reflected the client's needs. For example, the diag-

Inspection of Cardiopulmonary Status

Table 27-5

Abnormality	Cause
Eyes	
Xanthelasma (yellow lipid lesions on eyelids)	Associated with hyperlipidemia
Corneal arcus (whitish opaque ring around junction of cornea and sclera)	Abnormal finding in young to middle-age adults associated with hyperlipidemia (normal finding in older adults with arcus senilis)
Pale conjunctivae	Associated with anemia
Cyanotic conjunctivae	Associated with hypoxemia
Petechiae on conjunctivae	Associated with fat embolus or bacterial endocarditis
Skin	
Peripheral cyanosis	Vasoconstriction and diminished blood flow
Central cyanosis	Hypoxemia
Decreased skin turgor	Dehydration (normal finding in older adults as a result of decreased skin elasticity)
Dependent edema	Associated with right- and left-sided heart failure
Periorbital edema	Associated with kidney disease
Fingertips and Nail Beds	
Cyanosis	Decreased cardiac output or hypoxia
Splinter hemorrhages	Bacterial endocarditis
Clubbing	Chronic hypoxemia
Mouth and Lips	
Cyanotic mucous membranes	Decreased oxygenation (hypoxia)
Pursed-lip breathing	Associated with chronic lung disease
Neck Veins	
Distention	Associated with right-sided heart failure
Nose	
Flaring nares	Air hunger, dyspnea
Chest	
Retractions	Increased work of breathing, dyspnea
Asymmetry	Chest wall injury

Assessment of Abnormal Chest Wall Movement

Table 27-6

Abnormality	Cause
Retraction—visible sinking in soft tissues of chest between and around firmer tissue and cartilaginous and bony ribs; retractions having specific beginning point and worsening with need for increased inspiratory effort; possibly found at intercostal space, intra-clavicular space, trachea, and substernally*	Any condition that causes increased inspiratory effort (e.g., airway obstruction, asthma, tracheobronchitis)
Paradoxical breathing—asynchronous breathing; chest contraction during inspiration and expansion during expiration	Flail chest
Increased anteroposterior diameter	Senile emphysema or chronic obstructive pulmonary disease

*Infants can experience sternal and substernal retractions with only slight inspiratory effort because of chest pliability.

nosis of *ineffective airway clearance related to the presence of tracheobronchial secretions* is supported by objective findings including productive cough, breathlessness, crackles, tachypnea, changes in depth of respiration, and pleuritic pain. The ability of your client to bring up sputum is a crucial part of treatment for pneumonia. Pleuritic pain can interfere with a client's ability to rest and can impair the ability to cough and clear the airway, resulting in worsening infection.

Another example of a related nursing diagnosis is *activity intolerance related to imbalance between oxygen supply and demand.* The objective findings include an inability to move secretions, restlessness, tachycardia, breathlessness, use of accessory muscles, and hypoxia (PaO_2 less than 60 mm Hg). Clients will avoid physical effort because dyspnea may be precipitated by exercise. Consequently their level of fitness decreases, they become weak, and they have

Respiratory Pattern
Table 27-7

Type/Pattern	Rate (Breaths per Minute)	Clinical Significance	Type/Pattern	Rate (Breaths per Minute)	Clinical Significance
Eupnea	16-20	Normal	Kussmaul's	Usually >35, may be slow or normal	Tachypnea pattern associated with diabetic ketoacidosis, metabolic acidosis, or renal failure
Tachypnea	>35	Respiratory failure Response to fever Anxiety Shortness of breath Respiratory infection			
Bradypnea	<10	Sleep Respiratory depression Drug overdose Central nervous system (CNS) lesion	Cheyne-Stokes	Variable	Increasing and decreasing pattern caused by alterations in acid-base status; underlying metabolic problem or neurocerebral insult
Apnea	Periods of no respiration lasting >15	May be intermittent, such as in sleep apnea Respiratory arrest	Biot's	Variable	Periods of apnea and shallow breathing caused by CNS disorder; found in some healthy clients
Hyperpnea	16-20	Can result from anxiety or response to pain Can cause marked respiratory alkalosis, paresthesia, tetany, confusion	Apneustic	Increased	Increased inspiratory time with short grunting expiratory time; seen in CNS lesions of the respiratory center

From Weilitz PB: *Pocket guide to respiratory care,* St. Louis, 1991, Mosby.

Example of a Focused Client Assessment
Table 27-8

Factors to Assess	Questions and Approaches	Physical Assessment Strategies
Dependent edema	• Do your legs swell every day? • Are they swollen in the morning when you arise? • Do they get better if you put them up? • Do you have trouble getting your socks and shoes on and off?	• Palpate amount of edema: trace to 4+. • Observe for neck vein distention. • Observe for breathlessness at rest and on exertion. • Assess pedal and popliteal pulses. • Observe for bilateral or unilateral edema.
Breathing pattern	• When do you become short of breath? • Are you able to do your own personal hygiene? • How far can you walk without getting short of breath?	• Observe client perform activities of daily living. • Observe ambulating. Determine distance walked without shortness of breath. • Observe for use of pursed-lipped breathing. • Observe client in various positions.
Airway patency	• How often do you cough? • Do you bring up any mucus when coughing? • Is there anything that brings on your cough?	• Monitor sputum for color, consistency, amount, and odor.

difficulty with normal activities of daily living. As the level of exercise tolerance is increased, the degree of dyspnea and shortness of breath may actually diminish. Identifying the appropriate related factor can enable you to design nursing interventions to maximize the balance between the client's oxygen supply and demand.

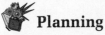

Planning
GOALS AND OUTCOMES. Clients with impaired oxygenation require a nursing care plan directed toward meet- ing the actual or potential oxygenation needs of the client. Individual goals are derived from your client-centered needs. Goals for your client may include providing a patent airway, improving oxygenation, and increasing the level of independence and tolerance for activity (see care plan, p. 660).

All goals must have a measurable outcome for you to be able to determine whether they have been met. These include objective data, such as arterial blood gases, laboratory findings, chest radiographs, ECG patterns, blood pressure, and pulse. Subjective findings, such as breathlessness or pain, need to be quantified.

It is important to include the family and client in all care planning. Alterations in oxygenation are often chronic problems that affect the client and the family. The client remains a member of the community despite the illness. Planning with the family and using community resources help clients adapt to activities of daily living. Many stores now provide motorized carts to assist clients with mobility while shopping. Handicapped parking includes clients who have alter-

ations in oxygenation and are not able to walk more than 50 feet without stopping.

SETTING PRIORITIES. Help the client and family set priorities for care based on the client's tolerance level. Ask the client how he or she is feeling today and then determine what aspects of care are most important. If the client is having pain, relief of pain is the priority over getting up in the chair or completing personal hygiene. Ask clients what they want to accomplish. If they are diaphoretic, they may appreciate clean sheets and a bath after being medicated for pain.

The decision to delegate responsibility to an assistive person should be based on your assessment of the client and care to be accomplished. You must consider what tasks are safe to delegate, within the skill set of the assistive personnel, and how the client will feel about the care that has been delegated. The priority is to maintain or improve the client's oxygenation and meet the client's needs.

CONTINUITY OF CARE. Impaired levels of oxygenation affect all aspects of your client's life, not just the

---

Nursing Diagnoses for
CARDIOPULMONARY DYSFUNCTION
Box 27-6

- Activity intolerance
- Airway clearance, ineffective
- Breathing pattern, ineffective
- Cardiac output, decreased
- Gas exchange, impaired
- Infection, risk for
- Fatigue

Case Study Nursing Care Plan **OXYGENATION**

ASSESSMENT

Mr. King is in respiratory distress as evidenced by **dyspnea, cough, prolonged expiration, audible expiratory wheezing, diminished breath sounds** over right lower lobe, **anxiety, sputum-producing cough, hyperresonance, cyanosis** of nail beds and mucous membranes, and use of **accessory muscles during breathing.** His vital signs are pulse rate 120, temperature 102° F, **respiratory rate 36,** and blood pressure 110/45.

*Defining characteristics are shown in bold type.

NURSING DIAGNOSIS

Impaired gas exchange related to increased pulmonary secretions.

PLANNING

GOAL

Client's excessive pulmonary secretions will return to baseline levels within 24 to 36 hours.

EXPECTED OUTCOMES

Client's sputum will be clear, white within 36 hours.
Client's adventitious lung sounds will disappear within 36 hours.
Client's respiratory rate will be between 16 and 24 within 24 hours.
Client will be able to clear airway by coughing in 24 hours.

IMPLEMENTATION

STEPS

1. Instruct client to deep breathe and cough every 2 hours while awake.

2. Encourage frequent position changes if on bed rest; if able, ambulate for 10 to 15 minutes every 8 hours and encourage client to sit up in chair as often as tolerated.

3. Increase fluid intake to greater than 2700 ml/24 hr if not contraindicated by cardiac condition. Avoid caffeinated beverages and alcohol; recommend water.

RATIONALE

Major complication of reduced mobility is retained pulmonary secretions, which predispose client to atelectasis and pneumonia (Phipps and others, 1999; St. John, 1999).
Ambulation, sitting upright, and frequent position changes are consistent with normal activities and promote normal lung function and mucociliary clearance (Meek, 2000; McCarley, 1999).
Intake of fluids more than 2700 ml/24 hr will help liquefy secretions for easy removal. Caffeinated and alcoholic beverages promote diuresis and dehydration. Water is the best expectorant on the market, easily available, and cost-effective (St. John, 1999).

EVALUATION

- Observe color of client's sputum.
- Auscultate client's lungs.
- Observe client's respirations.
- Observe client's cough.

physical component. Designing collaborative nursing interventions with physical and occupational therapy can improve your client's level of functioning. Respiratory therapy assists in designing measures to improve breathing and cough control. When planning care for clients with impaired oxygenation, be sensitive to the needs of the client as well as the family. Chronic illness changes the dynamics of family relationships. Roles may need to change, and the client and family may have difficulty coping. You may need to provide an empathic ear to the family as well as the client. Help them develop solutions that maintain the dignity of both parties and continue to support the family unit.

Social services assist in identifying resources within the community. These can include Better Breathing groups, the local American Lung Association, and support groups for specific disease processes.

Implementation

Nursing interventions for promoting and maintaining adequate oxygenation include actions such as health promotion and prevention behaviors, positioning, coughing techniques, and interdependent or dependent interventions, such as oxygen therapy, lung inflation techniques, hydration, medications, and chest physiotherapy.

HEALTH PROMOTION.   Maintaining the client's optimal level of health is important in reducing the number and severity of respiratory symptoms. Prevention of respiratory infections is foremost in maintaining optimal health. You provide health education to help clients make choices for improving health practices (Box 27-7). In addition, older adults present and respond differently from younger clients (Box 27-8).

INFLUENZA AND PNEUMOCOCCAL VACCINE.   Annual influenza vaccines are recommended for older clients and those with chronic illnesses. The value of vaccination for immunocompromised clients is unclear. HIV-positive clients may receive the flu vaccine. Persons with a known hypersensitivity to eggs, chickens, or feathers and adults with fever should not receive the vaccine (Centers for Disease Control and Prevention, 2000a).

The pneumococcal vaccine is given every 10 years for low-risk clients and every 5 years for those with multiple underlying conditions. Both the influenza vaccine and pneumococcal vaccine can be given to pregnant women after the first trimester. However, in all cases consult the client's obstetrician before administering either vaccine.

ENVIRONMENTAL MODIFICATIONS.   Avoiding exposure to secondhand smoke is important for clients with cardiopul-

---

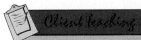

Client Teaching   Box 27-7

CARDIOPULMONARY HEALTH PROMOTION

- Educate the client about the importance of regular blood pressure checkups and taking blood pressure medications as prescribed.
- Educate the client about the importance of monitoring the serum cholesterol and triglyceride levels.
- Educate the client about the basic food groups and recommended servings of each.
- Educate the client about low-fat, low-salt, proper caloric diet, and provide sample menus.
- Educate the client about need for regular aerobic exercise 3 or 4 times per week for 30 to 40 minutes.
- Discuss strategies for minimizing and reducing stress in the client's life, such as setting realistic goals, relaxation and meditation techniques, and getting adequate amounts of rest, relaxation, and sleep.
- Discuss the importance and benefits of pneumococcal vaccine and annual influenza vaccine.
- Discuss the importance of monitoring pollution indexes and limiting exposure on days when the index is high.
- Discuss the need to avoid smoking and secondhand smoke exposure. If the client smokes, enroll him or her in a structured smoking cessation program.
- Discuss strategies to avoid or control secondary infection exposure, such as avoiding prolonged exposure to crowds during the flu season.
- Educate the client about the need to cover the mouth and nose with a scarf when going out into cold air.

Gerontological Nursing Practice   Box 27-8

- Risk factor modification is important in the older adult, including smoking cessation, weight reduction, a low-cholesterol diet, management of hypertension, and exercise.
- Coronary artery disease is the leading cause of death and disability in women older than 40 years of age. Women present with differing symptoms from men. Presenting symptoms may include epigastric distress, midsternal chest pain radiating to the back, and a choking feeling.
- Older adults have more atypical signs and symptoms of coronary artery disease (Lueckenotte, 2000).
- The incidence of atrial fibrillation increases with age and is the leading contributing factor for stroke in the older adult (Lueckenotte, 2000).
- It may be more difficult to get older adults to change long-term unhealthy habits; however, healthy behavior changes can slow or halt the progression of their disease (Lueckenotte, 2000).
- Mental status changes are often the first sign of respiratory problems in the older adult. These may include subtle increases in forgetfulness and irritability.
- The older adult may not complain of dyspnea until it impacts activities of daily living and then only if the activities are important to the older adult.
- Changes in the older client's cough mechanism may lead to retention of pulmonary secretions, plugged airways, and atelectasis if cough suppressants are not used with caution.
- Older adults with chronic lung disease can lead active productive lives with proper medical care and nursing management.
- Chronic illness in the older adult may result in unacceptable behavior patterns because of loss of control experienced with a chronic illness.

monary illnesses. Most public places and businesses have now adopted a no-smoking policy and may offer separate smoking areas. When a client lives with secondhand smoke in the home, you will need to provide counseling and support to help the smoker understand the effects of secondhand smoke on the client. The client, smoker, and you will need to develop a plan that takes into account the client's and smoker's needs.

ACUTE CARE.   Clients with acute pulmonary illnesses require nursing interventions directed toward halting the pathological process, such as a respiratory tract infection; shortening the duration and severity of the illness, such as hospitalization with pneumonia; and preventing complications from illness or treatments, such as nosocomial infection resulting from invasive procedures.

DYSPNEA MANAGEMENT.   Dyspnea is difficult to measure and treat. You need to individualize treatments for each client, and more than one therapy is usually implemented. The underlying processes that cause or worsen dyspnea must be treated and stabilized initially, and then four additional therapies should be administered:
1. Medications (e.g., bronchodilators, steroids, mucolytics, antianxiety drugs)
2. Oxygen therapy as indicated
3. Physical techniques (e.g., cardiopulmonary reconditioning, breathing techniques, cough control)
4. Psychosocial techniques (e.g., relaxation techniques, biofeedback, meditation) to lessen the sensation of dyspnea

MAINTENANCE OF A PATENT AIRWAY.   The airway is patent when the trachea, bronchi, and large airways are free from obstructions. You use three types of interventions to maintain a patent airway: coughing techniques, suctioning, and insertion of an artificial airway.

Coughing Techniques.   Coughing maintains a patent airway by removing secretions from both the upper and lower airways. Cough effectiveness is evaluated by sputum expectoration, the client's report of swallowed sputum, or clearing of adventitious lung sounds. Clients with chronic pulmonary diseases, upper respiratory tract infections, and lower respiratory tract infections are encouraged to deep breathe and cough at least every 2 hours while awake. Clients with a large amount of sputum should be encouraged to cough every hour while awake and may need to awaken to cough every 2 to 3 hours while asleep until the acute phase of sputum production has ended.

Cascade Cough.   With the cascade cough, the client takes a slow, deep breath and holds it for 2 seconds while contracting expiratory muscles. Then the client opens the mouth and performs a series of coughs throughout exhalation, thereby coughing at progressively lowered lung volumes. This technique promotes airway clearance and a patent airway in clients with large volumes of sputum.

Huff Cough.   The huff cough stimulates a natural cough reflex and is generally effective only for clearing central air-

ways. While exhaling, the client opens the glottis by saying the word *huff.* With practice the client inhales more air and may be able to progress to the cascade cough.

Quad Cough.   The quad cough technique is used for clients without abdominal muscle control, such as those with spinal cord injuries. While the client breathes out with a maximal expiratory effort, the client or you push inward and upward on the abdominal muscles toward the diaphragm, causing the cough.

Suctioning Techniques.   When a client is unable to effectively clear respiratory tract secretions with coughing, suctioning is initiated to clear the airways. The primary suctioning techniques are oropharyngeal and nasopharyngeal suctioning, orotracheal and nasotracheal suctioning, and tracheal suctioning through an artificial airway (Skill 27-1).

These techniques are based on common principles. Because the nasotrachea and trachea are considered sterile, sterile technique is required for suctioning. The mouth is considered clean, and therefore the suctioning of oral secretions should be performed after suctioning of the nasotrachea and trachea. Suctioning requires the use of a round-tipped, multiholed catheter. Frequency of suctioning is determined by clinical assessment. When secretions are identified by inspection or auscultation techniques, suctioning is required. Sputum is produced as a response to a pathological condition. There is no rationale for routine suctioning every 1 to 2 hours.

Oropharyngeal and Nasopharyngeal Suctioning.   Oropharyngeal or nasopharyngeal suctioning is used to assist the client who is able to cough effectively but is unable to clear secretions by expectorating or swallowing.

Orotracheal and Nasotracheal Suctioning.   Orotracheal or nasotracheal suctioning is necessary when the client is unable to cough and does not have an artificial airway (see Skill 27-1). A catheter is passed through the mouth or nose into the trachea. The nose is the preferred route because stimulation of the gag reflex is minimal. The procedure is similar to nasopharyngeal suctioning, but the catheter tip is into the trachea.

Tracheal Suctioning.   Tracheal suctioning is performed through an artificial airway, such as a tracheostomy tube or endotracheal tube. Two methods of suctioning are currently used. Open suctioning uses a freshly opened sterile suction catheter each time. Closed suctioning involves a multiple-use catheter that is encased in a plastic sheath and used for 24 to 48 hours. Closed suctioning is most often used for clients who require mechanical ventilation because it permits continuous delivery of oxygen during suctioning (Figure 27-3).

Artificial Airways.   An artificial airway is indicated for a client with decreased level of consciousness, airway obstruction, mechanical ventilation, and removal of tracheobronchial secretions (see Skill 27-1).

Oral Airway.   The oral airway, the simplest type of artificial airway, prevents obstruction of the trachea by displacement of the tongue into the oropharynx (Figure 27-4). The

Text continued on p. 670

Skill 27-1
SUCTIONING

DELEGATION CONSIDERATIONS

This skill requires problem solving and knowledge application unique to a professional nurse. When the client is assessed by the nurse to be stable, the skill of performing suctioning of an established tracheostomy can be delegated to assistive personnel and sometimes to the client in special situations. These situations include clients with permanent tracheostomy tubes after head and neck surgery and clients receiving mechanical ventilation at home.

EQUIPMENT

- Appropriate-size suction catheter or closed-suction catheter (smallest diameter that will remove secretions effectively) or Yankauer catheter (oral suction)
- Nasal or oral airway (if indicated)

- Two sterile gloves or one sterile and one nonsterile glove
- Clean towel or paper drape
- Portable or wall suction
- Mask or face shield
- 30-ml sterile saline ampules
- Connecting tube (6 feet)

Equipment that will be needed if not using closed-suction catheter:

- Small Y-adapter (if catheter does not have a suction control port)
- Water-soluble lubricant
- Sterile basin
- Sterile normal saline solution or water (about 100 ml)

STEPS	RATIONALE
1. Assess signs and symptoms of upper and lower airway obstruction requiring nasotracheal or orotracheal suctioning, including respiratory rate or adventitious sounds, nasal secretions, drooling, gastric secretions, or vomitus in mouth.	Physical signs and symptoms result from decreased oxygen to tissues as well as pooling of secretions in upper and lower airways.
Assess signs and symptoms associated with hypoxia and hypercapnia: apprehension, anxiety, decreased ability to concentrate, lethargy, decreased level of consciousness (especially acute), increased fatigue, dizziness, behavioral changes (especially irritability), increased pulse rate or rate of breathing, decreased depth of breathing, elevated blood pressure, cardiac dysrhythmias, pallor, cyanosis, and dyspnea.	
2. Determine factors that normally influence upper or lower airway functioning.	
a. Fluid status.	Fluid overload may increase amount of secretions. Dehydration promotes thicker secretions.
b. Lack of humidity.	The environment influences secretion formation and gas exchange, necessitating airway suctioning when the client cannot clear secretions effectively.
c. Infection.	Clients with respiratory infections are prone to increased secretions that are thicker and sometimes more difficult to expectorate.
d. Anatomy.	Abnormal anatomy can impair normal drainage of secretions. For example, nasal swelling, deviated septum, or facial fractures may impair nasal drainage. Tumors in or around the lower airway may impair secretion removal by occluding or externally compressing the lumen of the airway.
3. Assess client's understanding of procedure.	Reveals need for client instruction and encourages cooperation.
4. Obtain physician's order if indicated by agency policy.	Some institutions require a physician's order for tracheal suctioning.
5. Explain to client how procedure will help clear airway and relieve breathing problems. Explain that temporary coughing, sneezing, gagging, or shortness of breath is normal during the procedure. Encourage client to cough out secretions. Practice coughing, if able. Splint surgical incisions, if necessary.	Encourages cooperation and minimizes risks, anxiety, and pain of procedure.

STEPS	RATIONALE
6. Explain importance of and encourage coughing during procedure.	Facilitates secretion removal and may reduce frequency and duration of future suctioning.
7. Assist client to assume position comfortable for nurse and client (usually semi-Fowler's or sitting upright with head hyperextended, unless contraindicated).	Reduces stimulation of gag reflex, promotes client comfort and secretion drainage, prevents aspiration and nurse strain. Hyperextension facilitates insertion of catheter into trachea.
8. Place pulse oximeter on client's finger. Take reading and leave pulse oximeter in place.	Provides baseline SpO$_2$ to determine client's response to suctioning.
9. Place towel across client's chest, if needed.	Reduces transmission of microorganisms by protecting gown from secretions.

10. Perform appropriate suction technique.

    A. **Performing Nasopharyngeal and Nasotracheal Suctioning**

STEPS	RATIONALE
(1) Wash hands, and apply face shield if splashing is likely.	Reduces transmission of microorganisms.
(2) Connect one end of connecting tubing to suction machine, and place other end in convenient location near client. Turn suction device on, and set vacuum regulator to appropriate negative pressure.	Excessive negative pressure damages nasal pharyngeal and tracheal mucosa and can induce greater hypoxia.
(3) If indicated, increase supplemental **oxygen therapy** to 100% or as ordered by physician. Encourage client to do breathe deeply.	These measures reduce suction-induced hypoxemia. Oxygen-sensitive clients include those with chronic heart and lung conditions and those with pneumonia.

• *Critical Decision Point*

Oxygen must be readjusted as ordered by physician after procedure to avoid increased risk of oxygen toxicity and absorption, atelectasis from prolonged administration of high concentrations of oxygen, and increased carbon dioxide retention in clients with chronic obstructive lung diseases.

STEPS	RATIONALE
(4) Prepare suction catheter.	
a. Open suction kit or catheter with use of aseptic technique. If sterile drape is available, place it across client's chest or on the overbed table. Do not allow the suction catheter to touch any nonsterile surfaces.	Maintains asepsis and reduces transmission of microorganisms.
b. Unwrap or open sterile basin, and place on bedside table. Be careful not to touch inside of basin. Fill with about 100 ml sterile normal saline solution or water (see illustration).	Saline or water is used to clean tubing after each suction pass.
c. Open lubricant. Squeeze small amount onto open sterile catheter package without touching package.	Prepares lubricant while maintaining sterility. Water-soluble lubricant is used to avoid lipoid aspiration pneumonia. Excessive lubricant can occlude catheter.
(5) Apply sterile glove to each hand, or apply nonsterile glove to nondominant hand and sterile glove to dominant hand.	Reduces transmission of microorganisms and allows nurse to maintain sterility of suction catheter.
(6) Pick up suction catheter with dominant hand without touching nonsterile surfaces. Pick up connecting tubing with nondominant hand. Secure catheter to tubing (see illustration).	Maintains catheter sterility. Connects catheter to suction.
(7) Check that the equipment is functioning properly by suctioning small amount of normal saline solution from basin.	Ensures equipment function. Lubricates internal catheter and tubing.
(8) Lightly coat distal 6 to 8 cm (2 to 3 in) of catheter tip with water-soluble lubricant.	Lubricates catheter for easier insertion.

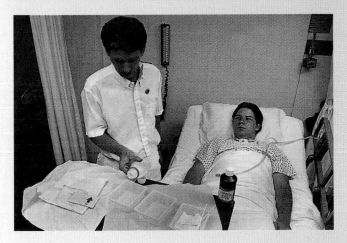

STEP 8A(4)B   Pouring sterile saline into tray.

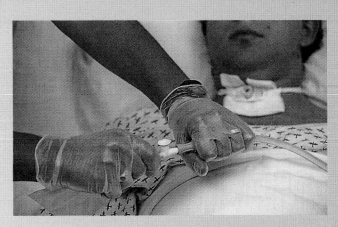

STEP 8A(6)   Attaching catheter to suction.

(9) Remove oxygen delivery device, if applicable, with nondominant hand. Without applying suction and using dominant thumb and forefinger, gently but quickly insert catheter into naris during inhalation and following natural course of the naris, slightly slant the catheter downward or through mouth. Do not force through naris (see illustration).

Application of suction pressure while introducing catheter into trachea increases risk of damage to mucosa and increases risk of hypoxia because of removal of entrained oxygen present in airways.

- **Critical Decision Point**
  *Be sure to insert catheter during client inhalation, especially if inserting catheter into trachea, because epiglottis is open. Do not insert during swallowing or catheter will most likely enter esophagus. **Never** apply suction during insertion. Client should cough. If client gags or becomes nauseated, catheter is most likely in esophagus and must be removed.*

  a. Pharyngeal suctioning: In adults, insert catheter about 16 cm (6 in); in older children, 8 to 12 cm (3 to 5 in); in infants and young children, 4 to 8 cm (2 to 3 in). Rule of thumb is to insert catheter distance from tip of nose (or mouth) to base of earlobe.

  b. Tracheal suctioning: In adults, insert catheter about 20 cm (8 in); in older children, 14 to 20 cm (5.5 to 8 in); and in young children and infants, 8 to 14 cm (3 to 5.5 in) (see illustration).

  c. Positioning option for tracheal suctioning: In some instances turning client's head to right helps nurse suction left mainstem bronchus; turning head to left helps nurse suction right mainstem bronchus. If resistance is felt after insertion of catheter for maximum recommended distance, catheter has probably hit carina. Pull catheter back 1 to 2 cm before applying suction.

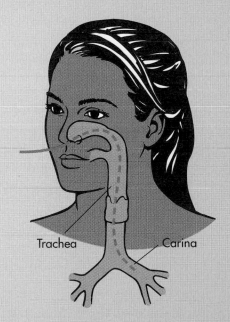

STEP 8A(9)   Pathway for nasotracheal catheter progression.

Trachea   Carina

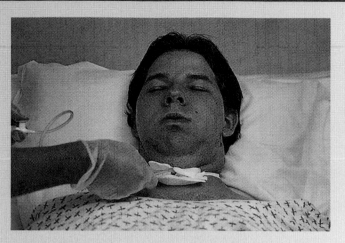

STEP 8A(9)B   Suctioning tracheostomy.

- **Critical Decision Point**
Use the nasal approach and perform tracheal suctioning before pharyngeal suctioning whenever possible. The mouth and pharynx contain more bacteria than the trachea does. If copious oral secretions are present before beginning the procedure, suction mouth with oral suction device.

(10) Apply intermittent suction for up to 10 seconds by placing and releasing nondominant thumb over vent of catheter and slowly withdrawing catheter while rotating it back and forth between dominant thumb and forefinger. Encourage client to cough. Replace oxygen device, if applicable.	Intermittent suction and rotation of catheter prevent injury to mucosa. If catheter "grabs" mucosa, remove thumb to release suction. Suctioning longer than 10 seconds can cause cardiopulmonary compromise, usually from hypoxemia or vagal overload.

- **Critical Decision Point**
While monitoring client's vital signs and oxygen saturation, note if the client's pulse drops more than 20 beats/min or increases more than 40 beats/min or if pulse oximetry falls below 90% or 5% from baseline, cease suctioning (Lewis and others, 2000).

(11) Rinse catheter and connecting tubing with normal saline or water until cleared.	Secretions that remain in suction catheter or connecting tubing decrease suctioning efficiency.
(12) Assess for need to repeat suctioning procedure. When possible, allow adequate time (1 to 2 minutes) between suction passes for ventilation and oxygenation. Assist client to deep breathe and cough.	Observe for alterations in cardiopulmonary status. Suctioning can induce hypoxemia, dysrhythmias, laryngospasm, and bronchospasm. Deep breathing reventilates and reoxygenates alveoli. Repeated passes clear the airway of excessive secretions but can also remove oxygen and may induce **laryngospasm.**
(13) When pharynx and trachea are sufficiently cleared of secretions, perform oral pharyngeal suctioning to clear mouth of secretions. Do not suction nose again after suctioning mouth.	Removes upper airway secretions. More microorganisms are generally present in mouth.
(14) When suctioning is completed, roll catheter around fingers of dominant hand. Pull glove off inside out so that catheter remains coiled in glove. Pull off other glove over first glove in same way to seal in contaminants. Discard in appropriate receptacle. Turn off suction device.	Reduces transmission of microorganisms.

STEPS	RATIONALE
(15) Remove towel, place in laundry or appropriate receptacle, and reposition client. (Nurse may need to wear clean gloves for personal care.)	Reduces transmission of microorganisms. Promotes comfort.
(16) If indicated, readjust oxygen to original level because client's blood oxygen level should have returned to baseline.	Prevents absorption atelectasis and oxygen toxicity while allowing client time to reoxygenate blood.
(17) Discard remainder of normal saline into appropriate receptacle. If basin is disposable, discard into appropriate receptacle. If basin is reusable, rinse it out and place it in soiled utility room.	Reduces transmission of microorganisms.
(18) Remove face shield, and discard into appropriate receptacle. Wash hands.	Reduces transmission of microorganisms.
(19) Place unopened suction kit on suction machine table or at head of bed.	Provides immediate access to suction catheter for next procedure.
(20) Assist client to a comfortable position, and provide oral hygiene as needed.	

B. Performing Artificial Airway Suctioning

STEPS	RATIONALE
(1) Wash hands, and apply face shield.	Reduces transmission of microorganisms.
(2) Connect one end of connecting tubing to suction machine, and place other end in convenient location. Turn suction device on, and set vacuum regulator to appropriate negative pressure (see manufacturer's directions).	Excessive negative pressure damages tracheal mucosa and can induce greater hypoxia.
(3) Prepare proper suction catheter.	Suction catheter's outer diameter should not exceed one-half of the internal diameter of the endotracheal tube (ET) or tracheostomy tube (St. Johns, 1999).
(4) Aseptically open suction catheter package. If sterile drape is available, place it across client's chest. Do not allow suction catheter to touch any nonsterile surface.	Prevents contamination of clothing and provides a sterile surface on which to lay suction catheter between passes, if needed. Prepares catheter and prevents transmission of microorganisms.
(5) Unwrap or open sterile basin, and place on bedside table. Be careful not to touch inside of basin. Fill with about 100 ml of sterile normal saline.	Normal saline is used to rinse catheter after suctioning.
(6) Apply one sterile glove to each hand, or apply nonsterile glove to nondominant hand and sterile glove to dominant hand.	Reduces transmission of microorganisms and allows nurse to maintain sterility of suction catheter.
(7) Pick up suction catheter with dominant hand without touching nonsterile surfaces. Pick up connecting tubing with nondominant hand. Secure catheter to tubing.	Maintains catheter sterility. Establishes suction.
(8) Check that equipment is functioning properly by suctioning small amount of saline from basin.	Ensures equipment function; lubricates catheter and tubing.
(9) Hyperinflate and/or hyperoxygenate client before suctioning, using manual resuscitation Ambu-bag connected to oxygen source or sigh mechanism on mechanical ventilator. Some mechanical ventilators have a button that when pushed delivers 100% oxygen for a few minutes and then resets to the previous value.	Hyperinflation decreases arterial oxygen desaturation and atelectasis caused by negative pressure of suctioning (St. Johns, 1999). Preoxygenation converts large proportion of resident lung gas to 100% oxygen to offset amount used in metabolic consumption while ventilator or oxygenation is interrupted, as well as to offset volume lost during suction procedure.

STEPS	RATIONALE
(10) If client is receiving mechanical ventilation, open swivel adapter or if necessary remove oxygen or humidity delivery device with nondominant hand.	Exposes artificial airway.

• **Critical Decision Point**

Be careful not to allow client to remain on high fraction of inspired oxygen (F_IO_2), such as 100%, too long. Atelectasis can develop.

(11) Without applying suction, gently but quickly insert catheter using dominant thumb and forefinger into artificial airway until resistance is met or client coughs, then pull back 1 cm. (Best to time catheter insertion during client inspiration.)	Application of suction pressure while introducing catheter into trachea increases risk of damage to tracheal mucosa, as well as increased hypoxia related to removal of entrained oxygen present in airways. Pulling back stimulates cough and removes catheter from mucosal wall so that catheter is not resting against tracheal mucosa during suctioning.

• **Critical Decision Point**

*If unable to insert catheter past the end of the ET tube, the catheter is probably caught in the Murphy eye (i.e., side hole at distal end of ET tube that allows for collateral air flow in event of mainstem **intubation**. If this happens, rotate the catheter to reposition it away from the Murphy eye, or withdraw it slightly and reinsert with the next inhalation. Usually the catheter meets resistance at the carina. One indication that the catheter is at the carina is acute onset of coughing because the carina contains many cough receptors. The catheter should be pulled back.*

(12) Apply intermittent suction by placing and releasing nondominant thumb over vent of catheter; slowly withdraw catheter while rotating it back and forth between dominant thumb and forefinger. Encourage client to cough. Watch for respiratory distress.	Intermittent suction and rotation of catheter reduce injury to tracheal mucosal lining. If catheter "grabs" mucosa, remove thumb to release suction (St. Johns, 1999).

• **Critical Decision Point**

If the client develops respiratory distress during the suction procedure, immediately withdraw the catheter and supply additional oxygen and breaths as needed. Oxygen can be administered directly through the catheter in an emergency. Disconnect suction and attach oxygen at prescribed flow rate through the catheter.

(13) If client is receiving mechanical ventilation, close swivel adapter or replace oxygen delivery device.	Reestablishes artificial airway.
(14) Encourage client to deep breathe, if able. Some clients respond well to several manual breaths from the mechanical ventilator or Ambu-bag.	Reoxygenates and reexpands alveoli. Suctioning can cause hypoxemia and atelectasis.
(15) Rinse catheter and connecting tubing with normal saline until clear. Use continuous suction.	Removes catheter secretions. Secretions left in tubing decrease suction and provide environment for microorganism growth. Secretions left in connecting tube decrease suctioning efficiency.
(16) Assess client's cardiopulmonary status (vital signs, oxygen saturation), secretion clearance, and complications. Repeat Steps 8B(9) through 8B(15) once or twice more to clear secretions. Allow adequate time (at last 1 full minute) between suction passes for ventilation and reoxygenation.	Suctioning can induce dysrhythmias, hypoxia, and bronchospasm and impair cerebral circulation or adversely affect hemodynamics (Kerr and others, 1999). Repeated passes with suction catheter clear airway of excessive secretions and promote improved oxygenation (Wood, 1998).
(17) Perform nasopharyngeal and oropharyngeal suctioning. After nasopharyngeal and oropharyngeal suctioning is performed, catheter is contaminated; do not reinsert into ET or tracheostomy tube.	Upper airway is considered "clean," and lower airway is considered "sterile." Therefore the same catheter can be used to suction from sterile to clean areas, but not from clean to sterile areas.

STEPS	RATIONALE
(18) Disconnect catheter from connecting tubing. Roll catheter around fingers of dominant hand. Pull glove off inside out so that catheter remains in glove. Pull off other glove over first glove in same way to contain contaminants. Discard into appropriate receptacle. Turn off suction device.	Reduces transmission of microorganisms. Clean equipment should not be touched with contaminated gloves.
(19) Remove towel and place in laundry, or remove drape and discard in appropriate receptacle.	
(20) Reposition client as indicated by condition. Nurse may need to reapply clean gloves for client's personal care.	Proper positioning based on client's condition promotes comfort and encourages secretion drainage and reduces risk of aspiration.
(21) Discard remainder of normal saline into appropriate receptacle. If basin is disposable, discard into appropriate receptacle. If basin is reusable, rinse and place in soiled utility room.	Solution is contaminated.
(22) Remove and discard face shield, and wash hands.	Reduces transmission of microorganisms.
(23) Place unopened suction kit on suction machine or at head of bed according to institution preference.	Provides immediate access to suction catheter for next procedure.
11. Compare client's vital signs and O_2 saturation before and after suctioning.	Identifies physiological effects of suction procedure to restore airway patency.
12. Ask client if breathing is easier and if congestion is decreased.	Provides subjective confirmation that airway obstruction is relieved with suctioning procedure.
13. Observe airway secretions.	Provides data to document presence or absence of respiratory tract infection.

UNEXPECTED OUTCOMES AND RELATED INTERVENTIONS

- Worsening respiratory status
  - Limit length of suctioning.
  - Determine need for more frequent suctioning, possibly of shorter duration.
  - Determine need for supplemental oxygen. Supply oxygen between suctioning passes.
  - Notify physician.
- Return of bloody secretions
  - Determine amount of suction pressure used. May need to be decreased.
  - Evaluate suctioning frequency.
  - Provide more frequent oral hygiene.
- Unable to pass suction catheter through first naris attempted
  - Try other naris or oral route.
  - Insert nasal airway, especially if suctioning through client naris frequently (St. Johns, 1999).
  - Follow naris floor to avoid turbinates.
  - If obstruction is mucus, apply suction to relieve obstruction, but do not apply suction to mucosa. If obstruction is thought to be a blood clot, consult physician.
  - Increase lubrication of catheter.

- Paroxysms of coughing
  - Administer supplemental oxygen.
  - Allow client to rest between passes of suction catheter.
  - Consult physician regarding need for inhaled bronchodilators or topical anesthetics.
- No secretions obtained
  - Evaluate client's fluid status.
  - Assess for signs of infection.
  - Determine need for chest physiotherapy.
  - Assess adequacy of humidification on oxygen delivery device.

RECORDING AND REPORTING

- Record the amount, consistency, color, and odor of secretions and client's response to procedure; document client's presuctioning and postsuctioning cardiopulmonary status.

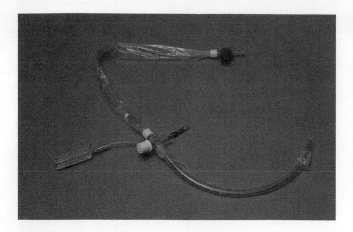

FIGURE **27-3** Ballard tracheal care closed suction.

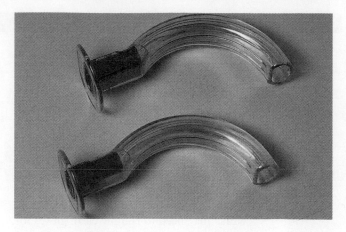

FIGURE **27-4** Artificial oral airways.

oral airway extends from the teeth to the oropharynx, maintaining the tongue in the normal position. The correct-size airway must be used. Proper oral airway size is determined by measuring the distance from the corner of the mouth to the angle of the jaw just below the ear. The length is equal to the distance from the flange of the airway to the tip. If the airway is too small, the tongue is not held in the anterior portion of the mouth; if too large, it may force the tongue toward the epiglottis and obstruct the airway.

The airway is inserted by turning the curve of the airway toward the cheek and placing it over the tongue. When the airway is in the oropharynx, turn it so the opening points downward. Correctly placed, the airway moves the tongue forward, away from the oropharynx, and the flange, the flat portion of the airway, rests against the client's teeth. Incorrect insertion merely forces the tongue back into the oropharynx.

Tracheal Airway. Tracheal airways include endotracheal, nasotracheal, and tracheal tubes. These allow easy access to the trachea for deep tracheal suctioning. Because of the artificial airway, the client no longer has normal humidification of the tracheal mucosa. Ensure that humidity is being supplied to the airway through nebulization or with the oxygen delivery system. This humidification is protective and helps reduce the risk of airway plugging.

MOBILIZATION OF PULMONARY SECRETIONS. The ability of a client to mobilize pulmonary secretions may make the difference between a short-term illness and a long recovery involving complications.

Hydration. Maintenance of adequate hydration promotes mucociliary clearance, the body's natural mechanism for removing mucus and cellular debris from the respiratory tract. In clients with adequate hydration, pulmonary secretions are thin, white, watery, and easily removable with minimal coughing. A fluid intake of 1500 to 2000 ml/day will help keep pulmonary secretions thin and easy to expectorate, unless contraindicated by cardiac condition.

Humidification. **Humidification** is necessary for clients receiving oxygen therapy at more than 4 L/min. A nasal catheter, nasal cannula, or face mask can be humidified by bubbling it through water. When humidity is used, ensure that sterile saline for inhalation is used for humidification and the solution is changed according to agency procedures. Humidification can be a source for nosocomial infections because the moist environment supports the growth of pathogens.

Nebulization. **Nebulization** uses the aerosol principle to suspend a maximum number of water drops or particles of the desired size in inspired air. The moisture added to the respiratory system through nebulization improves clearance and is often used for administration of bronchodilators and mucolytic agents.

MAINTENANCE OR PROMOTION OF LUNG EXPANSION. Nursing interventions to maintain or promote lung expansion include positioning, incentive spirometry, chest physiotherapy, and chest tube management.

Positioning. Healthy people maintain adequate ventilation and oxygenation by frequent position changes. When a person's illness or injury restricts mobility, there is an increased risk for respiratory impairment. Frequent position changes are a simple and cost-effective method for reducing the client's risk for pooled airway secretions and decreased chest wall expansion.

The most effective position for clients with cardiopulmonary diseases is the 45-degree semi-Fowler's position, using gravity to assist in lung expansion and reduce pressure from the abdomen on the diaphragm. Ensure that the client does not slide down in bed, causing reduced lung expansion. Clients with unilateral lung disease, such as a pneumothorax or atelectasis, should be positioned with the healthy lung down. This promotes better perfusion of the healthy lung, improving oxygenation. In the presence of pulmonary abscess or hemorrhage, place the affected lung down to prevent drainage toward the healthy lung.

Incentive Spirometry. **Incentive spirometry** is a method of encouraging voluntary deep breathing by provid-

Nursing care and selection of CPT skills are based on specific assessment findings. The following guidelines help you with physical assessment and subsequent decision making:

1. Know the client's normal range of vital signs. Conditions requiring CPT, such as atelectasis and pneumonia, can affect vital signs. The degree of change is related to the level of hypoxia, overall cardiopulmonary status, and tolerance to activity.
2. Know the client's medications. Certain medications, particularly diuretics and antihypertensives, cause fluid and hemodynamic changes. These may decrease the client's tolerance to positional changes and postural drainage. Long-term steroid use increases the client's risk of pathological rib fractures and often contraindicates rib shaking.
3. Know the client's medical history. Certain conditions, such as increased intracranial pressure, spinal cord injuries, and abdominal aneurysm resection, contraindicate the positional changes of postural drainage. Thoracic trauma or surgery may also contraindicate percussion, vibration, and rib shaking.
4. Know the client's level of cognitive function. Participation in controlled cough techniques requires the client to follow instructions. Congenital or acquired cognitive limitations may alter the client's ability to learn and participate in these techniques.
5. Be aware of the client's exercise tolerance. CPT maneuvers are fatiguing. When the client is not used to physical activity, initial tolerance to the maneuvers may be decreased. However, with gradual increases in activity and planned CPT, client tolerance to the procedure improves.

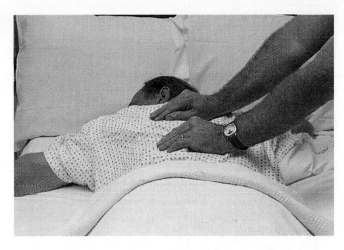

FIGURE **27-5**   Hand position for chest wall percussion during physiotherapy.

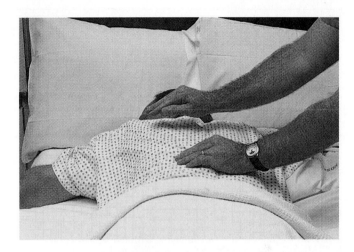

FIGURE **27-6**   Chest wall percussion, alternating hand motion against the client's chest wall.

ing visual feedback to clients about inspiratory volume. Incentive spirometry promotes deep breathing to prevent or treat atelectasis in the postoperative client. It encourages clients to breathe to their normal inspiratory capacities. A postoperative inspiratory capacity one half to three fourths of the preoperative volume is acceptable because of postoperative pain. Administration of pain medications before incentive spirometry will help the client achieve deep breathing by reducing pain and splinting. There is no clinical benefit to using incentive spirometry in place of early ambulation. Encourage your postoperative clients to ambulate as soon as possible.

Flow-oriented incentive spirometers consist of one or more plastic chambers that contain freely moving colored balls. The client inhales slowly with an even flow to elevate the balls and keep them floating as long as possible. This will allow a maximally sustained inhalation.

Volume-oriented incentive spirometry devices have a bellows that is raised to a predetermined volume by an inhaled breath. An achievement light or counter is used to provide feedback. Some devices will not turn the light on unless the bellows is held at a minimum desired volume for a specified period of time.

Chest Physiotherapy.   **Chest physiotherapy (CPT)** is used to mobilize pulmonary secretions (Box 27-9). CPT includes postural drainage, chest percussion, and vibration, followed by productive coughing or suctioning. CPT is recommended for clients who produce more than 30 ml of sputum per day or have evidence of atelectasis by chest x-ray film.

Chest Percussion.   **Chest percussion** involves striking the chest wall over the area being drained. The hand is positioned so that the fingers and thumb touch, and the hand is cupped (Figure 27-5). Percussion on the surface of the chest wall sends waves of varying amplitude and frequency through the chest, changing the consistency and location of the sputum. Chest percussion is performed by alternating hand motion against the chest wall (Figure 27-6). Percussion is performed over a single layer of clothing, not over buttons, snaps, or zippers. The single layer of clothing prevents slapping the client's skin. Thicker or multiple layers of material dampen the vibrations.

Caution should be taken to percuss the lung fields and not the scapular area, or trauma may occur to the skin and underlying musculoskeletal structures. Percussion is contraindicated in clients with bleeding disorders, osteoporosis, or fractured ribs.

Positions for Postural Drainage

Table 27-9

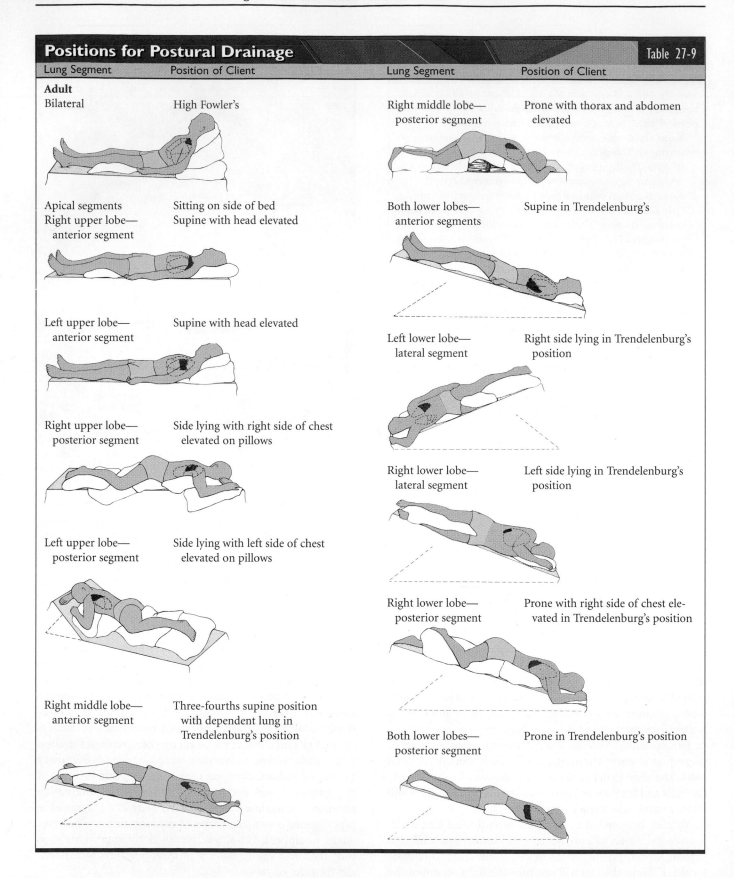

Lung Segment	Position of Client	Lung Segment	Position of Client
Adult			
Bilateral	High Fowler's	Right middle lobe—posterior segment	Prone with thorax and abdomen elevated
Apical segments Right upper lobe—anterior segment	Sitting on side of bed Supine with head elevated	Both lower lobes—anterior segments	Supine in Trendelenburg's
Left upper lobe—anterior segment	Supine with head elevated	Left lower lobe—lateral segment	Right side lying in Trendelenburg's position
Right upper lobe—posterior segment	Side lying with right side of chest elevated on pillows	Right lower lobe—lateral segment	Left side lying in Trendelenburg's position
Left upper lobe—posterior segment	Side lying with left side of chest elevated on pillows	Right lower lobe—posterior segment	Prone with right side of chest elevated in Trendelenburg's position
Right middle lobe—anterior segment	Three-fourths supine position with dependent lung in Trendelenburg's position	Both lower lobes—posterior segment	Prone in Trendelenburg's position

Positions for Postural Drainage—cont'd

Table 27-9

Lung Segment	Position of Client	Lung Segment	Position of Client
Child			
Bilateral—apical segments	Sitting on nurse's lap, leaning slightly forward flexed over pillow	Bilateral lobes— anterior segments	Lying supine on nurse's lap, back supported with pillow
Bilateral—middle anterior segments	Sitting on nurse's lap, leaning against nurse		

Vibration.   **Vibration** is a fine, shaking pressure applied to the chest wall only during exhalation. This technique is thought to increase the velocity and turbulence of exhaled air, facilitating secretion removal. Vibration increases the exhalation of trapped air and may shake mucus loose and induce a cough. Vibration is most often used in clients with cystic fibrosis and is not recommended in infants and young children.

Postural Drainage.   **Postural drainage** is the use of positioning techniques that drain secretions from specific segments of the lungs and bronchi into the trachea. The procedure for postural drainage can include most lung segments (Table 27-9). Because the client may not require postural drainage of all lung segments, the procedure is based on clinical assessment findings. For example, clients with left lower lobe atelectasis may require postural drainage of only the affected region, whereas a child with cystic fibrosis may require postural drainage of all segments.

Chest Tubes.   A **chest tube** is a catheter inserted through the thorax to remove air and fluids from the pleural space and to reestablish normal intrapleural and intrapulmonic pressures. Chest tubes are used after chest surgery and chest trauma and for pneumothorax or hemothorax to promote lung expansion (Skill 27-2).

A **pneumothorax** is a collection of air or other gas in the pleural space. The gas causes the lung to collapse because it obliterates the negative intrapleural pressure and a counterpressure is exerted against the lung, which is then unable to expand. There are a variety of mechanisms for a pneumothorax. It may occur spontaneously or from chest trauma.

A client with a pneumothorax usually feels pain as atmospheric air irritates the parietal pleura. The pain may be sharp and pleuritic. Dyspnea is common and worsens as the size of the pneumothorax increases.

Hemothorax is an accumulation of blood and fluid in the pleural cavity between the parietal and visceral pleurae, usually as the result of trauma. It produces a counterpressure and prevents the lung from full expansion. In addition to pain and dyspnea, signs and symptoms of shock can develop if blood loss is severe.

Disposable chest drainage systems, such as Thora-Sene III or Pleur-Evac chest drainage system (DeKental), are one-piece molded plastic units that are used to evaluate any volume of air or fluid with controlled suction (Figure 27-7). The first chamber provides a water seal to prevent air from being drawn back into the pleural space. The second chamber collects fluid or blood. The third chamber is for suction, to facilitate removal of chest drainage. The suction pressure causes gentle, continuous bubbling in the third chamber. Suction pressure is measured in centimeters of water and is equated with length of the long tube submerged in water. Usually 215 to 220 cm H_2O is used for adults. Children require lesser amounts of suction pressure.

The disposable units appear to be the system of choice because they are cost-effective and some facilitate autotransfusion, a common practice in open heart surgeries. Knowledge of the basics of chest tube management and troubleshooting maneuvers reduces the client's risk of complications.

The one-bottle system, used for smaller amounts of drainage, is the simplest closed drainage system because the single bottle serves as a collector and a water seal. This system is rarely used, except for the drainage of exudate from an empyema. During normal respiration the fluid should ascend with inspiration and descend with expiration.

Special Considerations.   Clamping chest tubes is contraindicated when the client is ambulating or being transported. You should handle the chest drainage unit carefully and maintain the drainage device below the client's chest.

Skill 27-2
CARE OF CLIENTS WITH CHEST TUBES

DELEGATION CONSIDERATIONS

This skill requires problem solving and knowledge application unique to a professional nurse and should not be delegated. For this skill, all staff should be informed of the following:

- Proper positioning of a client with chest tubes to facilitate drainage
- Appropriate setup of drainage equipment for the type of system to be used
- To inform the nurse of any changes in vital signs or excessive bubbling in water-seal chamber

- To notify the nurse immediately if disconnection of system, sudden bleeding, or sudden shortness of breath occurs

EQUIPMENT

- Disposable chest drainage system
- Suction source and setup (wall canister or portable)
- Nonsterile gloves
- 2-inch tape
- Sterile gauze sponges
- 2 shodded hemostats

STEPS	RATIONALE
1. Assess client for respiratory distress and chest pain, breath sounds over affected lung area, and stable vital signs (see Chapter 24).	Signs and symptoms should reflect improvement in respiratory distress and chest pain after insertion of chest tube. Signs and symptoms of increased respiratory distress and/or chest pain are decreased breath sounds over the affected and nonaffected lungs, marked cyanosis, asymmetrical chest movements, presence of subcutaneous emphysema around tube insertion site or neck, hypotension, and tachycardia. Notify physician immediately.
2. Observe:	
a. Chest tube dressing.	Ensures that dressing is intact, without air or fluid leaks.
b. Tubing for kinks, dependent loops, or clots.	Maintains a patent, freely draining system, preventing fluid accumulation in chest cavity. Ensures that tubing is patent.
c. Chest drainage system, which should be upright and below level of tube insertion.	System must be in this position to function properly.
3. Provide two shodded hemostats for each chest tube, attached to top of client's bed with adhesive tape. Chest tubes are only clamped under specific circumstances per physician order or nursing policy and procedure:	Shodded hemostats have a covering to prevent hemostat from penetrating chest tube once changed.
a. To assess air leak.	
b. To quickly empty or change drainage system; performed by a nurse who has received education in the procedure.	
c. To change disposable systems; have new system ready to be connected before clamping tube so that transfer can be rapid and drainage system reestablished.	
d. To assess if client is ready to have chest tube removed (which is done by physician's order); monitor the client for recurrent pneumothorax.	
4. Position the client.	Permits optimal drainage of fluid and/or air.
a. Semi-Fowler's position to evacuate air (pneumothorax).	Air rises to highest point in chest. Pneumothorax tubes are usually placed on the anterior aspect at midclavicular line, second or third intercostal space.
b. High Fowler's position to drain fluid (hemothorax).	Permits optimal drainage of fluid. Posterior tubes are placed on midaxillary line, eighth or ninth intercostal space.
5. Maintain tube connection between chest and drainage tubes intact and taped.	Secures chest tube to drainage system and reduces risk of air leak causing breaks in airtight system.
a. Water-seal vent must be without occlusion.	Permits displaced air to pass into atmosphere.
b. Suction-control chamber vent must be without occlusion when suction is used.	Provides safety factor of releasing excess negative pressure into atmosphere.
6. Coil excess tubing on mattress next to client. Secure with rubber band, safety pin, or plastic clamp.	Prevents excess tubing from hanging over edge of mattress in dependent loop. Drainage could collect in loop and occlude drainage system.

STEPS	RATIONALE
7. Adjust tubing to hang in straight line from top of mattress to drainage chamber. If chest tube is draining fluid, indicate time (e.g., 0900) that drainage was begun on drainage bottle's adhesive tape or on write-on surface of disposable commercial system.	Provides a baseline for continuous assessment of type and quality of drainage.
8. Strip or milk chest tube only if indicated (this means compressing the tube to encourage clots to press through the tube): Stripping—compression along length of the tubing beginning at client and continuing until drainage unit is reached. Milking—compressing and releasing the tube sequentially.	Stripping may cause complications because it creates excessive negative intrapleural pressure (over -100 cm H_2O pressure). Milking causes less of a pressure change.

- *Critical Decision Point*

Check your institutional policy before stripping or milking chest tubes. This practice is being discontinued at most institutions because it is believed that stripping the tube greatly increases intrapleural pressure, which could damage the pleural tissue and cause or worsen an existing pneumothorax.

9. Wash hands.	
10. Evaluate:	
a. Chest tube dressing.	Appearance of drainage may be due to tube occlusion, causing drainage to exit around tube.

- *Critical Decision Point*

Check the dressing carefully. It can come loose from the skin, although this may not be readily apparent.

b. Tubing should be free of kinks and dependent loops.	Straight and coiled drainage tube positions are optimal for pleural drainage. However, when dependent loop is unavoidable, periodic lifting and draining of the tube will also promote pleural drainage (Schmetz and others, 1999).
c. The chest drainage system should be upright and below level of tube insertion. Note presence of clots or debris in tubing.	System must be in this position to function and to facilitate proper drainage (Gordon and others, 1997).

- *Critical Decision Point*

Monitor the position of the system relative to the chest tube carefully, especially during client transport.

d. Water seal for fluctuations with client's inspiration and expiration.	
(1) Waterless system: diagnostic indicator for fluctuations with client's inspirations and expirations.	In the non–mechanically ventilated client, fluid should rise in the water seal or diagnostic indicator with inspiration and fall with expiration. The opposite occurs in the client who is mechanically ventilated. This indicates that the system is functioning properly (Lewis and others, 2000).
(2) Water-seal system: bubbling in the water-seal chamber.	When system is initially connected to the client, bubbles are expected from the chamber. These are from air that was present in the system and in the client's intrapleural space. After a short time, the bubbling stops. Fluid continues to fluctuate in the water seal on inspiration and expiration until the lung is reexpanded or the system becomes occluded.

STEPS	RATIONALE
e. Waterless system: bubbling is diagnostic indicator.	Indicates proper functioning of system.
f. Type and amount of fluid drainage: Nurse should note color and amount of drainage, client's vital signs, and skin color. What is the normal amount of drainage?	
(1) In the adult, less than 50 to 200 ml/hr immediately after surgery in a mediastinal chest tube (Johanson and others, 1988); approximately 500 ml in the first 24 hours (Duncan and others, 1987).	Dark-red drainage is expected only in the postoperative period, turning serous with time (Lewis and others, 2000).
(2) Between 100 and 300 ml of fluid may drain in a pleural chest tube in an adult during the first 2 hours after insertion. This rate decreases after 2 hours; 500 to 1000 ml can be expected in the first 24 hours. Drainage is grossly bloody during the first several hours after surgery and then changes to serous (Lewis and others, 2000). Remember that a sudden gush of drainage may be retained blood and not active bleeding. This increase in drainage can result from client position change.	Reexpansion of lungs forces drainage into the tube. Coughing can also cause large gushes of drainage or air. Excessive amounts and/or the continued presence of frank bloody drainage the first several hours after surgery should be reported to the physician, along with client's vital signs and respiratory status.
g. Water-seal system: bubbling in the suction control chamber (when suction is being used).	Suction control chamber has constant, gentle bubbling. Tubing to the suction source should be free of obstruction, and the suction source should be turned to the appropriate setting.
h. Waterless system: The suction control (float ball) indicates the amount of suction the client's intrapleural space is receiving.	The suction float ball dictates the amount of suction in the system. The float ball allows no more suction than dictated by its setting. If the suction source is set too low, the suction float ball cannot reach the prescribed setting. In this case the suction must be increased for the float ball to reach the prescribed setting.

UNEXPECTED OUTCOMES AND RELATED INTERVENTIONS

- Continuous bubbling is seen in water-seal chamber, indicating that leak is between client and water seal.
  - Tighten loose connections between client and water seal.
  - Cross-clamp chest tube close to client's chest. If bubbling stops, air leak is inside client's thorax or at chest tube insertion site. Unclamp tube, and notify physician immediately. Reinforce chest dressing. Leaving chest tube clamped causes a tension pneumothorax and mediastinal shift.
  - Tighten loose connections between client and water seal.
  - Gradually move clamps down drainage tubing away from client and toward drainage chamber, moving one clamp at a time. When bubbling stops, leak is in section of tubing or connection distal to the clamp. Replace tubing or secure connection and release clamp.
- Leak is in drainage system.
  - Change drainage system.

- Tension pneumothorax is present.
  - Determine that chest tubes are not clamped, kinked, or occluded. Obstructed chest tubes trap air in intrapleural space when air leak originates within client.
  - Notify physician immediately.
  - Prepare immediately for another chest tube insertion; obtain a flutter (Heimlich) valve or large-gauge needle for short-term emergency release of air in intrapleural space; have emergency equipment (e.g., oxygen, code cart) near client.
- Dependent loops of drainage tubing have trapped fluid.
  - Drain tubing contents into drainage bottle. Coil excess tubing on mattress, and secure in place or place in a straight line down the length of the bed.

RECORDING AND REPORTING

- Record in nurse's notes patency of chest tubes; presence, type, and amount of drainage; presence of fluctuations; client's vital signs; chest dressing status; amount of suction and/or water seal; and level of comfort.

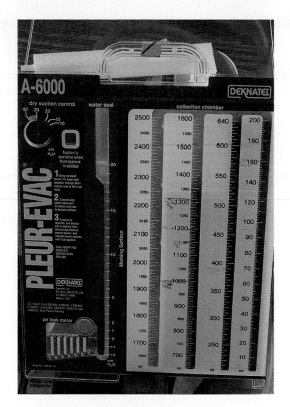

FIGURE **27-7**   Disposable, commercial chest drainage system.

If the tubing disconnects from the unit, instruct the client to exhale as much as possible and to cough. This maneuver rids the pleural space of as much air as possible. Then cleanse the tip of the tubing, and reconnect the tubing to the unit quickly. Clamping the chest tube is not recommended, because it may result in a tension pneumothorax, which is a life-threatening event.

Chest Tube Removal.   Removal of a chest tube requires client preparation. An analgesic administered before removal may help to minimize discomfort and anxiety. Generally the physician removes the tube. The most frequent sensations reported during removal of a chest tube include burning, pain, and a pulling sensation.

MAINTENANCE AND PROMOTION OF OXYGENATION.   Some clients require oxygen therapy to keep a healthy level of tissue oxygenation. The goal of oxygen therapy is to prevent or relieve hypoxia. Any client with impaired tissue oxygenation can benefit from controlled oxygen administration. Oxygen is not a substitute for other treatments, however, and should be used only when indicated. Oxygen is a drug. It is expensive and has dangerous side effects. As with any drug, the dosage or concentration of oxygen should be continuously monitored. Routinely check the physician's orders to verify that the client is receiving the prescribed oxygen concentration. The five rights of medication administration also pertain to oxygen administration (see Chapter 13).

Safety Precautions With Oxygen Therapy.   Oxygen is a highly combustible gas and fuels fire readily. Although it will

not spontaneously burn or cause an explosion, it can easily cause a fire to ignite in a client's room if it contacts a spark from a cigarette or electrical equipment.

With increasing use of home oxygen therapy, clients and health care professionals must be aware of these dangers of combustion. Promote safety by using the following measures:

1. Place "No smoking" signs on the client's room door and over the bed. The client, visitors, roommates, and all personnel should be informed that smoking is not permitted in areas where oxygen is in use.
2. Determine that all electrical equipment in the room is functioning correctly and is properly grounded (see Chapter 25).
3. Know the fire procedures and the location of the closest fire extinguisher.
4. Check the oxygen level of portable tanks before transporting to ensure there is enough oxygen in the tank.

Oxygen Supply.   Oxygen is supplied to the client's bedside either by oxygen tanks or through a permanent wall-piped system. Oxygen tanks are transported on wide-based carriers that allow the tank to be placed upright at the client's bedside. Regulators are used to control the amount of oxygen delivered. One common type is an upright flow meter with a flow-adjustment valve at the top. A second type is a cylinder indicator with a flow-adjustment handle.

Methods of Oxygen Delivery.   Oxygen can be delivered to the client by nasal cannula, nasal catheter, face mask, or mechanical ventilator (Table 27-10).

Home Oxygen.   Indications for home oxygen therapy include an arterial partial pressure (PaO_2) of 55 mm Hg or less or arterial oxygen saturation (SaO_2) of 88% or less on room air at rest, on exertion, or with exercise.

When home oxygen is required, it is usually delivered by nasal cannula. If your client has a permanent tracheostomy, a T tube or tracheostomy collar is necessary to provide humidification to the airway.

Three types of oxygen systems are used: compressed oxygen, liquid oxygen, and oxygen concentrators. The advantages and disadvantages of each type are assessed, along with the client's needs and community resources, before placing a certain delivery system in the home. In the home the major consideration is the oxygen delivery source.

Clients requiring home oxygen need extensive teaching to be able to continue oxygen therapy at home efficiently and safely. This includes oxygen safety, regulation of the amount of oxygen, and how to use the prescribed home oxygen delivery system. You will need to coordinate the efforts of the client and the family, home care nurse, home respiratory therapist, and home oxygen equipment vendor. The social worker usually assists with arranging the home care nurse and oxygen vendor.

RESTORATION OF CARDIOPULMONARY FUNCTIONING.   When hypoxia is severe and prolonged, cardiac arrest may result. A cardiac arrest is a sudden cessation of cardiac output and circulation. When this occurs, oxygen is not delivered to the tis-

Oxygen Delivery Systems

Table 27-10

Delivery System	Indications	O₂ Concentration (Flow Rate)	Considerations
Nasal cannula	Simple, comfortable device to deliver low-concentration O₂ (<6 L/min)	24% (1 L/min) 28% (2 L/min) 32% (3 L/min) 36% (4 L/min) 40% (5 L/min) 44% (6 L/min)	Flow rates more than 4 L/min often cause drying effect on mucosa; humidify oxygen; be alert for skin breakdown over ears and in nares; questionable efficiency in mouth breathers
Transtracheal O₂ (TTO)	For chronic lung diseases; small, IV-size catheter inserted directly into trachea	Flow requirements may be reduced to 60%-80%, which greatly increases amount of time available from portable source of O₂	No O₂ lost to atmosphere; clients achieve adequate oxygenation at lower rates (more efficient, less expensive, and produces fewer side effects); clients more likely to use O₂ because of mobility, comfort, and cosmetic improvement
Oxygen masks	Administer O₂, humidity, or heated humidity		
Simple face mask	Short-term O₂ therapy	30%-60% (6-8 L/min)	Contraindicated for clients with carbon dioxide retention; effective for mouth breathers (Figure 27-8)
Plastic face mask with a reservoir bag	Delivers high concentrations of O₂	80%-90% (10 L/min)	Frequently inspect the bag to make sure it is inflated (Figure 27-9) Mask must be removed when client eats (Figure 27-10)
Venturi mask	Can deliver precise, high-flow rates of O₂; adapters can be applied to increase humidification	24% (2 L/min) 28% (3 L/min) 30% (4 L/min) 35% (6 L/min) 40% (8 L/min) 45% (10 L/min) 55% (14 L/min)	

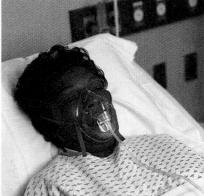

FIGURE **27-8** Simple face mask.

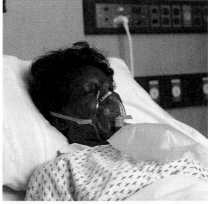

FIGURE **27-9** Plastic face mask with inflated reservoir bag.

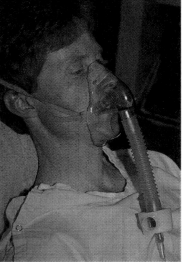

FIGURE **27-10** Venturi mask.

sues, carbon dioxide is not transported from tissues, tissue metabolism becomes anaerobic, and metabolic and respiratory acidosis occurs. Permanent heart, brain, and other tissue damage occurs within 4 to 6 minutes.

Cardiopulmonary Resuscitation. Cardiac arrest is characterized by an absence of pulse and respiration. If you determine that the client has experienced a cardiac arrest, **cardiopulmonary resuscitation (CPR)** must be initiated.

CPR is a basic emergency procedure of artificial respiration and manual external cardiac massage (Skill 27-3). The "ABCs" of CPR are to establish an airway, initiate breathing, and maintain circulation. When an airway cannot be established, reassess proper head position and assess for airway obstruction. The 2000 guidelines for CPR do not recommend lay rescuers perform blind sweeps of the mouth or abdominal thrusts (American Heart Association, 2000). The recommendation is to begin standard CPR.

Text continued on p. 684

Skill 27-3
CARDIOPULMONARY RESUSCITATION

DELEGATION CONSIDERATIONS

Properly trained assistive personnel can perform the skill of cardiopulmonary resuscitation.

- Caution the care provider to make certain the client is indeed pulseless or lacks signs of circulation, such as breathing, coughing, or movement in response to stimulation (American Heart Association, 2000) before initiating chest compressions.
- Review the procedures for opening the airway if the client has any risk for cervical neck trauma.

- Caution the provider regarding the differences among infants, children, and adults.

EQUIPMENT

- Manual resuscitator-bag or bag-mask device if available
- CPR pocket mask or barrier device if available
- Chest compression board if available
- Gloves if available
- Resuscitation cart if available
- Face shield if available

STEPS	RATIONALE
1. Determine if client is unconscious by shaking client and shouting, "Are you OK?"	Confirms that client is unconscious as opposed to intoxicated, sleeping, or hearing impaired. Unconsciousness can be caused by substance abuse, hypoglycemia, ketoacidosis, and shock.

- **Critical Decision Point**

  If unconscious person has adequate respirations and pulse, remain until further assistance is present. Place victim in recovery position. Continue to determine presence of respirations and pulse because respiratory or cardiopulmonary arrest is still possible.

STEPS	RATIONALE
2. Immediately activate emergency medical services (EMS) for adult client. If alone do CPR on infant or child for 1 minute, then activate EMS.	The majority of adult victims are in ventricular fibrillation and need immediate defibrillation when emergency personnel arrive (Lemmer and others, 2001).
3. Determine breathlessness and carotid or brachial (use with infants) pulse.	Presence of pulse and respirations contraindicates initiation of CPR.
a. To determine breathlessness, open airway using head tilt–chin lift or jaw-thrust maneuver. Look, listen, and feel for exchange of air (American Heart Association, 2000).	Tongue is most common cause of airway obstruction. Using these measures to open airway may alleviate cause of breathlessness.
4. Place victim on hard surface such as floor, ground, or backboard. Victim must be flat. If necessary, logroll victim to flat, supine position using spine precautions.	External compression of heart is facilitated. Heart is compressed between sternum and spinal vertebrae, which must be on hard and firm surface.
5. Assume correct and comfortable position.	Nurse may be administering CPR for extended period, particularly in community setting. Correct, comfortable position decreases skeletal muscle fatigue and promotes more effective compressions.
a. One-person rescuer:	
(1) Position to face victim, on knees, parallel to victim's sternum.	Allows rescuer to quickly move back and forth from victim's mouth to sternum.
b. Two-person rescuer:	
(1) One person faces victim, kneeling parallel to victim's head. Second person moves to opposite side and faces victim, kneels parallel to victim's sternum.	Allows one rescuer to maintain breathing while other maintains circulation, without getting in each other's way.
6. If available, apply gloves and face shield.	Reduces transmission of microorganisms.
7. Open airway:	
a. If no head or neck trauma, use head tilt–chin lift method (American Heart Association, 2000) (see illustration).	Spinal cord injury should be suspected with motor vehicle accident, falls, face or head injury or laceration, diving accident, or football or other contact sports injury. In these situations rescuer must use jaw-thrust maneuver. Tongue is most common cause of airway obstruction in unconscious client. Airway obstruction from tongue is relieved. If necessary, remove foreign body.

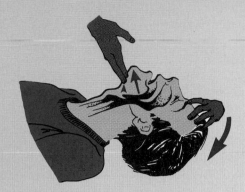

STEP 7A   Head tilt–chin lift.

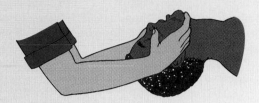

STEP 7B   Jaw thrust without head tilt.

   b. Jaw-thrust maneuver (see illustration) can be used by health professionals but is not taught to general public. Grasp angles of victim's lower jaw and lift with both hands, displacing mandible forward while tilting head backward.

When head and/or neck trauma is suspected, this maneuver opens airway while maintaining proper head and neck alignment, thus reducing risk of further damage to neck.

8. If readily available, insert oral airway.

Maintains tongue on anterior floor of mouth and prevents obstruction of posterior airway by tongue.

9. If victim does not resume breathing, administer artificial respiration:

Airtight seal is formed, and air is prevented from escaping through nose.

   a. Mouth-to-mouth:

• *Critical Decision Point*

CPR pocket masks with one-way valves are available as required by Occupational Safety and Health Administration (OSHA) guidelines (Occupational Health and Safety Act, 1992). Oral airways are readily available in hospital and extended care and outpatient settings. However, they are not available in all community settings. CPR can effectively be accomplished without oral airway or CPR pocket mask. However, rescuer must take appropriate measures to reduce transmission of infectious agents (e.g., hepatitis B, human immunodeficiency virus [HIV], herpes virus, tuberculosis) as proposed by Centers for Disease Control and Prevention (1989).

Adult

   (1) Pinch victim's nose with thumb and index fingers, and occlude mouth with nurse's mouth or use CPR pocket mask. Maintain head tilt–chin lift while administering breaths so air enters lungs and not stomach. Blow two slow full breaths into victim's mouth (each breath should take $1^1/_2$ to 2 seconds); allow victim to exhale between breaths. Continue giving 12 breaths per minute (American Heart Association, 2000).

Hyperventilation is promoted and assists in maintaining adequate blood oxygen levels. In most adults this volume is 800 to 1200 ml and is sufficient to make chest rise. Rescuer should take a breath after each ventilation; this maximizes oxygen content and minimizes carbon dioxide concentration in delivered breaths (American Heart Association, 2000).

• *Critical Decision Point*

An excess of air volume and fast inspiratory flow rates are likely to cause pharyngeal pressures that exceed esophageal opening pressures, allowing air to enter stomach and result in gastric distention, thereby increasing risk of vomiting and compromised respiration.

Child

   (1) Place nurse's mouth over child's mouth or use CPR pocket mask. For mouth-to-mouth resuscitation of child, administer two slow breaths lasting 1 to $1^1/_2$ seconds with a pause between. Continue giving 20 breaths per minute (American Heart Association, 2000).

Airtight seal is formed, and air is prevented from escaping from nose.

STEPS	RATIONALE

Infant

(1) Because infant's air passages are smaller and resistance to flow is quite high, making recommendations about force or volume of rescue breaths is difficult. Place nurse's mouth over infant's nose and mouth. However, three factors should be remembered: (1) rescue breaths are single most important maneuver in assisting nonbreathing child, (2) an appropriate volume is one that makes chest rise and fall, and (3) slow breaths provide an adequate volume at lowest possible pressure, thereby reducing risk of gastric distention.

b. Mouth-to-nose:

(1) Keep victim's head tilted with one hand on forehead. Use other hand to lift jaw and close mouth. Seal rescuer's lips around victim's nose, and blow. Allow passive exhalation.

In some victims (those whose mouth cannot be opened or whose jaws or mouth is seriously injured) mouth to nose can be a more effective method of ventilation.

• **Critical Decision Point**

It may be necessary to open victim's mouth on occasion to allow trapped exhaled air to escape.

c. Ambu-bag:

Adult and Child

(1) For Ambu-bag resuscitation use proper-size face mask and apply it under chin, up and over victim's mouth and nose.

Airtight seal is formed; as bag is compressed, oxygen enters client. Rescuer must squeeze bag fully to deliver 400 to 600 ml of air with supplemental oxygen or 700 ml of air without supplemental oxygen (American Heart Association, 2000). This avoids overinflation and erroneous gastric inflation.

(2) Observe for rise and fall of chest wall with each respiration. Listen for air escaping during exhalation, and feel for flow of air. If lungs do not inflate, reposition head and neck and check for visible airway obstruction, such as vomitus.

Repositioning ensures airway is properly opened and that artificial respirations are entering lungs.

10. Suction secretions if necessary, or turn victim's head to one side, unless contraindicated.

Suctioning prevents airway obstruction. Turning client's head to one side allows gravity to drain secretions.

11. Check for presence of carotid (adults and children) or brachial (infants) pulse after restoring breathing. Check pulse for 5 to 10 seconds.

Carotid artery pulse is most easily accessible and persists when other peripheral pulses are no longer palpable. Makes certain assessment is long enough to thoroughly assess absence of pulse. Following respiratory arrest, pulse may be very slow and weak. Brachial pulse is most accessible and accurate pulse site in infant.

Performing external cardiac compressions on victim who has a pulse may result in serious medical complications.

• **Critical Decision Point**

In the nonintubated victim in acute care setting it may be possible to use two rescue breathers with Ambu-bag. In this case one rescuer maintains seal, and other uses two hands to compress bag, thus delivering greater volumes.

12. If pulse is absent, initiate chest compressions:

a. Assume correct hand position:

Places hands and fingers over heart in proper position. Prevents xiphoid process and rib fracture, which can further compromise cardiopulmonary status.

STEPS	RATIONALE

Adult

(1) Place hands over lower half of sternum, being careful to avoid xiphoid process on sternum. Keep hands parallel to chest and fingers above chest. Interlocking fingers is helpful. Keep fingers off chest wall. Extend arms, and lock elbows. Maintain arms straight and shoulders directly over victim's sternum (see illustration A).

It is critical to keep hands off xiphoid process by marking that area with two fingers of one hand and then placing heel of other hand next to them. Hand marking xiphoid process can than be moved and placed on top of other hand.

Child

(1) Place heel of one hand on lower half of sternum above xiphoid process (see illustration B). Maintain head tilt with other hand if possible.

Proper placement ensures heart compression, maintains patent airway.

Infant

(1) Place index and middle fingers of one hand on lower half of sternum above xiphoid process. Fingers should be 1 cm below nipple line and perpendicular to sternum and not slanted (see illustration C).

Finger placement prevents abdominal injury.

(2) An alternative technique is to place both thumbs side by side over lower half of sternum about xiphoid process.

- **Critical Decision Point**
  Ensure fingers are off ribs.

b. Compress sternum to proper depth from shoulders and then release pressure, maintaining contact with skin to ensure ongoing proper placement of hands. Do not rock, but transmit weight vertically down.

(1) Adult and adolescent: 4 to 5 cm ($1\frac{1}{2}$ to 2 inches) (see illustration).

(2) Older child: 3 to 4 cm (1 to $1\frac{1}{2}$ inches).

Compression occurs only on sternum and is meant to squeeze heart between sternum and spine. Pressure necessary for external compression is created by nurse's upper arm muscle strength and upper body. When compression is released, heart fills.

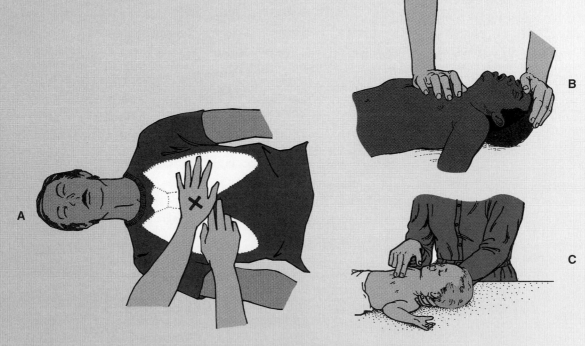

STEP 12A(1)   Proper hand position. **A,** Adult. **B,** Child. **C,** Infant.

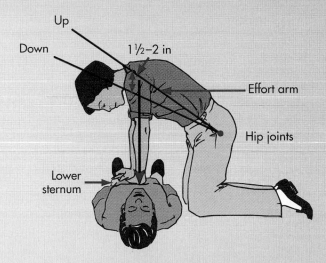

Up

Down

1½–2 in

Effort arm

Hip joints

Lower
sternum

STEP I2B(I)   Compression occurs only on sternum.
Pressure necessary for external compression is created by nurse's
upper arm muscle strength.

(3) Toddler and preschooler: 2 to 4 cm (³/₄ to 1¹/₂
inches).

(4) Infant: 1 to 2 cm (¹/₂ to 1 inch).

c. Maintain proper rate of compression:

(1) Adult and adolescent: 80 to 100 per minute
(count "one one-thousand; two one-thousand").

(2) Child: at least 100 per minute.

(3) Infant: at least 100 per minute.

Proper number of compressions per minute should be delivered to ensure adequate cardiac output.

• *Critical Decision Point*
*Ratio of compressions to breaths in adult CPR for both one rescuer and two rescuers is 15 to 2. Infant and child CPR is
performed at a ratio of 5 compressions to 1 breath.*

d. Continue mouth-to-mouth or Ambu-bag
ventilations:

(1) Adult and adolescent: every 5 seconds (12 per
minute).

(2) Older child: every 4 seconds (15 per minute).

(3) Child: every 3 seconds (20 per minute).

(4) Infant and toddler: every 3 seconds (20 per
minute).

Promotes adequate ventilations to excrete waste gas and supply oxygen.

13. Palpate for carotid or brachial pulse with each external
chest compression for first full minute (two-person
rescue). If carotid pulse is not palpable, compressions
are not strong enough or hand position is incorrect.

Assessment of pulse validates that adequate stroke volume is
achieved with each compression.

14. Continue CPR until relieved, until victim regains
spontaneous pulse and respirations, until rescuer is exhausted and unable to perform CPR effectively, or until physician discontinues CPR.

Artificial cardiopulmonary function is maintained.
CPR is interrupted when changing CPR personnel, during
defibrillation, or when transporting victim. During intubation, CPR may be interrupted for more than 5 seconds but
should not exceed 30 seconds. Nurse should remind nurse
team of number of seconds elapsing during intubation.

15. Remove and discard into appropriate receptacle:
gloves, face shield, and pocket mask.

Reduces transmission of microorganisms.

16. Palpate carotid pulse at least every 5 minutes after first
minute of CPR.

Documents adequacy of external cardiac compressions.

STEPS	RATIONALE
17. Observe for spontaneous return of respirations or heart rate.	Performance of CPR on client with a pulse is dangerous.
18. CPR is not interrupted for more than 5 seconds.	Maintains adequacy of oxygenation and circulation.

UNEXPECTED OUTCOMES AND RELATED INTERVENTIONS
- Client develops skeletal injury, such as fractured ribs or sternum, or internal organ injury, such as lacerated lung or liver.
  - Obtain appropriate diagnostic tests to document rib fracture.
  - Assess client's postarrest breathing for symmetry and pain.
  - Observe for hemoptysis or gastrointestinal bleeding.
  - Observe for distending abdomen.
- Client's CPR is unsuccessful.
  - Contact chaplain services.
  - Contact social worker.

- Complete postmortem care on client.
- Provide privacy for client's family to say their goodbyes to client.
- Rescurer is unassisted, tires, and is unable to continue.
  - Obtain assistance.

RECORDING AND REPORTING
- Immediately report arrest, indicating exact location of victim. In hospital setting, follow hospital policy. In community setting, dial 911 or other emergency number.
- Record in nurse's notes and appropriate code sheet onset of arrest, medication and other treatments given, procedures performed, and victim's response.

Defibrillation is recommended within 5 minutes for an out-of-hospital sudden cardiac arrest and within 3 minutes for an in-hospital victim (Hankley & others, 1997). The recommendation further states that in addition to health care providers, specific lay individuals, police, firefighters, security personnel, ski patrol members, ferryboat crews, and airline flight attendants be trained in CPR and the use of an automated external defibrillator (American Heart Association, 2000).

When an acute myocardial infarction (AMI) is determined by 12-lead ECG, clot-busting medications are indicated and may be administered in the prehospital setting. The medication must be administered within a few hours of the myocardial infarction or stroke (American Heart Association, 2000).

RESTORATIVE AND CONTINUING CARE. Restorative and continuing care may emphasize cardiopulmonary reconditioning as a structured rehabilitation program. **Cardiopulmonary rehabilitation** is actively assisting the client to achieve and maintain an optimal level of health through controlled physical exercise, nutrition counseling, relaxation and stress management techniques, prescribed medications, and oxygen administration. As physical reconditioning occurs, the client's physical symptoms, anxiety, depression, or somatic concerns should decrease. The client and the rehabilitation team define the goals of rehabilitation.

RESPIRATORY MUSCLE TRAINING. Respiratory muscle training improves strength and endurance, resulting in improved activity tolerance. Respiratory muscle training may prevent respiratory failure in clients with COPD.

Breathing Exercises. Breathing exercises include techniques to improve ventilation and oxygenation. The three

Case Study EVALUATION

Mary cares for Mr. King throughout his hospital stay. He is able to go home with improved activities of daily living. He does not require supplemental oxygen use at home. Because he participated in breathing exercises, he practices purse-lipped breathing, his breathing is more controlled, and his subsequent anxiety is relieved.

Mr. King is afebrile, white blood cells are within normal limits, and sputum cultures are negative at discharge. He is able to describe ways to prevent respiratory infections, since they aggravate airways and may precipitate an episode of acute respiratory failure.

While Mary observes Mr. King prepare for discharge, it is quite evident that Mr. King is using the various breathing techniques that they have worked on together. His wife even appears less anxious and states she feels as though for the first time they have taken a step (even though small) to improve the quality of their lives.

Documentation Note
Mr. King discharged to home. Able to state the purpose of breathing exercises and each medication, able to list causes and symptoms of respiratory tract infection. Has an appointment in 1 week with a community-based rehabilitation program. Scheduled to see his physician in 2 weeks. Prescriptions explained and given to client. Accompanied to the exit. Left with wife and son.

basic techniques are deep breathing and coughing exercises, pursed-lip breathing, and diaphragmatic breathing. Review coughing techniques on p. 662.

Pursed-lip breathing involves deep inspiration and prolonged expiration through pursed lips to prevent alveolar collapse. While sitting up, the client is instructed to take a deep breath and to exhale slowly through pursed lips. Clients need to gain control of the exhalation phase so that exhalation is longer than inhalation. The client is usually able to

Nursing Action	Client Response/Finding	Achievement of Outcome
Ask Mr. King to keep track of his fluid intake.	Accurate intake list is completed daily, averaging 2400 ml/hr. Coughing thin secretions.	Good daily fluid intake. Secretions are thin, white, and watery. Outcome has been met.
Ask Mr. King to ambulate for 10 minutes every 4 hours.	Mr. King ambulates once every 8 hours.	Mr. King has met the goal half of the time. Outcome not completely achieved.
Auscultate the chest.	Lung sounds are clear.	Outcome has been met.
Ask Mr. King to keep track of deep breathing every 2 hours while awake.	Diary completed for each day. Mr. King has documented deep breathing every 2 hours while awake 85% of the time.	Secretions are thinned, the lung is clear, and there is no evidence of infection. Outcome has been met.

perfect this technique by counting inhalation time and gradually increasing the count during exhalation.

Diaphragmatic breathing is more difficult and requires the client to relax intercostal and accessory respiratory muscles while taking deep inspirations. The client concentrates on expanding the diaphragm during controlled inspiration. The client is taught to place one hand flat below the breastbone above the waist and the other hand 2 to 3 cm below the first hand. The client is asked to inhale while the lower hand moves outward during inspiration. The client observes for inward movement as the diaphragm ascends. These exercises are initially taught with the client in the supine position and then practiced while the client sits and stands. The exercise is often used with the pursed-lip breathing technique.

 Evaluation

CLIENT CARE.   Nursing interventions and therapies are evaluated by comparing the client's progress to the goals and desired outcomes of the nursing care plan. When nursing measures directed to improve oxygenation are unsuccessful, modify the care plan by revising existing interventions or introducing new interventions. Do not hesitate to notify the physician about a client's deteriorating oxygenation status.

Prompt notification can avoid an emergency situation or even the need for CPR.

Management of the client with COPD depends on achieving three major goals: reduction of airflow obstruction, prevention or management of complications, and improvement in the client's quality of life.

Clients with chronic cardiopulmonary disease present a nursing challenge. They require frequent nursing interventions when they are acutely ill. Because this is a chronic disease, you cannot think in terms of recovery, but rather health maintenance. You are caring for clients with a debilitating disease. You will not see a dramatic cure. You will be assisting clients to improve the quality of their life in small but significant ways.

CLIENT EXPECTATIONS.   The goals that are set for the client must be individualized and realistic. Clients need to know how to cope with this chronic disease. Before any teaching program can be effective, the client must want to learn. Ask the client if he or she would like to know more about COPD and how to control it. Inform the client that it is possible to gain greater independence, improve mobility, decrease dyspnea, and decrease the frequency of acute respiratory infections. Presenting an individualized education program, based on assessment data, helps to ensure the client will comprehend, learn, use, and ultimately benefit from the education (Box 27-10).

Key Terms

accessory muscles, *p. 660*
afterload, *p. 647*
atelectasis, *p. 649*
atrioventricular (AV) node, *p. 646*
bundle of His, *p. 646*
cardiac index, *p. 647*
cardiac output, *p. 646*
cardiopulmonary rehabilitation, *p. 684*
cardiopulmonary resuscitation (CPR), *p. 678*
chest percussion, *p. 671*
chest physiotherapy (CPT), *p. 671*

chest tube, *p. 673*
cough, *p. 657*
cyanosis, *p. 660*
diaphragmatic breathing, *p. 685*
diffusion, *p. 647*
dyspnea, *p. 654*
dysrhythmias, *p. 650*
electrocardiogram (ECG), *p. 646*
hemoptysis, *p. 657*
hemothorax, *p. 673*
hypercapnia, *p. 649*
hyperventilation, *p. 648*
hypoventilation, *p. 648*
hypovolemia, *p. 648*

hypoxemia, *p. 649*
hypoxia, *p. 648*
humidification, *p. 670*
incentive spirometry, *p. 670*
intubation, *p. 668*
laryngospasm, *p. 666*
left-sided heart failure, *p. 650*
myocardial contractility, *p. 647*
myocardial infarction, *p. 650*
myocardial ischemia, *p. 650*
nebulization, *p. 670*
normal sinus rhythm (NSR), *p. 647*
orthopnea, *p. 656*
oxygen therapy, *p. 664*

Continued

Key Terms—cont'd

pneumothorax, *p. 673*
postural drainage, *p. 673*
preload, *p. 647*
productive cough, *p. 657*

Purkinje network, *p. 646*
pursed-lip breathing, *p. 684*
right-sided heart failure, *p. 650*
sinoatrial (SA) node, *p. 646*
stroke volume, *p. 646*
surfactant, *p. 653*

valvular heart disease, *p. 650*
ventilation, *p. 647*
vibration, *p. 673*
wheezing, *p. 656*

Key Concepts

- The primary function of the heart is to deliver deoxygenated blood to the lungs for oxygenation and to deliver oxygen and nutrients to the tissues.
- Cardiac output is altered by preload, afterload, contractility, and heart rate.
- Cardiac dysrhythmias are classified by cardiac activity and site of impulse origin.
- The primary function of the lungs is to transfer oxygen from the atmosphere into the alveoli and carbon dioxide out of the body as a waste product.
- Ventilation is the process of providing adequate oxygenation from the alveoli to the blood.
- Compliance, or the ability of the lungs to expand and contract, depends on the function of musculoskeletal and neurological systems and on other physiological factors.
- The process of inspiration (active process) and expiration (passive process) is achieved with lung changes in pressures and volumes.
- Respiration is controlled by the central nervous system and by chemicals within the blood.
- Decreased hemoglobin levels alter the client's ability to transport oxygen.
- Impaired chest wall movement reduces the level of tissue oxygenation.
- Hyperventilation is a respiratory rate greater than that required to maintain normal levels of carbon dioxide.

- Hypoventilation causes carbon dioxide retention.
- Hypoxia occurs if the amount of oxygen delivered to tissues is too low.
- The nursing assessment includes information about the client's cough, dyspnea, fatigue, wheezing, chest pain, environmental exposures, respiratory infection, cardiopulmonary risk factors, use of medications, and physical functioning.
- Pursed-lip breathing is an effective intervention to control breathing and increase oxygenation.
- Breathing exercises improve ventilation, oxygenation, and sensations of dyspnea.
- Relaxation techniques and imagery are valuable interventions in controlling dyspnea and anxiety in clients with chronic obstructive pulmonary disease.
- Nebulization delivers small drops of water or particles of medication to the airways.
- Chest physiotherapy includes postural drainage, percussion, and vibration to mobilize pulmonary secretions.
- Coughing and suctioning techniques are used to maintain a patent airway.
- Oxygen therapy is used to improve levels of tissue oxygenation and is delivered by nasal cannula, nasal catheter, or oxygen mask.
- Cardiac arrest requires the use of CPR.

Critical Thinking Activities

1. Mr. Jefferson has been assigned to you for the next 8 hours. He has COPD and is known to be difficult to work with, frequently refusing to participate in care. How would you approach his plan of care?
2. You have been assigned three clients on the cardiac care floor. Mrs. Miller is going home today. An acute myocardial infarction was ruled out; however, she does have angina, lives with her husband, and has been pain-free since entering the hospital. Mr. Ruiz has just moved out of the intensive care unit (ICU) following an acute myocardial infarction. He is anxious to go home. He is the head of his household and needs to get back to work. Mr. Silverstein has just been readmitted to the cardiac care unit. He has frequent episodes of chest pain, shortness of breath, and bradycardia. He is scheduled for a cardiac pacemaker today. How would you approach this assignment?

Review Questions

1. Risk factors for cardiopulmonary disease include:
    1. lack of exercise and poor nutrition.
    2. family history of coronary artery disease (CAD).
    3. family history of CAD, smoking, and obesity.
    4. age, gender, lack of exercise, high-fat diet, and obesity.
2. Assessment of your client with tachycardia should include:
    1. risk factors for CAD.
    2. consumption of caffeine and herbal substances.
    3. heart rate, blood pressure, and respiratory rate.
    4. nutritional assessment for high-fat foods and poor nutrition.
3. When assessing the client's oxygenation you would include:
    1. complete blood count (CBC) and chest x-ray.
    2. heart rate and respiratory rate.
    3. arterial blood gases (ABGs) and pulse oximetry.
    4. chest x-ray, heart rate, respiratory rate, and ABGs.
4. The most reliable physical assessment indicator of low oxygen in the blood (hypoxemia) is:
    1. cyanosis.

2. heart rate.
3. blood pressure.
4. cyanosis of the oral mucosa or conjunctiva of the eyes.

5. A normal-appearing electrocardiogram (ECG) tracing with a heart rate of 125 beats per minute would be considered:
   1. sinus rhythm.
   2. sinus bradycardia.
   3. sinus tachycardia.
   4. ventricular tachycardia.

6. Incentive spirometry is used to:
   1. promote coughing.
   2. replace the need for early ambulation.
   3. increase deep breathing and prevent atelectasis.
   4. keep the patient occupied postoperatively.

7. More precise oxygen concentrations can be achieved using a:
   1. nasal cannula.
   2. simple face mask.
   3. venturi mask system.
   4. plastic face mask with inflated reservoir bag.

8. In caring for the client with multiple rib fractures you must keep in mind that:
   1. a tight rib binder will reduce pain.
   2. pain medication should be administered every 4 hours.
   3. deep breathing should not be implemented until after the ribs are healed.
   4. impaired chest wall movement reduces the level of tissue oxygenation.

9. When caring for a client with a decreased hemoglobin level it is important to remember:
   1. the client is at risk for bleeding.

2. the client has altered oxygen transport.
3. the client is at risk for elevated carbon dioxide levels.
4. the client has alterations in the chemical regulators of respiration.

10. During assessment of a client with cardiopulmonary dysfunction you observe restlessness, anxiety, decreased ability to concentrate, increased heart rate, and elevated blood pressure. You would suspect:
    1. hypoxia.
    2. hypoxemia.
    3. right-sided heart failure.
    4. chronic obstructive pulmonary disease (COPD).

11. Contraction of the myocardium occurs:
    1. before the electrical activity (ECG).
    2. during the electrical activity (ECG).
    3. immediately after the electrical activity (ECG).
    4. between 3 and 4 seconds after the electrical activity (ECG)

12. You should remember that the diastolic blood pressure of children is determined:
    1. at 45 mm Hg.
    2. at 30 mm Hg.
    3. by the loss of sound.
    4. when the sound becomes muffled.

13. Clients are candidates for chest physiotherapy if:
    1. the client is receiving long-term steroids.
    2. the client has had abdominal surgery.
    3. the client has increased intracranial pressure.
    4. the client has good exercise tolerance and can follow instructions.

References

American Heart Association: Guidelines 2000 for cardiopulmonary resuscitation and emergency cardiovascular care: international consensus on science, *Circulation* 102:I-371, 2000.

Canobbio MM: *Cardiovascular disorders,* St. Louis, 1990, Mosby.

Caroll PF: What's new in chest-tube management, *RN* 54(5):34, 1991.

Centers for Disease Control and Prevention: Guidelines for prevention of transmission of human immunodeficiency virus and hepatitis B virus to health care and public safety workers, *MMWR Morb Mortal Wkly Rep* 38(suppl 6):1, 1989.

Centers for Disease Control and Prevention: Prevention and control of influenza: Recommendation of the advisory committee on immunization practices (ACIP), *Morb Mortal Wkly Rep* 49(RR03):1, 2000a.

Centers for Disease Control and Prevention: Reducing tobacco use: a report of the Surgeon General, *Morb Mortal Wkly Rep* 49(RR-16):1, 2000b.

Duncan C and others: Effect of chest tube management on drainage after cardiac surgery, *Heart Lung* 16(10):1, 1987.

Gordon PA and others: Positioning of chest tubes: effects on pressure and drainage, *Am J Crit Care* 6:33, 1997.

Hankley AJ and others: Single-rescuer adult basic life support: an advisory statement from the basic life support working group of the international liaison committee on resuscitation, *Circulation* 97(95):2174, 1997.

Johanson BC and others: *Standards for critical care,* ed 3, St. Louis, 1988, Mosby.

Kerr ME and others: Effect of endotracheal suctioning on cerebral oxygen in traumatic brain injured patients, *Crit Care Med* 27(12):2776, 1999.

Lemmer D and others: *Emergency care,* ed 9, Upper Saddle, NJ, 2001, Brady/Prentice Hall Health.

Lewis SL and others: *Medical surgical nursing: assessment and management of clinical problems,* ed 5, St. Louis, 2000, Mosby.

Lueckenotte AG: *Textbook of gerontologic nursing,* ed 2, St. Louis, 2000, Mosby.

McCarley S: A model of chronic dyspnea, *Image J Nurs Sch* 31(3):231, 1999.

Meek PM: Influence of attention and judgment on perception of breathlessness in healthy individuals and patients with chronic obstructive pulmonary disease, *Nurs Res* 49(1):11, 2000.

Occupational Health and Safety Act: *Occupational exposure to blood borne pathogens,* OSHA, 3127, 1992.

Pierson DJ: Effects of aging on the respiratory system. In Pierson DJ, Kacmarek RM, editors: *Foundations of respiratory care,* New York, 1992, Churchill Livingstone.

Phipps WJ and others: *Medical surgical nursing: concepts and clinical practice,* ed 6, St. Louis, 1999, Mosby.

Schmetz JO and others: Effects of position of chest drainage tube on volume drained and pressure, *Am J Crit Care* 8(5):319, 1999.

Seidel HM and others: *Mosby's guide to physical examination,* ed 4, St. Louis, 1999, Mosby.

St. Johns RE: Airway management, *Crit Care Nurse* 19(40):79, 1999.

Wilson SF, Thompson JM: *Mosby's clinical nursing series: respiratory disorders,* St. Louis, 1990, Mosby.

Wong D and others: *Nursing care of infants and children,* ed 6, St. Louis, 1999, Mosby.

Wood CJ: Endotracheal suctioning: a literature review, *Intensive Care Nurse* 14(930):124, 1998.

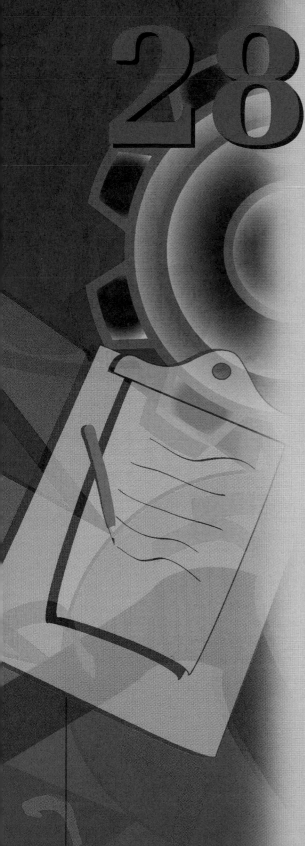

28

Sleep

Objectives

- Define key terms.
- Compare the characteristics of rest and sleep.
- Explain the effect the 24-hour sleep-wake cycle has on biological function.
- Discuss mechanisms that regulate sleep.
- Describe the normal stages of sleep.
- Explain the functions of sleep.
- Compare and contrast the characteristics of sleep for different age-groups.
- Identify factors that normally promote and disrupt sleep.
- Discuss characteristics of common sleep disorders.
- Gather a sleep history for a client.
- Describe interventions appropriate in promoting sleep for clients with various sleep disorders.
- Discuss differences in nursing interventions used for clients of different age-groups.
- Develop a teaching plan to improve a client's sleep hygiene.
- Describe ways to evaluate sleep therapies.

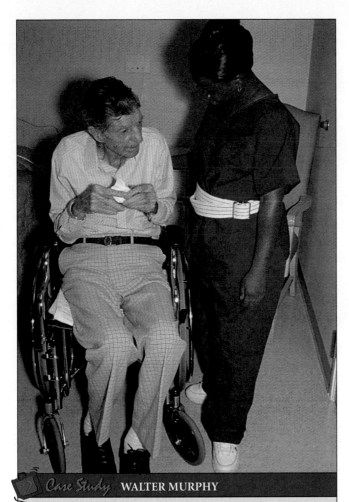

Case Study **WALTER MURPHY**

Walter Murphy is an 82-year-old client who has resided in the local nursing home for the last 3 months. His wife, Mary, still lives at home but visits Walter on a daily basis. Walter is confined to a wheelchair as a result of osteoarthritis and a mild stroke, experienced just 1 year ago. Even though he has physical limitations, he is alert and oriented. Over the last several weeks, Mary has found her husband to be very sleepy when she visits him just before lunchtime. Walter tells Mary that he has trouble falling asleep at night, and once he does fall asleep, he reawakens frequently during the night. Mary is concerned because her husband does not seem as alert or interested during her visit.

Anna is a 23-year-old junior student assigned to the nursing home for her second semester in nursing school. She has had experience in nursing homes, having worked in one center as a nurse assistant during the last two summers. Anna is assigned to care for Mr. Murphy over the next 4 weeks.

Physical and emotional health depend on adequate sleep and rest. Without proper amounts of rest and sleep, the ability to concentrate, make judgments, heal, and participate in daily activities decreases. To help a client gain needed rest and sleep, you as a nurse must understand the nature of sleep, the factors influencing it, and the client's sleep habits. Nurses care for clients who often have preexisting sleep disturbances and for clients who develop sleep problems as a result of illness or being in the health care environment. You must learn to use an individualized approach based on clients' personal sleep habits and pattern of sleep to provide effective sleep therapies.

SCIENTIFIC KNOWLEDGE BASE

Sleep and Rest

When people are at rest, they usually feel mentally relaxed, free from anxiety, and physically calm. They are in a state of mental and physical activity that leaves them feeling refreshed, rejuvenated, and ready to resume the activities of the day. Rest does not imply inactivity, although everyone often thinks of it as settling down in a comfortable chair or taking a brief nap. All persons have their own habits for obtaining rest, for example, reading a book, practicing a relaxation exercise (see Chapter 29), or taking a long walk.

Sleep is a recurrent, altered state of consciousness that occurs for sustained periods. When persons obtain proper sleep, they feel that their energy has been restored. Some experts believe that these feelings of energy restoration imply that sleep provides time for the repair and recovery of body systems for the next period of wakefulness.

Physiology of Sleep

Sleep is a cyclical physiological process that alternates with longer periods of wakefulness. The sleep-wake cycle influences and regulates body functions and behavioral responses.

CIRCADIAN RHYTHMS. People experience cyclical rhythms as part of their everyday life. The most familiar rhythm is the 24-hour, day-night cycle known as the diurnal or **circadian rhythm.** All circadian rhythms, including the sleep-wake cycle, are affected by light and temperature and external factors such as social activities and environmental stressors. All persons have **biological clocks** that synchronize their sleep cycles. Some people can fall asleep at 8 PM, whereas others go to bed at midnight or early in the morning. Different people also function best at different times of the day.

The biological rhythm of sleep frequently becomes synchronized with other body functions. Normal variations in body temperature, for example, correlate with sleep patterns (see Chapter 11). When the sleep-wake cycle becomes disrupted (e.g., by working rotating shifts), other physiological functions may change as well. For example, the person may experience a decreased appetite and lose weight. Failure to maintain one's usual sleep-wake cycle can adversely affect a person's overall health.

SLEEP REGULATION. Sleep involves a sequence of physiological states maintained by highly integrated central nervous system (CNS) activity that is associated with changes in the peripheral nervous, endocrine, cardiovascular, respiratory, and muscular systems (Guyton and Hall, 1997). Each sequence can be identified by specific physiological responses and patterns of brain activity. The control and regulation of sleep may depend on the interrelationship be-

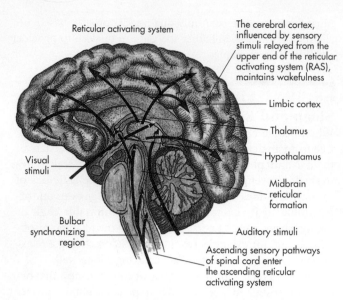

FIGURE **28-1**   The RAS and BSR control sensory input, intermittently activating and suppressing the brain's higher centers to control sleep and wakefulness.

tween two cerebral mechanisms that intermittently activate and suppress the brain's higher centers to control sleep and wakefulness (Figure 28-1). The **reticular activating system (RAS)** causes wakefulness, whereas the **bulbar synchronizing region (BSR)** causes sleep.

While persons try to fall asleep, they close their eyes, assume relaxed positions, and have the room dark, quiet, and at a comfortable temperature. Stimuli to the RAS in the upper brain stem decline. At some point the BSR takes over, causing sleep. Persons will generally not reawaken until their usual sleep cycle is finished or stimuli in the environment (e.g., traffic outside or chirping of birds) stimulate the RAS to awaken the individual.

STAGES OF SLEEP.   Normal sleep involves two phases: **nonrapid eye movement (NREM) sleep** and **rapid eye movement (REM) sleep** (Box 28-1). During NREM a sleeper progresses through four stages during a typical 90-minute sleep cycle. The quality of sleep from stage 1 through stage 4 becomes increasingly deep. Lighter sleep is characteristic of stages 1 and 2, when a person is more easily arousable. Stages 3 and 4 involve a deeper sleep called slow-wave sleep from which a person is more difficult to arouse. REM sleep is the phase at the end of each 90-minute sleep cycle.

SLEEP CYCLE.   Normally an adult's routine sleep pattern begins with a presleep period during which the person is aware only of a gradually developing sleepiness. This period normally lasts 10 to 30 minutes, but if a person has difficulty falling asleep, it may last an hour or more.

Once asleep, the person usually passes through four to six complete sleep cycles, each consisting of four stages of NREM sleep and a period of REM sleep. The cyclical pattern usually progresses from stage 1 through stage 4 of NREM,

Stages of the Sleep Cycle   Box 28-1

STAGE 1: NREM
Stage includes lightest level of sleep.
Stage lasts a few minutes.
Decreased physiological activity begins with gradual fall in vital signs and metabolism.
Person is easily aroused by sensory stimuli such as noise.
Awakened, person feels as though daydreaming has occurred.

STAGE 2: NREM
Stage is period of sound sleep.
Relaxation progresses.
Arousal is still relatively easy.
Stage lasts 10 to 20 minutes.
Body functions continue to slow.

STAGE 3: NREM
It involves initial stages of deep sleep.
Sleeper is difficult to arouse and rarely moves.
Muscles are completely relaxed.
Vital signs decline but remain regular
Stage lasts 15 to 30 minutes.

STAGE 4: NREM
It is deepest stage of sleep.
It is very difficult to arouse sleeper.
If sleep loss has occurred, sleeper will spend considerable portion of night in this stage.
Vital signs are significantly lower than during waking hours.
Stage lasts approximately 15 to 30 minutes.
Sleepwalking and enuresis may occur.

REM SLEEP
Vivid, full-color dreaming may occur. Less vivid dreaming may occur in other stages.
Stage usually begins about 90 minutes after sleep has begun.
It is typified by autonomic response of rapidly moving eyes, fluctuating heart and respiratory rates, and increased or fluctuating blood pressure.
Loss of skeletal muscle tone occurs.
Gastric secretions increase.
It is very difficult to arouse sleeper.
Duration of REM sleep increases with each cycle and averages 20 minutes.

followed by a reversal from stage 4 to 3 to 2, ending with a period of REM sleep (Figure 28-2).

With each successive cycle, stages 3 and 4 shorten, and the period of REM lengthens. REM sleep may last up to 60 minutes during the last sleep cycle. Not all people progress consistently through the usual stages of sleep. For example, a sleeper may fluctuate back and forth for short intervals between NREM stages 2, 3, and 4 before entering REM sleep. The amount of time spent in each stage varies. The number of sleep cycles depends on the total amount of time that the person spends sleeping.

Functions of Sleep

The purpose of sleep is still unclear. One theory suggests that sleep is a time of restoration and preparation for the next period of wakefulness (McCance and Huether, 2002). During

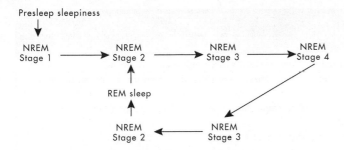

FIGURE **28-2**   The stages of the adult sleep cycle.

NREM sleep, biological functions slow. A healthy adult's normal heart rate throughout the day averages 70 to 80 beats per minute. However, during sleep the heart rate falls to 60 beats per minute, thus preserving cardiac function.

Sleep may also restore biological processes. During NREM stage 4 sleep, the body releases human growth hormone for the repair and renewal of epithelial and specialized cells such as brain cells (McCance and Huether, 2002; Jones, 2000). Protein synthesis and cell division for the renewal of tissues may also occur during rest and sleep.

REM sleep appears to be important for cognitive restoration. REM sleep is associated with changes in cerebral blood flow, increased cortical activity, increased oxygen consumption, and epinephrine release. This association may assist with memory storage and learning.

The benefits of sleep often go unnoticed until a person develops a problem resulting from sleep deprivation. A loss of REM sleep can lead to feelings of confusion. Various body functions (e.g., motor performance, memory, immune function) appear to be altered when prolonged sleep loss occurs.

DREAMS.   The dreams of REM sleep are more vivid and elaborate than those of NREM sleep and are believed to be functionally important to the consolidation of long-term memory (Lee, 1997). REM dreams may progress in content throughout the night from dreams about current events to emotional dreams of childhood or the past. Personality can influence the quality of dreams; for example, a creative person may have very vivid, unusual dreams, and a depressed person may dream of helplessness.

Dreams may help people sort out immediate concerns or erase certain fantasies or nonsensical memories. Since most dreams are forgotten, many people have little dream recall and do not believe they dream at all. To remember a dream, a person must consciously think about it on awakening. People who recall dreams vividly usually awaken just after a period of REM sleep.

▌ NURSING KNOWLEDGE BASE
Normal Sleep Requirements and Patterns
Sleep duration and quality vary among persons of all age-groups. The neonate up to the age of 3 months averages about 16 hours of sleep a day. Approximately 50% of this sleep is REM sleep, which stimulates the higher brain centers

(Wong and others, 1999). Infants usually develop a nighttime pattern of sleep by 3 months of age. The infant may take several naps during the day but usually sleeps an average of 9 to 11 hours during the night. About 30% of sleep time is spent in the REM cycle. Awakening commonly occurs early in the morning, although the infant may waken during the night.

By the age of 2 years, children usually sleep through the night and take daily naps. Total sleep averages 12 hours a day. Naps may be eliminated at 3 years. It is common for toddlers to awaken during the night. The percentage of REM sleep continues to fall. Toddlers may be unwilling to go to bed at night. A preschooler sleeps an average of 12 hours a night (about 20% is REM). By the age of 5, the preschooler rarely takes daytime naps (Wong and others, 1999) except in cultures where a siesta is the custom. The preschooler usually has difficulty relaxing or quieting down after long, active days. A preschooler also has problems with bedtime fears, waking during the night, and nightmares.

The school-age child usually does not require a nap. A 6-year-old averages 11 to 12 hours of sleep nightly, whereas an 11-year-old sleeps about 9 to 10 hours (Wong and others, 1999). The 6- or 7-year-old can usually be persuaded to go to bed by encouraging quiet activities. The older child often resists sleeping because of an unawareness of fatigue or a need to be independent. Typically teenagers get about $7\frac{1}{2}$ hours of sleep per night. At a time when sleep needs actually increase, the typical adolescent is subject to a number of changes that often reduce the time spent sleeping (Dahl and Carskadon, 1995). Usually parents no longer set a specific bedtime. School demands, after-school social activities, and part-time jobs may lessen time available for sleep. Teens go to bed later and rise earlier during the high school years. Because of lifestyle demands that shorten the time available for sleep and physiological needs, teens often experience excessive daytime sleepiness (EDS). School performance, vulnerability to accidents, behavioral problems, and increased use of alcohol and stimulants can be the result of EDS due to insufficient sleep (Mitler and others, 2000).

Most young adults average 6 to $8\frac{1}{2}$ hours of sleep a night, but this can vary. Young adults rarely take regular naps. Approximately 20% of sleep time is spent in REM sleep, which remains consistent throughout the remainder of life. Healthy young adults require adequate sleep to participate in the day's busy activities. However, lifestyle demands often interrupt usual sleep patterns, causing insomnia. During middle adulthood the total time spent sleeping at night begins to decline. The amount of stage 4 sleep begins to fall, a decline that continues with advancing age. Sleep disturbances are often initially diagnosed among people in this age range even when the symptoms of a disorder have been present for several years. Members of this age-group may rely on sleeping medications.

Complaints of sleeping difficulties increase with age. More than 50% of persons age 65 and older report regular problems with sleep (Ancoli-Israel, 1997). Older adults have less stage 3 and stage 4 NREM sleep; some older adults have

Illnesses and Conditions That Can Alter Sleep		Table 28-1
Illness/Condition	Nature of Sleep Alteration
Respiratory disease (e.g., emphysema, asthma, bronchitis, allergic rhinitis, common cold)	Shortness of breath requires use of two to three pillows to raise head. Rhythm of breathing may be altered. Nasal congestion and sore throat impair breathing and ability to relax.
Coronary heart disease with episodes of chest pain and irregular heart rates	Frequent awakenings and sleep stage changes during sleep and significant alterations in all stages of sleep.
Hypertension	Early morning awakening and fatigue.
Hypothyroidism	Decreases stage 4 sleep.
Hyperthyroidism	Takes more time to fall asleep.
Nocturia (reduced bladder tone, diabetes, urethritis, prostate disease)	Awakenings at night to urinate; difficulty returning to sleep.
Gastric reflux	Burning pain in lower esophagus; increases when lying flat in bed.
Depression	Awakenings in early morning with inability to return to sleep; worsened by anxiety or agitation.

almost no stage 4, or deep sleep. Episodes of REM sleep tend to shorten. Older adults awaken more often during the night, and it may take more time for them to fall asleep. Their sleep efficiency (the amount of time asleep given the amount of time in bed) is reduced, and the number of naps taken during the day is increased (Beck-Little and Weinrich, 1998). Tests show that older adults do not have an increased need for sleep, but the ability to sleep is reduced.

As people age, their circadian clock advances, causing **advanced sleep phase syndrome.** The syndrome is common in older adults and often is the reason behind the complaint of waking early in the morning and being unable to get back to sleep (Shneerson, 2000). People with the syndrome get sleepy early in the evening (e.g., 8 or 9 PM). If they were to go to bed at that time, they would sleep for about 8 hours and wake up around 4 or 5 AM. However, when people with advanced sleep phase syndrome stay up until their customary 10 or 11 PM, their bodies still awaken at 4 or 5 AM. They thus receive only 5 to 6 hours of sleep, the amount of time they are in bed before their advanced sleep-wake cycle wakes them up (Ancoli-Israel, 1997).

Factors Affecting Sleep

A number of factors (physical, psychological, and environmental) affect the quantity and quality of sleep. Often more than one factor combine to cause a sleep problem.

PHYSICAL ILLNESS.   Any illness or condition that causes pain, difficulty breathing, nausea, or mood problems such as anxiety or depression can result in sleep problems. Persons with such alterations may have trouble falling or staying asleep. Illnesses also may force clients to sleep in positions to which they are unaccustomed. Table 28-1 summarizes illnesses and conditions that have the potential for causing sleep alterations.

DRUGS AND SUBSTANCES.   A considerable number of drugs cause either sleepiness, insomnia, or fatigue as a side effect (Box 28-2). Medications prescribed for sleep often cause

more problems than benefits. L-Tryptophan is a natural protein found in foods such as milk, cheese, and meats and may help a person sleep. It is a precursor to the neurotransmitter serotonin, which has a role in the sleep-wake cycle.

LIFESTYLE.   A persons' daily routine may influence sleep patterns. An individual who alternately works day and night shifts, for example, often has difficulty adjusting to the altered sleep schedule. Other alterations in routine that can disrupt sleep patterns include performing unaccustomed heavy work or exercise, engaging in late-night social activities, and changing evening mealtime.

USUAL SLEEP PATTERNS AND EXCESSIVE DAYTIME SLEEPINESS.   On average, adults sleep just under 7 hours per night during the week, and 33% of adults sleep only $6^{1}/_{2}$ hours or less nightly (National Sleep Foundation, 2000). Many Americans are sleep deprived and experience excessive sleepiness during the day. EDS often results in impairment of waking function, poor work or school performance, accidents while driving or using equipment, and behavioral or emotional problems. Feelings of sleepiness are usually most intense upon awakening from or right before going to sleep and about 12 hours after the midsleep period.

Sleepiness becomes pathological when it occurs at times when persons need or want to be awake. Persons who temporarily experience sleep deprivation as a result of an active social evening or lengthened work schedule usually feel sleepy the next day. However, they may be able to overcome these feelings even though they have difficulty performing tasks and remaining attentive. Chronic lack of sleep is much more serious than temporary sleep deprivation and can cause serious alterations in the ability to perform daily activities. EDS is most difficult to overcome during sedentary tasks (e.g., driving).

EMOTIONAL STRESS.   Worry over personal problems or situations can disrupt sleep. Emotional stress causes tension and often leads to frustration when sleep does not come.

Drugs and Their Effect on Sleep

Box 28-2

HYPNOTICS
Interfere with reaching deeper sleep stages
Provide only temporary (1 week) increase in quantity of sleep
Eventually cause "hangover" feeling during day
May worsen sleep apnea in older adults

DIURETICS
Cause nocturia

ANTIDEPRESSANTS AND STIMULANTS
Suppress REM sleep
Decrease total sleep time

ALCOHOL
Speeds onset of sleep and disrupts REM sleep
Awakens person during night and causes difficulty returning to sleep

CAFFEINE
Prevents person from falling asleep
May cause person to awaken during night

BETA-ADRENERGIC BLOCKERS
Cause nightmares and insomnia
Cause awakening from sleep

BENZODIAZEPINES
Increase sleep time
Increase daytime sleepiness

NARCOTICS (OPIATES)
Suppress REM sleep
Cause increased daytime drowsiness

ANTIHISTAMINES
Cause drowsiness
Excess amounts can cause insomnia

NASAL DECONGESTANTS
Cause daytime sleepiness

Stress may also cause a person to try too hard to fall asleep, to awaken frequently during the sleep cycle, or to oversleep. Continued stress may cause poor sleep habits.

ENVIRONMENT. The physical environment in which a person sleeps has a significant influence on the ability to fall and remain asleep. Good ventilation, a comfortable temperature, and a darkened or softly lit room are essential for restful sleep. The size, firmness, and position of a bed can also affect sleep quality. Hospital beds are often harder than those at home. If a person usually sleeps with another individual, sleeping alone during times of illness can cause wakefulness. However, sleeping with a restless or snoring bed partner can also disrupt sleep.

SOUND. The level of noise needed to awaken a person depends on the stage of sleep (Webster and Thompson, 1986). Low noises are more likely to arouse a person from stage 1 sleep, whereas louder noises awaken a person in stage 3 or 4 sleep. Some persons require silence to fall asleep, whereas others prefer background noise such as soft music or television.

In health care facilities, noise creates a problem for clients. Noise in health care settings is usually new or strange to the client. This problem is greatest the first night a client stays in a hospital or other facility, when clients often experience increased total wake time, increased awakening, and decreased REM sleep and total sleep time. Nursing activities are a source of increased sound levels. The intensive care setting is one of the loudest, where close proximity of clients, noise from confused and ill clients, and ringing of alarm systems and telephones make the environment very unpleasant.

EXERCISE AND FATIGUE. A person who is moderately fatigued usually achieves restful sleep, especially if the fatigue results from enjoyable work or exercise. Completing rigorous exercise 2 hours or more before bedtime allows the body to cool down and maintains a state of fatigue that promotes

relaxation. However, excess fatigue resulting from exhausting or stressful work can make falling asleep difficult.

FOOD AND CALORIC INTAKE. Following good eating habits is important for proper health, including sleep. Eating a large, heavy, and/or spicy meal at night may result in indigestion that interferes with sleep. Alcohol consumed in the evening has insomnia-producing effects. Coffee, tea, cola, and chocolate contain caffeine and xanthines that cause sleeplessness as a result of CNS stimulation. Food allergies may cause insomnia. In infants, nighttime waking and crying may be caused by a milk allergy, requiring that breast milk or a nonmilk formula be used. Other foods that often result in an insomnia-producing allergy in children and adults include corn, wheat, nuts, chocolate, eggs, seafood, red and yellow food dyes, and yeast (Hauri and Linde, 1990).

Weight loss or gain influences sleep patterns. When a person gains weight, sleep periods become longer with fewer interruptions. Weight loss can cause short and fragmented sleep. Certain sleep disorders may be the result of the semi-starvation diets popular in a weight-conscious society.

Sleep Disorders

Sleep disorders are conditions that, if untreated, cause disturbed nighttime sleep that results in one of three problems: insomnia; abnormal movements or sensation during sleep or when awakening at night; or excessive daytime sleepiness (Aldrich and Naylor, 2000). The occurrence of sleep disorders is becoming a significant health problem especially for persons living in stressful environments. Sleep disorders have been classified into three major categories with one additional proposed category (American Sleep Disorders Association, 1997) (Box 28-3). The dyssomnias are primary disorders that have their origin in different body systems. the intrinsic sleep disorders include disorders of initiating and maintaining sleep. Extrinsic sleep disorders develop from external factors, which if removed, lead to res-

Classification of Select Sleep Disorders   Box 28-3

DYSSOMNIAS
Intrinsic Sleep Disorders
Psychophysiological insomnia
Narcolepsy
Obstructive sleep apnea syndrome
Periodic limb movement disorder

Extrinsic Sleep Disorders
Inadequate sleep hygiene
Insufficient sleep syndrome
Hypnotic-dependent sleep disorders
Alcohol-dependent sleep disorders

Circadian Rhythm Sleep Disorders
Time-zone change (jet lag) syndrome
Shift-work sleep disorder
Delayed sleep phase syndrome

PARASOMNIAS
Arousal Disorders
Sleepwalking
Sleep terrors

Sleep-Wake Transition Disorders
Sleeptalking
Nocturnal leg cramps

PARASOMNIAS—cont'd
Parasomnias Usually Associated With REM Sleep
Nightmares
REM sleep behavior disorder

Other Parasomnias
Sleep bruxism (teeth grinding)
Sleep enuresis (bed-wetting)
Sudden infant death syndrome

SLEEP DISORDERS ASSOCIATED WITH MEDICAL/PSYCHIATRIC DISORDERS
Associated With Psychiatric Disorders
Mood disorders
Anxiety disorders

Associated With Neurological Disorders
Dementia
Parkinsonism

Associated With Other Medical Disorders
Nocturnal cardiac ischemia
Chronic obstructive pulmonary disease

PROPOSED SLEEP DISORDERS
Menstruation-associated sleep disorders
Sleep choking syndrome

Data from American Sleep Disorders Association, Diagnostic Classification Steering Committee: *International classification of sleep disorders,* 1997. In Thorpy M: Classification of sleep disorders. In Kryger M and others, editors: *Principles and practice of sleep medicine,* ed 3, Philadelphia, 2000, WB Saunders.

olution of the sleep disorder. The circadian rhythm sleep disorders arise from a misalignment between the timing of sleep and what is desired by the individual or is a societal norm. The parasomnias are undesirable behaviors that occur usually during sleep. Many medical and psychiatric sleep disorders are associated with sleep and wake disturbances. These sleep disturbances are divided into those associated with psychiatric, neurological, or other medical disorders. The proposed sleep disorders are newly described disturbances still under study.

INSOMNIA.   **Insomnia** is a symptom experienced by clients who have chronic difficulty falling asleep, frequent awakenings from sleep, and/or a short sleep or nonrestorative sleep (Zorick and Walsh, 2000). The person with insomnia complains of EDS, as well as insufficient quantity and quality of sleep. Frequently, however, the client gets more sleep than is realized. Insomnia may signal an underlying physical or psychological disorder.

People may experience transient or temporary insomnia as a result of situational stresses such as work or family problems. Insomnia may recur, but between episodes the client is able to sleep well. A temporary case of insomnia caused by a stressful event can, however, lead to chronic difficulty in obtaining sufficient sleep. Insomnia is often associated with poor sleep habits. If the condition continues, the fear of not being able to sleep can be enough to cause wakefulness. During the day a person with chronic insomnia may feel sleepy, fatigued, depressed, and anxious.

Treatment such as improved sleep hygiene measures, biofeedback, and relaxation techniques can be directed at the symptoms. It is important to treat underlying emotional or medical problems that may be causing the insomnia.

SLEEP APNEA.   **Sleep apnea** is a disorder in which the individual cannot breathe and sleep at the same time (Ancoli-Israel, 1997). There is a lack of airflow through the nose and mouth for periods from 10 seconds to 1 to 2 minutes in length. There can be 10 or 15 to more than 100 respiratory events per hour of sleep (Ancoli-Israel, 1997). There are three types of sleep apnea: obstructive, central, and mixed apnea, which has both an obstructive and a central component.

The most common form, obstructive sleep apnea, is characterized by cessation of airflow despite the effort to breathe. It occurs when muscles or structures of the oral cavity or throat relax during sleep. The upper airway becomes partially or completely blocked, and nasal airflow is diminished (hypopnea) or stopped (apnea). The person tries to breathe because chest and abdominal movement continues, which often results in loud snoring sounds. When breathing is partially or completely diminished, each successive diaphragmatic movement becomes stronger until the obstruction is relieved. Structural abnormalities such as a deviated septum, nasal polyps, or enlarged tonsils may predispose a client to obstructive apnea.

EDS is the most common complaint of people with obstructive sleep apnea. Clients are at risk for cardiac dysrhythmias, right heart failure, pulmonary hypertension, angina attacks, stroke, and hypertension. A serious decline in the arterial oxygen level can occur (see Chapter 27).

Central sleep apnea is caused by cessation of diaphragmatic and intercostal respiratory effort as a result of dysfunction of the brain's respiratory control center. The impulse to breathe temporarily fails. Nasal airflow and chest wall movement cease, with oxygen saturation of the blood also falling. Central sleep apnea is seen in clients with brain stem injury, muscular dystrophy, and encephalitis, as well as in people who breathe normally during the day. It is the least common sleep apnea.

Treatment for sleep apnea includes therapy for underlying cardiac or respiratory complications and emotional problems. The treatment of choice is use of a nasal continuous positive airway pressure (CPAP) device at night. The CPAP machine pushes positive pressure into the airway in an attempt to reduce the apnea periods the client experiences during sleep. Improved sleep hygiene and a weight loss program may also be helpful.

NARCOLEPSY.   Narcolepsy is a CNS dysfunction of mechanisms that regulate sleep and wake states. EDS is the most common complaint associated with narcolepsy. During the day a person may suddenly feel an overwhelming wave of sleepiness and fall asleep. REM sleep can occur within 15 minutes of falling asleep. **Cataplexy,** or sudden muscle weakness during intense emotions such as anger or laughter, is a symptom of narcolepsy that may occur at any time during the day. If the cateplectic attack is severe, the client may lose voluntary muscle control and fall to the floor.

A person with narcolepsy often falls asleep uncontrollably at inappropriate times. Unless this disorder is understood, a sleep attack can easily be mistaken for laziness, lack of interest in activities, or drunkenness. Typically symptoms first occur in adolescence and may be confused with EDS. Narcoleptics are treated with stimulants that may only partially increase wakefulness and reduce sleep attacks. Medications that suppress cataplexy and the other REM-related symptoms may also be effective.

SLEEP DEPRIVATION.   **Sleep deprivation** is a problem many clients have as a result of the dyssomnias. Causes may include illness (e.g., fever, difficulty breathing, or pain), emotional stress, medications, environmental disturbances (e.g., frequent interruptions in sleep during nursing care), and variability in the timing of sleep as a result of shift work.

Hospitalization, especially in intensive care units, makes clients vulnerable to the extrinsic and circadian sleep disorders (Redeker, 2000). Sleep deprivation involves decreases in the quantity and quality of sleep as well as inconsistency in the timing of sleep. When sleep becomes interrupted or fragmented, changes in the normal sequencing of the sleep cycles occur. A cumulative sleep deprivation develops.

Individuals respond to sleep deprivation differently. Clients may experience a variety of physiological and psychological symptoms such as blurred vision, decreased reflexes, slow response time, cardiac arrythmias, confusion,

and irritability. The severity of symptoms is often related to the duration of sleep deprivation. The most effective treatment for sleep deprivation is elimination or correction of factors that disrupt the sleep pattern. Nurses play an important role in identifying treatable sleep deprivation problems.

PARASOMNIAS.   The parasomnias are sleep disorders that produce undesirable physical symptoms as a result of autonomic nervous system changes and skeletal muscle activity during sleep. They are more common in children than in adults. One common exception is sleep **bruxism** (tooth grinding), frequently seen in adults experiencing continuous stress. Sudden infant death syndrome (SIDS) is believed to be related to apnea, hypoxia, and cardiac arrhythmias caused by abnormalities in the autonomic nervous system that occur during sleep (Gillis, 2000). Specific treatment for these disorders varies based on the underlying cause. However, in all cases it is important to support clients experiencing a disorder and maintain their safety.

CRITICAL THINKING
Synthesis

It is not uncommon for almost any client to have experienced some type of sleep disorder. However, it is important not to overlook such a problem or consider it as normal. Use of a critical thinking approach helps you to correctly identify the nature of a sleep problem and then to initiate appropriate nursing care. You must apply your knowledge, experience, and appropriate critical thinking attitudes and standards to make the correct clinical judgments for clients.

KNOWLEDGE.   To make decisions about the nature and cause of a client's sleep problems, it is important for you to synthesize knowledge regarding the physiology and functions of sleep and factors that affect sleep. Knowledge of the pathophysiology of select disease processes further helps in understanding the mechanisms for certain sleep problems. In addition, you should have a good knowledge of pharmacological information because many of the medications clients receive can contribute to sleeping difficulties.

Another important area of knowledge to synthesize is that of a client's personal routine and cultural orientation. Infant care practices such as co-sleeping and the practice of regular siestas or naps are examples of cultural variations influencing sleep. You should anticipate how such cultural factors could ultimately influence an individual client's ability to sleep.

EXPERIENCE.   You know of factors that have either disrupted or promoted your own ability to sleep. This personal experience can be valuable when assessing clients' sleep problems or in selecting therapies for sleep promotion. Previous clinical experience with clients helps you to appreciate that environmental and lifestyle variations significantly affect the quality and quantity of sleep a client receives.

ATTITUDES.   When dealing with sleep problems, it may take a long time to find effective therapies. Chronic insomnia, for example, is not easily eliminated in a short period. Perseverance is an important critical thinking attitude to use if you are to help find effective solutions for the client. The problems posed by sleep disturbances also often require creative approaches. An original idea may be necessary, for example, to minimize or control environmental stressors in the client's sleep environment.

STANDARDS.   When learning about a client's sleep problem, you must use numerous intellectual standards in conducting the nursing assessment. Always conduct a detailed sleep assessment to understand the nature of the sleep problem and potential causes and solutions. A clear, precise, specific, and accurate assessment will also be very important so that an appropriate plan of care can be established. Use of a sleep diary is an accepted standard for gathering a complete history of the quality of sleep over time.

NURSING PROCESS

 Assessment

Assess a client's sleep pattern to gather information about factors that usually influence sleep. Because sleep is a subjective experience, only the client can report whether it is sufficient and restful. If a client admits to or you suspect a sleep problem, a more detailed history is needed. Aim your assessment at understanding the characteristics of any sleep problem and the client's usual sleep habits so that ways for promoting sleep can be incorporated into nursing care.

SOURCES FOR SLEEP ASSESSMENT.   Clients are your best resources for describing a sleep problem and any change from their usual sleep and waking patterns. Bed partners can offer information on clients' sleep patterns that may reveal the nature of certain disorders.

Obtain a child's sleep history from the parents. Older children often are able to relate their fears or worries that prevent them from falling asleep. If children frequently awaken in the middle of bad dreams, parents can identify the problem without necessarily knowing the meanings of the dreams. Parents can also describe typical behavior patterns that foster or impair sleep. With chronic sleep problems, parents can relate the duration of the problem, its progression, and children's responses. Parents of infants may need to keep a 24-hour log of their infant's waking and sleeping behavior over a period of several days.

SLEEP HISTORY.   You can obtain a brief sleep history from clients who report they enjoy adequate sleep. Determine usual bedtime, normal bedtime rituals, preferred environment for sleeping, and what time the client usually rises to plan care to support the client's positive sleep habits and patterns. You need to assess the quality and characteristics of sleep in greater depth when a sleep problem is suspected.

SLEEP PATTERN.   Begin the sleep history with the client's self-report of his or her sleep pattern. Most persons can give a reasonably accurate estimate of their sleep patterns, particularly if any changes have occurred. An effective, subjective method for you to use for assessing sleep quality is the visual analog scale (Closs, 1988). Draw a straight horizontal line about 100 mm (4 inches) long. Opposing statements such as "best night's sleep" and "worst night's sleep" are at each end of the line. Clients are asked to place a mark along the horizontal line at the point that best matches their perception of the previous night's sleep. The distance of the mark along the line in millimeters offers a numerical value for satisfaction with sleep. You can use the scale repeatedly to show change in sleep over time. You cannot use the scale to compare the quality of sleep for different clients.

It is important to have clients describe their usual sleep pattern should there be significant changes created by a sleep disorder. To assess the client's sleep pattern, ask the following questions:

1. What time do you usually get in bed?
2. What time do you usually fall asleep? Do you do anything special to help you fall asleep?
3. How many times do you awaken during sleep? Why do you think you awaken? What do you do about awakening?
4. What time do you typically wake up?
5. What time do you get out of bed and stay up once you have awakened?
6. What is the average number of hours you sleep?

Compare the assessment data with the pattern usually found for other clients of the same age, and look for patterns that might suggest problems. Clients with sleep problems may show patterns very different from their usual one, or the change may be relatively minor. Hospitalized clients usually need or want more sleep as a result of illness. However, some may require less sleep because they are less active. Clients who are ill may think that it is important to try to sleep more than what is usual for them, eventually making sleeping difficult.

DESCRIPTION OF SLEEPING PROBLEMS.   When a client admits to or you suspect a sleep problem, ask open-ended questions to help a client describe the problem more fully. A general description of the problem followed by more focused questions usually reveals specific sleep characteristics (Table 28-2).

You need to understand the nature of the sleep problem, its signs and symptoms, its onset and duration, its severity, predisposing factors or causes, and the overall effect on the client. Assessment questions might include the following:

1. *Nature of the problem:* Tell me what type of problem you have with your sleep. Tell me why you think you are not getting enough sleep. Describe for me a recent typical night's sleep. How is this sleep different from what you are used to?
2. *Signs and symptoms:* Have you been told that you snore loudly? Do you have headaches when awakening? Does your child awaken from nightmares? Ask bed partners or parents whether clients have restful sleep or problems such as going to the bathroom frequently.

Example of a Focused Client Assessment		Table 28-2
Factors to Assess	**Questions and Approaches**	**Physical Assessment Strategies**
Bedtime routines	Determine what the client does to prepare for sleep.	Observe for dark circles under client's eyes.
Bedtime environment	Ask the client to describe the bedroom sleeping condition (e.g., level of light, noise, temperature)	Observe the number of times the client yawns.
Current life events	Ask client about normal hours worked.	Observe for multiple client position changes.
	Determine if changes in job responsibilities have occurred.	Observe the client's ability to concentrate on the conversation.
	Ask client about social activities outside of work.	

3. *Onset and duration:* When did you notice the problem? How long has this problem lasted?
4. *Severity:* How long does it take you to fall asleep? How often during the week do you have trouble falling asleep or staying asleep?
5. *Predisposing factors:* Tell me what you do just before going to bed. Have you recently had any changes at work, school, or home? How would you describe your current mood, and have you noticed any recent changes? What medications or recreational drugs do you take regularly? Do you eat foods (e.g., spicy or greasy foods) or drink liquids (e.g., alcohol, caffeinated beverages) that might disrupt your sleep? If so, how much do you eat or drink daily?
6. *Effect on client:* How has the loss of sleep affected you? Do you feel excessively sleepy or irritable or have trouble concentrating? Do you have trouble staying awake, or have you fallen asleep at inappropriate times? Ask a family member or friend: Have you noticed any changes in the client's behavior since the sleep problem started?

SLEEP LOG.   In addition to the sleep history, a client and bed partner may be asked to keep a sleep-wake log for 1 to 2 weeks (Beck-Little and Weinrich, 1998). The log is completed daily to provide information on day-to-day variations in sleep-wake patterns over time. Entries in the log often include 24-hour information on waking and sleeping activities such as exercise, work activities, mealtimes, alcohol and caffeine intake, time and length of daytime naps, evening and bed routines, the time the client tries to fall asleep, time and number of awakenings, and the time of morning awakening. A partner can help to complete the sleep-wake log. The log is most helpful if the client is motivated to complete it thoroughly. Use of a tape recorder is a helpful option for clients with visual impairment or who have difficulty writing. The log is not used with acutely ill clients who have short hospital stays.

PHYSICAL ILLNESS.   Assess for any physical or psychological problems that may be affecting a client's sleep. Review of known medical conditions can reveal symptoms (e.g., pain, shortness of breath, or fear) that interfere with the client's normal sleep pattern. Assess the client's medication history, including over-the-counter and prescribed drugs. If a client takes medications for sleep, gather information about the type and amount of medication that is being used. If the client has recently undergone surgery, you can expect the client to experience some disturbance in sleep. The effect on sleep depends on the severity of pain experienced after surgery (Closs, 1992).

CURRENT LIFE EVENTS.   Changes in lifestyle can disrupt a client's sleep. A person's family situation or occupation may offer a clue to the nature of a sleep problem. Changes in job responsibilities, rotating shifts, or the recent birth of a child or loss of a family member can contribute to a sleep disturbance. Questions about social activities, recent travel, or mealtime schedules also help clarify the sleep assessment.

EMOTIONAL AND MENTAL STATUS.   If a client is anxious, fearful, or angry, mental preoccupations can seriously disrupt sleep. The client may be experiencing emotional stress related to illness or situational crises. Ask clients to explore feelings about family relationships, job, or other meaningful situations. When a sleep disturbance is related to an emotional problem, the key is to treat the primary problem, and its resolution should improve sleep (Ancoli-Israel, 1997).

BEDTIME ROUTINES.   Ask how the client prepares for sleep. Assess habits that are beneficial compared with those that have been found to disturb sleep. You may need to point out that a particular habit may be interfering with sleep and help clients find ways to change or eliminate habits that disrupt sleep. A client's activity or exercise pattern before bedtime offers additional information about sleep quality. Does the client perform strenuous exercise within 2 hours of going to sleep? Does the client usually spend 1 to 2 hours cooling down or relaxing before sleep?

BEDTIME ENVIRONMENT.   Ask the client to describe preferred bedroom conditions, for example, keeping the bedroom dark or softly lit and closing the door. The client may listen to a radio or watch TV or may prefer a quiet environment if noise prevents the client from falling asleep. Also ask about room temperature and ventilation.

Assess the type of bed in which the person sleeps. Does the client sleep in the same bed every night? Is the mattress comfortable? Does the client need several pillows or cushions in bed to sit up during sleep? Does the client use a lounge chair to sleep? Information about the sleeping environment helps you design better sleeping conditions.

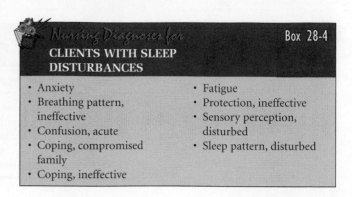

As Anna prepares to conduct an assessment of Mr. Murphy, she knows it is important to consider how sleep is altered in older adults. Because they typically have less deep sleep and more awakenings to begin with, it will be important to consider what factors in the nursing home environment may be disrupting sleep. In addition, she has learned that the pain of Mr. Murphy's osteoarthritis can be a contributing factor to any possible sleep disturbance. His immobility resulting from the stroke may add to any discomfort. Anna also plans to assess Mr. Murphy's medications carefully to determine if any drugs might be adding to a sleep alteration.

From Anna's experience in a nursing home, she knows that a resident's sleep is often fragmented. Furthermore, she has read in a journal article that multiple factors affect sleep in the nursing home client, including physical illness, dementia, depression, high prevalence of sleep-disordered breathing, chronic bed rest, circadian rhythm disturbances, and the noise and lighting of the nursing home environment (Ancoli-Israel, 1997). She wants to be sure that her assessment considers all potential factors influencing Mr. Murphy's sleep pattern. Anna plans to include Mr. Murphy's wife in the assessment to learn more about Mrs. Murphy's perceptions of changes in Mr. Murphy's behavior. A complete assessment must be clear and precise; thus Anna plans to talk with Mr. Murphy more than one time to gather the necessary information and to keep her client from becoming fatigued.

Box 28-4

Nursing Diagnoses for CLIENTS WITH SLEEP DISTURBANCES

- Anxiety
- Breathing pattern, ineffective
- Confusion, acute
- Coping, compromised family
- Coping, ineffective
- Fatigue
- Protection, ineffective
- Sensory perception, disturbed
- Sleep pattern, disturbed

In the health care setting, determine whether environmental stimuli are disrupting the client's sleep. A roommate who stays up late or has multiple visitors, the presence of electrical equipment at a client's bedside, and the likelihood of noise coming from an outside hallway are examples of factors to consider that can be reduced or controlled.

BEHAVIORS OF SLEEP DEPRIVATION.   Some clients may be unaware of how their sleep problems are affecting their behavior. Observe for behaviors such as irritability, disorientation (similar to a drunken state), and slurred speech. If sleep deprivation has lasted a long time, psychotic behavior such as delusions and paranoia may develop. For example, a client may report seeing strange objects or colors in the room. The client may act afraid when you or other health personnel enter the room.

CLIENT EXPECTATIONS.   After assessing the client's sleep history, determine the client's expectations regarding nursing care. Use a caring and skilled approach to assess the client's sleep needs. For example, you might ask, "Now that I understand more about your sleep habits and the recent problems you have had, what is it that you expect from us regarding your care?" or "In order to improve your sleep, what do you feel is most important that we do for you?" The client may have a different view on the relationship of sleep and health from your own. Examining client expectations helps to clarify any misconceptions you might have. In the hospital setting, clients might be more concerned about be-

ing sure you are checking their condition routinely than about whether they are awakened from sleep.

Nursing Diagnosis

Your assessment will reveal clusters of data that include defining characteristics for a sleep problem or other nursing diagnoses that result from disturbed sleep. If a sleep pattern disturbance is identified, it is helpful for you to specify the exact condition (Box 28-4). By specifying the nature of a sleep disturbance, you can design more effective interventions.

Your assessment should also identify the probable cause or related factor for the sleep disturbance, such as a noisy environment, a high intake of caffeine, or stress involving work. The cause becomes the focus of interventions for minimizing or eliminating the problem. For example, a hospitalized client who experiences insomnia as a result of a noisy sleeping environment might benefit from a reduction in hospital equipment noise or minimizing interruptions. If the insomnia is related to worry over a threatened marital separation, your interventions might involve introducing coping strategies. If the probable cause or related factors are incorrectly defined, the client may not benefit from your care.

Planning

GOALS AND OUTCOMES.   After identifying all relevant nursing diagnoses for a client, you develop a plan of care (see care plan). An individualized care plan can be developed only after you understand how the nursing diagnosis relates to the client's normal and current sleep pattern, the client's perception of the sleep problem, and the factors disrupting sleep. Together you and the client develop realistic goals and outcomes. For example, the goal of "Client establishes a healthy sleep pattern" will include outcomes such as "Client will fall asleep within $1/_2$ hour of planned time" and "Client will have less than two awakenings during the night." This will be realistic if you know from your assessment that it now takes the client an hour to fall asleep and that awakenings occur 3 to 4 times a night. The outcomes will serve as measurable guidelines to determine goal achievement. An effective plan includes outcomes established over a realistic time frame that focus on the goal of

Care Study Nursing Care Plan INSOMNIA

ASSESSMENT

Anna learns that Mr. Murphy usually slept from 10:30 PM to 6:00 AM when he was at home, usually awakening once or twice during the night to urinate. He rarely had difficulty falling asleep, but according to his wife, listening to music helped him relax. Since being in the nursing home he now reports, **"I have so much trouble falling asleep, it probably takes over an hour."** When asked if he awakens during the night, Mr. Murphy responds, "Are you kidding? No one can sleep here; something is always going on." Mr. Murphy admits to **awakening as many as 3 or 4 times during the night.** The client estimates he received maybe **4 hours of sleep the previous night.** He denies that he is having discomfort from the osteoarthritis but is **having difficulty** changing positions and **getting comfortable.** While Mr. Murphy describes his situation, he **yawns frequently** and states, **"I really feel tired."** Anna asks him to rate the quality of the previous night's sleep, and he places a **mark on the analog scale near "worst night's sleep."** Anna notices during the assessment that Mr. Murphy's roommate is frequently calling out to anyone who passes the room door. The roommate's television is also on.

*Defining characteristics are shown in bold type.

NURSING DIAGNOSIS

Disturbed sleep pattern related to excessive environmental stimuli.

PLANNING

GOAL	EXPECTED OUTCOMES
Client will obtain a sense of restfulness following sleep within 1 month.	Client will have fewer than two self-reported awakenings during the night within 2 weeks.
	Client will report being able to fall asleep within $1/_2$ hour of going to bed within 2 weeks.
	Client will obtain an average of 7 hours of sleep per night within 4 weeks.

IMPLEMENTATION

STEPS	RATIONALE
1. Have Mr. Murphy moved to a room at the end of the hall. Match with roommate who is also alert and oriented.	Matching roommates with similar nighttime behaviors and daytime routines can reduce sleep disruption (Ancoli-Israel, 1997).
2. Arrange for client to have a CD player with earphones, to play music of his choice when first going to sleep.	Soothing music blocks out sounds from environment and reduces anxiety, promoting relaxation (Pope, 1995).
3. Discourage frequent daytime napping. Replace it with regular exercise (e.g., have Mr. Murphy propel down hallways in wheelchair for 5 minutes, 4 times a day).	Increases likelihood of client feeling fatigued and ready for sleep at bedtime (Rogers, 1997).
4. Have an egg-crate mattress placed over bed mattress. Have staff position client with extra pillows.	Increases comfort of sleeping position, enhancing relaxation, which can promote a sleep state.
5. Encourage Mr. Murphy to decrease his fluids 2 to 4 hours before sleep.	Decreases number of times client awakens to urinate (Ancoli-Israel, 1997).

EVALUATION

- Ask Mr. Murphy to use a visual analog scale to rate the quality of his sleep at the end of each week.
- Ask Mrs. Murphy to evaluate her perceptions of Mr. Murphy's level of fatigue.
- Have Mr. Murphy report on the time he estimates falling asleep and the number of awakenings at night.
- Ask Mr. Murphy at the end of 4 weeks to keep a record for a week of the length of time he estimates sleeping.

---

improving the quality of sleep. This type of plan may require many weeks to accomplish.

SETTING PRIORITIES. Using the data you gathered about the nature of the client's problem, you need to identify priority strategies and interventions to promote sleep. Together, you and the client identify and select the strategies and interventions that are most likely to be beneficial in the home or health care setting. The plan of care should include priority strategies that support positive sleep habits and patterns that fit the client's living environment, cultural orientation, and lifestyle. For example, the client may decide that purchasing a new mattress to increase comfort is the first step toward improving sleep. In a health care setting, you can

plan treatments or routines to give the client more time to rest. For example, you might turn and reposition a client at the same time medication is given or a treatment such as suctioning is performed, to limit the number of nurse-client contacts. All staff caring for the client should know the plan so that they can cluster activities at times to reduce awakenings. In a nursing home rest periods may be planned around the activities of other residents.

CONTINUITY OF CARE. The nature of a sleep disturbance determines whether referrals to additional health care providers are necessary. For example, if a sleep problem is related to a situational crisis or emotional problem, you may refer the client to a psychiatric clinical nurse specialist, pas-

SLEEP-WAKE PATTERN
- Maintain a regular rising time.
- Eliminate naps unless they are a routine part of the schedule.
- If naps are used, limit to 20 minutes or less twice a day.
- Avoid extremes of sleep, that is, becoming excessively sleepy on the weekends.
- Go to bed when sleepy.
- Use relaxation techniques to promote sleep.
- If unable to sleep in 15 to 30 minutes, get out of bed.

ENVIRONMENT
- Sleep where you sleep best.
- Keep noise to minimum; use soft music to mask noise if necessary.
- Use night-light and keep path to bathroom free of obstacles.
- Set room temperature to preference; use blankets and socks to promote warmth.

MEDICATIONS
- Use sedatives and hypnotics as last resort and then only short term if needed.
- Adjust medications being taken for other conditions, and look for drug interactions that may cause insomnia or EDS.

DIET
- Limit alcohol, caffeine, and nicotine in late afternoon and evening.
- Drink warm milk as a light snack before bedtime.
- Decrease fluids 2 to 4 hours before sleep.

PHYSIOLOGICAL/ILLNESS FACTORS
- Elevate head of bed and provide extra pillows as preferred.
- Use analgesics 30 minutes before bed to ease aches and pains.
- Use prescribed medications to control symptoms of chronic conditions.

SLEEP HYGIENE HABITS
- Caution client against sleeping long hours during weekends or holidays to prevent disturbances of normal sleep-wake cycle.
- Explain that if possible, the bedroom should not be used for intensive studying, snacking, or other nonsleep activity, besides sex.
- Explain that client should try to avoid worrisome thinking when going to bed and should use relaxation exercises.
- If client has trouble falling asleep, advise to get out of bed and do some quiet activity until feeling sleepy enough to go back to bed.
- Instruct client to avoid heavy meals for 3 hours before bedtime; a light snack may help.

a light, warm blanket. Healthy infants should be placed on their side or back when being put to sleep (American Academy of Pediatrics, 1992). This position reduces the incidence of SIDS. Children and adults vary more in regard to comfortable room temperature but usually sleep best in cooler environments. Some prefer to sleep without covers. Older adults may require extra blankets or covers or may sleep wearing socks (Box 28-5).

Eliminate or reduce distracting noise so that the bedroom is as quiet as possible. In the home the TV or the ringing of the telephone may disrupt a client's sleep. The family becomes important participants in care when each has different schedules for going to sleep. It may require the cooperation of several people living with the client to reduce noise. Some clients sleep better with familiar inside noises, such as the hum of a ceiling fan.

The bed and mattress should provide support and comfortable firmness. A bed board can be placed under the mattress to add support. Sometimes extra pillows help a person to position more comfortably in bed. The position of the bed in the room may also make a difference for some clients.

For any client prone to confusion or falls, safety is critical. In the home a small night-light might assist the client in orienting to the room environment before arising to go to the bathroom. Beds set lower to the floor may reduce the risk of falls when a person stands. Clutter should be removed from the path a client uses to walk from the bed to the bathroom. If a client needs help in ambulating from the bed to the bathroom, a small bell at the bedside can be used to call family members.

Clients vary in regard to the amount of light that they prefer at night. Infants and older adults sleep best in softly lit rooms. Light should not shine directly on their eyes. Small table lamps or night-lights prevent total darkness. For older adults this reduces the chance of confusion when arising from bed. If streetlights shine through windows or when clients nap during the day, heavy shades, drapes, or slatted blinds are helpful.

toral care professional, or clinical psychologist for counseling. This helps to ensure that the client's problems are attended to not only in the health care setting but in the home as well. When chronic insomnia is the problem, a medical referral or referral to a sleep center can be beneficial.

Implementation

Your nursing interventions for improving the quality of a person's sleep are largely focused on health promotion. In an acute care setting, you focus on managing the environment and trying to support the client's normal sleep habits. When clients enter long-term care or nursing home environments, special considerations are needed to promote adequate sleep and rest.

HEALTH PROMOTION.   Clients need adequate sleep and rest to maintain active and productive lifestyles. Your specific interventions will promote a person's normal sleep and rest pattern.

ENVIRONMENTAL CONTROLS.   All clients require a sleeping environment with a comfortable room temperature and proper ventilation, minimal noise, a comfortable bed, and proper lighting. Infants sleep best when the room temperature is 18° to 21° C (64° to 70° F) and they are covered with

PROMOTING BEDTIME ROUTINES.   Bedtime routines relax clients in preparation for sleep. It is important for persons to go to sleep when they feel fatigued or sleepy. To develop good sleep habits at home, clients and their bed partners should learn techniques that promote sleep and conditions that interfere with sleep (Box 28-6).

Newborns and infants benefit from quiet activities such as holding them snugly in blankets, talking or singing softly, and gently rocking. A bedtime routine (e.g., same hour for bedtime or quiet activity) used consistently helps toddlers and preschool children avoid delaying sleep. Patterns of preparing for bedtime need to be reinforced. Reading stories, allowing children to sit in a parents' lap while listening to music or prayer, and coloring are routines that can be associated with preparing for bed.

Adults need to avoid excessive mental stimulation just before bedtime. Reading a light novel, watching a relaxing television program, or listening to music helps a person relax. Relaxation exercises and praying can induce calm (see Chapter 29).

PROMOTING COMFORT.   People fall asleep only after feeling comfortable and relaxed. You can recommend and use several measures to promote comfort, such as encouraging the client to wear loose-fitting nightwear and to void before bedtime. Family members can give a relaxing back rub. Minor irritants can keep persons awake. Diapers should be changed before placing infants in bed. An extra blanket can prevent chilling when one tries to fall asleep.

Clients who suffer painful illnesses can try a variety of measures at home to promote comfort. Application of dry or moist heat, use of supportive dressings or splints (see Chapter 34), and proper positioning with the use of extra pillows for support can be very helpful. For clients with temporary acute pain (e.g., following surgery), it may be advantageous to the client and bed partner to let the client sleep alone until the pain subsides.

You can help clients with physical illness learn ways to control symptoms that disrupt sleep. For example, a client with respiratory abnormalities should sleep with two pillows or in a semisitting position to ease the effort to breathe. The client may benefit from taking prescribed bronchodilators before sleep to prevent airway obstruction.

PROMOTING ACTIVITY.   In the home encourage clients to stay physically active during the day so that they are more likely to sleep at night. Increasing daytime activity lessens problems with falling asleep. Rigorous exercise should always be planned at least several hours before bedtime.

Exercise is believed to be beneficial to older adults by improving nighttime sleep. However, individuals with chronic diseases that influence their functional abilities are likely to have limited activity (Lueckenotte, 2000). You must recommend activities that are safe for older clients to perform. Walking, swimming, and cycling on a stationary bike are excellent for those clients with limited physical impairment. Repetitions of sit-to-stand or transferring and up to 5 minutes of walking or wheelchair propulsion are excellent for those with physical limitations (Alessi and others, 1995). Weight lifting using light weights (e.g., 2 to 5 lb) is also excellent to build upper body strength and endurance.

STRESS REDUCTION.   When clients feel emotionally upset, they should be urged to try not to force sleep. Otherwise, insomnia often develops, and soon bedtime is associated with the inability to relax. Encourage a client who has difficulty falling asleep to get up and pursue a relaxing activity rather than staying in bed and thinking about sleep. When the emotional problem is ongoing and the client finds little relief, encourage referral to an appropriate counselor.

Children often have problems going to bed and falling asleep. After nightmares, parents should enter children's rooms immediately and talk to them briefly about their fears to provide a cooling-down period. Comforting children while they lie in their own bed can be reassuring. Keeping a light on in the room may also help. Usually experts do not recommend that a child be allowed to sleep with parents; however, cultural traditions may cause families to approach sleep practices differently. For examples, Hispanic and Asian families often practice co-sleeping, in which children are allowed to sleep with parents or siblings to lessen the child's anxiety and promote a sense of security.

BEDTIME SNACKS.   Some persons enjoy bedtime snacks, whereas others cannot sleep after eating. A dairy product snack such as warm milk, which contains L-tryptophan may help to promote sleep. A full meal before bedtime can often cause gastrointestinal upset and interfere with the ability to fall asleep.

Clients should avoid drinking excess fluids or ingesting caffeine before bedtime. Coffee, tea, cola, and chocolate will cause a person to stay awake or awaken throughout the night. Alcohol can interrupt sleep cycles and reduce the amount of deep sleep. Coffee, tea, colas, and alcohol act as diuretics, causing **nocturia.**

PHARMACOLOGICAL APPROACHES TO PROMOTING SLEEP.   Many of the drugs clients take to manage symptoms can cause insomnia. CNS stimulants such as amphetamines, nicotine, terbutaline, theophylline, and pemoline should be used sparingly and under medical management (McKenry and Salerno, 1998). Withdrawal from CNS depressants such as alcohol, barbiturates, and tricyclic antidepressants can also cause insomnia and must be managed carefully.

Sleep medications can help a client if used correctly. **Sedatives** and **hypnotics** are groups of drugs used to induce and/or maintain sleep. However, long-term use of these drugs can disrupt sleep and lead to more serious problems. One group of drugs considered to be relatively safe is the benzodiazepines (Table 28-3). These medications do not cause general CNS depression as sedatives or hypnotics do. A low dose of a short-acting benzodiazepine for short-term use (no longer than 2 to 3 weeks) is recommended (Ancoli-Israel, 1997; Neubauer, 1999).

The use of benzodiazepines in the older adult population is potentially dangerous because of the drug's tendency to remain active in the body for a longer time. This means the drugs can potentially interact with other agents (Lueckenotte, 2000). Short-acting benzodiazepines (e.g., oxazepam, lorazepam, or temazepam) at the lowest possible dose are recommended. Initial doses should be small, and

Pharmacology of Antiinsomnia Agents   Table 28-3

Generic Name	Trade Name	Onset of Action (min)	Oral Dosage (mg)	Indications
Alprazolam	Xanax	15-60	0.25-0.5 (3 times daily)	Anxiety
Diazepam	Valium	15-45	5-10 at bedtime	Sleep disorder
Flurazepam	Dalmane Apo-Flurazepam	15-45	15-30 at bedtime	Sleep disorder
Lorazepam	Ativan Apo-Lorazepam	15-60	1-2 at bedtime	Anxiety, sleep disorder
Oxazepam	Serax Zapex	45-90	10-30 (3-4 times daily)	Anxiety
Temazepam	Restoril	30-45	15-30 at bedtime	Sleep disorder
Triazolam	Halcion	15-30	0.125-0.25 at bedtime	Sleep disorder
Zolpidem	Ambien	15-45	10-20 at bedtime	Sleep disorder

increments are added gradually, based on client response, for a limited time.

Melatonin is a hormone produced in the brain that helps control circadian rhythms (Ancoli-Israel, 1997). It is a popular nutritional supplement in the United States used to aid sleep. Melatonin is usually sold in 3-mg tablets, but the body produces less than 0.5 mg. Because of the lack of large-scale studies on its safety, you should caution clients about the timing of ingestion and the dose taken (Ancoli-Israel, 1997).

The use of nonprescription sleeping medications is not advisable. Over the long term, these drugs can lead to further sleep disruption even when they initially seem effective. Caution older adults about using over-the-counter antihistamines because of their long duration of action that can cause confusion, constipation, and urinary retention (Neubauer, 1999). You can help clients with interventions that do not require the use of drugs.

Regular use of any sleep medication can lead to tolerance, and withdrawal can then cause rebound insomnia. All clients should understand the possible side effects of sleep medications. Routine monitoring of client response to sleeping medications is important.

MANAGING SPECIFIC SLEEP DISTURBANCES.   Clients who suffer specific sleep disturbances will likely benefit from the health promotion strategies discussed so far. Weight loss can be effective for the client with obstructive sleep apnea. It is important for the client to follow an appropriate weight reduction plan (see Chapter 30). In milder cases of obstructive sleep apnea, body position during sleep can be effective. Ancoli-Israel (1997) recommends a simple measure of having clients keep off their backs during sleep by sewing a pocket into the back of their nightshirt and inserting a tennis ball into the pocket.

ACUTE CARE.   The nursing interventions described for health promotion are applicable to a client requiring acute care. The nature of the acute care setting requires you to be creative in finding ways to maintain the client's normal sleep pattern.

Control of Noise in the Hospital   Box 28-7

Close doors to the client's room when possible.
Keep doors to work areas on unit closed when in use.
Reduce volume of nearby telephone and paging equipment.
Wear rubber-soled shoes. Avoid clogs.
Turn off bedside oxygen and other equipment that is not in use.
Turn down alarms and beeps on bedside monitoring equipment.
Turn off room TV and radio unless client prefers soft music.
Avoid abrupt loud noise such as flushing a toilet or moving a bed.
Keep necessary conversations at low levels, particularly at night.
Conduct conversations and reports in private areas away from client rooms.

MANAGING ENVIRONMENTAL STIMULI.   A challenge for you in the hospital is controlling noise. Because many clients spend only a short time in hospitals, it is easy to forget the importance of establishing good sleep conditions. Box 28-7 outlines options for you to use in reducing room noise.

In the hospital setting, plan care to avoid awakening clients. Try to schedule assessments, treatments, procedures, and routines for times when clients are awake. Group nursing activities before the client receives sleeping medication or begins to fall asleep. For example, a client who has had surgery should have the surgical dressing changed, be repositioned, receive a pain medication, and have a set of vital signs completed before retiring for the night. Medications should be given and blood drawn during waking hours when possible. Plan with other departments and services to schedule therapies at intervals that give clients time to rest. Whenever it becomes necessary to awaken a client, it should be done as soon as possible so that the client can fall back to sleep quickly.

SAFETY.   Safety precautions are important for clients who awaken during the night to use the bathroom and for those with excessive daytime sleepiness. Beds should be set lower to the floor to lessen the chance of the client's falling when first standing. Clutter should be removed and equipment moved from the path a client uses to walk from the bed to the bathroom. If a client needs assistance in ambulating from the bed to the bathroom, the call light should always be within the client's reach. Be sure the client knows how to turn the light on correctly.

Clients who experience daytime sleepiness can fall asleep while sitting up in a chair or wheelchair. Position clients so that they will not fall out of the chair when sleeping. Elevating the client's feet on an ottoman or small bench may assist in positioning the client safely. A pillow placed in the client's lap might offer some support. If a client enjoys leaning over an over-bed table while sitting in a chair, be sure the table is locked and secure. Use of safety belts is considered to be a restraint and should be avoided (see Chapter 25).

COMFORT MEASURES.   You can make the client more comfortable in an acute setting by providing personal hygiene before bedtime. A warm bath or shower can be very relaxing. Clients restricted to bed should be offered the opportunity to wash their face and hands. Toothbrushing and care of dentures also help to prepare the client for sleep. Clients should void before retiring so they are not kept awake by a full bladder. While a client prepares for bed, help to position the client off any potential pressure sites. Offering a back rub or massage may help relax the client.

Removal of irritating stimuli is another way you can improve the client's comfort for a restful sleep. Changing or removal of moist dressings, repositioning drainage tubings, reapplying wrinkled thromboembolic hose, and changing tape on nasogastric tubes eliminate constant irritants to the client's skin. When an intravenous (IV) site becomes irritated and painful, reinsertion of the IV is usually recommended (see Chapter 14). Clients who are incontinent should have the perineal or anal area cleaned thoroughly. Diaphoretic clients will benefit from a cool sponging.

RESTORATIVE AND CONTINUING CARE.
The quality of sleep in a long-term care or nursing home environment is often fragmented. Residents of a nursing home often suffer chronic disease, incontinence, and dementia and take multiple medications, all of which can disrupt sleep. Psychotropic medications are commonly used in nursing homes, with some evidence of a change in normal diurnal variation in sleep (Alessi and others, 1995). Noise, light, and repositioning of nursing home residents during linen changes are factors that can cause clients to awaken. Besides care activities, nursing home residents themselves can be very disruptive by crying out loudly to roommates or nursing staff.

In the long-term care environment many clients require rehabilitation or supportive care. The nature of their illnesses and treatment requirements can disrupt sleep. For example, clients who are ventilator dependent will likely get brief periods of sleep throughout the day rather than prolonged sleep because of disruptions from ventilator alarm sounds and the need for occasional suctioning.

MAINTAINING ACTIVITY.   General recommendations to improve sleep in older adults have often suggested increasing daytime activity or exercise (Neubauer, 1999). Stevenson and Topp (1990) studied the effects of long-term exercise in older adults residing in the community and found improved self-reported sleep. However, in a study of extremely frail older adults residing within a nursing home, Alessi and others (1995) did not find an improvement in sleep as a result of physical activity. Alessi and others (1995) acknowledged that the clients in their study suffered from complex problems, all of which could have negated the benefits of exercise. The general benefits of activity and exercise—improved activity endurance, improved mobility, and improved sense of well-being—may prove to be beneficial to those older adults who are not institutionalized and thus not exposed to repetitive environmental distractions.

In the restorative care setting try to limit the time clients spend in bed. In the nursing home meals should be served in the resident dining area. Otherwise clients should be up in a chair for meals and for personal hygiene activities. It is also important to keep the residents involved in social activities planned at the nursing home (e.g., card playing or arts and crafts). Regular exercise keeps the clients active and stimulated. It is also ideal to limit naps to once a day for 30 minutes or less (Ancoli-Israel, 1997).

Clients with dementia often have disrupted sleep-wake cycles. They often become easily fatigued and experience periods of insomnia (Lueckenotte, 2000). In this situation activities and visits may need to be shortened to allow the client to maintain an adequate energy level. If the client awakens during the night, keeping the lights at a low level and using soothing techniques such as quiet music or a back rub can promote sleep.

REDUCING SLEEP DISRUPTION.   Knowing the many factors that can disrupt sleep in restorative care settings, you must find ways to make the environment more conducive to sleep. Noise control is critical. Often staff within a nursing home naturally speak louder because of residents' difficulties with hearing. Walking up close to a client and talking in a normal but clear voice will likely improve the client's hearing and reduce the chance of awakening a nearby roommate. Training assistive personnel to be more sensitive to the sources of noise that disrupt clients' sleep can be very useful.

 Evaluation

CLIENT CARE.   Evaluation of therapies designed to promote sleep and rest must be individualized. Clients in relatively good health may not need as much sleep as clients whose physical conditions are poor.

If you have established realistic goals of care, the expected outcomes become guidelines for evaluating the client's progress and response to interventions (Box 28-8). Evaluative measures may be used shortly after a therapy has been tried. Use other evaluative measures after a client awakens from sleep (e.g., asking a client to describe the number of awakenings during the night). Together the client and bed partner can usually provide accurate information. If the client lives or sleeps alone, reliability of evaluation can be questioned.

Outcome Evaluation for MR. MURPHY · Box 28-8

Nursing Action	Client Response/Finding	Achievement of Outcome
Encourage Mr. Murphy to decrease fluid intake 2 to 4 hours before sleep	Mr. Murphy drinks 8 oz of milk at his evening meal at 6 PM No further fluid is consumed after dinner.	Mr. Murphy is obtaining an average of 7 hours of uninterrupted sleep per night.
Have an egg-crate mattress placed over bed mattress. Have staff position Mr. Murphy with extra pillows.	Mr. Murphy feels more comfortable lying on his side with pillows behind his back.	Mr. Murphy reports two self-awakenings during the night; less than two self-reported awakenings per night have not been achieved.
Arrange for Mr. Murphy to have a CD player with earphones to play music of his choice when first going to bed.	Within 20 minutes, Mr. Murphy's eyes are closed and his breathing is deep and even, at a rate of 12 breaths per minute.	Mr. Murphy is falling asleep within $\frac{1}{2}$ hour of going to bed.

Case Study EVALUATION

After 4 weeks at the nursing home, Anna has been able to have Mr. Murphy transferred to a new room and has been monitoring his progress. He has been in the new room for 2 weeks. Anna asks Mr. Murphy, "Tell me how our plan to improve your sleep has been working. Have the music and headphones been helpful?" Mr. Murphy replies, "Well, it has helped to be down here at the end of the hall. It still is a bit noisy, especially if the nurses are working with people across the way. I have used the headphones the last 2 weeks, and they have helped me relax and fall asleep in about 20 or 30 minutes." Anna questions Mr. Murphy further and learns that he is awakening 2 or 3 times during the night. However, during the last week he estimated getting about 6 hours of sleep, an improvement from a month ago. Mr. Murphy also reports that the staff has usually been good about reminding him to do his daily exercises with the wheelchair. He dislikes staying in his room and has tried to exercise as much as possible.

Anna decides to revise the care plan, adding an intervention for placing a sign on the client's door at night asking staff to keep the door closed. Mr. Murphy's sleep is improving, and Anna selects an additional measure aimed at reducing awakenings.

Anna wants to know Mr. Murphy's level of satisfaction with her care. She asks, "Have I met your expectations so far? If not, tell me how I can better help you." Mr. Murphy replies, "You've been great. I know you can't make this place like home. There is so much to think about when you are here. I think about my wife a lot." Anna responds, "Tell me more. What do you mean there is so much to think about?" Anna recognizes that psychological and physical stressors can alter sleep. She decides to reassess Mr. Murphy to determine if additional nursing interventions might be appropriate.

Documentation Note
Client reports some improvement in overall sleep quality. Able to fall asleep within 20 to 30 minutes using headphones with music. Reports sleeping approximately 6 hours per night. Continues to experience reawakenings, resulting from noise in outside hallway. Recommend closing room door at night to reduce noise further. Client has begun to admit thinking about his wife and possibly other concerns. Will explore further with him.

When expected outcomes are not met, revise the nursing measures based on the client's needs or preferences. Document the client's response to sleep therapies so that a continuum of care can be maintained.

CLIENT EXPECTATIONS. Review the progress in the plan of care with the client, and determine if the client's expectations were met. Does the client believe your interventions were helpful and useful? Did you incorporate the client's typical sleep routine into the plan of care? For the hospitalized client, were unnecessary interruptions avoided to give the client a chance to rest? The client's perceptions are valuable sources of information regarding the overall success in improving the quality of the client's sleep.

Key Terms

advanced sleep phase syndrome, p. 692
biological clocks, p. 689
bruxism, p. 695
bulbar synchronizing region (BSR), p. 690

cataplexy, p. 695
circadian rhythm, p. 689
hypnotics, p. 701
insomnia, p. 694
narcolepsy, p. 695
nocturia, p. 701
nonrapid eye movement (NREM) sleep, p. 690

rapid eye movement (REM) sleep, p. 690
reticular activating system (RAS), p. 690
sedatives, p. 701
sleep, p. 689
sleep apnea, p. 694
sleep deprivation, p. 695

Key Concepts

- Sleep is believed to provide physiological and psychological restoration.
- The 24-hour sleep-wake cycle is a circadian rhythm that influences physiological function and behavior.
- The control and regulation of sleep depends on a balance between CNS regulators.
- During a typical night's sleep a person passes through four to six complete sleep cycles. Each sleep cycle contains three NREM stages of sleep and a period of REM sleep.
- The number of hours of sleep needed by each person to feel rested is variable.
- Long-term use of sleeping pills may lead to difficulty in initiating and maintaining sleep.
- The hectic pace of a person's lifestyle, emotional and psychological stress, and alcohol ingestion disrupt the sleep pattern.
- An environment with a darkened room, reduced noise, comfortable bed, appropriate temperature, and good ventilation promotes sleep.

- The most common type of sleep disorder is insomnia, which is characterized by the inability to fall asleep, to remain asleep during the night, or to go back to sleep after awakening earlier than is desired.
- Only a client can report whether sleep is restful.
- When using environmental controls to promote sleep, you should consider the usual characteristics of the client's home environment and normal lifestyle.
- Noise can disrupt sleep and enhance pain perception.
- A bedtime routine of relaxing activities prepares a person physically and mentally for sleep.
- Pain or other symptom control is essential to promote the ability to sleep.
- One of the most important nursing interventions for promoting sleep is establishing periods for uninterrupted sleep and rest.

Critical Thinking Activities

1. Mrs. Riley is a 66-year-old woman who comes to the community health clinic every 6 months for management of her hypertension. During this visit she reports the following to the nurse: "I am having more difficulty falling asleep. During the last month I bet I got up at least twice every night. My husband is convinced something is wrong. I still go to bed about the same time, around 10 PM, and I awaken around 6 AM." What would your analysis be of this client's assessment? How might you proceed further?

2. Edward Pena is a 34-year-old businessman who comes to the physician's office complaining of being very sleepy during the day. He has noticed the problem for about 3 months. He states, "If I'm lucky, I get about 4 or 5 hours of sleep each night." He spends most of the workweek flying to various cities across the country. His day begins at 5 AM and often does not end until 7 PM or later. He admits that his eating habits are erratic; sometimes he does not

have a meal until 8 or 9 at night. He drinks coffee during the day to keep him going. Mr. Pena likes to play golf on weekends but exercises little during the week. Last month his boss had a long talk with Mr. Pena after hearing that he had fallen asleep during a business meeting. This was the second time it had occurred. Mr. Pena is asking if he might be able to try a sleeping pill to help him sleep. What might be Mr. Pena's problem? What recommendations might you make to help him sleep?

3. As a nurse you are asked to present a program on "Good Sleep Habits in Young Children" to parents of children attending the local preschool. What general information should be included in the program?

4. Mrs. Thompson, age 50, is a client on your nursing unit recovering from colon surgery 2 days ago. She tells you she is having difficulty sleeping since surgery. What interventions should you include on a plan of care to promote sleep for Mrs. Thompson?

Review Questions

1. When assessing a client for obstructive sleep apnea, you know the most common symptom is:
   1. headache.
   2. early wakening.
   3. impaired reasoning.
   4. excessive daytime sleepiness.
2. You understand that a client should not use prescription sleeping medications for longer than:
   1. 1 week.
   2. 6 weeks.
   3. 2 to 3 weeks.
   4. 4 to 5 weeks.

3. A priority nursing intervention to promote sleep in the hospitalized client is to:
   1. turn television on low to late night programming.
   2. coordinate laboratory draws for blood to be completed at 5:00 AM.
   3. give client his prescribed sleeping medication by 11:00 PM.
   4. encourage client to continue to follow regular bedtime routines.
4. An older client complains about difficulty falling asleep. A priority nursing goal for the client is to:
   1. sleep for 7 hours each night.
   2. limit napping during the day to three or four naps.
   3. decrease awakenings to two or three a night.
   4. fall asleep within 20 minutes of getting in bed.

Continued

Review Questions—cont'd

5. You explain to a client that the most vivid dreaming occurs during:
   1. REM sleep.
   2. stage 1 NREM sleep.
   3. stage 4 NREM sleep.
   4. transition from NREM to REM sleep.

6. You teach a client that the beta-adrenergic blockers he is taking for hypertension may interfere with normal sleep patterns by:
   1. causing nocturia.
   2. increasing daytime sleepiness.
   3. causing awakenings from sleep.
   4. increasing difficulty falling asleep.

7. You are developing a care plan for an older client who is having difficulty sleeping. An intervention to include on the plan is to:
   1. nap during the day to make up lost sleep.
   2. exercise in the evening to increase fatigue.
   3. allow the client to sleep as late as possible.
   4. decrease fluids 2 to 4 hours before going to bed.

8. A mother tells the nurse that her 3-year-old is having sleep problems. When gathering assessment data related to this problem, an important issue you should question the mother about is:
   1. the age of other siblings in the home.
   2. usual bedtime practices for the child.
   3. growth and development patterns for the child.
   4. the type of preschool the child attends during the day.

9. A client in the community clinic becomes upset after learning he has narcolepsy. He asks you what this means. Your best response is that narcolepsy is:
   1. a sudden muscle weakness during periods of stress.
   2. stopping breathing for very short periods while sleeping.
   3. frequent awakenings during the night with difficulty falling back asleep.
   4. a dysfunction in which the client falls asleep uncontrollably at inappropriate times.

10. A nursing measure to promote sleep in young children is to:
    1. make sure the room is dark and quiet.
    2. allow children to fall asleep in parents' bed.
    3. increase evening activities to promote fatigue.
    4. encourage reading a story just before bedtime.

References

Aldrich M, Naylor M: Approach to the patient with disordered sleep. In Kryger M and others, editors: *Principles and practice of sleep medicine*, ed 3, Philadelphia, 2000, WB Saunders.

Alessi CA and others: Does physical activity improve sleep in impaired nursing home residents? *J Am Geritar Soc* 43:1098, 1995.

American Academy of Pediatrics: Positioning and SIDS: AAP Task Force on Infant Positioning and SIDS, *Pediatrics* 79:1122, 1992.

Ancoli-Israel, S: Sleep problems in older adults: putting myths to bed, *Geriatrics* 52(1):20, 1997.

Beck-Little R, Weinrich S: Assessment and management of sleep disorders in the elderly, *J Gerontol Nurs* 24(4):21, 1998.

Close SJ: Assessment of sleep in hospital patients: a review of methods, *J Adv Nurs* 13:501, 1988.

Close SJ: Post-operative patients' views of sleep, pain, and recovery, *J Clin Nurs* 1(2):83, 1992.

Dahl R, Carskadon M: Sleep and its disorders in adolescence. In Ferber R, Kryger M: *Principles and practice of sleep medicine in the child*, Philadelphia, 1995, WB Saunders.

Gillis AM: Cardiac arrhythmias. In Kryger MH and others, editors: *Principles and practice of sleep medicine*, ed 3, Philadelphia, 2000, WB Saunders.

Guyton A, Hall J: *Human physiology and mechanisms of disease*, ed 6, Philadelphia, 1997, WB Saunders.

Hauri P, Linde S: *No more sleepless nights*, New York, 1990, Wiley.

Jones B: Basic mechanisms of sleep-wake states. In Kryger M and others, editors: *Principles and practice of sleep medicine*, ed 3, Philadelphia, 2000, WB Saunders.

Lee KA: An overview of sleep and common sleep problems, *ANNA J* 24(6):614, 1997.

Lueckenotte A: *Gerontologic nursing*, ed 2, St. Louis, 2000, Mosby.

McCance K, Huether S: *Pathophysiology: the biologic basis for disease in adults and children*, ed 4, St. Louis, 2002, Mosby.

McKenry LM, Salerno E: *Mosby's pharmacology in nursing*, ed 20, St. Louis, 1998, Mosby.

Mitler H and others: Sleep medicine, public policy and public health. In Kryger M and others, editors: *Principles and practice of sleep medicine*, ed 3, Philadelphia, 2000, WB Saunders.

National Sleep Foundation: 2000 omnibus sleep in America poll, retrieved October 17, 2000, http:www.sleepfoundation.org/pressarchives/new_stats.html.

Neubauer D: Sleep problems in the elderly, *Am Fam Physician* 59(9):2551, 1999.

Pope DS: Music, noise, and the human voice in the nurse-patient environment, *Image J Nurs, Sch* 27(4):291, 1995.

Redeker N: Sleep in acute care settings: an integrative review, *Image J Nurs Sch* 32(1):31, 2000.

Rogers A: Nursing management of sleep disorders. II. Behavioral interventions, *ANNA J* 24(6):672, 1997.

Shneerson J: *2000 Handbook of sleep medicine*, Cambridge, UK, 2000, Blackwell Science.

Stevenson JS, Topp R: Effects of moderate and low intensity long-term exercise by older adults, *J Res Nurs Health* 13:209, 1990.

Thorpy M: Classification of sleep disorders. In Kryger M and others, editors: *Principles and practice of sleep medicine*, ed 3, Philadelphia, 2000, WB Saunders.

Webster RA, Thompson DR: Sleep in hospital, *J Adv Nurs* 11:447, 1986.

Wong DL and others: *Whaley and Wong's nursing care of infants and children*, ed 6, St. Louis, 1999, Mosby.

Zorick F, Walsh J: Evaluation and management of insomnia: an overview. In Kryger MH and others, editors: *Principles and practice of sleep medicine*, ed 3, Philadelphia, 2000 WB Saunders.

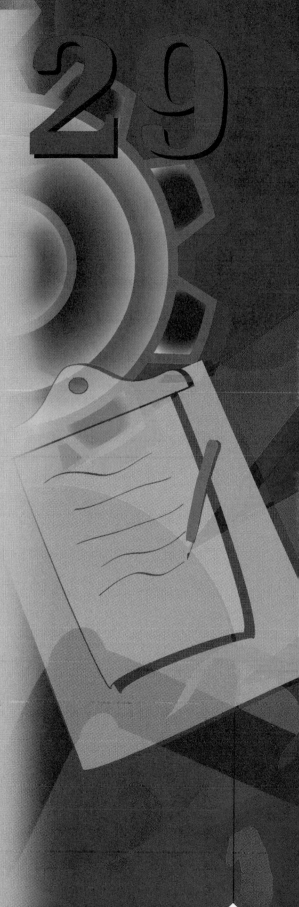

Promoting Comfort

Objectives

- Define key terms.
- Discuss common misconceptions about pain.
- Describe the physiology of pain.
- Identify components of the pain experience.
- Discuss the three phases of behavioral responses to pain.
- Explain how the gate control theory relates to selecting nursing thera-pies for pain relief.
- Assess a client experiencing pain.
- Develop appropriate nursing diagnoses for a client in pain.
- Describe guidelines for selecting and individualizing pain therapies.
- Describe applications for use of nonpharmacological pain therapies.
- Discuss nursing implications for administering analgesics.
- Differentiate the nursing implications associated with managing cancer pain versus noncancer pain.
- Describe interventions for the relief of acute pain following operative or medical procedures.
- Describe the sequence of treatments recommended in pain management for cancer clients.
- Evaluate a client's response to pain therapies.

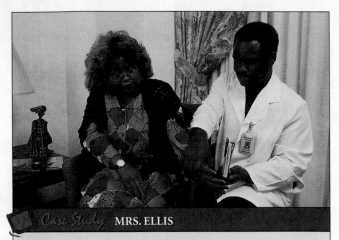

Case Study   MRS. ELLIS

Mrs. Ellis is a 70-year-old black woman with hypertension, diabetes, and rheumatoid arthritis. She has been receiving home visits following a recent hospitalization for the control of her diabetes. Her current health priority is the discomfort and disability associated with her rheumatoid arthritis. Her hands and feet are severely deformed by the arthritis. The pain in her feet has become so severe that Mrs. Ellis can often only walk short distances. The pain interferes with sleep and reduces her energy both physically and emotionally; as a result, she does not leave her home often. She has lived alone since her husband's death 6 years ago.

Jim is a 26-year-old sophomore nursing student assigned to do home visits with the community health nurse. Jim has had the opportunity to conduct assessments, perform procedures, and teach health promotion with a variety of clients with various illnesses over the past 6 weeks. This is Jim's first experience with a client with severe chronic pain.

SCIENTIFIC KNOWLEDGE BASE

Comfort

The provision of comfort is a concept central to the art of nursing. Each individual brings physiological, sociocultural, spiritual, psychological, and environmental characteristics that influence how comfort is interpreted and experienced. An understanding of comfort gives you as a nurse a larger range of choices when selecting pain therapies. Pain management is more than administering analgesics. You must first understand how the pain experience affects a client's comfort level and then use therapies that meet the unique needs of clients (Hall, 2000).

Nature of Pain

Pain is more than a single physiologic sensation caused by a specific stimulus. It is subjective and highly individualized. The person experiencing pain is the only authority on it. According to McCaffery (1979), "Pain is whatever the experiencing person says it is, existing whenever he says it does." Acute pain is a physiological mechanism that protects the individual from a harmful stimulus. For example, a client with a sprained ankle avoids bearing full weight on the foot to prevent further injury. Pain can also be a warning of tissue damage, which should be your first concern when assessing pain. (International Association for the Study of Pain [IASP], 1992;

Hall, 2000). Clients unable to feel sensations, such as after spinal cord injury, are unaware of pain-inducing injuries. Special precautions must be taken to protect these individuals from additional injury.

Health care providers often have prejudices about clients in pain. Unless clients have objective signs of pain, nurses may not believe they are experiencing pain. The extent to which you make assumptions about clients in pain influences your nursing assessment and can seriously limit your ability to offer pain relief (Watt-Watson and others, 2000). Too often, nurses allow misconceptions about pain (Box 29-1) to affect their willingness to provide pain relief (McCaffery and Ferrell, 1996; McCaffery and Pasero, 1999). Many nurses even avoid acknowledging a client's pain because of their own fear of the outcome of their interventions and denial that the client is having pain. These misconceptions may lead to mistrust between the nurse and client, increased client recovery time, increased complications and mortality, increased psychological problems, and increased cost (Hall, 2000; Mayer and others, 2001).

The failure of health care providers to assess pain accurately and consistently results in poor pain management and increased client suffering. Efforts have been made by national and international organizations to correct this problem (AHCPR, 1992; IASP, 1992; Mayer and others, 2001). The Joint Commission for Accreditation of Health Care Organizations (JCAHO) (2000) has a pain standard that requires that all clients be assessed for pain on a regular basis. Many health care institutions have adopted this standard by recommending that staff include pain as a "fifth vital sign." It is important that you develop a "pain conscience" when you care for clients and learn to asses for pain in each client, select proper pain therapies, and evaluate the effects of your actions in relieving clients' pain.

Physiology of Pain

Pain is complex. An understanding of the three components of pain, **reception, perception,** and **reaction,** will help you recognize factors that cause pain, symptoms that accompany pain, and the rationale and actions of therapies.

Examples of Physical Sources of Pain

Table 29-1

Type of Stimulus	Source	Pathophysiological Process
Mechanical	Alteration in body fluids	Edema distending body tissues
	Duct distention	Overstretching of duct's narrow lumen (e.g., passage of kidney stone through ureter)
	Space-occupying lesion (tumor)	Irritation of peripheral nerves by growth of lesion within confined space.
Chemical	Perforated visceral organ	Chemical irritation by secretions on sensitive nerve endings (e.g., ruptured appendix, duodenal ulcer)
Thermal	Burn (heat or extreme cold)	Inflammation or loss of superficial layers of epidermis, causing increased sensitivity of nerve endings
Electrical	Burn	Skin layers burned with muscle and subcutaneous tissue injury, causing injury to nerve endings

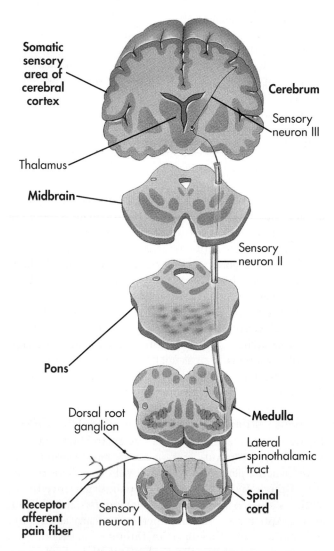

Somatic sensory area of cerebral cortex

Cerebrum

Sensory neuron III

Thalamus

Midbrain

Sensory neuron II

Pons

Dorsal root ganglion

Medulla

Lateral spinothalamic tract

Spinal cord

Receptor afferent pain fiber

Sensory neuron I

FIGURE **29-1**   Spinothalamic pathway that conducts pain stimuli to the brain.

RECEPTION.   Any cellular damage caused by thermal, mechanical, chemical, or electrical stimuli (Table 29-1) releases pain-producing substances. Exposure to painful stimuli releases substances such as histamine, bradykinin, and potassium, which combine with receptor sites on **nocicep-**

tors (receptors that respond to harmful stimuli) to initiate the neural transmission associated with pain (McCaffery and Pasero, 1999).

Painful stimuli produce nerve impulses that travel along afferent peripheral nerve fibers. There are primarily two types of peripheral nerve fibers that conduct painful stimuli: the fast, myelinated A-delta fibers and the small, slow unmyelinated C fibers. The A fibers send sharp, localized, and distinct sensations. The small C fibers relay slower impulses that are poorly localized, visceral, and persistent (Willens, 1996). For example, after stepping on a nail, a person initially feels a sharp localized pain, which is the result of A-fiber transmission. Within a few seconds the whole foot aches from C-fiber stimulation.

A-delta and C fibers transmit impulses from the periphery to the dorsal horn of the spinal cord, where an excitatory neurotransmitter, substance P, is released. This causes a synaptic transmission from the afferent (sensory) peripheral nerve to spinothalamic tract nerves. Pain stimuli travel through nerve fibers in the spinothalamic tracts, cross to the opposite side of the spinal cord, and then travel up the spinal cord. Figure 29-1 shows the normal pain reception pathway. After the pain impulse ascends the spinal cord, information is sent quickly to higher centers in the brain.

A protective reflex response also occurs with pain reception (Figure 29-2). When a person is injured, a noxious stimulus from the skin travels along sensory neurons to the dorsal horn of the spinal cord where it synapses with spinal motor neurons. The impulse continues to travel along the spinal nerve to the skeletal muscle, causing the person to withdraw from the source of the pain.

Pain reception requires an intact peripheral nervous system and spinal cord. Common factors that disrupt pain reception include trauma, drugs, tumor growth, and metabolic disorders.

NEUROREGULATORS.   Neuroregulators are substances that affect the sending of nerve stimuli (Box 29-2). **Neurotransmitters** such as substance P send electrical impulses across the synaptic cleft between two nerve fibers. They either excite or inhibit nerve transmission. **Neuromodulators** such as **endorphins** modify neuron activity without directly

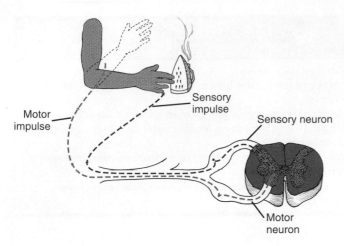

FIGURE **29-2** Protective pain reflex. Sensory impulse directly stimulates motor nerves, bypassing the brain, causing withdrawal from pain stimulus.

transferring a nerve signal through a **synapse.** They are believed to act indirectly by increasing and decreasing the effects of neurotransmitters. Pain perception is influenced by the balance of neurotransmitters and the descending pain-control fibers originating from the cerebral cortex.

GATE CONTROL THEORY OF PAIN.   Researchers know there is no specific pain center in the nervous system. The gate control theory gives you a way to understand pain-relief measures. The gate control theory of Melzack and Wall (1996) suggests that pain impulses can be regulated or even blocked by gating mechanisms along the central nervous system. The gating mechanism occurs within the spinal cord, thalamus, reticular formation, and limbic system (Melzack and Wall, 1996). The theory suggests that pain impulses pass through when the gate is open and not while it is closed. Closing of the gate is the basis for pain-relief therapies. For example, distraction, counseling, and massage techniques are ways to release endorphins, which close the gate. This prevents or reduces the client's perception of pain (Freeman and Lawlis, 2001).

PERCEPTION.   Perception is the point at which a person is aware of pain. A client's neurological function can influence the pain experience. Any factor that interrupts or influences normal pain reception or perception, such as normal fatigue or pain therapies, affects the client's awareness and response to pain. For example, analgesics, sedatives, and anesthetics depress the central nervous system. Assess the neurological status of clients at risk for being insensitive to pain (e.g., clients with spinal cord injury, stroke, or diabetic neuropathy) and provide preventive care.

REACTION.   The reaction to pain is the physiological and behavioral responses that occur after pain is perceived (e.g., crying, or moving away from the painful stimulus).

PHYSIOLOGICAL RESPONSES.   When acute and chronic pain impulses travel up the spinal cord toward the brain stem and thalamus, the autonomic nervous system is stimulated as

---

Neurophysiology of Pain: Neuroregulators Box 29-2

NEUROTRANSMITTERS
Substance P
Found in the pain neurons of the dorsal horn (excitatory peptide)
Needed to transmit pain impulses from the periphery to higher brain centers
Causes vasodilation and edema

Serotonin
Released from the brain stem and dorsal horn to inhibit pain transmission

Prostaglandins
Increase sensitivity to pain

NEUROMODULATORS
Endorphins and Dynorphins
Body's natural supply of morphinelike substances
Activated by stress and pain
Located within the brain, spinal cord, and gastrointestinal tract
Cause analgesia when they attach to opiate receptors in the brain

Bradykinin
Released from plasma that leaks from surrounding blood vessels at the site of tissue injury
Binds to receptors on peripheral nerves, increasing pain stimuli

---

part of the stress response. Pain of low-to-moderate intensity and superficial pain cause the fight-or-flight response of the general adaptation syndrome. Stimulation of the sympathetic branch of the autonomic nervous system results in the physiological responses summarized in Table 29-2. If pain is unrelenting, severe, or deep, typically involving visceral organs, the parasympathetic nervous system goes into action. Sustained physiological responses to pain could cause serious harm. Except in cases of severe traumatic pain, which may place a client into shock, most clients quickly adapt, with physical signs, such as vital signs, returning to normal. Thus a client in pain will not always have physical signs (McCaffery and Ferrell, 1996).

BEHAVIORAL RESPONSES.   The phases of a pain experience are anticipation, sensation, and aftermath (Meinhart and McCaffery, 1983). Anticipation occurs before pain is perceived when a person knows pain will occur. This is a result of the individual's own prior pain experience or oftentimes the result of what a person has heard from others. Anticipation allows a person to learn about pain and methods of relieving pain through instruction and support. Of course not all pain has an anticipatory phase. However, you can help clients anticipate pain through instruction and support. For example, you may explain the stinging sensation of a needlestick. Proper explanation helps clients control their anxiety. In cases in which clients are too fearful, anticipation of pain can heighten pain perception.

Sensation of pain occurs when pain is felt. People react to pain in different ways. A person's **tolerance** to pain is the point at which there is an unwillingness to accept pain of

Physiological Reactions to Pain

Table 29-2

Response	Cause or Effect
Sympathetic Stimulation*	
Dilation of bronchial tubes and increased respiratory rate	Provides increased oxygen intake
Increased heart rate	Provides increased oxygen transport
Peripheral vasoconstriction (pallor, elevation in blood pressure)	Elevates blood pressure with shift of blood supply from periphery and viscera to skeletal muscles and brain
Increased blood glucose level	Provides additional energy
Diaphoresis	Controls body temperature during stress
Increased muscle tension	Prepares muscles for action
Dilation of pupils	Affords better vision
Decreased gastrointestinal motility	Frees energy for more immediate activity
Parasympathetic Stimulation†	
Pallor	Causes blood supply to shift away from periphery
Muscle tension	Results from fatigue
Decreased heart rate and blood pressure	Results from vagal stimulation
Rapid, irregular breathing	Causes body defenses to fail under prolonged stress of pain
Nausea and vomiting	Causes return of gastrointestinal function
Weakness or exhaustion	Results from expenditure of physical energy

*Pain of low to moderate intensity and superficial pain.
†Severe or deep pain.

greater severity or duration. Tolerance depends on attitudes, motivation, and values. The client with high pain tolerance is willing to endure severe pain without assistance. Often you must encourage such a client to accept pain-relieving measures. In contrast, a client with low tolerance may seek relief before pain occurs. Nurses are often more than willing to attend to the client whose pain tolerance is high. Yet it is unfair to ignore the needs of a client unable to tolerate even minor pain (Watt-Watson and other, 2000).

Typical body movements and facial expressions that indicate acute pain during movement and rest include clenching the teeth, facial grimacing, holding or guarding the painful part, and bent posture. You will soon learn to recognize patterns of behavior that reflect pain, including moaning, alterations in sleep, agitation, lack of conversation, withdrawal, or hypersensitivity to touch (Victor, 2001). However, lack of pain expression does not mean a client is not having pain. Unless a client openly reacts to pain, it is difficult to assess the nature and extent of the discomfort. You must help a client communicate the pain response effectively.

The aftermath phase occurs when pain is reduced or stopped. Even though the source of pain is controlled, a client may still require your attention. During the aftermath, clients may have physical symptoms such as chills, nausea, vomiting, anger, or depression. If a client has pain again and again, aftermath responses can become serious health problems.

NURSING KNOWLEDGE BASE
Acute and Chronic Pain

Pain is the most common reason that clients seek health care (Taylor, 1999; Mayer and others, 2001). The most common types of pain you will observe in clients include acute, chronic cancer, and chronic noncancer pain.

ACUTE PAIN. Acute pain usually has an identifiable cause following acute injury, disease, or types of surgery. It has a rapid onset, varies in intensity (mild to severe), and lasts briefly. Acute pain warns people of impending injury or disease. It eventually resolves after a damaged area heals. Clients in acute pain are frightened, anxious, and expect relief quickly. The time sequence of acute pain usually results in a willingness by health team members to treat acute pain aggressively. However, conflict between you and the client may arise if you do not provide quick relief. Acute pain is self-limiting, and the client therefore knows an end is in sight.

Acute pain seriously threatens a client's recovery by hampering the client's ability to become active and involved in self-care. It may cause complications such as physical and emotional exhaustion, immobility, sleep deprivation, delayed wound healing, and pulmonary complications (Hall, 2000). Client education and rehabilitation may be delayed and hospitalization prolonged if acute pain is not controlled. If not adequately controlled, acute pain can progress to chronic pain. After acute pain is relieved, the client can direct full attention toward recovery.

CHRONIC PAIN. Chronic pain is prolonged, varies in intensity, and usually lasts longer than is typically expected or predicted (Fulton, 1996; McCaffery and Pasero, 1999). Chronic pain caused by uncontrolled cancer or conditions such as diabetic neuropathy or phantom limb is called **intractable pain,** which can last until death.

Chronic noncancer pain such as low back pain often results from nonprogressive or healed tissue injury. Frequently there may be no identifiable cause. The pain is ongoing and often does not respond to treatment. In chronic pain, endorphins either cease to function or are reduced.

Health care workers are usually less willing to treat chronic pain as aggressively as acute pain. However, the Agency for Health Care Policy and Research (AHCPR) reports that up to 90% of the 8 million Americans who have cancer can have their pain managed effectively (Jacox and others, 1994). Too often these clients are undertreated.

Clients with chronic pain often have periods of **remissions** (partial or complete disappearance of symptoms) and **exacerbations** (increases in severity). This unpredictability frustrates the client, often leading to depression. Chronic pain is a major cause of psychological and physical disability, leading to problems such as job loss, inability to perform simple daily activities, sexual dysfunction, and social isolation. The client with chronic pain often does not show overt symptoms and does not adapt to the pain but seems to suffer more with time because of physical and mental exhaustion. Symptoms of chronic pain include fatigue, insomnia, anorexia, weight loss, withdrawal, depression, hopelessness, and anger.

Caring for the client with chronic pain is a challenge. You should not become frustrated or offer false hope for a cure. You must help the client identify ways to cope and to minimize the client's perception of pain.

Factors Influencing Pain

To accurately assess and then treat a client's pain you must understand the various factors that influence the pain experience.

AGE.   Developmental differences influence how children and older adults react to pain. Young children have trouble understanding pain and the procedures that you administer that may cause pain. Young children without full vocabularies also have difficulty verbally describing and expressing pain to parents or caregivers. Children's temperaments affect how they cope with pain. Children often describe treatments and procedures as the most difficult part of being sick or in the hospital.

Children are grossly undermedicated for pain. When comparing children with adults having the same medical diagnoses, children received fewer medication doses. In addition, analgesic doses are often too small or given too infrequently to be effective (Ochsenreither and Cubina, 1996). You must understand a child's response to pain. If a child is too young to speak, you may observe behavioral changes such as irritability, loss of appetite, unusual quietness, disturbed sleep patterns, restlessness, and rigid posturing as signs of pain (Jacox and others, 1994; McIntosh, 1997). If a behavior such as crying changes after a child receives an analgesic, it was probably caused by pain.

Pain is not a natural part of aging. Likewise, pain perception does not decrease with age. However, older adults often suffer acute and chronic painful disease, which is frequently taken for granted or underestimated by the person, the family, and health care providers. They may use words such as *hurting* or *aching* instead of using the word *pain* to describe their pain. This may be the reason that older adults are con-

sistently prescribed and receive lower doses of pain medication (Celia, 2000; Victor, 2001). Older adults can suffer serious loss of functional status as a result of pain. Mobility, self-care activities, socialization, and activity tolerance can all be reduced (McCaffery and Pasero, 1999). A client with cognitive impairment may have trouble communicating pain and providing a detailed description (Eiman and others, 1996; AGS Panel on Chronic Pain in Older Persons, 1998; Memran and others, 1998). Yet pain can be assessed accurately in most clients using physical and behavioral cues (AGS Panel on Chronic Pain in Older Persons, 1998).

The ability of older adults to interpret pain can be complicated by multiple diseases and vague symptoms affecting similar parts of the body. When older clients have more than one source of pain, you must gather detailed assessments. Different diseases can cause similar symptoms. For example, a client who has had a below-knee amputation may continue to perceive pain from the foot that has been amputated (phantom pain) and have suture-line pain from the surgery. A stroke client may experience pain in the paralyzed arm and in areas of the body unaffected by the stroke (Mattson, 2000).

GENDER.   Generally men and women do not differ significantly in pain responses. However, cultural influences on gender may affect pain expression (e.g., making it acceptable for a little boy to be brave and not cry, whereas a little girl in the same situation may cry). Although the pain experience has been found to be similar in men and women, research has indicated that men tend to receive a larger initial dose and more frequent doses of pain medication (Celia, 2000).

CULTURE.   Culture influences how people perceive the causes of and learn to react to and express pain. Italian, Jewish, black, and Spanish-speaking persons smile readily and use facial expressions and gestures to communicate pain or displeasure (Giger and Davidhizar, 1995). In contrast, Irish, English, and Northern European persons tend to have less facial expression and are less responsive, especially to strangers such as professional caregivers. Understanding cultural background and personal characteristics will help you to more accurately assess pain and its meaning for clients (Celia, 2000; Hall, 2000).

MEANING OF PAIN.   The meaning a client associates with pain affects the pain experience. Clients perceive pain differently if it suggests a threat, loss, punishment, or challenge. The degree and quality of pain perceived by a client are related to the meaning of pain (Bozeman, 1996; Celia, 2000).

ATTENTION.   The degree to which a client focuses on pain influences pain perception. Increased attention has been associated with increased pain, whereas distraction has been associated with decreased pain. This concept is applied when you use pain-relief therapies such as listening to music and rhythmical breathing. By focusing a client's attention and concentration on other stimuli, you place pain on the periphery of awareness. Usually, increased tolerance for pain lasts only during the time of distraction (McCaffery and Pasero, 1999).

ANXIETY. Elevated anxiety levels increase pain perception. In addition, pain may also cause anxiety. Autonomic arousal patterns are similar in pain and anxiety. A stressful environment, such as a hospital, or the attitude of a nurse may increase clients' anxiety and decrease their tolerance to pain (Hall, 2000).

FATIGUE. Fatigue heightens pain perception. This intensifies pain and decreases coping abilities (Hall, 2000). Pain is often experienced less after restful sleep than at the end of a tiring day.

PREVIOUS EXPERIENCE. Previous pain experience does not necessarily mean a client will accept pain more easily in the future. Frequent episodes of pain without relief or bouts of severe pain may produce anxiety or fear. In contrast, experiences with the same type of pain that has successfully been relieved may make it easier for the client to interpret the pain sensation. As a result, the client is better prepared to take steps to relieve the pain. A client who has had no experience with a particular type of pain may have an impaired ability to cope with it. You should prepare such a client with a clear explanation of the type of pain that will be experienced and methods to reduce it (Kettelman, 2000).

COPING STYLE. The experience of pain can be lonely. Frequently clients feel a loss of control over their environments or the outcome of events. Coping style thus influences the ability to deal with pain. Clients with internal loci of control perceive themselves as having personal control over their environments and the outcome of events. They ask questions, desire information, and like choices of treatment. In contrast, clients with external loci of control perceive other factors in their environments, such as nurses, as being responsible for the outcome of events. These clients tend to be less demanding, follow directions, and take a passive stance in managing their pain. They want specific instructions but may become anxious if too much information is given (Courts, 1996). Those with internal loci of control report less severe pain than those with external loci. This concept is applied in the use of **patient-controlled analgesia (PCA).**

FAMILY AND SOCIAL SUPPORT. Clients depend on the support and assistance of spouses, family, or friends when coping with pain. Family members may have misconceptions about pain and pain management. They may think the client should wait as long as possible before receiving pain medication and fear the possibility of addiction. It is your responsibility to educate the client, family, and public about the importance of early assessment and treatment of pain (Ferrell and others, 2000). The presence of a loved one can minimize loneliness and fear when a client is experiencing pain. Clients of different sociocultural groups have different expectations of people to whom they report their pain.

Absent family or friends can often make the pain experience more stressful. The presence of parents is especially important for children in pain.

CRITICAL THINKING
Synthesis
Because the experience of pain is both unique and dynamic, critical thinking requires synthesis of knowledge about pain, previous experience, intellectual attitudes, and professional standards in order for you to partner with clients in an attempt to ease the client's suffering.

KNOWLEDGE. It is important for you to apply knowledge regarding the physiology of pain, along with the physiology of any underlying disease processes, to understand the client's pain response and the types of interventions needed for pain management. Knowledge and application of communication skills will enhance the thoroughness of a pain assessment. Once you have a clear picture of the physiological nature of a client's condition, synthesis of knowledge regarding the client's psychological and sociocultural perspective becomes critical for an individualized approach to care. In addition, an understanding of pharmacological and non-pharmacological therapies will help you to work with the client and physician in selecting certain pain therapies (Benzaia, 1999; McCaffery and Pasero, 1999).

EXPERIENCE. Caring for clients who have pain is an important part of a nurse's clinical experience. Because pain is so common, you soon learn that clients vary widely in their expressions of pain, the degree pain affects their behaviors, and the actions they take to find relief. Such experience should sensitize you to the personal nature of pain. Furthermore, your own experience with pain emphasizes the importance of having someone who is supportive and understanding. Reflecting on the experiences of caring for those in pain helps you to search for better approaches for each new client encountered.

ATTITUDES. Critical thinking attitudes ensure that you make decisions that are fair and responsible. When a client is in pain, perseverance is often needed to find an approach that will offer the client some degree of relief. Quick solutions often can simply aggravate a client's discomfort. You must learn as much as possible about the client's pain, try various interventions, and continue different creative approaches until an effective one is discovered.

STANDARDS. The application of intellectual standards is particularly important when attempting to acquire an accurate pain assessment. A clear, precise, and accurate description of the client's pain is essential. You should make sure that information related to factors influencing the client's pain is relevant and complete. You must also have an open mind and listen to all sources, including client, family, and friends, who have been affected by the client's experience to

Example of a Focused Client Assessment		Table 29-3
Factors to Assess	Questions and Approaches	Physical Assessment Strategies
Location of pain	Ask client, "Show me where you are feeling the pain." Have client use hand to locate area where pain originates and then spreads.	Depending on area of pain, use inspection to determine if body part is swollen, discolored, or warm to touch. Use light palpation over area identified by client.
Aggravating factors	Ask client to describe what factors increase the pain, "When you feel the pain, what worsens it or makes you more uncomfortable?"	When pain is aggravated by positioning of body part, determine if range of motion is altered. Observe client's facial expression when activity that typically aggravates pain is attempted.

gain a clear picture of what pain means for the client (Victor, 2001).

Professional standards, such as those developed by the Agency for Health Care Policy and Research (AHCPR), the World Health Organization (WHO), the American Society of Pain Management Nurses (ASPMN), and JCAHO, provide valuable guidelines for pain management. These standards have been established by nursing and other health care experts to improve the quality of care to those in pain. You must apply these standards when making decisions about pain therapies.

NURSING PROCESS

Assessment

The assessment of pain is aimed at trying to find the cause of a person's pain and to evaluate the effect of pain on the individual. Accurate and factual pain assessment is necessary for determining clients' progress and response, arriving at proper nursing diagnoses, and selecting appropriate therapies (Table 29-3). Pain assessment is one of the most common and one of the most difficult activities you will perform. Always assess the pain experience from the client's perspective. It is important to carefully interpret pain cues and remember that psychological and physical components of pain influence the reaction to it.

The AHCPR (1992) has established specific guidelines for assessing clients who are to have surgery or other procedures. The focus is planning successful pain-management therapies before pain is experienced. It emphasizes the importance of assessing the resources available for pain management, completing a preoperative client assessment, and developing a collaborative plan for postoperative pain management with the physician, client, and family members. Clients must understand that reporting their pain is valuable and necessary if the health care team is to manage pain in an individualized and effective way.

You must be sensitive to a client's level of discomfort. If pain is acutely severe, it is unlikely the client can provide a detailed description. During an episode of acute pain, assess how a client feels, as well as the location, severity, and quality of pain. A more thorough pain assessment takes time and should be done when the client becomes more alert and attentive.

Routine Clinical Approach to Pain Assessment and Management "ABCDE"	Box 29-3

A *Ask about pain regularly.*
   Assess pain systematically.
B *Believe the client and family in their report of pain and what relieves it.*
C *Choose pain control options appropriate for the client, family, and setting.*
D *Deliver interventions in a timely, logical, and coordinated fashion.*
E *Empower clients and their families.*
   Enable them to control their course to the greatest extent possible.

From Jacox A and others: *Management of cancer pain,* Clinical practice guideline No. 9, AHCPR Pub No. 94-0592, Rockville, Md, March 1994, AHCPR, USDHHS, PHS.

For clients with chronic pain, assessment may be best focused on the emotional impact and the meaning of the pain experience, as well as on its history and context (National Institute of Health Consensus Development Panel, 1986). In addition, assessment should include level of function, because it may be impossible to achieve complete pain relief. The AHCPR recommends that families of cancer clients learn how to assess pain so as to promote continuity of effective pain management (Jacox and others, 1994). In the home setting, family members' involvement in pain assessment offers the client and family control over the pain experience (Box 29-3). You should be aware of possible errors in pain assessment. Bias (overestimating or underestimating level of pain), vague or unclear assessment questions, and use of unreliable or invalid pain-assessment tools will not provide accurate data (McCaffery and Ferrell, 1996; Willens, 1996).

CLIENT'S EXPRESSION OF PAIN.   Clients often fail to report or discuss pain (McCaffery and Ferrell, 1996). To complicate assessment, nurses frequently believe that clients will report pain if they have it. Regularly ask clients about pain. A client must trust you and perceive your willingness to help before discussing pain openly. Learn the verbal or nonverbal ways that the client communicates discomfort.

Implications of Pain Assessment for Nursing Interventions — Table 29-4

Assessment Criteria	Nursing Interventions
Onset and duration	Administer analgesics so that peak action occurs when pain is most acute (e.g., during dressing change or exercise therapy).
Location	Position client off affected area. Apply local treatments (e.g., elastic bandage, cold, heat, splinting) directly over painful site.
Severity	Change or revise interventions, depending on success of one intervention in reducing severity.
Precipitating or aggravating factors	Avoid activities that cause or aggravate pain. Teach client or family to avoid same activities.
Relief measures	Use measures that client uses to relieve pain, as long as they are safe and appropriate.

Clients unable to communicate effectively often require special attention during assessment. Children, developmentally delayed persons, aphasic clients, psychotic clients, clients with dementia, clients receiving neurological-blocking medications, and non–English-speaking clients all require different approaches. Cognitively impaired clients require simple assessment approaches involving close observation of behavior, especially changes in behavior. If a client speaks a different language, a family member or interpreter may be needed. Clients in pain often confide in only one person (Willens, 1996). Clients receiving medications that paralyze their muscles, preventing them from being able to communicate their pain verbally or behaviorally, must be closely monitored. Often proxy pain ratings, the rating of pain by family members or friends who stay with clients and observe their behavior, are useful.

CLASSIFICATION OF THE PAIN EXPERIENCE.   It helps to know the phase of pain clients are undergoing, because it influences not only clients' symptoms but also the types of therapies most likely to relieve pain. Clients in the anticipatory phase, such as those scheduled for invasive procedures, may appear anxious or fearful, or they may ask questions about upcoming pain. Studies have shown that providing clients with physiological coping (positioning and deep breathing), sensory information (description of discomforts to be expected), and procedural information leads to clients with fewer complications, reporting less pain, and using less analgesia (AHCPR, 1992; McCaffery and Pasero, 1999).

Clients who are sensing pain, especially severe pain, want fast relief. These clients may demonstrate more intense responses to the pain, such as crying, nausea, or guarding the painful area. After the pain has been relieved, you must assess carefully for physical and psychological effects.

Assess if a client's pain is acute or chronic. Conduct a detailed assessment of pain characteristics if the pain is acute in nature. With chronic pain determine if it is intermittent, persistent, or limited.

CHARACTERISTICS OF PAIN.   Characteristics of pain can be described only by the client. Client self-report to assess pain characteristics is the single most reliable indicator of the existence and intensity of pain and any related discomfort (McCaffery and Pasero, 1999). Each pain characteristic presents implications for how you will help to manage clients' pain (Table 29-4).

ONSET AND DURATION.   Ask questions to determine the onset, duration, and time sequence of pain. When did the pain begin? How long has it lasted? Does it occur at the same time each day? How often does it recur?

It may be easier to diagnose the nature of pain by identifying time factors. The onset of sudden and severe pain is easier to assess then gradual, mild discomfort. Knowing the time cycle of a client's pain helps you to intervene before the pain occurs or worsens. For example, a client with rheumatoid arthritis may always awaken in the morning with stiffness and pain in the joints. Part of your recommendations may include having the client use heat or warm baths upon awakening.

LOCATION.   To assess pain location, ask the client to point to all areas of discomfort. To localize the pain more specifically, have the client trace the area from the most severe point outward. This is difficult to do if pain is diffuse, involves several sites, or involves large parts of the body. A drawing showing the location of pain can be used as a baseline if the pain changes. Use anatomical landmarks and descriptive terminology to record the pain location (e.g., "Pain is in the right upper abdominal quadrant"). Pain classified by location may be superficial or cutaneous, deep or visceral, localized or diffuse, or referred or radiating (Table 29-5).

SEVERITY.   The most subjective characteristic of pain may be its severity or intensity. Clients are often asked to describe pain as mild, moderate, or severe. However, the meaning of these terms differs for you and the client. Descriptive scales attempt to measure pain severity objectively (Figure 29-3). Use a scale to measure the current severity of the client's pain. In addition, ask the client to rate what was the worst pain experienced in the past 12 hours. You may also ask how severe is the pain at its best. This helps to determine an average pain intensity that allows you to see trends.

A verbal descriptor scale (VDS) consists of a line with three to six word descriptors equally spaced along the line. Show the client the scale and ask the client to choose the descriptor that best represents the severity of pain. A numerical rating scale (NRS) requires clients to rate pain on a scale of 0 to 10, with 0 representing no pain and 10 representing the worst pain a client has ever felt. The scales work best when assessing an individual client's pain intensity before and after therapeutic interventions to determine if relief is achieved. When scales are used to rate pain, a 10-cm (4-inch)

Classification of Pain by Location
Table 29-5

Location	Characteristics	Examples of Causes
Superficial or Cutaneous Pain resulting from stimulation of skin	Pain is of short duration and is localized. It usually is sharp sensation.	Needle stick; small cut or laceration
Deep Visceral Pain resulting from stimulation of internal organs	Pain is diffuse and may radiate in several directions. Duration varies, but it usually lasts longer than superficial pain. Pain may be sharp, dull, or unique to organ involved.	Crushing sensation (e.g., angina pectoris); burning sensation (e.g., gastric ulcer)
Referred Common in visceral pain because many organs themselves have no pain receptors; entrance of sensory neurons from affected organ into same spinal cord segment as neurons from areas where pain is felt	Pain is felt in part of body separate from source of pain and may assume any characteristic.	Myocardial infarction, which may cause referred pain to jaw, left arm, and left shoulder; kidney stones, which may refer pain to groin
Radiating Sensation of pain extending from initial site of injury to another body part	Pain feels as though it travels down or along body part. It may be intermittent or constant.	Low back pain from ruptured intravertebral disk; pain radiates down leg from sciatic nerve irritation

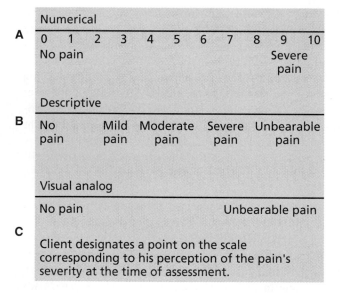

FIGURE **29-3**   Sample pain scales. **A,** Numerical. **B,** Descriptive. **C,** Visual analog.

baseline is recommended. You may also choose to have clients verbally identify their pain intensity on a scale of 0 to 10 instead of using a printed scale or line (AHCPR, 1992; Willens, 1996; Victor, 2001).

A visual analog scale (VAS) consists of a straight line without labeled subdivisions. The straight line shows a continuum of intensity and has labeled endpoints. A client indicates pain by marking the appropriate point on the VAS. This scale gives the client total freedom to identify pain severity. The VAS may be a more sensitive measure of pain severity but

does not provide information on the emotional and sensory qualities of the client's pain (Mattson, 2000). For this reason, the VAS has been found to be more useful for research than in the clinical setting (Ferrell and others, 2000).

Several pain scales have been developed to assess pain in children. Wong and Baker (1988b) developed the FACES Pain Rating Scale to assess pain in children (Figure 29-4). The scale consists of six cartoon faces ranging from a very happy, smiling face for "no pain" to increasingly less happy faces to a final sad, tearful face for "worst pain." Children as young as 3 years of age can use the scale. The advantage is that clients do not have to interpret the meaning of numbers or adjectives. The faces more clearly and quickly depict the concept of pain or discomfort (Willens, 1996).

A unique tool designed to measure pain intensity in children is the Oucher pain scale (Beyea and others, 1992). The Oucher consists of two separate scales: a 0 to 100 scale on the left for older children and a six-picture photographic scale on the right for younger children (Figure 29-5). There are Oucher scales for Caucasians, African-Americans, and Hispanics. Photographs of the face of a child (in increasing levels of discomfort) are designed to cue children into understanding what pain is and its severity. A child merely points to the selection, thus simplifying the task of describing the pain.

A pain scale should be easy to use and not time consuming. If a client can easily read and understand a scale, the description of pain should be more accurate. If clients use a hearing aid or glasses, be sure they are using them when answering pain assessment questions or marking a pain scale (Victor, 2001). Descriptive scales are useful in assessing pain severity and in evaluating changes in a client's condition. Do not use pain scale ratings to compare one client with another.

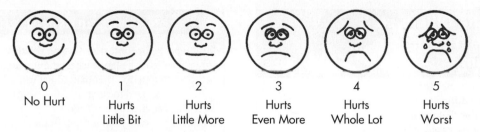

0	1	2	3	4	5
No Hurt	Hurts Little Bit	Hurts Little More	Hurts Even More	Hurts Whole Lot	Hurts Worst

FIGURE **29-4**   Wong-Baker FACES Pain Rating Scale. (From Wong DL and others: *Wong's essentials of pediatric nursing,* ed 6, St. Louis, 2001, Mosby.)

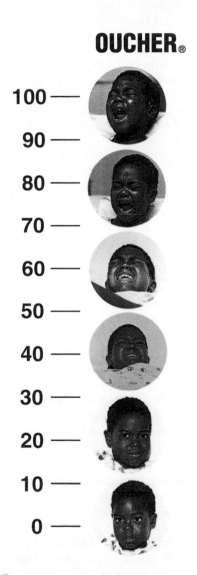

FIGURE **29-5**   Oucher pain scale. (©Beyea, Denyes, 1990. Used with permission.)

QUALITY.   Assessment of the quality of pain helps to identify somatic, visceral, or neuropathic pain. When assessing the quality of pain, do not provide descriptive words for the client. Assessment is more accurate if a client can describe the sensation in his or her own words after open-ended questions. For example, you might say, "Tell me what your pain feels like." The only time you might offer to list de-

scriptive terms is when the client cannot describe pain. The qualities of pricking, burning, and aching are useful to describe pain initially (McCaffery and Pasero, 1999). Later the client may choose more descriptive terms.

There is some consistency in the way clients describe certain types of pain. The pain of a myocardial infarction (heart attack) is often described as crushing or viselike, whereas the pain of a surgical incision is often described as sharp and stabbing. When the descriptions fit the pattern forming in your assessment, a clearer analysis can be made of the nature and type of pain. If descriptions do not fit, it does not mean that the client's pain is not real.

PAIN PATTERN.   Many factors affect the character of pain. It helps to assess specific events or conditions that precipitate or aggravate pain. Ask the client to describe activities that cause pain, such as physical activity, coffee or alcohol ingestion, urination, swallowing, or emotional stress. Ask the client to demonstrate actions that cause painful responses such as coughing or turning in a certain manner. After identifying specific factors, it is easier to plan interventions to avoid worsening the pain (Willens, 1996).

RELIEF MEASURES.   You should know if a client has an effective way for relieving pain such as changing position, using ritualistic behavior (pacing, rocking, or rubbing), eating, or applying heat or cold to the painful site. In the home determine if relief measures are used safely. Assessment of relieving factors should also include identifying practitioners (e.g., internist, chiropractor, or faith healer) whose services the client has sought. Clients with chronic pain are more likely to try alternative health care methods (Courts, 1996).

CONCOMITANT SYMPTOMS.   Concomitant symptoms are those that often occur with pain, including nausea, headache, dizziness, urge to urinate, constipation, depression, and restlessness. Certain types of pain have predictable symptoms. For example, severe rectal pain often causes constipation. These symptoms can be as much a problem to a client as the pain itself.

PHYSICAL SIGNS AND SYMPTOMS.   When a client has pain, conduct a focused physical examination and observe for autonomic nervous system involvement (see Table 29-2,

Assessing the Influence of Pain on Activities of Daily Living

Box 29-4

SLEEP

Does the client have difficulty in falling asleep?

Does pain awaken the client at night?

Are sleeping pills or other aids needed?

HYGIENE

Does pain hinder the client's ability to bathe, dress, or perform other hygiene measures independently?

Are family members or friends available or needed to assist?

EATING

Is client able to manipulate eating utensils?

Can client chew and swallow without discomfort?

SEXUAL FUNCTIONING

Do physical conditions such as arthritis or back pain prevent the client from assuming usual positions during intercourse?

Does pain or fatigue reduce the client's desire for sex?

Are clients fearful that pain will increase as a result of intercourse?

HOME MANAGEMENT AND WORK ACTIVITIES

Is the client able to perform usual housework chores?

Is physical activity required in the job, and is activity now limited by pain?

If pain is related to emotional stress, does the job involve tension-filled decision making?

Must the client stop activities momentarily to relieve pain?

SOCIAL ACTIVITIES

Does the client regularly socialize?

To what extent has pain disrupted activities?

Case Study SYNTHESIS IN PRACTICE

Jim prepares for tomorrow's home health visit with Mrs. Ellis. He reviews what he has learned about pain physiology and the pathophysiology for rheumatoid arthritis. This allows him to anticipate the need to carefully assess to what extent pain limits Mrs. Ellis's ability to perform activities of daily living and walk. Jim plans to assess the location, duration, and aggravating and relieving factors influencing Mrs. Ellis's pain, as well as any behavioral symptoms he might observe. He also wants to use a VAS to establish a baseline for the severity of the pain, as well as any behavioral symptoms he observes. Because Mrs. Ellis is 70, Jim reviews gerontological principles and knows he must take time to establish a trusting relationship with the client so as to encourage a complete description of the pain experience. Jim recalls previous experience with clients n pain and interventions used to relieve pain. He also remembers his own experiences with pain after suffering a broken arm during a soccer game. This experience will sensitize him to the personal and dynamic nature of each individual's pain experience.

Jim considers the AHCPR guidelines for the management of chronic pain. He wants to be careful in clarifying with Mrs. Ellis the extent to which the chronic arthritic pain and the acute exacerbations have affected her life. If Jim is to help her with pain relief and health promotion activities, he must learn as much as he can about Mrs. Ellis's lifestyle and the support systems that are available for her. If she is reportedly living alone, Jim wants to assess if family or friends who can offer assistance live nearby.

---

p. 711). Physiological signs can reveal pain in a client who tries not to complain or is unable to report pain due to cognitive or neurological impairments. At the first onset of acute pain, the heart and respiratory rates and blood pressure may increase. Compare vital sign values with baseline measurements recorded before onset. A change in vital signs is significant, but you should take into account all signs and symptoms before determining that pain is the cause. Do not confuse signs and symptoms of pain with other pathological changes. Base the assessment on the client's pain history. Examine the painful area to see if palpation or manipulation of the site increases pain (Jacox and others, 1994). During a general overview, observe for cues indicating pain (e.g., posturing, restricting limb movements or guarding a painful area). If pain is unrelieved, look for signs of physical exhaustion.

BEHAVIORAL EFFECTS. A verbal report of pain is a vital part of assessment. You must be willing to listen to verbal and nonverbal messages and understand what the client has to say. Many clients cannot verbalize discomfort because of an inability to communicate or decreased levels of consciousness. In these cases you must be alert for subtle behaviors that indicate pain. When clients have pain, also assess their vocal response (e.g., moaning, crying, or gasping), facial movements (e.g., grimacing, clenched teeth, or tightly closed eyes), and body movements (e.g., restlessness, increased hand and finger movements, or pacing), or inactivity. Also assess social interaction. Does the client avoid conversation or social contacts? Does the client have a reduced attention span?

INFLUENCE ON ACTIVITIES OF DAILY LIVING. Pain is a stressful event that can alter lifestyle and psychological well-being. By recognizing the effects of pain on a client, you can identify more clearly the nature and implications of the pain. Clients who live with daily pain are less able to participate in routine activities. Assessment reveals the extent of the disability and the adjustments that will be necessary for participation in self-care (Box 29-4).

CLIENT EXPECTATIONS. Clients rely on their caregivers to recognize and alleviate their physical discomfort. This may involve using a skilled and caring approach, trying a variety of comfort measures, and serving as an advocate for the client. A caring nurse is one perceived to tailor care to the individual's needs. You should always ask clients what they expect regarding their comfort needs. This might include asking clients not only what interventions they might prefer but also how they should be administered. It is also important to understand if clients expect full pain relief or if they simply hope to have their discomfort reduced. When your clients ask for assistance because of pain, they expect you to respond promptly (Taylor, 1999).

DOCUMENTATION.   You must carefully assess and routinely document your client's report of pain and the effectiveness of interventions. Use the assessment tool that is appropriate for your client, and use the same tool to reassess the client's pain after implementing any treatments (Acello, 2000a).

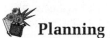

Nursing Diagnosis

Identification of accurate nursing diagnoses for clients in pain result from thorough data collection and analysis. An accurate diagnosis is made after reviewing all of the assessment data and identifying the defining characteristics (Box 29-5). In the example of the diagnosis of *acute pain,* you may assess the client's withdrawal from communication, rigid posturing, moaning, and verbalization of discomfort. In contrast, the diagnosis of *anxiety* may be made by observing a client's facial tension and appearance, poor eye contact, restlessness, and verbalization of feeling scared. The two diagnoses have similar defining characteristics, but you must sort out patterns to reveal *pain* versus *anxiety.*

The related factor for the diagnostic statement focuses on the specific nature of the client's problem. *Pain related to physical trauma* and *pain related to natural childbirth processes* require very different nursing interventions. Successful identification of related factors ensures that nursing therapies will be directed toward relieving the client's discomfort.

Planning

GOALS AND OUTCOMES.   Develop an individualized plan of care for each nursing diagnosis identified (see care plan). Work with the client to set realistic expectations for pain relief and the degree of pain relief to expect. The client should understand that complete pain relief cannot be guaranteed, but it will be attempted. Goals for pain relief and levels of function are to be individualized and realistic with measurable outcomes (Loeb and Pasero, 2000). For example, if a client's baseline assessment reveals a pain severity consistently between 7 and 8 on a VAS, a realistic goal is for the client to achieve improved comfort with the outcome of reaching a reduction in pain severity to a 2 or 3 on the scale. "Pain ratings of 4 or higher on a scale of 0 to 10 are unacceptable unless they are short term" (Loeb and Pasero, 2000).

In the home, plan to use the client's remedies, as long as they are safe. You should assess the home environment carefully to be sure there are no obvious risks to the client. For example, a client might wish to use a heating pad, but the electrical cord is frayed and damaged.

It is always important to remember that a successful plan of care requires development of a therapeutic relationship with the client and a focus on education regarding pain. Helping clients learn how to manage their pain is an important goal of care. You can best help by seeing the client as a total person, listening carefully to concerns, attending promptly to his or her needs, and respecting any response to pain. In a successful nurse-client relationship, the nurse rec-

Box 29-5

Nursing Diagnoses for CLIENTS WITH PAIN

- Anxiety
- Coping, ineffective
- Fatigue
- Hopelessness
- Injury, risk for
- Mobility, impaired physical
- Nausea
- Pain, acute
- Pain, chronic
- Self-care deficit; bathing/hygiene, dressing/grooming, feeding, toileting
- Sexual dysfunction
- Sleep pattern, disturbed

ognizes that the client knows more about his or her own pain and its relief.

SETTING PRIORITIES.   When developing the care plan, you and the client should work together to select priorities based on the client's level of pain and its effect on the client's condition (Taylor, 1999). For acute severe pain, it is important to provide quick relief. Analgesics can be very effective. After a client gains some relief from pain, you should plan other therapies such as client education, use of relaxation exercises, or the application of heat to enhance the effect of analgesics.

CONTINUITY OF CARE.   A comprehensive plan of care should involve the resources of a client's family and friends. The family may need to administer care in the home and thus be prepared to assess the client's pain and administer therapies safely. Discharge teaching in an acute care setting prepares the client and family to understand the nature and extent of the client's pain, the choice of therapies, and how to safely administer therapies. Family members or friends who show a disinterest or prejudice toward pain can impede the client's recovery. Additional resources in planning care include nurse specialists, physical therapists, and occupational therapists. An oncology nurse specialist knows therapies for chronic cancer pain. Physical therapists can plan exercises that strengthen muscle groups and lessen pain. Occupational therapists may devise splints to support painful body parts. If an agency does not have the resources to manage the client's pain, the client must be referred to a health care provider or agency that can provide the care needed (Acello, 2000a). Document all discharge teaching and referrals implemented.

Implementation

The nature of pain and the extent to which it affects an individual's physical and psychosocial well-being determine the choice of pain-relief therapies. You are responsible for administering and monitoring therapies ordered by physicians for pain relief and independently providing pain-relief measures that complement those prescribed by a physician. Client remedies are often most successful, especially when the client has already had experience with pain. Generally the least invasive and safest therapy should be tried first.

Case Study Nursing Care Plan   **CHRONIC PAIN**

ASSESSMENT

When Jim enters Mrs. Ellis's four-room apartment, he finds the home to be in some disarray. Mrs. Ellis is sitting in a recliner in her living room, with clothing on the floor and soiled dishes on a nearby table. Mrs. Ellis reports that the **pain** she has been experiencing has **made it** very **difficult to use her hands and walk between rooms.** She is able to get to the bathroom, but it does cause her to become fatigued. Her **pain is constant and localized in the joints of her hands and knees.** When Jim shows her a VAS, Mrs. Ellis **rates the pain at the level of 5 on a scale of 0 to 10.** Jim asks how she would rate the **pain when** it is **most severe,** and Mrs. Ellis **rates the pain at 9.** She currently takes aspirin for the pain. The pain continues to **prevent her from being able to fall asleep,** and when she does fall asleep, she **often reawakens at night.** She has begun to have some "burning in the stomach" when she takes the aspirin. Jim asks her to stand and walk with him to the kitchen. She **has difficulty standing** and has an **unsteady gait.** Jim asks if Mrs. Ellis has friends or neighbors available who can assist her, and Mrs. Ellis responds, "I hate to be a bother, although my next door neighbor has offered to help in the past."

*Defining characteristics are shown in bold type.

NURSING DIAGNOSIS

Chronic pain related to joint inflammation.

PLANNING

GOAL

Client will achieve a sense of pain relief within 1 week.

Client will ambulate with less discomfort on self-report within 14 days.

EXPECTED OUTCOMES

Client will report pain at 3 on a scale of 0 to 10 following relaxation therapy and heat application.

Client will demonstrate ability to rise to standing position without assistance within 1 week.

Client will demonstrate ability to walk from room to room with steady gait in 2 weeks.

Client will be able to perform activities of daily living such as dishwashing and cleaning.

IMPLEMENTATION

STEPS

1. Confer with client's physician regarding possibility of nonsteroidal antiinflammatory drugs (NSAIDs) for pain relief.

2. Have client take analgesics approximately 30 minutes before client begins ambulation, self-care activities, or goes to sleep. Instruct client to take medication with a light snack or meal and a full glass of water. During instruction, tell client the drug will relieve pain.

3. Have client place a sturdy stool in shower stall and run warm water continuously over joints of hands and feet.

4. Have client apply moist, warm compresses to joints of hands 3 times a day.

5. Refer client to physical therapist to determine possible use of a walker or other assistive devices.

RATIONALE

Aspirin can cause irritation of gastric mucosa with bleeding or ulceration. Replacement with NSAID provides better analgesic and antiinflammatory properties with fewer gastrointestinal disturbances. Caution is necessary with older adults.

Medication will exert peak effect when client begins activities. Administration with meals and water reduces chance of gastrointestinal upset. An added placebo effect is brought into play when client's attention is focused on action and purpose of analgesic. Then medication is taken with assurance that it will work (Salerno, 1996).

Heat reduces pain by improving blood flow and reducing stiffness of inflamed tissues.

Cutaneous stimulation may activate mechanoreceptor A-beta fibers, thus inhibiting transmission of pain by releasing inhibitory neurotransmitters.

Physical therapist can teach effective exercise and ambulation techniques to reduce pain and conserve energy.

EVALUATION

- Observe client's ability to stand and walk from living room to kitchen.
- Ask if client experiences discomfort during dressing and bathing activities.
- Observe client perform dressing and/or bathing as appropriate, noting range of motion.
- Ask client to rate pain on a scale of 0 to 10 after each nursing therapy and compare with baseline assessment.

Regardless of the type of therapies used, your ability to show caring toward a client can maximize pain control (see Chapter 15). Pain can be minimized through caring behaviors such as gentle handling and touch (Mayer and others, 2001). Two types of touching, task-oriented and affective, can be effective with clients. Task-oriented touching occurs when a nurse takes a client's blood pressure or helps the client walk. Affective is less routine and is intended to show concern, such as holding the client's hand during a procedure. You can combine task-oriented and affective touching (e.g., placing a hand on the client's shoulder while administering a tablet). Simply sitting and holding a client's hand, allowing clients to

Guidelines for Individualized Pain Therapy
Box 29-6

Use different types of pain-relief measures. This produces an additive effect in reducing pain and allows for changes in the character of pain.

Provide pain-relief measures before pain becomes severe. It is easier to prevent severe pain than try to relieve it after it occurs.

Use measures the client believes are effective. The client's beliefs may make pain therapy successful, so include those remedies unless they are harmful.

A client may have ideas about measures to use and times to use them. Consider the client's ability or willingness to participate in pain-relief measures.

Suggest measures that require little physical effort for clients unable to actively assist with pain therapy because of fatigue or altered levels of consciousness. Do not force participation.

Choose pain-relief measures on the basis of client behavior that reflects the severity of pain. Never administer a potent analgesic for mild pain. Only the client can determine the potency of an effective therapy.

If a therapy is ineffective at first, encourage the client to try it again before abandoning it. Client anxiety or doubt may prevent therapy from relieving pain, or the measure may require adjustment or practice to become effective.

Keep an open mind about ways to relieve pain. Rejecting nonconventional therapy leads to mistrust. Be sure all therapies are safe.

Keep trying. When efforts at pain relief fail, do not abandon the client but reassess the situation and consider alternative therapies.

Protect the client. Pain therapy should not cause more distress than the pain itself; you want to relieve pain without disabling the client mentally, emotionally, or physically.

Educate the client about pain. Explain the cause of pain, times when analgesics can be given, and alternative therapies.

---

move at their own speed, speaking in a soft tone of voice, and staying with a client for a time after a procedure are all caring behaviors. Your use of nonverbal expressions to reinforce words of encouragement and support also convey caring. When you successfully convey compassion, maintain the client's dignity, and consistently strive to minimize discomfort, pain-relieving measures will be more successful.

HEALTH PROMOTION. When providing pain-relief measures, choose therapies suited to the client's unique pain experience. Box 29-6 includes guidelines that McCaffery (1979) suggests for individualizing pain therapy.

MAINTAINING WELLNESS. Measures that promote a sense of well-being to minimize or avoid discomfort include warm baths, thorough personal hygiene measures, and a schedule of adequate rest. Chapter 28 discusses the effect pain can have on a client's sleep pattern and ways to promote better sleep habits. Also help the client find ways to plan rest periods before participating in exhausting activities. Clients with chronic pain should rest before any social activities in the home.

Pain can disable and immobilize a person enough to impair the ability to perform self-care activities. As a result

the client might also experience social isolation, depression, and changes in self-concept. Change in function can mean a significant loss to a client. Help clients and families learn to discuss their feelings about the loss so as to find ways to cope with pain and the lifestyle it imposes (see Chapter 22).

Pain from an injury or disabling illness may limit a client's mobility. In this case health promotion is aimed at retaining function. Instruct clients and families on the safe and proper use of elastic bandages, braces, and splints that protect body parts. When a client has chronic, disabling pain it can be helpful for you to instruct family members on proper positioning techniques and ways to assist the client with ambulation.

You may refer clients who have difficulty eating, bathing, grooming, and dressing to an occupational therapist. Some agencies may require a physician's order to begin occupational therapy. Devices designed to maintain function, even when finger movement or grasp is impaired, can help. The therapist can attach eating utensils, a comb, or a toothbrush to extension devices that have enlarged handles or splints for easy use. Clothing fasteners made of Velcro tape allow clients to remove or apply clothing by themselves.

A client with pain may avoid sexual activity. The need for sexual warmth is not negated by pain. Clients can learn to express themselves sexually by assuming alternative positions during intercourse and learning more about ways to make their partner feel sexually stimulated. You should caution clients that some pain medications can decrease libido and potency.

NONPHARMACOLOGICAL PAIN-RELIEF MEASURES. One of the most basic nursing responsibilities is protecting the client from harm. A number of nonpharmacological or complementary therapies are used for pain relief, including massage, imagery, music, biofeedback, meditation, hypnosis, exercise, therapeutic touch, acupuncture, and relaxation techniques (Freeman and Lawlis, 2001). Several of these therapies require special training to perform, including biofeedback and acupuncture. Other therapies, such as massage, imagery, and relaxation techniques that lessen the reception and perception of pain, can be used by nurses in a variety of health care settings. These therapies can and should be used in combination with pharmacological measures. The AHCPR guidelines for acute pain management (1992) cite nonpharmacological interventions to be appropriate for clients who:

Find such interventions appealing

Express anxiety or fear

May benefit from avoiding or reducing drug therapy

Are likely to experience and need to cope with a prolonged interval of postoperative pain

Have incomplete pain relief with use of pharmacological therapies

You are responsible for evaluating the effects of nonpharmacological measures to ensure pain relief occurs so that clients are not excluded from use of pharmacological therapies.

Reducing Pain Reception and Perception. A simple way to promote comfort is by removing or preventing painful stimuli. For example, tighten and smooth wrinkled bed linen and be sure to position clients off tubing and other equipment. Change wet dressings or bed linen immediately. Do not allow tubing from a Foley catheter to become kinked; bladder distention is uncomfortable. When repositioning clients, lift them in bed, do not pull, and position them in correct anatomical alignment. Avoid exposing the skin to irritants such as diarrheal stool or wound drainage. Many of these measures are easy for family members to learn. Removing noxious stimuli is especially important for clients who are immobilized. Pain can also be prevented by anticipating painful activities (e.g., ambulation, turning). Before performing a procedure consider the client's condition, aspects of the procedure that are painful, and ways to avoid causing pain. It takes only simple consideration of the client's comfort and a little extra time to avoid pain-producing situations.

Anticipatory Guidance. Modifying anxiety directly associated with pain relieves pain and adds to the effects of other pain-relief measures. The AHCPR (1992) reports that giving clients detailed descriptions of all medical procedures, expected postoperative discomfort, and instruction aimed at decreasing treatment- and mobility-related pain can decrease self-reported pain, analgesic use, and postoperative length of stay. Provide clients sufficient procedural and sensory information (e.g., prick of a needle during blood draw or burning during urinary catheter insertion) to satisfy their interest and enable them to assess, evaluate, and communicate pain (McCaffery and Pasero, 1999).

Distraction. With meaningful sensory stimuli, a client can ignore or become unaware of pain. Pleasurable sensory stimuli reduces pain perception by the release of endorphins. Distraction directs a client's attention to something else and thus can reduce the awareness of pain and even increase tolerance. Distraction may work best for short, intense pain lasting a few minutes such as during an invasive procedure or while waiting for an analgesic to work. Useful forms of distraction include singing, praying, listening to music, describing photos out loud, telling jokes, and playing games.

Cutaneous Stimulation. **Cutaneous stimulation** is the stimulation of the skin to relieve pain. A massage, warm bath, ice bag, and **transcutaneous electrical nerve stimulation (TENS)** are simple ways to reduce pain perception. The mode of action for cutaneous stimulation is unclear, but it may release endorphins. The gate control theory suggests that cutaneous stimulation activates larger, faster A-beta sensory nerve fibers that are sensitive to touch, pressure, and warmth. This decreases pain transmission through small-diameter A-delta and C fibers. Synaptic gates close to the transmission of pain impulses (Freeman and Lawlis, 2001).

An advantage to cutaneous stimulation is that the measures can be used in the home, giving clients and families

---

Procedural Guidelines for MASSAGE   Box 29-7

1. Based on client assessment, decide on performing massage on one or more body parts.
2. Help client to assume comfortable lying or sitting position.
3. Dim room lights and/or turn on soft music.
4. Massage each body part at least 10 minutes.
   Hands: Make contact with the client's skin, first with one hand and then the other. Using both hands, slowly open the client's palm, gliding your fingers over the palmar surface. While supporting the hand, use both thumbs to apply friction to the palm and use them in a circular motion to stretch the palm outward. Massage each finger outward and then separately, using a corkscrewlike motion from base of finger to the tip. With thumb and finger, knead each small muscle in the client's fingers. Glide hands smoothly from fingertips to wrists. Repeat for other hand.
   Arms: Use a gliding stroke to massage from the client's wrist to forearm. With thumb and forefinger of both hands, knead muscles from forearm to shoulder. Continue kneading biceps, deltoid, and triceps muscles. Finish with gliding strokes from the wrist to the shoulder.
   Neck: Support the neck at the hairline with one hand and massage up it with a gliding stroke. Knead muscles on one side. Switch hands to support neck and knead other side. Stretch the neck slightly, with one hand at the top and the other at the bottom.
   Back: Begin at sacral area and massage in circular motion (see Figure 29-6) while moving upward from buttocks to shoulders. Use a firm, smooth stroke over the scapula. Continue in one smooth stroke to upper arms and laterally along sides of back down to iliac crests. Use long, gliding strokes along muscles of spine. Knead any muscles that feel tense or tight.
5. At end of massage have client relax, taking slow, deep breaths.

---

some control over pain symptoms and treatment. The proper use of cutaneous stimulation can reduce pain perception and help to reduce muscle tension that might otherwise increase pain. When using cutaneous stimulation methods, eliminate sources of environmental noise, help the client to assume a comfortable position, and explain the purpose of the therapy. Cutaneous stimulation should not be used directly on sensitive skin areas (e.g., burns, bruises, skin rashes, inflammation, or underlying bone fractures) (Freeman and Lawlis, 2001).

Massages have been used by nurses as a safe and effective way to produce physical and mental relaxation, reduce pain, and enhance the effectiveness of pain medication for many years (Box 29-7 and Figure 29-6). Massaging the back and shoulders or the hands and feet for 3 to 5 minutes can help relax muscles and promote sleep (Grealish and others, 2000). Massages communicate caring and can be easily taught to family members (McCaffery and Pasero, 1999).

Cold and heat applications relieve pain and promote healing. The choice to use heat or cold should be based on the origin of the pain and the client's past preferences and past experience with pain relief using these methods. When using any form of heat or cold application, you must instruct the client to avoid injury to the skin. For example, when us-

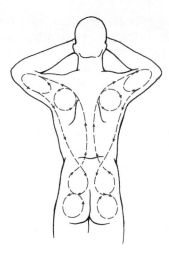

FIGURE **29-6**   Back massage pattern.

ing a heating pad for an extended period, the control must be set on a low temperature and the pad wrapped in a towel to avoid injury. Never allow a client to sleep lying on a heating pad. Clients at risk for burns from heating pads or other devices are those with spinal cord or other neurological injury, older adults, and confused clients.

TENS is a form of cutaneous stimulation that involves stimulation of the skin with a mild electrical current passed through external electrodes. It requires a physician's order. The TENS unit consists of a battery-powered transmitter, lead wires, and electrodes. The electrodes are placed directly over or near the site of pain. Hair or skin preparations should be removed before attaching the electrodes. When a client feels pain, the transmitter is turned on and a buzzing or tingling sensation is created. The tingling sensation can be applied until pain relief is achieved. TENS may be useful in managing postoperative pain and in reducing pain caused by postoperative procedures (e.g., removing drains) (Courts, 1996). It is safe, noninvasive, inexpensive, and easy to use.

Relaxation.   The ability to relax physically promotes mental relaxation. **Relaxation** techniques provide clients with self-control when pain occurs, reversing the physical and emotional stress of pain. Clients who use relaxation techniques successfully go through physiological and behavioral changes (e.g., decreased pulse and blood pressure and decreased muscle tension). Relaxation strategies include simple relaxation, imagery, and music-assisted relaxation. Relaxation and imagery techniques have been successful in reducing self-reported pain and analgesic use (McCaffery and Pasero, 1999). The techniques require periodic reinforcement through encouragement and coaching (AHCPR, 1992).

For effective relaxation the client needs to participate and cooperate. Relaxation techniques are taught only when the client is not in acute discomfort and thus is able to concentrate. Explain the technique in detail, and note that it may take several training sessions before clients can effectively minimize pain. Relaxation training can be practiced indefinitely and usually has no side effects. Remove any noises or

other irritating stimuli, such as bright lights, from the environment. Have the client sit in a comfortable chair in good alignment or lie in bed. A light sheet or blanket keeps the client warm and comfortable. Describe common sensations that the client may experience (e.g., a decrease in temperature, a feeling of heaviness, or numbness of a body part). The client uses these sensations as feedback. Acting as a coach, guide the client slowly through the steps of the exercise. Relaxation may be done alone or with guided imagery.

In **guided imagery** the client creates an image in the mind, concentrates on that image, and gradually becomes less aware of pain. Initially ask the client to think of a pleasant scene or experience that promotes using all senses. The client describes the image, and you record it so that it can be used later. You should use only specific information given by the client and make no changes in the image. The following is an example of a portion of a guided imagery exercise:

> Imagine yourself lying on a cool bed of grass with the sounds of water trickling over stones in a nearby stream. It's a warm day. You turn to see a patch of blue wildflowers in bloom and can smell their fragrance.

You should sit close enough to the client to be heard but not be intrusive. A calm, soft voice helps the client to focus more completely on the suggested image. While relaxing, the client focuses on the image, and it becomes unnecessary for you to speak continuously. If the client shows signs of agitation, restlessness, or discomfort, stop the exercise and begin later when the client is more at ease.

Progressive relaxation exercises involve a combination of controlled breathing exercises and a series of contractions and relaxation of muscle groups. The client begins by breathing slowly and diaphragmatically, allowing the abdomen to rise slowly and the chest to expand fully. Often a client closes the eyes to focus on the exercise. When the client establishes a regular breathing pattern, you should coach the client to locate any area of muscular tension, think about how it feels, gently tense the muscles, and then completely relax them. This creates the sensation of removing all discomfort and stress. Gradually the client can relax the muscles without first tensing them. After the client achieves full relaxation, pain perception is lowered, and anxiety toward the pain experience becomes minimal. If the client becomes agitated or uncomfortable, stop the exercise. If the client reports having difficulty relaxing only part of the body, you should slow the progression of the exercise and concentrate on the tensed body part. If the client complains of increased pain, focus on relaxing areas of muscle tension instead of consciously tensing the muscle. The client may stop the exercise at any time. With practice the client can learn to perform relaxation exercises independently. Relaxation techniques are particularly effective for chronic pain, labor pains, and relief of procedure-related pain. The techniques are less effective for episodes of acute or severe pain.

ACUTE CARE.   In the acute care setting the additional effects of other symptoms and multiple treatments can make pain management complex. Your ability to make appropriate decisions depends on a critical thinking approach.

PHARMACOLOGICAL PAIN THERAPY.   All pharmacological agents require a physician's order. Your judgment in the use of medications with or without other pain therapies ensures the best pain relief possible. A systematic approach ensures quick response on the part of caregivers to client discomfort.

Analgesics.   Analgesics are the most common method of pain relief (Jacox and others, 1994). Although analgesics can effectively relieve pain, nurses and physicians tend to undertreat clients because of incorrect drug information, concerns about addiction, anxiety over errors in judgment while using narcotic analgesics, and administration of less medication than was ordered (Watt-Watson and others, 2000). You must understand the drugs available for pain relief and their pharmacological effects (McCaffery and Ferrell, 1996). Clients need to be reassured that fears of addiction are unfounded. Agency policies must be reviewed and updated regularly to support and guide health care providers in providing maximum pain relief to clients with acute and chronic pain and pain at the end of life (Ferrell and others, 2000).

The three types of analgesics are nonopioids, opioids, and adjuvants. Nonopioid analgesics, including acetaminophen, tramadol (Ultram), and nonsteroidal antiinflammatory drugs (NSAIDs), are effective in treating mild to moderate pain. One exception is ketorolac (Toradol), which is an injectable analgesic NSAID that is comparable to morphine in efficacy. NSAIDs act by inhibiting the synthesis of **prostaglandins** and by inhibiting the cellular responses during inflammation. Most NSAIDs act on peripheral nerve receptors to diminish transmission and reception of pain stimuli. Acetaminophen acts on central nervous system prostaglandins.

Opioid analgesics are generally used for severe pain. They are legally distinct from **narcotics;** therefore opioids should no longer be referred to as narcotics. Opioid analgesics include codeine, morphine, hydromorphone (Dilaudid), fentanyl, oxycodone, propoxyphene (Darvon), and other natural and synthetic medications. Meperdine HCl (Demerol) is no longer a drug of choice and is rarely used because of the potential to cause seizures and severe side effects of nausea and vomiting. Opioids act on the central nervous system to produce a combination of depressing and stimulating effects. Opioid analgesics such as morphine act on higher centers of the brain and spinal cord by binding with opiate receptors to modify perception of and reaction to pain. Morphine is a derivative of opium. It raises the pain **threshold** (reducing pain perception), reduces anxiety and fear (components of the reaction to pain), and induces sleep. Morphine and other opioid analgesics can depress vital nervous system functions such as respirations, although this is rare. Clients may also have side effects such as nausea, vomiting, constipation, and altered mental processes (McCaffery and Pasero, 1999; Reiff and Niziolek, 2001).

Adjuvants such as sedatives, anticonvulsants, steroids, antidepressants, antianxiety agents, and muscle relaxants enhance pain control or relieve other symptoms associated with pain, such as anxiety, depression, and nausea. They may be given alone or with analgesics (McCaffery and Pasero, 1999).

The proper use of analgesics requires careful assessment, application of pharmacological principles, and common sense (Box 29-8). Responses to analgesics are highly individualized. An NSAID may be as effective as a potent opioid for some clients, or an orally administered analgesic may bring the same relief as an injectable form. You must remain familiar with comparative doses of different analgesics

---

Nursing Principles for Administering Analgesics   Box 29-8

KNOW THE CLIENT'S PREVIOUS RESPONSE TO ANALGESICS
Determine whether relief was obtained.
Ask whether a nonnarcotic was as effective as a narcotic.
Identify previous doses and routes of administration to avoid undertreatment.
Determine whether the client has allergies.

SELECT PROPER MEDICATIONS WHEN MORE THAN ONE IS ORDERED
Use NSAIDs or milder opioids for mild to moderate pain.
The concurrent use of opioids and NSAIDs often provides for more effective analgesia than either drug class alone.
Use of NSAIDs can help reduce opioid side effects.
In older adults, avoid combinations of opioids.
Remember that morphine and hydromorphone are the opioids of choice for long-term management of severe pain.
Know that injectable medications act quicker and can relieve severe, acute pain within 1 hour and that oral medication may take as long as 2 hours to relieve pain.
For chronic pain, give an oral drug for longer, more sustained relief.

KNOW THE ACCURATE DOSAGE
Remember that doses at the upper end of normal are generally needed for severe pain.

Adjust doses, as appropriate, for children and older clients.
Dosage typically requires adjustment over time.
Know the comparative potencies of analgesics (refer to drug manual or pharmacy) in oral and injectable form.

ASSESS THE RIGHT TIME AND INTERVAL FOR ADMINISTRATION
Administer analgesics as soon as pain occurs and before it increases in severity.
Do not give analgesics only on "as needed" schedules. An around-the-clock administration schedule is best.
Given analgesics before pain-producing procedures or activities.
Know the average duration of action for a drug and the time of administration so that the peak effect occurs when pain is most intense.

CHOOSE THE RIGHT ROUTE
Intravenous and oral routes are preferred.
Intramuscular and subcutaneous administration should be avoided because those routes can be painful and absorption is not reliable.

(equianalgesics). This information is readily available from your agency pharmacy. In addition, nurses on succeeding shifts must know the route of administration most effective for a client so that controlled, sustained pain relief is achieved. Repetitive intramuscular or subcutaneous injections of medications should be avoided.

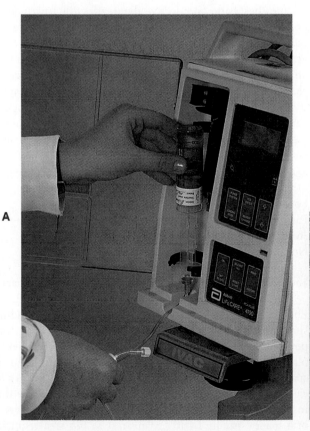

Gerontological Nursing Practice   Box 29-9

- In older adults there is fear that pain will result in crippling and forced dependency.
- Older adults are at high risk for pain-inducing situations.
- Several pain-producing conditions may coexist.
- The potential for lowered pain tolerance exists with diminished adaptive capacity.
- Changes in peripheral vascular function, skin, and transmission of pain impulses place the older adult at risk for being unable to sense pain (Ebersole and Hess, 1994).
- When administering analgesics, you should confer with physicians regarding proper dosing. Clients may be susceptible to side effects of opioids because of changes in serum proteins, liver and renal function, and a reduction in cardiac output.
- The risk for gastric and renal toxicity from NSAIDs is increased among older adults.
- Older adults are more sensitive to the analgesic effects of opioid drugs because they experience a higher peak and longer duration of pain relief.
- Pain is *not* normal with aging. Presence of pain requires aggressive assessment and management.

Children require careful calculation of drug doses. Equianalgesia charts that convert recommended adult doses to children's doses are available. These charts consider age and body size. Older adults also require special considerations (Box 29-9).

Patient-Controlled Analgesia. Clients benefit from having control over pain therapy. Patient-controlled analgesic (PCA) is a safe method for postoperative, traumatic, labor and delivery, sickle cell crisis, cancer, and end-of-life pain management that most clients prefer to intermittent injections (Tye and Gell-Walker, 2000; Reiff and Niziolek, 2001). It is a drug-delivery system that allows clients to administer pain medications when they want them. It has been an effective form of pain management with older adults and with children as young as 10 years of age. Systemic PCA usually involves intravenous drug administration, but it can also be given subcutaneously. PCA uses portable infusion pumps containing a chamber for a syringe (Figure 29-7, *A* and *B*) that delivers a small preset dose of medication (usually morphine or Dilaudid). To receive a dose the client pushes a button attached to the PCA device. The system is designed to deliver no more than a specified number of doses either every hour or every 4 hours (depending on pump) to avoid overdoses. A typical PCA prescription relies on a series of "loading" doses (e.g., 3 to 5 mg of morphine, repeated every 5 minutes until initial postoperative pain diminishes). A low-dose basal infusion (0.5 to 1 mg/hr) at night allows uninterrupted sleep. On-demand doses typically add 1 mg of morphine every 6 minutes, with a total hourly limit of 10 mg (American Pain Society, 1999). Most pumps have locked safety systems to prevent tampering.

Benefits of PCA include the following: clients have control over pain, pain relief does not depend on nurses' availability, clients tend to take less medication, and small doses of opioids delivered at short intervals stabilize serum drug concentrations for sustained pain relief. Client preparation and teaching are critical to the safe and effective use of PCA (Box 29-10). Surgery clients should receive teaching and demonstration of the PCA pump before surgery if the physician orders PCA use. Clients must be able to understand the use of

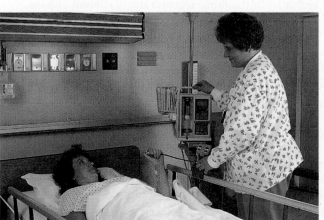

FIGURE **29-7**   **A,** PCA pump with syringe chamber. **B,** Patient learns to use PCA pump.

PREPARATION FOR PATIENT-CONTROLLED ANALGESIA

- Teach the use of PCA so that the client can understand how to use it. For surgical patients provide instruction during the preoperative period. (Confused and unresponsive clients; clients with a history of narcotic abuse, neurological disease, or impaired renal or pulmonary function; and those unable to press the delivery button are not candidates for PCA.)
- Instruct clients in the purpose of PCA, operating instructions, expected pain relief, precautions, and potential side effects (Intravenous Nurses Society, 1990), emphasizing that the client controls medication therapy.
- Explain that the pump prevents risks of overdose.
- Tell family members or friends that they should not operate the PCA device for the client.
- Have the client demonstrate use of the PCA delivery button.

the equipment and be physically able to locate and press the button to deliver the dose (Tye and Gell-Walker, 2000).

Check the client's intravenous line and PCA device regularly to ensure proper functioning. Certain pumps keep track of cumulative dosage and print out the information on demand. Drug doses must be carefully documented, and any opioids that are wasted or unused must be recorded. Successful implementation of PCA into nursing practice requires that you accept pain as a subjective and personal experience (Fulton, 1996). You must monitor the client for drug side effects, as well as pain management effectiveness (Tye and Gell-Walker, 2000). Use of PCA gives you and the client more flexibility in pain management. Family members should be taught the importance of the client's pushing the button to administer the medication. This will prevent the client's receiving more medication than is needed for pain relief (Reiff and Niziolek, 2001).

Placebo Effect.   **Placebos** are dose forms that contain no pharmacologically active ingredients (e.g., normal saline injection or sugar pill). Use of placebos is considered highly unethical and against policy in many hospitals even with a physician's order. However, a nurse can use a "placebo effect" when administering analgesics by telling clients that the drug will act to reduce pain. Belief that a medication will work and trust in the nurse increase the likelihood of pain relief (McCaffery and Pasero, 1999; Salladay, 2000).

Local Anesthetics.   **Local anesthesia** is the loss of sensation to a localized body part. Physicians provide local anesthesia by injecting a medication (e.g., lidocaine, Marcaine, or Naropin) into tissues, near major nerves, or intraspinally before suturing a wound, moving a painful body part, delivering an infant, and performing some surgery. Local anesthetics have fewer risks than general anesthetics, which cause loss of consciousness and depress vital functions. The drugs produce temporary loss of sensation by inhibiting nerve conduction; they also block motor and autonomic functions when administered as nerve blocks. Typically a client loses sensation in small sensory nerves before losing motor function; conversely, motor activity returns before sensation.

After administration of a local anesthetic you need to protect the client from injury until full sensory and motor function return. Clients can easily injure themselves without knowing it. You need to provide emotional support to clients receiving local anesthesia by explaining insertion sites and warning clients that they will temporarily lose sensory function. Autonomic function (bowel and bladder control) may also be temporarily lost. To reassure the client, explain application of the anesthetic and the sensations the client might experience. Injection can be painful unless the physician first numbs the injection site. Prepare clients for such discomfort. Before a client receives an anesthetic, you must check for allergies. To monitor systemic effects, assess vital signs.

Topical local anesthetics are absorbed through the skin or mucous membranes to produce anesthesia. The amount of time it takes for the medication to take effect and the duration of the effect vary according to the client and the medication. Topical anesthetics are available in spray, liquid, gel, and cream forms. Sprays (e.g., Americaine, Cetacaine) may be used for procedures such as bronchoscopy and sigmoidoscopy. Other topical anesthetics may be used to reduce pain from other procedures including venous, arterial, finger, and heel punctures; suturing; removal of sutures; and wound cleaning (McCaffery and Pasero, 1999). Topical anesthetics can cause side effects, depending on their absorption. Itching, burning of the skin, and a localized rash are common. Application to vascular mucous membranes may cause systemic effects such as a change in heart rate.

Epidural Analgesia.   Epidural analgesia is a form of local anesthesia and an effective therapy for the treatment of postoperative, traumatic, chronic noncancer, and cancer pain (Kingsley, 2001). It permits control or reduction of severe pain without the sedative effects of opioids. Epidural analgesia can be short or long term, depending on the client's condition and life expectancy. Short-term therapy is used for pain after intrathoracic, abdominal, and orthopedic surgery. Long-term therapy is used for intractable pain in the lower part of the body. The advantages of epidural analgesia include the following:

Production of excellent analgesia
Occurrence of minimal sedation
Longer-lasting pain relief with fewer opioid doses
Facilitation of early ambulation
Avoidance of repeated injections
No significant effect on sensation
Little effect on blood pressure or heart rate
Fewer pulmonary complications, or improved pulmonary function

Epidural analgesia is administered into the spinal epidural space usually while the client is in the operating room, postanesthesia care unit, or intensive care unit. The client is placed in the fetal position (lateral decubitus) to open the space between the vertebrae. The physician administers a local anesthetic into the skin at the needle insertion site then inserts the catheter and advances it to the level of the vertebral space (usually L4 to L5) nearest to the area requiring analgesia. Once the catheter is advanced into the epidural

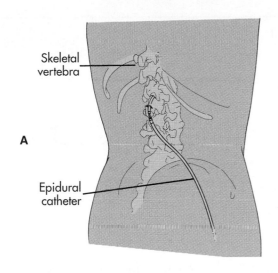

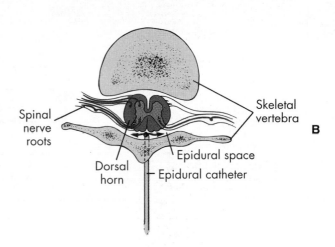

FIGURE **29-8**   **A,** Epidural catheter inserted into L4 and L5 space. **B,** Anatomical drawing of epidural space.

Nursing Care of Clients With Epidural Infusions — Table 29-6

Goal	Actions
Prevent catheter displacement	Secure catheter (if not connected to implanted reservoir) carefully to outside skin.
Maintain catheter function	Check external dressing around catheter site for dampness or discharge. (Leak of cerebrospinal fluid may develop.)
	Use transparent, adhesive dressing to aid inspection.
	Inspect catheter for breaks.
Prevent infection	Use strict aseptic technique when caring for catheter.
	Do not routinely change dressing over site.
	Change tubing every 24 hours.
Monitor for respiratory depression	Monitor vital signs, especially respirations, per policy.
	Pulse oximetry and apnea monitoring may be used.
Prevent undesirable complications	Assess for pruritus (itching) and nausea and vomiting.
	Administer antiemetics as ordered.
Maintain urinary and bowel function	Monitor intake and output.
	Assess for bladder and bowel distention.
	Assess for discomfort, frequency, and urgency.

space (Figure 29-8) and the needle is removed, the remainder of the catheter is secured with an occlusive dressing and taped up the back of the client. A temporary catheter can be connected to tubing positioned along the spine and over the client's shoulder. The end of the catheter can then be placed on the client's chest for easier access. Permanent catheters may be tunneled through the skin and exit at the client's side. Assessment of the insertion site and patency of the tubing is an important nursing responsibility (Kingsley, 2001).

The epidural catheter is connected to a continuous **epidural infusion** pump, a port, or a reservoir, or it is capped off for bolus injections. In many hospitals only anesthesiologists can administer epidural anesthesia or registered nurses are required to be certified. To reduce the risk of accidental epidural injection of drugs intended for intravenous use, it helps to place a brightly colored intermittent injection cap on the catheter tubing. Labeling the catheter "epidural catheter" also helps. Continuous infusions must be administered through electronic infusion devices for proper control. Because of the catheter location, strict surgical aseptic tech-

nique is needed to prevent a potentially fatal infection. Notify the physician immediately if any signs or symptoms of infection or pain at the insertion site develop (Kingsley, 2001).

Medications used commonly for epidural analgesia include preservative-free morphine sulfate, fentanyl, sufentanil citrate, and methadone. Morphine has a long-lasting effect but also causes more side effects. The medications block transmission of pain stimuli in the spinal cord.

Nursing implications for managing epidural analgesia are numerous (Table 29-6). Monitoring for drug effects differs, depending on if infusions are intermittent or continuous. Complications of epidural narcotic use include respiratory depression (rare), nausea and vomiting, urinary retention, constipation, orthostatic hypotension, and pruritus. Clients usually do not receive any other form of opioid, sedative, or hypnotic while receiving epidural analgesia. When clients are started on epidural analgesia, monitoring occurs as often as every 15 minutes, including assessment of respiratory rate, respiratory effort, and skin color. Pulse oximetry may be used. If a client remains stable, monitoring can move to

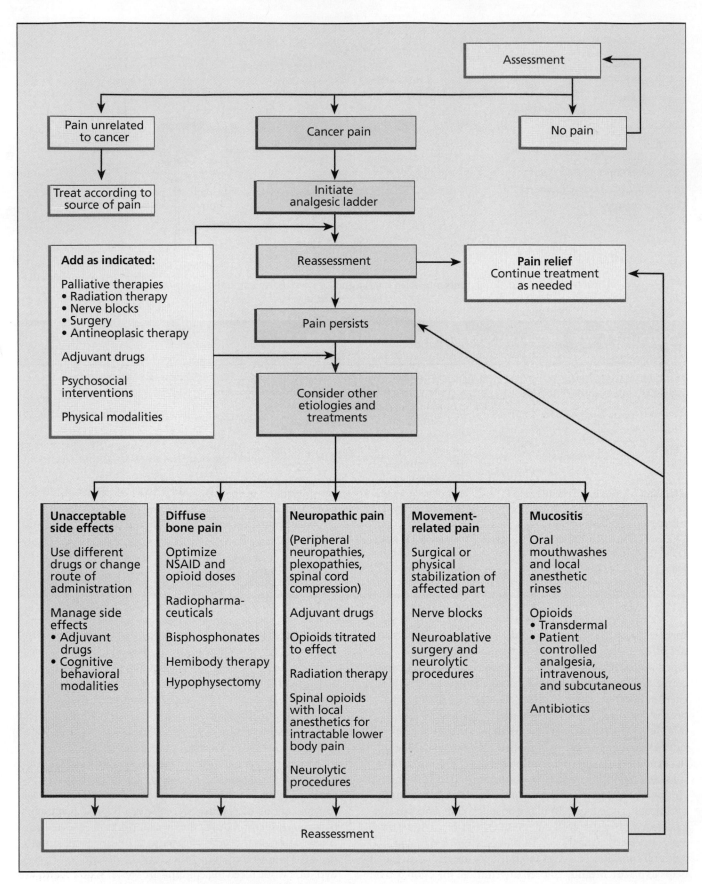

FIGURE **29-9** Flowchart: continuing pain management in patients with cancer. (From Jacox A and others: *Management of cancer pain*, Clinical practice guideline No. 9, AHCPR Pub No. 94-0592, Rockville Md, March 1994, AHCPR, USDHHS, PHS.)

every hour. Inform clients about the potential for respiratory depression and instruct them to notify you if breathing difficulty develops. If respiratory depression develops, the infusion is turned off immediately (Kingsley, 2001).

CLIENTS WITH INTRACTABLE PAIN. Intractable pain cannot be permanently relieved. It can become so debilitating that clients will try anything to gain relief. The AHCPR released clinical practice guidelines for the management of cancer pain (Jacox and others, 1994). The guidelines are designed to treat cancer pain in a more comprehensive and aggressive manner. Similarly, they provide clients and families more options for pain relief. Figure 29-9 is a flowchart depicting cancer pain management from assessment to various treatment measures. The best choice of treatment often changes when the client's condition and the characteristics of pain change. Both nonpharmacological and pharmacological therapies can be beneficial (McCaffery and Pasero, 1999).

Administering analgesics to treat cancer-related pain requires applying principles different from those used to treat acute pain. The WHO (1990) recommends a three-step approach to managing cancer pain (Figure 29-10). Therapy begins with NSAIDs and/or adjuvants and then progresses to strong opioids if pain persists. When a client with cancer first has pain, it is best to begin with a higher dosage than will be needed for relief. The physician can slowly decrease the dosage to the amount needed, thus giving the client immediate relief. Side effects of analgesia are aggressively treated so analgesia can be continued. Terminally ill clients with prolonged pain may develop a tolerance to analgesics. They thus require higher dosages to attain pain relief. Higher dosages are not lethal, because clients also develop tolerance to life-threatening side effects (McCaffery and Pasero, 1999). However, tolerance does not prevent the side effect of constipation. When constipation develops, clients require stimulant laxatives and not just stool softeners.

For clients with cancer, the aim of drug therapy is to anticipate and minimize pain rather than cure it. It is therefore necessary to give required dosages regularly, even when pain, nausea, and other symptoms subside. Regular administration maintains blood levels for ongoing pain control. However, clients may still have exacerbations of pain or "breakthrough pain" that requires additional bolus doses of medication (rescue doses). A decrease in the duration of pain relief provided by the regular analgesia therapy and the need for an increased number of rescue doses are indications that an increased titration of the opioid dose is needed (McCaffery and Pasero, 1999).

Transdermal drug systems administer drugs over predetermined rates for 48 to 72 hours. This is useful when clients are unable to take drugs orally. Self-adhesive patches release the drug slowly over time, achieving effective analgesia throughout the day and night. Hyperthermia causes more rapid drug absorption. For this reason clients should be warned to avoid external heat such as heating pads, hot showers, and prolonged exposure to the sun while using a patch. Inform clients that it may take 12 to 16 hours for

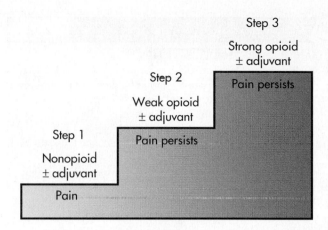

FIGURE **29-10** WHO analgesic ladder is a three-step approach to using drugs in cancer pain management. ± *adjuvant*, With or without adjuvant medications. (From World Health Organization: *Cancer pain relief and palliative care*, Report of a WHO expert committee, WHO Technical Report Series No. 804, Geneva, Switzerland, 1990, WHO.)

analgesia to take effect when they first begin to use an analgesic patch (Acello, 2000b).

Another measure to treat severe intractable cancer pain is morphine given by continuous intravenous drip or intermittently by a PCA pump. Continuous infusions provide uniform pain control at lower dosages. Thus there are fewer side effects. Continuous-drip morphine is given in acute care settings and the home. Morphine mixed in intravenous solution is delivered by an infusion control pump to ensure safe and accurate administration. Each agency has guidelines for morphine dose and infusion rates. The drug can cause numerous side effects that require your ongoing assessment. Adjuvant drugs may be needed to enhance pain control and prevent side effects (Jacox and others, 1994).

When a client is first placed on continuous-drip morphine, it is essential that an intravenous access is patent and the intravenous site is without complications. To prevent overdose and central nervous system depression, record baseline blood pressure and respiratory rates before the infusion begins. After the infusion starts, monitor vital signs as often as every 15 to 30 minutes for the first few hours until the client gains relief at a constant dosage. If blood pressure or respirations decrease, the infusion rate is reduced according to the physician's order or agency policy. If the client shows signs of severe respiratory depression, the physician will order the infusion discontinued. The narcotic antagonist naloxone (Narcan) should be available to reverse respiratory depression but not pain relief (Salerno, 1996).

RESTORATIVE AND CONTINUING CARE. Clients in need of restorative care for pain usually are suffering chronic or intractable pain that is unrelenting. You should continue to use nonpharmacological measures that are effective for individual clients. However, additional pharmacological measures are designed to give a client better long-term pain

AMBULATORY INFUSION PUMPS

- Tell client and family to observe for the following side effects: dizziness or fainting, nausea, vomiting, slow and shallow respirations, constipation, mood changes, euphoria, inability to empty bladder fully, dry mouth, weakness, agitation, tremors, strange dreams.
- Instruct family on how to administer naloxone (Narcan) intramuscularly to reverse respiratory depression.
- Teach client and family how to keep central venous catheter patent, maintain pump flow rate, and irrigate the catheter routinely with heparin flush.
- Tell client how to prevent air from entering central venous catheter and to clamp catheter when infusion has stopped.
- Explain how to prevent infection at catheter site and to keep site clean with soap and water.
- Have client follow a preventive bowel routine using stool softeners, laxatives, dietary fiber, hydration, and routine exercise.
- Warn client against wearing pump in shower or submerging in bathtub. Device can be temporarily disconnected during shower or placed in a plastic bag hung outside shower or tub.
- During sleep, keep the pump on the bed or adjacent nightstand. During lovemaking, the pump can be set to the side so it does not interfere with closeness and intimacy.
- Instruct the client and family on the purpose of the pump alarms and how to respond when they sound.
- Keep a 24-hour emergency telephone number nearby.

control. The focus in restorative care is to use a comprehensive approach in supporting the client and family.

MORPHINE INFUSIONS. In the home or extended care settings, clients may use ambulatory infusion pumps for narcotic infusions. The pumps are lightweight, compact, and allow free movement. The pump is battery powered and worn in a pouch attached to a belt or harness. The bag of medication and intravenous fluid fits inside the pump. A dose of morphine, delivered continuously over 24 hours, is usually slowly infused into a peripherally inserted central catheter (PICC) or a subclavian placed catheter (see Chapter 14). Both catheters can be left in place for an extended period of time. The pumps differ from PCA devices, which deliver only small, preset doses of medication. The client and family learn to manage the pump, observe for drug side effects, and maintain function of the central venous catheter (Box 29-11). Because the client is initially managed on morphine in the hospital before going home, the risk of side effects is not as great unless the client or family member increases dosages. A home health nurse makes routine visits to be sure the client manages the pump correctly.

HOSPICE. Hospices are programs to care for the terminally ill. The programs help terminally ill clients continue to live at home in comfort and privacy with the help of a health care team. Pain control is a priority. Families learn to monitor the client's symptoms and become primary caregivers. Chapter 22 discusses hospice in more detail.

PAIN CLINICS. Pain clinics have evolved to provide pain management for a variety of clients. A comprehensive pain center can treat clients in the hospital or in outpatient clinics. A multidisciplinary team collaborates to find the most effective pain-relief therapies. Diverse therapies and research into new treatments are among the center's services (Miller and others, 1996).

END-OF-LIFE CARE. Family members and clients need to be taught and reassured about the use of analgesics and end-of-life (EOL) issues. Emphasize the need to provide maximum pain relief by increasing (titrating) the dosage of medication to meet the client's pain-control needs. Opioids may be increased by 25% to 50% depending on the client's response. If the maximum dose ordered by the physician is ineffective, you are responsible for notifying the physician. The dosage needed to relieve the client's pain may exceed the normal dosage range published in printed drug information. The fastest route of medication administration should be used until pain is under control. Once pain is controlled, use the least invasive technique possible including oral, rectal, transdermal, or sublingual routes. Remember, a combination of opioid, nonopioid, adjunct, and nonpharmacological therapy may be needed to provide adequate pain relief.

 Evaluation

CLIENT CARE. With regard to pain management, the client is the source for evaluating outcomes. The client is the only one who will know if the severity of pain has lessened and which therapies bring most relief. To evaluate the effectiveness of nursing interventions, compare baseline pain assessments before treatments with ongoing assessment findings after treatment. Similarly, evaluate whether the client's response to pain (e.g., positioning and body movements or ability to socialize or perform self-care) has changed. Outcomes are compared with expected outcomes to determine the client's health status (McCaffery and Pasero, 1999; Loeb and Pasero, 2000) (Box 29-12). Continuous evaluation allows you to determine whether new or revised therapies are required and if new nursing diagnoses have developed. It is important to discuss the client's ongoing pain management needs with the family members and health care providers who will be involved in the client's care upon discharge or transfer.

CLIENT EXPECTATIONS. Subtle behaviors often indicate the level of a client's satisfaction. For example, a gentle smile, a sigh of relief, or reaching out for your hand can convey the client's gratitude. However, it is also important for you to *ask* clients if their expectations have been met. If a client's expectations have not been met, then you need to spend more time understanding the client's desires. Working closely with the client will enable you to redefine expectations that can be realistically met within the limits of the client's condition and treatment.

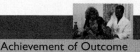

Outcome Evaluation for MRS. ELLIS
Box 29-12

Nursing Action	Client Response/Finding	Achievement of Outcome
Have Mrs. Ellis tell you, on a scale of 0 to 10, how her pain feels when it is most severe.	Mrs. Ellis rates pain at a 5.	Most severe level of pain has reduced from a 9 to a 5. Improved pain relief achieved.
Ask Mrs. Ellis to describe how the pain is affecting her ability to perform daily chores such as bathing and dressing and washing the dishes.	Mrs. Ellis reports less stiffness in hands; able to wash dishes and says warm water is soothing. States she still has some difficulty putting on clothes, "My hands really hurt when I have to reach behind my back to pull a zipper." She reports that getting up to walk to bathroom and kitchen still creates discomfort in knees and hips, although she has less pain while she walks through her home.	She is able to perform limited ADLs, showing some improvement by being able to wash dishes. Joint pain continues to affect ability to dress self. Pain persists during standing, but has less of an effect during walking. Continue plan of care, suggest use of heat compresses before dressing. Also suggest use of Velcro closures on clothes.

Case Study EVALUATION

After 2 weeks, Jim returns to evaluate Mrs. Ellis's progress. Mrs. Ellis reports that she has seen her physician and has been referred to physical therapy for supportive hand splints. In addition, the physician has prescribed NSAIDs for pain control and to reduce gastrointestinal irritation caused by her aspirin. Mrs. Ellis reports that she is falling asleep more easily if she takes her medication 30 minutes before going to bed. Jim gets the chance to observe Mrs. Ellis use a warm compress on her hands and wrist. Afterward he asks her to rate her pain on a scale of 0 to 10. Mrs. Ellis rates it as a 3. During the visit Mrs. Ellis gets up to walk to the kitchen. Jim notes that although it takes her time to stand, her gait is more steady. She is ambulating with a walker that the physical therapist recommended. Jim asks if Mrs. Ellis has found someone she can call when she needs assistance. The client mentions that she has talked with her neighbor, who has offered to help her with shopping and to take her to church.

Documentation Note

Client reports improved satisfaction with pain control, able to fall asleep more easily. After using warm compress, rates pain at 3 on a scale of 0 to 10. Appears less fatigued and is ambulating with steadier gait, using walker. Has initiated social contact with neighbor as support system. Will evaluate effectiveness of supportive devices and ongoing NSAID effectiveness at next visit.

Key Terms

analgesics, p. 724
cutaneous stimulation, p. 722
endorphins, p. 709
epidural infusion, p. 727
exacerbations, p. 712
guided imagery, p. 723
intractable pain, p. 711
local anesthesia, p. 726

narcotics, p. 724
neuromodulators, p. 709
neurotransmitters, p. 709
nociceptors, p. 709
pain, p. 708
patient-controlled analgesia (PCA), p. 713
perception, p. 708
placebos, p. 726
prostaglandins, p. 724

reaction, p. 708
reception, p. 708
relaxation, p. 723
remissions, p. 712
synapse, p. 710
threshold, p. 724
tolerance, p. 710
transcutaneous electrical nerve stimulation (TENS), p. 722

Key Concepts

- Acute pain, a protective mechanism that warns a person of tissue injury, is completely subjective.
- Misconceptions about pain can lead to undertreatment.
- Knowledge of the three components of the pain experience—reception, perception, and reaction—provide you with guidelines for determining relief measures.
- The pain experience is influenced by a client's age, sex, anxiety, culture, and experience and the meaning of pain.

- A client's pain tolerance influences your perceptions of the seriousness of the discomfort.
- The difference between acute and chronic pain involves the duration of discomfort, physical signs and symptoms, and the client's perceptions regarding relief.
- Pain scales attempt to objectively evaluate the severity of pain and the effectiveness of pain therapies.
- The client's family and friends can be a key resource in pain assessment.

Continued

Key Concepts—cont'd

- You individualize pain therapy by collaborating closely with the client, using assessment findings, trying a variety of therapies, and maintaining the client's well-being.
- Eliminating sources of painful stimuli is a basic nursing measure for promoting comfort.
- Nonpharmacological cutaneous therapies are effective in altering client perception of pain, promoting muscle relaxation, and giving the client control over pain experienced.
- Using a regular schedule for analgesic administration is more effective than an as-needed schedule.

- A PCA device gives clients pain control with a low risk of overdose.
- Your primary role in caring for a client who receives local anesthesia is protecting the client from injury.
- The aim of therapy for clients with chronic pain is to anticipate and prevent pain rather than to treat it.
- A serious but rare side effect of morphine infusions is respiratory depression, which can be reversed with intravenous Narcan.
- Evaluation of pain therapy requires consideration of the changing character of pain, response to therapy, and the client's perceptions of a therapy's effectiveness.

Critical Thinking Activities

1. Mr. Jasper and Mr. Stern are clients experiencing back pain. Mr. Jasper's pain resulted from a fall from a ladder 48 hours ago. Mr. Stern's pain has been bothering him for more than 8 months with no known cause. In caring for both clients, how might your assessment and treatment differ?
2. Ms. Rogers is receiving morphine by way of a PCA device following abdominal surgery for a hysterectomy. During your assessment you note that Ms. Rogers is more drowsy and her respirations have decreased from 16 per minute to 10. What actions should you take?
3. Mr. Lake is a 45-year-old man who experienced a traumatic injury to his left arm following an industrial accident 24 hours ago. His arm is in a very bulky dressing, and pain is aggravated when he lies on his left side. He has an intravenous line with a continuous infusion of intravenous fluids in his right arm. What nonpharmacological pain-relief measures might be helpful for Mr. Lake?
4. Ms. Johns had coronary surgery and is complaining of severe incisional pain. After you administer her morphine intravenously, she tells you that she just does not think it is going to do much good because she is so tense. You offer to give her a back massage. What explanation would you provide Ms. Johns for offering this complementary intervention at this time? How would you teach her husband to do the procedure?

Review Questions

1. One of the reasons that many nurses avoid acknowledging a client's pain is:
   1. inadequate pain management skills.
   2. insufficient time to respond to the client.
   3. fear that the intervention may cause addiction.
   4. inability to manage their increased client load.
2. An 82-year-old client with Alzheimer's disease is restless and moaning. The client's daughter states the client did not sleep well most of the night and she usually sleeps at least 6 hours each night. Your first response would be to:
   1. restrain the client.
   2. obtain a psychiatric consultation.
   3. administer Tylenol, 2 tabs by mouth.
   4. carefully assess and document physical and behavioral data.
3. According to the WHO, treatment of cancer-related pain is different from acute pain. Therefore when caring for a client with cancer pain, you should:
   1. begin with opioids to ensure pain relief.
   2. administer pain medication with caution.
   3. administer lower doses of opioids to prevent tolerance and side effects.
   4. begin with higher doses of prescribed medications to ensure pain relief.
4. Your client requested medication for her abdominal incision pain, which she rates as a 5 (scale of 0 to 10, with 10 the worst pain). One hour after administration of her pain medications, she was able to walk in the hall for 10 minutes and rated her pain as a 7. This indicated that the dosage of pain medication was:
   1. adequate.
   2. excessive.
   3. insufficient.
   4. unnecessary.
5. One of the reasons that PCA morphine pumps are frequently used for postoperative pain management is to:
   1. increase client satisfaction.
   2. decrease the frequency of client complaints.
   3. control client use of narcotics and reduce the chance of addiction.
   4. encourage the use of pain medications before the client experiences severe pain.
6. Thirty minutes after administering a complementary treatment such as heat therapy or back massage, you should:
   1. turn and reposition the client.
   2. document the pain assessment data.
   3. evaluate the effectiveness of the treatment.
   4. administer the prescribed pain medication.
7. A preventative approach for acute pain relief means that analgesic medications are given:
   1. before the pain is experienced.
   2. with complementary therapies.
   3. before the pain becomes severe.
   4. when the pain tolerance level is exceeded.

References

Acello B: Meeting JCAHO standards for pain control, *Nursing* 30(3):52, 2000a.

Acello B: Controlling pain: switching to the patch, *Nursing* 30(8):72, 2000b.

AGS Panel on Chronic Pain in Older Persons: Clinical practice guidelines: the management of chronic pain in older persons, *J Am Geriatr Soc* 46:635, 1998.

AHCPR: Acute pain management guideline panel: *Acute pain management in infants, children and adolescents: operative or medical procedures and trauma.* Clinical practice guideline, AHCPR Pub No. 92-0032, Rockville, Md, February 1992, AHCRP, PHS, USDHHS.

American Pain Society: *Principles of analgesic use in the treatment of acute and cancer pain,* ed 4, Glenview, Ill, 1999, American Pain Society.

Benzaia D: The new breed of pain killers, *Remedy* 6(2):14, 1999.

Beyer JE and others: The creation, validation, and continuing development of the Oucher: a measure of pain intensity in children, *J Pediatr Nurs* 7(5):335, 19992.

Bozeman M: Cultural aspects of pain management. In Salerno E, Williams J, editors: *Pain management handbook: an interdisciplinary approach,* St. Louis, 1996, Mosby.

Celia B: Age and gender differences in pain management following coronary artery bypass surgery, *J Gerontol Nurs* 26(5):7, 2000.

Courts N: Nonpharmacologic approaches to pain. In Salerno E, Williams J, editors: *Pain management handbook: an interdisciplinary approach,* St. Louis, 1996, Mosby.

Dalton J, Youngblood R: Clinical application of the World Health Organization analgesic ladder, *J Intravenous Nurs* 23(2):118, 2000.

Eiman M and others: Geriatric pain management. In Salerno E, Williams J, editors: *Pain management handbook: an interdisciplinary approach,* St. Louis, 1996, Mosby.

Ferrell B and others: Analysis of pain content in nursing textbooks, *J Pain Symptom Manage* 19(3):216, 2000.

Freeman L, Lawlis G: *Mosby's Complementary and alternative medicine: a research-based approach,* St. Louis, 2001, Mosby.

Fulton T: Nurses' adoption of a patient-controlled analgesia approach, *West J Nurs Res* 18(4):383, 1996.

Giger JN, Davidhizar RE: *Transcultural nursing: assessment and intervention,* ed 2, St. Louis, 1995, Mosby.

Grealish L and others: Foot massage: a nursing intervention to modify the distressing symptoms of pain and nausea in patients hospitalized with cancer, *Cancer Nurs* 23(3):237, 2000.

Hall J: Learning curve: the nature of pain . . . the first of a five-part series, *Am J Nurs* 100(5):22, 2000.

Hekmat N and others: Preventive pain management in the postoperative hand surgery patient, *Orthop Nurs* 13(3):37, 1994.

Intravenous Nurses Society: Intravenous nursing standards of practice, *J Intravenous Nurs* 5:70, 1990.

International Association for the Study of Pain: *Management of acute pain: a practical guide,* Seattle, 1992, IASP Publications.

Jacox A and others: *Management of cancer pain,* Clinical practice guideline No. 9, AHCPR Pub No. 94-0592, Rockville, Md, March 1994, AHCPR, USDHHS, PHS.

JCAHO: *Comprehensive accreditation manual for hospital standards: the official handbook,* 1999.

Kettleman K: Controlling pain: soothing the ache of joint surgery, *Nursing* 30(7):14, 2000.

Kingsley C: Epidural analgesia: your role, *RN* 64(3):53, 2001.

Loeb J, Pasero C: JCAHO standards in long-term care: tools and techniques for putting the standards into practice, *Am J Nurs* 100(5):22, 2000.

Mattson J: The language of pain, *Reflection on Nursing Leadership* 26(4):10, 2000.

Mayer D and others: Speaking the language of pain, *Am J Nurs* 101(2):44, 2001.

McCaffery M: *Nursing management of the patient with pain,* ed 2, Philadelphia, 1979, Lippincott.

McCaffery M, Ferrell B: Correcting misconceptions about assessment and use of opioid analgesics: educational strategies aimed at public concerns, *Nurs Outlook* 44(4):184, 1996.

McCaffery M and Pasero C: *Pain: clinical manual,* ed 2, St. Louis, 1999, Mosby.

McIntosh N: Pain in the newborn, a possible new starting point, *Eur J Pediatr* 156:173, 1997.

Meinhart N, McCaffery M: *Pain a nursing approach to assessment and analysis,* Norwalk, Conn, 1983, Appleton-Century-Crofts.

Melzack R, Wall P: *The challenge of pain,* ed 2, London, 1996, Penguin.

Memran N and others: Management of post operative pain in the elderly, *Semaine des Hospitaux* 74:700, 1998.

National Institutes of Health Consensus Development Panel: New gains against pain, *Emerg Med,* November 1986.

Ochsenreither J, Cubina M: Pediatric pain management. In Salerno E, Williams J, editors: *Pain management handbook: an interdisciplinary approach,* St. Louis, 1996, Mosby.

Reiff P, Niziolek M: Troubleshooting tips for PCA, *RN* 64(4):33, 2001.

Salerno E: Pharmacologic approaches. In Salerno E, Williams J, editors: *Pain management handbook: an interdisciplinary approach,* St. Louis, 1996, Mosby.

Salladay S: Ethical problems: limited role for placebos, *Nursing* 30(7):65, 2000.

Taylor A: Complementary/alternative therapies in the treatment of pain. In Spencer J, Jacob J, editors: *Complementary/alternative medicine: an evidenced-based approach,* St. Louis, 1999, Mosby.

Tye T, Gell-Walker V: Patient-controlled analgesia . . . the second of a five-part series, *Nurs Times* 96(2):38, 2000.

Victor K: Properly assessing pain in the elderly, *RN* 64(5):45, 2001.

Watt-Watson J and others: The impact of nurses' empathetic responses on patients' pain management in acute care, *Nurs Res* 49(4):191, 2000.

Willens J: Introduction to pain management. In Salerno E, Williams J, editors: *Pain management handbook: an interdisciplinary approach,* St. Louis, 1996, Mosby.

Wong DL, Baker CM: Pain in children: comparison of assessment scales, *Oklahoma Nurs* 33(1):8, 1988a.

Wong DL, Baker CM: Pain in children: comparison of assessment scales, *Pediatr Nurs* 14(1):9, 1988b.

Wong DL and others: *Whaley and Wong's nursing care of infants and children,* ed 6, St. Louis, 1999, Mosby.

World Health Organization: *Cancer pain relief and palliative care,* Report of a WHO expert committee, WHO technical Report Series No. 804, Geneva, Switzerland, 1990, WHO.

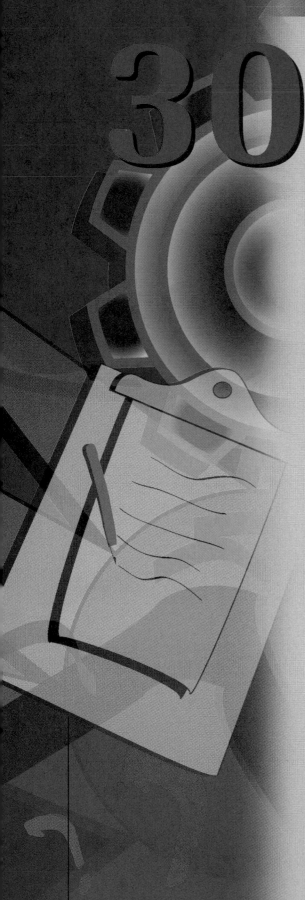

30

Nutrition

Objectives

- Define key terms.
- Explain the importance of a balance between energy intake and output.
- List the end products of carbohydrate, protein, and lipid metabolism.
- Explain the significance of saturated, unsaturated, and polyunsaturated lipids in nutrition.
- Describe the basic food groups (using the food guide pyramid) and their value in planning meals for good nutrition.
- Explain dietary referenced intakes (DRIs).
- Discuss the major areas of nutritional assessment.
- Identify nutritional problems and describe a client at risk for these problems.
- Establish a plan of care to meet the nutritional needs of the client.
- Describe the procedure for initiating and maintaining tube feedings.
- Describe the procedure for initiating and maintaining total parenteral nutrition.

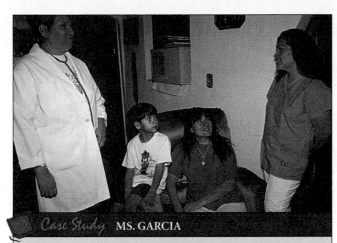

Case Study MS. GARCIA

Ms. Garcia is a 24-year-old Hispanic single mother who has inflammatory bowel disease (IBD) and has recently had an operation to remove a segment of her small intestine. Ms. Garcia has had IBD for 10 years, but this is her first surgical procedure. She lives with a roommate and her 5-year-old son in a second-story apartment. Ms. Garcia's roommate works part time and helps with child care for Ms. Garcia in exchange for buying their groceries and preparing meals. Ms. Garcia's parents live in another state, and her father has had a stroke. Although Ms. Garcia's mother came to visit during her hospitalization for the surgery, she had to return home to care for Ms. Garcia's father. Ms. Garcia works at a fast-food restaurant, from which she has taken several weeks off for her surgery. Ms. Garcia's physician has ordered home nursing visits to assess the status of her abdominal wound and to determine how well she is eating. Ms. Garcia's weight had dropped by 15 lb before the operation, and she is currently about 10% below her ideal weight.

Shawneen Bott is a senior nursing student who is in her home health nursing rotation. Shawneen is single and 22 years of age. She has seen other home care patients with her preceptor, but Ms. Garcia is the closest to her own age. Shawneen is a little nervous about this visit because she will be performing her first independent assessment and treatment with observation by her nursing preceptor.

*N*utrition is a basic component of health and is essential for normal growth and development, tissue maintenance and repair, cellular metabolism, and organ function. An adequate supply of nutrients is needed for essential functions of cells.

Scientific principles regarding nutrition and the role of various nutrients in metabolism and health form a basis for the nutritional plan of care that you develop with your clients. Disease processes, age, gender, and activity can affect utilization of nutrients and nutritional requirements. Pharmaceutical agents prescribed to treat disease can also interact with nutrients and foods.

SCIENTIFIC KNOWLEDGE BASE
Principles of Nutrition

The body requires food to provide energy for all functions, including movement, maintenance of body temperature, growth and development, cellular metabolism, synthesis and repair of tissues, and organ function. The gastrointestinal system comprises a number of organs and structures that enable the body to nourish itself through the ingestion of food. Each organ or structure in the gastrointestinal (GI) tract has a specific function aimed toward preparing food for the digestion and absorption of its nutrients.

Nutrients

Found in foods, **nutrients** provide the substances necessary for body function. Energy needs are met by the metabolism of carbohydrates, lipids, and, if necessary, protein. Vitamins and minerals do not provide energy, but they are necessary in the chemical reactions that produce energy. Water is essential to life, acting as a chemical fluid to transport substances, providing fullness to tissues, and helping to maintain body temperature.

CARBOHYDRATES.   **Carbohydrates** are composed of carbon, hydrogen, and oxygen. They are starches and sugars obtained mainly from plant foods, with the exception of lactose, which is found in milk (milk sugar). Carbohydrates may contribute as much as 90% of the total caloric intake in parts of the world where grains are a major food source. Carbohydrates can be used as a source of energy, providing 4 kilocalories per gram (kcal/g).

Some polysaccharides cannot be digested because humans do not have enzymes capable of breaking them down (e.g., insoluble fibers of cellulose, hemicellulose, and lignin), whereas soluble fibers, such as pectin, and mucilage are broken down. Fiber is a useful dietary factor in the prevention of diarrhea in tube-fed clients.

PROTEINS.   Amino acids are the building blocks of **proteins** and are made of hydrogen, oxygen, carbon, and nitrogen. **Amino acids** are the most important components of proteins in the human body, and they are essential for synthesis of body tissue in growth, maintenance, and repair. Some amino acids, essential amino acids, cannot be synthesized by the body and can be obtained only from daily food sources. Proteins can be used as a source of energy, providing 4 kcal/g.

The required daily intake of protein varies according to age. For example, infants under 6 months of age require 2.2 g/kg daily. Adolescents require 1 g/kg daily. Most healthy people require only about 0.8 g/kg of body weight per day. In disease, protein requirements can double or triple, such as for major burns. Pregnant women require an additional 30 g and lactating women an additional 20 g above the usual daily need.

Nutrition experts believe that the intake of protein in America is generally greater than required. Protein foods are expensive to buy and produce, and meats, whole milk, cheese, and eggs contain significant amounts of saturated fatty acids and cholesterol. Nutritional guidelines recommend reducing saturated fats and cholesterol in the diet along with increasing complex carbohydrates from fruits, vegetables, and whole grains (U.S. Department of Health and Human Services [USDHHS], 2000).

LIPIDS.   **Lipid** is a comprehensive term applied to compounds that are insoluble in water but soluble in organic solvents such as ethanol and acetone; and at room temperature, these include solid fats and liquid oils. Lipids are composed of carbon, hydrogen, and oxygen. As with the other nutrients, lipids can be used as a source of energy, providing 9 kcal/g.

Approximately 98% of the lipids in foods and 90% of the lipids in the human body are in the form of triglycerides. High blood levels of certain lipoproteins have been linked to cardiovascular diseases.

A **saturated fatty acid** contains as much hydrogen as it can hold. An **unsaturated fatty acid** can take up another hydrogen atom, and a **polyunsaturated fatty acid** can take up many more hydrogen atoms and become hydrogenated fat. Ingestion of saturated fatty acids appears to increase blood cholesterol levels. Ingestion of unsaturated fatty acids has a minimal effect on blood cholesterol. Polyunsaturated fatty acids appear to lower blood cholesterol levels. Fatty acids are usually not purely saturated, unsaturated, or polyunsaturated. Most animal fats have high proportions of saturated fatty acids; most vegetable fats have higher amounts of unsaturated and polyunsaturated fatty acids (e.g., safflower oil is about 75% polyunsaturated, olive oil about 25%).

Fat is the body's form of stored energy. The metabolism of 1 g of lipid yields 9 kcal (38 J), more than twice the energy provided by carbohydrates or proteins. Lipids account for 35% to 45% of the American diet. Nutritional guidelines recommend a reduction of lipid intake to about 30% (10% saturated lipids and 20% polyunsaturated lipids) of the total caloric intake (American Heart Association, 1996a, 1996b).

VITAMINS.   **Vitamins** are organic substances present in small amounts in foods and are essential for normal metabolism because they serve as coenzymes in cellular enzyme reactions. The body is unable to synthesize vitamins in the required amounts and depends on dietary intake. The Food and Nutrition Board reviews ongoing research and periodically revises the recommended allowances for vitamins and other nutrients. Although contained in many foods, vitamins are affected by processing, storage, and preparation. Vitamin content is usually highest in foods that are fresh and used quickly after minimal exposure to heat, air, or water. Vitamins are classified as water soluble and fat soluble.

Water-soluble vitamins are stored in only a limited amount for short periods, necessitating daily consumption. It was once assumed that water-soluble vitamins were not toxic, due to limited storage capacity. However, megadoses of vitamin C and vitamin B_6 may result in toxicity. Vitamins are used as catalysts in biochemical reactions. When there is enough of a vitamin to meet the catalyst demands, the remaining serum level of the vitamin supply acts as a free chemical and may be toxic to the body.

Fat-soluble vitamins can be stored in the body for longer periods; however, dietary intake is still required. Vitamin K is found within dark leafy green vegetables but is also produced within the large intestine. In addition, vitamin D is produced within the body as a response to sunlight exposure. Toxicity to some fat-soluble vitamins can occur, usually related to megadoses of synthetic vitamins, especially vitamin A.

Controversy exists over the safety and need for vitamin supplementation. In general, vitamin needs appear to be modestly increased in the following conditions: pregnancy and lactation (A, C, D, B complex including folate), oral contraceptive use (B complex, C), aging (C, thiamine, riboflavin, pyridoxine), weight reduction diets less than 1200 kcal, strenuous exercise (riboflavin), smoking (vitamin C), alcohol consumption (B complex, C), and caffeine consumption (B complex, C). Diseases can produce increased needs or the inability to store or excrete certain vitamins.

MINERALS.   **Minerals** are inorganic elements that act as catalysts in biochemical reactions. Minerals are classified as macrominerals when the daily requirement is 100 mg or more and microminerals when less than 100 mg is needed daily. Because the required amount of microminerals is usually very small or a trace, they are also called trace elements. In addition to the microminerals, arsenic, nickel, silicon, tin, vanadium, boron, aluminum, and cadmium play unidentified roles in nutrition.

WATER.   Water is an important nutrient because the function of cells depends on a fluid environment. A lean person's body contains a higher percentage of water than an obese person's body. Infants have the greatest percentage of total body weight as water; older adults have the least. Infants and older adults are most vulnerable to water deprivation or water loss.

The human body requires 1.5 ml of water for every kilocalorie of energy used. Fluid needs are met by the ingestion of liquids and solid foods such as fresh fruits and vegetables and by water produced when food is oxidized during digestion.

Thirst is a protective mechanism that alerts the oriented person to the need for fluids. Thirst is a less reliable guide for infants and confused clients. These clients are usually unable to communicate that they are thirsty.

Digestion

The process of **digestion** begins in the mouth, where mastication, or chewing, breaks down food into smaller particles, and amylase in saliva begins to break down starches. Mucus lubricates food particles for their passage through the esophagus into the stomach. Churning movements of the stomach mix food particles with hydrochloric acid. The most significant absorption of nutrients occurs in the small intestine. Digestive proteins in the gastrointestinal system act on food particles to break them into a simpler form. Most nutrients are digested and absorbed in the small intestine; the large intestine absorbs electrolytes and water, thus helping to maintain the body's electrolyte balance (see Chapter 14).

ABSORPTION.   The small intestine is the primary site of **absorption** of simple nutrients. It is lined with villi, which project into the lumen and greatly increase the surface area available for absorption. Cholesterol, vitamins E and K, folic acid, riboflavin, and thiamin are absorbed in the upper duodenum. Glucose, amino acids, minerals, and fats are absorbed in the lower duodenum and upper jejunum, and sucrose, lactose, and maltose are absorbed in the lower jejunum and ileum.

Intestinal contents move by peristaltic action into the large intestine. Water is the only nutrient absorbed from the large intestine. Other nutrients remaining in the intestinal contents when they reach the large intestine are excreted as waste products. When intestinal motility is increased, such as in diarrhea, the body loses nutrients that move through the small intestine too quickly for complete absorption.

METABOLISM.   Nutrients are transported through the circulatory system to body tissues. Through **metabolism,** nutrients are converted into necessary substances for cell function. Metabolism refers to all of the biochemical and physiological processes by which the body maintains itself.

Carbohydrates, protein, and fat produce chemical energy and maintain a dynamic balance of tissue buildup and breakdown. The chemical energy produced by metabolism is converted to other types of energy by different tissues. Muscle contraction involves mechanical energy, the nervous system involves electrical energy, and the mechanisms of heat production involve thermal energy. These forms of energy all originate in metabolism.

Absorbed nutrients are carried to the liver, where major metabolic processes occur. The liver also regulates energy through its control of glucose metabolism. **Glucose** is the primary fuel for the body. The liver and muscles store glucose in the form of **glycogen** via a process called **glycogenesis. Lipogenesis** stores excess glucose as fat. Insulin and glucagon act as regulatory hormones to promote glucose storage or use. Insulin promotes glucose use, and glucagon promotes glucose storage. During states where energy needs exceed glycogen storage, the body breaks down fat and amino acids for conversion to glucose via a process called **gluconeogenesis.**

The basal metabolic rate (BMR) represents the energy needs of a person at rest after awakening. Energy balance occurs when energy requirements equal energy intake. In general, when a person's energy needs are exceeded or are insufficient, the person gains weight or loses weight, respectively.

The two basic types of metabolism are anabolism and catabolism. **Anabolism** is the production of more-complex chemical substances by synthesis of nutrients. **Catabolism** is the breakdown of body tissues into simpler substances. Although catabolism produces some energy, both processes require energy, which must be provided from food or stored sources.

STORAGE.   The body stores energy as adipose tissue. Glycogen is stored in small reserves in liver and muscle tissue, and protein is stored in muscle mass. When the body's energy demands exceed dietary sources, stored (fat) energy is used; unused energy is stored, principally in fat.

Fat-soluble vitamins are also stored in limited reserves (6 to 8 months) and are released to meet the body's needs

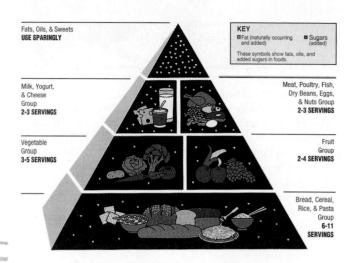

FIGURE **30-1**   Food guide pyramid. (From U.S. Department of Agriculture: *USDA's food guide pyramid,* USDA Human Nutrition Information Service, Pub No. 249, Washington, DC, 1996, U.S. Government Printing Office.)

when dietary intake is insufficient. Water-soluble vitamins are minimally stored (3 to 5 days).

ELIMINATION.   The intestinal contents move through the large intestine by peristalsis (see Chapter 32). As the material moves toward the rectum, water is reabsorbed through the mucosa. The end products of digestion include cellulose and similar fibrous substances the body is unable to digest. Sloughed cells from the intestinal walls, mucus, digestive secretions, water, and microorganisms are also eliminated.

Foundations of Nutrition

A number of agencies and organizations in the United States regularly publish and update dietary guidelines. The guidelines change as nutritional research discovers new knowledge. Some guidelines are intended to provide information and education for the general public about a healthful diet.

FOOD GUIDE PYRAMID.   The pyramid was designed as a basic guide for buying food and meal preparation (Figure 30-1). This basic plan provides for diets ranging from 1600 to 2800 kcal/day (U.S. Department of Agriculture [USDA], 1996). The pyramid suggests that an individual choose most of the day's selections from the grain group (6 to 11 servings), the vegetable group (3 to 5 servings), and the fruit group (2 to 4 servings). Selections should include 2 to 3 servings per day from the milk group and from the meat group (which includes dry beans and nuts). The fats, oils, and sweets group is to be used sparingly.

DIETARY REFERENCED INTAKES.   The Food and Nutrition Board of the National Academy of Sciences has published recommended daily allowances (RDAs) since 1943. In 1997 these recommendations were renamed **dietary referenced intakes (DRIs)** in response to the increased public use of nutritional supplements. The DRIs broaden the base of information on

Nutrition Objectives for Healthy People 2010   Box 30-1

Healthy weight

Reduction of obesity in adults

Reduction of obesity in children (6 to 11) and adolescents (12 to 19)

Decrease in growth retardation to <10% in low-income children <5 years

Decrease in fat intake to <30% daily intake

Decrease in saturated fat intake to <10% daily intake

Vegetable and fruit intake of five daily servings in 75% of people

Grain products intake of six daily servings in 80% of people

Calcium DRI met in 90% of people

Sodium daily intake no more than 2400 mg in 65% of people

Reduction of prevalence of iron deficiency in children and child-bearing women

Reduction of prevalence of anemia in pregnant women to <23%

Nutrient-dense meals and snacks at school for children and adolescents

Nutrition education required in elementary schools

Nutrition education required in middle/junior high schools

Nutrition education required in senior high schools

Work-site nutrition education and weight management programs

Nutrition assessment and individualized planning at primary care sites

Nutritional education and counseling services for diabetics at primary care sites

Increase in prevalence of food security to 94% of households

Data from U.S. Department of Health and Human Services: *Healthy people 2010 objectives: draft for public comment,* 1998, www.health.gov/healthypeople.

each vitamin or mineral to reflect a range of minimum to maximum amounts that avert deficiency or toxicity.

OTHER DIETARY GUIDELINES.   In 1997 the U.S. Department of Health and Human Services (USDHHS) and the Public Health Service (PHS) began a consensus process that resulted in the updated publication of *Healthy People 2010: Understanding and Improving Health* (see Chapter 1). The report defines national goals or objectives to be met in this decade to increase the proportion of Americans who live long, healthy lives. Nutrition-related goals for the year 2010 include increasing intake of fruits, vegetables, and grain products and reducing fat and sodium consumption. There continues to be an effort to integrate these goals with the food guide pyramid, the nutrition facts label, and the healthy index recommended by the USDA (USDHHS, 2000) (Box 30-1).

NURSING KNOWLEDGE BASE

We celebrate holidays and events with food, bring food to those who are grieving, use food for medicinal purposes, recognize cultural food differences, incorporate food into family traditions and rituals, associate appearance with eating behaviors, abstain from or recognize foods in religious beliefs and practices, and associate certain foods and dining practices with socioeconomic status.

For most people, food has sociological and psychological significance, which varies with each individual. In attempting to affect eating patterns, you must understand how client's values, beliefs, and attitudes about food affect food purchase, preparation, and intake. You must also be cognizant of their own values, beliefs, and attitudes about food.

Nutritional requirements vary according to clients' developmental needs. Individuals differ in caloric and nutrient requirements by stage of development, activity levels, conditions such as pregnancy and lactation, and the presence of disease. A summary of factors that influence dietary patterns and needs is presented in Box 30-2.

Alternative Food Patterns

Many people follow special patterns of food intake based on religion, cultural background, ethics, health beliefs, personal preference, or concern for the efficient use of land to produce food. Such special diets are not necessarily more or less nutritional than diets based on the food guide pyramid or other nutritional guidelines because good nutrition depends on a balanced intake of all required nutrients. A common dietary pattern is the vegetarian diet, which is the consumption of a diet consisting predominantly of plant foods. Vegetarians may be ovolactovegetarians, who avoid meat, fish, and poultry but eat eggs and milk, or lactovegetarians, who drink milk but avoid eggs. Vegans eat only foods of plant origin and should supplement their diets with vitamin B_{12} and carefully choose foods to ensure ingestion of essential amino acids. Knowledge of complete versus incomplete protein sources is necessary to assure adequate protein intake.

Developmental Needs

Nutrient and kilocalorie needs are unique to the individual's developmental stage. Maturation of the gastrointestinal system, periods of rapid growth and development, alterations in digestion and absorption, activity level, and pregnancy affect nutrient and energy needs (see Chapter 18).

In addition, when rapid growth periods end, as with the young and middle adult, the energy needs decline and the risk of weight gain increases. If unchecked, this weight gain can result in obesity. Increased physical exercise, a healthy dietary intake that is low in fat and high in fresh fruits and vegetables, and moderate use of convenience foods all help to reduce the risk of weight gain.

CRITICAL THINKING
Synthesis

Critical thinking enables you to synthesize information gathered from knowledge, experience, attitudes, and standards. The end result of critical thinking will be your clinical judgment of the client's nutritional problems and subsequent nursing interventions.

KNOWLEDGE.   Application of knowledge from nutritional principles and the basic and social sciences forms your knowledge base related to nutritional care. Information de-

Factors Influencing Dietary Patterns and Needs
Box 30-2

DEVELOPMENTAL STAGE

Infants, toddlers, children, pregnant women, adolescents, and older adults have nutritional needs that are unique to their developmental stage.

HEALTH STATUS

Illness can have minor effects on dietary patterns, such as appetite or amount ingested, or it can have major effects, such as impaired digestion or absorption.

Nutritional assessment is an important part of a total health assessment.

CULTURE AND RELIGION

Cultural, ethnic, and religious dietary patterns may affect health or the client's acceptance of dietary recommendations.

Special foods and diet should be incorporated into the dietary recommendations when possible.

SOCIOECONOMIC STATUS

Food preferences, selection, and purchase are influenced by socioeconomic status.

SOCIOECONOMIC STATUS

Dietary recommendations should take into account the client's food budget, the availability of foods, and the client's knowledge of food preparation techniques.

PSYCHOLOGICAL FACTORS

Body image, media messages about food, and beliefs, values, and attitudes affect dietary patterns.

Food and dietary patterns may have symbolic meanings (such as meat symbolizing strength).

ALCOHOL AND DRUGS

Alcohol and other drugs can affect appetite, nutrient absorption, and metabolism.

Alcohol and other drugs can affect organ function.

MISINFORMATION AND FOOD FADS

Nutrition misinformation or unproven theories are prevalent because of the current focus on disease prevention and health enhancement.

Fad diets are especially prevalent because many Americans are overweight.

---

rived from interviewing and observing the client and the responses obtained during nursing interventions will guide you toward application of knowledge. For example, the client may report a dietary pattern of avoiding a food such as cabbage. This pattern could arise from physiological discomfort (gas-forming food), psychological issues (forced to eat cabbage as a child), sociological reasons (associated with lower socioeconomic class), ethnicity (not readily available in the country of origin), teaching- or learning-related reasons (never taught how to prepare cabbage), or mythology (a food that contains harmful chemicals).

EXPERIENCE.   People's dietary patterns are based on multiple factors. Just as your clients are influenced by multiple factors to develop dietary practices, you have also been influenced. Individuals who have nutritional or health problems often need to change their long-standing dietary practices to enhance health. In assisting a client in changing dietary patterns, draw on examples from your own experience. Perhaps you attempted to change a dietary practice or have a family member who requires a special diet. Previous experiences with therapeutic diets or behavioral changes may assist in the identification of nursing interventions that will be successful for the client.

ATTITUDES.   Open-mindedness is a required critical thinking skill that is beneficial during nutritional assessment and counseling. Although you may encounter clients whose dietary practices are dramatically different from yours, you assist those clients in attaining a nutritionally balanced diet. In addition, you encounter clients whose dietary patterns are not healthful, but whose beliefs and values about food are dramatically different from yours. To develop effective interventions for these clients, recommend practices that would be quite effective for the client.

STANDARDS.   When assisting clients to adjust to changes in nutritional patterns, incorporate standards from the DRIs, American Heart Association (AHA), American Society of Parenteral and Enteral Nutrition (ASPEN), or other professional organizations. Because food holds strong symbolic values and is closely associated with nurturing, ethical issues in health care have arisen around the withdrawal or withholding of specialized feeding (Burck, 1996). As part of an advance directive, clients are asked if they wish to have nutrition or hydration as a means of life support. Advance directives make the client's wishes known and have become a standard area of assessment for clients in the hospital and in the home care setting.

NURSING PROCESS

 Assessment

Nutritional screening is part of your initial assessment of the client. If the client is found to be at risk for nutritional problems, conduct a more in-depth nutritional assessment with the assistance of a nutritionist. The intent of the nutritional assessment, as outlined by ASPEN (1993, 1996), is as follows:

1. Establish baseline subjective and objective nutrition parameters.
2. Identify specific nutritional deficits.
3. Determine nutritional risk factors.
4. Establish nutritional needs.
5. Identify medical and psychosocial factors that may influence the prescription and administration of nutritional support.

The nutritional assessment consists of nursing health assessment and physical examination, observation, medical record review (if available), and laboratory data.

Example of a Focused Client Assessment		Table 30-1
Factors to Assess	Questions and Approaches	Physical Assessment Strategies
Chewing	Ask if client has difficulty chewing. If client has dentures, ask if client has areas of gum discomfort.	Observe client eating a meal; determine client's ability to eat all types of foods. Inspect condition of teeth, gums, and mouth.
Diet	Ask client about eating habits. Ask client about food preferences. Determine if client has religious or cultural dietary practices.	Observe fit of dentures and observe gums for sores or pressure areas. Obtain a 3-day meal diary from client.
Muscle mass	Determine if client has noticed weight gain or loss. Was weight gain or loss an expected change? Determine client's exercise patterns. Determine client's perception of ideal weight.	Weigh client. Perform anthropometric measurements. Review laboratory values (e.g., CBC, albumin).

Information in a Diet History   Box 30-3

Name
Age
Present weight
Usual weight
Recent weight changes
Height
Number of meals and snacks a day
Person who prepares meals
Food preferences, allergies, and aversions
Foods that cause indigestion, diarrhea, or gas
Chewing or swallowing difficulties
Use of dentures
Usual bowel movements
Dietary problems
Use of medications
    Prescribed
    Over-the-counter (including herbs and nutritional support)
    Recreational
History of diseases, surgeries, or weight problems
Level of physical activity
Appetite changes
Type, time, and size of usual meals
Emotional crises
Personal crises

In addition to the general nursing health assessment and physical examination (see Chapter 12), obtain a more specific diet history to assess the client's actual or potential nutritional needs (Table 30-1).

DIET HISTORY.   The diet history focuses on habitual intake of food and liquids and information about preferences, allergies, and digestive problems (Box 30-3). When interviewing the client about dietary practices, ask open-ended questions that encourage the client to elaborate. For example, you may ask a client who reports that she avoids dairy products, "What caused you to avoid dairy products?" The client's answer to this question may lead to physiological, psychological, sociological, religious, cultural, or food preference factors that can be further explored.

A detailed record can be kept of food intake over 3 days that represents the client's typical pattern, including a weekend day. This record allows you to calculate the client's nutritional intake and to compare it with the RDIs. Carefully instruct the client how to record the specific type of food and the amount ingested. Also gather information to determine the client's activity level and metabolic status to estimate energy needs. For example, a client who has a fever or has suffered severe trauma has high caloric demands even though the activity level is limited. The estimated energy need is compared to actual caloric intake, through calorie counts. You may need to consult with a registered dietician to determine exact calorie count or requirements.

MEDICATION HISTORY.   Prescribed and over-the-counter medications have the potential for a drug-nutrient interaction. Knowing what medications your clients are taking is important when meeting nutritional needs. Consultation with a pharmacist can determine specific risks for nutrient/drug interactions for your clients.

CLIENTS AT RISK FOR NUTRITIONAL PROBLEMS.   A client with a condition that interferes with the ability to ingest, digest, or absorb adequate nutrients should be considered at risk. Congenital anomalies and surgical revisions of the gastrointestinal tract interfere with normal function. Clients fed only by intravenous infusion of 5% to 10% dextrose are at risk for nutritional deficiencies. Older adults (Figure 30-2), infants, or the malnourished are at greatest risk. Common conditions and pathophysiology that place clients at nutritional risk are summarized in Box 30-4.

PHYSICAL EXAMINATION.   Examine the client for signs of actual or potential nutritional alterations (Table 30-2). The skin and hair are primary areas that reflect nutrient deficiencies. Be alert for rashes, dry scaly skin, poor skin turgor, skin lesions, hair loss, easily pluckable hair, hair without luster, and an unhealthy scalp.

ANTHROPOMETRY.   Anthropometry is a systematic measurement of the size and makeup of the body at specific body sites. Unless contraindicated, height and weight measure-

DETERMINE YOUR NUTRITIONAL HEALTH

The Warning Signs of poor nutritional health are often overlooked. Use this checklist to find out if you or someone you know is at nutritional risk.

Read the statements below. Circle the number in the yes column for those that apply. For each yes answer, score the number in the box. Total the nutritional score.

	YES
I have an illness or condition that made me change the kind and/or amount of food I eat.	2
I eat fewer than 2 meals per day.	3
I eat few fruits or vegetables, or milk products.	2
I have 3 or more drinks of beer, liquor or wine almost every day.	2
I have tooth or mouth problems that make it hard for me to eat.	2
I don't always have enough money to buy the food I need.	4
I eat alone most of the time.	1
I take 3 or more different prescribed or over-the-counter drugs a day.	1
Without wanting to, I have lost or gained 10 pounds in the last 6 months.	2
I am not always physically able to shop, cook and/or feed myself.	2
TOTAL	

Total Your Nutritional Score. If it's –

0–2   **Good!** Recheck your nutritional score in 6 months.

3–5   **You are at moderate nutritional risk.** See what can be done to improve your eating habits and lifestyle. Your office on aging, senior nutrition program, senior citizens center or health department can help. Recheck your nutritional score in 3 months.

6 or more   **You are at high nutritional risk.** Bring this checklist the next time you see your doctor, dietitian or other qualified health or social service professional. Talk with them about any problems you may have. Ask for help to improve your nutritional health.

These materials developed and distributed by the Nutritional Screening Initiative, a project of:

AMERICAN ACADEMY OF FAMILY PHYSICIANS

THE AMERICAN DIETETIC ASSOCIATION

NATIONAL COUNCIL ON THE AGING

Remember that warning signs suggest risk, but do not represent diagnosis of any condition.

FIGURE **30-2** Nutrition screening tool for older adult. (Reprinted with permission by the Nutrition Screening Initiative, a project of the American Academy of Family Physicians, the American Dietetic Association, and the National Council of the Aging, Inc, and funded in part by a grant from Ross Products Division, Abbott Laboratories, Inc.)

Nutritionally at-Risk Adult Clients   Box 30-4

Involuntary loss or gain of ≥10% of usual body weight within 6 months

or

≥5% of usual body weight in 3 months
20% over or under ideal body weight
Presence of chronic disease or increased metabolic requirements
Altered diets or diet schedules
Inadequate nutrient intake or NPO for >5-7 days

Data from ASPEN Board of Directors: Standards of practice: nutrition support nurses, *Nutr Clin Pract* 11(3):127, 1996.

Case Study   **SYNTHESIS IN PRACTICE**

As Shawneen prepares to assess Ms. Garcia, she recalls information about nutrition and its effect on wound healing. She will focus assessment on Ms. Garcia's weight, recent weight loss elimination patterns, and discomfort. Shawneen knows that it is important to assess for fluid balance as well.

Shawneen knows that consulting with a dietitian to further assess Ms. Garcia's nutritional status and assist with nutritional interventions will be beneficial. The dietitian will use data from Shawneen's initial nursing assessment and assist Shawneen in collecting further nutritional-related information.

Experience has taught Shawneen that economic and cultural preferences will also affect how food is chosen, purchased, and prepared. She will need to be creative in teaching Ms. Garcia to adjust to a new diet.

---

ments should be obtained during admission to any health care setting. If the client is unable to stand, height may be estimated from length while lying supine in bed, using a tape measure, and bed scales may be used for weight. Height and weight are then compared with usual measurements and standard norms for normal height-weight relationships. Body mass index (BMI) is used as an indicator of the relationship of height to weight. It is calculated by dividing weight in kilograms (kg) by height in meters squared (m²). A BMI range of 20 to 27 is recommended for optimal health.

When possible, weigh the client about the same time each day, on the same scale, and with the same amount of clothing. In some clients, weight changes of 2 lb in 24 hours may be significant because 1 lb is roughly equivalent to 500 ml of fluid.

LABORATORY VALUES.   Laboratory values useful in nutritional assessment include complete blood count (CBC), albumin, transferrin, prealbumin, electrolytes, blood urea nitrogen, creatinine, glucose, and triglycerides. A low red blood cell count and depressed hemoglobin value may indicate anemia. The hemoglobin, hematocrit, and blood urea nitrogen values also help to reflect the state of hydration. Decreased serum levels of albumin and transferrin identify malnutrition.

Urinary nitrogen excretion is obtained by collecting a 24-hour urine sample for nitrogen. Nitrogen excretion measured in the urine plus a factor added for nitrogen losses from the gastrointestinal and pulmonary systems can be used to estimate the amount of protein needed to achieve a positive **nitrogen balance.**

CLIENT EXPECTATIONS.   Clients who require assistance with nutritional problems have a variety of expectations. Clients with impairments in upper arm mobility may expect assistance with a range of activities, such as preparing the meal, setting up the meal tray or plate, or being fed. Another client may expect information on the availability and use of assistive devices, used to increase a client's independence with meals. Clients who have impaired vision need to be taught how to feed themselves. It is also important for you to learn what the client expects in terms of resuming a normal diet or learning to adjust to a therapeutic diet.

Nursing Diagnosis

Following assessment, cluster relevant defining characteristics to determine whether actual or potential nutritional problems exist (Box 30-5). An alteration can occur when a nutrient is not ingested in sufficient quantity, is poorly digested, or is incompletely absorbed or when total daily caloric needs are deficient or excessive.

The overweight client can actually have nutrient deficiencies and may require supplements or specialized nutritional support during episodes of acute illness. The assessment should elicit dietary patterns that have contributed to the **obesity** and will require careful scrutiny for adequacy of all food groups. Patterns such as inadequate fruit and vegetable intake can be present. The nursing diagnosis should be as precise as possible. Related factors must be accurate so that appropriate

interventions are selected. For example, a diagnosis of *deficient fluid volume related to vomiting* will require different interventions than *deficient fluid volume related to anorexia*.

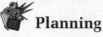 **Planning**

Goals, expected outcomes, and priorities reflect the client's physiological, therapeutic, and individualized needs. In addition, the client's nutritional needs extend well beyond the hospital setting, and it is important that you consider poten-

Clinical Signs of Nutritional Status   Table 30-2

Body Area	Signs of Good Nutrition	Signs of Poor Nutrition
General appearance	Alert, responsive	Listless, apathetic, cachectic
Weight	Normal for height, age, body build	Overweight or underweight (special concern for underweight)
Posture	Erect, arms and legs straight	Sagging shoulders, sunken chest, humped back
Muscles	Well-developed, firm, good tone, some fat under skin	Flaccid, poor tone, undeveloped, tender, "wasted" appearance, cannot walk properly
Nervous control	Good attention span, not irritable or restless, normal reflexes, psychologic stability	Inattentive, irritable, confused, burning and tingling of hands and feet (paresthesia), loss of position and vibratory sense, weakness and tenderness of muscles (may result in inability to walk), decrease or loss of ankle and knee reflexes
Gastrointestinal function	Good appetite and digestion, normal regular elimination, no palpable (perceptible to touch) organs or masses	Anorexia, indigestion, constipation or diarrhea, liver or spleen enlargement
Cardiovascular function	Normal heart rate and rhythm, no murmurs, normal blood pressure for age	Rapid heart rate (above 100 beats per minute, tachycardia), enlarged heart, abnormal rhythm, elevated blood pressure
General vitality	Endurance, energetic, sleeps well, vigorous	Easily fatigued, no energy, falls asleep easily, looks tired, apathetic
Hair	Shiny, lustrous, firm, not easily plucked, healthy scalp	Stringy, dull, brittle, dry, thin and sparse, depigmented, can be easily plucked
Skin (general)	Smooth, slightly moist, good color	Rough, dry, scaly, pale, pigmented, irritated, bruises, petechiae
Face and neck	Skin color uniform, smooth, healthy appearance, not swollen	Greasy, discolored, scaly, swollen, skin dark over cheeks and under eyes, lumpiness or flakiness of skin around nose and mouth
Lips	Smooth, good color, moist, not chapped or swollen	Dry, scaly, swollen, redness and swelling (cheilosis), or angular lesions at corners of the mouth or fissures or scars (stomatitis)
Mouth, oral membranes	Reddish pink mucous membranes in oral cavity	Swollen, boggy oral mucous membranes
Gums	Good pink color, healthy, red, no swelling or bleeding	Spongy, bleed easily, marginal redness, inflamed, receding
Tongue	Good pink color or deep reddish in appearance, not swollen or smooth, surface papillae present, no lesions	Swelling, scarlet and raw, magenta color, beefy (glossitis), hyperemic and hypertrophic papillae, atrophic papillae
Teeth	No cavities, no pain, bright, straight, no crowding, well-shaped jaw, clean, no discoloration	Unfilled caries, absent teeth, worn surfaces mottled (fluorosis), malpositioned
Eyes	Bright, clear, shiny, no sores at corner of eyelids, membranes moist and healthy pink color, no prominent blood vessels or mound of tissue or sclera, no fatigue circles beneath	Eye membranes pale (pale conjunctivae), redness of membrane (conjunctival injection), dryness of infection, Bitot's spots, redness and fissuring of eyelid corners (angular palpebritis), dryness of eye membrane (conjunctival xerosis), dull appearance of cornea (corneal xerosis), soft cornea (keratomalacia)
Neck (glands)	No enlargement	Thyroid enlarged
Nails	Firm, pink	Spoon-shaped (koilonychia), brittle, ridged
Legs and feet	No tenderness, weakness, or swelling; good color	Edema, tender calf, tingling, weakness
Skeleton	No malformations	Bowlegs, knock-knees, chest deformity at diaphragm, beaded ribs, prominent scapulas

Data from Williams SR: *Nutrition and diet therapy,* ed 9, St. Louis, 1997, Mosby.

tial restorative and continuing care interventions when you initially establish the plan of care.

GOALS AND OUTCOMES.   In general the goal in caring for clients with nutritional alterations is to improve the

---

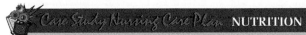

CLIENTS WITH NUTRITIONAL ALTERATIONS — Box 30-5
• Aspiration, risk for
• Body image, disturbed
• Diarrhea
• Fatigue
• Fluid volume, deficient
• Fluid volume, excess
• Nutrition, imbalanced: less than body requirements
• Nutrition, imbalanced: more than body requirements
• Nutrition, risk for imbalanced: more than body requirements
• Self-care deficit, feeding
• Tissue perfusion, ineffective: gastrointestinal

---

client's nutritional status. If the nutritional diagnosis is *imbalanced nutrition: less than body requirements,* the outcome will be for the client to gain weight or to ingest adequate nutrients in a certain category. If a client is obese, a goal of care will be to safely achieve weight reduction. Specific, individualized goals are determined by identifying client behaviors that have led to the nutritional alteration (see nursing care plan). The goals are achieved through a prescribed diet, patient education, and assisting the client in developing new behaviors that will enable the client to achieve an adequate nutritional status. Professionals who may assist in providing care include the nutritionist, nutritional support clinical nurse specialist, pharmacists, and physicians.

Weight gain or loss of $1/2$ to 1 lb/wk is a realistic level for clients who are underweight or overweight. Clients often have unrealistic expectations about nutritional repletion or dieting in reference to weight gain or loss. Assist clients in understanding this concept by asking them to reflect on their rate of weight gain or loss. Changes in weight usually have occurred over months or years unless an acute illness has occurred. When clients do not see rapid achievement of

---

Case Study Nursing Care Plan **NUTRITION**

ASSESSMENT

Ms. Garcia's diet history reveals that she is **below her estimated caloric requirement by 800 kcal/day** and **protein intake is 10 g below her required need.** She tries to eat three meals a day but cannot because of **the feeling of fullness. Milk and milk products cause abdominal cramping and diarrhea.** Ms. Garcia enjoys foods from her **Hispanic heritage, such as beans, corn, tortillas, tomatoes, soups, yellow vegetables, and rice.** On physical examination Ms. Garcia does exhibit some signs of nutritional deficiency. Her **albumin, transferrin, and prealbumin levels are slightly below normal, she is 10% below ideal body weight, and she complains of feeling weak.** She would like to gain weight and has requested assistance in identifying appropriate foods.

*Defining characteristics are shown in bold type.

NURSING DIAGNOSIS

Imbalanced nutrition: less than body requirements related to inadequate intake of calories and proteins.

PLANNING

GOAL

Client will achieve ideal body weight (8 to 12 weeks).

EXPECTED OUTCOMES

Client will gain $1/2$ to 1 lb/wk.

Client will not report cramping or diarrhea.

Client's albumin, transferrin, and prealbumin will begin to return to normal.

IMPLEMENTATION

STEPS

1. Use lactose-free oral supplements, $1 1/2$ kcal/ml, between or with meals. Choose flavors that appeal. Take three cans per day.

2. Ms. Garcia will provide her roommate with a list of "favorite foods" so that these can be included in the food purchases.
3. Ms. Garcia will eat six small meals instead of trying to eat three large ones.
4. Monitor Ms. Garcia for weight gain and improved laboratory values.

RATIONALE

The formula is lactose free and is available in multiple flavors. The oral supplement will also provide supplemental protein and vitamins. Three cans per day will provide 750 to 1125 extra calories.

Appealing foods are more likely to be ingested.

Spreading intake out over the day may assist client to ingest more.

Weight gain should be slow and progressive.

Serum albumin level >4.0 g/dl and total leukocyte count >1500/mm³ are within normal limits (Grodner and others, 2000).

EVALUATION

- Weigh Ms. Garcia on a weekly basis.
- Review Ms. Garcia's use of the oral supplements and frequent meals.
- Measure laboratory values at 6-week intervals.

Hospital Therapeutic Diets   Table 30-3

Diet	Description
Clear liquid	Broth, gelatin, clear fruit juices, popsicles—easily absorbed; short-term use after vomiting, diarrhea, or surgery
Full liquid	Addition of some dairy products and cream soups; provides more sustenance, used after surgery or for acutely ill
Pureed	Addition of scrambled eggs, pureed meats, vegetables, fruits, mashed potatoes with gravy; after surgery, for chewing difficulty, disorders of head and neck
Mechanical soft	Addition of ground meat, flaked fish, cottage cheese, rice, bananas, peanut butter, and all soups; used for dysphagia (supervision), difficulty chewing, or stomatitis
Soft/low residue	Addition of low-fiber, easily digested foods such as pasta, casseroles, moist tender meats, and canned cooked fruits and vegetables; for exacerbations of bowel disease (ulcerative colitis, diverticulitis)
High fiber	Addition of fresh uncooked fruits, steamed vegetables, bran, oatmeal and dried fruits; for remissions of diverticulosis, irritable bowel syndrome, or ulcerative colitis
Low sodium	4-g (no added salt), 2-g, 1-g, or 500-mg sodium diets; for congestive heart failure, renal, liver dysfunction, or hypertension
Low cholesterol	300 mg/day cholesterol, in keeping with AHA guidelines for serum lipid reduction with coronary artery disease
Diabetic	In diabetes mellitus, recommended food exchanges by the American Diabetic Association; new diabetic clients require teaching and blood glucose monitoring to evaluate effect
Regular	Full client choice, with no specific restrictions

weight goals, they may become discouraged. Remember that correction of poor dietary patterns is a long-term rather than a short-term goal. Short-term goals may involve achieving calorie or nutrient targets on a daily or weekly basis.

SETTING PRIORITIES. The identification of clients at risk for nutritional problems results in a care plan to prevent or minimize nutritional problems. Although changes in the client's weight may be gradual, a priority is to improve your client's nutritional intake.

The client and family need to collaborate in the care plan and share priorities as well. Because food purchase and preparation may involve family members, the nutritional plan of care might not succeed without their commitment to, involvement in, and understanding of nutritional goals. A list of diets commonly used for hospitalized clients is provided in Table 30-3.

CONTINUITY OF CARE. Client nutritional needs extend beyond the acute, hospital setting and into the home or rehabilitation care setting. Some clients with physiological conditions causing more severe cases of malnutrition may require enteral tube feeding or parenteral nutrition to meet fluid, electrolyte, and nutritional needs.

Enteral tube feeding can be administered into the stomach or intestines via a tube inserted through the nose (nasogastric or nasointestinal). Alternatively, a gastroenterologist may insert a percutaneous endoscopic gastrostomy (PEG) or jejunostomy (PEJ) tube. Both of these enteral feedings are provided in restorative and continuing care settings, as well as in acute care settings.

When **parenteral nutrition (PN),** a solution consisting of glucose, amino acids, lipids, minerals, electrolytes, trace elements, and vitamins, is needed, it is given through an indwelling peripheral or central venous catheter.

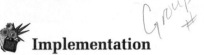

Group #2

Implementation

HEALTH PROMOTION.   You play a major role in promoting healthy dietary practices. Using tools such as the food guide pyramid, assist clients with food choices, menu planning, and dietary patterns. You can also educate clients about food labels and their meaning. An area of particular importance is education about product claims that can be misleading: "reduced fat" foods may still have significant amounts of fat, "lite" foods may still contain considerable calories, and "low cholesterol" may not mean low fat.

An increasing percentage of Americans are overweight, and many people who attempt to lose weight are unsuccessful, regaining lost weight (plus additional pounds) after completing a diet. Fad diets abound, and bookstores are filled with best-selling diet books. Some weight reduction methods lack scientific validity, and some are dangerous.

Principles of food safety are important considerations for health promotion. Contaminated and undercooked food products, especially eggs and meats, can result in severe debilitating and even fatal illnesses (Table 30-4). Client education is one method of improving safe food practices for clients and their families (Box 30-6).

ACUTE CARE.   Ill or debilitated clients usually have poor appetites. It is important that you provide monitoring of the client's nutritional status, identify influences that reduce appetite, and plan interventions to increase intake.

One of the most disruptive influences on intake in acute care is diagnostic testing. Some blood and radiographic studies require the client to fast. Therefore the client's food is usually withheld until the client returns from the test or the testing is completed. Mealtimes are disrupted, and sometimes clients are too fatigued to eat or experience discomfort related to the test. Stress also influences intake. Clients who are worried about their families, finances, employment, or

Food Safety

Table 30-4

Food-Borne Disease	Organisms	Food Source	Symptoms
Botulism	*C. botulinum*	Improperly home-canned foods, smoked and salted fish, ham, sausage, shellfish	Symptoms are varied from mild discomfort to death in 24 hours, initially nausea, dizziness, progressing to motor (respiratory) paralysis
Escherichia coli	*Escherichia coli* 0157:H7	Undercooked meat (ground beef)	Severe cramps, nausea, vomiting, diarrhea (may be bloody), renal failure. Appears 1-8 days after eating, lasts 1-7 days
Listeriosis	*Listeria* *L. monocytogenes*	Soft cheese, meat (hot dogs, pate, lunch meats), unpasteurized milk, poultry, seafood	Severe diarrhea, fever, headache, pneumonia, meningitis, endocarditis. Appears 3-21 days after infection
Perfringens enteritis	*Clostridium* *C. perfringens*	Cooked meats, meat dishes held at room or warm temperature	Mild diarrhea, vomiting. Appears 8-24 hours after eating, lasts 1-2 days
Salmonellosis	*Salmonella* *S. typhi* *S. paratyphi*	Milk, custards, egg dishes, salad dressings, sandwich fillings, polluted shellfish	Mild to severe diarrhea, cramps, vomiting. Appears 12 to 24 hours after ingestion, lasts 1-7 days
Shigellosis	*Shigella* *S. dysenteriae*	Milk, milk products, seafood, salads	Mild diarrhea to fatal dysentery. Appears 7-36 hours after ingestion. Lasts 3-14 days
Staphylococcus	*Staphylococcus* *S. aureus*	Custards, cream fillings, processed meats, ham, cheese, ice cream, potato salad, sauces, casseroles	Severe abdominal cramps, pain, vomiting, diarrhea, perspiration, headache, fever, prostration. Appears 1-6 hours after ingestion, lasts 1-2 days

From Williams SR: *Nutrition and diet therapy,* ed 9, St. Louis, 1997, Mosby.
*Symptoms are generally most severe for youngest and oldest age-groups.

Client Teaching

Box 30-6

FOOD SAFETY
- Food safety is an important public health issue. The very young, older adults, clients with chronic illness, and those clients who are immunosuppressed are at risk for food-borne illnesses (see Table 30-4).
- Teach precautionary measures to avoid food-borne illnesses:
  - Wash hands with hot soapy water before food preparation.
  - Cook meat, poultry, fish, eggs until they are well done.
  - Wash fresh fruits and vegetables thoroughly.
  - Do not eat raw meat or unpasteurized milk or juices.
  - Do not use food past expiration date.
  - Keep foods properly refrigerated.
  - Discard food that you suspect is spoiled.
  - Do not use wooden cutting boards. Instead use plastic laminate or solid surface cutting boards that can be disinfected.
  - Wash dishrags, dish towels, sponges regularly, or use paper towels.
  - Clean inside of refrigerator and microwave regularly.

Modified from Keithly JK, Swanson M: Minimizing HIV/AIDS malnutrition, *Medsurg Nurs* 7(5):256, 1998.

illness may not be able to eat or eat enough to compensate for the effect of stress on metabolism.

Medications also affect intake and in some cases the use of nutrients. Medications can affect the sensations of taste or smell, and as a result food is not appetizing. Medications can also cause nausea or vomiting; the client is anorexic as a result of the nausea, or the nutrients are lost. In addition, medications such as insulin, glucocorticoids, and thyroid hor-

mones can affect metabolism. Keep these factors in mind when designing measures to promote nutrition.

Food presentation is a factor in appetite. Hot foods that are cold or cold foods that are warm are not appetizing. Overcooked or undercooked foods are unappealing. A meal tray precariously balanced on a crowded, soiled over-bed table does not enhance the meal. Clients who are bothered by food odors may need you to remove the cover from hot food before the tray is brought into the room. Attention to details in food presentation, meal scheduling, and the client's difficulties with food may enhance a client's intake. You can help to stimulate a client's appetite through environmental adaptations, consultation with a diet therapist, special diets and food preferences, and client and family counseling.

PROVIDING A COMFORTABLE ENVIRONMENT.   Provide an environment conducive to eating. The client's room should be free of reminders of treatments and odors. Mouth care should be provided when necessary to remove unpleasant tastes. The client should be positioned comfortably so that the meal can be more enjoyable. If a client refuses a portion of the meal, every effort should be made to replace it with a suitable alternative.

ASSISTING CLIENTS WITH FEEDING.   You can improve client feeding by carefully protecting clients' dignity and actively involving them. Any material used to protect clothing should be referred to as a napkin, not a bib. Allow the client time to empty the mouth after every spoonful, attempting to match the speed of feeding to the client's readiness and asking frequently about the rate. Encourage clients to direct the order in which they wish to eat food items. Mealtime is a good time to instruct clients and their families about the selection of appropriate foods and the importance of a balanced diet.

DISABLED CLIENTS. Clients with disabilities that interfere with independent food intake should be allowed to do as much as possible for themselves. When necessary, prepare the tray, cutting food into bite-sized pieces, buttering bread, and pouring liquids. Use special eating utensils. Some disabled clients may become tired from their efforts to feed themselves. Determine whether this client is still hungry and needs assistance. Evaluate the results of self-feeding on the basis of food intake. Success should be recognized and commended.

PROVIDING ENTERAL TUBE FEEDINGS. **Enteral nutrition (EN)** refers to nutrients given via the intestinal tract. Enteral formulas are usually one of four types. Polyermic (1.0 to 2.0 kcal/ml) includes milk-based blenderized foods prepared by hospital dietary staff or at the client's home and commercially prepared whole nutrient formulas. The gastrointestinal tract must be able to absorb whole nutrients. Modular (3.8 to 4.0 kcal/ml) formulas contain a single macronutrient (e.g., protein, glucose, polymers, or lipids) and are not nutritionally complete. Modular formulas are added to other food for meeting special needs. Elemental (1.0 to 1.3 kcal/ml) formulas contain predigested nutrients that are easier for a partially dysfunctional gastrointestinal tract to absorb. Specialty (1.0 to 2.0 kcal/ml) formulas are specifically designed to meet nutritional needs in certain disease states (e.g., liver or hepatic failure, pulmonary disease, or HIV infection). These formulas are expensive and are used only when indicated (Grodner and others, 1996). Oral diets provide a safe and economical method of meeting nutritional needs and are the preferred method if the client's gastrointestinal tract is functional. For clients with eating difficulties, EN may be indicated.

Studies have demonstrated a beneficial effect of enteral feedings over parenteral routes. Postoperative feeding by the enteral route can help reduce sepsis and enhance the immune response, and EN is also preferable to total parenteral nutrition (TPN) in protecting intestinal mucosal cells (Bowers, 1996).

TUBE FEEDINGS. When the client cannot ingest, chew, or swallow food but can digest and absorb nutrients, a feeding tube is placed nasally into the stomach or small intestine or surgically into the stomach or jejunum (Skills 30-1 and 30-2). Intestinal tubes may reduce the risk of aspiration of formula into the lungs during enteral feeding and may be necessary when gastric emptying is delayed.

Aspiration of enteral formula into the lungs irritates the bronchial mucosa, resulting in decreased blood supply to affected pulmonary tissue. This can lead to pneumonia. The high glucose content of formula serves as a medium for bacterial growth, promoting infection. Adult respiratory distress syn-

drome (ARDS) is also an outcome associated with aspiration of gastric contents and enteral formulas (Goodwin, 1996).

Traditional bedside methods of testing placement of feeding tubes, such as injection of air, are ineffective. The "gold standard" is radiographic confirmation of feeding tube location, but this is costly. pH testing is now recommended (Box 30-7). For accurate pH measurements, 30 ml of air is injected into the feeding tube before aspiration of gastric contents. Flushing with air clears out formula, medications, or flush solutions. Only 5 to 10 ml of gastric fluid is needed for pH testing. A client who takes acid-inhibitor medications will usually have an acidic pH at values ranging from 4.0 (after 4 hours of fasting) to 6.0 (with continuous EN infusion). By contrast, intestinal aspirate has a pH of 7.8 to 8.0. More precise indicators are needed to help differentiate the source of tube feeding aspirate, such as bilirubin test strips (Metheny and others, 2000).

Some enterally fed clients have a more permanent device, such as a gastrostomy tube or a jejunostomy tube, placed for EN (Skill 30-3). A **gastrostomy feeding tube** is inserted into the stomach during surgery or by endoscopic placement (PEG) (Figure 30-3). Similarly, a **jejunostomy tube** is surgically inserted into the jejunum or by endoscopy as a PEJ.

The formula used for tube feedings must be nutritionally adequate, tolerated by the client, and delivered at an appropriate rate and volume for the site of feeding delivery within the gastrointestinal tract. A wide variety of commercial products are available for tube feedings. The formulas differ in osmolarity, digestibility, caloric density, viscosity, nutrient content, and electrolyte content. Generally physicians prescribe EN formulas after conferring with the registered dietician. Relevant considerations include disease states that may require more or less of some substrate (i.e., lipids or carbohydrates) or amino acid variation for protein needs (e.g., clients with hepatic or renal disease, diabetes, critical illnesses, or burns).

Clients may be maintained indefinitely on tube feedings, which can provide all the essential nutrients. Although cramping and diarrhea are associated with tube feedings, these symptoms usually subside when the flow rate of the solution is reduced, the formula strength is diluted with water, or a formula containing fiber is used. More than three liquid stools per day is an indication that the client is experiencing diarrhea. The addition of free water is necessary to adequately hydrate the tube-fed client and prevent constipation. Observation and documentation of bowel elimination is an important aspect of monitoring the client's response to enteral nutrition therapy.

PROVIDING PN. Parenteral nutrition is a specialized nutrition support that provides daily nutritional requirements by the intravenous route. PN is selected when the gastrointestinal tract cannot be used or cannot absorb nutrients in sufficient amounts to provide adequate nutrition. The client is reevaluated daily for continued need for PN. The goal is to move toward the use of the gastrointestinal tract for enteral nutrition and eventual normal oral intake (ASPEN, 1996).

Text continued on p. 758

Skill 30-1
INSERTING A SMALL-BORE NASOENTERIC TUBE FOR ENTERAL FEEDINGS

DELEGATION CONSIDERATIONS

This skill requires problem solving and knowledge application unique to a nurse. For this reason, delegation of this skill to assistive personnel is inappropriate.

EQUIPMENT

- Nasogastric (NG) or nasointestinal (NI) tube (8 to 12 Fr) with guide wire or stylet
- Stethoscope
- 60-ml or larger Luer-Lok or catheter-tip syringe
- Hypoallergenic tape and tincture of benzoin
- pH indicator strip
- Glass of water and straw
- Emesis basin
- Safety pin
- Rubber band
- Towel
- Facial tissues
- Clean gloves
- Suction equipment in case of aspiration
- Penlight to check placement in nasopharynx
- Tongue blade

STEPS	RATIONALE
1. Assess client for the need for enteral tube feeding: nothing by mouth (NPO) or insufficient intake for more than 5 days, functional gastrointestinal (GI) tract, unable to ingest sufficient nutrients.	Identifying clients who need tube feedings before they become nutritionally depleted may help to prevent complications related to malnutrition.
2. Assess client for appropriate route of administration:	
a. Close each nostril alternately, and ask client to breathe.	Evaluates nares for patency. Nares may be obstructed.
b. Assess for gag reflex.	Identifies ability to swallow and risk of aspiration.
c. Inspect nares for any irritation or obstruction.	Assessment determines which naris to use.
d. Review client's medical history for nasal problems and risk of aspiration.	You may seek physician's order to change route of nutritional support or to place tube past the stomach into the intestine with increased risk of aspiration.
3. Assess for bowel sounds. Consult physician if bowel sound are absent.	Absence of bowel sounds may indicate decreased or absent peristalsis and increased risk of aspiration or abdominal distention.
4. Wash hands.	Reduces transmission of microorganisms.
5. Explain procedure to client.	Increases client's cooperation with intubation procedure.
6. Explain to client how to communicate during intubation by raising index finger to indicate gagging or discomfort.	It is important for client to have a way of communicating to alleviate stress.

- **Critical Decision Point**

NG or NI feeding tubes may be inserted in clients with decreased level of consciousness, but risk of inadvertent respiratory placement is increased if there is an impaired gag reflex.

STEPS	RATIONALE
7. Position client in sitting or high-Fowler's position. If client is comatose, place in semi-Fowler's position.	Reduces risk of pulmonary aspiration in event client should vomit.
8. Examine feeding tube for flaws: rough or sharp edges on distal end and closed or clogged outlet holes.	Flaws in feeding tube hamper tube intubation and can injure client.
9. Determine length of tube to be inserted and mark with tape or indelible ink (see illustration).	Being aware of proper length to intubate determines approximate depth of insertion.

- **Critical Decision Point**

Tip of tube must reach stomach. Measure distance from tip of nose to earlobe to xyphoid process of sternum (see illustration). Add additional 20 to 30 cm (8 to 12 inches) for nasointestinal tube (Welch, 1996; Hanson, 1979).

STEPS	RATIONALE
10. Prepare NG or NI tube for intubation:	
a. Plastic tubes should *not* be iced.	Tubes will become stiff and inflexible, causing trauma to mucous membranes.
b. Wash hands.	Reduces spread of microorganisms.
c. Inject 10 ml of water from 30-ml or larger Luer-Lok or catheter-tip syringe into the tube.	Aids in guide wire or stylet insertion.

STEPS	RATIONALE
d. Make certain that guide wire is securely positioned against weighted tip and that both Luer-Lok connections are snugly fitted together.	Promotes smooth passage of tube into GI tract. Improperly positioned stylet can induce serious trauma.
11. Cut adhesive tape 10 cm (4 inches) long, or prepare tube fixation device.	
12. Put on clean gloves.	Reduces transmission of microorganisms.
13. Dip tube with surface lubricant into glass of water.	Activates lubricant to facilitate passage of tube into naris to GI tract.
14. Hand client a glass of water with straw or glass with crushed ice (if able to swallow).	Client will be asked to swallow water to facilitate tube passage.
15. Gently insert tube through nostril to back of throat (posterior nasopharynx). May cause client to gag. Aim back and down toward ear (see illustration).	Natural contours facilitate passage of tube into GI tract.
16. Have client flex head toward chest after tube has passed through nasopharynx.	Closes off glottis and reduces risk of tube entering trachea.

• ***Critical Decision Point***
Encourage client to swallow by giving small sips of water or ice chips when possible. Advance tube as client swallows. Rotate tube 180 degrees while inserting. Swallowing facilitates passage of tube past oropharynx. Rotating tube decreases friction.

17. Emphasize need to mouth breathe and swallow during the procedure.	Helps facilitate passage of tube and alleviates client's fears during the procedure.
18. When tip of tube reaches the carina (about 25 cm [10 inches] in an adult), stop and listen for air exchange from the distal portion of the tube.	If air can be heard, tube could be in respiratory tract; remove tube and start over (Metheny, 2000).
19. Advance tube each time client swallows until desired length has been passed.	Reduces discomfort and trauma to client.

• ***Critical Decision Point***
Do not force tube. If resistance is met or client starts to cough, choke, or become cyanotic, stop advancing the tube and pull tube back.

20. Check for position of tube in back of throat with penlight and tongue blade.	Tube may be coiled, kinked, or entering trachea.

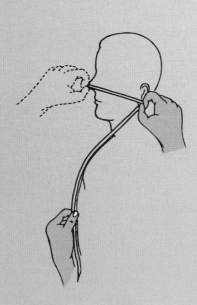

STEP 9   Determine length of tube to be inserted.

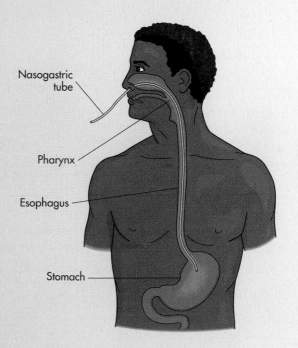

STEP 15   Nasogastric tube inserted through nose and esophagus into stomach.

STEPS	RATIONALE
21. Check placement of tube (see Box 30-7).	Proper position is essential before initiating feedings.
22. After gastric aspirates are obtained, anchor tube to nose and avoid pressure on nares. Mark exit site with indelible ink. Use one of following options for anchoring:	A properly secured tube allows the client more mobility and prevents trauma to nasal mucosa.
A. Apply Tape	
(1) Apply tincture of benzoin or other skin adhesive on tip of client's nose and allow it to become "tacky."	Helps tape adhere better. Protects skin.
(2) Remove gloves, and split one end of the adhesive tape strip lengthwise 5 cm (2 inches).	
(3) Wrap each of the 5-cm strips around tube as it exits nose (see illustration).	Tape minimizes movement and displacement of tube.
B. Apply Tube Fixation Device Using Shaped Adhesive Patch	
(1) Apply wide end of patch to bridge of nose (see illustration).	Device minimizes movement and displacement of tube.
(2) Slip connector around feeding tube as it exits nose (see illustration).	
23. Fasten end of nasogastric tube to client's gown by looping rubber band around tube in slip knot. Pin rubber band to gown (see illustration).	Reduces traction on the naris if tube moves.

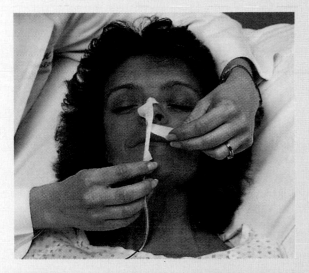

STEP 22A(3)   Wrapping tape to anchor nasoenteral tube.

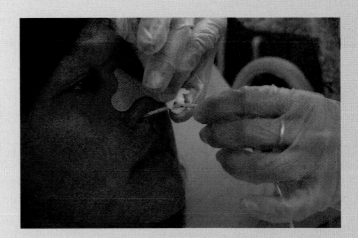

STEP 22B(2)   Slip connector around feeding tube.

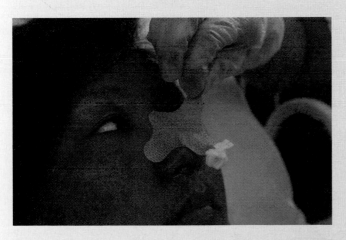

STEP 22B(1)   Applying patch to bridge of nose.

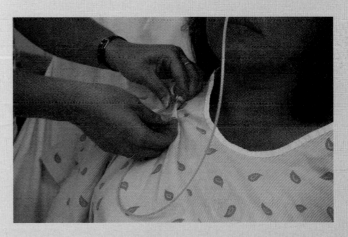

STEP 23   Fastening feeding tube to client's gown.

STEPS	RATIONALE
24. For intestinal placement, position client on right side when possible until radiological confirmation of correct placement has been verified. Otherwise, assist client to a comfortable position.	Promotes passage of the tube into the small intestine (duodenum or jejunum).

- **Critical Decision Point**
  Leave guide wire or stylet in place until correct position is ensured by x-ray film. Never attempt to reinsert partially or fully removed guide wire or stylet while feeding tube is in place.

STEPS	RATIONALE
25. Obtain x-ray film of chest/abdomen.	Placement of tube is verified by x-ray examination (Metheny, 1988).
26. Apply gloves, and administer oral hygiene (see Chapter 26). Cleanse tubing at nostril with washcloth dampened in soap and water.	Promotes client comfort and integrity of oral mucous membranes.
27. Remove gloves, dispose of equipment, and wash hands.	Reduces transmission of microorganisms.
28. Observe client to determine response to NG or NI tube intubation:	
a. Persistent gagging	Indicates prolonged irritation and stimulation of client's gag reflex. Can result in vomiting and increased risk of aspiration.
b. Paroxysms of coughing	May indicate presence of NG or NI tube in client's airway.
29. Confirm x-ray results.	Verifies tube position.
30. Routinely note location of external exit site marking on the tube.	Can reveal if end of tube has migrated position.

UNEXPECTED OUTCOMES AND RELATED INTERVENTIONS

- Aspiration of stomach contents into respiratory tract (immediate response), evidenced by coughing, dyspnea, cyanosis, auscultation of crackles or wheezes.
  - Position client on side.
  - Suction nasotracheally or orotracheally.
  - Consult physician immediately to order a chest x-ray examination for confirming aspiration.
- Aspiration of stomach contents into respiratory tract (delayed response), evidenced by auscultation of crackles or wheezes, dyspnea, fever.
  - Consult physician to obtain order for chest x-ray examination.
  - Prepare for possible initiation of antibiotics.
- Displacement of feeding tube to another site (i.e., from duodenum to stomach), may occur when client coughs or vomits.
  - Aspirate GI contents and measure pH (Metheny and others, 1993a).
  - Remove displaced tube, and insert new tube.
- Clogging of feeding tube.
  - Assess patency of tube by aspirating.
  - Irrigate as needed.
- Nasal mucosa becomes inflamed, tender, and/or eroded.
  - Retape tube to relieve pressure on mucosa.
  - Consider removal of tube and reinsertion in opposite naris (physician's order required).

RECORDING AND REPORTING

- Record and report type and size of feeding tube placed, location in centimeters of distal tip of tube, client's tolerance to procedure, and confirmation of tube position by x-ray examination.

Skill 30-2
ADMINISTERING ENTERAL FEEDINGS VIA NASOENTERIC TUBES

DELEGATION CONSIDERATIONS

Administration of enteral tube feeding via nasogastric tube is a procedure that can be delegated to assistive personnel.

- Verify tube placement before the feeding (Box 30-7, p. 755) and establish patency of the tube by flushing it with water.
- Ensure that the client is sitting upright in a chair or in bed, and instruct the assistive personnel to infuse the feeding slowly.
- Assistive personnel should be instructed to report any difficulty infusing the feeding or any discomfort voiced by the client.

EQUIPMENT

- Disposable feeding bag and tubing or ready-to-hang system
- 30-ml or larger Luer-Lok or catheter-tip syringe
- Stethoscope
- pH indicator strip
- Infusion pump (required for intestinal feedings); use pump designed for tube feedings
- Prescribed enteral feedings
- Gloves
- Equipment to obtain blood glucose by finger stick

STEPS	RATIONALE
1. Assess client's need for enteral tube feedings: impaired swallowing, decreased level of consciousness, head or neck surgery, facial trauma, surgeries of upper alimentary canal.	Identify clients who need tube feedings before they become nutritionally depleted.
2. Auscultate for bowel sounds before feeding.	Absent bowel sounds may indicate decreased ability of GI tract to digest or absorb nutrients.
3. Obtain baseline weight and laboratory values. Assess client for fluid volume excess or deficit, electrolyte abnormalities, and metabolic abnormalities such as hyperglycemia.	Enteral feedings are to restore or maintain a client's nutritional status. Provides objective data to measure effectiveness of feedings.
4. Verify physician's order for formula, rate, route, and frequency. Laboratory data and bedside assessments, such as finger-stick blood glucose measurement, are also ordered by the physician.	Tube feedings, laboratory tests, and bedside tests must be ordered by physician.
5. Explain procedure to client.	Well-informed client is more cooperative and at ease.
6. Wash hands.	Reduces transmission of microorganisms.
7. Prepare feeding container to administer formula continuously:	
a. Check expiration date on formula and integrity of can or bottle.	Ensures GI tolerance of formula. Prevents leakage of tube feeding.
b. Have tube feeding at room temperature.	Cold formula may cause gastric cramping and discomfort because the liquid is not warmed by mouth and esophagus.
c. Connect tubing to container as needed or prepare ready-to-hang container.	Tubing must be free of contamination to prevent bacterial growth.
d. Shake formula container well, and fill container with formula (see illustration). Open stopcock on tubing, and fill tubing with formula to remove air. Hang on intravenous (IV) pole.	Filling the tubing with formula prevents excess air from entering gastrointestinal tract once infusion begins.
8. For intermittent feeding have syringe ready and be sure formula is at room temperature.	Cold formula causes gastric cramping.
9. Place client in high-Fowler's position or elevate head of bed at least 30 degrees.	Elevated head helps prevent aspiration.
10. Determine tube placement (see Box 30-7). Consider together the results from pH testing and the aspirate's appearance.	On occasion, color alone may differentiate gastric from intestinal placement. Because most intestinal aspirates are stained by bile to a distinct yellow color, and most gastric aspirates are not, the difference can often distinguish the sites (Metheny and others, 1999). The pH of an aspirate offers valuable data as well in tracking advancement of a feeding tube (Metheny and others, 1998b).

STEPS	RATIONALE

11. Check for gastric residual (see illustration).
    a. Connect syringe to end of feeding tube, pull back evenly to aspirate gastric contents.
    b. Return aspirated contents to stomach unless the volume exceeds 100 ml (check agency policy).
12. Flush tubing with 30 ml water.
13. Initiate feeding:
	Residual volume indicates if gastric emptying is delayed. Delayed gastric emptying may be reflected by 100 ml or more remaining in the client's stomach (McClave and others, 1999). Return of aspirate prevents fluid and electrolyte imbalance.
	Ensures tube is clear and patent.

A. Syringe or Intermittent Feeding
      (1) Pinch proximal end of feeding tube.
      (2) Remove plunger from syringe and attach barrel of syringe to end of tube.
      (3) Fill syringe with measured amount of formula (see illustration). Release tube, and elevate syringe to no more than 18 inches (45 cm) above insertion site, and allow it to empty gradually by gravity. Refill until prescribed amount has been delivered to client.
      (4) If feeding bag is used, attach gavage tubing to end of feeding tube. Set rate by adjusting roller clamp on tubing. Allow bag to empty gradually over 30 to 60 minutes (see illustration). Label bag with tube-feeding type, strength, and amount. Include date, time, and initials.
	Prevents air from entering client's stomach.
	Barrel receives formula for instillation.
	
	Height of syringe allows for safe, slow, gravity drainage of formula.
	
	Gradual emptying of tube feeding by gravity from syringe or feeding bag reduces risk of abdominal discomfort, vomiting, or diarrhea induced by bolus or too-rapid infusion of tube feedings.

B. Continuous-Drip Method
      (1) Hang feeding bag and tubing on IV pole.
 	
      (2) Connect distal end of tubing to proximal end of feeding tube.
	Continuous-feeding method is designed to deliver prescribed hourly rate of feeding. This method reduces risk of abdominal discomfort. Clients who receive continuous-drip feedings should have residuals checked every 8 to 12 hours and tube placement verified.

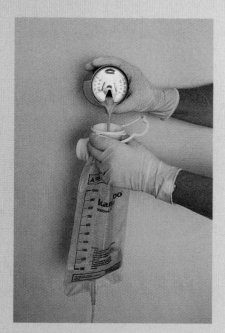

STEP 7D   Pour formula into feeding container.

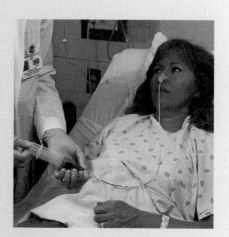

STEP 11   Check for gastric residual (small-bore tube).

STEPS	RATIONALE

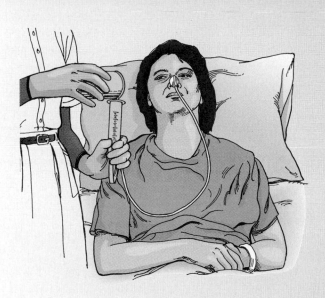

STEP 13A(3)   Fill syringe with formula.

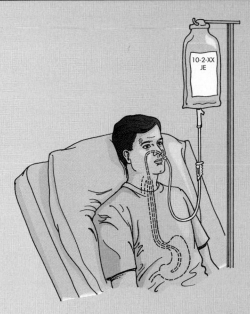

STEP 13A(4)   Administer feeding.

(3) Connect tubing through infusion pump, and set rate (see manufacturer's directions) (see illustration).	Delivers continuous-drip feeding.

• **Critical Decision Point**
  Maximum hang time for formula is 8 hours in an open system, 24 hours in closed, ready-to-hang system.

14. Advance rate of concentration of tube feeding gradually (Box 30-8).	Prevents diarrhea and gastric intolerance to formula.
15. Following intermittent infusion or at end of continuous infusion, flush nasoenteral tubing with 30 ml of water, using irrigating syringe. Repeat every 4 to 6 hours around the clock (Simon and Fink, 1999). Have registered dietitian recommend total free water requirement per day.	Provides client with source of water to help maintain fluid and electrolyte balance. Clears tubing of formula.
16. When tube feedings are not being administered, cap or clamp the proximal end of the feeding tube.	Prevents air from entering stomach between feedings.
17. Rinse bag and tubing with warm water whenever feedings are interrupted.	Rinsing bag and tubing with warm water clears old tube feedings and reduces bacterial growth.
18. Change bag and tubing every 24 hours.	Reduces incidences of bacterial growth.
19. Measure amount of aspirate (residual) every 8 to 12 hours.	Evaluates tolerance of tube feeding.
20. Monitor finger-stick blood glucose every 6 hours until maximum administration rate is reached and maintained for 24 hours.	Alerts nurse to client's tolerance of glucose. May require physician to revise type of formula administered.
21. Monitor intake and output every 8 hours (Metheny and others, 2000).	Intake and output are indications of fluid balance or fluid volume excess or deficit.

STEPS	RATIONALE
22. Weigh client daily until maximum administration rate is reached and maintained for 24 hours, then weigh client 3 times per week.	Weight gain is indicator of improved nutritional status; however, sudden gain of more than 2 lb in 24 hours usually indicates fluid retention.
23. Observe return of normal laboratory values.	Improving laboratory values (i.e., albumin, transferrin, pre-albumin) indicate an improved nutritional status.

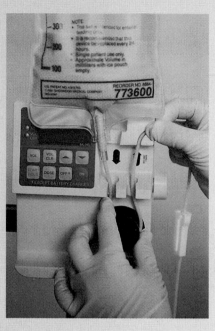

STEP 13B(3)   Connect tubing through infusion pump.

UNEXPECTED OUTCOMES AND RELATED INTERVENTIONS

- Gastric residual exceeds 100 ml. (See agency policy.)
  - Hold feeding.
  - Notify physician.
  - Maintain client in semi-Fowler's or at least have head of bed elevated 30 degrees.
  - Recheck residual in 1 hour.
- Client aspirates formula when tube inappropriately placed or client is positioned flat in bed.
  - Position client in Fowler's position, suction, and notify physician immediately.
  - Prepare for chest x-ray examination.
- Client develops diarrhea 3 times or more in 24 hours, indicating intolerance.
  - Notify physician, and confer with dietitian to determine need to modify type of formula, concentration, or rate of infusion.
- Consider change of antibiotic.

RECORDING AND REPORTING

- Record amount and type of feeding, client's response to tube feeding, patency of tube, and any side effects.
- Record volume of formula and any additional water on intake and output form.
- Report type of feeding status of feeding tube, client's tolerance, and adverse effects.
- Client develops nausea and vomiting.
  - May indicate gastric ileus. Withhold tube feeding, and notify physician.
  - Be sure tubing is patent, aspirate for residual.

Procedural Guidelines for   Box 30-7

OBTAINING GI FLUID FOR pH MEASUREMENT: LARGE- AND SMALL-BORE NASOGASTRIC TUBES: BOLUS AND CONTINUOUS FEEDING

1. Perform measures to verify placement of tube:
   a. For intermittently fed clients, test placement immediately before feeding (usually a period of at least 4 hours will have elapsed since previous feeding). More frequent checking has been associated with increased clogging of small-bore tubes (Powell and others, 1993). To avoid clogging, flush tube with 30 ml water after aspirating for the residual volume (Edwards and Metheny, 2000).
   b. For continuously tube-fed clients, test placement at least once every 12 hours.
   c. Wait at least 1 hour after medication administration by tube or mouth.
2. Draw up 30 ml of air into syringe, then attach to end of feeding tube. Flush tube with 30 ml of air before attempting to aspirate fluid. It will likely be more difficult to aspirate fluid from the small intestine than from the stomach. Repositioning the client from side to side may be helpful. More than one bolus of air through the tube may be needed in some cases. Burst of air aids in aspirating fluid more easily (Metheny and others, 1993b).
3. Draw back on syringe and obtain 5 to 10 ml of gastric aspirate. Observe appearance of aspirate (see illustration).

4. Gently mix aspirate in syringe. Then expel a few drops into a clean medicine cup. Dip the pH strip into the fluid or by applying a few drops of the fluid to the strip (see illustration). Compare the color of the strip with the color on the chart provided by the manufacturer (Metheny and others, 1998b).
   a. Gastric fluid from client who has fasted for at least 4 hours usually has pH range of 1 to 4 (Metheny and others, 1998a).
   b. Fluid from nasointestinal tube of fasting client usually has pH greater than 6 (Metheny and others, 1989).
   c. Client with continuous tube feeding may have pH of 5 or higher.
   d. pH of pleural fluid from the tracheobronchial tree is generally greater than 6.

CRITICAL DECISION POINT

If after repeated attempts, it is not possible to aspirate fluid from a tube that was originally established by x-ray examination to be in desired position, and (a) there are no risk factors for tube dislocation, (b) tube has remained in original taped position, and (c) client is not experiencing difficulty, assume tube is correctly placed (Metheny and others, 1993a).

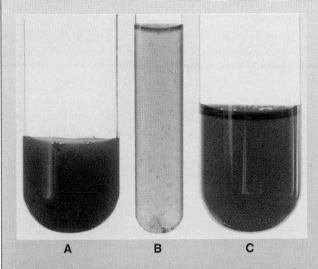

STEP 3   Gastrointestinal contents: **A,** Stomach. **B,** Stomach. **C,** Intestinal. (Courtesy Dr. Norma Metheny, Professor, St. Louis University School of Nursing.)

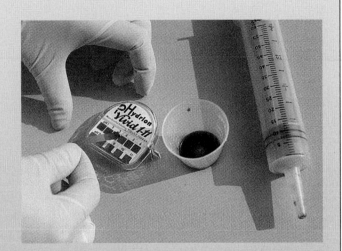

STEP 4   Comparing pH strip with color chart.

Advancing the Rate of Tube Feeding   Box 30-8

INTERMITTENT
1. Start formula at full strength for isotonic formulas (300 to 400 mOsm) or at ordered concentration.
2. Infuse bolus of formula over at least 20 to 30 minutes via syringe or feeding container.
3. Begin feedings with no more than 150 to 250 ml at one time. Increase by 50 ml per feeding per day to achieve needed volume and calories in six to eight feedings. (NOTE: Concentrated formulas at full strength may be infused at slower rate until tolerance is achieved.)

CONTINUOUS
1. Start formula at full strength for isotonic formulas (300 to 400 mOsm) or at ordered concentration. Usually hypertonic formulas are also started at full strength but at a slower rate.
2. Begin infusion rate at designated rate.
3. Advance rate slowly (e.g., 10 to 20 ml/hr per day) to target rate if tolerated (tolerance indicated by absence of nausea and diarrhea, and low gastric residuals).

Skill 30-3

ADMINISTERING ENTERAL FEEDINGS VIA GASTROSTOMY OR JEJUNOSTOMY TUBE

DELEGATION CONSIDERATIONS

Administration of enteral tube feeding via a gastrostomy or jejunostomy tube or a jejunal tube is a procedure that can be delegated to assistive personnel.

- Verify tube placement before the feedings, and establish patency of the tube by flushing it with water.
- Ensure that the client is sitting upright in a chair or in bed, and instruct the assistive personnel to infuse the feeding slowly.
- Assistive personnel should be instructed to report any difficulty infusing the feeding or any discomfort voiced by the client.

EQUIPMENT

- Disposable feeding container or ready-to-hang bag
- 30-ml or larger Luer-Lok or catheter-tip syringe
- Formula
- Infusion pump: use pump designed for tube feedings
- pH indicator strips
- Stethoscope
- Gloves
- Equipment to obtain blood glucose by finger stick

STEPS	RATIONALE
1. Assess client's need for enteral tube feedings (see Skill 30-1, p. 747): impaired swallowing, decreased level of consciousness, surgeries of upper alimentary tract, need for long-term enteral nutrition.	Identifies clients who need tube feedings before they become nutritionally depleted. Enteral feedings preserves the function and mass of the gut, promotes wound healing, diminishes hypermetabolism in burn injuries, and may decrease infection in critically ill clients (Zaloga, 1994).
2. Auscultate for bowel sounds before feeding. Consult physician if bowel sounds are absent.	Absence of bowel sounds may indicate decreased or absent peristalsis and increased risk of aspiration or abdominal distention.
3. Obtain baseline weight and laboratory values.	Enteral feedings are to restore or maintain nutritional status. Provides objective data to measure effectiveness of feedings.
4. Verify physician's order for formula, rate, route, and frequency.	Tube feedings must be ordered by physician.
5. Assess gastrostomy/jejunostomy site for breakdown, irritation, or drainage.	Infection, pressure from gastrostomy tube, or drainage of gastric secretions can cause skin breakdown.
6. Explain procedure to client.	Well-informed client is more cooperative and feels more at ease.
7. Wash hands.	Reduces transmission of microorganisms.
8. Prepare feeding container to administer formula continuously:	
a. Have tube feeding at room temperature.	Cold formula may cause gastric cramping and discomfort because the liquid is not warmed by mouth and esophagus.
b. Connect tubing to container as needed or prepare ready-to-hang container.	Tubing must be free of contamination to prevent bacterial growth.
c. Shake formula well. Fill container and tubing with formula.	Filling tubing with formula prevents excess air from entering gastrointestinal tract.
9. For intermittent feeding have syringe ready and be sure formula is at room temperature.	Cold formula causes gastric cramping.
10. Elevate head of bed 30 to 45 degrees.	Elevating client's head helps prevent chance of aspiration.
11. Apply gloves, and verify tube placement:	
A. **Gastrostomy Tube**	
(1) Attach syringe and aspirate gastric secretions, observe their appearance, and check pH. Return aspirated contents to stomach unless the volume exceeds 100 ml. If the volume is greater than 100 ml on several consecutive occasions, hold feeding and notify physician (McClave and others, 1999).	Fluid from gastric tube of client who has fasted for at least 4 hours usually has pH range of 1 to 4, especially when client is not receiving a gastric-acid inhibitor. Continuous administration of tube feedings may elevate the pH (Metheny and others, 1999). Gastric residual determines if gastric emptying is delayed. Delayed gastric emptying may be indicated by 100 ml or more remaining in client's stomach from previous feeding.

STEPS	RATIONALE
B. Jejunostomy Tube	
(1) Aspirate intestinal secretions, observe their appearance and check pH.	
12. Flush with 30 ml water.	Ensures tube is clear and patent.
13. Initiate feedings:	
A. Syringe Feedings	Gastrostomy and jejunostomy feedings are given continuously to ensure proper absorption. However, initial feedings may be given by bolus to assess client's tolerance (see Box 30-8, p. 755).
(1) Pinch proximal end of the gastrostomy/jejunostomy tube.	Prevents excessive air from entering the client's stomach or leaking of gastric contents.
(2) Remove plunger, and attach barrel of syringe to end of tube, then fill syringe with formula.	
(3) Release tube, and elevate syringe. Allow syringe to empty gradually by gravity, refilling until prescribed amount has been delivered to the client.	Gradual emptying of tube feedings by gravity reduces the risk of diarrhea induced by bolus tube feedings.
B. Continuous-Drip Method	
(1) Fill feeding container with enough prescribed formula for 4 hours of feeding.	
(2) Hang container on IV pole, and clear tubing of air.	Allows for gravity flow of formula. Prevents accumulation of air in stomach.
(3) Thread tubing into feeding pump according to manufacturer's directions.	
(4) Connect end of feeding tubing to proximal end of gastrostomy/jejunostomy tube.	
(5) Begin infusion at prescribed rate.	Continuous-feeding method is designed to deliver a prescribed hourly rate of feeding. This method reduces the risk of diarrhea. Clients who receive continuous-drip feedings should have residuals checked every 8 to 12 hours.
14. Administer water via feeding tube as ordered with or between feedings.	Provides client with source of water to help maintain fluid and electrolyte balance.
15. Flush tube with 30 ml of water every 4 to 6 hours around the clock and before and after administering medications via the tube (Simon and Fink, 1999).	Maintains patency of tube and provides client with some free water. Small jejunal tubes are very prone to clogging and are difficult to replace.
16. When tube feedings are not being administered, cap or clamp the proximal end of the gastrostomy/jejunostomy tube.	Prevents excess air from entering the gastrointestinal tract between feedings and prevents leakage of gastric contents.
17. Rinse container and tubing with warm water after all intermittent feedings.	Rinsing container and tube with warm water clears old tube feedings and prevents bacterial growth.

• *Critical Decision Point*
  Advance tube feeding rate gradually (see Box 30-8, p. 755). Tube feedings should be advanced gradually to prevent diarrhea and gastric intolerance of formula.

STEPS	RATIONALE
18. The gastrostomy/jejunostomy exit site is usually left open to air. However, if a dressing is needed because of drainage, change dressing daily or as needed and report the drainage to the physician; inspect exit site every shift.	Leakage of gastric drainage may cause irritation and excoriation. Skin around feeding tube should be cleansed daily with warm water and mild soap; a small precut gauze dressing may be applied to exit site.
19. Dispose of supplies, and wash hands.	Reduces transmission of microorganisms.
20. Evaluate client's tolerance of tube feeding. Check amount of aspirate (residual) every 8 to 12 hours.	Tolerance of tube feeding is evaluated by checking.
21. Monitor finger-stick blood glucose every 6 hours until maximum rate of administration is reached and maintained for 24 hours.	Alerts nurse to client's tolerance of glucose or fluid volume excess.
22. Monitor intake and output every 8 hours.	Intake and output are indications of fluid balance.

STEPS	RATIONALE
23. Weigh client daily until maximum administration rate is reached and maintained for 24 hours, then weigh client 3 times per week.	Weight gain is indicator of improved nutritional status; however, a sudden gain of more than 2 lb in 24 hours usually indicates fluid retention.
24. Observe return of normal laboratory values.	Improving laboratory values (i.e., albumin, transferrin, prealbumin) indicate return to normal nutritional status.
25. Observe stoma site for skin integrity.	Gastric secretions can cause injury and necrosis at stoma site.

UNEXPECTED OUTCOMES AND RELATED INTERVENTIONS
■ Client aspirates formula when gastric emptying is delayed or formula is administered too rapidly and produces vomiting.
  • Position client in side-lying position, and suction airway to keep it clear. Do not initiate gagging during suctioning.
  • Notify physician; obtain chest x-ray film.
■ Client develops diarrhea: diarrhea or liquid stools (3 times or more in 24 hours) indicate intolerance. Antibiotics and medications containing sorbitol may also induce diarrhea.
  • Decrease rate of feeding, review medications, and notify physician.
  • Type of formula may be altered, and antidiarrheal agents may be ordered.

■ Skin surrounding gastrostomy site breaks down.
  • Provide appropriate wound care (see Chapter 34).

RECORDING AND REPORTING
■ Record amount and type of feeding, client's response to feeding, patency of tube, any untoward effects, and condition of gastrostomy/jejunostomy site in nurses' notes.
■ Record amount of feeding on intake and output form.
■ Report to oncoming nursing staff: type of feeding, status of gastrostomy tube, client's tolerance, and adverse effects.

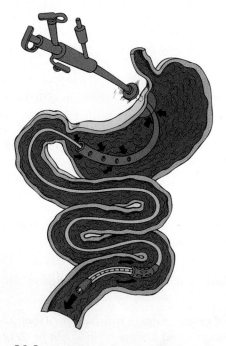

FIGURE **30-3** Endoscopic insertion of jejunostomy tube.

The complications of PN can be reduced by meticulous aseptic care of the central venous access device, a gradual increase in the administration rate of PN over several hours or days, careful monitoring of laboratory results for metabolic or electrolyte abnormalities, and assessment of fluid balance.

PN solutions that contain 10% dextrose or greater are hyperosmolar (i.e., highly concentrated) and irritate small peripheral veins. As a result, PN at this concentration must be infused through central venous lines. Each day PN is prescribed by the physician and mixed in the pharmacy. This prescribed solution reflects the client's most recent laboratory values and nutritional needs. The solution itself is tailored to the client's specific nutritional needs, containing amino acids, dextrose, lipids, vitamins, minerals (electrolytes), and water. This mixture is referred to as total parenteral nutrition (TPN) and is given over a 24-hour period.

Because the mixture includes lipid emulsions, it should not be used if oil droplets or if an oily or creamy layer is observed on the surface of the solution. Some clients receive no lipids or receive lipids only 2 to 3 times per week. Lipid emulsion may be co-infused peripherally or centrally using a Y connector, below an in-line filter. Infusion rate is 0.5 to 1.0 ml/min for the first 30 minutes. Reactions to lipid infusion can include dyspnea, cyanosis, vomiting, headache, and/or chest pain. Stop the infusion, and notify the physician. If the client tolerates the slow lipid infusion, advance the rate as ordered by the physician.

Initiating PN. PN therapy requires a central venous catheter (CVC) inserted into the jugular or subclavian vein. Nurses assist with this procedure for inserting a central venous catheter. Specially trained nurses insert peripherally inserted central catheters (PICCs) (see Chapter 14). A chest x-ray film is used to confirm the location of the central venous

Outcome Evaluation for **MS. GARCIA**		Box 30-9
Nursing Action	**Client Response/Finding**	**Achievement of Outcome**
Ask Ms. Garcia to describe meals.	Ms. Garcia admits to skipping meals occasionally.	Ms. Garcia's body weight has improved, but weekly weight gain is less than $1/_2$ lb/wk.
Ask her how much of the meal is eaten.	She states that when she has a meal she eats all of it.	
	Ms. Garcia ingests nutritional supplement as ordered.	
Ask Ms. Garcia to complete 3-day dietary history.	Ms. Garcia completed diet history.	Laboratory values such as albumin, transferrin, and CBC have remained the same. However, they did not decline.
	Diet is improved but remains high in carbohydrates and fats.	
Ask Ms. Garcia about any abdominal symptoms.	Ms. Garcia denies any diarrhea and reports more regular bowel movements.	Cramping and diarrhea have resolved.

catheter. Clients may have a long-term central venous access device, such as a tunneled catheter or an implanted port.

Before beginning an infusion, verify the physician's order. An infusion pump is always used. Beginning infusion at 40 to 60 ml/hr is recommended. The rate is gradually increased until the client's complete nutrition needs are supplied. Clients receiving PN at home frequently administer the entire daily solution over 12 hours at night. This allows the client to disconnect from the infusion each morning, flush the central line, and have independent mobility during the day.

Caring for the Client Receiving PN. Nursing care for the client receiving PN is based on four major nursing goals: (1) preventing infection; (2) maintaining the PN system, (3) preventing metabolic, electrolyte, or fluid balance complications, and (4) assessing the client's readiness for EN or discharge planning for home PN.

Primary methods to prevent infection include asepsis during insertion and care of the central venous catheter, use of an in-line IV filter and maintaining secure, uncontaminated tubing connections. PN solutions should not exceed their 24-hour infusion limit.

Clients receiving PN have laboratory measurements monitored regularly. Capillary blood glucose testing or urine glucose testing occurs during the initiation of PN to assess for metabolic tolerance. Be alert for changes in vital signs or fluid balance and abnormal laboratory results that would indicate infection, **hyperglycemia,** glucosuria, or electrolyte imbalance (Andris and Krzywda, 1999; Souba, 1997). Report any unusual symptoms to the physician. An increased temperature may be an early sign of infection and should be reported to the physician.

RESTORATIVE AND CONTINUING CARE

DIET THERAPY IN DISEASE MANAGEMENT. Clients discharged from a hospital with diet prescriptions often need dietary education to plan meals that meet specific therapeutic requirements. Restorative care includes immediate postsurgical care, posthospitalization care, and routine medical care. Therefore preparation for the restorative aspect of client care may be integrated within the acute care setting.

Dietary intake patterns that result in good nutrition must often be modified for clients with specific diseases. These include gastrointestinal diseases, such as irritable bowel syndrome and malabsorption syndromes; metabolic disorders, such as diabetes mellitus and hypoglycemia; cardiovascular diseases; renal diseases; and cancers. Diet modifications are necessary to correspond with the body's ability to metabolize certain nutrients, to correct nutritional deficiencies, and to eliminate harmful foods from the diet. In all cases, work with the physician and diet therapist when planning and implementing modified diets.

HOME CARE. Specialized nutrition therapies, such as EN and PN, may need to be continued beyond the hospital setting to the home care setting. In home care you are often the only care provider who sees the client on a regular basis. As a home care nurse you teach clients or caregivers how to administer PN or EN, assess the client for tolerance of the nutrition prescription, and evaluate the client's progress toward nutritional goals.

 Evaluation

CLIENT CARE. The value of your activities in meeting the client's nutritional needs is measured by an ongoing evaluation. Adequate time should be allowed to test a nursing approach to a problem.

Evaluation of clinical progress can include objective data, such as weight gain or improved laboratory parameters, or subjective data, such as the client's reporting improvement in food choices or in self-reporting improved intake (Box 30-9). When clinical progress does not occur, determine whether the interventions were not effective, were not done or accepted by the client, were not realistic or appropriate, or were affected by unanticipated or unidentified factors.

If outcomes are not met, reassess the client to determine if important data were missed. Clients may need reeducation

Case Study EVALUATION

Shawneen sees Ms. Garcia on a home visit 3 weeks after her teaching session. She contacted Ms. Garcia and asked her to keep a 3-day food intake record before the visit. During the home visit, Shawneen notes that Ms. Garcia has gained 4 lb. Her 3-day food intake indicates use of the nutritional supplement and improved protein intake. Ms. Garcia tells Shawneen that her appetite has improved and that she is usually able to finish a small meal. She is still bothered by milk products if she has more than 8 oz at a time.

Shawneen advises Ms. Garcia to continue the current plan of care and emphasizes that her slow, consistent weight gain is appropriate. She consults with Ms. Garcia about a visit in another 3 weeks and asks Ms. Garcia to call her if Ms. Garcia's symptoms return or her weight gain stops.

Documentation Note
Ms. Garcia visited in her home. Weight gain of 4 lb in 3 weeks. Counseled to continue with new eating habits and to continue to avoid more than 8 oz of milk products. Rescheduled visit in 3 weeks.

if essential skills or knowledge has been forgotten or misunderstood. Also attempt to validate that the client is in agreement with the goals and is willing and able to follow the nutritional plan of care.

CLIENT EXPECTATIONS. Often entry into the health care system is associated with some type of illness and occasionally results in changes in independence. Nutritional interventions often depend on the client's willingness and ability to change behavior patterns and learn new patterns. If the client is not fully committed to the expected changes, the interventions may not be successful. The client may also find it difficult to change behavior and may be less motivated with the passage of time.

Most clients respond well to the opportunity to make informed choices. Your explanations of the reasons for the behavioral change and providing the client options for how the change may be achieved assist the client in making the change. Education may need to be provided in several brief sessions to maximize retention of information.

Key Terms

absorption, *p. 736*
amino acids, *p. 735*
anabolism, *p. 737*
anthropometry, *p. 740*
carbohydrates, *p. 735*
catabolism, *p. 737*
dietary referenced intake (DRIs), *p. 737*
digestion, *p. 736*

enteral nutrition (EN), *p. 746*
gastrostomy feeding tube, *p. 746*
gluconeogenesis, *p. 737*
glucose, *p. 737*
glycogen, *p. 737*
glycogenesis, *p. 737*
hyperglycemia, *p. 759*
jejunostomy tube, *p. 746*
lipid, *p. 736*
lipogenesis, *p. 737*
metabolism, *p. 737*

minerals, *p. 736*
nitrogen balance, *p. 741*
nutrients, *p. 735*
obesity, *p. 742*
parenteral nutrition (PN), *p. 744*
polyunsaturated fatty acid, *p. 736*
proteins, *p. 735*
saturated fatty acid, *p. 736*
unsaturated fatty acid, *p. 736*
vitamins, *p. 736*

Key Concepts

- Nutrients needed by the body to carry out vital functions are water, carbohydrates, proteins, lipids, vitamins, and minerals.
- Body weight is maintained when food intake equals energy requirements.
- Proteins are essential for growth, maintenance, and repair.
- Digestion is the mechanical and chemical process by which food is broken down into its simplest form for absorption. Digestion and absorption occur mainly in the small intestine.
- Dietary referenced intakes (DRIs), another basis for diet selection, were formulated for population groups, not individuals.
- Guidelines for dietary change advocate reduced intake of fat, saturated fat, salt, refined sugar, and cholesterol and increased intake of complex carbohydrates and fiber.
- Age affects the requirements for essential nutrients. Periods of rapid growth increase the need for protein, vitamins, and minerals.

- Because improper nutrition can affect all body systems, nutritional assessment includes a review of the total physical assessment.
- Proper feeding techniques can protect the dependent client from loss of dignity and self-esteem.
- Special hospital diets alter the composition, texture, digestibility, and residue of foods to suit the client's particular needs.
- Tube feedings can be used for clients who are unable to ingest food but are able to digest and absorb foods.
- Enteral nutrition may protect intestinal structure and function and enhance immunity.
- Total parenteral nutrition supplies essential nutrients in appropriate amounts to support life through the introduction of a concentrated nutrient solution into a large central vein or the right atrium of the heart.
- Evaluation of the outcomes of nursing intervention in the area of nutritional support is essential to revise, update, or continue nursing activities.

Critical Thinking Activities

1. You are completing a nursing history for a 24-year-old client who has diabetes. The client is slightly underweight and tells you that he is vegetarian and eats no animal products, including fish, eggs, and milk. What information about his diet would you need to determine whether it is adequate in calories and protein? What laboratory tests would reflect protein status? What physical assessment findings might suggest inadequate protein intake?

2. Mrs. Evans is 75 years of age and lives alone. She receives a social security check, which pays for her rent and utilities with about $100 a month left over. She has arthritis, takes aspirin, and has difficulty ambulating more than about 50 feet at a time. How might Mrs. Evans's situation affect her nutritional status?

3. While giving Mr. Orzo a bath, you notice that his PN solution looks odd. There is a small yellow layer at the top of the bag. Mr. Orzo is receiving lipids, amino acids, and dextrose in a single solution. What could this layer indicate, and what should you do first?

Review Questions

1. Positive nitrogen balance would occur in:
   1. infection.
   2. starvation.
   3. burn injury.
   4. pregnancy.
2. The nutrient that provides the body's most preferred energy source is:
   1. fat.
   2. protein.
   3. vitamin.
   4. carbohydrate.
3. The nutrient that is preferred to repair tissue is:
   1. fat.
   2. protein.
   3. vitamin.
   4. carbohydrate.
4. When feeding tubes are first positioned, verification is done by:
   1. auscultation.
   2. x-ray confirmation.
   3. pH testing of gastric contents.
   4. confirmation of distal mark on feeding tube.
5. The most accurate method for bedside confirmation of feeding tube placement is:
   1. auscultation.

2. x-ray confirmation.
3. pH testing for gastric contents.
4. confirmation of distal mark on feeding tube.
6. Parenteral nutrition is used when the client is:
   1. NPO.
   2. critically ill.
   3. recovering from abdominal surgery.
   4. experiencing a condition resulting in gastrointestinal dysfunction.
7. Assessment of glucose balance in a patient receiving parenteral nutrition is most accurate with:
   1. fasting blood glucose.
   2. urine testing for ketones.
   3. urine testing for glucose.
   4. serum glucose monitoring.
8. You have been working with an overweight client to achieve weight reduction. The client is adhering to his diet but wants faster results. You tell the client that he is having a steady weight loss progression. Ideal weight loss is:
   1. 0.5 lb/wk.
   2. 1 to 2 lb/wk.
   3. 2 to 3 lb/wk.
   4. more than 3 lb/wk.

References

Andris DA, Krzywda EA: Central venous catheter occlusion: successful management strategies, *Medsurg Nurs* 8(4):229, 1999.

American Society for Parenteral and Enteral Nutrition (ASPEN): Guidelines for use of parenteral and enteral nutrition in adult and pediatric patients, *JPEN J Parenter Enteral Nutr* 17(4)(suppl):ISA, 1993.

American Society for Parenteral and Enteral Nutrition (ASPEN): Standards of practice: nutrition support nurses, *Nutr Clin Pract* 11(3):127, 1996.

American Heart Association Science Advisory and Coordinating Committee: Dietary guidelines for Americans, *Circulation* 94:1795, 1996a.

American Heart Association Science Advisory and Coordinating Committee: Fish consumption, fish oil, lipids, and coronary heart disease, *Circulation* 94:2347, 1996b.

Bowers S: Tubes: a nurse's guide to enteral feeding devices, *Medsurg Nurs* 5(5):313, 1996.

Burck R: Invited review: feeding, withdrawing, and withholding—ethical perspectives, *Nutr Clin Pract* 11(6):243, 1996.

Edwards S, Metheny N: Measurement of gastric residual volume: state of the science, *Medsurg Nurs* 9(3):125, 2000.

Goodwin RS: Prevention of aspiration pneumonia: a research-based protocol, *Dimens Crit Care Nurs* 15(4):58, 1996.

Grodner M and others: *Foundations and clinical applications of nutrition: a nursing approach,* ed 2, St. Louis, 2000, Mosby.

Hanson RL: Predictive criteria for length of nasogastric tube insertions for tube feeding, *JPEN J Parenter Enteral Nutr* 3:160, 1979.

Keithly J, Swanson M: Minimizing HIV/AIDS malnutrition, *Medsurg Nurs* 7(5):256, 1998.

McCalve SA and others. Enteral tube feeding in the intensive care unit: factors impeding adequate delivery, *Crit Care Med* 27(7):1252, 1999.

Metheny N: Measures to test placement of nasogastric and enteral feeding tubes: a review, *Nurs Res* 37(6):323, 1988.

Metheny N and others: Effectiveness of pH measurements in predicting feeding tube placement, *Nurs Res* 38(5):285, 1989.

Metheny N and others: Effectiveness of pH measurements in predicting feeding tube placement: an update, *Nurs Res* 42:324, 1993a.

Metheny N and others. How to aspirate fluid from small-bore feeding tubes, *Am J Nurs* 93(5):86, 1993b.

Metheny N and others: Detection of improperly positioned feeding tubes, *Health Risk Manage* 18(3):37, 1998a.

Metheny N and others: pH, color, and feeding tubes, *RN* 61(1):27, 1998b.

Metheny N and others: pH and concentration of bilirubin in feeding tube aspirate as a predictor of tube placement, *Nurs Res* 48:189, 1999.

Metheny NA and others: Development of a reliable and valid bedside test for bilirubin and its utility for improving prediction of feeding tube location, *Nurs Res* 49(6):302, 2000.

Nutrition Screening Initiative: *Nutrition screening tool for older adults,* a project of the American Academy of Family Physicians, the American Dietetic Association, and the National Council of the Aging, Inc, and funded in part by a grant from Ross Products Division, Abbott Laboratories, 1998.

Ponell KS and others: Aspirating gastric residuals causes occlusion of small bore feeding tubes, *J Paren Enteral Nutr* 17:243, 1993.

Simon T, Fink AS: Current management of endoscopic feeding tube dysfunction, *Surg Endosc* 13:403, 1999.

Souba WW: Nutritional Support, *N Engl J Med* 336(1):41, 1997.

U.S. Department of Agriculture: *USDA's food guide pyramid,* USDA Human Nutrition Information Service Pub No. 249, Washington, DC, 1996, U.S. Government Printing Office.

U.S. Department of Health and Human Services: *Healthy people 2010 objectives: draft for public comment,* 1998, www.health.gov/healthypeople.

U.S. Department of Health and Human Services: *Healthy people 2010 objectives,* 2000, www.health.gov/healthypeople.

Welch SK: Certification of staff nurses to insert enteral feeding tubes, using a research-based procedures, *Nutr Clin Pract* 11(1):21, 1996.

Williams SR: *Nutrition and diet therapy,* ed 9, St. Louis, 1997, Mosby.

Zaloga G: Frontiers in critical care nutrition, *New Horizons* 2(2):121, 1994.

Urinary Elimination

Objectives

- Define key terms.
- Explain the function of each organ in the urinary system.
- Describe the process of urination.
- Identify factors that commonly influence urination.
- Compare and contrast common alterations in urination.
- Obtain a nursing history from a client with an alteration in urination.
- Describe physical assessment techniques used to assess urinary elimination.
- Describe characteristics of normal and abnormal urine.
- Describe nursing implications of common diagnostic tests of the urinary system.
- Identify nursing diagnoses relevant to the urinary system.
- Discuss nursing measures to assist the client with urinary elimination.
- Describe nursing measures to control incontinence.
- Discuss nursing measures to reduce urinary tract infections.
- Apply or insert an external or indwelling catheter.

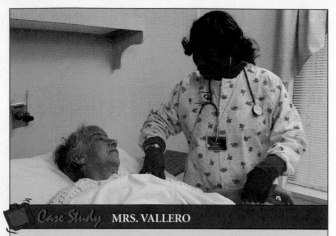

Case Study　MRS. VALLERO

Mrs. Vallero is an 85-year-old woman who is lying in her hospital bed. It is 9:30 AM. She has been in the hospital for 4 days for congestive heart failure with pulmonary edema. At the 7 AM report you learned her catheter and intravenous (IV) line were removed yesterday at 4 PM after she was taking fluids and her urinary output totaled 2000 ml. Her total input yesterday was 3400 ml: 2000 ml IV and 1400 ml oral. At 12 AM Mrs. Vallero was found to be incontinent of a small amount of urine and was complaining of lower abdominal pain. She was catheterized at 1 AM for 1100 ml of pale, clear yellow urine after the physician was called. The physician ordered "single catheterization now and times one." Today at 8 AM, she ate one slice of toast, half of her scrambled eggs, and 400 ml of fluids. She says she has not gone to the bathroom this morning but has "dribbled some."

Mrs. Stone is a 43-year-old divorced mother of two daughters. Mrs. Stone is a sophomore nursing student in her sixth week of clinical rotation at a community hospital. She was in the hospital as a client at the birth of her daughters. At the birth of her second child a year ago she had a cesarean section and had a urinary catheter in for 2 days.

*N*ormal elimination of urinary wastes is a function most people take for granted. When the urinary system fails to function properly, virtually all body systems can be affected. Clients with alterations in urinary elimination may also be affected by resulting body image problems.

SCIENTIFIC KNOWLEDGE BASE

Knowledge from the biological and social sciences helps to identify actual and potential urinary tract problems that the client might encounter. A thorough understanding of related information helps you to provide complete and competent care to the client with altered elimination.

Urinary Elimination

Urinary elimination depends on the function of the kidneys, ureters, bladder, and urethra. The kidneys remove wastes from the blood and urine. The ureters transport urine from the kidneys to the bladder. The bladder holds urine until the urge to urinate develops and urine leaves the body through the urethra. All these organs must be intact and functional

for the successful removal of urinary wastes. The normal range of urine production is 1 to 2 L/day (Huether and McCance, 2000). Fluid intake and body temperature may affect urine production. Urine is usually 95% water and 5% solutes. These solutes include electrolytes and organic solutes such as urea, uric acid, creatinine, and ammonia.

KIDNEYS. The kidneys are reddish brown, bean-shaped organs that lie on either side of the vertebral column behind the abdominal peritoneum and against the deep muscles of the back. The kidneys are level with the twelfth thoracic and third lumbar vertebrae. The functional units, **nephrons,** remove waste products from the blood and regulate water and electrolyte concentrations in body fluids. The kidneys can efficiently filter the blood of waste products in part because of their high blood flow, which represents approximately 25% of the cardiac output.

A cluster of capillaries forms the **glomerulus,** which is the initial site of urine formation. These capillaries filter water and glucose, amino acids, urea, uric acid, creatinine, and major electrolytes. Protein does not normally filter through the glomerulus. Therefore protein in the urine, **proteinuria,** is a sign of glomerular injury.

However, not all glomerular filtrate is excreted as urine. Approximately 99% is reabsorbed into the plasma. When the filtrate leaves the glomerulus, it passes through a system of tubules in which water and glucose, amino acids, uric acid, sodium, potassium, and bicarbonate ions are selectively reabsorbed into plasma. Hydrogen and potassium ions and ammonia are secreted into the tubules and become a part of the urine.

URETERS. A ureter is attached to each kidney pelvis and carries urinary wastes into the bladder. Urine draining from the ureters to the bladder is sterile. Peristaltic waves cause the urine to enter the bladder in spurts rather than steadily. To prevent urine from returning to the ureters, a small flaplike fold of mucous membrane acts as a valve and covers the juncture of the ureters and bladder.

BLADDER. The urinary bladder is a hollow, distensible, muscular organ that is a reservoir for urine. When empty, the bladder lies in the pelvic cavity behind the symphysis pubis. In the male the bladder rests against the rectum posteriorly, and in the female it rests against the anterior wall of the uterus and vagina.

The bladder's shape changes as it fills with urine. When the bladder is full, its superior surface expands up into a dome and pushes above the symphysis pubis. A greatly distended bladder may reach the umbilicus. In a pregnant woman the fetus pushes against the bladder, causing a feeling of fullness and reducing its capacity.

URETHRA. Urine travels from the bladder through the urethra and passes to the outside of the body through the urethral meatus. Mucous membrane lines the urethra, and urethral glands secrete mucus into the urethral canal. The

Factors Influencing Urinary Elimination   Box 31-1

GROWTH AND DEVELOPMENT

Infants and young children cannot concentrate urine and reabsorb water effectively.

Children cannot control urination voluntarily until 18 to 24 months.

A child must be able to recognize the feeling of bladder fullness, to hold urine for 1 to 2 hours, and to communicate the sense of urgency to a parent.

With age, the ability to concentrate urine declines and the frequency of urination increases.

The process of aging may impair micturition.

Problems of mobility sometimes make it difficult for older adults to reach the toilet or bedside commode in time.

SOCIOCULTURAL FACTORS

Cultural and gender norms vary on the privacy or publicness of urination. North Americans expect toilet facilities to be private, whereas some European cultures accept communal toilet facilities.

Social expectations (e.g., school recesses) influence the time of urination.

PSYCHOLOGICAL FACTORS

Anxiety and stress do not affect the characteristics of urine but may affect a sense of urgency and increase the frequency of urination.

Anxiety may prevent complete urination because tension makes it difficult to relax abdominal muscles.

PERSONAL HABITS

Privacy and adequate time to urinate are usually important to most people. Some people need distractions to relax.

MUSCLE TONE

Weak abdominal and pelvic floor muscles impair bladder contraction and control of the external sphincter.

Decreased muscle tone may be caused by immobility, childbirth, or trauma.

Muscle tone may also be lost with continuous drainage of urine through an indwelling catheter.

FLUID INTAKE

If fluids, electrolytes, and solutes are balanced, increased fluid intake increases urine production.

Alcohol stops the release of antidiuretic hormones, thus promoting urine production.

FLUID INTAKE—cont'd

Fluids containing caffeine increase urinary output frequency.

Foods with high fluid content, such as fruits and vegetables, may increase urine production.

PATHOLOGICAL CONDITIONS

Diabetes mellitus and multiple sclerosis cause neuropathies that alter bladder function.

Rheumatoid arthritis, degenerative joint disease, and parkinsonism slow or hinder physical activity and interfere with urination.

Chronic diseases, such as stroke, alter urinary patterns.

Acute renal disease reduces urine volume; chronic renal disease initially increases volume of poorly concentrated urine.

Febrile conditions reduce the amount of urine but increase its concentration.

Spinal cord injuries interrupt voluntary bladder emptying.

SURGICAL PROCEDURES

The stress response to surgery reduces the amount of urinary output to increase circulatory fluid volume.

Anesthetics and pain-killing drugs slow the filtration rate and reduce urinary output.

Local trauma during lower abdominal and pelvic surgery may obstruct urine flow, so indwelling catheters may be needed.

MEDICATIONS

Diuretics prevent reabsorption of water and certain electrolytes, and urinary output increases.

Some drugs also change the color of urine (e.g., amitriptyline turns it blue-green, and methyldopa turns it red; warfarin sodium turns it orange, and indomethacin turns it green).

Medications may affect the ability to relax and empty the bladder.

DIAGNOSTIC EXAMINATIONS

Following intravenous pyelograms, monitor client for complications such as hypersensitivity reactions and acute renal failure.

Cystoscopy may cause localized edema of the urethral passageway and bladder sphincter spasm, resulting in urinary retention and the passing of red or pink urine.

---

external urethral sphincter, located about halfway down the urethra, permits voluntary flow of urine.

Act of Urination

Urination, **micturition,** and **voiding** are all terms for the process by which urine is expelled from the urinary bladder. The desire to urinate can be sensed when the bladder contains only a small amount of urine (150 to 200 ml in an adult and 50 to 100 ml in a child). As the volume of urine increases, the bladder wall stretches. Normally a person is conscious of the need to urinate. If the person chooses not to void, the external urinary sphincter remains contracted, and the reflex is inhibited. However, when a person is ready to void, the external sphincter relaxes, the micturition reflex stimulates the detrusor muscle to contract, and urination occurs.

Factors Influencing Urination

Normal urinary elimination can be affected by physiological factors, psychosocial conditions, and diagnostic or treatment-induced factors (Box 31-1). Knowledge of these factors enables you to anticipate possible elimination problems.

Common Urinary Elimination Problems

The most common urinary problems involve disturbances in urination. These disturbances result from impaired bladder function, obstruction to urine outflow, or an inability to voluntarily control micturition. Some clients may have permanent or temporary changes in the normal pathway of urination. For example, the client with a **urinary diversion** may have special problems because urine drains through an artificial opening (stoma) on the abdominal wall.

URINARY RETENTION.   **Urinary retention** is an accumulation of urine in the bladder because the bladder is unable to partially or completely empty. The client who retains at least 25% of total bladder capacity is experiencing urinary retention. Urine collects in the bladder, stretching its walls and causing feelings of pressure, discomfort, tenderness over the symphysis pubis, restlessness, and diaphoresis. These findings along with an absence of urinary output over several hours and a distended bladder may indicate urinary retention. In urinary retention the bladder may hold more than 1000 ml of urine.

Eventually retention with overflow may develop. Pressure in the bladder builds so that the external urethral sphincter is unable to hold back urine. The sphincter opens to allow a small volume of urine (25 to 60 ml) to escape, after which the bladder pressure falls enough to allow the sphincter to close. The client may void or be incontinent of small amounts of urine 2 or 3 times an hour with no relief of distention or discomfort. Retention with incontinence is sometimes referred to as overflow incontinence (Fantl and others, 1996).

Decreased urine production can cause retention by filling the bladder gradually, thus preventing activation of the stretch receptors. After distending beyond a certain point, the bladder cannot contract. Retention can occur because of many other factors (Table 31-1).

URINARY TRACT INFECTIONS.   Urinary tract infections account for 36% to 40% of hospital-acquired (**nosocomial**) infections in the United States (Steed, 1999). Most of these infections are directly due to catheterization. **Bacteriuria** (bacteria in the urine) is often inevitable once a retention catheter is inserted (Warren, 1997). The catheter is a source of injury to the mucosa, thus allowing bacterial invasion. It is important to keep catheterization at a minimum because bacteriuria may lead to the spread of organisms into the bloodstream (**urosepsis**) and kidneys, especially in the severely ill client.

Microorganisms can enter the urinary tract through the urethral meatus or the bloodstream. However, the ascending route through the urethra is more common. Bacteria inhabit the vagina in women and the distal urethra and external genitalia in men and women. Organisms enter the urethral meatus easily and travel up the inner mucosal lining to the bladder. Women are more susceptible to urinary tract infection because of the proximity of the anus to the urethral meatus and because of a short urethra. In the male the length of the urethra and the antibacterial substance in prostatic secretions reduce the risk of urinary tract infection.

Normally organisms are flushed out during voiding. However, bladder distention reduces blood flow to the mucosal and submucosal layer, and tissues become more susceptible to bacteria. **Residual urine,** urine that remains in the bladder after urination, is an ideal site for microorganism growth. Table 31-1 summarizes the causes of lower urinary tract infection.

Clients with urinary tract infections often have pain or burning urination (**dysuria**) and urgency. An irritated bladder also causes a frequent and urgent sensation of the need to void. Fever, chills, nausea and vomiting, and malaise may develop. Irritation to bladder and urethral mucosa may result in blood-tinged urine (hematuria). The urine appears concentrated and cloudy because of bacteria. If infection spreads to the kidneys (pyelonephritis), fever, flank pain, tenderness, and chills are common symptoms. The older adult with urinary tract infection with an accompanying fever may also exhibit an alteration in mental status such as acute confusion (Foreman and Zane, 1996).

Formulation of Nursing Diagnoses

Table 31-1

Disorder	Causes
Urinary Retention Urine flow is obstructed; urine accumulates in bladder. Low fluid intake can lead to retention.	Prostate gland enlargement, fecal impaction, pregnancy in third trimester, urethral stricture or edema after childbirth, and urethral edema after surgery or diagnostic examination may obstruct urine flow. Spinal cord and peripheral nerve trauma and degeneration of peripheral nerves (e.g., diabetic neuropathy) alter sensory and motor innervation. Emotional anxiety and muscle tension may alter ability to relax sphincters. Medications (anesthetics and narcotics).
Lower Urinary Tract Infection Microorganisms may be introduced resulting in bacterial spread, causing inflammation of bladder muscle.	Kinked or blocked urethral catheter and urinary retention can cause obstruction of urine flow. Poor perineal hygiene, frequent sexual intercourse, ingredients in bubble baths, improperly handled diagnostic instruments, improperly sterilized instruments, and contaminated urine receptacles can cause spread of bacteria.
Urinary Incontinence Incontinence involves incompetent or weakened sphincter and loss of control of voiding.	Multiple childbirths, pelvic organ surgery, and removal of prostate gland can weaken sphincter. Mental confusion, sedatives or analgesics, spinal cord injury, bladder spasm, and bladder atrophy can cause loss of voiding control.

URINARY INCONTINENCE.   **Urinary incontinence** is the loss of control over voiding. It may be temporary or permanent. The client cannot control the external urethral sphincter. Leakage may be continuous or intermittent. You may be the first or only professional to whom clients will reveal their incontinence. Therefore be sensitive to this problem, which is thought to occur in some settings such as nursing homes in 33% to 50% of the population (Nicolle, 1997). There are five types of incontinence (Table 31-2). The causes of incontinence vary by type.

Incontinence is a common problem that can develop in people of every age. It is a myth that incontinence is caused by aging. The annual cost of incontinence for clients in the community and in nursing homes is over $10 million annually (Fantl and others, 1996). Urinary incontinence has an impact on body image and social interaction. Clothing becomes wet with urine, and the accompanying odor adds to embarrassment. Clients with this problem often avoid physical and social activities (Steeman and Defever, 1998).

Older adults are more susceptible to incontinence because of functional limitations and the environment in which they live. An older person with restricted mobility has a greater chance of being incontinent because of the inability to reach toilet facilities in time. Low-set chairs and high beds may be additional obstacles for the older adult who must get up to reach a toilet. An older adult who has difficulty undoing buttons or manipulating zippers faces another obstacle. The older adult with chronic health problems may lack the energy to walk very far at one time, and if there is only one toilet in the home, the distance may be too far for the client with urge incontinence (Lueckenotte, 2000). Continued episodes of incontinence can create skin breakdown. Acidic urine is irritating to the skin. The client who has frequent incontinence is especially at risk for pressure ulcers (see Chapter 34).

Urinary Diversions

With surgery it is possible to divert the drainage of urine from a diseased or dysfunctional bladder. There are two

Types of Urinary Incontinence

Table 31-2

Description	Causes	Symptoms
Total		
Total uncontrollable and continuous loss of urine	Neuropathy of sensory nerves Trauma or disease of spinal nerves or urethral sphincter	Constant flow of urine at unpredictable times Nocturia Lack of awareness of bladder filling or incontinence
Functional		
Involuntary unpredictable passage of urine in client with intact urinary and nervous systems	Fistula between bladder and vagina Change in environment Sensory, cognitive, or mobility deficits	Strong urge to void with loss of urine before reaching appropriate receptacle
Stress		
Increased intraabdominal pressure causing leakage of small amount of urine	Coughing, laughing, vomiting, or lifting with full bladder Obesity Full uterus pressing against bladder during third trimester of pregnancy Incompetent bladder outlet Weak pelvic musculature	Dribbling of urine with increased intraabdominal pressure Urinary urgency Frequency
Urge		
Involuntary passage of urine after strong sense of urgency to void	Decreased bladder capacity Irritation of bladder stretch receptors Alcohol or caffeine ingestion Increased fluid intake	Urinary urgency Abnormal frequency (more often than every 2 hours) Bladder contracture or spasm Nocturia Voiding in small (less than 100 ml) or in large (more than 550 ml) amounts
Reflex		
Involuntary loss of urine occurring at somewhat predictable intervals when specific bladder volume is reached	Upper spinal cord injury or disease involving area above reflex arc, blocking cerebral awareness Lower spinal cord injury blocking impulses to reflex arc	Lack of awareness of bladder filling No urge to void Uninhibited bladder contraction or spasm or regular interval

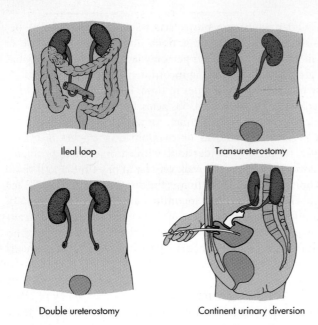

Ileal loop

Transureterostomy

Double ureterostomy

Continent urinary diversion

FIGURE **31-1**   Types of incontinent and continent urinary diversions.

classifications for urinary diversions: continent and incontinent. A **ureterostomy** (an incontinent diversion) is any surgical procedure that creates stomas on the outer abdominal wall for continuous urine drainage. Typically the client with a ureterostomy has had the bladder removed surgically because of a malignant growth, birth defects, or a spinal cord injury. A ureterostomy may be the preferred treatment for chronic incontinence. Figure 31-1 illustrates several types of ureterostomies. The ileal loop or conduit, which has been commonly used for the last 40 years, involves separating a loop of intestinal ileum with its blood supply intact. A ureterostomy involves bringing the end of one or both ureters to the abdominal surface. To avoid the need for two collecting devices, a transureterostomy connects the ureters and brings one out through the abdominal wall.

Surgery for continent diversion creates an internal pouch where urine is stored. Clients do not need to wear an external ostomy pouch over the urinary stoma. Instead they are taught to insert a catheter into their stoma to drain urine periodically throughout the day. A urinary diversion poses threats to body image. The client with an incontinent diversion may wear an artificial device to collect urine and must learn to manage it. The client with a urinary diversion can wear normal clothing, engage in any physical activity, travel, and have sexual relations.

█ NURSING KNOWLEDGE BASE

Urinary elimination is a natural and often private process that may require physiological and psychological assistance. Therefore providing nursing care for a client with

potential or actual urinary problems requires an understanding beyond anatomy and physiology. You must be knowledgeable about concepts such as infection control, hygiene measures, growth, and development and also be sensitive to the client's psychosocial needs when a urinary problem develops.

Infection Control and Hygiene

The urinary tract is a common site for infection, and therefore principles of infection control are used to prevent the onset and spread of urinary tract infections and to promote the treatment of infections that do occur (see Chapter 10). Urinary tract infections are often caused by *Escherichia coli*, and the infections can occur anywhere along the urinary tract from the urethra to the kidneys. Urinary tract infections that occur after admission to a health care facility are called nosocomial infections. The major reason for most nosocomial infections is lack of hand washing (Steed, 1999).

Principles of medical and surgical asepsis must be meticulously followed when carrying out procedures involving the urinary tract or external genitalia. Any instrumentation used on the urinary tract such as catheterization requires the use of sterile technique. Procedures that involve manipulation of the perineum, such as perineal care or examination of the genitalia, require the use of medical asepsis.

Developmental Considerations

The neonate should void within 24 hours after birth. In the neonate and infant, urination is a voiding response and is produced when the bladder fills. As the child reaches the age of 2 or 3, the neuromuscular and cognitive functions develop to the point where the child can begin to control voiding (see Chapter 18).

As we age, changes occur in both the male and female that may contribute to the development of voiding problems. In the male, prostate enlargement may start after age 40 and continue until the 80s, thus producing problems with increased frequency. In the female, childbearing and hormonal levels may influence urination. Changes associated with pregnancy often produce urinary frequency and urgency. With repeated deliveries or hormone changes after menopause, temporary or permanent changes can occur that result in decreased perineal muscle tone. These changes may lead to urgency and stress incontinence (see Table 31-2, p. 767). Hormonal changes may also contribute to an increased susceptibility to infection. Decreased levels of estrogen tend to cause the urethral mucosa to become thinner and more fragile and consequently more easily traumatized and infected (Haus, 1998).

Psychosocial Implications

Self-concept, culture, and sexuality are all closely related concepts that may be affected when a client has elimination problems. Self-concept changes over our life span and includes one's body image, self-esteem, roles, and identity (see Chapter 19). Little children may not want to urinate on the toilet because they don't want to flush part of themselves away. Gender influences the position we use to urinate. Males tend to stand to urinate, and females assume a sitting position. Culture may influence how urination is talked about and how much privacy is needed. It may be considered improper in some cultures for a male to ask a female client about private matters such as urination.

CRITICAL THINKING

Synthesis

In caring for clients with altered patterns of elimination, you need to synthesize knowledge, draw from experience, apply critical thinking attitudes, and be knowledgeable about the standards of practice. Practical experience and knowledge from scientific and nursing domains assist in providing individualized nursing care for these clients.

KNOWLEDGE.   It is important that you understand changes in normal urinary elimination caused by pathological conditions and changes associated with age, gender, and improper hygiene practices. A comprehensive view of your client's situation allows you to make the most accurate decisions about client care. Information regarding a client's fluid balance and knowledge of medication will further complement your knowledge base.

When clients have changes in their fluid balance, this also affects elimination patterns. In addition, these changes can increase the clients' risks for impairments in urination related to infection, incontinence, or retention.

EXPERIENCE.   Previous and personal experience can provide a basis for determining elimination needs. Perhaps you have cared for a previous client who was incontinent. Perhaps you or a close personal friend has had personal experience of a Foley catheter insertion, or you or a friend had a urinary tract infection and experienced frequency, burning, urgency, and hesitancy. Last, when caring for previous clients, experience has taught you that voiding patterns are individual and to find out about voiding patterns you must ask clients about their usual patterns of elimination.

ATTITUDE.   Elimination needs of clients are individual and very personal. Flexibility and creativity are needed to establish elimination schedules and interventions. You must always consider the client's preferences first in setting elimination practices and priorities. Perseverance and client advocacy enables you to respond promptly to the client's need to adapt to altered urinary elimination.

STANDARDS.   Because urination is often a private matter, you must protect the client's privacy. In addition, it is important that you adhere to the standards of medical and sur-

gical asepsis. Some of the interventions you select to restore urinary elimination may be invasive. Adherence to standards of asepsis reduces risk of infection.

NURSING PROCESS

Assessment

You need to complete a nursing history, perform a physical assessment, assess the client's urine, and review information from laboratory and diagnostic tests to identify a urinary elimination problem.

NURSING HISTORY.   Information from the scientific and the nursing knowledge base assist you in completing a nursing history. The nursing history includes a review of the client's elimination patterns and symptoms of urinary alterations and assessment of factors that may be affecting the ability to urinate normally.

PATTERN OF URINATION.   Ask the client about daily voiding patterns, including frequency and times of day, normal volume at each voiding, and history of recent changes. Frequency varies among individuals. Most people void an average of 5 or more times a day. The client who voids frequently during the night may have renal or cardiovascular disease. Information about the pattern of urination is necessary to establish a baseline of comparison.

SYMPTOMS OF URINARY ALTERATIONS.   Certain symptoms of alterations may occur in more than one type of urinary disorder. During assessment ask the client about the presence of symptoms listed in Table 31-3. Also determine whether the client is aware of conditions or factors that precipitate or aggravate symptoms.

FACTORS AFFECTING URINATION.   Focused assessment enables you to gather data relevant to your client's elimination pattern (Table 31-4). In addition, there are important factors in the client's history that normally affect urination. These factors include the following:

1. Medications, including prescribed, over-the-counter, and herbal supplements, may affect fluid and electrolyte balance. Diuretics are successfully used to regulate fluid balance; however, side effects can further potentiate fluid and electrolyte imbalances. Narcotic analgesics may cause urinary retention. Anesthetics can temporarily depress renal function.
2. Consider the client's mobility status as it influences access to toileting facilities. Assessments that should be made include use of walking aids, distance to the toilet, ability to remove clothing or to get in and out of the bathroom, and lighting.
3. Environmental barriers in the home or health care setting may prevent the client from accessing the toilet.

Common Symptoms of Urinary Alterations

Table 31-3

Description	Causes or Associated Factors
Urgency Feeling of the need to void immediately	Full bladder Inflammation or irritation to bladder mucosa from infection Incompetent urethral sphincter Psychological stress
Dysuria Painful or difficult urination	Bladder inflammation Trauma or inflammation of urethra
Frequency Voiding at frequent intervals	Increased fluid intake Bladder inflammation Increased pressure on bladder (e.g., pregnancy or psychological stress)
Hesitancy Difficulty in initiating urination	Prostate enlargement Anxiety Urethral edema
Polyuria Voiding large amount of urine	Excess fluid intake Diabetes mellitus or insipidus Use of diuretics
Oliguria Diminished urinary output in relation to fluid intake	Dehydration Renal failure Urinary tract obstruction Increased secretion of antidiuretic hormone (ADH)
Nocturia Urination, particularly excessive, at night	Excess intake of fluids (especially coffee or alcohol before bedtime) Renal disease Cardiovascular disease
Dribbling Leakage of urine despite voluntary control of micturition	Urine retention from incomplete bladder emptying Stress incontinence
Hematuria Presence of blood in urine	Neoplasms of kidney, certain glomerular diseases, infections of kidneys or bladder, traumatic injury to urinary structure, calculi, blood dyscrasia
Retention Accumulation of urine in bladder, with inability of bladder to empty	Urethral obstruction, bladder inflammation, decreases in sensory activity, neurogenic bladder, prostate enlargement after anesthesia, side effects of certain medications (e.g., anticholinergics, antispasmodics, antidepressants)
Residual Urine Volume of urine remaining in bladder after voiding (volumes of 100 ml or more)	Inflammation or irritation of bladder mucosa from infection, neurogenic bladder, prostatic enlargement, trauma or inflammation of urethra

The client may need an elevated toilet seat, grab bars, or a portable commode (Smith, 1994).

4. Sensory restrictions (e.g., clients with visual problems who may have trouble reaching toilet facilities) may hamper self-toileting. If the client has difficulty with hand coordination, assess the type of clothing and the client's ease in using clothing fasteners.

5. Past illness such as urinary tract infection or surgery increases the risk for recurrent problems. Chronic diseases (e.g., multiple sclerosis) that impair bladder function require you to consider preventive care measures. Clients returning from surgery often have difficulty voiding the first few hours until the effects of anesthesia diminish.

6. Clients recovering from major surgery and suffering critical illness or disability often have an indwelling catheter to aid urinary drainage and provide a measurement of urinary output. A catheter places a client at risk for infection.

Example of a Focused Client Assessment		Table 31-4
Factors to Assess	**Questions and Approaches**	**Physical Assessment Strategies**
Fluids	Determine if client has any fluid restrictions. Ask if client is able to obtain fluids independently. Ask what client's usual 24-hour intake equals.	Observe skin and mucous membranes. Obtain intake and output.
Urinary elimination	In ambulatory clients: Ask client about ability to use toileting facilities. For clients with restricted mobility: Determine client's frequency and needs in using toileting facilities with assistance. Ask client what type of assistance was used at home.	Observe client's ability to use toileting facilities. Observe assistance with transfer and ambulation to and from the toilet area.
Bladder	Ask or determine when client last voided, noting amount of urine. Ask client about perception of urge to void. Ask client if bladder feels empty after voiding.	Palpate bladder.

7. The presence of urinary diversion will directly affect urinary elimination. If the client has a urinary diversion, assess its type, location, and function. The condition of surrounding skin and usual methods for management (presence of appliance or pouch, type of skin care products and application) should also be assessed. If the client has an incontinent diversion, assess the methods and frequency of appliance changes and the type of nighttime drainage system. In addition, in the client with a continent urinary diversion (CUR) the frequency and type of catheters used to drain urine must be determined.

8. Personal habits may inhibit urination or put the client at risk for infection. If a client is hospitalized, assess the extent to which personal habits are altered. Privacy is often difficult to accomplish in a health care setting, particularly if a client must use a bedpan (see Chapter 32) or a urinal. Determine the client's knowledge and practices of perineal hygiene (see Chapter 26).

9. Fluid intake is directly related to urinary output. A client's physical condition affects the frequency with which you monitor fluid intake (see Chapter 14). Regular intake and output (I&O) measurements help to assess a client's overall fluid balance. Clients who have urinary tract infections and are experiencing urgency, burning, and frequency may mistakenly decrease their fluid intake to try to fix the symptoms.

10. Consider the client's age when assessing micturition habits. Toilet training and enuresis are concerns that arise in the toddler and preschooler. In the adult increasing age may bring disease and physiological changes that predispose to incontinence.

CLIENT EXPECTATIONS.   Note the client's responses to questions about urination. Does the client seem hesitant or embarrassed? Psychosocial factors such as culture or sexuality may be influencing the client's response. In addition, ask the client what he or she expects from care. Does the client expect the infection to be resolved? Does the woman who has stress incontinence expect this condition to be relieved?

Because urination is often considered a private matter, clients may find it difficult to be asked about their voiding habits. The postoperative client or client taking medications that affect urination may become concerned that something is wrong when asked every couple of hours if they have voided. Clients receiving intravenous (IV) fluids may not realize that they may have an increased need for urination. Urinary catheters may indicate to some that the client is very ill; they may not recognize that urinary catheters are used for diagnosis and monitoring for a variety of clients.

PHYSICAL ASSESSMENT

SKIN AND MUCOSA.   Assess the skin's hydration status by noting texture and turgor. Observe the skin around periurethral tissues and stomas for excoriation, drainage, and tenderness. Urinary incontinence, fluid imbalance, and electrolyte disturbances increase the risk for skin breakdown. Observation of the oral mucosa also reveals whether hydration is adequate.

KIDNEYS.   If the kidneys become infected or inflamed, flank pain typically develops. You can assess for tenderness early in the disease by gently percussing the costoveretbral angle (the angle formed by the spine and twelfth rib). Inflammation of the kidney results in pain on percussion.

BLADDER.   Normally the bladder rests below the symphysis pubis and cannot be examined. When distended, the bladder rises above the symphysis pubis at the midline of the abdomen and just below the umbilicus. When you apply light pressure to the bladder, the client may feel tenderness or even pain. Palpation may also cause the urge to urinate.

URETHRAL MEATUS.   The female client assumes a dorsal recumbent position to provide full exposure of the genitalia. Using the gloved nondominant hand retract the labial folds to observe the urethral meatus. There is normally no discharge from the meatus. Drainage may indicate infection. Be sure you note the color and consistency of drainage.

The male's urethral meatus is normally a small opening at the tip of the penis. To inspect the meatus for discharge and inflammation, it may be necessary for you to retract the foreskin in uncircumcised males. Following inspection of the meatus, return foreskin over the meatus.

ASSESSMENT OF URINE.   The assessment of urine involves measuring the client's fluid intake and urinary output and observing the characteristics of the urine.

Intake and Output.   When clients have altered or impaired urinary elimination, their I&O is measured to help monitor fluid and electrolyte balance. Although often written as part of a physician's order, placing a client on I&O may be a nurse's or a physician's judgment. Placing a client on I&O measurements requires cooperation and assistance from the client and family. Intake measurements must include all oral liquids and semiliquids; all enteral feedings through nasogastric, gastrostomy, or jejunostomy tubes; and all parenteral fluids such as intravenous solutions, blood components, and parenteral nutrition (see Chapter 14).

You are responsible for accurate recording. Measurements are kept throughout the day and totaled every 8 hours, but you may determine that more frequent measurements are required. Marking the I&O when the client has voided or eaten is often a task that is delegated. Before delegating this task, inform the care provider what the metric conversions are for common liquid-holding containers such as coffee cups and milk cartons and ensure that the care provider knows aseptic principles relating to body fluids. In addition, caution the care provider to be sensitive to the privacy needs of the clients and clarify what should be reported to you about I&O, such as changes in color, amount, or odor of urine or presence and frequency of incontinence. If the client needs assistance, inform the care provider about the amount of assistance the client requires to use the urinal or bedpan and if standing or bathroom privileges are permitted.

Urinary output is a key indicator of kidney function. A change in urine volume is a significant indicator of fluid imbalance, kidney dysfunction, or decreased blood volume. For example, in a catheterized postoperative client, hourly urinary output provides an indirect measure of circulating volume. If the urinary output falls below 30 ml/hr, notify the physician and assess for other signs of blood loss.

Assess urine volume by measuring with a **graduated measuring container** (receptacle for volume measurement) the output that has been collected in a bedpan, urinal, **urine hat** (a receptacle that fits inside the commode), or catheter bag. It is critical that each client have an individual measuring container with name and room number marked on it and that only one graduate be used for each client. Transmission of microorganisms occurs when equipment is used for other clients.

Special **urometers** attach to catheter drainage tubing and are a convenient means of measuring small urine volume on a regular basis. A urometer holds 100 to 200 ml of urine. After measuring urine from a urometer, drain the cylinder into the urinary drainage bag or into a receptacle for disposal.

If a precise measurement of fluid intake is needed from the client who is at home, you may need to ask the client to show a commonly used glass or cup on which the intake estimate is based.

Characteristics.   Inspect the client's urine for color, clarity, and odor. Monitor and document any changes. In a client with a known urinary tract infection who has had a slight sediment in the urine, this information would be monitored for improvement and recorded.

Color.   Normal urine ranges in color from a pale straw color to amber, depending on its concentration. Urine is usually more concentrated in the morning. As the person drinks more fluids, it becomes less concentrated.

Unexpected changes such as the appearance of blood in the urine (**hematuria**) should alert you to assess for associated signs and symptoms and report the information to the physician. Bleeding from the kidneys or ureters usually causes urine to become dark red; bleeding from the bladder or urethra usually causes a bright red urine.

Drugs can also change the urine's color. Beets, rhubarb, and blackberries may cause red urine. Special dyes used in intravenous diagnostic studies are eventually excreted by the kidneys and discolor the urine. Dark amber urine may be the result of high concentrations of bilirubin (urobilinogen) in clients with liver disease. Report unexpected color changes to the physician.

Clarity.   Normal urine appears transparent at the time of voiding. Urine that stands several minutes in a container becomes cloudy. Freshly voided urine in clients with renal disease may appear cloudy because of protein concentration. Urine also appears thick and cloudy as a result of bacteria.

Odor.   Urine has a characteristic ammonia odor. The more concentrated the urine, the stronger the odor. As urine remains standing (e.g., in a collection device), more ammonia breakdown occurs, and the odor becomes stronger.

LABORATORY AND DIAGNOSTIC TESTING.   You may be responsible for collecting urine specimens for laboratory testing. The type of test determines the method of collection. Label all specimens with the client's name, date, and time of collection. Table 31-5 lists routine urinary analysis and specific nursing interpretations for each type of measurement.

SPECIMEN COLLECTION.   You may collect several types of urine specimens for testing.

Urinalysis Sample.   A simple urinalysis does not require a sterile urine specimen. The laboratory performs urinalysis on a routine or clean-voided specimen or on a specimen obtained from a catheter. The urinalysis is a screening test for renal disease, metabolic disorders, lower urinary tract alterations, and fluid imbalances (see Table 31-5). For a quick screening, you can perform certain portions of the urinalysis with special reagent strips. Dip the strip into the urine and watch for a color change, which indicates the presence of protein, blood, sugar, ketones, and other solutes. You can

Routine Urinalysis Values

Table 31-5

Measurement (Normal Value)	Interpretation
pH (4.6 to 8.0)	pH level helps to indicate acid-base balance. Urine that stands for several hours becomes alkaline from bacterial invasion. If pH is alkaline, selected antibiotics (e.g., neomycin and streptomycin) are more effective against urinary tract infections.
Protein (up to 8 mg/100 ml)	Protein is normally not present in urine. It is seen in renal disease because damage to glomerular membrane allows protein to enter urine. However, temporary presence of protein can occur after strenuous exercise, exposure to cold, or psychological stress.
Glucose (not normally present)	Diabetic clients have glucose in urine because of inability of tubules to reabsorb high serum glucose concentrations (over 180 mg/100 ml). Ingestion of high concentrations of glucose may cause some to appear in urine of healthy persons.
Ketones (not normally present)	With poor control of diabetes, clients experience breakdown of fatty acids. End product of fatty acid metabolism is ketones. Clients with dehydration, starvation, or excessive aspirin ingestion also have ketonuria.
Blood (up to two red blood cells)	Damage to glomerulus or tubules may cause blood cells to enter urine. Trauma or disease of lower urinary tract also causes hematuria.
Specific gravity (1.01 to 1.03)	Specific gravity tests measure concentration of particles in urine. High specific gravity reflects concentrated urine, and low specific gravity reflects diluted urine. Dehydration, reduced renal blood flow, and increase in ADH secretion elevate specific gravity. Overhydration and inadequate ADH secretion reduce it.

also perform a specific gravity test in the clinic or hospital unit.

The client may void into a clean urine cup, a urinal, or a bedpan. The client must void before defecating so that feces do not contaminate the specimen. If a woman is menstruating, make note of this on the specimen requisition in case red blood cells appear. Transfer the urine to the proper container, and send it to the laboratory.

Clean-Voided or Midstream Specimen. To obtain a specimen relatively free of the microorganisms growing in the lower urethra, you need to instruct the client on the method for obtaining a clean-voided specimen. Female and male clients are given a sterile urine cup, sterile disinfectant wipes, and clean gloves. The cup and disinfectant wipes are often prepackaged together. The package usually contains instructions, but the client should be instructed on how to wash and how to collect the specimen. Anxiety, difficulty or inability to read, or language barriers may prohibit the client from fully comprehending the instructions independently.

The woman should wipe from the meatus toward the rectum. The man cleans the meatus in a circular motion moving from the meatus up the glans penis. Caution the client against wiping repeatedly with the contaminated cloth. The client receives a sterile urine cup. Tell your client to start and discard the initial stream into a toilet or bedpan. This cleans or flushes the urethral orifice and meatus of resident bacteria. During the midstream, or middle portion of voiding, collect the specimen. Immediately after obtaining the specimen, place a sterile top securely over the container and send it to the laboratory for testing. Urine specimens must reach the laboratory within 1 hour of collection or be refrigerated. Urine that stands in a container at room temperature can grow bacteria.

Sterile Specimen. Another method for collecting a sterile urine specimen for culture is by catheterizing a client or by obtaining the specimen from an indwelling catheter. Urine specimens should not be collected for culture from urine drainage bags unless it is the first urine drained into a new sterile bag. Bacteria grow rapidly in drainage bags, and the specimen would give a false measurement of bacteria.

During catheterization collect the specimen as soon as urine flows from the catheter's end. After filling the sample container, you can withdraw the catheter or connect the newly inserted indwelling catheter to a drainage tube (see Skill 31-1, p. 781).

If a client already has an indwelling catheter, use a sterile syringe to withdraw urine. Most urine drainage tubes have special ports referred to as sampling ports to withdraw specimens. Some companies have mass-produced catheters with a sampling port that accepts most plastic or blunt cannulas (needle less) to reduce the risk of needle stick. Read the manufacturer's instructions to determine if the catheter tubing in use accepts blunt cannulas.

First, clamp the tubing about 3 inches below the sampling port, allowing fresh sterile urine to collect in the tube. Then wipe the port with a disinfectant swab. Using the needleless device or the agency-recommended procedure, withdraw 3 ml for a culture. While aspirating urine, be careful not to raise the tubing, which would cause urine to return (backflow) to the bladder.

After obtaining the specimen, transfer the urine into a sterile container using sterile aseptic technique and place it in a plastic pouch or bag per agency policy for transportation to the laboratory. The laboratory requisition should indicate the way the specimen was collected. The site from which the specimen was obtained should be inspected periodically to check that the catheter is not leaking.

Twenty-Four-Hour Urine Specimen. Some tests of renal function and urine composition require a 24-hour collection of urine. You must indicate the starting time on the gallon container and on the laboratory requisition. **Always discard the first sample.** The 24-hour collection period begins after the first specimen is discarded. The client then collects all urine voided in 24 hours. Any missed specimens make the results inaccurate, and the test must be restarted. You should remind the client to void before defecating so that feces do not contaminate urine. If there is fecal contamination, consult the laboratory for instructions. The client should void the last specimen as close as possible to the end of the 24-hour period.

Common Urine Tests. In addition to urinalysis, other tests that may be performed are measurement of specific gravity, urine culture, and glucose and ketone levels. Your role in collecting specimens is that of teaching. You should identify what preparation (if any) is needed before the test, what is expected of the client during the test, and any post-test care.

Specific Gravity. To measure specific gravity you use a urinometer and cylinder. The urinometer has a specific gravity scale at the top and a weighted mercury bulb at the bottom. Pour a urine specimen into a clean dry cylinder and suspend the weighted urinometer in it. The concentration of dissolved substances in the urine determines the depth at which the urinometer will float. The point the level of urine reaches on the urinometer scale is the specific gravity measurement.

Urine Culture. A urine culture simply requires a sterile sample of urine. It takes approximately 72 hours before the laboratory can report significant findings of bacterial growth. If bacteria are present, an additional test for sensitivity determines the antibiotics that will be effective or ineffective.

DIAGNOSTIC EXAMINATIONS. The urinary system is one of the few organ systems amenable to accurate diagnostic study by radiographic techniques. The two approaches for visualizing urinary structures, namely direct and indirect techniques, can be quite simplistic or very complex, requiring extensive nursing interventions. These procedures are further subdivided into invasive and noninvasive categories.

Noninvasive Procedures

Abdominal Roentgenogram. Abdominal roentgenogram, also referred to as plain film, KUB, or flat plate of the abdomen, is commonly used to assess the gross structures of the urinary tract for abnormalities. It can be used to determine size, parity, shape, and location of the kidneys, ureters, and bladder structures. It is also useful in visualizing calculi or tumors in these organs.

Intravenous Pyelogram. To view the entire urinary system and to assess some renal function, excretory urogram or intravenous pyelogram (IVP) is done. Although these procedures are noninvasive, the IVP does require that the client receive an intravenous injection of a radiopaque dye. Because the kidneys and ureters lie behind the intestines, it is necessary that the client receive a bowel preparation before the procedure.

Nursing implications before the test include recognizing clients at risk for alterations in renal function as a result of the intravenous injection of the contrast material. Any client with preexisting renal insufficiency is at risk. Older adults in particular are prone to the nephrotoxic effects of these substances because of their risk for volume depletion during bowel preparation. Appropriate nursing assessment of fluid volume status before this procedure is of utmost importance (see Chapter 14).

Additional nursing implications before the test are as follows:
1. Assess the client for allergy: intravenous contrast materials; shellfish or iodine allergy, which may predict allergies to the IVP dye.
2. If ordered, have the client complete bowel preparation the evening before the test.
3. Explain that the client is usually allowed nothing by mouth (NPO) after midnight.
4. Explain that an intravenous infusion for dye injection is started before the test.
5. Explain that facial flushing is normal during dye injection and that the client may feel dizzy, warm, or nauseous.
6. Explain that the test involves x-ray studies taken at several intervals and that the client will void near the end of the test.

Nursing implications after the test are as follows:
1. Ensure that the client resumes a normal diet.
2. Encourage fluid intake to minimize dehydration caused by fasting and to avoid the potential nephrotoxic effects of the contrast material.
3. Remind the client to watch for itching, rash, or hives, which indicate delayed hypersensitivity to IVP dye.
4. Monitor I&O, or explain to the client to report decreased or absent urination.

Renal Scan. Renal scans allow indirect visualization of urinary tract structures after an intravenous injection of radioactive isotopes. Except for the venipuncture, the procedure is painless. The scanning procedure is completed in approximately 1 hour. Information pertaining to renal blood flow, anatomical structures, and their excretory function can be obtained from this procedure. This procedure is indicated for clients unable to receive IVP dyes.

Nursing implications before the test include the following:
1. Explain that the radioisotope is injected intravenously through an existing IV line or needle.
2. Explain that the client will feel no discomfort but must lie still.
3. Explain that there is no risk of radioactive exposure.

Computerized Axial Tomography. Computerized axial tomography is used to visualize abnormal pathologic conditions such as tumors, obstructions, retroperitoneal masses, and lymph node enlargement. Although this procedure is noninvasive, in some examinations oral and/or intravenous contrast material is used to enhance the areas under study.

Renal Ultrasound. Ultrasonography is a painless, noninvasive diagnostic tool in the assessment of urinary disorders. The ultrasound is used to identify gross renal anatomy and structural abnormalities of the kidneys or lower urinary tract.

Invasive Procedures

Endoscopy. Endoscopy is the visualization of organs with the aid of a telescope or fiber-optic imaging. To view the interior of the bladder and urethra, the physician performs a cystoscopy. The cytoscope looks like a urinary catheter, although it is not as flexible. It is inserted through the urethra. The procedure is painful during instrument insertion. Unless the client lies still, the bladder may be perforated. Local, spinal, or general anesthesia may be administered. Because the test requires insertion of a foreign object into a sterile cavity, the client receives large amounts of fluids (intravenously or orally) before and during the procedure to maintain a continuous urine flow and to flush out bacteria. Antibiotics may also be administered intravenously. During the test, urine and tissue specimens may be collected.

Nursing implications before the test include the following:

1. Observe the client signing an informed consent form.
2. Perform a bowel preparation or enema, or administer a cathartic on the evening before the test.
3. If local anesthetic will be used, encourage intake of oral fluids.
4. In general anesthetic is to be used, ensure that the client is NPO after midnight.
5. Because this procedure is considered a minor surgical procedure, a preoperative checklist may need to be completed (see Chapter 36).
6. Explain that insertion of the cystoscope is similar to insertion of a urethral catheter.
7. Explain the importance of lying still during the test.
8. Explain that an intravenous line will be started to give fluids during the test.
9. Administer a sedative or analgesic per the physician's orders.

Nursing implications after the test include the following:

1. Instruct the client to remain in bed as ordered.
2. Assess for signs of urinary retention and first voiding.
3. Observe characteristics of urine, noting bloody or cloudy urine.
4. Encourage increased fluid intake, and monitor I&O.
5. Observe for fever, dysuria, or a change in blood pressure.
6. Administer medications to alleviate bladder spasms and/or lower back pain.

In addition to complete visual inspection of the bladder and urethra through the cystoscope, retrograde pyelography may also be performed. During this procedure the physician passes a small catheter through the cystoscope into the bladder that allows catheterizing of the ureters and renal pelvis. Urine specimens are then collected separately from each ureter. Radiopaque dye can be instilled into the renal pelvis while serial x-ray films are taken to examine the filling of the renal collecting system.

Invasive examinations to visualize the bladder and urethra include retrograde cystograms, voiding cystourethrogram, and cystourethrogram. All of these studies involve the instillation of a radiopaque fluid into the bladder via a catheter (urethral or suprapubic). Serial x-ray films taken during this procedure will provide information regarding abnormalities. Nursing implications for this procedure are the same as those for the cystoscopy procedure.

Arteriogram (Angiogram). The renal angiogram is an invasive radiographic procedure with radiopaque contrast material that outlines the vascular supply to the kidneys. Most frequently this procedure evaluates the arterial system; however, techniques to investigate the venous system (venogram) are available. Pretest nursing implications are similar to those for the IVP. Clients may be given a narcotic or antianxiety agent for relaxation before the examination.

Nursing implications after the angiogram include the following:

1. Monitor the client's vital signs hourly until stability is verified, and then advance the intervals to every 2 hours, then every 4 hours.
2. Ensure that the client maintains bed rest for 4 to 8 hours.
3. Check pulses and assess the circulation in the cannulated extremity.
4. Observe for bleeding, increased tenderness, or hematoma formation at the catheter insertion site for 24 hours.
5. Maintain a pressure dressing over the site for 24 hours.
6. Observe the client for possible delayed allergic reactions to the contrast material.
7. Monitor the client's I&O, and report abnormalities in urine volume to the physician.

Urodynamic Testing. Urodynamic testing is a group of tests that measure transport, elimination, and storage of urine in the lower urinary tract. The tests do not cause much pain, but they do require catheterization. A contraindication to testing is a urinary tract infection. Care after the procedures includes teaching the client the signs and symptoms of

SYNTHESIS IN PRACTICE

Case Study

As Mrs. Stone prepares to assess the client, she remembers that urinary problems are common in older adults but that age alone does not cause incontinence. She recalls that clients with urinary retention may leak urine and therefore be misdiagnosed as incontinent. She knows clients generally should void at least every 6 to 8 hours and that Mrs. Vallero's problems last night with urination, her recent catheterization, and her decreased mobility since hospitalization could predispose her to retention or incontinence. In addition, she knows she will need to assess if Mrs. Vallero feels the urge to urinate, if she has gone to the bathroom to try to urinate, and to find out more about her normal urination patterns at home.

Previous clinical experience has taught Mrs. Stone that palpation of the abdomen can cause some discomfort. Mrs. Vallero grimaces slightly when her abdomen is palpated and says she's only got a little "dolor."

Because pneumonia and bed rest have left Mrs. Vallero in a weakened state, Mrs. Stone must be flexible and creative in designing a plan of care to meet the client's elimination needs. This plan needs to incorporate scheduled voiding, oral fluids, and increased physical activity.

infection and to report to the physician if any of those signs and symptoms appears.

Nursing Diagnosis

Thorough assessment of the client's urinary function may identify defining characteristics that support actual or risk for elimination problems. Identification of the defining characteristics leads you to select an appropriate diagnostic label. It is very helpful to read the definition of the diagnosis and to examine whether there is a match between the data you collected and the defining characteristics.

There are five recognized diagnoses for incontinence (Box 31-2), and it is not easy for the beginning student to make a decision without looking for a match between data and defining characteristics. The differentiation between stress and urge incontinence is a common problem. In both, the client has an involuntary loss of urine, but the accuracy of data collection helps to identify the correct diagnosis. If the client loses urine after sneezing or coughing, then the diagnosis is stress incontinence. If the client reports that there was a strong urge to urinate just before the incontinence occurred, then the diagnosis is urge incontinence.

Associated problems require interventions that often have no direct effect on urinary elimination. For example, when the client has the diagnosis *toileting self-care deficit related to limited lower extremity mobility,* appropriate nursing interventions provide the client a means of easy access to toileting facilities. However, if you identify the related factor in the aforementioned example to be loss of voluntary control of micturition, interventions would be selected to prevent incontinence. It is important to identify the correct related factors for a given nursing diagnosis because this will affect the selection of the appropriate nursing interventions.

Planning

GOALS AND OUTCOMES. Client-centered goals and outcomes should be established in collaboration with the client and family. A realistic client goal may be that the client has normal micturition with complete bladder emptying within 1 month. To achieve this goal a number of outcomes may be identified; for example, the client will ingest at least 2000 ml of fluids per day, empty the bladder within 1 hour of drinking, and have less than 50 ml of residual urine. Problems develop when the goal and outcomes are established without adequate assessment and collaboration with the client.

You and the client work together to establish ways of maintaining client involvement in nursing care and to maintain normal elimination patterns when possible (see care plan). Reinforcement of good health habits that are already followed improves the likelihood for compliance with the plan of care. Determine the client's educational needs. Return demonstrations of psychomotor and self-care skills are performed by the client to ensure adherence to procedures and accuracy in their performance.

Box 31-2
Nursing Diagnoses for CLIENTS WITH ALTERATIONS IN URINARY ELIMINATION

- Body image, disturbed
- Incontinence, functional urinary
- Incontinence, reflex urinary
- Incontinence, stress urinary
- Incontinence, total urinary
- Incontinence, urge urinary
- Infection, risk for
- Knowledge, deficient
- Pain, acute
- Pain, chronic
- Self-care deficit, toileting
- Skin integrity, risk for impaired
- Urinary elimination, impaired
- Urinary retention

SETTING PRIORITIES. It is important to establish priorities of care based on client's immediate physical and safety needs, client expectations, and readiness to perform some self-care activities. For example, a client with a long-term continent urinary diversion admitted with a severe urinary tract infection expects to resume his or her self-care routine. However, due to the severity of the infection, all care for the client's urinary diversion must be done with sterile technique. In this case the priorities are to treat the infection, prevent reinfection, and teach the client how to perform sterile techniques.

CONTINUITY OF CARE. In the hospital, planning for care also includes preparations for discharge. The need for home health services should be explored and appropriate referrals made. Planning should include consideration of the client's home environment and normal elimination routines. Determine if there is a need to enlist the assistance of other disciplines in this planning process (e.g., social services) to explore family financial resources or other influences that may affect the discharge process. Community resources, such as ostomy support groups for clients with incontinent diversions, may be used.

Significant others are also included in discharge planning and in teaching sessions. Identify who will be involved with the care of the client at home. Your active and thoughtful role in planning these interventions will result in the client's progress toward improved urinary elimination.

Implementation

Clients should know basic mechanisms for urine production and voiding. Your care is focused in three general areas, health promotion, acute care, and restorative and continuing care. The specific interventions include client education, normal micturition, complete bladder emptying, prevention of infection, skin integrity, and comfort.

HEALTH PROMOTION. Success of therapies aimed at optimizing normal urinary elimination depends in part on successful client education (Box 31-3). Instruct clients about their specific elimination problems. For example, a client who practices poor hygiene will benefit from learning about normal sterility of the urinary tract and ways to prevent bac-

Case Study Nursing Care Plan   URINARY RETENTION

ASSESSMENT

Mrs. Vallero is **unable to void after catheter removal.** She has been catheterized once and 1100 ml of urine obtained. She complains of **dribbling** and being unable to urinate. She was **incontinent** on the last shift of a **small amount of urine.** The nursing assessment reveals a **distended bladder.**

*Defining characteristics are shown in bold type.

NURSING DIAGNOSIS

Urinary retention related to detrusor inadequacy secondary to catheterization.

PLANNING

GOAL

Client will have normal micturition with complete bladder emptying in 2 days.

EXPECTED OUTCOMES

Client will void within 8 hours.
Client will void 300 ml or more with each voiding.
Client's urine remains clear yellow.
Client is free of discomfort during voiding.
Client's bladder remains nondistended.

IMPLEMENTATION

STEPS

1. Have client attempt voiding at regularly scheduled times.
2. Have client use bladder compression (Credé's method) during voiding.
3. Allow client to sit on toilet for 15 minutes to encourage second voiding.
4. Encourage fluids of 2000 ml/day.

RATIONAL

Training bladder can help reduce dribbling (Dowd and others, 2000).
Credé's method helps to stimulate micturition and promotes bladder emptying.
Sitting on the toilet facilitates the use of the abdominal muscles and gravity to promote voiding.
Adequate fluids are necessary to ensure perfusion of the kidneys.

EVALUATION

- Measure and observe color of each voided specimen.
- Palpate client's bladder every 4 hours and after each voiding.
- Ask client about sensation to void, bladder fullness, and discomfort when voiding.

Urinary Elimination Health Promotion/Restoration Activities   Box 31-3

ADEQUATE HYDRATION

A client with normal renal function who does not have heart disease or alterations requiring fluid restriction should drink 2000 to 2500 ml of fluid daily (Marchiondo, 1998).

MICTURITION HABITS

Ensure client comfort and privacy.
Allow sufficient time to void (at least 30 minutes).
Integrating the client's habits into the care plan fosters a more normal voiding pattern.
Offer the client use of toilet facilities if possible, avoiding bedpans.
Ensure access to toilet facilities.
Assist the client in the appropriate position for voiding (i.e., females—sitting, males—standing).

PERSONAL HYGIENE

Instruct female clients to cleanse the perineum and urethra from front to back after each voiding and bowel movement.
Clients prone to urinary tract infections should be encouraged to shower instead of bathe (Marchondo, 1998).

COMPLETE BLADDER EMPTYING

Clients who have difficulty starting or stopping the urine stream may benefit from exercises to strengthen pelvic muscles (Johnson, 2000).
Credé's method of manual bladder compression helps to stimulate urination and manually expels urine when bladder tone is reduced.

COMPLETE BLADDER EMPTYING—cont'd

Drug therapy alone or in conjunction with other therapies can be useful for treating problems of incontinence and retention (Johnson, 2000).

INFECTION PREVENTION

Ensure adequate fluid intake.
Encourage good hand washing.
Prevent breaks in closed catheter drainage systems.
Follow tips for preventing infection in catheterized clients.
Teach client how to keep urine acidic. Acid urine tends to inhibit growth of microorganisms. Meats, eggs, whole-grain breads, cranberries, and prunes increase urine acidity (Marchiondo, 1998).

SKIN INTEGRITY

The skin is the first barrier of defense.
The normal acidity of urine is irritating to the skin.
Washing with mild soap and warm water is the best way to remove urine from the skin.
After performing hygiene, dry clothing should be applied immediately on incontinent client.
Clients with external urinary devices should receive assistance in selecting appliances that fit appropriately. They should also be taught preventive skin care measures.

URINARY ELIMINATION PROBLEMS
- Instruct client or caregiver about observations to make regarding urinary output.
- Provide clients with pertinent signs and symptoms of infection.
- Frequently remind ambulatory clients about intake and output measurements.
- Reinforce correct perineal hygiene measures to reduce the risk of urinary tract infection.
- Determine client's knowledge of medications and provide instruction on medications that affect urination, color of urine, and urine volume.
- Instruct client and caregiver regarding health promotion measures to prevent infection.

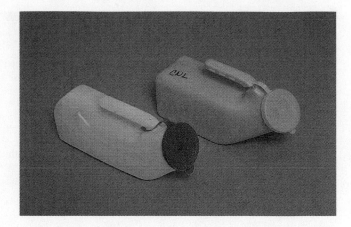

FIGURE **31-2** Types of male urinals.

terial invasion of the urinary tract. It may also be useful to discuss the basic mechanism for urine production and voiding for clients with elimination alterations. Knowledge of factors that promote normal urine production and voiding can also help. Health promotion skills should always be the initial focal point of teaching (Box 31-4).

You can easily incorporate teaching during delivery of care. For example, if you are attempting to increase the client's fluid intake, a good time to discuss benefits is while giving fluids with medications or meals. You may be more successful in teaching about perineal hygiene during a bath or while giving catheter care. When possible, include family members in these discussions.

NORMAL MICTURITION

Stimulating the Micturition Reflex.   The client's ability to void depends on feeling the urge to urinate, on being able to control the urethral sphincter, and on being able to relax. You can foster relaxation and stimulate the reflex to void by helping clients to assume the normal position for voiding.

Females are better able to void in a squatting position. This position promotes contraction of the pelvic and intraabdominal muscles that assist in sphincter control and bladder contraction. If the client cannot use a toilet, position her on a bedpan or bedside commode.

The male client voids more easily in the standing position. At times it may be necessary for one or more nurses to assist the male client to stand. If the client cannot reach a toilet, he may stand at the bedside and void into a **urinal** (a plastic or metal receptacle for urine) (Figure 31-2). Always determine mobility status before standing a client to void.

If the client is unable to stand at the bedside, you may need to assist him to use the urinal in bed. When possible, the client should hold the urinal and position the penis in the urinal. If the client needs assistance, position the penis completely within the urinal and hold the urinal in place or assist the client in holding the urinal. Make sure the penis is placed completely within the urinal to avoid urine spills.

Once the client has finished voiding, remove the urinal and wash and dry the penis to prevent growth of microorganisms and to aid in preventing skin breakdown.

Other measures to promote normal micturition include the use of sensory stimuli (e.g., turning on running water, putting a client's hand in a pan of warm water, or stroking the female client's inner thigh). Each tends to promote relaxation and the reflex to void.

Maintaining Elimination Habits.   Many clients follow set routines of normal voiding. In a hospital or long-term care facility, routines may conflict with those of the client. Integrating the client's habits into the care plan fosters a more normal voiding pattern.

The client should be given privacy and not be rushed. Privacy is essential for normal voiding. If the client cannot reach the bathroom, make sure the bedside area is private. In the home, the debilitated client may prefer using a bedside commode enclosed behind a partition or room divider. Some clients are embarrassed by the sound of voiding. Running water or flushing the toilet masks the sound effectively. Young children are often unable to void in the presence of persons other than parents.

Assess the times when a client normally voids, and offer the opportunity to use a toilet at those times. Respond in a timely manner to the client's urge to urinate. Delay in assisting the client to the bathroom may interfere with normal micturition. Research has shown that promptly assisting clients to toileting facilities reduces incontinence when the clients were able to perceive the urge to void (Fantl and others, 1996). Older adults may also require other special interventions owing to the aging process (Box 31-5).

Comfort is an important factor in facilitating voiding. Therefore activities that increase client comfort may aid urination. If the client typically uses special measures to void (e.g., reading or listening to music), encourage their continued use at home and, when possible, in the health care setting. Toilet seat extenders are used for clients with arthritis or after a total hip replacement to aid the client in sitting and in rising off the toilet.

Encourage and if needed provide appropriate personal hygiene, including hand washing and perineal care (see Chapter 26). Nosocomial genitourinary infections are second only to respiratory infections (see Chapter 10). Bacteria

- The older client may experience urinary incontinence problems as a result of mobility problems or neurological impairments. You should be aware of these problems and arrange scheduled toileting and promote access to toileting facilities.
- Older clients may be prone to physiological urinary retention as a result of diminished bladder muscle tone, capacity, and contractility. This may increase their risk toward large postvoid residuals with a concomitant risk of frequent infections. Teaching sessions should include techniques to stimulate the voiding reflex and to provide for complete bladder emptying and prevention of infections (Steeman and Defever, 1998).
- Older clients may also experience delayed sensations to void, resulting in urgency. Educate the client regarding any factor that interferes with the client's perceptions of sensation to void (e.g., medications, emotional disturbances, decreased fluid intake).
- Older adults experience the following physiological changes that make them more prone to incontinence. During teaching sessions, consider these normal physiological changes to plan appropriate interventions:
    Decreased renal blood flow secondary to decreased cardiac output
    Decreased ability to concentrate urine secondary to decrease in nephron mass
    Decreased tone of the pelvic floor muscles
- Older adults in institutionalized settings (e.g., hospitals, nursing homes) are at the greatest risk for experiencing incontinence problems.
- Older adults may also experience sensory alterations such as diminished vision, which may delay attempts to locate toilet facilities. During teaching sessions, orient clients to their environment with special emphasis on the location of toileting facilities, bedpans or urinals, and assistive devices (e.g., walkers, call light).

Treatment Options for Incontinence   Table 31-6

Type	Treatments
Total	Protective undergarments
	Indwelling and external catheters
	Artificial sphincter
Functional	Bladder training
	Protective undergarments
	Environmental alterations
	Indwelling and external catheters
	Skin care
Stress	Conditioning (Kegel) exercises
	Estrogen replacement
	Alpha-adrenergic agonists
	Surgery
	Intravaginal electrical stimulation
	Bladder neck suspension surgery
	Artificial sphincter
	Penile clamp
Urge	Anticholinergic drug therapy
	Biofeedback
	Treatment of associated urinary tract infection
	Treatment of associated vaginitis
	Incontinence garments
Reflex (upper motoneuron lesion)	Intermittent self-catheterization
	Bladder training
	Electrical stimulation

client should work together to design interventions that promote continence or control wetness (Table 31-6).

Strengthening Pelvic Floor Muscles. Clients who have difficulty starting and stopping the urine stream may benefit from exercises to strengthen pelvic muscles. The client may practice Kegel exercises anytime and anywhere. The client first learns to feel the pelvic muscles. The client does this with each voiding.

Then while sitting or standing, the client tries to tighten the muscles around the anus without tensing leg, buttock, or abdominal muscles. This maneuver allows the client to identify the posterior muscles of the pelvic floor (Kolcaba and others, 2000).

Modified sit-ups may also aid bladder control by strengthening the abdominal muscles. Starting with a few at a time and gradually increasing the number of repetitions will improve pelvic muscle strength.

Manual Bladder Compression. By manually compressing the walls of the bladder, a person can improve bladder emptying. Credé's method helps to stimulate micturition and manually expels urine when bladder tone is reduced. Instruct the client to place both hands flat on the abdomen below the umbilicus and above the symphysis pubis with the fingers pointed down toward the bladder's dome. The client

are the most common cause of these infections, and *E. coli* invasion through the urethra is the most frequent organism and route (Steed, 1999).

Maintaining Adequate Fluid Intake. A simple method of promoting normal micturition is maintenance of a good fluid intake. A client with normal renal function who does not have heart disease or alterations requiring fluid restriction should drink 2000 to 2500 ml of fluid daily. When fluid intake is increased, excreted urine flushes out solutes or particles that may collect in the urinary system. Because a client probably is not accustomed to drinking 2500 ml of water daily, offer fluids the client prefers. At home it may help to set a schedule for drinking fluids (e.g., with meals or medications). A simple trick is to encourage the client to drink a cup of water after voiding. Voiding becomes a natural cue to drinking fluids. A rigid schedule is not needed. To prevent nocturia, fluids should be avoided 2 hours before bedtime.

PROMOTION OF BLADDER EMPTYING. Clients with urinary retention and incontinence are frequently unable to empty the bladder. Incontinence is a major nursing challenge. Choosing from a variety of treatment options, you and the compresses the hands downward against the bladder's walls while tightening the perineum, contracting the abdominal wall, and holding the breath. When urine is in the bladder, Credé's compression causes the sensation of bladder fullness. The maneuver also promotes bladder emptying by relaxing the urethral sphincter.

Drug Therapy. Drug therapy alone or in conjunction with other therapies can be useful for treating problems of incontinence and retention. Drugs are used to increase bladder emptying (e.g., retention), bladder capacity (e.g., urge incontinence), and sphincter tone (e.g., stress incontinence).

When the bladder empties, the detrusor muscle contracts in response to stimulation. Incomplete bladder emptying results from impaired innervation or weakness of the detrusor muscle. As a result, the client experiences retention and overflow incontinence. Therapy with cholinergic drugs is aimed at increasing bladder contraction and improving emptying. Bethanechol (Urecholine) stimulates nerves to increase bladder wall contraction and relax the sphincter. It can be given subcutaneously or orally. Alpha-adrenergic agents such as phenoxybenzamine can also be used to improve bladder emptying. Using Credé's method or other measures for stimulating micturition can augment the effect of the drug.

If urine is in the bladder, urge incontinence may occur as a result of hyperactivity of the bladder muscle that suddenly increases pressure. Local irritants such as stones or infection may cause uncontrolled bladder contractions. Anticholinergic drugs (e.g., propantheline) reduce incontinence by blocking contractility of the bladder. These drugs should be used with caution in clients with heart disease, glaucoma, high blood pressure, kidney and liver disease, and urinary retention. Direct smooth-muscle relaxants (e.g., oxybutynin) may also be used. These drugs work by decreasing the contractility of the bladder. Client instructions are similar to those for propantheline (Fantl and others, 1996).

To treat stress incontinence, alpha-adrenergic drugs may be used. Phenylpropanolamine is the drug commonly used. This medication along with pelvic strengthening exercises has been found to work in some women. Estrogen therapy has also been used to decrease stress incontinence (Fantl and others, 1996).

ACUTE CARE. Often clients need care in hospitals, clinics, or their homes for urinary conditions of sudden onset. One of the most frequent treatments is urinary catheterization.

CATHETERIZATION. **Catheterization** of the bladder involves introducing a rubber or plastic tube through the urethra and into the bladder. The catheter provides a continuous flow of urine in clients unable to control micturition or in clients with obstructions. Because bladder catheterization carries a high risk of urinary tract infection, first try other interventions to empty the bladder.

Types of Catheterization. Intermittent catheterizations and indwelling catheterization are the two forms of catheter

insertion. With the intermittent technique, a single-use straight catheter is introduced for a short period to drain the bladder (5 to 10 minutes). When the bladder is empty, remove the catheter. Intermittent catheterization can be repeated as necessary. An indwelling or Foley catheter remains in place until a client is able to void completely and voluntarily. It may be necessary to change indwelling catheters periodically.

The single-use straight catheter has a single lumen with a small opening approximately 1.3 cm ($^1/_2$ inch) from the tip. Urine drains from the tip, through the lumen, and to a receptacle. An indwelling Foley catheter has a small inflatable balloon that encircles the catheter just below the tip. When inflated, the balloon rests against the bladder outlet to anchor the catheter in place. The indwelling catheter also has as many as two or three separate lumens within the body of the catheter. One lumen drains urine through the catheter to a collecting tube. A second lumen carries sterile water to and from the balloon when it is inflated or deflated. A third (optional) lumen may be used to instill fluids or drugs into the bladder. A three-lumen catheter is most often inserted when irrigations of the catheter are anticipated. These three-way catheters are often used with male clients who have had a transurethral resection of the prostate.

Indications for Use. Intermittent catheterization is preferred for short-term use or to minimize infection in clients who are chronically unable to void. Intermittent catheterization is indicated in the following situations:

1. For immediate relief of acute bladder distention
2. For long-term management of clients with incompetent bladders
3. To obtain a sterile urine specimen
4. To assess for residual urine after voiding
5. To instill a medication

Done correctly, intermittent catheterization has a lower risk of infection than indwelling catheterization. However, if a client requires frequent intermittent catheterization, an indwelling catheter may be preferable. Indwelling catheterization is indicated in the following situations:

1. Obstruction to urine outflow
2. Clients undergoing surgical procedures involving the urinary tract or surrounding structures
3. To prevent urethral obstruction from blood clots
4. To accurately record output in critically ill or comatose clients
5. To prevent skin breakdown in incontinent comatose clients
6. To provide continuous or intermittent bladder irrigations

Catheter Insertion. Urethral catheterization requires a physician's order. Insert the catheter using strict sterile technique. The steps for inserting an indwelling and a single-use straight catheter are the same. The difference lies in the procedure taken to inflate the indwelling catheter balloon and secure the catheter. You can collect needed specimens while inserting either catheter. Skill 31-1 lists steps for performing female and male urethral catheterization.

Text continued on p. 787

Skill 31-1

INSERTING A STRAIGHT OR INDWELLING CATHETER

DELEGATION CONSIDERATIONS

The skill of urinary catheterization is not usually delegated to assistive personnel. The use of assistive personnel for inserting urinary catheters may occur in some settings (e.g., ER), but it has not become routine practice. However, assistive personnel may assist with positioning the client, focusing lighting for the procedure, and aiding in the client's comfort during the procedure by measures such as holding the client's hand or keeping the client warm.

EQUIPMENT

- Catheterization kit containing the following sterile items:
  Gloves (extra pair optional)
  Drapes, one fenestrated
  Lubricant
  Antiseptic cleansing solution
  Cotton balls
  Forceps
  Prefilled syringe with sterile water to inflate balloon of indwelling catheter
  Catheter of correct size and type for procedure (i.e., intermittent or indwelling)
  Sterile drainage tubing with collection bag and multipurpose tube holder or tape, safety pin, and elastic band for securing tubing to bed if client is bed-bound (for indwelling catheter)
  Receptacle or basin (usually bottom of catheterization tray)
  Specimen container
- Blanket

STEPS	RATIONALE
1. Assess status of client:	
a. Time of last urination by asking client, checking I&O flow sheet, or palpating the bladder.	Bladder fullness may be detected with deep palpation above the symphysis pubis.
b. Level of awareness or developmental stage.	Reveals client's ability to cooperate and level of explanation needed.
c. Mobility and physical limitations of client.	Affect way that nurse positions client.
d. Client's gender and age. *8-10 child* *14-16 women* *16-18 male*	Determines catheter size: 8 to 10 Fr is generally used for children, 14 to 16 Fr is indicated for women, 12 Fr may be considered for young girls, and 16 to 18 Fr is used for male clients unless larger size is ordered by physician.
e. Distended bladder.	Causes pain. Can indicate need to insert catheter if client is unable to void independently.
f. Assess perineum for erythema, drainage, and odor.	Determines condition of perineum.
g. Assess for any pathological condition that may impair passage of catheter (e.g., enlarged prostate gland in men).	Obstruction prevents passage of catheter through urethra into bladder.
h. Allergies to antiseptic (e.g., povidone-iodine [Betadine]), tape, latex, lubricant, and shell-fish.	Betadine allergies are common. Exposure to agents may cause local reaction at urinary meatus or even anaphylaxis.
2. Review client's medical record, including physician's order and nurses' notes.	Determines purpose of inserting catheter: preparation for surgery, urinary irrigations, collection of sterile urine specimen, or measurement of residual urine. Assess for previous catheterization, including catheter size, response of client, and time of last catheterization.
3. Assess client's knowledge of the purpose for catheterization.	Reveals need for client instruction.
4. Explain procedure to client.	Promotes cooperation.
5. Arrange for extra nursing personnel to assist as necessary.	Client may be unable to assume positioning for procedure.
6. Wash hands.	Reduces transmission of microorganisms. Infection is common after catheterization. Foley catheter systems are often colonized with bacteria within 48 hours of catheterization (Suchinski and others, 1999).
7. Close curtain or door.	Offers privacy, reduces embarrassment, and aids in relaxation during procedure.
8. Raise bed to appropriate working height.	Promotes use of proper body mechanics.

STEPS	RATIONALE
9. Facing client, stand on left side of bed if right-handed (on right side if left-handed). Clear bedside table and arrange equipment.	Successful catheter insertion requires nurse to assume comfortable position with all equipment easily accessible.
10. Raise side rail on opposite side of bed, and put side rail down on working side.	Promotes client safety.
11. Place waterproof pad under client.	Prevents soiling of bed linen.
12. Position client:	Provides good visualization of perineal structures.
A. Female Client	
(1) Assist to dorsal recumbent position (supine with knees flexed). Ask client to relax thighs so the hip joints can be externally rotated.	Legs may be supported with pillows to reduce muscle tension and promote comfort.
(2) Position female client in side-lying (Sims') position with upper leg flexed at knee and hip if unable to be supine. If this position is used, nurse must take extra precautions to cover rectal area with drape during procedure to reduce chance of cross contamination.	This alternate position is used if client cannot abduct leg at hip joint (e.g., if client has arthritic joints). Also, this position may be more comfortable for client. Support client with pillows if necessary to maintain position.
B. Male Client	
(1) Assist to supine position with thighs slightly abducted.	Comfortable position for client that aids in visualization.
13. Drape client:	Avoids unnecessary exposure of body parts and maintains client's comfort.
A. Female Client	
(1) Drape with bath blanket. Place blanket diamond fashion over client, with one corner at client's neck, side corners over each arm and side, and last corner over perineum.	
B. Male Client	
(1) Drape upper trunk with bath blanket and cover lower extremities with bed sheets, exposing only genitalia.	
14. Wearing disposable gloves, wash perineal area with soap and water as needed; dry and dispose of gloves (see Chapter 26).	Reduces microorganisms near urethral meatus and allows further opportunity to visualize perineum and landmarks.
15. Position lamp to illuminate perineal area. (When using flashlight, have assistant hold it.)	Permits accurate identification and good visualization of urethral meatus.
16. Open package containing drainage system; place drainage bag over edge of bottom bed frame and bring drainage tube up between side rail and mattress.	Prepares bag for attachment to catheter.

• *Critical Decision Point*
This step is necessary only if indwelling catheter is to be inserted and drainage system is not part of the catheterization kit.

STEPS	RATIONALE
17. Open catheterization kit according to directions, keeping bottom of container sterile.	Prevents transmission of microorganisms from table or work area to sterile supplies. The materials in the kit are ordered in sequence of use.
18. Place plastic bag that contains kit within reach of work area to use as waterproof bag to dispose of used supplies.	
19. Apply sterile gloves (see Chapter 10).	Allows nurse to handle sterile supplies without contamination.

• *Critical Decision Point*
If underpad is first item in kit, place the pad plastic side down under the client, touching only the edges so as to maintain sterility. Then apply sterile gloves (see Chapter 10, sterile fields).

STEPS	RATIONALE
20. Organize supplies on sterile field. Open inner sterile package containing catheter. Pour sterile antiseptic solution into correct compartment containing sterile cotton balls. Open packet containing lubricant. Remove specimen container (lid should be loosely placed on top) and prefilled syringe from collection compartment of tray and set them aside on sterile field if needed.	Maintains principles of surgical asepsis and organizes work area.
21. Before inserting indwelling catheter, a common practice is to test balloon by injecting fluid from prefilled syringe into balloon port (see illustrations).	Checks integrity of balloon. Do not use the catheter if the balloon does not inflate or leaks. This is a controversial step. Follow manufacturer's recommendations. Checking the balloon in this way may stretch the balloon and cause increased trauma on insertion.
22. Lubricate catheter 2.5 to 5 cm (1 to 2 inches) for women and 12.5 to 17.5 cm (5 to 7 inches) of men. NOTE: Some catheter kits will have a plastic sheath over the catheter that must be removed prior to lubrication. (Optional: Physician may order use of lubricant containing local anesthetic.)	Eases insertion of catheter through urethral canal.
23. Apply sterile drape, keeping gloves sterile: 　**A. Female Client** 　　(1) Allow top edge of drape to form cuff over both hands. Place drape down on bed between client's thighs. Slip cuffed edge just under buttocks, taking care not to touch contaminated surface with gloves.	Outer surface of drape covering hands remains sterile. Sterile drape against sterile gloves is sterile.
(2) Pick up fenestrated sterile drape and allow it to unfold without touching an unsterile object. Apply drape over perineum, exposing labia and being sure not to touch contaminated surface.	Maintains sterility of work surface.
B. Male Client: Two Methods Are Used for Draping, Depending on Preference.	Maintains sterility of work surface.
(1) First method: Apply drape over thighs and under penis without completely opening fenestrated drape.	

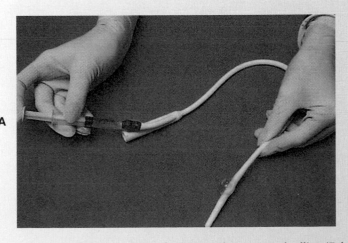
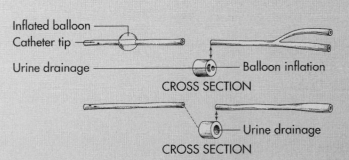

STEP 21   Types of urinary catheters. **A,** Indwelling (Foley) catheter. **B,** Cross section of indwelling and straight catheters.

STEPS	RATIONALE
(2) Second method: Apply drape over thighs just below penis. Pick up fenestrated sterile drape, allow it to unfold, and drape it over penis with fenestrated slit resting over penis.	
24. Place sterile tray and contents on sterile drape between legs. Open specimen container. NOTE: Client's size and positioning will dictate exact placement. This method works best with flexible, average-size clients.	Provides easy access to supplies during catheter insertion. Maintains aseptic technique during procedure.

25. Cleanse urethral meatus.
   A. **Female Client**
      (1) With nondominant hand, carefully retract labia to fully expose urethral meatus. **Maintain position of nondominant hand throughout procedure.**
	Full visualization of urethral meatus is provided. Full retraction prevents contamination of urethral meatus during cleansing.

• *Critical Decision Point*
Closure of labia during cleansing requires that the procedure be repeated because the area has become contaminated.

(2) Using forceps in sterile dominant hand, pick up cotton ball saturated with antiseptic solution and clean perineal area, wiping front to back from clitoris toward anus. Using a new cotton ball for each area, wipe along the far labial fold, near labial fold, and directly over center of urethral meatus.	Cleansing reduces number of microorganisms at urethral meatus (Asci and Beyea, 1996). Use of single cotton ball for each wipe prevents transfer of microorganisms. Preparation moves from areas of least contamination to that of most contamination. Dominant hand remains sterile.
B. **Male Client** (1) If client is not circumcised, retract foreskin with nondominant hand. Grasp penis at shaft just below glans. Retract urethral meatus between thumb and forefinger. Maintain nondominant hand in this position throughout procedure.	Accidental release of foreskin or dropping of penis during cleansing requires process to be repeated because area has become contaminated.

• *Critical Decision Point*
If the foreskin does not remain retracted during insertion, then the cleansing procedure must be repeated because the area has become contaminated.

(2) With dominant hand, pick up cotton ball with forceps and clean penis. Move it in circular motion from urethral meatus down to base of glans. Repeat cleansing three more times, using clean cotton ball each time.	Reduces number of microorganisms at urethral meatus and moves from areas of least to most contamination. Dominant hand remains sterile.
26. Pick up catheter with gloved dominant hand 7.5 to 10 cm (3 to 4 inches) from catheter tip. Hold end of catheter loosely coiled in palm of dominant hand (Optional: May grasp catheter with forceps). Place distal end of catheter in urine tray receptacle if straight catheterization is being done.	

• *Critical Decision Point*
Hold catheter near tip because it allows easier manipulation during insertion into urethral meatus and prevents distal end from striking contaminated surface.

27. Insert catheter:
   A. **Female Client**
      (1) Ask client to bear down gently as if to void and slowly insert catheter through urethral meatus (see illustration).
	Relaxation of external sphincter aids in insertion of catheter.

STEPS   RATIONALE

    (2) Advance catheter a total of 5 to 7.5 cm (2 to 3 inches) in adult or until urine flows out catheter's end. When urine appears, advance catheter another 2.5 to 5 cm (1 to 2 inches). Do not force against resistance. Place end of catheter in urine tray receptacle.

Female urethra is short. Appearance of urine indicates that catheter tip is in bladder or lower urethra. Advancement of catheter ensures bladder placement.

• **Critical Decision Point**
If no urine appears, check if catheter is in vagina. If misplaced, leave catheter in vagina as landmark indicating where not to insert, and insert another sterile catheter.

    (3) Release labia and hold catheter securely with nondominant hand.

Bladder or sphincter contraction may cause accidental expulsion of catheter.

B. Male Client

    (1) Lift penis to position perpendicular to client's body and apply light traction (see illustration).

Straightens urethral canal to ease catheter insertion.

    (2) Ask client to bear down as if to void and slowly insert catheter through urethral meatus.

Relaxation of external sphincter aids in insertion of catheter.

    (3) Advance catheter 17.5 to 22.5 cm (7 to 9 inches) in adult or until urine flows out catheter's end. If resistance is felt, withdraw catheter; do not force it through urethra. When urine appears, advance catheter another 2.5 to 5 cm (1 to 2 inches). **Do not use force to insert a catheter.**

The adult male urethra is long. It is normal to meet resistance at the prostatic sphincter. When resistance is met, nurse should hold catheter firmly against sphincter without forcing catheter. After few seconds, sphincter relaxes and catheter is advanced. Appearance of urine indicates catheter tip is in bladder or urethra. Further advancement of catheter ensures proper placement.

    (4) Lower penis and hold catheter securely in nondominant hand. Place end of catheter in urine tray receptacle.

Catheter may be accidentally expelled by bladder or urethral contraction. Collection of urine prevents soiling and provides output measurement.

    (5) Reduce (or reposition) the foreskin.

Paraphimosis (retraction and constriction of the foreskin behind the glans penis) secondary to catheterization may occur if foreskin is not reduced.

28. Collect urine specimen as needed. Fill specimen cup or jar to desired level (20 to 30 ml) by holding end of catheter in dominant hand over cup.

Allows sterile specimen to be obtained for culture analysis.

29. Allow bladder to empty fully unless institution policy restricts maximal volume of urine drained with each catheterization (about 800 to 1000 ml).

Retained urine may serve as reservoir for growth of microorganisms.

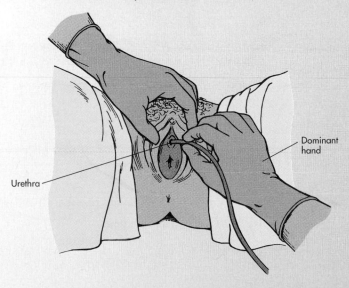

STEP 27A(1)   Inserting the catheter.

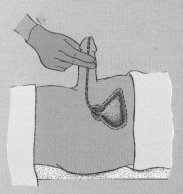

STEP 27B(1)   Position penis perpendicular to body for catheter insertion.

• *Critical Decision Point*
If a straight, single-use catheter was inserted, withdraw catheter slowly but smoothly until removed.

STEPS	RATIONALE
30. Inflate balloon fully per manufacturer's recommendations, and then release catheter with nondominant hand and pull gently to feel resistance (see accompanying box).	Inflation of balloon anchors catheter tip in place above bladder outlet to prevent removal of catheter. Note the size of balloon on the catheter. Most commonly a 5-ml balloon is used, but a 30-ml balloon may be ordered. A prefilled syringe may be included with the kit; use only the amount included. Do not overinflate or underinflate the balloon.

• *Critical Decision Point*
If resistance is noted to inflation or the client complains of pain, the balloon may not be entirely within the bladder. Stop inflation; aspirate any fluid injected into the balloon and advance the catheter a little more before reattempting to inflate.

STEPS	RATIONALE
31. Attach end of catheter to collecting tube of drainage system (see illustration). Drainage bag must be below level of bladder; do not place bag on side rails of bed.	Establishes closed system for urine drainage. Raising bag on side rail will cause backflow of urine into bladder.
32. Anchor catheter:	
A. Female Client	
(1) Secure catheter tubing to inner thigh with strip of nonallergenic tape (commercial multipurpose tube holders with a Velcro strap are available). Allow for slack so movement of thigh does not create tension on catheter (see illustration).	Anchoring catheter to inner thigh reduces pressure on urethra, thus reducing possibility of tissue injury in this area (Evans, 1999).
B. Male Client	
(1) Secure catheter tubing to top of thigh or lower abdomen (with penis directed toward chest). Allow slack in catheter so movement does not create tension on catheter (see illustration).	Anchoring catheter to lower abdomen reduces pressure on urethra at junction of penis and scrotum, thus reducing possibility of tissue injury in this area.

• *Critical Decision Point*
Be sure there are no obstructions in tubing. Coil excess tubing on bed and fasten it to bottom sheet with clip from kit or with rubber band and safety pin.

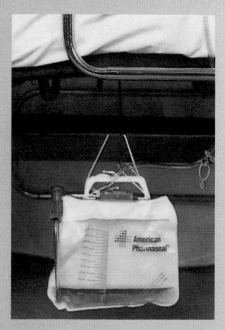

STEP 31   Drainage bag below level of bladder.

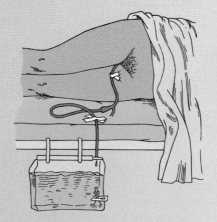

STEP 32A(1)   Securing the female indwelling catheter.

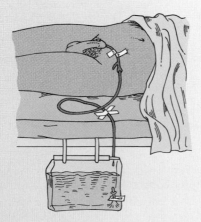

STEP 32B(1)   Securing the male indwelling catheter.

Inflation of Balloon for Indwelling Catheter

Inflate balloon of indwelling catheter with amount of fluid recommended by the manufacturer.

a. While holding catheter with nondominant hand at urethral meatus, take end of catheter and place it between first two free fingers of nondominant hand.

b. With free dominant hand, attach syringe to injection port at end of catheter.

c. Slowly inject total amount of solution. If client complains of sudden pain, aspirate solution and advance catheter farther.

d. After inflating balloon, release catheter and pull gently to feel resistance. Then move catheter slightly back into bladder. Inflation of balloon anchors catheter tip in place above bladder outlet to prevent removal of catheter (see illustrations).

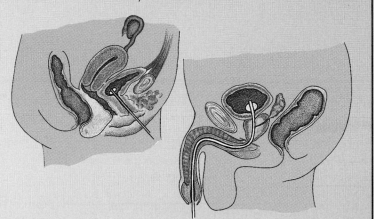

33. Assist client to comfortable position. Wash and dry perineal area as needed.	Maintains comfort and security.
34. Remove gloves and dispose of equipment, drapes, and urine in proper receptacles.	Reduces transmission of microorganisms.
35. Wash hands.	Reduces spread of microorganisms.
36. Palpate bladder.	Determines if distention is relieved.
37. Ask about client's comfort.	Determines if client's sensation of discomfort or fullness has been relieved.
38. Observe character and amount of urine in drainage system.	Determines if urine is flowing adequately.
39. Determine that there is no urine leaking from catheter or tubing connections.	Prevents injury to client's skin and ensures a closed sterile system.

UNEXPECTED OUTCOMES AND RELATED INTERVENTIONS

- Urethral or perineal irritation is present.
  - Observe for leaking, and replace catheter if necessary.
  - If catheter is present, ensure that indwelling catheter is anchored.
  - If securing catheter does not help or if catheter has been removed, notify physician of urethral irritation.
- Client has fever and/or odor is present, or client experiences small, frequent voidings or any burning or bleeding.
  - Monitor vital signs and urine, but report findings to physician because any of these symptoms/signs may indicate a UTI.
- Client experiences urinary retention and is unable to void after catheter removal.
  - Ensure adequate intake and privacy, and facilitate urination by relaxation.
  - If client unable to void within 6 to 8 hours of catheter removal, notify physician.

RECORDING AND REPORTING

- Ensure that times for catheter care are set in the care plan. Clients with indwelling catheters should receive perineal and catheter care every 8 hours and after bowel movements.
- Record in nurses' notes when catheter care was given, removal of catheter and assessment of urethral meatus, and character of urine.

Closed Drainage Systems. After an indwelling catheter is inserted, it is necessary to maintain a closed urinary drainage system to minimize the risk of infection. Urinary drainage bags are plastic and can hold approximately 2000 ml of urine. The bag should hang on the lower bed frame without touching the floor. Some urinary drainage bags have special urometers between the collection tubing and bag. When the client ambulates, instruct client or caregiver to carry the bag below the level of the client's bladder. Never raise a drainage bag and tubing above the level of the client's bladder. Urine in the bag and tubing is a medium for bacteria, and infection can develop if urine is allowed to reflux (return to the bladder).

Most drainage bags contain an antireflux valve to prevent urine from reentering the drainage tubing and contaminating the bladder. A spigot at the base of the bag provides a means to empty the bag. The spigot should always be clamped, except during emptying, and tucked into the protective pouch at the bag's side.

To keep the drainage system patent, check for kinks or bends in the tubing, avoid positioning the client on drainage tubing, prevent tubing from becoming dependent, and observe for clots or sediment that may occlude the tubing.

Routine Catheter Care. Clients with indwelling catheters require specific perineal hygiene care to reduce the risk of urinary tract infection. Any secretions or encrustation at the catheter insertion site must be completely removed. Perineal care and the cleansing of the first 2 inches of the catheter every 8 hours are minimally expected. These measures are often referred to as catheter care. The use of powders or lotions on the perineum is contraindicated because of the risk of growth of microorganisms, which may ascend the urinary tract. Clients who are catheterized and who are incontinent of stool will need cleaning after bowel movements.

Provide perineal care (see Chapter 26), and observe the urethral meatus and surrounding tissues for inflammation, swelling, and discharge. Note the amount, color, odor, and consistency of discharge to determine local infection and status of hygiene.

Replace, as necessary, the adhesive tape or multipurpose tube holder that anchors the catheter to the client's leg or abdomen, and remove adhesive residue from the skin. Secure the catheter, thus reducing the risk of the catheter's being pulled on and exposing the portion that was in the urethra. This also prevents drag on the catheter and avoids pressure from the balloon on the bladder floor. Replace the urinary tubing and collection bag if necessary, adhering to principles of surgical asepsis. The urinary tubing and collection bag should be changed if there are signs of leakage, odor, or sediment buildup. Check the drainage tubing and bag to ensure that no tubing loops hang below the level of the bladder, the tube is coiled and secured onto the bed linen, the tube is not kinked or clamped, and the drainage bag is positioned on the bed frame.

Removal of Indwelling Catheter. Removal of a retention catheter is a skill requiring clean technique. If the retention catheter balloon is not fully deflated, its removal can result in trauma and subsequent swelling of the urethral meatus, and urinary retention can occur. If the catheter was in place for more than several days, the client may experience dysuria resulting from inflammation of the urethral canal. Because of decreased bladder muscle tone, the client may urinate frequently or experience urinary retention.

Before removing a catheter, check agency policy or the physician's orders to determine if a sterile specimen is required. To remove a catheter, use a clean disposable towel,

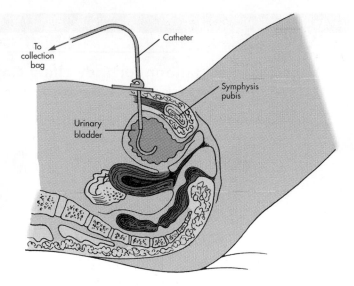

FIGURE **31-3** Placement of suprapubic catheter above the symphysis pubis.

clean gloves, and a sterile syringe the same size as the volume of solution within the catheter's inflated balloon. The end of each catheter contains a label that denotes the volume of solution (5 to 30 ml) within a balloon. Position the client in the same position as during catheterization.

Remove the adhesive tape or Velcro tube anchoring the catheter. Cleanse any residue from the skin, and insert the hub of the syringe into the inflation valve (balloon port). Aspirate the entire amount of fluid used to inflate the balloon, and then pull the catheter out smoothly and slowly to prevent trauma to urethral mucosa. If resistance is met as the catheter is pulled, stop because the balloon is probably still inflated. Remove additional fluid from the balloon, do not attempt to remove catheter until you are sure the balloon is deflated. Wrap the contaminated catheter in a waterproof pad, and unhook the collection bag and drainage tubing from the bed. Provide perineal care following removal, and document the removal.

The catheter causes inflammation of the urethral canal. It is important for you to note the time and amount of the client's first void after catheter removal. Often the client's I&O are monitored until voiding is established. If more than 8 hours elapse before the client voids, it may be necessary to catheterize the client again to determine if there is a blockage, retention, or suppression of urine. If the volume of urine voided is small, residual urine may be in the bladder.

ALTERNATIVES TO URETHRAL CATHETERIZATION.   To avoid the risks associated with catheters inserted through the urethra, alternatives for urinary drainage exist. **Suprapubic catheters** are inserted surgically into the bladder through the lower abdomen above the symphysis pubis (Figure 31-3). Although most successfully used for short periods with clients who have had gynecological and bladder surgery, the suprapubic catheter may be used in older adult males who require a long-term alternative to urinary catheterization. As with in-

---

Procedural Guidelines for
APPLYING A CONDOM CATHETER

Box 31-6

1. Check physician's order.
2. Obtain equipment:
   a. Condom catheter (may come with self-adhesive or an elastic adhesive).
   b. Collection bag
   c. Basin with warm water
   d. Towel and washcloth
   e. Clean gloves
   f. Scissors
3. Wash hands.
4. Raise bed to working height and raise far upper side rail.
5. Using sheet, drape client so only genitalia are exposed.
6. Prepare condom catheter and drainage (see manufacturer's directions).

7. Apply gloves and provide perineal care.
   a. If needed, clip hair at base of penile shaft.
8. Apply skin prep to penile shaft, and allow to dry.
9. Holding penis in nondominant hand, apply condom by rolling smoothly onto penis. NOTE: Leave a 2.5- to 5-cm (1- to 2-inch) space between tip of penis and end of catheter (see illustration).
10. Secure condom catheter:
    a. If using elastic adhesive, wrap the strip of adhesive over the condom to secure it in place by using a spiral technique (see illustration). NOTE: Adhesive tape must never be used.
    b. For self-adhesive catheter, follow manufacturer's directions.
11. Attach catheter to drainage bag and attach drainage bag to lower bed frame.
12. Make client comfortable.
13. Observe urinary drainage, drainage tube patency, condition of penis, and tape placement.

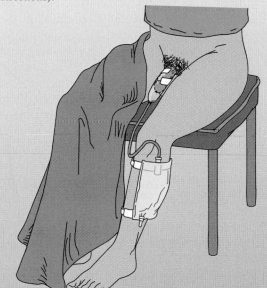

STEP 9   Distance between end of penis and tip of condom.

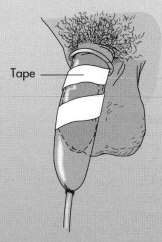

Tape

STEP 10A   Elastic tape is applied in spiral fashion to secure the condom catheter to the penis.

---

dwelling urinary catheters, the suprapubic catheter predisposes the client to urinary tract infections, but the incidence may be lower. Spread of infection to the kidneys may require removing the catheter. The advantages of a suprapubic catheter for clients are that they may void naturally when the catheter is clamped and it is more comfortable (Warren, 1997). Daily care will depend on policy, but the cleaning and dressing of the site are similar to care of any surgical drain (see Chapter 36).

The condom catheter is suitable for incontinent or comatose male clients who still have complete and spontaneous bladder emptying (Box 31-6). The condom catheter poses little risk of infection. Local infections, however, can result from buildup of secretions around the urethra, trauma to the urethral meatus, or buildup of pressure in the outflow tubing.

It is necessary to remove the condom catheter daily to check for skin irritation. Clean the urethral meatus and penis thoroughly with each condom catheter change. Twisting

of the condom at the drainage tube attachment irritates the skin and obstructs urine outflow. The drainage tubing must be checked frequently for patency. For a man with a retracted foreskin, maintaining the intactness of a conventional condom catheter may prove difficult. Special devices are available to help alleviate this problem. Manufacturer's guidelines for product application should be reviewed.

External incontinence devices and pelvic floor support devices for women are more difficult to design and fit (Johnson, 2000). Women may wear the newer absorbent pads and adult disposable undergarments. However, wearers of these disposable undergarments report skin irritation, odor, and increased infection rate. For the active incontinent woman, these devices are options that can promote more independence.

RESTORATIVE AND CONTINUING CARE. Returning to normal micturition often means preventing complications from treatment. Many restorative functions are related to pre-

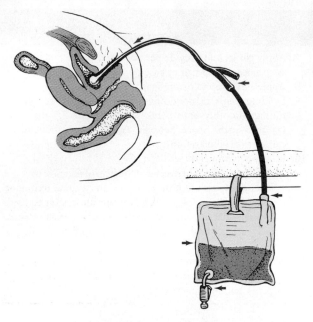

FIGURE **31-4**   Potential sites for introduction of infection.

venting infection after catheterization, promoting comfort, and preventing skin breakdown if the client is incontinent.

PREVENTING INFECTION.   Maintaining a closed urinary drainage system is important in infection control. A break in the system can lead to introduction of microorganisms. Sites at risk are at the place of catheter insertion, drainage bag, spigot, tube junction, and junction of tube and bag (Figure 31-4). In addition, monitor the patency of the system to prevent pooling of urine. Urine in the drainage bag is an excellent medium for microorganism growth. Bacteria can travel up drainage tubing to grow in pools of urine. Therefore it is important to prevent the abnormal backward flow of urine (**urinary reflux**). If this urine flows back into the bladder, an infection will probably develop. Box 31-7 gives suggestions for ways to prevent infections in catheterized clients.

PROMOTION OF COMFORT.   Clients with urinary alterations can be uncomfortable as a result of the symptoms of urinary problems. Frequent or unpredictable voiding, dysuria, and painful distention are sources of discomfort.

The incontinent client gains comfort from having clean, dry clothing. When incontinence is the problem, a protective pad or sanitary belt offers protection against soiling. Wet clothing adheres to the skin and can cause rubbing and irritation.

Giving urinary analgesics that act on the urethral and bladder mucosa may relieve dysuria. Phenazopyridine helps to relieve dysuria, burning, and itching. It is available in combination with sulfonamide antibiotics in preparations such as Axo Gantanol and Azo Gantrisin. The sulfonamide provides additional antibacterial action. Clients taking drugs with phenazopyridine should be aware that their urine may appear orange and their clothing may be stained. They must drink large amounts of fluids to prevent toxicity from the sulfonamides and to maintain optimal flow through the urinary system. Always ask clients about allergies to sulfa before giving these drugs.

If the client has local discomfort from an inflamed urethra, a warm sitz bath may provide pain relief. The warm water soothes inflamed tissues near the urethral meatus by improving blood supply. The client is often relaxed after a sitz bath, so voiding occurs easily.

The pain of distention cannot be relieved unless the client is able to empty the bladder. Methods for stimulating micturition or intermittent catheterization may be the only sources of pain relief.

MAINTENANCE OF SKIN INTEGRITY.   The normal acidity of urine is irritating to the skin. When urine becomes alkaline, encrustation or precipitate collects on the skin, fostering breakdown. Continuous exposure of the skin to urine leads to gradual maceration and excoriation. Washing and mild soap and warm water is the best way to remove urine from the skin. Body lotion keeps the skin moisturized and provides a barrier to the urine. Clients who wet their clothing should receive a clean set of clothes after each voiding.

When the skin becomes irritated or inflamed, the physician may prescribe a cream or spray containing steroids to reduce inflammation (e.g., triamcinolone [Kenalog]). If fungal growth develops, the antifungal drug nystatin (Mycostatin), available in cream or powder form, is effective.

The client with a ureterostomy has a special hygiene problem because urine drains from the ostomy site continuously. The drainage pouch or appliance frequently becomes moist and slips from the skin. Continual oozing of urine around the stoma causes skin breakdown. Skin barriers provide a layer of protection between the skin and ostomy pouch. When urine leaks, it frequently covers the outer skin barrier. An enterostomal therapist can help the client select an ostomy appliance that fits snugly against the skin's surface around the stoma (see Chapter 32).

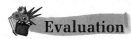 **Evaluation**

CLIENT CARE.   To evaluate the care plan use the expected outcomes developed during planning to determine whether interventions were effective (Box 31-8). This evaluation process is a dynamic one. You use this information to monitor the client's progress and to direct future interventions. The optimal goal is the client's ability to urinate voluntarily without dysuria, urgency, or frequency. The client's urine should be an amber color, clear, without abnormal constituents, and within the normal range of pH and specific gravity.

You can also evaluate specific outcomes designed to demonstrate normal urinary function and prevent complications of urinary alterations. Has the client's intake been at least 2000 ml? Is the bladder distended? Is there less than 50 ml of residual urine on the second voiding? Does urinary output equal fluid intake? Are there a reduced number of in-

Tips for Preventing Infection in Catheterized Clients   Box 31-7

Follow good hand-washing techniques.

Do not allow the spigot on the drainage bag to touch a contaminated surface.

Do not open the drainage system at connection points to obtain specimens or measure urine.

If the drainage tubing becomes disconnected, do not touch the ends of the catheter or tubing. Wipe the ends of the tube with antiseptic solution before reconnecting.

Each client should have a separate receptacle for measuring urine to prevent cross contamination.

Prevent pooling of urine and reflux of urine into the bladder. Avoid raising the drainage bag above the level of the bladder.

Avoid allowing any dependent loops of tubing.

If it is necessary to raise the bag during transfer of the client to a bed or stretcher, clamp the tubing.

Before client exercises or ambulates, drain all urine from tubing into bag.

Avoid prolonged clamping or kinking of the tubing (except during bladder conditioning).

Empty the drainage bag at least every 8 hours.

Remove the catheter as soon as possible after conferring with physician.

Tape the catheter to secure it in place, noting specific guidelines regarding the male client's taping procedure.

Perform routine perineal hygiene every shift and after defecation.

Outcome Evaluation for MRS. VALLERO   Box 31-8

Nursing Action	Client Response/Finding	Achievement of Outcome
Measure and observe color of each voided specimen.	Mrs. Vallero's fluid intake was 800 ml in 6 hours. Mrs. Vallero voided twice in 6 hours and voided 250-300 ml with each void. She noted that bladder felt empty.	Mrs. Vallero is ingesting and voiding fluid appropriately, indicating normal micturition.
Palpate bladder.	Bladder nondistended upon palpation following voiding. Mrs. Vallero did not perceive increased urge to void during palpation.	Complete bladder emptying achieved.
Ask Mrs. Vallero about voiding, sensations, fullness, and discomfort during voiding.	Mrs. Vallero stated that there was no pain with voiding. She did not perceive any sensations of fullness.	Mrs. Vallero is free of discomfort during voiding.

Case Study EVALUATION

Mrs. Stone and her instructor talk with Mrs. Vallero and explain that she probably needs to be catheterized again. She asks to try to "go" and nods to the bathroom. Mrs. Stone suggests that she sit for at least 15 minutes and leave the water running in the sink. The nurse also shows Mrs. Vallero how to push on her abdomen after she is sitting in the bathroom. Mrs. Vallero was able to void after 5 minutes.

Documentation Note

Client moved slowly to the bathroom. Her gait was steady, slow, and slightly stooped. Breathing was even and nonlabored, and as she sat on the toilet, she said, "I'm ready." Mrs. Vallero used manual bladder compression and turned the water on in the sink. She voided 1300 ml of clear, pale yellow urine. Stated that she felt her bladder was empty. Client returned to bed. No bladder distention to palpation.

continent episodes? Is the urine culture showing negative bacterial growth? Does the client use correct hand-washing techniques? Are there any areas of skin breakdown around the perineum, stoma, or condom?

Be systematic in evaluating the client's response to care. Nursing research is being conducted to validate the effectiveness of nursing interventions. Evidence-based practice will improve the quality of care you provide.

CLIENT EXPECTATIONS.   Control over urination is taken for granted until it is lost. Clients report that it is degrading and they feel like a baby when they lose control over voiding. Therefore evaluation of care from the incontinent client's standpoint centers around maintaining a level of dryness that is personally satisfactory. Clients want to have control, and to achieve that outcome they should have confidence in utilizing triggering mechanisms to initiate voiding.

In clients who have a urinary tract infection, pain, urgency, and frequency rule their life. Clients who have an infection will be satisfied with their care if they can report an absence or decrease in their symptoms. Can the client void without dysuria? Can the client sleep and carry out activities of daily living with lessened or no discomfort?

For all clients with urinary problems, lack of privacy is a potential issue. Did they feel that staff were considerate, and did the staff protect their privacy? Clients will also evaluate whether they were included in the planning of their care. Were they able to tell you the important information about their habits? Did you consider that information when you suggested a plan of care or implemented an intervention?

Key Terms

bacteriuria, *p. 766*
catheterization, *p. 780*
dysuria, *p. 766*
glomerulus, *p. 764* *capillaries that filter*
graduated measuring container, *p. 772*
hematuria, *p. 772*

micturition, *p. 765*
nephrons, *p. 764* *kidney wastes acquired from blood infect in hos*
nosocomial, *p. 766*
proteinuria, *p. 764*
residual urine, *p. 766*
suprapubic catheter, *p. 788* *endwelling*
ureterostomy, *p. 768*
urinal, *p. 778* *container*

urinary diversion, *p. 765* *three stoma accid*
urinary incontinence, *p. 767*
urinary reflux, *p. 790*
urinary retention, *p. 766* *can't void*
urine hat, *p. 772*
urometer, *p. 772* *measure small*
urosepsis, *p. 766*
voiding, *p. 765* *voiding*

Key Concepts

- Micturition or voiding is influenced by voluntary control from higher brain centers and involuntary control from the spinal cord.
- Symptoms common to urinary disturbances include urgency, dysuria, polyuria, oliguria, and difficulty in starting the urinary stream.
- When collected properly, a clean-voided urine specimen does not contain bacteria picked up from the urethral meatus.
- A client can better understand the importance of perineal hygiene by knowing that the urinary tract is normally sterile.
- Methods of promoting the micturition reflex assist clients in sensing the urge to urinate and controlling urethral sphincter relaxation.

- An increased fluid intake results in urine formation that flushes particles and solutes from the urinary system.
- Incontinence is classified as total, urge, stress, reflex, or functional. Each type of incontinence has specific nursing interventions.
- An indwelling urinary catheter remains in the bladder for an extended period, making the risk of infection greater than with intermittent catheterization.
- Closed drainage systems deliver sterile solutions and medication to the bladder. Strict asepsis is necessary when caring for a client with a closed bladder drainage system.
- Because urine drains almost continuously from a ureterostomy, there is risk of skin breakdown around a stoma site.
- A primary function of the elimination process is fluid balance.

Critical Thinking Activities

1. Six hours after removal of an indwelling catheter you are checking on your client and she states her bladder feels full. She says she has only minimal incision discomfort (1 on pain scale of 0 to 10) but demands client-controlled analgesia of morphine. The client is 1 day post total abdominal hysterectomy and bilateral salpingo-oophorectomy. Her I&O balanced in the first 24 hours. She has no intravenous fluids and has had 1000 ml of oral intake this day. At 11 AM when her Foley catheter was removed, there was 700 ml in the bag. She has a midline dressing on her lower abdomen and no drainage tubes. What assessments would you make to determine bladder status? What interventions would you implement to enhance urination?

2. You are caring for an athletic 16-year-old girl who has frequent urinary tract infections, and when she gets an infection, she does not appear to recognize the signs and symptoms. What information are you going to provide to help her reduce the incidence of these infections and seek early treatment when an infection occurs?

3. You are on a home visit to a client who is using a condom catheter. His wife, who is the caregiver, tells you the "darn thing never stays on." What problems might cause the condom not to stay on? What assessments of the client do you need to make to determine the cause? If the wife applied the catheter incorrectly, what steps can be taken to ensure she understands how to do the procedure?

Review Questions

1. An adult client has not voided in 12 hours and complains about a continued perception of the urge to pee. Your initial action is to:
   1. notify the physician.
   2. insert a straight catheter.
   3. palpate the client's bladder.
   4. increase client's fluid intake.
2. Identification of a "2 plus hematuria" in your female client with a urinary tract infection indicates:
   1. a response to the antibiotic therapy.
   2. a ruptured vessel within the bladder.
   3. irritation of the bladder mucosa from the pathogen.
   4. the result of a straight catheter used to obtain a sterile specimen.

3. Your client is 3 hours postoperative from bladder surgery. The nurse assistant reports to you that the client has just started draining "bright red urine" in his catheter drainage bag. Your first action would be to:
   1. notify the physician.
   2. obtain client's vital signs and assess his renal output.
   3. irrigate the Foley catheter with normal saline until clear.
   4. delegate the assistant to monitor the vital signs every 15 minutes until the client's physician appears.
4. When applying a condom catheter, it is important to secure the catheter to the penile shaft in such a manner that the:
   1. catheter is tight and draining well.
   2. catheter is dependent and draining well.

3. catheter is secured with adhesive tape applied in a circular pattern.
4. catheter is snug and secure, but does not cause constriction to blood flow.
5. Patients with urinary tract infections experience:
   1. only pain on urination.
   2. decreased frequency, burning, and pain.
   3. increased frequency, hesitancy, and pain.
   4. increased frequency, hesitancy, burning, and pain on urination.
6. Maintaining a Foley catheter drainage bag in the dependent position prevents:
   1. urinary reflux.
   2. urinary retention.
   3. reflex incontinence.
   4. urinary incontinence.
7. The purpose of instructing the client to begin and discard the initial stream of urine when obtaining a midstream urine specimen is to:
   1. allow for client comfort.
   2. allow sufficient urine to be obtained for the culture specimen.

3. allow the initial urine to wash bacteria from the external genitalia.
4. allow the initial urine to drain from the bladder to avoid inaccurate urine cultures.
8. Hospital-acquired urinary tract infections are called:
   1. viral.
   2. funal.
   3. bacterial.
   4. nosocomial.
9. Hospital-acquired urinary tract infections are most frequently caused by inadequate handwashing and:
   1. urinary drainage bags.
   2. poor perineal hygiene.
   3. catheterization procedures.
   4. poor hand-washing techniques.

References

Asci J, Beyea S: Urologic update: indwelling urinary catheters—an integrative review of the literature, *Online J Knowledge Synthesis Nurs* 3(2):1, 1996.

Dowd T and others: Using cognitive strategies to enhance bladder control and comfort, *Holist Nurs Pract* 14(2):91, 2000.

Evans E: Indwelling catheter care: dispelling the misconceptions, *Geriatr Nurs* 20(2):85, 1999.

Fantl JA and others: *Urinary incontinence in adults: acute and chronic management,* Clinical practice guideline, No. 2, AHCPR Pub No. 96-0682, Rockville, Md, March 1996, Agency for Health Care Policy and Research, Public Health Services, U.S. Department of Health and Human Services.

Foreman M, Zane D: Nursing strategies for acute confusion in elders, *Am J Nurs* 96(4):44, 1996.

Haus E: Urinary tract infections in the homebound elderly, *Home Healthc Nurse* 16(5):323, 1998.

Huether S, McCance KL: *Understanding pathophysiology,* ed 2, St. Louis, 2002, Mosby.

Kolcaba K and others: Kegel exercises, *Am J Nurs* 100(11):59, 2000.

Johnson ST: From incontinence to confidence, *Am J Nurs* 100(2):69, 2000.

Lueckenotte AG: *Gerontologic nursing,* ed 2, St. Louis, 2000, Mosby.

Marchiondo K: A new look at urinary tract infection, *Am J Nurs* 98(3):34, 1998.

Nicolle LE: Asymptomatic bacteriuria in the elderly, *Infect Dis Clin North Am* 11(3): 647, 1997.

Steed CJ: Common infections acquired in the hospital: the nurse's role in prevention, *Nurs Clin North Am* 34(2):443, 1999.

Suchinski G and others: Treating urinary infections in the elderly. *Dimens Crit Care Nurs* 18(1):21, 1999.

Steeman E, Defever M: Urinary incontinence among elderly persons who live at home: a literature review, *Nurs Clin North Am* 33(3):441, 1998.

Urinary Incontinence Guideline Panel: *Urinary incontinence in adults: clinical practice guidelines,* AHCPR Pub No. 92-0038, Rockville, Md, March 1992, Agency for Health Care Policy and Research, Public Health Services, U.S. Department of Health and Human Services.

Warren J: Catheter-associated urinary tract infections, *Infect Dis Clin North Am* 11(3):609, 1997.

32

Bowel Elimination

Objectives

- Define key terms.
- Explain the physiology of digestion, absorption, and bowel elimination.
- List and discuss physiological and psychological factors that influence bowel elimination.
- Describe common physiological alterations in bowel elimination.
- Assess a client's bowel elimination pattern.
- Perform a fecal occult blood test.
- List nursing diagnoses related to alterations in bowel elimination.
- Describe nursing implications for common diagnostic examinations of the gastrointestinal tract.
- Administer an enema.
- List nursing measures aimed at promoting normal elimination and defecation.
- Describe nursing care required to maintain structure and function of a bowel diversion.

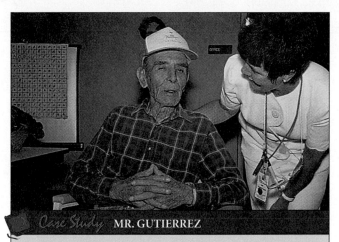

Case Study MR. GUTIERREZ

Residing in the assisted living wing of one of the four local long-term care centers, Mario Gutierrez busies himself in his small garden plot. He is 82 years old, widowed, and has lived in this particular area of the care center for over 3 years. His family, with whom he is quite close, is scattered across the country. One niece lives in the same town. Mr. Gutierrez feels he is in good health. He believes as long as he eats green chili peppers every day, he will remain healthy. His diet consists of flour and corn tortillas, beans, and rice. He likes most meats, but he prefers chicken and asado (pork). For breakfast he usually has huevos rancheros. He has been hospitalized only twice, once for the flu and once for placement of a pacemaker. He presently takes only three medications: digoxin, Zestril, and Metamucil.

This afternoon Mr. Gutierrez has telephoned his niece for the fourth time. The complaint is always the same: Mr. Gutierrez's bowels are "locked up and haven't moved in the last 2 days." He ate a big meal the previous evening and now reports feeling "all bloated." His niece tried to explain about eating, bowel habits, and methods of facilitating bowel movements, but in exasperation reminded Mr. Gutierrez that the nursing student was coming later this afternoon and he could talk to the student about his problem.

Vickie, a 45-year-old married mother of two sons, is Mr. Gutierrez's nursing student. Vickie's oldest son is a freshman at the same community college she is attending; the other is a sophomore in high school. Her husband, Roger, is very supportive of her being in school. Vickie has been seeing Mr. Gutierrez once a week for 5 weeks as a portion of a home health clinical experience. They have developed a good rapport. Mr. Gutierrez's self-identified problems with his bowels are a frequent topic of conversation.

*R*egular bowel elimination is essential for the maintenance of a healthy body state. Although often considered a common and expected occurrence in the older adult, individuals of any age can experience changes in intestinal elimination. These changes may be the result of illness, diagnostic testing, the aging process, or surgical intervention. Alterations in intestinal elimination respond to both preventive and supportive nursing care.

SCIENTIFIC KNOWLEDGE BASE

Anatomy and Physiology of the Gastrointestinal Tract

The gastrointestinal (GI) tract is a series of hollow mucous membrane–lined muscular organs that begin at the mouth and end at the anal orifice. The functions of the GI tract are to prepare food products for use by the body's cells and to promote the absorption of fluid and nutrients. The GI tract is a complex system, and changes in any one area can alter total body functioning.

MOUTH.   The mouth mechanically and chemically breaks down nutrients into usable size and form. The teeth **masticate** food, breaking it down into a size suitable for swallowing. Saliva, produced by the salivary glands in the mouth, dilutes and softens the food in the mouth for easier swallowing. Digestion begins in the mouth and ends in the small intestine.

ESOPHAGUS.   As food enters the upper esophagus, it passes through the upper esophageal sphincter, a circular muscle that prevents air from entering the esophagus and food from refluxing into the throat. The bolus of food travels down the esophagus and is pushed along by **peristalsis,** which propels food through the length of the GI tract.

The food moves down the esophagus and reaches the cardiac sphincter, which lies between the esophagus and the upper end of the stomach. The sphincter prevents reflux of stomach contents back into the esophagus.

STOMACH.   The stomach performs three tasks: the storage of the swallowed food and liquid; the mixing of food, liquid, and digestive juices; and the emptying of its contents into the small intestine. The stomach produces and secretes hydrochloric acid (HCl), mucus, the enzyme pepsin, and intrinsic factor. Pepsin and HCl facilitate the digestion of protein. Mucus protects the stomach mucosa from acidity and enzyme activity. The intrinsic factor is essential in the absorption of vitamin B_{12}.

SMALL INTESTINE.   Movement within the small intestine, occurring by both **segmentation** and peristalsis (Figure 32-1), facilitates both digestion and absorption. Approximately 7 to 10 L of liquid **chyme** moves through on an average day. Reabsorption in the small intestine is so efficient that by the time the chyme reaches the end of the small intestine, it is pastelike in consistency, with a volume of 600 to 800 ml (Phipps and others, 1999). The small intestine is divided into three sections: the duodenum, the jejunum, and the ileum.

The duodenum is approximately 2 feet long and continues to process the chyme from the stomach. The second section, the jejunum, is approximately 9 feet long and has the primary function of absorption of carbohydrates and proteins. The ileum, which is approximately 12 feet long, specializes in the absorption of water, fats, and bile salts. Most nutrients and electrolytes are absorbed in the small intestine,

Segmentation

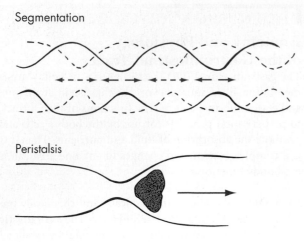

Peristalsis

FIGURE 32-1   Segmented and peristaltic waves.

specifically by the duodenum and jejunum. The ileum absorbs certain vitamins, iron, and bile salts.

If small intestine function is impaired, the digestive process is greatly altered. Conditions such as inflammation, surgical resection, or obstruction can disrupt peristalsis, reduce the area of absorption, or block the passage of chyme. Electrolyte and nutrient deficiencies then develop.

LARGE INTESTINE.   The lower GI tract is called the large intestine (**colon**) because it is larger in diameter than the small intestine. However, its length (1.5 to 1.8 m [5 to 6 feet]) is much shorter. The larger intestine is divided into the cecum, colon, and rectum. The large intestine is the primary organ of bowel elimination.

Chyme enters the large intestine by waves of peristalsis through the ileocecal valve, a circular muscle layer that prevents regurgitation. The colon is divided into the ascending, transverse, descending, and sigmoid colons. The colon's muscular tissue allows it to accommodate and eliminate large quantities of waste and gas (**flatus**). The colon has three functions: absorption, secretion, and elimination. A large volume of water (up to 1.5 L) and significant amounts of sodium and chloride are absorbed by the colon daily (Doughty, 2000b). The amount of water absorbed from chyme depends on the speed at which colonic contents move. Chyme is normally a soft, formed mass. If peristalsis is abnormally fast, there is less time for water to be absorbed and the stool will be watery. If peristaltic contractions slow down, water continues to be absorbed and a hard mass of stool forms, resulting in constipation.

The secretory function of the colon aids in electrolyte balance. Bicarbonate is secreted in exchange for chloride. About 4 to 9 mEq of potassium is also excreted daily. Serious alterations in colon function (e.g., diarrhea) can cause severe electrolyte disturbances.

Slow peristalic contractions move contents through the colon. Intestinal content is the main stimulus for contraction. Mass peristalsis pushes undigested food toward the rectum. These mass movements occur only three or four times daily, with the strongest during the hour after mealtime.

The rectum is the final portion of the large intestine. Normally the rectum is empty of waste products (**feces**) until just before defecation. The rectum contains vertical and transverse folds of tissue that may help to temporarily hold fecal contents during **defecation.** Each fold contains an artery and veins that can become distended from pressure during straining. This distention can result in hemorrhoid formation.

ANUS.   Feces and flatus are expelled from the rectum through the anal canal and anus. Contraction and relaxation of the internal and external sphincters, innervated by sympathetic and parasympathetic stimuli, aid in the control of defecation. The anal canal is richly supplied with sensory nerves that help to control continence.

DEFECATION.   The physiological factors critical to bowel function and defecation include normal GI tract function, sensory awareness of rectal distention and rectal contents, voluntary sphincter control, and adequate rectal capacity and compliance (Doughty, 2000a). Normal defecation begins with movement in the left colon, moving stool toward the anus. When stool reaches the rectum the distention causes relaxation of the internal sphincter, and an awareness of the need to defecate. At the time of defecation, the external sphincter relaxes and abdominal muscles contract, increasing intrarectal pressure and forcing the stool out (Doughty, 2000a). Pressure can be exerted to expel feces through a voluntary contraction of the abdominal muscles while maintaining forced expiration against a closed airway. This is termed **Valsalva maneuver.** This will assist in stool passage. Clients with cardiovascular disease, glaucoma, increased intracranial pressure, or a new surgical wound can be placed at further risk, such as cardiac irregularities or elevated blood pressure, with this maneuver and should be cautioned to avoid straining to pass the stool. Normal defecation is painless, resulting in passage of soft, formed stool. See Box 32-1 for other factors influencing elimination and defecation.

Common Bowel Elimination Problems

Alteration in bowel elimination results from a variety of factors. Some of the more common alterations are discussed below.

CONSTIPATION.   **Constipation** is defined as having fewer bowel movements than normal with the difficult passage of hard, dry feces (Lueckenotte, 2000). Common causes of constipation include changes in diet, medications, inflammation, environmental factors (e.g., unavailability of toilet facilities, lack of privacy), and lack of knowledge about regular bowel habits. In the older adult (Box 32-2), constipation is usually diet related, most commonly a lack of fiber (Gibson and others, 1995). Regardless of etiology, intestinal motility slows, causing prolonged exposure of the fecal mass to the intestinal walls. Fecal water continues to be absorbed, leaving the stool hard and underlubricated (Lueckenotte, 2000).

Constipation can be a significant threat to well-being. Straining during defecation is contraindicated for clients

Factors Influencing Bowel Elimination

Box 32-1

AGE

Infants have a smaller stomach capacity, less secretion of digestive enzymes, and more rapid intestinal peristalsis. The ability to control defecation does not occur until 2 to 3 years of age.

Adolescents experience rapid growth of the large intestine and increased secretion of HCl.

Older adults have decreased chewing ability. Partially chewed food is not digested as easily. Peristalsis declines, and esophageal emptying slows. Absorption by the intestinal mucosa is impaired. Muscle tone in the perineal floor and anal sphincter weakens, causing difficulty in controlling defecation (see Box 32-2, p. 798).

DIET

Regular daily food intake promotes peristalsis.

High-fiber foods, raw fruits, cooked fruits, greens, raw vegetables, and whole grains (cereals and breads) promote peristalsis and defecation by creating bulk.

Low-fiber foods (pasta, lean meats, and milk) slow peristalsis.

Gas-producing foods (broccoli, cauliflower, onions, and dried beans) can stimulate peristalsis.

Persons with lactose intolerance lack the enzyme lactose, which is needed to digest the simple sugars in milk. Such intolerance can lead to diarrhea and cramping.

POSITION DURING DEFECATION

Squatting allows a person to lean forward, exert intraabdominal pressure, and contract thigh muscles to normally defecate.

Older adults or those with arthritis may be unable to rise from a toilet seat.

Immobilized clients, required to use a bedpan while lying, cannot contract muscles to defecate.

PREGNANCY

As pregnancy advances and the fetus enlarges, pressure is exerted on the rectum. Constipation commonly occurs.

DIAGNOSTIC TESTS

Certain examinations involving visualization of GI structures require the emptying of bowel contents. Nothing by mouth (NPO) status, bowel evacuants, and enema administration to cleanse the bowel before a test, which are factors that interfere with normal elimination.

Barium examinations require ingestion of barium, a mixture that can harden and cause serious constipation unless eliminated soon after a test.

FLUID INTAKE

Fluid liquefies intestinal contents for easier passage.

Hot beverages and fruit juices soften stool and increase peristalsis.

Large quantities of milk may slow peristalsis and cause constipation.

ACTIVITY

Immobilization depresses colon motility, and regular physical exercise promotes peristalsis.

PSYCHOLOGICAL FACTORS

Stress, anxiety, or fear can initiate parasympathetic impulses, causing acceleration of digestion and peristalsis. Diarrhea and gaseous distention may result.

Emotional depression can decrease peristalsis and lead to constipation.

PERSONAL HABITS

Personal habits such as failing to respond to the need to defecate and lack of privacy interfere with normal elimination patterns and can lead to constipation.

Hospitalized clients often share toilet facilities or use bedpans or bedside commodes. The resulting embarrassment can cause them to ignore the urge to defecate.

PAIN

Hemorrhoids, rectal surgery, and abdominal surgery may cause a client to suppress defecation because of pain; constipation develops.

MEDICATIONS

Laxatives and cathartics soften stool and promote peristalsis.

Antidiarrheal agents inhibit peristalsis.

Narcotic analgesics, opiates, and anticholinergic drugs depress peristalsis and can cause constipation.

Antibiotics alter normal bowel flora and can produce diarrhea.

Drugs that contain iron may turn the stool black. Antacids may cause a white discoloration. Anticoagulants may result in frank or occult blood in the stool.

SURGERY AND ANESTHESIA

General anesthetics may cause slowing or halting of peristalsis.

Surgery involving bowel manipulation temporarily stops peristalsis (paralytic ileus) for 24 to 48 hours.

---

with cardiovascular problems or for those who have had recent abdominal or rectal surgery. Clients who exert effort to pass a stool experience Valsalva maneuver. The action traps the blood in the chest; upon relaxing, blood rushes to the heart, overloading the heart. This increased cardiac workload can lead to cardiac dysrhythmias or angina. It also increases intraabdominal pressure, leading to stress on suture lines.

IMPACTION.   **Fecal impaction,** resulting from unrelieved constipation, is a collection of hardened feces, wedged in the rectum, that cannot be expelled. Clients at greatest risk for impaction include those who are confused or unconscious, badly constipated, or those who have experienced an interruption in nerve supply to the bowel. An obvious sign of impaction is the inability to pass a stool for several days, despite

a repeated urge to defecate. Frequently the first sign of impaction is overflow diarrhea, in which liquid stool seeps around the fecal mass, causing diarrhea. **Anorexia,** abdominal distention and cramping, and rectal pain may also occur.

DIARRHEA.   **Diarrhea** is an increased frequency in the passage of loose stools (Table 32-1). Fluid and electrolyte imbalances can result from diarrhea. Older adults and the very young are at the greatest risk for electrolyte imbalance. Because of the irritating effects of the intestinal contents, persistent diarrhea readily leads to skin breakdown in the perianal region.

The aim of treatment is first to maintain adequate hydration (Lueckenotte, 2000). Parenteral replacement of fluids may be necessary when the client is at risk for fluid and elec-

- Maintenance of a proper diet, including the appropriate intake of fluid and bulk. Fiber (4 to 6 g, which is equal to 3 to 4 tablespoons of bran per day) is recommended to reduce the risk of constipation.
- Proper body position to facilitate bowel evacuation.
- Education concerning the dangers of excessive laxative/cathartic use for bowel elimination. Excessive use of these medications may cause an atony of the colon, further contributing to chronic constipation (Lueckenotte, 2000). Instruct clients that if their stool is soft and passes easily, it is not necessary to have a bowel movement daily. If clients should miss a daily movement, it does not mean that they are constipated and require a laxative.
- Instruct clients that changes in dietary intake can cause transient changes in bowel elimination patterns. Also, changes in dietary reference intake (RDI) include a decrease in calories because of a decrease in metabolic rate and an increase in calcium. Clients should also avoid tobacco products and large amounts of alcohol (Lueckenotte, 2000).

Conditions That Cause Diarrhea   Table 32-1

Condition	Physiological Effects
Emotional stress (anxiety)	Increased intestinal motility
Intestinal infection (streptococcal or staphylococcal enteritis)	Inflammation of intestinal mucosa, increased mucus secretion in colon
Food allergies	Reduced digestion of food elements
Food intolerance (greasy foods, coffee, alcohol, spicy foods)	Increased intestinal motility, increased mucus secretion in colon
Tube feedings	Hyperosmolarity of some enteral solutions results in diarrhea, because hyperosmolar fluids draw fluids into the gastrointestinal tract
Medications	
Iron	Irritation of intestinal mucosa
Antibiotics	Suprainfection allowing overgrowth of normal flora, inflammation and irritation of mucosa
Laxatives (short term)	Increased intestinal motility
Inflammatory bowel disease (colitis, Crohn's disease)	Inflammation and ulceration of intestinal walls, reduced absorption of fluids, increased intestinal motility
Surgical alterations	
Gastrectomy	Loss of reservoir function of stomach, improper absorption because food is moved into duodenum too quickly
Colon resection	Reduced size of colon, reduced amount of absorptive surface

trolyte imbalance. Intervention is then aimed at identifying and correcting causative factors. Depending on the cause, antispasmodic or antidiarrheal medications may be used to slow peristalsis.

INCONTINENCE.   **Fecal incontinence** is the involuntary passage of stool. Any condition that impairs function or control of the anal sphincter may cause fecal incontinence. Conditions creating frequent, loose, large-volume, watery stools also predispose to incontinence.

In many situations the client is mentally alert but physically unable to avoid defecation. Loss of control over intestinal elimination may be associated with feelings of inadequacy or guilt. Like diarrhea, incontinence predisposes the client to skin breakdown.

FLATULENCE.   Flatulence is one of the most common GI disorders. It refers to a sensation of bloating and abdominal distention that is accompanied by excess gas. The accumulation of gas forces the diaphragm up and reduces lung expansion (Phipps and others, 1999).

HEMORRHOIDS.   **Hemorrhoids** are made up of a mass of dilated blood vessels that lie beneath the lining of the skin in the anal mucosa. Increased venous pressure resulting from straining at defecation, pregnancy, and chronic illnesses, such as congestive heart failure and chronic liver disease, can lead to hemorrhoids. Passage of hard stool can cause hemorrhoid tissue to stretch and bleed. Hemorrhoid tissue can become inflamed and tender, and clients may complain of itching, and burning. Because pain worsens during defecation, the client may ignore the urge to defecate. Constipation can result.

BOWEL DIVERSIONS.   Certain diseases prevent the normal passage of intestinal contents throughout the small and large bowel. The treatment for these disorders may result in the need for a temporary or permanent artificial opening (**stoma**) in the abdominal wall. Surgical openings may be created in the ileum (ileostomy) or colon (colostomy) with the end of the intestine brought through the abdominal wall to create the stoma.

The standard bowel diversion creates a stoma, or the client has reconstructive surgery that uses the native sphincter. The reconstructive surgery includes a continent stoma procedure, which is rarely done anymore, or reconstructive surgery, the ileoanal pouch anastomosis, which is described in a later section (Colwell and others, 2001).

OSTOMIES.   The location of the **ostomy** determines stool consistency. For example, an ileostomy bypasses the entire large intestine, creating frequent, liquid stools. The sigmoid colostomy emits near-normal stool. The location of an ostomy depends on the client's medical problem and general condition.

Loop colostomies are usually temporary large stomas constructed in the transverse colon (Figure 32-2). The sur-

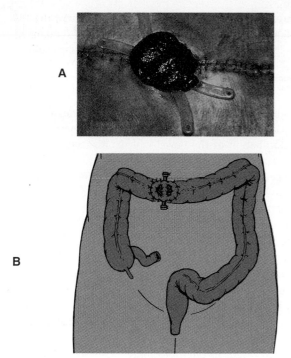

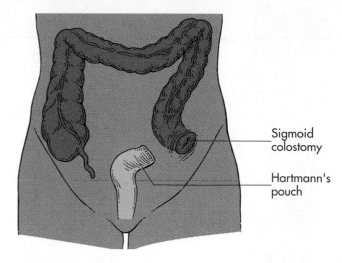

FIGURE **32-3**   Sigmoid colostomy. Distal bowel is oversewn and left in place to create Hartmann's pouch. (From Hampton BG, Bryant RA: *Ostomies and continent diversions: nursing management,* St. Louis, 1992, Mosby.)

FIGURE **32-2**   **A,** A temporary transverse loop colostomy supported with a flexible red rubber catheter. (Courtesy Hollister, Inc., Libertyville, Ill.) **B,** Abdominal view of loop colostomy in transverse colon. (From Hampton BG, Bryant RA: *Ostomies and continent diversions: nursing management,* St. Louis, 1992, Mosby.)

geon pulls a loop of bowel onto the abdomen. A plastic rod, bridge, or rubber catheter is temporarily placed under the bowel loop to keep it from slipping back. The surgeon then opens the bowel and sutures it to the skin of the abdomen. The loop ostomy has two openings through the stoma. The proximal end drains stool, and the distal portion drains mucus.

The end colostomy consists of one stoma formed from the proximal end of the bowel with the distal portion of the GI tract either removed or sewn closed (called Hartmann's pouch) and left in the abdominal cavity. End colostomies are a surgical treatment for colorectal cancer. In such cases the rectum may also be removed. Clients with diverticulitis often have a temporary end colostomy constructed with a Hartmann's pouch (Figure 32-3).

Unlike the loop colostomy, the bowel is surgically severed in a double-barrel colostomy (Figure 32-4) and the two ends are brought out onto the abdomen. The double-barrel colostomy consists of two distinct stomas: the proximal functioning stoma and the distal nonfunctioning stoma (mucous fistula).

A stoma that produces frequent passage of liquid stool (e.g., an ileostomy) creates a management challenge. Skin protection is important because of the liquid and caustic nature of the output. A pouch with a skin barrier is fitted around the stoma, and the pouch is emptied several times a day. The pouching system is changed approximately every 3 to 5 days depending upon the type of system utilized.

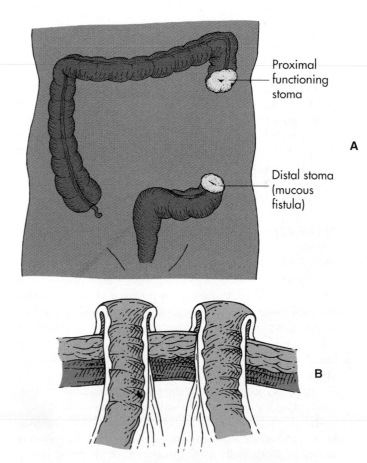

FIGURE **32-4**   Double-barrel colostomy. **A,** Double-barrel colostomy in the descending colon. **B,** Cross-sectional view of double-barrel stoma. (From Hampton BG, Bryant RA: *Ostomies and continent diversions: nursing management,* St. Louis, 1992,

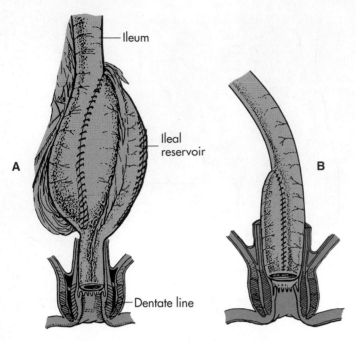

FIGURE **32-5**   Ileoanal reservoirs (IARs). **A,** S-shaped configuration. **B,** J-shaped configuration. (From Hampton BG, Bryant RA: *Ostomies and continent diversions: nursing management,* St. Louis, 1992, Mosby.)

A colostomy located in the descending or sigmoid portion of the colon may discharge stool only once a day. The client may choose to use a pouch that can be removed and discarded rather than empty the pouch. An option for the client with a sigmoid stoma is to irrigate the stoma, training the bowel to empty stool at a specific time. A person who irrigates the stoma may use a small cap over the stoma for protection (Colwell and others, 2001).

ALTERNATIVE PROCEDURES.   The ileoanal pouch anastomosis is a newer surgical procedure that is an option for some clients who need to undergo a colectomy, removal of the colon, for treatment of ulcerative colitis or familial polyposis. In this procedure the colon is removed, a pouch is created from the end of the small intestine, and the pouch is attached to the anus (Figure 32-5). The ileoanal pouch provides for collection of waste material in a similar fashion to the rectum. Stool is evacuated from the anus; the client is continent of stool. When the ileal pouch is created, a temporary ileostomy is created to allow the pouch anastomosis to heal. The temporary ileostomy is usually closed 3 months later.

The Kock continent ileostomy is created using the small intestine to create a pouch. The Kock continent ileostomy is indicated occasionally for the treatment of ulcerative colitis. The pouch has a continent stoma, a type of nipple valve that can only be drained when an external catheter is placed intermittently into the stoma. The client empties the pouch several times a day. The stoma is covered with a protective dressing or stoma cap (Colwell and others, 2001).

Low anterior resection is a procedure performed for a client with a low rectal cancer. The cancer is removed, and a low anastomosis is performed. To protect this new anastomosis a temporary loop ileostomy is created and remains in place for approximately 3 months (Colwell and others, 2001).

NURSING KNOWLEDGE BASE

Any alteration in bowel elimination can be embarrassing for a client. Because of the sensitivity many clients experience regarding elimination of the bowel with its associated sounds and odors, you must be very sensitive to communication techniques, especially nonverbal. Changes in facial expression or gagging can be perceived as disgust by the client. Awareness of the client's need for privacy should also be addressed.

Clients with a chronic disease of the GI system have endured numerous hospitalizations, perhaps multiple surgeries, and significant changes in eating habits and lifestyles. They are often on complicated medication regimens that are taxing both physically and financially. Their desire for wellness may lead them to consider alternative forms of medical treatment. It is important for you to remain accepting of client's health care choices.

An ostomy causes serious body image changes, with clients losing control over a very basic body function. Even though clothing conceals the ostomy, the client feels different. The idea of being different or not a whole person can affect the client's social interaction with others, resulting in isolation. Some clients experience difficulty in maintaining or initiating normal sexual relations. One important factor in the client's acceptance of this change in body functioning is the ability to control fecal secretions. Foul odors, spillage, leakage of liquid stools, and the inability to regulate bowel movements further place the client at risk for loss of self-esteem.

CRITICAL THINKING
Synthesis

As you begin the problem-solving process of caring for a client experiencing elimination problems, it becomes important to reflect on the knowledge, experience, and standards of care that will improve client outcomes. Assuming the proper attitudes of critical thinking will also ensure a well-designed, individualized approach to care.

KNOWLEDGE.   You need to reflect on knowledge regarding normal anatomy and physiology of the GI tract, as well as knowledge regarding specific GI alterations. This information will help you more accurately focus the nursing assessment and identify alterations when they exist. Even insignificant alterations in bowel elimination can produce significant health problems for the client. For example, diarrhea can lead to electrolyte imbalances, dehydration, and rectal soreness.

Abdominal pain is one of the most common complaints of clients who seek health care. You must apply knowledge of the nature of pain (see Chapter 29) and pain assessment to accurately analyze elimination problems.

Functional bowel disorders make up the most frequently reported GI complaints. Understand and consider the psychological aspects associated with these diseases to provide appropriate care.

The intake of certain foods also reflects the client's culture or beliefs. Foods in various cultures have different status relating to religion, availability, cost, and tradition. For example, among Hispanic Americans certain hot foods (e.g., chocolate, cheese, and eggs), are utilized for conditions producing fever, and cold foods (e.g., fresh vegetables, dairy foods, and honey), are used for disorders such as cancer or headache (Giger and Davidhizar, 1999). You should understand the client's cultural heritage and the role diet plays in health promotion and maintenance.

A final area of knowledge is understanding those changes occurring as a result of the aging process. Far too often an older adult's problems with intestinal elimination are discounted as an everyday complaint. Remember that what might appear at the outset to be quite insignificant can be a major problem to the client physically and psychologically.

EXPERIENCE.   Elimination alterations are common for many clients who seek health care. In the acute care environment numerous variables, including diet changes, medications, fluid restrictions, decreased activity, and diagnostic tests, can cause major alterations to bowel function. You can provide better care to clients by reflecting on your previous experiences involving clients with similar alterations and similar lifestyle habits affecting elimination.

ATTITUDES.   Apply all of the attitudes of critical thinking when caring for a client with elimination problems. Creativity comes into play, especially when adjustments are needed in the client's diet and exercise planning. Similarly, perseverance is important in selecting effective diet therapies and in finding the best appliances for ostomy clients. Confidence is an important factor in providing care to clients with bowel diversions or resections. Often these clients are very ill and in significant pain. Your confidence with moving and positioning the client, handling stomal supplies, and managing pain will place the client at ease and facilitate the recovery process.

STANDARDS.   To establish regular bowel habits, clients require consistency in bowel care and training. It is possible to establish regular bowel habits by setting standards for appropriate nutritional and elimination support. Regardless of age or disease state, maintenance of bowel function and integrity is essential to well-being.

When assessing a client's abdominal pain, findings should be specific, clear, precise, and accurate. Although the intellectual standards for critical thinking apply to all symptoms, thorough pain assessment is critical. A multitude of problems can be detected on the basis of the nature of abdominal pain. Physicians will collaborate with you on your assessment to identify the appropriate medical diagnosis.

Clients with alterations in bowel elimination, especially incontinence, can be at risk for ridicule and shame on the part of some health care providers. This may be especially true for providers with limited educational experience, to whom the

task of client hygiene is often delegated. It is your responsibility to make certain such individuals understand the needs of these clients and attend to their needs in a respectful way.

NURSING PROCESS

The needs and problems of clients experiencing alterations in bowel elimination are distinct and numerous. Incorporate assessment skills and utilize appropriate communication techniques throughout the entire care planning process.

 Assessment

Assessment of bowel elimination requires you to review any complaints the client may have affecting the GI system. Because the client's chewing ability, recent intake of both solids and liquids, personal eating habits, and level of stress all influence bowel function, this information should be included in the review (Norton and Chelvanayagam, 2000).

HEALTH HISTORY.   In determining the client's bowel habits, remember "normal" is unique to each individual. Apply this knowledge in preparing questions for the client interview to determine the presence and extent of GI alterations. Family members can help if the client is unable to provide necessary information.

Areas typically assessed in the history include the following (Norton and Chelvanayagam, 2000):

1. Determine the frequency of bowel elimination and if any changes in elimination patterns have occurred. Ask client to make suggestions about the basis for any change.
2. Client's description of usual characteristics of stool. Determine whether the stool is normally watery or formed, soft or hard, and the typical color. Ask the client to describe a normal stool's shape and the number of stools per day.
3. Appetite, recent change in eating patterns, and change in weight (amount of loss or gain).
4. Identification of routines followed to promote normal elimination. Examples are drinking hot liquids, laxatives, eating specific foods, or taking time to defecate during a certain part of the day.
5. Assessment of the use of artificial aids at home, for example, the use of enemas, laxatives, or special foods before having a bowel movement. Ask how often the client uses them.
6. Presence and status of artificial orifices. If the client has an ostomy, assess the frequency of fecal drainage, character of feces, type of appliance used, and methods used to maintain the ostomy function.
7. Daily diet history, including the client's dietary preferences. Is mealtime regular or irregular, and are certain foods eaten infrequently?
8. Description of daily fluid intake. This includes the type and amount of fluid. The client may have to estimate the amount using common household measurements.

		Table 32-2
Factors to Assess	**Questions and Approaches**	**Physical Assessment Strategies**
Chewing	Ask if client has difficulty chewing. Ask if client has dentures.	Inspect condition of teeth, gums, and mouth. Observe for fit of dentures, observing for sores or pressure areas from dentures. Observe client eating meal, determine client's ability to eat all types of foods.
Mobility	**In Ambulatory Clients** Ask client about activity/exercise patterns.	Observe client's gait.
	For Clients With Restricted Mobility Determine client's frequency in using toileting facilities independently. Ask client and family how much assistance is needed for toileting.	Observe client's ability to assist with transfer, positioning, and activity.
Anal sphincter function	Ask if client is able to sense bowel distention, because an inability to sense bowel distention impairs client's ability to evacuate bowel.	Palpate abdomen for signs of distention or discomfort. Inspect anal sphincter at rest, and perform digital examination while asking client to contract and relax sphincter. NOTE: A small amount of stool is normal; large amount or hard stool may indicate impaired emptying of bowel.
Abdominal muscle contractility	Instruct client to "bear down" while lightly palpating the abdominal wall	Palpate lower abdomen for muscle contraction and distention.

Example of a Focused Client Assessment

9. History of surgery or illnesses affecting the GI tract. This information can often help to explain symptoms, the potential for maintaining or restoring a normal elimination pattern, and whether there is a family history of cancer involving the GI tract.
10. Medication history. Determine whether the client takes medications that might alter defecation or fecal characteristics.
11. Emotional state. Observe client's emotional state, including tone of voice and mannerisms, which can reveal significant behaviors indicating stress.
12. History of exercise. Obtain a description of the type, frequency, and amount of daily exercise.
13. History of pain or discomfort. Ask the client whether there is a history of abdominal or anal pain. The location and nature of pain can help to locate the source of a problem (see Chapter 29).
14. Social history. If the client is not independent in bowel management, determine methods and degree of assistance required.

PHYSICAL ASSESSMENT.   Assess the status of GI function to detect factors that may affect elimination, and gather data regarding the client's elimination problems. Table 32-2 summarizes some of the assessments to include in the examination of bowel function (Doughty, 2000a). You will need to conduct an examination of the oral cavity, abdomen, and anus and rectal canal (see Chapter 12).

When a digital examination is necessary, inspect the fecal material on the glove for several characteristics (Table 32-3).

If there are no feces on the glove, ask the client to describe a typical stool, noting recent changes. The client or primary caregiver is the most knowledgeable about changes. You should also determine whether the client passes an unusual amount of or little flatus.

LABORATORY AND DIAGNOSTIC EXAMINATIONS
LABORATORY TESTS.   Several laboratory tests are available to assist in diagnosing problems with the GI system, including the following blood tests:

Total bilirubin—a degraded product of hemoglobin excreted in the bile. Obstruction in the biliary tract contributes primarily to a rise in direct values.

Alkaline phosphatase—an enzyme found in many tissues. Obstructive biliary tract disease may cause significant elevation.

Amylase—an enzyme secreted by the pancreas. Damage to these cells causes the enzyme to be absorbed into the blood.

Protein—a measure of nutrition. Malnourished clients have greatly deceased levels of blood protein.

Carcinoembryonic antigen (CEA)—a protein. It is typically elevated in persons with colorectal tumors.

Analysis of fecal contents can also detect alterations in GI functioning. Bacteria can easily be acquired by a person who handles a specimen improperly. Standard precautions must be followed for anyone coming in contact with the specimen (see Chapter 10). The client is often capable of obtaining the specimen without assistance if properly instructed. The client must understand that feces cannot be mixed with

Fecal Characteristics

Table 32-3

Characteristic	Normal	Abnormal	Abnormal Cause
Color	Infant: yellow; adult: brown	White or clay	Absence of bile
		Black or tarry (melena)	Iron ingestion or upper GI bleeding
		Red	Lower GI bleeding, hemorrhoids, ingestion of beets
		Pale with fat	Malabsorption of fat
		Translucent mucus	Spastic constipation, colitis, excess straining
		Bloody mucus	Neoplasm or inflammation
Odor	Pungent; affected by food type	Noxious change	Blood in feces or infection
Consistency	Soft, formed	Liquid	Diarrhea, reduced absorption
		Hard	Constipation
Frequency	Varies: infant 5 to 8 times daily (breast-fed) or 1 to 3 times daily (bottle fed); adult daily or 2 to 3 times a week	Infant more than 6 times daily or less than once every 1 to 2 days; adult more than 3 times a day or less than once a week	Hypomotility or hypermotility
Amount	150 g per day (adult)		
Shape	Resembles diameter of rectum	Narrow, pencil shaped	Obstruction, rapid peristalsis
Constituents	Undigested food, dead bacteria, fat, bile pigment, cells lining intestinal mucosa, water	Blood, pus, foreign bodies, mucus, worms	Internal bleeding, infection, swallowed objects, irritation, inflammation
		Excess fat	Malabsorption syndrome, enteritis, pancreatic disease, surgical resection of intestine

urine or water. The client defecates into a clean, dry bedpan or special container that is placed under the toilet seat.

Laboratory tests for blood in the stool and stool cultures require only a small sample. Minimum abrasions of the intestinal mucosa are thought to cause blood loss of 1 to 3 ml daily in feces (Norton and Chelvanayagam, 2000). Blood loss of over 50 ml appears as **melena.** To detect quantities less than 50 ml of blood, laboratory analysis is needed. Collect approximately an inch of formed stool or 15 to 30 ml of liquid diarrheal stool. Tests for measuring the output of fecal fat require the client to collect stools for 3 to 5 days. All fecal material must be saved throughout the test period. Some tests require a chemical preservative.

After obtaining a specimen, tightly seal the container, complete laboratory requisition forms, and record all specimen collections in the client's medical record. Avoid delays in sending specimens to the laboratory. Some tests require the stool to be warm. When stool specimens are allowed to stand at room temperature, bacteriological changes that alter test results can occur.

A common test is the **fecal occult blood test,** or guaiac test, which measures microscopic amounts of blood in the feces (Box 32-3). It is a useful diagnostic screening test for colon cancer (Box 32-4). One positive result does not confirm GI bleeding. The test should be repeated at least 3 times while the client refrains from ingesting foods and medications that can cause a false-positive result. Examples of these foods and medications include red meat, poultry, fish, some raw vegetables, vitamin C, and aspirin (Ransohoff and Lang, 1997). Clients on anticoagulants are at risk for developing GI bleeding and should be regularly screened with this test.

Case Study   SYNTHESIS IN PRACTICE

When Vickie prepared to conduct an assessment of Mr. Gutierrez, she reflected back on experiences with other clients in the home setting. She recalled one client in particular who had elimination problems resulting from a diet consisting mainly of high-fat and high-carbohydrate foods. She thought that her involvement with that client would likely help in the care of Mr. Gutierrez.

Vickie also reviewed her class notes on the anatomy and physiology of the GI system. Given Mr. Gutierrez's age, Vickie focused on reviewing the physiological changes that aging produces within the GI system. These changes include loss of teeth, taste bud atrophy, decreased secretion of gastric acid, and a slight decrease in small intestine motility (Lueckenotte, 2000).

Vickie will need to do a thorough assessment of Mr. Gutierrez's dietary intake over the last few days. Being familiar with Mr. Gutierrez's Hispanic heritage, Vickie anticipates certain food preferences and will need to assess these. Vickie knows Mr. Gutierrez does not like the food served at the long-term care center and frequently requests "home cooked" tortillas and green chili peppers from his niece.

The symptoms Mr. Gutierrez exhibits, no bowel movement in 2 days and a feeling of bloating, can be associated with several different problems. Vickie plans the assessment to be thorough and precise, being sure to rule out any abdominal discomfort or other symptoms that can be expected from elimination problems. Because problems with bowel elimination have been an ongoing concern for Mr. Gutierrez, Vickie will need perseverance while she begins to identify nursing diagnoses and outline goals of care. Vickie will need to avoid preconceived ideas regarding constipation in older adults. She must remain open to all the possibilities concerning changes in GI functioning.

Procedural Guidelines for
Measuring Fecal Occult Blood

Box 32-3

1. Explain purpose of test and ways client can assist. Client can collect own specimen if possible.
2. Wash hands.
3. Apply clean, disposable gloves.
4. Use tip of wooden applicator (see illustration) to obtain a small portion of uncontaminated stool specimen.

7. Wash hands.
8. Record results of test; note any unusual fecal characteristics.

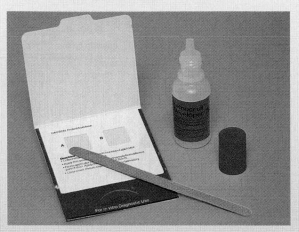

STEP 4

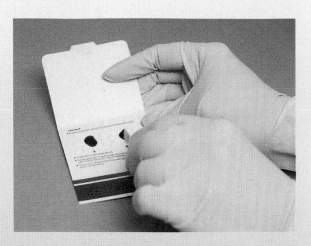

STEP 5A

5. Perform hemoccult slide test:
   a. Open flap of slide and, using a wooden applicator, thinly smear stool in first box of the guaiac paper. Apply a second fecal specimen from a different portion of the stool to slide's second box (see illustration).
   b. Close slide cover and turn the packet over to reverse side (see illustration). Open cardboard flap and apply two drops of developing solution on each box of guaiac paper. A blue color indicates a positive guaiac, or presence of blood.
   c. Assess the color of the guaiac paper after 30 to 60 seconds.
   d. Dispose of test slide in proper receptacle.
6. Wrap wooden applicator in paper towel, remove gloves, and discard in proper receptacle.

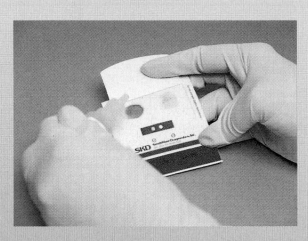

STEP 5B

Screening for Colon Cancer

Box 32-4

RISK FACTORS
- Age: over 50
- Family history: colorectal cancer or polyps
- History of inflammatory bowel disease (colitis or Crohn's disease)
- Personal history of polyps
- Diet: high intake of animal fats and low fiber intake
- Obesity and inactivity

WARNING SIGNS
- Change in bowel habits
- Rectal bleeding
- A sensation of incomplete evacuation

SCREENING TESTS
- Digital rectal examination every year after age 40
- Fecal occult blood test every year after age 50
- Endoscopy every 3 to 5 years after age 50, after two annual negative examinations

From American Cancer Society: *Colon and rectal cancer—2001,* Atlanta, 2000, The Society (www3.cancer.org).

Radiologic and Diagnostic Tests
Box 32-5

PLAIN FILM OF ABDOMEN/KIDNEYS, URETER, BLADDER
A simple x-ray film of the abdomen requiring no preparation.

UPPER GI/BARIUM SWALLOW
An x-ray examination using an opaque contrast medium (barium) to examine the structure and motility of the upper GI tract, including pharynx, esophagus, and stomach.
Client must be NPO after midnight the night before the examination.
Client must remove all jewelry or other metallic objects.
After the test, client must increase fluids to facilitate passage of barium.

UPPER ENDOSCOPY
An endoscopic examination of the upper GI tract allowing more direct visualization through a lighted fiber-optic tube that contains a lens, forceps, and brushes for biopsy.
Preparation is similar to that of the upper GI.
Light sedation is required.

BARIUM ENEMA
An x-ray examination using an opaque contrast medium to examine the lower GI tract.
Preparation includes NPO after midnight, a bowel prep such as magnesium citrate, and in some instances enemas to empty out any remaining stool particles.

ULTRASOUND
A technique that uses high-frequency sound waves to echo off body organs, creating a picture.
Preparation depends on the organ to be visualized and may include NPO or no prep.

COLONOSCOPY
An endoscopic examination of the entire colon with the use of colonoscopy inserted into the rectum.

COLONOSCOPY—cont'd
Preparation is similar to that of barium enema: clear liquids the day before and then some form of bowel cleanser, such as GoLytely. Enemas until clear may also be ordered. Light sedation is required.

FLEXIBLE SIGMOIDOSCOPY
An examination of the interior of the sigmoid colon through the use of a flexible or rigid lighted tube.
Preparation is similar to that of a barium enema or colonoscopy. Light sedation is required.

COMPUTERIZED TOMOGRAPHY SCAN
An x-ray examination of the body from many angles utilizing a scanner analyzed by a computer.
Preparation may be NPO, or nothing may be required.
The client must be informed of the need to lie very still. If claustrophobia is a problem, light sedation may be utilized.

MAGNETIC RESONANCE IMAGING
A noninvasive examination that uses magnet and radio waves to produce a picture of the inside of the body.
Preparation is NPO 4 to 6 hours before examination.
No metallic objects are allowed in the room, including metal objects on clothes.

ENTEROCLYSIS
Introduction of contrast material to jejunum, allowing entire small intestine to be studied.
Preparation is 24 hours of clear liquid diet and colon cleansing, such as a GoLytely or enemas until clear.

DIAGNOSTIC EXAMINATIONS. A variety of radiological and diagnostic tests are used with the client experiencing alterations in the GI system. The preparation and the test itself are often quite unpleasant for the client. See Box 32-5 for an explanation of these tests.

CLIENT EXPECTATIONS. When you assess the client's expectations of care, it may be helpful to anticipate the client's need for privacy and respect. Bowel elimination problems can be embarrassing. You should be able to ask the client what is important to ensure that care is given in a personal and professional way.

Because there is a direct link between nutrition and bowel elimination, consider the client's cultural choices of foods and fluids. Concessions may need to be made on certain food selections. Methods of preparation may also be a concern, especially if tradition and cost are deciding factors.

When determining the client's expectations, consider his or her normal bowel pattern. The client may wish to have activities planned so that normal routines can be maintained. If what is "normal" to the client is unhealthy or could promote negative health practices, you must first meet the client's educational needs.

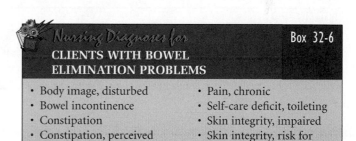

Nursing Diagnoses for
CLIENTS WITH BOWEL ELIMINATION PROBLEMS
Box 32-6

- Body image, disturbed
- Bowel incontinence
- Constipation
- Constipation, perceived
- Diarrhea
- Pain, acute
- Pain, chronic
- Self-care deficit, toileting
- Skin integrity, impaired
- Skin integrity, risk for impaired

Nursing Diagnosis

Gather data from the nursing assessment, and analyze clusters of defining characteristics to identify relevant nursing diagnoses (Box 32-6). Reflecting on each of the data sources is necessary in determining the correct diagnosis. Selected defining characteristics can apply to more than one diagnosis, so you must be clinically skillful in seeing the patterns that reveal the diagnosis that best fits the client's situation. For example, a client may report not having a bowel movement for several days. This defining characteristic may apply

Care Study Nursing Care Plan   BOWEL ELIMINATION

ASSESSMENT

From their first visit, Vickie and Mr. Gutierrez have been able to communicate without difficulty. Mr. Gutierrez complains of feeling **"full of gas"** but has not "passed any wind," perhaps in the last 2 days. Because of the feeling of fullness Mr. Gutierrez also states, "I really **haven't felt like eating today** and I need to move my bowels. I took a laxative last night, and I think I need an enema." Vickie confirms that Mr. Gutierrez had his **last bowel movement 3 days ago.** The **stool was brown in color and hardformed.** On examination of the abdomen Vicki finds **hypoactive bowel sounds** in all four quadrants. His abdomen is soft but slightly distended. A medication history shows that Mr. Gutierrez frequently resorts to taking laxatives. An assessment of Mr. Gutierrez's diet reveals a high intake of corn tortillas and cheese and a low intake of fruits. His stove has not been working well, and he has been unable to prepare rice and beans. On the basis of the nursing history, Vickie estimates Mr. Gutierrez normally drinks about 1200 ml of fluid daily.

*Defining characteristics are shown in bold type.

NURSING DIAGNOSIS

Constipation related to less than adequate fluid and dietary intake and chronic laxative use.

PLANNING

GOAL

Client will establish and maintain a normal defecation pattern within 1 month.

EXPECTED OUTCOMES

Client will have a bowel movement within 48 hours.

Client's abdomen will be soft, nondistended, and nontender within 24 hours.

Client will pass soft, formed stools at least every 3 days.

IMPLEMENTATION

STEPS

1. Instruct client on a weekly menu plan, including foods high in fiber: posole, beans and rice, tomatoes, and wheat tortillas.

2. Consult with client's niece and long-term care center to have client's stove repaired.

3. Educate client about use of liquids to promote softening of stool and defecation; have client drink fluids of choice (1 glass every 2 hours during the day).

4. Have client take time to defecate 1 hour after breakfast or other meal, until a regular time becomes established.

RATIONALE

High-fiber foods increase, peristalsis, improving movement of intestinal contents through the GI tract. The need for laxatives is also reduced (Colwell and others, 2000).

Cooking facilities are necessary for preparation of selected food preferences.

Fluids keep fecal mass soft and increase stool bulk, causing increase in colon peristalsis (Phipps and others, 1999).

Gastrocolic reflex normally occurs approximately 1 hour after breakfast, resulting in mass movement of colon contents (Lueckenotte, 2000).

EVALUATION

* Ask client to keep a diary of foods and fluids ingested for 1 week, and review.
* Ask client to describe the effect fluids and high-fiber foods have on elimination.
* Ask client to describe frequency and character of stool.
* Palpate abdomen for distention and tenderness.

---

to the diagnosis of *constipation* and *perceived constipation*. The difference is that on examination the client with *constipation* has a dry, hard stool with abdominal or rectal fullness. In contrast, the client with *perceived constipation* has expectation of having a stool daily, and in fact the stools can be quite normal.

It is important to establish the correct "related to" factor for a diagnosis. For example, with the diagnosis of *constipation* you must distinguish between nutritional imbalance, exercise, medications, and emotional problems as causative factors. Selection of the correct etiology for the diagnosis ensures that the appropriate nursing interventions will be implemented.

Planning

GOALS AND OUTCOMES.   After nursing diagnoses are identified, you and the client set goals and expected outcomes to direct interventions. When possible, these goals

and outcomes should incorporate the client's elimination routines or habits as much as possible and reinforce those that promote health. In addition, preexisting health concerns are also considered. For example, if the client is at risk for the development of congestive heart failure, an expected outcome of increasing fluid intake must be tailored to the client's cardiac function to safely handle the volume of fluid.

The goals and expected outcomes you establish must be realistic. The outcomes provide measurable behaviors or physiological responses that indicate progress toward the goal of a normal bowel elimination pattern. Nursing interventions are designed to achieve the outcomes of care.

Setting Priorities

Defecation patterns vary among individuals. For this reason you and the client work together to plan effective interventions to meet the client's elimination needs and priorities (see care plan). What may be a realistic time frame to estab-

Dietary Recommendations for Elimination Problems

Box 32-7

CONSTIPATION

Increase intake of high-fiber foods. Added fluids should accompany increase in fiber intake.

Vegetables (dried beans, brussels sprouts, corn, peas, and potatoes)

Fruits (apples with peels, raisins, and prunes)

Cereals (bran and whole wheat) and whole grain breads

For the older adult with poor dentition, offer chopped, not pureed, foods. Add extra chopped vegetables to soups.

Persons with difficulties in swallowing need mashed, not pureed, foods. Liquids such as fruit juices and hot tea are beneficial.

DIARRHEA

Avoid spicy or high-fiber foods.

If client is lactose intolerant, avoid the use of milk and milk products.

Increase intake of low-fiber foods: chicken, fish, lean beef, pasta, bananas, and rice.

DIARRHEA—cont'd

If diarrhea causes serious fluid loss, replace with water, weak tea, gelatin, plain soda, and bouillon.

FLATULENCE

Avoid gas-producing foods: cauliflower, broccoli, brussels sprouts, onions, dried beans and lentils, and beer.

OSTOMIES

The location of an ostomy determines the type of diet needed for regular evacuation. Initially place clients on low-fiber diets to avoid stomal obstruction. Slowly add high-fiber foods one at a time over a period of several weeks. Maintain a high fluid intake.

Avoid foods that may cause blockage: oranges, apples with tough skins, corn, Chinese vegetables in large amounts, popcorn, and uncooked mushrooms.

---

lish a normal defecation pattern for one client might be very different for another. In addition, if the client has a new ostomy resulting from cancer, the priority of coping with cancer and its treatment may precede the client's need to independently manage care of the bowel diversion. In addition, when a bowel diversion is necessary, coping with changes in body image is a high priority for both the client and family.

CONTINUITY OF CARE.   Other health care team members are important resources for the client and family. You may refer a client with chronic constipation to a dietitian to plan a nutritionally balanced diet that incorporates the client's food preferences and lifestyle.

Involvement of the family in the plan of care is important. When clients are disabled or debilitated, family members often become the primary caregivers. Client and family education is important to promote understanding of ways to establish normal bowel function. If access to proper nutrition is a concern, community organizations that deliver meals to the home or that provide transportation for clients can be beneficial.

A clinical nurse specialist or wound, ostomy, and continence nurse specialist can provide guidance in the care and management of ostomy sites and problems involving incontinence or skin breakdown. In many institutions, members of the health care team collaborate in developing a critical pathway for client care.

Implementation

HEALTH PROMOTION.   The factors that normally promote bowel elimination are appropriate interventions for helping clients develop normal bowel habits.

DIET.   Depending on the client's elimination problem, specific foods are recommended to ensure proper nutrient intake and normal defecation (Box 32-7). There is increasing evidence indicating that low fat intake and increases in dietary fiber and bulk-forming foods reduce the client's risk of colorectal cancers, digestive diseases, and other cancers. Assisting clients and their families in different food selection and preparation practices can help to reduce the risks of GI disease. Consideration must be given to whether a client can afford the foods recommended. In addition to solid foods, you encourage the client to drink 2000 to 3000 ml of fluids daily, if not contraindicated by other medical conditions.

EXERCISE.   An age-related exercise program also assists clients in maintaining a healthy bowel pattern. Regular exercise, 3 to 5 times a week, promotes normal GI motility. Examples of exercise include walking, cycling, or swimming. A client experiencing a period of immobilization from illness should ambulate as soon as possible. Ambulation promotes peristalsis and a return to normal bowel function.

TIMING AND PRIVACY.   One of the most important habits a nurse can teach a client regarding bowel habits is to take time for defecation. Ignoring the urge to defecate and not taking time to defecate completely are common causes of constipation. To establish regular bowel habits, a client must respond to the urge to defecate. Prompt response may help the client to reduce episodes of constipation.

Defecation is most likely to occur an hour after meals. If attempts are made to defecate during the time when mass colonic peristalsis occurs, the chances of success are great. If a client is restricted to bed or requires assistance in ambulating, you should recommend use of a bedside commode or a bedpan or have a caregiver help the client reach the bathroom. Prompt assistance is needed before the urge disappears.

Clients may have previously established routines to assist them with defecation. When clients become hospitalized, health promotion habits can become disrupted. Encourage clients to maintain as many of these regular practices as possible. Privacy is often a concern for clients. Health care providers often walk in and out of rooms without knocking, and many clients may reside in semiprivate rooms or living areas. You must remain acutely aware of the client's need for modesty and privacy.

PROMOTION OF NORMAL DEFECATION. To help clients evacuate contents normally and without discomfort, recommend interventions that stimulate the defecation reflex or increase peristalsis. One way to promote defecation is by having the client assume a squatting position during defecation. Squatting increases pressure on the rectum and facilitates use of intraabdominal muscles. Clients who have difficulty in squatting because of muscular weakness or mobility limitations benefit from the use of elevated toilet seats. Regular toilets are too low for clients unable to lower themselves to a squatting position because of joint or muscle-wasting diseases or for those who have had abdominal surgery. With an elevated seat, less effort is needed to sit or stand.

ACUTE CARE. When clients become acutely ill, the GI system is often one of the first systems to be affected. Simple changes in activity levels, sleeping patterns, diet, and medications directly affect regular bowel habits. Surgical intervention can create additional elimination problems for the acute care client (e.g., discomfort from an abdominal incision, absent or decreased gastrointestinal peristalsis, or increased accumulation of intestinal gas following surgery). Sensitivity to the client's need for the provision of as much self-care as possible will assist the client in coping with the changes.

MEDICATIONS. Medications can initiate and facilitate stool passage. **Cathartics** and **laxatives** have the short-term action of emptying the bowel. These agents are also used in bowel evacuation for clients undergoing GI tests and abdominal surgery. While the terms *cathartic* and *laxative* are often used interchangeably, cathartics have a stronger and more rapid effect on the intestines.

Although the oral route is more commonly used, cathartics prepared as suppositories are more effective because of their stimulant effect on the rectal mucosa. Cathartic suppositories such as bisacodyl (Dulcolax) may act within 30 minutes. Give the suppository shortly before the client's usual time to defecate or immediately after a meal. Teach clients about the potential harmful effects of repeated use of laxatives. The client should understand that laxatives and cathartics are not meant for long-term maintenance of bowel function.

Cathartics are classified by the method by which the agent promotes defecation. Stimulant cathartics cause local irritation to the intestinal mucosa and inhibit reabsorption of water in the large intestine. Intestinal irritation increases intestinal motility. The rapid movement of feces causes retention of water in the stool. The drugs can cause formation of a soft to fluid stool in 6 to 8 hours. Clients tend to abuse stimulants more than other cathartics. Overuse leads to loss of intestinal tone.

Saline or osmotic agents contain a salt preparation not absorbed by the intestines. The cathartic draws water into the fecal mass. This osmotic action increases the bulk of the intestinal contents and enhances lubrication. Rapid bowel evacuation may occur in 1 to 3 hours. Magnesium hydroxide (milk of magnesia) and sodium phosphate (Phospho-soda) are saline cathartics. Clients with impaired kidney function should avoid using these drugs because of the toxic buildup of magnesium.

Wetting agents or stool softeners are detergents that lower the surface tension of feces, allowing penetration by water and fat. These drugs also inhibit absorption of water by the intestines. The fecal mass becomes large and soft, preventing the client from straining during defecation. Commonly used wetting agents are dioctyl sodium sulfosuccinate (Colace) and dioctyl calcium sulfosuccinate (Surfak).

Bulk-forming cathartics consist of cellulose and polysaccharides that absorb water and increase solid intestinal bulk. The fecal bulk stretches the intestinal walls, stimulating peristalsis. Passage of stool will occur in 12 to 24 hours. Bulk-forming laxatives are the least irritating and safest of all cathartics. Clients should be encouraged to take bulk cathartics with plenty of liquids.

Lubricants soften the fecal mass, thus easing the strain of defecation. Clients with painful hemorrhoids particularly benefit from a lubricant. The only lubricant laxative available is mineral oil. Regular use of mineral oil interferes with absorption of the fat-soluble vitamins A, D, E, and K. The drug can also cause a dangerous form of pneumonia if aspirated.

For clients with diarrhea, the most effective antidiarrheal agents are opiates. Antidiarrheal agents decrease intestinal muscle tone to slow the passage of feces. As a result, more water is absorbed by intestinal walls. Antidiarrheal agents should be used with caution because opiates are habit forming.

ENEMAS. An **enema** is an instillation of a preparation into the rectum and sigmoid colon. An enema is given primarily to promote defecation by stimulating peristalsis. The volume of fluid instilled breaks up the fecal mass, stretches the rectal wall, and initiates the defecation reflex. Enemas are also given as a vehicle for drugs that exert a local effect on rectal mucosa.

The most common use for an enema is temporary relief of constipation. Other indications include removing impacted feces; emptying the bowel before diagnostic tests, surgery, or childbirth; and beginning a program of bowel training. Clients should be discouraged from relying on enemas to maintain bowel regularity. Enemas do not treat the cause of constipation. As with laxative abuse, frequent use destroys normal defecation reflexes.

Cleansing enemas promote complete evacuation of feces from the colon. They act by stimulating peristalsis through the infusion of a large volume of solution or through local irritation of the colon's mucosa. Cleansing enemas include tap water, normal saline, low-volume hypertonic saline, and soapsuds solution. Each solution exerts a different osmotic effect, causing the movement of fluids between the colon and interstitial spaces beyond the intestinal wall. Infants and children can tolerate only normal saline because they are at risk for fluid imbalance.

Tap water is hypotonic and exerts a lower osmotic pressure than fluid in interstitial spaces. After infusion into the colon, tap water escapes from the bowel lumen into interstitial spaces. The net movement of water is low; the infused volume stimulates defecation before large amounts of water leave the bowel. Tap water enemas should not be repeated, because water toxicity or circulatory overload can develop if large amounts of water are absorbed.

Physiologically, normal saline is the safest solution to use because it exerts the same osmotic pressure as fluids in interstitial spaces around the bowel. The volume of infused saline stimulates peristalsis. Giving saline enemas does not create the danger of excess fluid absorption.

Hypertonic solutions infused into the bowel exert osmotic pressure that pulls fluids out of interstitial spaces. The colon fills with fluid, and the resultant distention promotes defecation. Clients unable to tolerate large volumes of fluid benefit most from this type of enema. A hypertonic solution of 120 to 180 ml (4 to 6 oz) is usually effective. The Fleet enema is most commonly used.

Soap solution may be added to tap water or saline to create the additional effect of intestinal irritation. Only pure castile soap is safe. Harsh soaps or detergents can cause serious bowel inflammation.

A physician may order a high or low cleansing enema. The terms *high* and *low* refer to the height from which and hence the pressure with which the fluid is delivered. High enemas are given to cleanse the entire colon. A low enema cleans only the rectum and sigmoid colon. After the enema is infused, the client is asked to turn from the left lateral to the dorsal recumbent, then over to the right lateral position. The position change helps fluid to reach the large intestine.

Oil-retention enemas lubricate the rectum and colon. The feces absorb the oil and become softer and easier to pass. To enhance action of the oil, the client retains the enema for several hours if possible.

Certain enemas or enema administrations contain drugs. An example is sodium polystyrene sulfonate (Kayexalate), used to treat clients with dangerously high serum potassium levels. Skill 32-1 outlines the steps for enema administration.

The physician often orders "enemas till clear," which means that the enema is repeated until the client passes fluid that is clear and contains no fecal material. Excess enema seriously depletes fluids and electrolytes. If the enema fails to return a clear solution after 3 times, the physician should be notified. When an enema is given to a child, it helps to have a parent assist. The child should be able to see the equipment for the procedure.

Giving an enema to a client who is unable to contract the external sphincter can cause difficulties. Give the enema with

Skill 32-1
Administering a Cleansing Enema

DELEGATION CONSIDERATIONS

The skill of administering an enema can be delegated to assistive personnel. Inform and assist care provider in proper way to position clients who have mobility restrictions. Instruct care provider about how to position clients who also have therapeutic equipment present, such as drains, intravenous catheters, or traction. Be sure care provider knows signs and symptoms of client not tolerating the procedure, and when it must be stopped.

EQUIPMENT
- Disposable gloves
- Water-soluble lubricant
- Waterproof, absorbent pads
- Bath blanket
- Toilet tissue
- Bedpan, bedside commode, or access to toilet
- Wash basin, washcloths, towel, and soap
- IV pole

Enema Bag Administration
- Enema container
- Tubing and clamp (if not already attached to container)
- Appropriate-size rectal tube:
    - Adult: 22 to 30 Fr
    - Child: 12 to 18 Fr
- Correct volume of warmed solution:
    - Adult: 750 to 1000 ml
    - Child:
        - 150 to 250 ml, infant
        - 250 to 350 ml, toddler
        - 300 to 500 ml, school-age child
        - 500 to 700 ml, adolescent

Prepackaged Enema
- Prepackaged enema container with rectal tip

STEPS	RATIONALE
1. Assess status of client: last bowel movement, normal bowel patterns, hemorrhoids, mobility, external sphincter control, abdominal pain.	Determines factors indicating need for enema and influencing the type of enema used.
2. Assess for presence of increased intracranial pressure, glaucoma, or recent rectal or prostate surgery.	These conditions contraindicate use of enemas.
3. Determine client's level of understanding of purpose of enema.	Allows you to plan for appropriate teaching measures.
4. Check client's medical record to clarify the rationale for the enema.	Determines purpose of enema administration: preparation for special procedure or relief of constipation.

Steps	Rationale
5. Review physician's order for enema.	Order by physician is required. Determines number and type of enema to be given.

• *Critical Decision Point*
"Enemas until clear" order means that enemas are repeated until client passes fluid that is clear of fecal matter. Check agency policy, but usually client should receive only three consecutive enemas to avoid disruption of fluid and electrolyte balance.

Steps	Rationale
6. Collect appropriate equipment.	
7. Correctly identify client and explain procedure.	Information promotes client cooperation and reduces anxiety.
8. Assemble enema bag with appropriate solution and rectal tube.	
9. Wash hands, and apply gloves.	Reduces transmission of microorganisms.
10. Provide privacy by closing curtains around bed or closing door.	Reduces embarrassment for client.
11. Raise bed to appropriate working height for nurse: raise side rail on opposite side.	Promotes good body mechanics and client safety.
12. Assist client into left side-lying (Sims') position with right knee flexed. Children may also be placed in dorsal recumbent position.	Allows enema solution to flow downward by gravity along natural curve of sigmoid colon and rectum, thus improving retention of solution.

• *Critical Decision Point*
If client is suspected of having poor sphincter control, position on bedpan. Client will have difficulty retaining enema solution.

Steps	Rationale
13. Place waterproof pad under hips and buttocks.	Prevents soiling of linen.
14. Cover client with bath blanket, exposing only rectal area, clearly visualizing anus.	Provides warmth, reduces exposure of body parts, and allows client to feel more relaxed and comfortable.
15. Place bedpan or commode in easily accessible position. If client will be expelling contents in toilet, ensure that toilet is free. (If client will be getting up to bathroom to expel enema, place client's slippers and bathrobe in easily accessible position.)	Used in case client is unable to retain enema solution.
16. Administer enema:	
A. **Enema Bag**	
(1) Add warmed solution to enema bag: warm tap water as it flows from faucet, place saline container in basin of hot water before adding saline to enema bag, and check temperature of solution by pouring small amount of solution over inner wrist.	Hot water can burn intestinal mucosa. Cold water can cause abdominal cramping and is difficult to retain.
(2) Raise container, release clamp, and allow solution to flow long enough to fill tubing.	Removes air from tubing.
(3) Reclamp tubing.	Prevents further loss of solution.
(4) Lubricate 6 to 8 cm (3 to 4 inches) of tip of rectal tube with lubricating jelly.	Allows smooth insertion of rectal tube without risk of irritation or trauma to mucosa.
(5) Gently separate buttocks and locate anus. Instruct client to relax by breathing out slowly through mouth.	Breathing out promotes relaxation of external anal sphincter.
(6) Insert tip of rectal tube slowly by pointing tip in direction of client's umbilicus (see illustration). Length of insertion varies: Adult: 7.5 to 10 cm (3 to 4 inches) Child: 5 to 7.5 cm (2 to 3 inches) Infant: 2.5 to 3.75 cm (1 to $1\frac{1}{2}$ inches)	Careful insertion prevents trauma to rectal mucosa from accidental lodging of tube against rectal wall. Insertion beyond proper limit can cause bowel perforation.
(7) Hold tubing in rectum constantly until end of fluid instillation.	Bowel contraction can cause expulsion of rectal tube.

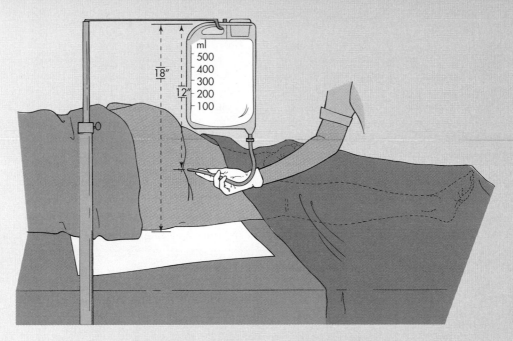

STEP 16A(6)   Insertion of rectal tube into rectum.

(8) Open regulating clamp, and allow solution to enter slowly with container at client's hip level.	Rapid instillation can stimulate evacuation of rectal tube.

- *Critical Decision Point*

If tube does not pass easily, do not force. Consider allowing a small amount of fluid to infuse and then try reinserting tube slowly.

(9) Raise height of enema container slowly to appropriate level above anus: 30 to 45 cm (12 to 18 inches) for high enema, 30 cm (12 inches) for regular enema, 7.5 cm (3 inches) for low enema. Instillation time varies with volume of solution administered (e.g., 1 L/10 min) (see illustration step 16A[6]).	Allows for continuous, slow instillation of solution; raising container too high causes rapid instillation and possible painful distention of colon. High pressure can cause rupture of bowel in infant.
(10) Lower container or clamp tubing if client complains of cramping or if fluid escapes around rectal tube.	Temporary cessation of instillation prevents cramping, which may prevent client from retaining all fluid, altering effectiveness of enema.
(11) Clamp tubing after all solution is instilled.	Prevents entrance of air into rectum.

B. Prepackaged Disposable Container

(1) Remove plastic cap from rectal tip. Tip is already lubricated, but more jelly can be applied as needed.	Lubrication provides for smooth insertion of rectal tube without causing rectal irritation or trauma.
(2) Gently separate buttocks and locate rectum. Instruct client to relax by breathing out slowly through mouth.	Breathing out promotes relaxation of external rectal sphincter.
(3) Insert tip of bottle gently into rectum toward the umbilicus.	Gentle insertion prevents trauma to rectal mucosa.

     Adult: 7.5 to 10 cm (3 to 4 inches)
     Child: 5 to 7.5 cm (2 to 3 inches)
     Infant: 2.5 to 3.75 cm (1 to $1\frac{1}{2}$ inches)

STEPS	RATIONALE
(4) Squeeze bottle until all of solution has entered rectum and colon. Instruct client to retain solution until the urge to defecate occurs, usually 2 to 5 minutes.	Hypertonic solutions require only small volumes to stimulate defecation.
17. Place layers of toilet tissue around tube at anus and gently withdraw rectal tube.	Provides for client's comfort and cleanliness.
18. Explain to client that feeling of distention is normal, as well as some abdominal cramping. Ask client to retain solution as long as possible while lying quietly in bed. (For infant or young child, gently hold buttocks together for few minutes.)	Solution distends bowel. Length of retention varies with type of enema and client's ability to contract rectal sphincter. Longer retention promotes more effective stimulation of peristalsis and defecation.
19. Discard enema container and tubing in proper receptacle, or rinse out thoroughly with warm soap and water if container is to be reused.	Reduces transmission and growth of microorganisms.
20. Assist client to bathroom or help to position client on bedpan.	Normal squatting position promotes defecation.
21. Observe character of feces and solution (caution client against flushing toilet before inspection).	
22. Assist client as needed in washing anal area with warm soap and water (if you administer perineal care, use gloves).	Fecal contents can irritate skin. Hygiene promotes client's comfort.
23. Remove and discard gloves, and wash hands.	Reduces transmission of microorganisms.
24. Inspect color, consistency, amount of stool, and fluid passed.	Determines if stool is evacuated or fluid is retained. Note abnormalities such as presence of blood or mucus.
25. Assess condition of abdomen; cramping, rigidity, or distention can indicate a serious problem.	Determines if distention is relieved. Excess volume can distend or perforate the bowel.

UNEXPECTED OUTCOMES AND RELATED INTERVENTIONS
- Abdomen becomes rigid and distended.
  - Stop enema if fluid is still being instilled.
  - Notify physician.
- Abdominal pain or cramping develops.
  - Slow rate of instillation.
- Bleeding develops.
  - Stop enema administration.
  - Notify physician.
  - Remain with client, and obtain vital signs.

RECORDING AND REPORTING
- Record type and volume of enema given, time administered and character of results.
- Record client tolerance to procedure.
  - Report failure of client to evacuate stool or contents of enema, presence of tenderness and/or distention, or newly absent bowel sounds.

the client positioned on the bedpan. Giving the enema with the client sitting on the toilet is unsafe because the curved rectal tubing can abrade the rectal wall.

IMPACTION REMOVAL.   For clients with an impaction, the fecal mass may be too large to be passed voluntarily. If enemas fail, you must break up the fecal mass digitally and remove it in sections. The procedure can be very uncomfortable for the client. Excess rectal manipulation may cause irritation to the mucosa, bleeding, and stimulation of the vagus nerve, which can result in a reflex slowing of the heart rate. Because of the procedure's potential complications, in some institutions only physicians are allowed to remove impactions digitally. Before you perform the procedure, check agency policy regarding a physician's order (Box 32-8).

POSITIONING ON BEDPAN.   A client restricted to use of a bedpan for defecation will usually need assistance. Sitting on a bedpan can be uncomfortable and awkward. Help position the client comfortably. Two types of bedpans are available. The regular bedpan, made of metal or hard plastic, has a curved smooth upper end and a sharp-edged lower end and is about 5 cm (2 inches) deep. A fracture pan, designed for clients with body or leg casts or for whom the semi-Fowler's position is contraindicated, has a shallow upper end about 1.3 cm ($1/_2$ inch) deep (Figure 32-6).

The upper end of either pan fits under the buttocks toward the sacrum, with the lower end just under the upper thighs. The pan should be high enough so that feces enter it. The most important element for you to consider in positioning the client is preventing muscle strain and dis-

Procedural Guidelines for	Box 32-8

DIGITAL REMOVAL OF STOOL

1. Explain the procedure, and help the client to lie on the left side with knees flexed and back toward you.
2. Assess heart rate in the beginning as baseline to determine tolerance to procedure.
3. Drape the trunk and lower extremities with a bath blanket, and place a waterproof pad under the buttocks. Keep a bedpan next to the client.
4. Apply disposable gloves, and lubricate the index finger of dominant hand with lubricating jelly.
5. Gently insert the index finger into the rectum and advance the finger slowly along the rectal wall toward the umbilicus.
6. Gently loosen the fecal mass by massaging around it. Work the finger into the hardened mass.
7. Work the feces downward toward the end of the rectum. Remove small pieces at a time and discard into bedpan.
8. Reassess the client's heart rate and look for signs of fatigue. Stop the procedure if the heart rate drops significantly or the rhythm changes.
9. Continue to remove feces, and allow the client to rest at intervals.
10. After completion, wash and dry the buttocks and anal area.
11. Remove bedpan and dispose of feces. Remove gloves by turning them inside out, then discard.
12. Assist client to toilet or clean bedpan if urge to defecate develops.
13. Wash hands. Record results of disimpaction by describing fecal characteristics and amount.
14. Follow procedure with enemas or cathartics as ordered by physician.

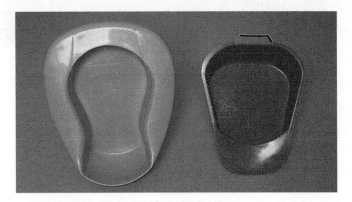

FIGURE **32-6** Types of bedpans: *From left,* regular bedpan and fracture pan.

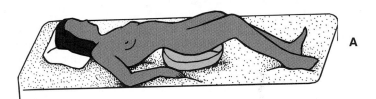

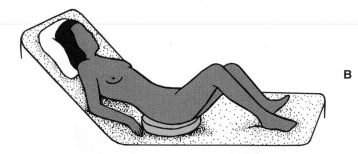

FIGURE **32-7** Positions on a bedpan. **A,** Improper positioning of a client. **B,** Proper position reduces client's back strain.

comfort. A client should never be placed on a bedpan and then left with the bed flat unless activity restrictions demand it. This forces the client to hyperextend the back to lift the hips onto the pan (Figure 32-7, *A*). It may be necessary to have the bed flat when placing the client on a bedpan. The nurse should then raise the head of the bed 30 to 45 degrees (Figure 32-7, *B*). Clients who have overhead trapeze frames can easily lift themselves by grasping the trapeze bar. Box 32-9 describes steps in assisting a client with a bedpan.

For the more mobile client, a bedside commode can be a safe, effective alternative to a bedpan. Its use is less exhausting and allows the client to assume a more "normal" or "familiar" position for defecation.

CONTINUING AND RESTORATIVE CARE. As the client recovers and is able to return home or to an extended care facility, establishment of regular elimination patterns must begin. Bowel retraining is one essential step in regaining independence.

BOWEL TRAINING. A bowel training program can help some clients, especially those who still have some neuromuscular control, to achieve normal defecation. The training program involves setting up a daily routine. By attempting to defecate at the same time each day and using measures that promote

defecation, the client gains control of bowel reflexes. The program requires time, patience, and consistency. The physician determines the client's physical readiness and ability to benefit from bowel training.

OSTOMY CARE. A client with a temporary or permanent bowel diversion has unique elimination needs. The client wears a pouch or appliance to collect stool emitted from the stoma. Meticulous skin care is needed to prevent liquid stool from irritating skin around a stoma (Box 32-10).

Some clients irrigate their left-sided colostomies to establish regular bowel elimination. The muscular quality of the colon allows it to be safely irrigated with a relatively large volume of water or saline. The irrigation acts like an enema, distending the bowel and stimulating peristalsis. Only specific equipment for irrigating an ostomy should be used. *Never* use an enema set to irrigate an ostomy.

A special cone-tipped irrigating kit (Figure 32-8) is used to prevent bowel penetration and to prevent backflow of the irrigating solution. The client sits on the toilet and wears an irrigating sleeve (Figure 32-9) that extends into the com-

1. Assess the client's level of mobility, strength, ability to help, and presence of any condition (e.g., orthopedic) that may interfere with use of a bedpan.
2. Explain the technique you will use in turning and positioning to the client.
3. Offer the bedpan at a time that coincides with the duodenocolic or mass peristaltic reflex.
4. Wash and dry hands, and apply disposable gloves.
5. Close the room curtain for privacy.
6. If metal bedpan is used, hold it under warm running water for a couple of minutes, then dry.
7. Raise the bed to a comfortable working height and be sure client is positioned high in bed with head elevated 30 degrees (unless contraindicated). Raise the side rail opposite the side where you are standing.
8. Fold back top linen to client's knees.
9. Assist with positioning: Instruct client to bend knees and place weight on heels. Place your hand, palm up, under client's sacrum, resting elbow on mattress. Then have client lift hips while you slip bedpan into place with other hand.
10. Dependent client: Lower head of bed flat and have client roll onto side opposite nurse. Apply powder lightly to lower back and buttocks (optional). Place bedpan firmly against buttocks and push down into mattress with open rim toward client's feet. Keeping one hand against bedpan, place other hand around client's forehip (see illustration). Ask client to roll onto pan, flat on bed. With client positioned comfortably, raise head of bed 30 degrees.

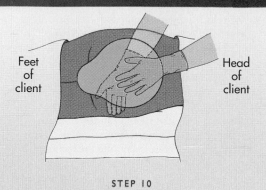

STEP 10

11. Place rolled towel under lumbar curve of client's back.
12. Place call light and toilet tissue within client's reach, and keep side rails up as needed.
13. Remove bedpan as client lifts hips up or as client carefully rolls off pan and to side. Hold pan firmly as client moves.
14. Assist in cleansing anal area. Wipe from pubic area toward anus. Replace top covers.
15. If a specimen or intake and output are collected, do not dispose of tissue in bedpan.
16. Have client wash and dry hands.
17. Empty pan's contents, dispose of gloves, and wash hands.
18. Inspect stool for color, amount, consistency, odor, or presence of abnormal substances.

Client Teaching

Box 32-10

STOMA CARE (CONVENTIONAL INCONTINENT ILEOSTOMY)

- Teach the client that the drainage from the stoma site is very irritating to skin and contact should be avoided if at all possible. If contact occurs, thorough cleansing with soap and water should be performed as soon as possible.
- Instruct the client to wash skin with mild soap and water or plain water and dry the skin thoroughly.
- Tell the client not to use creams or ointments on peristomal skin because they prevent the pouch from adhering to the skin.
- Teach the client to routinely inspect the appearance of the stoma and surrounding skin. (The stoma should be moist, shiny, and dark pink to red.) Bleeding around the stoma should be minimal. Tell the client to report excess bleeding, abnormal color, or edema to the nurse or physician.
- Teach the client how to select and apply a skin barrier and pouch. Include length of wear.
- Teach the client how to empty and change the pouch. It should be emptied when one-third to one-half full.
- Teach the client methods of reducing odor. Commercial deodorants are available.
- Tell the client to carry ostomy supplies at all times.
- If yeast infections develop, instruct the client to wash thoroughly but gently, pat dry, and apply medically prescribed Kenalog spray and Mycostatin topical powder to irritated skin.

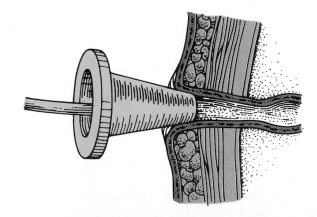

FIGURE 32-8   Ostomy irrigation cone inserted into stoma.

mode. The amount and type of solution used is ordered by the physician and is generally 500 to 700 ml of tap water. The solution is introduced slowly into the stoma via the lubricated irrigation cone tip, finishing the instillation of the solution in 5 to 10 minutes. The cone tip is removed, and the client waits 30 to 45 minutes for the solution and feces to drain. Once the drainage stops, the client applies a stoma cap.

Ostomies require a pouch to collect feces. An effective pouching system protects the peristomal skin, contains feces, and is odorproof and concealable. A person wearing a pouch

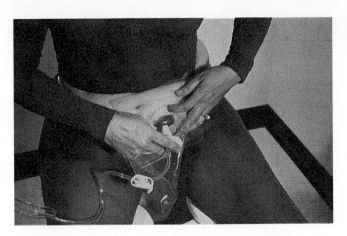

FIGURE **32-9** Client irrigating ostomy using irrigation sleeve.

should feel secure enough to participate in any activity. A variety of pouching systems are available.

A pouching system consists of a pouch and skin barrier. Pouches come in disposable or reusable one- and two-piece systems. Skin barriers include wafers, pastes, powders, and a liquid film that is applied to the skin around the stoma. A good skin barrier protects the skin and prevents irritation from repeated pouch removal.

The pouch is changed when there is little drainage from the ostomy (e.g., before meals or at bedtime). The client should participate in the procedure as much as possible. The client must learn to recognize the normal appearance of a stoma. Skill 32-2 describes the steps for pouching an ostomy.

A client with an ostomy can suffer a change in body image. The appearance of the stoma and accompanying body odors can cause psychological stress. For the client with a new ostomy, it is important for you to promote independence and acceptance of the ostomy. Early involvement in self-care promotes the client's independence. Even simple tasks such as holding pieces of equipment during stomal pouching can help the client begin to adjust to bodily changes. Many clients benefit from the information and encouragement from ostomy support groups.

CARE OF HEMORRHOIDS. Many clients experience discomfort from alterations in elimination. The client with hemorrhoids has pain when hemorrhoidal tissues are directly irritated from passage of hard stool. The primary goal for the client with hemorrhoids is soft-formed stools. Treatment includes proper diet, fluids, and regular exercise. Local heat provides temporary relief to swollen hemorrhoids. A sitz bath is the most effective means of heat application.

When hemorrhoids are present, it is important to prevent trauma to tissues. Use caution when inserting rectal thermometers, suppositories, or rectal tubes. A generous amount of lubricating jelly reduces friction. Often the client is better able to insert an object safely into the rectum. You should

Skill 32-2
POUCHING AN OSTOMY

DELEGATION CONSIDERATIONS
The skill of pouching an ostomy, especially a newly established ostomy, requires problem solving and knowledge application unique to a nurse. Delegation is inappropriate. Pouching of an established ostomy can be delegated to assistive personnel.
- Assist care provider in selecting appropriate pouch and skin barrier.
- Inform care provider of the signs of stomal and peristomal skin changes that should be reported to an RN.
- Have care provider monitor and report characteristics and volume of ostomy output.

EQUIPMENT
- Pouch, clear drainable colostomy/ileostomy in correct size for two-piece system or custom cut-to-fit one-piece type with attached skin barrier
- Pouch closure device, such as clamp
- Clean disposable gloves
- Deodorant
- Gauze pads or washcloth
- Towel or disposable waterproof barrier
- Basin with warm tap water
- Scissors/pen

STEPS	RATIONALE
1. Auscultate for bowel sounds.	Documents presence of peristalsis. Absence may indicate problem.
2. Observe skin barrier and pouch for leakage and length of time in place. Depending on type of pouching system used (such as with an opaque pouch), the nurse may have to remove the pouch to fully observe the stoma. Clear pouches permit the viewing of the stoma without their removal.	May indicate need for different type of pouch or sealant.

- *Critical Decision Point*
  Intact skin barriers with no evidence of leakage do not need to be changed daily and can remain in place for 3 to 5 days (Ayello, 2000).

STEPS	RATIONALE
3. Observe stoma for color, swelling, trauma, and healing; stoma should be moist and reddish pink. Assess type of stoma. Stomas can be flush with the skin or be a bud-like protrusion on the abdomen (see illustration for a normal bud stoma).	Stoma characteristics should be one of the factors to consider when selecting an appropriate pouching system.
4. Measure the stoma with each pouching change. Follow pouch manufacturer's directions and measuring guide as to which pouch to use based on client's stoma size.	Determines correct size equipment, preventing trauma to stoma.
5. Observe abdominal incision (if present).	Relationship to stoma determines proper placement of pouch.
6. Observe effluent from stoma, and keep a record of intake and output. Ask client about skin tenderness.	

7. Assess abdomen for best type of pouching system to use. Consider:
  a. Contour and peristomal plane
  b. Presence of scars, incisions
  c. Location and type of stoma
	Determines pouching system selection and need for other equipment.

8. Assess the client's self-care ability to determine the best type of pouching system to use.	Clients who have difficulty using their hands or who have limited vision may find a one-piece system or a precut pouch and skin barrier more desirable to use; others prefer being able to keep the skin barrier in place for several days, changing just the pouch, and therefore prefer the two-piece system.
9. After skin barrier and pouch removal, assess skin around stoma, noting scars, folds, skin breakdown, and peristomal suture line if present.	Determines need for barrier paste to increase adherence of pouch to skin or to fill in irregularities.
10. Determine client's emotional response and knowledge and understanding of an ostomy and its care.	Assists in determining extent to which client is able to participate in care and need for teaching and information clarification.
11. Explain procedure to client; encourage client's interaction and questions.	Lessens anxiety and promotes client's participation.
12. Assemble equipment, and close room curtains or door.	Organization saves time and optimizes use of time; conserves client's and your energy. Provides privacy.
13. Position client either standing or supine, and drape. If seated, position client either on or in front of toilet.	When client is supine, there are fewer skin wrinkles, which allows for ease of application of pouching system; maintains client's dignity.
14. Wash hands, and apply disposable gloves.	Reduces transmission of microorganisms.
15. Place towel or disposable waterproof barrier under client.	Protects bed linen.
16. Remove used pouch and skin barrier gently by pushing skin away from barrier. An adhesive remover may be used to facilitate removal of skin barrier.	Reduces skin trauma. Improper removal of pouch and barrier can irritate client's skin and can cause skin tears.
17. Cleanse peristomal skin gently with warm tap water using gauze pads or clean washcloth; do not scrub skin; dry completely by patting skin with gauze or towel.	Stool is alkaline, and this irritates skin; fecal bacteria can colonize on skin and increase risk of infection. Avoid use of soap because it leaves a residue on skin that interferes with pouch adhesion to skin. Skin must be as dry as skin barrier; pouch does not adhere to wet skin. If blood appears on gauze pad, do not be alarmed. If rubbed, stoma may ooze some blood as a result of cleaning process. Bleeding into pouch is abnormal. Stoma's surface is highly vascular mucous membrane.

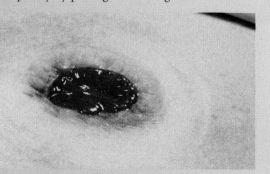

STEP 3   Normal bud stoma. (Courtesy, Hollister, Inc., Libertyville, Ill.)

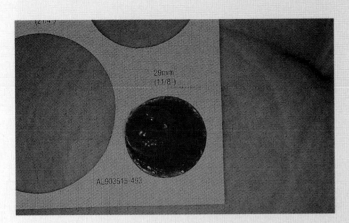

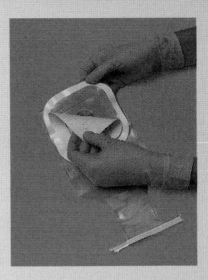

STEP 18   Measuring a stoma.   STEP 19   Preparing an ostomy pouch.

18. Measure stoma for correct size of pouching system needed using the manufacturer's measuring guide (see illustration).	Ensures accuracy in determining correct pouch size needed. Stoma shrinks and does not reach usual size for 6 to 8 weeks.
19. Select appropriate pouch for client based on client assessment. With a custom cut-to-fit pouch, use an ostomy guide to cut opening on the pouch $^1/_{16}$ to $^1/_8$ inch larger than stoma before removing backing. Prepare pouch by removing backing from barrier and adhesive (see illustration). With ileostomy, apply thin circle of barrier paste around opening in pouch; allow to dry.	Size of pouch opening keeps drainage off skin and lessens risk of damage to stoma during peristalsis or activity. Pouch and skin barrier are changed whenever leaking. Paste facilitates seal and protects skin. Change when client is comfortable; before a meal is better because this avoids increased peristalsis and chance of evacuation during pouch change. Can also be changed before or after tub bath or shower.

- **Critical Decision Point**
  If client has large amount of liquid stool from an ileostomy, consider using a "high-output" pouch that will contain this effluent and reduce frequency of pouch emptying.

20. Apply skin barrier and pouch. If creases next to stoma occur, use barrier paste to fill in; let dry 1 to 2 minutes.	Paste creates flat surface for pouch application.
A. For One-Piece Pouching System	
(1) Use skin sealant wipes on skin directly under adhesive skin barrier or pouch; allow to dry. Press adhesive backing of pouch and/or skin barrier smoothly against skin, starting from the bottom and working up and around sides.	Ensures smooth, wrinkle-free seal.
(2) Hold pouch by barrier, center over stoma, and press down gently on barrier; bottom of pouch should point toward client's knees (see illustration).	
(3) Maintain gentle finger pressure around barrier for 1 to 2 minutes.	
B. If Using Two-Piece Pouching System	
(1) Apply barrier-paste flange (barrier with adhesive) as in steps above for one-piece system. Then snap on pouch and maintain finger pressure (see illustration).	Creates wrinkle-free, secure seal; decreases irritation from adhesive on skin. Some two-piece pouching systems may have a snapping or clicking sound that occurs when attaching pouch to skin barrier.
C. For Both Pouching Systems Gently Tug on Pouch in a Downward Direction	Determines that pouch is securely attached.

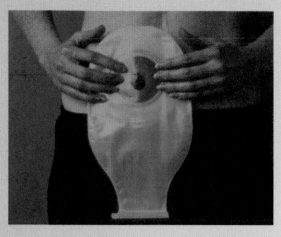

STEP 20A(2)   Applying a one-piece pouch. (Courtesy ConvaTec, Princeton, NJ.)

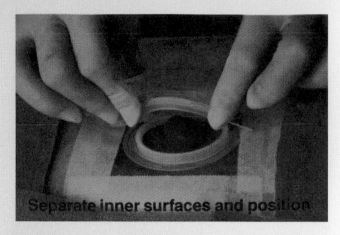

STEP 20B(1)   Application of barrier-paste flange. (Courtesy ConvaTec, Princeton, NJ.)

STEPS	RATIONALE
21. Apply nonallergenic paper tape around pectin skin barrier in a "picture frame" method. Half of the tape should be on skin barrier and half on client's skin. Some clients may prefer a belt attached to the pouch for extra security rather than tape.	"Picture framing" pectin skin barrier adds to security of keeping pouch system attached securely.

- *Critical Decision Point*
  Make sure client who chooses to wear an ostomy belt does not have the belt too tight. To check for appropriate tightness, two fingers should fit comfortably placed between belt and client's skin.

STEPS	RATIONALE
22. Although many ostomy pouches are odorproof, some nurses and clients like to add a small amount of ostomy deodorant into pouch. Do not use "home remedies," which can harm stoma, to control ostomy odor. Do not make a hole in pouch to release flatus.	Causes damage to pouch and defeats purpose of odorproof pouch.
23. Fold bottom of drainable open-ended pouches up once, and close using a closure device such as a clamp (or follow manufacturer's instructions for closure).	Maintains secure seal to prevent leaking.
24. Properly dispose of old pouch and soiled equipment. Client may also request spraying of room air freshener in room if needed.	Lessens odors in room.
25. Remove gloves, and wash hands.	Reduces transmission of microorganisms.
26. Change one- or two-piece pouch every 3 to 7 days unless leaking; pouch can remain in place for tub bath or shower; after bath, pat adhesive dry.	Avoids unnecessary trauma to skin from too-frequent changes. Drying ensures adhesion of pouch.
27. Ask if client feels discomfort around stoma.	Determines presence of skin irritation.
28. Note appearance of stoma around skin and existing incision (if present) while pouch is removed and skin is cleansed. Reinspect condition of skin barrier and adhesive.	Determines condition of tissues and progress of healing. Determines presence of leaks.
29. Auscultate bowel sounds, and observe characteristics of stool.	Determines return of peristalsis and bowel elimination.
30. Observe client's nonverbal behaviors as pouch is applied. Ask if client has any questions about pouching.	May indicate emotional response to stoma and readiness for teaching. Determines level of understanding of procedure.

STEPS	RATIONALE

UNEXPECTED OUTCOMES AND RELATED INTERVENTIONS

- Client experiences irritation and burning of peristomal skin.
  - Observe skin for breaks in integrity, skin inflammation, maceration, or infection.
  - Determine if mucosal layer of stoma has separated from skin.
  - Observe for allergic reaction, which can manifest as erythema and blistering, which is usually localized to the area immediately near the allergen (e.g., pouch, adhesive).
- Stoma becomes necrotic manifested as purple or black color, dry instead of moist, failure to bleed, or tissue sloughing.
  - Assess circulation to stoma.
  - Observe for excessive edema or tension on bowel suture line.
  - Report immediately to physician.

RECORDING AND REPORTING

- Client refuses to view stoma or participate in care.
  - Obtain information about ostomy support groups.
  - Refer client and family to ostomate volunteers in the community.
- Record condition of peristomal skin, size of stoma, and integrity of sutures, if present.
- Record amount and appearance of stool or drainage, color, and consistency.
- Record type of pouch and skin barrier applied.
- Document bowel sounds, abdominal distention, and tenderness.
- Record client's level of participation and need for teaching.
- Report any of the following:
  - Abnormal appearance of stoma, peristomal skin, sutures
  - Abnormal output
  - Presence of tenderness and/or distention
  - Absence of bowel sounds

never attempt to force a thermometer or suppository into the rectum without full view of the anus.

MAINTENANCE OF SKIN INTEGRITY. The client with diarrhea or fecal incontinence is at risk for skin breakdown when fecal contents remain on the skin. The same problem exists for the client with an ostomy that drains liquid stool. Liquid stool is usually acidic and contains digestive enzymes. Irritation from repeated wiping with toilet tissue aggravates skin breakdown. Cleansing the skin after soiling helps but may result in more breakdown unless the skin is thoroughly dried (Colwell and others, 2001).

Instruct the client about cleansing the anal area with mild soap and water after each passage of stool. When caring for a debilitated, incontinent client who is unable to ask for assistance, you should check frequently for defecation. The anal areas can be protected with petrolatum jelly, zinc oxide, or other barrier ointments that hold moisture in the skin and protect the skin from irritation. Yeast infections of the skin can develop easily. Baby powder or cornstarch should not be used because they have no medicinal properties and they frequently cake on the skin and become difficult to remove.

Evaluation

CLIENT CARE. For the client with alterations in bowel elimination, the effectiveness of nursing interventions is measured by success in meeting the client's expected outcomes and goals of care. Optimally the client will be able to eliminate soft-formed stools regularly. In addition, the client

will gain the information necessary to establish a normal elimination pattern (Box 32-11).

Evaluate success of the plan by having the client describe his or her elimination pattern following therapy. Focus on evaluating the character of the client's stool. A return to a more normal, regular elimination pattern can take time. Periodically reevaluate the client. A soft, nondistended abdomen is a desirable finding.

Evaluate an ostomy client's success at self-care. Inspect the client's peristomal skin, looking for impairment in skin integrity. Your evaluation might also include observing the client change and empty an ostomy pouch or perform an irrigation. Evaluate the output or functioning of the ostomy or reservoir as well. In addition, the client's self-esteem must be considered and can be evaluated by the client's response to and willingness to care for the ostomy.

CLIENT EXPECTATIONS. Using client expectations identified during assessment, determine the client's level of satisfaction with nursing care. Does the client feel that you provided care respectfully, offering privacy and support when necessary? Is the client satisfied with the elimination pattern established? Are stools easier to manage?

Your goal for the ostomy client is to achieve a realistic level of self-care and to maintain or reinforce a healthy body image. When discussing these issues with the client, determine if the client's participation in care helped the client accept the ostomy. Were expectations of the client unrealistic? Did the client feel like a partner in care? Learning about the client's level of satisfaction with care can go a long way toward helping future clients.

Outcome Evaluation for   **MR. GUTIERREZ**   Box 32-11

Nursing Action	Client Response/Finding	Achievement of Outcome
Review Mr. Gutierrez's diary of foods and ask him about his intake as well.	Mr. Gutierrez described likes and dislikes, but admits to eating high-fat foods and little fruits and vegetables.	Mr. Gutierrez's intake of high-fiber foods is still limited.
Ask him about pattern of elimination over the last 2 weeks and laxative use.	Mr. Gutierrez says, "I still go about the same" but states that he thinks he now goes about every 2 days.	He has bowel movements approximately every 2 days.
	Mr. Gutierrez has not used any laxatives. Bowel sounds are normal. Abdomen is soft and nontender with no distention.	His abdomen is less distended.
Ask Mr. Gutierrez about type and amount of fluid intake.	Mr. Gutierrez says he is drinking more water each day, "about 6 glasses."	Mr. Gutierrez's fluid intake is improving.

Case Study   **EVALUATION**

Vickie returns to see Mr. Gutierrez 2 weeks later. Vickie is eager to determine if Mr. Gutierrez has made any changes in his diet and how his problems with bowel elimination have been progressing. Vickie is also anxious to learn if the niece has assisted in having Mr. Gutierrez's stove repaired.

Mr. Gutierrez tells Vickie that he has been eating bran cereal in the morning, has been eating rice and/or beans for dinner, and has added one fruit each day to his diet. He has been walking twice a day through the long-term care center. Although he does not have a bowel movement each day, his stools are much softer and easier to pass and he says he is less concerned. He has not taken a laxative for a stool since last talking with Vickie.

Documentation Note
Client's problem with bowel elimination is improving. The client's abdomen is soft and nondistended; bowel sounds normal and audible in all quadrants. Per teaching plan, client has altered eating habits to include more fiber, fruit, and fluids. Niece assisted in having stove repaired. Although client's concern over bowel habits has not ceased, the client does state he feels "in better control" and has decreased laxative use.

Key Terms

anorexia, *p. 797*
cathartics, *p. 808*
chyme, *p. 795*
colon, *p. 796*
constipation, *p. 796*
defecation, *p. 796*

diarrhea, *p. 797*
enema, *p. 808*
fecal impaction, *p. 797*
fecal incontinence, *p. 798*
fetal occult blood test, *p. 803*
feces, *p. 796*
flatus, *p. 796*
hemorrhoids, *p. 798*

laxatives, *p. 808*
masticate, *p. 795*
melena, *p. 803*
ostomy, *p. 798*
peristalsis, *p. 795*
segmentation, *p. 795*
stoma, *p. 798*
Valsalva maneuver, *p. 796*

Key Concepts

- Mechanical breakdown of food elements, GI motility, and selective absorption and secretion of substances by the large intestine influence the character of feces.
- Food high in fiber content and an increased fluid intake keep feces soft.
- Regular use of laxatives can lead to constipation.
- The greatest danger from diarrhea is fluid and electrolyte imbalance.
- The location of an ostomy influences the consistency of stool.
- Assessment of an elimination pattern should focus on bowel habits, an analysis of factors that normally influence defecation, a review of recent changes in elimination, and a physical examination.

- A fecal occult blood test is recommended for clients who take anticoagulants, who have a bleeding disorder or GI disorder causing bleeding, or who are at risk for colon cancer.
- Indirect and direct visualization of the lower GI tract requires cleansing of the bowel before the procedure.
- You should consider frequency of defecation, fecal characteristics, and effect of foods on GI function when selecting a diet promoting normal elimination.
- The client's usual time of defecation should be considered in the administration of cathartics or laxatives.
- Proper administration of an enema is the slow instillation of the proper volume of a warm solution.
- A continent ostomy provides control over when fecal material exits.

- Irrigation of an ostomy follows the same principles as an enema administration, except that a special irrigating tube is needed and the client cannot control passage of feces.

- Dangers during digital removal of stool include traumatizing the rectal mucosa and promoting vagal stimulation.
- Skin breakdown can occur after repeated exposure to liquid stool. This is especially true in clients with a stoma.

Critical Thinking Activities

1. While fulfilling your community service responsibility of taking blood pressure measurements at the senior citizens' center, one of the clients tells you that this morning after he had a bowel movement, he noticed bright red blood on the toilet tissue. What further data would you need to gather?

2. An older adult woman with complaints of constipation tells you high-fiber foods are just too expensive. What would you advise?

3. This is your first day of caring for a 68-year-old woman who is 2 days postoperative for a bowel resection for cancer. She has a temporary ostomy. What are your priorities of care?

Review Questions

1. Most nutrients and electrolytes are absorbed in the:
   1. colon.
   2. stomach.
   3. esophagus.
   4. small intestine.
2. During assessment your client reveals that he has diarrhea and cramping every time he has ice cream. He attributes this to the cold nature of the food. However, you begin to suspect that these symptoms might be associated with:
   1. food allergy.
   2. irritable bowel.
   3. lactose intolerance.
   4. increased peristalsis.
3. You are assessing a 55-year-old client who is in the clinic for a routine physical. You will only instruct the client to obtain a fecal occult blood specimen:
   1. when there is a family history of polyps.
   2. if client reports rectal bleeding.
   3. if a palpable mass is detected on digital examination.
   4. as part of a routine examination, in accordance with American Cancer Society guidelines.
4. Diarrhea that occurs with a fecal impaction is the result of:
   1. a clear liquid diet.
   2. irritation of the intestinal mucosa.
   3. seepage of stool around the impaction.
   4. inability of the client to form a stool.
5. You are caring for a client with an ostomy, which is 5 years old. The client manages her colostomy on her own. However, she is now complaining of peristomal irritation. To determine the cause of this irritation, you must assess:
   1. circulation to stoma and fit of pouch.
   2. quantity and consistency of fecal drainage in pouch.
   3. presence of signs of infection at the stoma or peristomal skin.
   4. circulation to stoma, quantity and consistency of fecal drainage, allergic response to ostomy products, fit of pouch, and presence of infection.
6. A cleansing enema is ordered for a 55-year-old client before intestinal surgery. The maximum amount given is:
   1. 150 to 200 ml.
   2. 200 to 400 ml.
   3. 400 to 750 ml.
   4. 750 to 1000 ml.
7. During the enema your client begins to complain of pain. You note blood in the return fluid and rectal bleeding. Your actions are to:
   1. stop the instillation.
   2. slow down the rate of instillation.
   3. stop the instillation and obtain vital signs.
   4. tell the client to breathe slowly and relax.

References

American Cancer Society: *Colon and rectum cancer resource center—2001*, Atlanta, 2001, The Society (www3.cancer.org).

Ayellow EA: The ABCDs of stoma assessment and pouching, personal correspondence, 2000.

Colwell J and others: The state of the standard diversion, *J Wound Ostomy Continence Nurs* 28:6, 2001.

Doughty D: A physiologic approach to bowel training, *J Wound Ostomy Continence Nurs* 23(1):46, 2000a.

Doughty D: *Urinary and fecal incontinence nursing*, ed 2, St. Louis, 2000b, Mosby.

Gibson CJ and others: Effectiveness of bran supplement on the bowel management of elderly rehabilitation clients, *J Gerontol Nurs* (10):21, 1995.

Giger JN, Davidhizar RE: *Transcultural nursing: assessment and intervention*, ed 3, St. Louis, 1999, Mosby.

Hampton BG, Bryant RA: *Ostomies and continent diversions: nursing management*, St. Louis, 1992, Mosby.

Lueckenotte AG: *Gerontologic nursing*, ed 2, St. Louis, 2000, Mosby.

Norton C, Chelvanayagam S: A nursing assessment tool of adults with fecal incontinence, *J Wound Ostomy Continence Nurs* 27:279, 2000.

Phipps WJ and others: *Medical-surgical nursing*, ed 6, St. Louis, 1999, Mosby.

Ransohoff DF, Lang CA: Screening for colorectal cancer with the fecal occult blood test: a background paper, *Ann Intern Med* 126:881, 1997.

33

Immobility

Objectives

- Define key terms.
- Describe mobility and immobility.
- Discuss the benefits and hazards of bed rest.
- Identify changes in metabolic rate associated with immobility.
- Describe physical changes associated with immobility.
- Describe musculoskeletal changes associated with immobility.
- Discuss factors that contribute to pressure ulcer formation.
- Describe psychosocial and developmental effects of immobilization.
- Complete a nursing assessment of an immobilized client.
- Develop a nursing care plan for an immobilized client.
- List appropriate nursing interventions for an immobilized client.
- State evaluation criteria for the immobilized client.

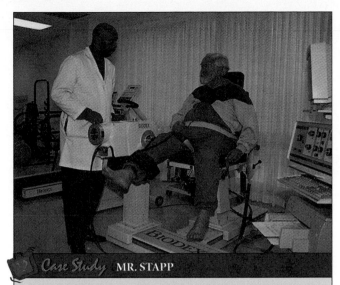

Case Study MR. STAPP

Bob Stapp is a 54-year-old man who is being admitted to the rehabilitation center after a bilateral total knee replacement 3 days ago. Mr. Stapp is expecting to be at the center about 10 days, when he will go home and continue therapy on an outpatient basis. He says his health is good, except he has a "bit of sugar" and "can't seem to lose that 50 pounds the doc wants me to." He plans to return to work in the steel mill, where he has worked for 28 years, as soon as he gets the physician's okay. His postoperative course has been as expected.

Mark Weber is a 52-year-old nursing student who is completing the second half of his first clinical experience in nursing. He is a retired fireman, divorced, and has a son who is also in nursing school at a nearby college. It is his first day at the center; he spent the first half of his clinical experience on an orthopedic unit in a community hospital. Mark has never taken care of someone who is the same age as he is.

SCIENTIFIC KNOWLEDGE BASE
Mobility

Mobility is a person's ability to move around freely in his or her environment. It serves many purposes, including expressing emotion, self-defense, attaining basic needs, performing recreational activities, and completing **activities of daily living (ADLs),** those activities of physical self-care such as bathing, dressing, and eating. In addition, mobility assists in maintaining the body's normal physiological activities. To maintain normal physical mobility, the nervous, muscular, and skeletal systems of the body must be intact, functioning, and used regularly.

A decline in a client's mobility status may result from many types of health problems. Clients with certain illnesses, injuries, or surgeries may experience a period of immobilization as a result of changes in medical and physical status. Factors that contribute to the amount of disability include the degree of **immobility** (inability to move around freely), length of immobilization, severity of the illness, emotional state of the client, and the client's premorbid physical condition. Immobilization can also be used therapeutically to limit

the movement of the whole body or a body part, and clients may have ambulation restrictions. You may see clients at any point on the mobility-immobility continuum.

BED REST. **Bed rest** is an intervention in which the client is restricted to bed for therapeutic reasons. It is important that you discuss with the physician or other health care provider the limitations on mobility. The duration of bed rest depends on the type and nature of the illness or injury and the client's prior state of health. You must explain the limitations to the client and family to ensure adherence.

Immobility

Immobility occurs when a client is unable to independently move or change positions, or movement is restricted for medical reasons. Physical inactivity may occur as a response to severe pain or as a result of sensory changes reducing the physical stimulus to move. Immobility may also be a result of cognitive-emotional changes, such as depression, or a result of a treatment, such as prescribed bed rest. Physical restriction or limitation of movement, such as by cast, traction, or restraints, also results in an imposed reduction of movement.

No body system is immune to the hazardous effects of immobility (Mahoney, 1998; McCance and Huether, 1998). The greater the extent and the longer the duration of immobility, the more pronounced the consequences. Your nursing care and client education are directed toward minimizing these hazards because it is easier to prevent the complications than to treat or cure them.

PHYSIOLOGICAL EFFECTS. Each body system is at risk for impairments resulting from immobility (Box 33-1). The severity of the impairment depends on the client's age, overall mental and physical health, and the degree of immobility. For example, frail older adult clients with chronic illnesses develop pronounced effects of immobility more quickly than do younger clients (Mahoney, 1998). Whether young or old, these effects are evident in the client's respiratory system, metabolic rate, metabolism, fluid and electrolyte balance, gastrointestinal tract, cardiovascular system, musculoskeletal system, integument, and urinary elimination.

RESPIRATORY CHANGES. With immobility there is decreased lung expansion, generalized respiratory muscle weakness, and stasis of secretions. These changes contribute to the development of **atelectasis** (collapse of alveoli) and **hypostatic pneumonia** (inflammation of the lung from stasis or pooling of secretions).

With decreased lung expansion and weakened respiratory muscles, secretions stagnate or pool in the dependent lung regions (Figure 33-1). In atelectasis a bronchiole or a bronchus becomes blocked by secretions and the distal lung tissue (alveoli) collapses. In addition, there is a decline in the client's ability to cough due to generalized muscle weakness. Ultimately mucus accumulates, particularly when the client is in the supine, prone, or lateral position (Figure 33-2), pro-

Pathophysiology of Immobility   Box 33-1

PHYSIOLOGICAL OUTCOMES
- ↓ Basal metabolic rate (BMR)
- ↓ Gastrointestinal motility
  - ↓ Nutrients/fluids
  - ↓ Appetite
  - Shift in electrolyte balance
- ↓ O_2 availability/ischemia
  - ↓ O_2/CO_2 exchange
  - ↑ Respiratory muscle weakness
  - ↓ Lung expansion
  - ↑ Atelectasis/hypostatic pneumonia
- ↓ Cardiac output
  - ↑ Cardiac workload
  - ↑ Oxygen demand
  - ↑ Dependent edema
  - ↑ Clot formation (DVT)
- ↑ Muscle atrophy
  - ↓ Strength/flexibility/endurance
  - ↑ Joint contractures
- ↑ Disuse osteoporosis
  - ↑ Bone resorption

PSYCHOLOGICAL OUTCOMES
- ↑ Stressors
- ↑ Depression
- ↓ Self-identity
- ↓ Self-esteem
- ↑ Behavioral changes
- ↑ Changes in sleep/wake cycles
- ↓ Coping successes
- ↑ Isolation
- ↑ Passive behaviors
- ↑ Sensory deprivation/overload

DEVELOPMENTAL OUTCOMES
- ↑ Dependence
- ↑ Regression in development

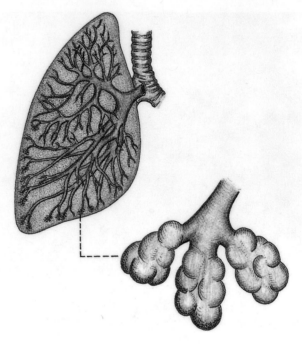

FIGURE **33-1**   Pooling of secretions in dependent regions of lungs in supine position.

viding an excellent medium for bacterial growth, and hypostatic pneumonia may result.

CHANGES IN METABOLIC RATE.   Decreased mobility results in a decrease in the basal metabolic rate (BMR). Your client's BMR falls in response to the decreased energy requirement of body cells, which is directly related to cellular oxygen demands. However, fever or wound healing may increase the BMR because these conditions increase cellular oxygen requirements (McCance and Huether, 1998). Therefore a balance must be maintained between energy consumption and demand.

CHANGES IN METABOLISM OF CARBOHYDRATES, FATS, AND PROTEINS.   While bed rest continues, pancreatic activity decreases, as does the body's ability to tolerate glucose. Insulin production is not enough to lower serum glucose levels. As proteins are metabolized, nitrogen is produced as an end product. Nitrogen balance provides a reliable indicator of protein use by the body. A **negative nitrogen balance** exists when the excretion of nitrogen from the breakdown of protein exceeds intake. A negative nitrogen balance predisposes your client to problems with wound healing and normal tissue growth. Decreased mobility results in increased percentage of body fat and the loss of lean body mass.

FLUID AND ELECTROLYTE BALANCES.   Because your client is in a recumbent position, major shifts in blood volume occur. **Diuresis** (increased urine excretion) occurs as a result of the changes of increased blood flow to the kidneys and the expanded circulating blood volume. Electrolytes, such as potassium and sodium, are lost due to diuresis. Serum calcium levels are also affected. Immobility causes an increase in calcium resorption (loss) from bones, causing a release of excess calcium into the circulation. Potentially this can lead to **hypercalcemia** if the kidneys are unable to respond appropriately (Beare and Myers, 1998).

GASTROINTESTINAL CHANGES.   Activity stimulates peristalsis. The immobile client is at risk for constipation from lack of activity and from hypercalcemia, which depresses peristalsis. Constipation may be so severe that fecal impaction may occur (see Chapter 32). Left untreated, a partial or complete bowel obstruction may occur (Phipps and others, 1999).

CARDIOVASCULAR CHANGES.   Orthostatic hypotension occurs in the client on bed rest, but it may also occur in clients after prolonged sitting. **Orthostatic hypotension** is a drop of 15 mm Hg or more in systolic blood pressure when the client rises from a lying or sitting position to a standing position. In the immobilized client there is decreased circu-

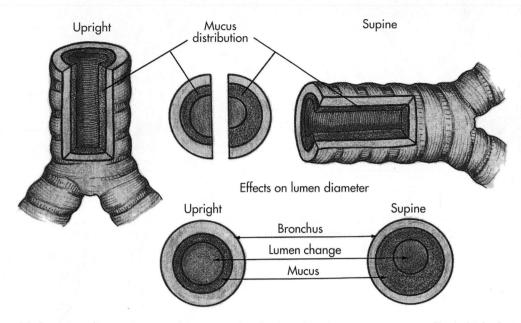

FIGURE **33-2**   Effect of recumbency and gravity on distribution of respiratory tract mucus of bronchiolar lumen.

lating fluid volume, pooling of blood in the lower extremities, and decreased autonomic response (Kihara and others, 1998). These result in decreased venous return, central venous pressure, and stroke volume and a drop in systolic blood pressure when the client stands (McCance and Huether, 1998).

Increased cardiac workload is demonstrated by rate changes. Prolonged bed rest increases the resting heart rate 4 to 15 beats per minute. When the immobilized client is asked to do physical activity such as with range-of-motion (ROM) exercises or ADLs, this increased rate is more pronounced. As the workload of the heart increases, so does its oxygen consumption. The heart therefore works harder and less efficiently during prolonged rest.

Immobile clients are at risk for deep venous thrombosis (DVT). A **thrombus** is an accumulation of platelets, fibrin, clotting factors, and cellular elements of the blood attached to the interior wall of a vein or artery, sometimes occluding the lumen of the vessel (Figure 33-3). Since DVT usually occurs during a client's recovery phase, you need to incorporate various interventions to try to prevent this potentially fatal complication (Blondin and Titler, 1996; Phipps and others, 1999).

Three factors predispose your client to venous thrombi; they are commonly referred to as Virchow's triad. These factors are hypercoagulability of the blood, venous wall damage, and stasis of blood flow (Phipps and others, 1999). In addition, the weight of the legs on the bed compresses the blood vessels of the calves, causing stasis and injury to vessel linings. Another problem in the venous system is the loss of the pumping action of the skeletal muscles. Normally calf muscles aid venous return by pumping blood through the

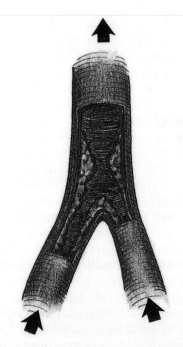

FIGURE **33-3**   Thrombus formation in vessel.

legs back to the heart. However, this mechanism is reduced when the client is on bed rest or has a cast on a leg.

Venous thrombi put the client at risk for pulmonary emboli, a life-threatening complication. Pulmonary emboli are clots that have moved in the venous system, blocking a portion of the pulmonary artery system and thus disrupting blood flow to the lungs. Immobilized surgical and older adult clients are at high risk for developing pulmonary emboli (Brough, 1998).

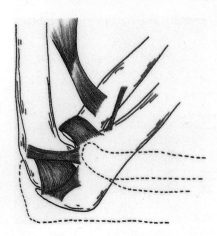

FIGURE **33-4** Flexion contracture of elbow resulting in permanent flexion of joint. Normally the elbow is able to extend to a 90-degree angle *(dotted line)* and to a 180-degree angle *(not shown)*.

MUSCULOSKELETAL CHANGES. Restricted mobility leads to loss of strength and endurance, decreased muscle mass, and decreased stability or balance. Muscle strength is lost when muscles are inactive. The rate of decline will vary with the degree of immobility but may be rapid while mobility and weight bearing are restricted (Kasper and others, 1996). These effects can be devastating to clients who are marginally functioning at their ADLs.

Reduced endurance results when clients are immobile from changes in muscle strength and altered cardiovascular functioning. Because of the increased cardiac workload, muscle endurance is decreased as a result of the decreased ability of the cardiopulmonary system to meet the oxygen needs of the tissue. In addition, because of the metabolic changes, the client loses lean body mass, which is composed partially of muscle. Therefore the reduced muscle mass is unable to sustain prolonged activity without fatigue.

As immobility continues and the muscles are not exercised, muscle mass continues to decrease. The muscle atrophies, and the size of the muscle decreases. The leg muscles appear to be the most affected by immobility, which accounts in part for the difficulty the older client may have in getting up out of a chair after periods of bed rest.

Immobilization causes two skeletal changes. A **joint contracture** is abnormal and may result in permanent contraction of a joint characterized by flexion and fixation. It is caused by disuse, atrophy, and shortening of muscle fibers and surrounding joint tissues. When a contracture occurs, the joint cannot maintain its full range of joint motion, leaving it in a nonfunctional position (Figure 33-4). Footdrop contracture (Figure 33-5) results in the foot being permanently fixed in plantar flexion. As a result, ambulation is extremely difficult at best with the foot in this position.

The second skeletal change is **disuse osteoporosis,** a disorder characterized by **bone resorption** secondary to immobility. Osteoporosis is the result of impaired calcium metabolism. Because immobilization results in bone resorption, bone tissue is less dense, and osteoporosis results. Your client

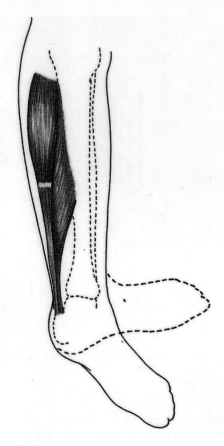

FIGURE **33-5** Footdrop. Ankle is fixed in plantar flexion.

is at risk for **pathological fractures,** a type of fracture that occurs as a result of bone weakness.

INTEGUMENT CHANGES. The direct effect of pressure on the skin by immobility is compounded by the changes in metabolism. Older adult clients and clients with paralysis have a greater risk for developing pressure ulcers (see Chapter 34). Pressure affects cellular metabolism by decreasing or obliterating tissue circulation. When a client lies in bed or sits in a chair, the weight of the body is on bony prominences. The longer the pressure is applied, the longer the period of **ischemia** and therefore the greater the risk of skin breakdown (see Figure 34-1, p. 843, and Figure 34-10, p. 860). Any break in the skin's integrity is difficult to heal in the immobilized client.

URINARY ELIMINATION CHANGES. Urine flows out of the renal pelvis and into the ureter and bladder because of gravitational forces when the client is upright. When the client in recumbent, the kidneys and ureters move toward a more level plane, and urine formed by the kidney must enter the bladder against gravity. Because the peristaltic contractions of the ureters are insufficient to overcome gravity, the renal pelvis may fill before urine enters the ureters (Figure 33-6). This condition, called urinary stasis, increases the client's risk of urinary tract infection and renal calculi. **Renal calculi** are calcium stones that lodge in the renal pelvis and pass through the ureters (Figure 33-7).

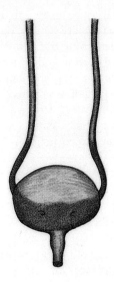

FIGURE **33-6**   Stasis of urine.

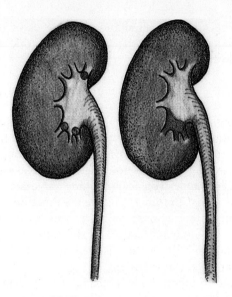

FIGURE **33-7**   Renal calculi in renal pelvis.

NURSING KNOWLEDGE BASE

Monitoring or assisting clients with mobility is basic to nursing. Concepts that relate to mobility such as movement, exercise and rest, and posture are soundly grounded in many nursing theories. Immobilization may lead to a variety of psychosocial responses and influence the development of the client. Because mobility is a function of intact neurological and musculoskeletal systems, you draw upon assessment skills to fully understand the client's initial condition and to monitor and evaluate care (see Chapter 12).

Psychosocial Effects

Immobilization may lead to changes in emotional, intellectual, sensory, and sociocultural responses. The most common emotional changes are depression, behavioral changes, sleep-wake disturbances, and impaired coping.

The immobilized client can become depressed because of changes in self-concept, independence, and other factors (see Chapter 19). Depression is an affective disorder characterized by exaggerated feelings of sadness, melancholy, dejection, worthlessness, emptiness, and hopelessness.

The immobilized client requires constant nursing care. Because of physiological hazards, your client may not be allowed to sleep for 8 hours without a change of position or other nursing care. Disruption of normal sleeping patterns can cause further behavioral changes. Nursing and medical interventions should be clustered together as much as possible to ensure the client receives sufficient sleep (see Chapter 28).

Long-term immobility or bed rest can affect usual coping patterns. Such a client may withdraw and become passive. The passive client allows you to provide care but is not interested in increasing independence or involvement in care. Early in the care of an immobilized client you should assess the client's normal coping mechanisms. Then design a nursing care plan that will allow the client to continue to use these coping abilities or will help the client develop new ones.

Developmental Effects

More developmental changes tend to be associated with immobility in the very young and in the older adult. The immobilized young or middle-age adult may experience few, if any, developmental changes. However, there are exceptions, such as a mother who has complications at childbirth and as a result cannot interact with the newborn as expected.

When the infant, toddler, or preschooler is immobilized, it is usually because of trauma or the need to correct a congenital skeletal abnormality. Prolonged immobilization can delay the child's motor skill and intellectual development. When caring for immobilized children you should plan activities that provide physical and psychosocial stimuli (Wong and others, 1999).

Immobilization of older adult clients increases their physical dependence on others and accelerates functional losses in physiological systems (Mahoney, 1998). Immobilization of an older adult client usually results from a degenerative disease, neurological trauma, or a chronic illness. For some clients immobilization occurs gradually and progressively, whereas for others—especially those who have had a stroke—immobilization is sudden. When providing care for an older adult client, develop a care plan that encourages the client to perform as many self-care activities as possible, thereby maintaining the highest level of functional mobility.

CRITICAL THINKING
Synthesis

You draw information from a variety of sources when caring for your client. The client's needs are multiple. Integrating your knowledge and experience makes it possible to determine the physiobiological needs of the client and to focus on the nonphysiological areas that affect the client and family.

KNOWLEDGE. Drawing on previous information from pathophysiology enables you to anticipate the types of limitations in mobility clients may have. These limitations may be the direct results of musculoskeletal alteration or may be the results of deconditioning resulting from a chronic health problem. Knowledge of physical assessment techniques enables you to determine the exact extent of any limitations. To fully anticipate the functional needs of the client with impaired mobility, you must assess the client's developmental stage to determine current functional and mobility status, as well as to determine the health care needs of the client.

The use of proper body mechanics is important for you and the client alike to assist the client in turning positioning, and transferring safely. Knowledge from physiology enables you to observe for complications of immobility and intervene appropriately. Further, teaching principles are important to apply in the rehabilitation process because the client's rehabilitation work needs to be vigorously maintained when returning home.

EXPERIENCE. You may have taken care of other clients who have had mobility restrictions. These experiences help you to anticipate the client's need for pain control, positioning, and support of activities of daily living. Visits to a physical therapy unit in the hospital or in a community setting can increase your experiential base. In addition, you can use experience from a personal exercise plan to help the client improve mobility status during health promotion activities, acute care, or rehabilitation.

ATTITUDE. You must be creative in designing solutions to improve the client's mobility status. Confer with other health care providers to determine the setting in which the care is best provided. Collaboration and creativity establish an individualized rehabilitation program. Reflect on your own perceptions of the client's mobility status. Self-reflection enables you to act as a client advocate to encourage the client's motivation to improve mobility status and to identify ways in which the family can also participate.

STANDARDS. At all times promote the client's independence while adhering to the prescribed rehabilitation plan and maintaining client safety. Recognize the client's physical limitations and the emotional stress associated with impaired mobility. Your genuine concern and compassion for the client helps to establish and maintain the client's self-confidence, independence, and self-respect.

Synthesis of knowledge, experience, attitudes, and standards into the plan of care for a client with impaired mobility is important in developing an individualized care plan for the client. Such a plan of care will help to prevent complications, promote rehabilitation, and promote a timely return of clients to their home.

NURSING PROCESS

Assessment

The assessment includes the client's present mobility, information about preillness functioning, and the potential effects of immobility. Table 33-1 presents focused examples of factors to assess related to immobility, questions and approaches, and physical assessment strategies.

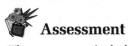

		Table 33-1
Factors to Assess	Questions and Approaches	Physical Assessment Strategies
Range of motion (ROM)	Ask if client has limited movement in joints. Ask if client has a history of connective tissue disorders, fractures, and/or damage to ligaments or tendons.	Observe client's gait and ability to carry out ADLs. Inspect joints for deformity. Measure ROM of affected joints.
Pain	Ask if client experiences pain or discomfort on movement. Ask if client needs pain medication before ambulating (with assistance), particularly after surgical procedure.	Observe for objective signs of pain such as grimacing, moaning, increasing respiratory rate, pulse, and blood pressure. (NOTE: These objective signs may not always be present, and it is best to ask the client if pain is present.) Inspect joints for redness or swelling, indicating potential inflammatory process.
Endurance and activity tolerance	Ask if client feels fatigued. Ask if client is experiencing difficulty with ADLs because of muscle weakness. Ask if client is experiencing shortness of breath, palpitations, light-headedness, or dizziness.	Observe for signs of fatigue. Observe client's performance of ADLs. Observe client for pallor; obtain baseline vital signs.

Example of a Focused Client Assessment

MOBILITY.   Assessment of the client's **mobility** focuses on range of motion, muscle strength, activity tolerance, gait, and posture. Chapter 24 describes the normal ROM for all joints in the body. In addition, observing the client's posture while sitting and standing and assessing gait helps you to determine the type of assistance the client may require to change positions or transfer from bed to chair. This information also helps you to assess the client's overall level of mobility and coordination.

RISKS AND INDICATORS OF IMMOBILITY.   A head-to-toe physical assessment (see Chapter 12) allows you to assess for the physiological hazards of immobility. In addition, keep in mind the potential negative impact of immobility on the psychosocial and developmental dimensions of the client.

PHYSIOLOGICAL CONDITION.   Assess those body systems most likely to be affected by immobility. During this assessment you must know normal functioning to detect adverse effects of immobility and expected changes attributable to the client's developmental stage.

RESPIRATORY SYSTEM.   A respiratory assessment should be performed at least every 2 hours for acutely ill clients with restricted activity. Inspect chest wall movements and auscultate the lungs to identify regions of diminished breath sounds. Auscultation for adventitious lung sounds should focus on the dependent lung field because pulmonary secretions tend to move to these lower regions. If a client has an atelectatic area, breath sounds may be asymmetrical. A complete respiratory assessment identifies the presence of secretions and can be used to determine nursing interventions necessary to maintain optimal respiratory function.

METABOLIC SYSTEM.   When assessing the client's metabolic functioning, you may use **anthropometric measurements** (body measures of height, weight, and skinfolds) to evaluate muscle atrophy. Intake and output records and laboratory data assist in evaluating fluid and electrolyte status. A client's nutritional status is assessed to determine risk for nitrogen imbalance. A client whose mobility is restricted may have a reduced appetite, altered gastrointestinal function, and a reduced capacity to self-feed.

Anorexia occurs commonly in immobilized clients. Assess food intake and the environment for unpleasant odors or noises that may interfere with appetite. Nutritional imbalances can be avoided if you learn the client's previous dietary patterns and food preferences early in the immobilization (see Chapter 30).

Anthropometric measurements include height, weight, mid–upper-arm circumference, and triceps skinfold measurements. Ideally this assessment should be done early in the period of immobilization and should be repeated at regular intervals. Assessment of height and weight is discussed in Chapter 12. A decrease in mid–upper-arm circumference, measured in centimeters, or triceps skinfold, measured in millimeters, indicates a decline in muscle mass. After the initial assessment this measurement may be done every 2 to 4 weeks depending on the client's age, premorbid condition, and the amount of immobility.

If an immobilized client has a wound, the speed of healing indicates how well nutrients are delivered to the tissues for use (see Chapter 34). The normal progression of wound healing indicates that the metabolic needs of the injured tissues are being met.

CARDIOVASCULAR SYSTEM.   The cardiovascular assessment of the immobilized client includes monitoring blood pressure, apical and peripheral pulses, and observing the venous system. Because of the risk for orthostatic hypotension, blood pressure should be measured, particularly when the client switches from lying to a sitting or standing position. In this way the client's ability to tolerate postural changes can be assessed.

Recumbency increases the cardiac workload and results in an increased pulse rate. In some clients, particularly the older adult, the heart may not be able to tolerate the increased workload, and a form of cardiac failure may develop. The absence of a peripheral pulse, particularly one that was previously present, should be documented and reported after a complete circulatory assessment is made (see Chapter 12).

Edema may indicate the heart's inability to handle the increased workload. Because fluid moves to dependent body regions, assessment of the immobilized client should include the sacrum, legs, feet, and hips. If the heart is unable to tolerate the increased cardiac workload, the peripheral body regions such as the hands, feet, nose, and earlobes will be colder than the central body regions.

Finally assess the venous system for DVT. To assess for DVT, remove the client's elastic stockings once every 8 hours and observe the calves for redness, warmth, and tenderness. Ask the client about calf pain. In addition, calf and thigh circumferences should be measured daily in clients at high risk for developing thrombi. DVT can also occur in the thigh. It is important to remember that half of all clients with DVT may not show any signs or symptoms. If DVT is suspected, report the finding and prepare the client for Doppler ultrasound studies (Brough, 1998).

MUSCULOSKELETAL SYSTEM.   The major musculoskeletal abnormalities identified during assessment include decreased muscle strength, loss of muscle tone and mass, and contractures. Clients with musculoskeletal injuries or chronic conditions require careful palpation of joints and extremities to reduce discomfort. Because immobilized clients are weakened, you must determine if difficulty in moving joints is the result of fatigue or decreased range of joint motion.

SKIN INTEGRITY.   Continually assess the skin for signs of pressure ulcer formation. The client with sensorimotor impairments, the chronically ill client in long-term care, the client with diminished mental status, the incontinent client in any setting, the orthopedic client, and the multiple-trauma client are at high risk for developing pressure ulcers (see Chapter 34).

ELIMINATION SYSTEM. The client's elimination status should be assessed on each shift, and the total intake and output should be assessed every 24 hours (see Chapter 14). Assessment of elimination should also include auscultation for bowel sounds, the frequency and consistency of bowel movements, and the client's usual urine and bowel elimination patterns. Accurate assessment and documentation enables you to intervene before fecal impaction occurs and may also prevent urine incontinence. Elimination assessment should be done at the beginning and at the end of each shift and as you deem necessary.

PSYCHOSOCIAL CONDITION. Changes in psychosocial status usually occur slowly. Observe for changes in emotional status (e.g., depression) and behavioral changes (e.g., cooperative clients who become argumentative or modest clients who begin to expose themselves repeatedly). Continual communication with the family is vital because they may identify and report changes in personality that you may not recognize.

Changes in the client's sleep-wake cycle, such as difficulty falling asleep or frequent awakenings, must be identified and corrected (see Chapter 28). Many sleep disruptions can be prevented or minimized with an assessment of prior sleep habits and early intervention when problems are suspected. Finally, observe for changes in the use of normal coping mechanisms to adapt to immobilization. Decreasing coping ability may cause the client to become disoriented, confused, or depressed or to experience other behavioral changes.

DEVELOPMENT. Assessment of the immobilized client should include developmental considerations. With a young child, first determine the child's developmental stage before immobilization. Development may regress or be slowed because of immobilization. By identifying a child's overall developmental needs, you can design nursing therapies to maintain normal development (Wong, and others, 1999). When developmental delays occur, you need to reassure the parents that these are usually temporary.

Developmental assessment is also important with the older adult. The nursing assessment enables you to determine the older adult client's ability to meet needs independently. A decline in developmental functioning prompts investigation to determine the reasons the change occurred and the interventions necessary to restore the client to an optimal level of function (see Chapter 18).

CLIENT EXPECTATIONS. Clients with impaired mobility may have certain expectations of the care provider. For example, some clients may expect to be challenged to improve their level of independence. This is particularly true of clients in the rehabilitative phase of their illness or injury. On the other hand, your client's physiological condition may

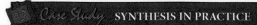

Case Study **SYNTHESIS IN PRACTICE**

As Mark prepares for an assessment on Mr. Stapp, he reviews the pathophysiology regarding the hazards of immobility. He gathers knowledge about knee replacement surgery and the expected postoperative physical therapy and rehabilitative measures. During a previous clinical experience, Mark cared for a client who was recently diagnosed with diabetes mellitus. He knows that the presence of diabetes mellitus can affect Mr. Stapp's postoperative status in several ways. Wound healing is slower in clients with diabetes. In addition, because Mr. Stapp will be participating in a physical exercise program to increase knee mobility, his caloric requirements may need to change and his blood sugar levels need to be monitored.

Mark knows that he needs to respect Mr. Stapp's need to be independent and desire to participate in rehabilitation. Although Mark and his client are close in age, he knows that Mr. Stapp has his own life goals. He approaches this clinical experience with energy and creativity; he plans to implement individualized care to increase Mr. Stapp's mobility status and progression through rehabilitation.

contraindicate such independence in function. Clients may agree or disagree with their physical limitations and expect their caregivers to do the same. In knowing the client's expectations, you are able to identify when care may be modified to meet these expectations, to know when teaching is needed to explain why care cannot be modified, or to be a compassionate listener to clients who cannot be as mobile as they wish.

Nursing Diagnosis

Assessment reveals clusters of data that indicate whether a client is at risk or if a mobility problem exists. Assessment also identifies pertinent defining characteristics that support the diagnostic label and probable cause of the diagnosis. Locating the probable cause of the diagnosis, based on assessment data, is important to planning client-centered goals and subsequent nursing interventions that will best help the client.

An immobilized or partially immobilized client may have one or more nursing diagnoses (Box 33-2). The two diagnoses most directly related to mobility problems are *impaired physical mobility* and *risk for disuse syndrome*. *Impaired physical mobility* is used for the client who demonstrates functional limitations but is not completely immobile. On the other hand, for the client who is immobile and is at risk for multisystem pathophysiology because of the unavoidable inactivity the diagnosis should be *risk for disuse syndrome*. Beyond these diagnoses the list of potential diagnoses is extensive because immobility affects multiple body systems. Many alterations in physiological, sociocultural, and developmental functioning are related to immobility. Often these problems are interrelated, and it is imperative that nursing care focus on all dimensions.

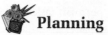

Nursing Diagnoses for
CLIENTS WITH IMMOBILITY

Box 33-2

- Activity intolerance
- Airway clearance, ineffective
- Breathing pattern, ineffective
- Constipation, risk for
- Coping, ineffective
- Disuse syndrome, risk for
- Fluid volume, risk for deficient
- Gas exchange, impaired
- Infection, risk for
- Mobility, impaired physical
- Skin integrity, risk for impaired
- Sleep pattern, disturbed
- Social isolation
- Tissue perfusion, ineffective
- Urinary elimination, impaired

Planning

Immobility may lead to serious complications such as pulmonary emboli or pneumonia. If these conditions develop, you will collaborate with the physician or nurse practitioner for prescribed therapy to intervene. Be alert for these potential complications, and work to prevent them.

GOALS AND OUTCOMES.   Clients at risk for hazards of immobility require nursing care plans directed at meeting their actual and potential needs (see care plan). In addition, it is important to develop client-centered goals aimed at preventing or reducing the hazards of immobility. Goals, like diagnoses, are mutually set with the client and family. A family who does too much or too little in an attempt to help the client may seriously impede the progress of the client. Watching a family member walk slowly and using effort may

---

Case Study Nursing Care Plan   IMMOBILITY

ASSESSMENT

Mr. Bob Stapp, a 54-year-old client, is admitted to the rehab hospital after bilateral **total knee replacement (TKR).** He has a history of smoking. He is **50 lb overweight.** He does not use his incentive spirometer. He is to **start physical therapy this afternoon.** He is able to **transfer himself with help to a chair from the bed and can stand on his own with the aid of a walker.** He has **50-degree flexion of his knee.**

*Defining characteristics are shown in bold type.

NURSING DIAGNOSIS

Impaired physical mobility related to mobility restrictions secondary to bilateral TKR.

PLANNING

GOAL	EXPECTED OUTCOMES
Client will remain free of complications of immobility.	Client's calf diameters will remain within 1 cm of baseline by 3/12. Client's lung fields will remain clear. Client's skin will remain dry and intact.

IMPLEMENTATION

STEPS	RATIONALE
1. Administer low-dose heparin as ordered.	Administration of low-dose heparin has shown reductions in risk of vein thrombosis (Brough, 1998).
2. Apply intermittent compression stockings, and remove them each shift for hygiene.	Application increases venous tone, improving venous return, and reduces venous stasis (Blondin and Titler, 1996; Collier, 1999; Phipps and others, 1999).
3. Reinforce antiembolic leg exercises hourly while awake.	Improves venous return.
4. Reinforce use of incentive spirometer every 2 hours while awake.	Promotes lung expansion.
5. Instruct client to shift position every $1/2$ hour while awake.	Prevents formation of pressure ulcer.
6. Ask client to report any numbness or burning over pressure areas such as the heels of the feet.	May be early warning sign of ischemia.
7. Keep heels off the bed by placing a pad under the lower legs.	Using a thin pad under the lower legs raises the heel just enough so that a paper can slide between the heels and the bed, reducing the pressure on the heels, so that blood flow is optimized (Agency for Health Care Policy and Research, 1994).

EVALUATION

- Measure calves daily; report any increases in dimensions.
- Perform circulatory assessment to extremities every shift.
- Auscultate lung fields every shift.
- Observe skin condition daily.

seem cruel, so the family may excessively perform tasks that clients need to learn how to do for themselves.

SETTING PRIORITIES.   Care planning is individualized to the client, taking into consideration the client's most immediate needs. The immediacy of any problem is determined by the effect the problem has on the client's mental and physical health. Because many of the skills associated with care of the immobile are delegated, such as turning and applying elastic stockings, it may be easy to overlook the potential complications of immobility until they occur. Therefore you must be vigilant in monitoring the client, reinforcing prevention techniques, and supervising assistive personnel in carrying out activities aimed at preventing immobility complications.

CONTINUITY OF CARE.   You may need the help of another health team member such as physical or occupational therapist when considering mobility needs. These factors are important for clients in institutional and home settings. Discharge planning is begun when a client enters the health care system. Anticipating the client's discharge from an institution, a referral may be necessary to help the client remain mobile or regain mobility at home.

 ## Implementation

Nursing interventions for the completely or partially immobilized client focus on health promotion and prevention of the hazards of immobility. In the acute care setting, specific interventions are designed to reduce the impact of immobility on the client and thus reduce complications of immobility to the body systems. In restorative and continuing care, interventions are directed at regaining and maximizing functional mobility and independence.

HEALTH PROMOTION.   Structured exercise programs for immobile clients can enhance their feelings of well-being, as well as their endurance, strength, and health. Exercise is recommended preoperatively for clients expected to have mobility restrictions after surgery.

Disuse and disease may account for much of the functional decline in the older adult population. Therefore the older adult client need not accept muscle deterioration as inevitable (Box 33-3). You must be alert to prevent further disuse while the older adult is ill.

You can contribute to promoting health for many types of clients by encouraging or starting managed exercise programs (Box 33-4). Even hospitalized clients can be encouraged to do stretching, ROM, and light walking within the limits of their condition. Distances walked should be measured in feet and yards instead of "walked to the nurses' station and back to room."

RESPIRATORY SYSTEM.   Your interventions for the respiratory system are aimed at promoting expansion of the chest and lungs, preventing stasis of pulmonary secretions, and maintaining a patent airway.

Promoting Expansion of the Chest and Lungs. Changing the client's position allows the dependent lung to expand. This maintains the elastic recoil property of the lungs and clears the dependent lung of pulmonary secretions. The minimum suggested timing for turning is every 2 hours, but that may not be enough. You must assess the client to determine the frequency of position changes (see Chapter 34).

Preventing Stasis of Pulmonary Secretions. Stagnant secretions accumulating in the bronchi and lungs of the immobilized or bed-bound client may lead to the growth of bacteria and the subsequent development of pneumonia. The stagnation of secretions can be reduced by changing the client's position at least every 2 hours, thus rotating the dependent lung and mobilizing the secretions.

Gerontological Nursing Practice   **Box 33-3**

- It is never too late to begin an exercise program (Huddleston, 1998). The older adult should consult a health care provider before beginning an exercise program, particularly in the presence of heart or lung disease and other chronic illnesses.
- Encourage the older adult to avoid prolonged sitting, to get up and stretch. Frequent stretching decreases joint contractures.
- Older adults should avoid sudden twisting movements, rapid movements, and rapid transitions from one movement to the next.
- Instruct older adults to stop exercising if angina, premature ventricular contractions, palpitations, light-headedness, or excessive breathlessness occurs.
- Older adults may engage in brisk walking for 10 to 15 minutes to tone the extremities and provide aerobic activity (Ebersole and Hess, 1998).
- Older adults may perform both strenuous and less strenuous activities. Activities may range from gardening to chair-based activities and tai chi (Ebersole and Hess, 1998).

Procedural Guidelines for   **Box 33-4**
ASSISTING CLIENTS WITH BASIC CARE

1. Teach clients breathing skills to help reduce anxiety and to fully oxygenate tissues and expand lungs.
2. Always know client's limitations.
3. Do not force a muscle or a joint during exercise.
4. Let each client move at own pace.
5. Keep a record of the client's progress, and provide feedback as client exercises.
6. Posture, body alignment, and good body mechanics should be maintained during exercise.
7. Monitor vital signs before, during, and after exercise.
8. Stop exercising if client has pain, shortness of breath, or a change in vital signs.
9. Clients should wear shoes and comfortable clothing.
10. Know what the client's mobility skills were prior to hospitalization.
11. Be aware of any medical limitations (e.g., weight-bearing status, untreated fracture, cardiovascular disease).

The immobile client should take in a minimum of 2000 ml/day, if not contraindicated, to help keep mucociliary clearance normal. In clients free from infection and with adequate hydration, pulmonary secretions will appear thin, watery, and clear. The client can easily remove the secretions with coughing. Without adequate hydration the secretions are thick and tenacious and difficult to remove. One method for removing pulmonary secretions is **chest physiotherapy.** The use of positioning techniques drains secretions from specific segments of the bronchi and lungs into the trachea and helps the client expel the secretions by coughing (see Chapter 27).

METABOLIC SYSTEM.   A dietary plan of carbohydrates, proteins, and fats is designed to meet the client's needs. Carbohydrates are needed to meet energy requirements. Proteins are necessary for tissue repair. Fats prevent further breakdown of nutritional stores. The specific caloric and diet prescription is determined from the nutritional assessment in collaboration with a registered dietitian (see Chapter 30).

CARDIOVASCULAR SYSTEM.   Nursing therapies are designed to minimize or prevent orthostatic hypotension, increased cardiac workload, and thrombus formation.

Reducing Orthostatic Hypotension.   After bed rest, clients usually have an increased pulse rate, a decrease in pulse pressure, and reduced stroke volume and cardiac output in response to a tilting or an erect posture (Lee and others, 1997). Attempts must be made to get the client out of bed as soon as the physical condition allows it, even if the move is only to a chair. This activity maintains muscle tone and increases venous return. **Isometric exercises,** those activities that involve muscle tension without muscle shortening, do not have any beneficial effect on preventing orthostatic hypotension but may improve activity tolerance (see Chapter 24).

When getting the client from a supine position into a chair, move the client gradually. First obtain baseline blood pressure and pulse with the client in the supine position (Roper, 1996). Then raise the client to a high-Fowler's position, and measure blood pressure and pulse again to detect decreases in blood pressure or elevations in pulse. Leave the client in this position for a few moments to allow the body to adapt. Monitor the client for dizziness or light-headedness and whether spots are seen. Now the client is ready to sit at the side of the bed with the feet on the floor. If there is no dizziness, assist the client to a chair. When getting an immobile client up for the first time, get the assistance of at least one other person.

Preventing Thrombus Formation.   Proper positioning used with other therapies (e.g., heparin and elastic stockings) helps reduce thrombus formation. When positioning clients, use caution to prevent pressure on the posterior knee and deep veins in the lower extremities. Teach clients to avoid crossing the legs, sitting for prolonged periods of time, wearing tight clothing that constricts the legs or waist, putting pillows under the knees, and massaging the legs.

Range-of-joint-motion exercises reduce the risk of contractures but may also aid in preventing thrombi (see Chapter 24). Activity causes contraction of the skeletal muscles, which in turn exerts pressure on the veins to promote venous return, thereby reducing venous stasis. Specific exercises that help prevent thrombophlebitis are ankle pumps, foot circles, hip rotation, and knee flexion. Ankle pumps, sometimes called calf pumps, include alternating plantar flexion and dorsiflexion. Foot circles require the client to rotate the ankle. Inward and outward rotation of the hip can be done while the client is supine (lying on back) or sitting. Knee flexion involves alternately extending and flexing the knee. These exercises that are aimed at preventing thrombus are sometimes referred to as antiembolic exercises and should be done hourly while awake.

MUSCULOSKELETAL SYSTEM.   The immobilized client must exercise to prevent excessive muscle atrophy, decreased endurance, and joint contractures. The amount of activity required to prevent physical disuse syndromes may be only about 2 hours in a 24-hour period, but it should be scheduled regularly throughout the day based on individual client needs. The best method to prevent complications from impaired mobility is to encourage ambulation.

If the client is unable to move any part or all of the body, perform passive range-of-joint-motion exercises for all immobilized joints at least 3 or 4 times a day unless contraindicated medically. If one extremity is paralyzed, the client can be taught to perform self-ROM. Clients on bed rest should have active range-of-joint-motion exercises incorporated into the daily schedule (see Chapter 24). These exercises can be incorporated into ADLs (Box 33-5).

The best nursing intervention is establishing an individualized progressive exercise program. A progressive exercise program gradually increases the client's physical activity to reverse the deconditioning associated with immobility. Teaching is an important aspect for clients with limited mobility (Box 33-6). Depending on the setting and resources available, you may want to refer the client for physical therapy to assist in setting up the exercise program.

SKIN INTEGRITY.   Early identification of high-risk client aids you in preventing pressure ulcers. Interventions aimed at prevention are positioning, skin care, and the use of pressure-relief devices. The immobilized client's position should be changed according to the client's activity level, perceptual ability, and daily routines (see Chapter 34). The time a client sits uninterrupted in a chair should be limited to 1 hour or less, but this time interval is individualized. Teach clients who are able to shift their weight every 15 minutes. Chair-bound clients should have a pressure-reducing device for the chair.

ELIMINATION SYSTEM.   Your interventions for maintaining optimal urinary functioning are directed toward keeping the client well hydrated without causing bladder distention and the reflux of urine into the ureters and, in some instances, the renal pelvis. Adequate hydration helps to prevent renal calculi and urinary tract infections. The client should void dilute urine that is comparable to the amount of intake.

Incorporating Active Range-of-Motion Exercises Into Activities of Daily Living

Box 33-5

Nodding head "yes" exercises *neck* (flexion).

Shaking head "no" exercises *neck* (rotation).

Moving right ear to right shoulder exercises *neck* (lateral flexion).

Moving left ear to left shoulder exercises *neck* (lateral flexion).

Reaching to turn on overhead light exercises *shoulder* (extension).

Reaching to bedside stand for book exercises *shoulder* (extension).

Scratching back exercises *shoulder* (hyperextension).

Rotating shoulders toward chest exercises *shoulder* (abduction).

Rotating shoulders toward back exercises *shoulder* (adduction).

Eating, bathing, shaving, and grooming exercise *elbow* (flexion and extension).

All activities requiring fine motor coordination, such as writing and eating, exercise *fingers* and *thumb* (flexion, extension, abduction, adduction, and opposition).

Walking exercises *hip* (flexion, extension, and hyperextension).

Moving to side-lying position exercises *hip* (flexion, extension, and abduction).

Moving from side-lying position exercises *hip* (extension and adduction).

Rolling feet inward exercises *hip* (internal rotation).

Rolling feet outward exercises *hip* (external rotation).

Walking exercises *knee* (flexion and extension).

Moving to and from a side-lying position exercises *knee* (flexion and extension).

Walking exercises *ankle* (dorsiflexion and plantar flexion).

Moving toe toward head of bed exercises *ankle* (dorsiflexion).

Moving toe toward foot of bed exercises *ankle* (plantar flexion).

Walking exercises *toes* (extension and hyperextension).

Wiggling toes exercises *toes* (abduction and adduction).

Client Teaching

Box 33-6

LIMITED MOBILITY

- Explain the need for position changes at regular intervals based on client needs.
- Demonstrate passive and active range-of-joint-motion exercises.
- Describe the risk factors for pressure sores.
- Describe early warning signs of immobility (e.g., continued erythema over a bony prominence) so interventions can be developed to prevent worsening of the condition.
- Discuss activities to reduce the psychosocial problems of immobilization.
- Encourage the client's participation in care and decision making.
- Explain the need to maintain fluid and nutrition intake.
- Explain the need for isometric and isotonic exercises while on bed rest.

Monitor the frequency and amount of urinary output to prevent bladder distention. A client who continually dribbles urine and whose bladder is distended has reflex incontinence. If the immobilized client does not have voluntary control of bladder elimination, bladder retraining may be necessary. If the client experiences bladder distention, you may be required to insert a straight catheter or an indwelling Foley catheter (see Chapter 31).

Record the frequency and consistency of bowel movements. A diet rich in fruits and vegetables can help to facilitate normal peristalsis. If a client is unable to maintain normal bowel patterns, you may initiate a bowel training program and the physician may order stool softeners, cathartics, or enemas (see Chapter 32).

PSYCHOSOCIAL PROBLEMS. Anticipate changes in psychosocial status, and intervene with preventive measures. Provide routine and informal socialization for the client. Activities are planned to give the client opportunities to interact with the staff. If possible, the client should be placed in a room with other mobile clients. If the client must remain in a private room, staff members are asked to visit with the client periodically throughout the client's waking hours. Provide stimuli to maintain the client's orientation and to entertain the client.

Encourage clients to wear their glasses or artificial teeth and to shave or apply makeup. These are normal activities through which people maintain body image. In addition, the client should be encouraged to perform as much self-care as possible. Hygiene and grooming articles should be kept within easy reach so the client can attend to personal needs.

Nursing care between 10 PM and 7 AM should be scheduled to minimize sleep interruptions. The balance between rest and the physiological effects of bed rest must be weighed. Assessments may be kept to a minimum in a stable client who is able to turn in bed unassisted. More seriously ill clients may need medications, assessments, and skin care during the night. Coordinate to prevent as many interruptions as possible.

Finally, observe the client for failure to cope with restricted mobility. If the nursing care plan is not improving the client's coping patterns, outside assistance may be required. Recommendations of consultants should be incorporated into the care plan.

DEVELOPMENTAL CHANGES. Your care should stimulate the client mentally as well as physically, particularly with a young child. Play activities can be incorporated into the nursing care plan. Puzzles, for example, can help to develop fine motor skills. Place an immobilized child in a room with children of the same age who are not immobilized, unless a contagious disease is present (Wong and others, 1999).

Immobilization or restricted mobility of an older adult may require complex care and innovative approaches. Inactive older adults are at risk for cognitive changes and depression as a result of immobilization, chronic illnesses, and medications. Therefore focus on activities to promote cognitive awareness of the client's surroundings (see Chapter 35). Explanations should be given before starting care and the client encouraged to make decisions about care. Plan nursing care to allow the older adult client to perform as many ADLs as possible. Not only are older adults more susceptible to the hazards of immobility, but the consequences of immobility appear more quickly and become severe more rapidly.

ACUTE CARE.   Clients in acute care settings may demonstrate more rapid and pronounced complications of immobility due to the presence of multisystem pathologic conditions. In these clients nursing interventions are designed to reduce the impact of immobility on body systems and prepare the client for restorative and continuing care. These interventions are used in combination with those outlined in the health promotion section to return the client to an optimal level of function.

RESPIRATORY SYSTEM.   Encourage the client to deep breathe and cough every 1 to 2 hours while awake. This action expands all lobes of the lungs and prevents atelectasis. Coughing reduces the stasis of pulmonary secretions. Some immobile clients, particularly after surgery, should use an incentive spirometer to aid in deep breathing (see Chapter 27).

Postoperative clients who have undergone anesthesia need to cough and deep breathe to prevent atelectasis and stasis of secretions. Timely pain management for incisional discomfort is essential. With less pain the client coughs more normally. If a client becomes drowsy from medication, actively reinforce coughing and deep breathing. Encourage early ambulation.

Maintaining a Patent Airway.   Immobilized clients and those on bed rest are generally weakened. If the weakness progresses, the cough reflex gradually becomes inefficient. If the client is too weak or unable to cough up secretions, you must maintain the client's airway by using suctioning techniques (see Chapter 27). This may involve oral or nasotracheal suctioning and suctioning of artificial airways. Suspect hypostatic bronchopneumonia if client develops a productive cough with greenish-yellow sputum, fever, and pain on breathing.

Cardiovascular System.   Nursing interventions are directed at reducing cardiac workload. When a client moves up in bed or strains on defecation, a Valsalva maneuver occurs. When using this maneuver, the client holds the breath and strains, increasing intrathoracic pressure, which decreases venous return and cardiac output. When the strain is released, venous return and cardiac output immediately increase, and systolic blood pressure and pulse pressure rise. These pressure changes produce a reflex bradycardia that may be associated with sudden cardiac death particularly in clients with heart disease. Teach the client to breathe out while moving or being lifted up in bed to avoid straining.

Interventions that reduce the risk of thrombus formation in the immobilized client include leg exercises, encouraging fluids, and position changes. Preoperative clients are instructed in exercise before surgery (see Chapter 36). Other interventions such as intermittent pneumatic compression devices and antiembolic elastic stockings require a physician's order.

When DVT is suspected, do not massage the area. Report your suspicions immediately. The leg should be elevated, with no pressure on the area of the leg with the suspected thrombus. Prepare the client for radiological studies such as a venous Doppler study or venogram (Brough, 1998; Collier, 1999).

Elastic stockings aid in maintaining pressure on the muscles of the lower extremities and are believed to promote venous return. The stockings must be applied properly (Skill 33-1) and removed and reapplied at least every 8 hours.

Skill 33-1
APPLYING ELASTIC STOCKINGS

DELEGATION CONSIDERATIONS
The following information is needed when delegating the application of elastic stockings to nursing staff or family members:
- Avoid activities that promote venous stasis (e.g., crossing legs, wearing garters, elevating legs on pillows).
- When possible, elevate legs to improve venous return.
- Do not massage legs.
- Elevate legs before applying stockings.
- Avoid wrinkles in the stockings.
- Observe for allergic reactions, skin irritation, and thrombophlebitis.

EQUIPMENT
- Tape measure
- Talcum powder
- Elastic support stockings

STEPS	RATIONALE

1. Assess client for risk factors in Virchow's triad:
  a. *Hypercoagulability:* all clients with clotting disorders, fever, dehydration, pregnancy and first 6 weeks postpartum if the woman was confined to bed, and oral contraceptive use (especially if client smokes)
  b. *Venous wall abnormalities:* local trauma, orthopedic surgeries, major abdominal surgery, varicose veins, atherosclerosis
  c. *Blood stasis:* immobility, obesity, pregnancy
	Potential candidates for elastic stockings are clients who have an alteration in one of the elements of Virchow's triad (Blondin and Titler, 1996; Collier, 1999; Phipps and others, 1999).

STEPS	RATIONALE

- **Critical Decision Point**

  Discourage clients from activities that promote venous stasis (e.g., crossing legs, wearing garters, elevating legs on pillows). When possible, elevate legs to improve venous return.

2. Observe for signs, symptoms, and conditions that might contraindicate use of elastic stockings. Signs and symptoms include:	
a. Dermatitis or open skin lesion	Elastic stockings may aggravate skin condition or cause it to spread. Also, physician may want medication and dressing applied to lesion.
b. Recent skin graft	Recent skin grafts are delicate and should not be dislodged (Phipps and others, 1999).
c. Disproportionately large thighs	Elastic stockings may not fit correctly, causing excessive pressure and constriction around thighs acting as a tourniquet, thereby reducing venous return as well as decreasing circulation (Blondin and Titler, 1996; Collier, 1999).
d. Decreased circulation in lower extremities as evidenced by cyanotic, cool extremities, gangrenous conditions affecting the lower limb(s).	Elastic stockings may further impede circulation (Phipps and others, 1999).
3. Obtain physician's order.	Protects nurse, physician, and client. May be needed for legal or reimbursement reasons.
4. Assess client's or caregiver's understanding of application of elastic stockings.	Identifies potential educational needs of client or caregiver.
5. Assess and document the condition of client's skin and circulation to the legs (i.e., presence of pedal pulses, edema, discoloration of the skin, temperature, lesions, or cuts).	Identifies a baseline for skin integrity and quality of peripheral pulses in lower extremities.

- **Critical Decision Point**

  Thrombophlebitis can develop in lower extremity. Clinical manifestations of thrombophlebitis vary according to size and location of thrombus. Signs and symptoms of superficial thrombosis include palpable vein and the surrounding area being tender to touch, reddened, and warm. There may be slight temperature elevation. Edema of extremity may or may not occur. Signs and symptoms of DVT include swollen extremity; pain; warm, cyanotic skin; and temperature elevation.

6. Assess client's or caregiver's understanding of proper care of elastic stockings.	Identifies potential educational needs of client or caregiver.
7. Explain procedure and reasons for applying stockings.	Reduces anxiety and encourages client cooperation.
8. Use tape measure to measure client's legs to determine proper stocking size.	Stockings must be measured according to manufacturer's directions. Elastic stockings come in two lengths: knee length and thigh length. The choice of length depends on physician's order.

- **Critical Decision Point**

  Compare client's measurements with the manufacturer's sizing chart. If too large, stockings will not adequately support extremities. If too small, stockings may impede circulation. The optimum stocking pressure is 20 to 30 mm Hg at the ankle, decreasing to 8 mm Hg at the middle to upper thigh. This change in pressure produces the greatest increase in venous flow velocity that is both safe and practical (Collier, 1999; Phipps and others, 1999).

9. Wash hands.	Reduces transmission of microorganisms.
10. Position client in supine position. Elevate head of bed to comfortable level.	Promotes good body mechanics for nurse. Client position eases application. Also, the stockings should be applied before standing to prevent stagnation of blood in lower extremities.
11. After legs are cleansed, apply small amount of talcum powder to legs and feet, provided client does not have sensitivity to talcum powder.	Talcum powder reduces friction and allows for easier application of stockings.

STEPS	RATIONALE

12. Apply stockings:

a. Turn elastic stocking inside out up to the heel. Place one hand into sock, holding heel. Pull top of sock with other hand inside out over foot of sock.

Allows easier application of stocking.

b. Place client's toes into foot of elastic stocking, making sure that sock is smooth (see illustration).

Wrinkles in sock can cause constrictions and impede circulation to lower region of extremity (Collier, 1999).

c. Slide remaining portion of sock over client's foot, being sure that the toes are covered. Make sure the foot fits into the toe and heel position of the sock. Sock will now be right side out (see illustration).

If toes remain uncovered, they will become constricted by elastic and their circulation can be reduced.

d. Slide top of sock up over client's calf until sock is completely extended. Be sure sock is smooth and no ridges or wrinkles are present particularly behind the knee (see illustration).

e. Instruct client not to roll socks partially down.

Rolling sock partially down has a constricting effect and can impede venous return.

13. Reposition client to position of comfort, and wash hands.

Maintains proper body alignment and promotes comfort. Reduces transmission of microorganisms.

14. Remove stockings at least once per shift.

Maintains natural venous return.

15. Inspect stocking to make sure there are no wrinkles or binding at top of stocking.

Wrinkles lead to increased pressure and alter circulation.

16. Observe circulatory status of lower extremities. Observe color, temperature, and condition of skin.

Ensures circulatory status in lower extremities has not been compromised.

17. Observe client's reaction to stockings.

Ensures client is adapting to stockings and is not experiencing any discomfort from stockings.

18. Observe client or caregiver apply stockings.

Determines ability to perform skill accurately.

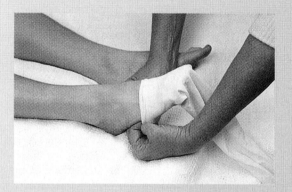

STEP 12B   Place toes into foot of stocking.

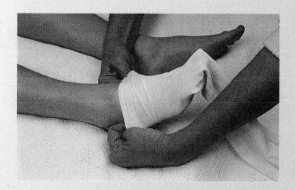

STEP 12C   Slide heel of sock over foot.

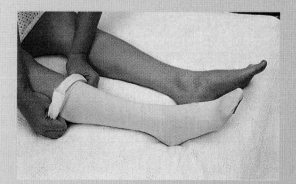

STEP 12D   Slide sock up leg until completely extended.

STEPS	RATIONALE

UNEXPECTED OUTCOMES AND RELATED INTERVENTIONS

- Skin reaction to elastic stockings develops.
  - Observe for evidence of redness, skin lesions, and client's subjective complaint of itching or burning. Some clients may have skin reaction to material used in elastic socks and may indicate allergic reaction. Leave stockings off. Contact physician.
- Decrease in circulation in lower extremities develops (e.g., coolness in lower extremities, cyanosis, decrease in pedal pulses, decrease in blanching, numbness or tingling sensation).
  - Check that elastic stockings are not too small or have wrinkles or folds that impede circulation.
  - Reevaluate size, and reorder elastic stockings as indicated.
  - Signs and symptoms may indicate obstruction of arterial blood flow. Notify physician immediately.
- Development of deep vein thrombosis is suspected.
  - Because clinical signs may be vague, an order for more sensitive radiology tests should be obtained from a physician. Doppler ultrasound, a noninvasive test, may be carried out to rule out the presence of thrombosis (Brough, 1998).
  - Lower extremities should not be massaged because of potential for dislodging thrombus.

- Pulmonary embolism develops. Signs and symptoms include tachypnea, shortness of breath, anxiety, pleuritic chest pain, cough, hemoptysis, tachycardia, and signs of right ventricular failure (i.e., distended neck veins) (Phipps and others, 1999).
  - Stay with client or call for another licensed personnel to remain at bedside monitoring vital signs and oxygenation status.
  - Call the physician immediately.
  - Administer supplemental oxygen as ordered.

RECORDING AND REPORTING

- Report and record the following:
  - Stocking length and size
  - Time of stocking application and condition of skin before application
  - Circulatory status of lower extremities before stocking application
  - Time stockings are removed during shift
  - Condition of skin and circulatory status after removal
  - Calf or thigh circumferences (daily if client is at risk for thrombophlebitis)
- Immediately report signs of thrombophlebitis or impeded circulation in lower extremities to charge nurse or physician.

Intermittent pneumatic compression (IPC), also referred to as sequential compression devices (SCDs), consist of sleeves or stockings wrapped around the legs. The plastic sleeves are connected to an air pump that alternately inflates and deflates, providing rhythmic, external extremity compression (Box 33-7). Use of the IPC on the legs decreases venous stasis by increasing venous return. In postoperative clients these compression stockings are kept on until the client is ambulatory.

Immobilized clients are frequently placed on low-dose heparin therapy to minimize the risk of venous thromboembolism. Heparin is an anticoagulant and thus suppresses clot formation. This therapy requires a physician's order. The medication is usually administered every 8 to 12 hours. The usual route of administration is subcutaneous injection. Because of the action of this medication, monitor the client for signs of bleeding (e.g., increased bruising, guaiac-positive stools, and bleeding gums).

Musculoskeletal System. Some orthopedic and neurological conditions require more frequent passive ROM exercises to restore the injured joint or extremity to maximal function. Clients with such conditions may use automatic equipment for passive range-of-joint-motion exercises. The machine referred to continuous passive motion (CPM), moves the extremity within a prescribed range for a specific

Procedural Guidelines for	Box 33-7

APPLICATION OF SEQUENTIAL COMPRESSION STOCKINGS

1. Measure client for proper-size stocking by measuring around the largest part of the client's thigh.
2. Place a protective stockinette over the client's leg.
3. Wrap the stocking around the leg, starting at the ankle, with the opening over the patella (see illustration). Secure with Velcro.
4. Attach the stockings to the insufflator and verify that the intermittent pressure is between 35 and 45 mm Hg.

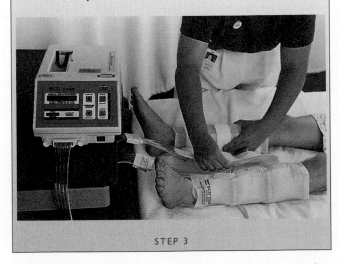

STEP 3

Outcome Evaluation for MR. STAPP

Box 33-8

Nursing Action	Client Response/Finding	Achievement of Outcome
Measure calves daily; report any increases in dimensions.	Bilateral calf diameters continue at 14.5 cm on first postoperative day. Mr. Stapp denies pain or feeling of tightness in calves. No reddened or warm areas noted on calves.	Mr. Stapp's calf diameters remained within 1 cm of baseline (baseline = 14 cm). Outcome met.
Perform circulatory assessment to extremities every shift.	Mr. Stapp is able to wriggle toes. Capillary refill is less than 3 seconds. He has strong pedal pulses. Toenail beds are pink. Feet are warm to touch.	Outcome met. Circulation appears adequate to lower extremities.
Auscultate lung fields every shift.	Mr. Stapp is using incentive spirometer every 2 hours. Small amount of clear, thin sputum noted after cough and deep breathing exercises performed.	Outcome met. Mr. Stapp's lungs remained clear.
Observe skin condition daily.	Mr. Stapp denies any numbness or burning over pressure areas. Slight redness noted on heels.	His skin remained intact, but outcome not fully achieved.

period. This method is beneficial when the client must gradually increase ROM of a particular joint.

RESTORATIVE AND CONTINUING CARE. The goal of restorative and continuing care for the client who is immobile is to maximize functional mobility and independence and to reduce residual functional deficits such as impaired gait and decreased endurance. The focus is not only on ADLs that relate to physical self-care but also on **instrumental activities of daily living (IADLs).** IADLs are activities that are necessary to be independent in society beyond eating, grooming, transferring, and toileting and include such skills as shopping, preparing meals, banking, and taking medications.

You will use many of the same interventions as described in the health promotion and acute care sections, but the emphasis is on working collaboratively with clients and their significant others and with other health care professionals. Intensive specialized therapy such as occupational or physical therapy is common. Your role is to work collaboratively with these professionals and reinforce exercises and teaching. Common items used to help adapt to mobility limitations include walkers, canes, wheelchairs, and assistive devices such as toilet seat extenders, reaching sticks, special silverware, and clothing with Velcro closures.

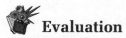

Evaluation

CLIENT CARE. All of your interventions for reducing the risks of immobility are evaluated by comparing the client's actual response to the expected outcomes for each goal (Box 33-8). If expected outcomes are not achieved, you will need to revise the care plan. The success in meeting each outcome is based on the use of evaluative measures such as ROM status, exercise tolerance, and fluid intake.

You will also evaluate specific outcomes designed to demonstrate normal function of specific subsystems and to prevent complications in those systems. Are the lungs clear?

Case Study EVALUATION

It has been 2 weeks since Mark Weber began to care for Mr. Stapp. Mr. Stapp's independence has increased greatly. He now has 110 degrees of flexion and 100 degrees of extension in his knees, and he is able to transfer independently and do his ROM exercises. He is planning to go home over the weekend. He is scheduled to return to his surgeon's office in 1 week.

During rehabilitation Mr. Stapp concentrated on increasing his exercise while monitoring his caloric intake. During the acute and restorative care he lost a total of 15 lb. He has worked out a diet with the dietitian at the center and will show this to his private medical physician, whom he is scheduled to visit in 1 month. Mr. Stapp has set a 30-lb goal for weight loss.

Documentation Note

Mr. Stapp discharged today. He received his prescriptions and follow-up appointments with his orthopedic surgeon and private medical physician. He received instruction on specific exercises to increase his knee mobility. He was met by his son and escorted by wheelchair to his son's car.

Is the client performing leg exercises regularly? Are bowel sounds present? Are bowels remaining soft, formed, and regular? Are there any areas of soft breakdown around pressure points? Does the client remain injury free?

CLIENT EXPECTATIONS. Movement is often taken for granted until it is lost. Clients who are immobile and dependent on others for some or all of their needs can become overly dependent or try to do too much themselves too early. It is a difficult task finding the interdependent balance between independence and dependence. Clients will want control over their mobility that is personally satisfactory. For clients who are completely dependent on others for care, control over how and when things are done may be very important. Do they feel they are treated with dignity? Do caregivers treat them as adults?

Clients who are dependent on others for care may see their demands as the only control they have over their life.

For most clients with mobility problems, lack of control is often a major issue. Do they feel staff were considerate, and did staff protect their privacy? Were their preferences taken into consideration when planning care? Did caregivers talk to them or ignore them? It is helpful to remember that lack of movement is often associated with punishment in our society. Children are given "time-outs," teens are "grounded," and criminals are jailed. It is therefore important to recognize that immobility may lead to fear, anger, grief, withdrawal, or hostility. Whether you are sensitive to these reactions and help the client work through them or respond negatively to the client can make a big difference in the client's outcome.

Key Terms

activities of daily living (ADLs), *p. 823*
anthropometric measurements, *p. 829*
atelectasis, *p. 823*
bed rest, *p. 823*
bone resorption, *p. 826*
chest physiotherapy, *p. 833*

disuse osteoporosis, *p. 826*
diuresis, *p. 824*
hypercalcemia, *p. 824*
hypostatic pneumonia, *p. 823*
immobility, *p. 823*
instrumental activities of daily living
  (IADLs), *p. 839*
ischemia, *p. 826*

isometric exercises, *p. 833*
joint contracture, *p. 826*
mobility, *p. 823*
negative nitrogen balance, *p. 824*
orthostatic hypotension, *p. 824*
pathological fracture, *p. 826*
renal calculi, *p. 826*
thrombus, *p. 825*

Key Concepts

- Normal physical mobility depends on intact and functioning nervous and musculoskeletal systems.
- The risk of disabilities related to immobilization depends on the extent and duration of the immobilization.
- Immobility may result from illness or trauma or may be prescribed for therapeutic reasons; in any case it presents hazards in the physiological, psychological, and developmental dimensions.
- Pressure ulcers, although preventable, are one of the most common physiological hazards of immobility.
- Effects of immobility include depression, behavioral changes, changes in the sleep-wake cycle, decreased coping abilities, and developmental effects.

- Assessment focuses on range of joint motion, musculoskeletal status, and complete physical examination for potential adverse effects in all body systems, as well as psychosocial and developmental effects.
- After identifying nursing diagnoses, plan and implement interventions to prevent or minimize the hazards and complications of immobilization.
- Adequate hydration measures can reduce immobility-related complications in the respiratory and elimination systems.
- The primary evaluation criterion for nursing care in the developmental dimension for immobilized clients is the prevention of any measurable decline in functioning or delay in development.
- Early mobilization helps to decrease the effects of bed rest.

Critical Thinking Activities

1. The client you are caring for is on complete bed rest. After removing the client's elastic support hose, you note an area of the right leg that is reddened and warm to touch. What could these signs signify, and what steps should you take immediately?
2. You are caring for an 80-year-old woman who was admitted to your floor 3 days ago for repair of a fractured hip. You are performing your morning assessment, and you note that she seems rather anxious and her heart rate has increased considerably over baseline. She complains of shortness of breath and pleuritic chest pain. What do these signs and symptoms indicate? What are the appropriate nursing interventions at this time?
3. A 77-year-old man with a history of chronic obstructive pulmonary disease (COPD) has been admitted to your unit for repair of bilateral fractured femurs due to a motor vehicle accident. It is expected that he will be on bed rest for at least 1 week. Describe at least two nursing interventions to help minimize the effects of immobility on the pulmonary system (keep in mind his past medical history).

Review Questions

1. A physiological risk associated with prolonged immobility is:
   1. decreased bone resorption.
   2. increased cardiac workload.
   3. decreased serum calcium levels.
   4. increased hemoglobin formation.

2. The client at greatest risk for developing adverse effects of immobility is a:
   1. 3-year-old with a fractured femur.
   2. 48-year-old woman following a thyroidectomy.
   3. 78-year-old man in traction for a broken hip.
   4. 38-year-old woman undergoing a hysterectomy.

3. The most important objective of bed rest for a client with bilateral pneumonia would be to:
    1. allow this client uninterrupted sleep.
    2. reduce the oxygen needs of the body.
    3. decrease the need for pain medications.
    4. prevent the client from falling due to an unsteady gait.
4. A client has been on bed rest for several days. The client stands, and you note that the client's systolic blood pressure drops 20 mm Hg. This is referred to as:
    1. rebound hypotension.
    2. orthostatic hypotension.
    3. positional hypotension.
    4. central venous hypotension.
5. A client has been immobilized for 5 days because of extensive abdominal surgery. When getting this client out of bed for the first time, a nursing diagnosis related to the *safety* of this client would be:
    1. pain.
    2. impaired skin integrity.
    3. altered tissue perfusion.
    4. risk for activity intolerance.
6. You are instructing a client who has been diagnosed with stable angina pectoris about an exercise program. A statement indicating that learning has occurred is:
    1. "I will start my exercise program by jogging 30 minutes per day."
    2. "I will exercise until my muscles become fatigued. You know—no pain, no gain."
    3. "I will stop exercising and rest if I become short of breath."
    4. "I know I have exercised enough if my heart rate goes at least 50 beats over my baseline."
7. The purpose of elastic stockings after a surgical procedure is to:
    1. prevent varicose veins.
    2. prevent muscular atrophy.
    3. ensure joint mobility and prevent contractures.
    4. facilitate the return of venous blood to the heart.
8. You suspect that a client has a deep vein thrombosis in the left lower leg. The priority intervention at this time would be to:
    1. check for Homans' sign immediately.
    2. massage the area to promote circulation to the area.
    3. prepare the client for radiological studies such as a Doppler study.
    4. apply elastic stockings and intermittent pneumatic compression device.
9. A client has been admitted for a fractured hip and is expected to remain on bed rest for at least 1 week because of complications. A past history of chronic obstructive pulmonary disease (COPD) is noted. A priority nursing intervention related to this client's past medical history would be to instruct the client to:
    1. increase fluid intake.
    2. perform leg exercises at least every hour.
    3. perform incentive spirometry every hour while awake.
    4. ask for pain medication at the very onset of discomfort.
10. A client complains of sudden onset of severe chest pain upon inspiration, and increasing shortness of breath is noted. You suspect pulmonary emboli. Your *first* nursing intervention is to:
    1. call the physician immediately.
    2. place the client in Fowler's position and assess oxygenation status.
    3. encourage the client to take a deep breath to promote lung expansion.
    4. place the client in a supine position to prevent dislodgement of the clot into the left ventricle.

References

Agency for Health Care Policy and Research: *Treating pressure sores: consumer guide,* Clinical practice guidelines, No. 15, Rockville, Md, 1994, U.S. Department of Health and Human Services.

Beare PG, Myers JL: *Adult health nursing,* ed 3, St. Louis, 1998, Mosby.

Blondin M, Titler M: Deep vein thrombosis and pulmonary embolism: prevention—what role do nurses play? *Medsurg Nurs* 5(3):205, 1996.

Brough E: Deep vein thrombosis, *Prof Nurse* 13(10):687, 1998.

Collier M: Brevet tx: anti-embolism stockings for prevention and treatment of DVT, *Br J Nurs* 8(1):44, 1999.

Ebersole P, Hess P: *Toward healthy aging: human needs and nursing response,* ed 5, St. Louis, Mosby, 1998.

Huddleston JL: Exercise. In Edelman CL, Mandle CL, editors: *Health promotion throughout the lifespan,* ed 4, St. Louis, 1998, Mosby.

Kasper C and others: Alterations in skeletal muscle related to short-term impaired physical mobility, *Res Nurs Health* 19:133, 1996.

Kihara M and others: Autonomic dysfunction in elderly bedfast patients, *Age Ageing* 27:551, 1998.

Lee S and others: Upright exercise or supine lower body negative pressure exercise maintains exercise responses after bedrest, *Med Sci Sports Exer* 29(7):892, 1997.

Mahoney J: Immobility and falls, *Clin Geriatr Med* 14(4):699, 1998.

McCance K, Huether S: *Pathophysiology: the biologic basis for disease in adults and children,* ed 3, St. Louis, 1998, Mosby.

Phipps W and others: *Medical-surgical nursing: concepts and clinical practice,* ed 6, St. Louis, 1999, Mosby.

Roper M: Back to basics: assessing orthostatic vital signs, *Am J Nurs* 96(8):43, 1996.

Wong D and others: *Whaley & Wong's nursing care of infants and children,* ed 6, St. Louis, 1999, Mosby.

34

Skin Integrity and Wound Care

Objectives

- Define key terms.
- Describe risk factors for pressure ulcer development.
- List the four stages of pressure ulcers.
- Discuss the body's response during each phase of the wound healing process.
- Describe the wound assessment criteria: anatomical location, size, type and percentage of wound tissue, volume and color of wound drainage and condition of surrounding skin.
- Differentiate healing by primary and secondary intention.
- Discuss common complications of wound healing.
- Explain factors that impair or promote normal wound healing.
- Describe the purposes of and precautions taken with applying bandages and binders.
- Describe the mechanism of action of wound care dressings.
- Describe the differences in therapeutic effects of heat and cold.
- Complete an assessment for a client with impaired skin integrity.
- List nursing diagnoses associated with impaired skin integrity.
- Develop a nursing care plan for a client with impaired skin integrity.
- State evaluation criteria for a client with impaired skin integrity.

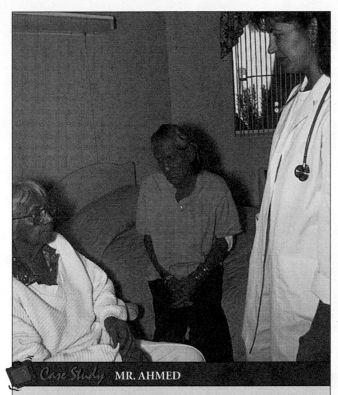

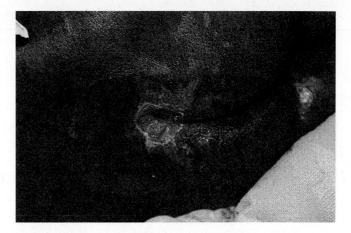

FIGURE **34-1**   Pressure ulcer with tissue necrosis.

Case Study   MR. AHMED

Mr. Omar Ahmed, a 76-year-old accountant, has once again been admitted to the hospital, this time for treatment of pneumonia. Before admission he had been unable to eat and had lost more than 20 lb over the last 2 months. Three years ago he had coronary artery bypass surgery. As a precaution, he has been put on telemetry monitoring. He also has hypertension and type 2 diabetes mellitus. His mobility is limited because of his weakness, difficulty breathing, and acutely ill state. Mr. Ahmed is retired. He lives in a one-family home with his wife, Natalie. Their children and grandchildren live nearby and visit often. On admission his skin is intact. He complains that his "bottom hurts" from lying in bed.

Lynda Abraham is a junior nursing student who is doing 2 days a week of her clinical experience for her medical-surgical nursing course on Mr. Ahmed's medical nursing unit. This is her first hospital-based clinical practice.

SCIENTIFIC KNOWLEDGE BASE
Pressure Ulcers

Pressure ulcer (formerly called *pressure sore, decubitus ulcer,* or *bedsore*) is the preferred term used to describe impaired skin integrity (Figure 34-1) resulting from pressure (Agency for Health Care Policy and Research [AHCPR], 1992, 1994; Pieper, 2000). A client experiencing decreased mobility, inadequate nutrition, decreased sensory perception, or decreased activity can be at risk for pressure ulcer development.

Tissue ischemia occurs when capillary blood flow is obstructed by pressure. When pressure is relieved in a relatively short time a phenomenon called reactive hyperemia occurs. **Reactive blanching hyperemia** is a mechanism that causes the blood vessels to dilate in the area of injury and can pre-

vent tissue trauma. The injured area appears red and warm. The area blanches (turns lighter in color) with fingertip pressure (Figure 34-2). In clients with dark skin this will be harder to assess; the discoloration appears as a deepening of normal ethnic color or a purple hue to the skin (Bates-Jensen and Wethe, 1998). This hyperemia should resolve without tissue loss if pressure is reduced or relieved (Pieper, 2000).

Nonblanching reactive hyperemia indicates tissue damage. When a finger is pressed against the red or purple area, it does not turn lighter in color, indicating tissue damage. Deep tissue damage is present and is commonly the first stage of pressure ulcer development. This stage of skin injury may also be reversible if the pressure is relieved and the tissue protected (Figure 34-3).

CONTRIBUTING FACTORS TO PRESSURE ULCER FORMATION.   In addition to pressure, other factors can increase the client's risk for developing pressure ulcers. The external factors include shear, friction, and moisture, and internal factors include nutrition, infection, and age.

SHEAR.   **Shear** is the force exerted against the skin while the skin remains stationary and the bony structures move. For example, when the head of the bed is elevated, gravity causes the bony skeleton to pull towards the foot of the bed, while the skin remains against the sheets (Figure 38-4). The underlying tissue blood vessels are stretched and angulated, and blood flow is impeded to the deep tissue. Ulcers occur with large areas of undermined damage and less damage at the skin surface.

FRICTION.   **Friction** is an injury to the skin that has the appearance of an abrasion. Friction results from two surfaces rubbing against one another. The body surfaces most at risk for friction are the elbows and heels because abrasion of these surfaces can occur when they are rubbed against the sheets during repositioning. Injury from friction is shallow without necrosis and is limited to the epidermis (Bryant and others, 2000).

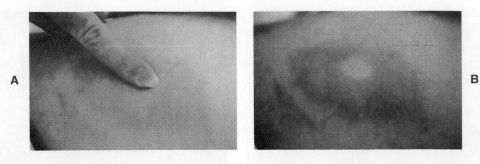

FIGURE **34-2**   **A,** Blanching reactive hyperemia. **B,** Blanches with fingertip pressure.

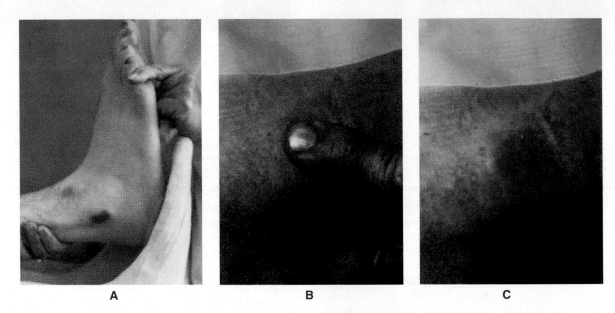

FIGURE **34-3**   **A,** Nonblanching reactive hyperemia. **B** and **C,** In nonblanching reactive hyperemia the area is much darker than the surrounding skin and does not blanch with fingertip pressure.

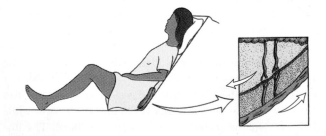

FIGURE **34-4**   Shear exerted against sacral area.

MOISTURE.   Moisture on the skin increases the risk of ulcer formation. Moisture reduces the skin's resistance to other physical factors such as pressure or shear. Moisture can originate from wound drainage, perspiration, and/or fecal and urinary incontinence. The susceptibility to pressure ulcer formation increases with the duration of the exposure to moisture (Jeter and Lutz, 1996).

NUTRITION.   Poor nutrition, specifically severe protein deficiency, can cause soft tissue to become susceptible to break-

down. Low protein levels cause edema, which contributes to problems with oxygen transport and the transport of nutrients (Pieper, 2000).

Poor nutrition alters fluid and electrolyte balance. In clients with severe protein loss, hypoalbuminemia (serum albumin level below 3 g/100 ml) leads to a shift of fluid from the extracellular fluid volume to the tissues, resulting in edema (Breslow and others, 1993). **Edema** increases the affected tissue's risk for pressure ulcer formation. The blood supply to the edematous tissue is decreased, and waste products remain because of the changing pressures in the capillary circulation and capillary bed.

Cachexia is generalized ill health and malnutrition, marked by weakness and emaciation. Basically the cachectic client has lost the adipose tissue necessary to protect bony prominences from pressure.

INFECTION.   Infection results from the presence of pathogens in the body. A client with an infection usually has a fever. Infection and fever increase the metabolic needs of the body, making already hypoxic tissue more susceptible to ischemic injury. In addition, fever results in diaphoresis and increased skin moisture, which further predispose the client to skin breakdown.

AGE.   Skin structure changes with age, causing a loss of dermal thickness and an increase in the risk of skin tears. Older adults are at highest risk for development of pressure ulcers; 60% to 90% of all pressure ulcers occur in clients over 65 years of age (Boynton and others, 1999).

Pathogenesis of Pressure Ulcers

Pressure ulcers are caused by pressure exerted against the skin surface; the skin is compressed by two surfaces, generally a bony prominence and the bed surface. However, pressure ulcers can occur on any skin surface where pressure applied against the skin exceeds capillary closure pressure. Normal capillary pressure, the amount of pressure needed to keep the capillary open, is thought to be in the range of 12 to 32 mm Hg, depending on the location in the capillary (Landis, 1930). When the intensity of the pressure exerted to the capillary exceeds 12 to 32 mm Hg, the vessel is occluded, causing ischemic injury to the tissues it normally feeds. However, pressure to the tissue will not routinely result in pressure ulceration. Two other concepts, duration of the pressure and tissue tolerance, play a role.

High pressure over a short time and low pressure over a long time can cause skin breakdown. Thus duration influences the effects of pressure. Tissue tolerance also plays an important role in pressure ulcer development. The integrity of the skin and the supporting structures can influence the skin's ability to redistribute the pressure. The factors mentioned above—shear, friction, moisture and the internal factors such as nutrition, infection, and age—can alter the ability of the skin and supporting tissue to respond to the pressure (Pieper, 2000).

Wound Classification

One method to classify pressure ulcers is to stage the ulcer according to tissue layer involvement. The National Pressure Ulcer Advisory Panel (NPUAP) (1999) supports the following staging system:

Stage I: An observable pressure ulcer related to alteration of intact skin whose indicators as compared to the adjacent or opposite area on the body may include changes in one or more of the following: skin temperature (warmth or coolness), tissue consistency (firm or boggy feel), and/or sensation (pain, itching). The ulcer appears as a defined area of persistent redness in lightly pigmented skin, whereas in darker skin tones, the ulcer may appear with persistent red, blue, or purple hues (Figure 34-5, A).

Stage II: Partial-thickness skin loss involving epidermis, dermis, or both. Ulcer is superficial and presents clinically as an abrasion, blister, or shallow crater (Figure 34-5, B).

Stage III: Full-thickness skin loss involving damage to, or necrosis of, subcutaneous tissue that may extend down to, but not through, underlying fascia. Ulcer presents clinically as a deep crater with or without undermining of adjacent tissue (Figure 34-5, C).

Stage IV: Full-thickness skin loss occurs with extensive destruction, tissue necrosis, or damage to muscle, bone, or supporting structures (e.g., tendon or joint capsule). Undermining and sinus tracts may also be associated with stage IV (Figure 34-5, D).

Although this staging system can be used, one drawback of the system is that a wound covered with necrotic tissue cannot be adequately staged.

Wound assessment (regardless of etiology) should include the following parameters: anatomical location, size (dimensions and depth of wound), type (viable or nonviable) and percentage of wound tissue (the proportion of tissue type), volume and color of wound drainage, and condition of surrounding skin (Cooper, 2000). These parameters will assist in evaluating the progress of the wound, will drive decision making, and will provide assessment to evaluate wound healing.

Wound Healing Process

The process of wound healing involves an orderly series of integrated physiological responses. Multiple factors promote or impede wound healing (Box 34-1). A wound with little or no tissue loss, such as a clean surgical incision, heals by **primary intention.** The skin edges **approximate,** or close together, and the risk of infection developing is slight. In contrast, a wound involving loss of tissue such as a severe laceration or a chronic wound such as a pressure ulcer heals by **secondary intention.** The edges do not close, increasing the risk for infection and loss of tissue function. There are also instances in which a surgical wound is initially closed in the deep tissue layers; however, the subcutaneous fat and skin layers are left open. This method of wound closure is called *delayed primary closure.* The wound heals with a layer of **granulation tissue** at the edges and base, and several days after the initial wounding the wound edges are brought together with sutures or adhesive closures. The wound then heals by primary intention. An example of a wound closure by delayed primary closure occurs when a client has a ruptured appendix. The surgeon may be unsure if the appendix had microperforations and subsequent spilling of the intestinal contents into the abdomen and wound. Thus the incision may be left open for up to 4 days following surgery. The wound is assessed, and, if after 4 days no clinical signs of infection are noted, the wound is closed with either Steri-strips or sutures.

Wounds heal by one of two mechanisms: partial-thickness repair or full-thickness repair. Partial-thickness repair is required when there is loss of the epidermis and/or part of the dermis, such as wound healing by primary intention. Full-thickness repair is required when there is loss of the epidermis, dermis, and possible extension into subcutaneous layers, bone, and/or muscle.

PARTIAL-THICKNESS WOUND REPAIR.   Wounds that heal by primary intention and shallow wounds that only involve loss of the epidermis and perhaps some of the dermis are repaired by resurfacing of the wound with new epider-

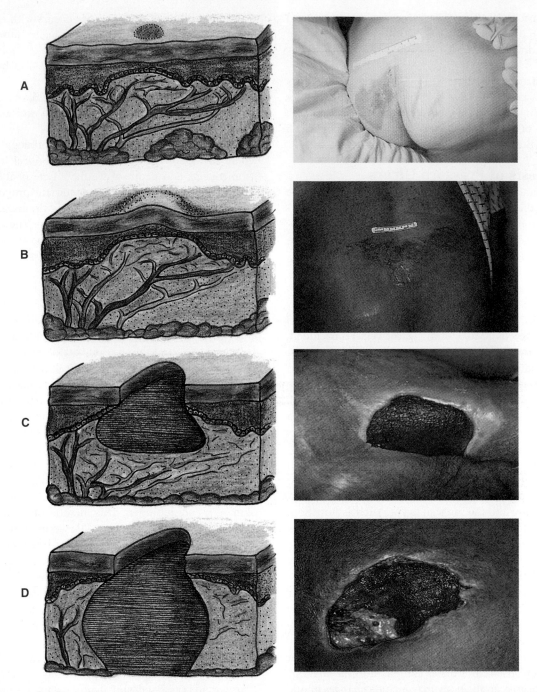

FIGURE 34-5   A, Stage I pressure ulcer. B, Stage II pressure ulcer. C, Stage III pressure ulcer. D, Stage IV pressure ulcer. (Courtesy Laurel Wiersema-Bryant, RN, MSN, Clinical Nurse Specialist, Barnes Hospital, St. Louis.)

mal cells (Sussman, 1998). The wounds go through several phases of wound healing.

INFLAMMATORY RESPONSE.   Erythema and edema are the initial response, bringing to the site white blood cells. The wounded area appears red and swollen. If the exudate that brings the white blood cells to the area is allowed to dry, a scab will form. This response occurs for approximately 24 hours (Waldrop and Doughty, 2000).

EPIDERMAL REPAIR.   Epidermal cells begin migration across the wound, originating from the epidermal cells at the wound edges or the epidermal appendages. Peak epithelial proliferation occurs within 24 to 72 hours after injury. Wounds kept in a moist environment will heal in approximately 4 days (as opposed to 7 days when kept dry) because new epithelial cells migrate across a moist surface. If a wound is kept dry, the cells must find moisture below the skin surface (Waldrop and Doughty, 2000).

Factors Influencing Wound Healing
Box 34-1

AGE

Blood circulation and oxygen delivery to the wound, clotting, inflammatory response, and phagocytosis may be impaired in the very young and older adults. Risk of infection is greater.

Cell growth and differentiation in reconstruction are slower with advancing age.

Scar tissue never regains the tensile strength of noninjured skin, increasing the risk of altered body part function in older adults.

Age affects all phases of wound healing. A decline in the number of white blood cells places older adults at greater risk for a wound infection. A slowdown is seen in the deposition of collagen in reepithelization.

NUTRITION

Tissue repair and infection resistance depend on balanced diet. Surgery, severe wounds, serious infections, and preoperative nutritional deficits increase nutritional requirements.

Nutrients provide raw materials needed for cellular activities that contribute to wound healing.

INFECTION

Wound infection prolongs the inflammatory phase, delays collagen synthesis, and prevents epithelialization.

OBESITY

The less abundant supply of blood vessels in fatty tissue impairs delivery of nutrients and cellular elements needed for healing.

EXTENT OF WOUND

Wounds with extensive tissue loss heal by secondary intention and remain open for a prolonged period of time to heal.

TISSUE PERFUSION

Oxygen fuels the cellular function essential to the repair process. Chronic tissue hypoxia has been associated with impaired collagen synthesis and reduced tissue resistance to infection.

SMOKING

Functional hemoglobin levels decrease; oxygen release in the tissues is impaired.

IMMUNOSUPPRESSION

Cortisone suppresses the inflammatory response, increasing the wound's vulnerability to infection.

Because steroids decrease the inflammatory response, you may not detect early signs of inflammation or infection.

Chemotherapeutic drugs and certain cancerous diseases interfere with leukocyte production and the immune response.

Immunosuppressive therapy impairs wound healing by preventing normal progression of the phases of wound healing.

DIABETES MELLITUS

The diabetic client has small vessel disease that impairs tissue perfusion; thus oxygen delivery may be poor.

An elevated blood glucose level impairs macrophage function.

Risk of infection is increased because of poor wound healing.

Clients with diabetes demonstrate the following problems with wound healing: reduced collagen synthesis, decreased wound strength, and impaired white blood cell functioning. These adverse effects are at least in part due to poor glycemic control.

RADIATION

Radiation therapy, which eventually results in fibrosis and vascular scarring, interferes with postoperative wound healing when surgery is delayed more than 4 to 6 weeks and irradiated tissues have become fragile and poorly perfused.

WOUND STRESS

Sustained stress (e.g., vomiting, abdominal distention, coughing) disrupts wound layers and tissue repair.

Modified from: Waldrop J, Doughty D: Wound healing physiology in acute and chronic wounds. In Bryant RA, editor: *Acute and chronic wounds: nursing management*, ed 2, St. Louis, 2000, Mosby.

DIFFERENTIATION. The epidermis thickens, anchors to adjacent cells, and resumes normal function. The new epidermis is pink, dry, and fragile. If dermal repair is necessary, dermal repair occurs concurrently with epidermal repair.

FULL-THICKNESS REPAIR. Full-thickness wounds involve tissue loss and are more commonly seen in chronic wounds such as pressure ulcers. Three phases are involved in healing a full-thickness wound.

INFLAMMATION PHASE. The key events in the inflammatory phase are control of bleeding and the provision of a clean wound environment for wound healing. The first event in this phase is hemostasis. Platelets cause coagulation and vasoconstriction. The platelets break down and release growth factors, which appear to initiate the entire wound-healing cascade (Waldrop and Doughty, 2000). The inflammatory response brings white blood cells to the area, cleaning up the site and releasing additional growth factors. This phase lasts approximately 3 days in an acute clean wound, such as a surgical incision.

PROLIFERATIVE PHASE. The key events in the proliferative phase are production of new tissue, epithelialization, and contraction. New capillary networks form to provide oxygen and nutrients for new tissue and contribute to the synthesis of collagen. As collagen fibers and capillary networks continue to synthesize and increase in size, the wound begins to contract. The last component of this phase is epithelialization, in which the epithelial cells migrate and cover the defect. It is important to note that epithelialization occurs faster in a moist environment, supporting the role of moist wound dressings in wound care.

REMODELING PHASE. The remodeling phase, which can last up to 1 year, reorganizes the collagen to produce a more elastic, stronger collagen for the scar tissue. The tensile strength of the scar tissue is never more than 80% of the tensile strength in nonwounded tissue (Waldrop and Doughty, 2000).

The phases of wound healing overlap depending upon the client's ability to heal and the type of wound. Acute wounds (most surgical wounds, for example) typically heal following the phases noted above; however, chronic wounds (some pressure ulcers, for example) appear to fail to negotiate one or more of the phases of wound healing.

Complications of Wound Healing

Wound healing is not without complications. When caring for clients with wounds, you must observe the healing process while observing for complications.

HEMORRHAGE.   Bleeding from an acute wound is normal during and immediately after initial trauma, but **hemostasis,** which is cessation of bleeding by vasoconstriction and coagulation, usually occurs within several minutes. Hemorrhage occurring later indicates a slipped surgical suture, a dislodged clot, infection, or the erosion of a blood vessel by a foreign object (e.g., a drain). Hemorrhage may be external or internal. Symptoms of internal bleeding are hypovolemic shock and swelling of the affected body part. A **hematoma,** a collection of clotted blood, is a localized collection of blood underneath tissues, often appearing as a bluish swelling or mass. External hemorrhaging may be more obvious because dressings covering the wound soon become saturated with blood. Surgical drains also drain blood. A decrease in the client's hemoglobin level and hematocrit will be noted.

INFECTION.   Bacterial wound infection inhibits healing by increasing tissue damage and altering the healing process. The chances of wound infection are greater when the wound contains dead or necrotic tissues, when foreign bodies are in or near the wound, and when the blood supply and local tissue defenses are reduced.

A contaminated or traumatic wound infection may develop within 2 to 3 days; a surgical wound infection may develop within 4 to 5 days. Locally drainage may be yellow, green, or brown and may be odorous, depending on the causative organism. The wound edges may appear tense, swollen, and painful, with redness extending beyond the immediate wound edge. Systemic signs include fever, general malaise, and an elevated white blood cell count.

DEHISCENCE.   When an acute wound fails to heal properly, the layers of skin and tissue may separate. This most commonly occurs before collagen formation (3 to 11 days after injury). **Dehiscence** is the partial or total separation of layers of skin and tissue above the fascia in a wound that is not healing properly. Obese clients have a high risk for dehiscence because of constant strain on their wounds and the poor vascularity of fatty tissue. Dehiscence occurs most often in abdominal surgical wounds after a sudden strain such as coughing, vomiting, or sitting up in bed. Clients often report feeling as though something has given way. When serosanguineous drainage increases from a wound, you should be alert for dehiscence.

EVISCERATION.   **Evisceration** occurs when wound layers separate below the fascial layer, and visceral organs may protrude through the wound opening. It is a medical emergency requiring placement of sterile towels soaked in sterile saline over the extruding tissues to reduce chances of bacterial invasion and drying before surgical repair occurs.

FISTULAS.   A **fistula** is an abnormal opening between two organs or between an organ and the outside of the body. Fistulas can result from wound-healing problems associated with trauma, infection, radiation exposure, or disease such as cancer. Fistulas increase the risks of infection, fluid and electrolyte imbalances, and skin breakdown from chronic drainage.

NURSING KNOWLEDGE BASE

A major aspect of nursing care is the maintenance of skin integrity and wound care. Impaired skin integrity can occur from prolonged pressure, shear, friction, and/or moisture, leading to the development of pressure ulcers.

Prediction and Prevention

Prevention and treatment of pressure ulcers are major nursing priorities. In 1992 the Agency for Health Care Policy and Research (AHCPR) developed guidelines for care of adult clients at risk for pressure ulcers. Predictive instruments for pressure ulcer development identify those clients at highest risk for pressure ulcers. Clients with little risk for pressure ulcer development are spared the unnecessary expense of preventive treatments and the risk of complications.

One reliable predictive tool is the Braden Scale. The Braden Scale is composed of six subscales: sensory perception, moisture, activity, mobility, nutrition, and friction and shear (Table 34-1). A hospitalized adult with a score of 16 or below is considered at risk for pressure ulcer development. In older clients, a score of 17 or 18 may be a more efficient prediction of risk (Bergstrom and others, 1998). This instrument is highly reliable in the identification of clients at greatest risk for pressure ulcers (Bergstrom and others, 1987a, 1987b, 1998; Ramundo, 1995).

Additional instruments, such as the Gosnell, Knoll, and Norton Scales, are also effective in identifying clients at risk for the development of pressure ulcers. The overall objective of predictive instruments is to effectively and efficiently identify those clients with the greatest risk for pressure ulcer development.

CRITICAL THINKING
Synthesis

Clients who have pressure ulcers or chronic wounds require competent nursing care that integrates information from all health-related sciences. Nurses are able to draw from knowledge and experience and incorporate appropriate standards of practice into the management of the client's wound.

KNOWLEDGE.   Performing a pressure ulcer risk assessment requires you to use one of the validated risk assessment

Braden Scale for Predicting Pressure Sore Risk

Table 34-1

	1 Point	2 Points	3 Points	4 Points
Sensory Perception Ability to respond meaningfully to pressure-related discomfort	**Completely limited:** Unresponsive (does not moan, flinch, or grasp) to painful stimuli due to diminished level of consciousness or sedation. **or** Limited ability to feel pain over most of body surface.	**Very limited:** Responds only to painful stimuli. Cannot communicate discomfort except by moaning or restlessness. **or** Has a sensory impairment that limits the ability to feel pain or discomfort over half of body.	**Slightly limited:** Responds to verbal commands but cannot always communicate discomfort or need to be turned. **or** Has some sensory impairment, which limits ability to feel pain or discomfort in 1 or 2 extremities.	**No impairment:** Responds to verbal commands. Has no sensory deficit that would limit ability to feel or voice pain or discomfort.
Moisture Degree to which skin is exposed to moisture	**Constantly moist:** Skin is kept moist almost constantly by perspiration, urine, etc. Dampness is detected every time patient is moved or turned.	**Moist:** Skin is often, but not always, moist. Linen must be changed at least once a shift.	**Occasionally moist:** Skin is occasionally moist, requiring an extra linen change approximately once a day.	**Rarely moist:** Skin is usually dry; linen requires changing only at routine intervals.
Activity Degree of physical activity	**Bedfast:** Confined to bed.	**Chairfast:** Ability to walk severely limited or nonexistent. Cannot bear own weight and/or must be assisted into chair or wheelchair.	**Walks occasionally:** Walks occasionally during day, but for very short distances, with or without assistance. Spends majority of each shift in bed or chair.	**Walks frequently:** Walks outside the room at least twice a day and inside room at least once every 2 hours during waking hours.
Mobility Ability to change and control body position	**Completely immobile:** Does not make even slight changes in body or extremity position without assistance.	**Very limited:** Makes occasional slight changes in body or extremity position but unable to make frequent or significant changes independently.	**Slightly limited:** Makes frequent though slight changes in body or extremity position independently.	**No limitations:** Makes major and frequent changes in position without assistance.
Nutrition Usual food intake pattern	**Very poor:** Never eats a complete meal. Rarely eats more than one third of any food offered. Eats 2 servings or less of protein (meat or dairy products) per day. Takes fluids poorly. Does not take a liquid dietary supplement. **or** Is NPO and/or maintained on clear liquids or IVs for more than 5 days.	**Probably inadequate:** Rarely eats a complete meal and generally eats only about half of any food offered. Protein intake includes only 3 servings of meat or dairy products per day. Occasionally will take a dietary supplement. **or** Receives less than optimal amount of liquid diet or tube feeding.	**Adequate:** Eats over half of most meals. Eats a total of 4 servings of protein (meat, dairy products) each day. Occasionally will refuse a meal, but will usually take a supplement if offered. **or** Is on a tube-feeding or TPN regimen that probably meets most of nutritional needs.	**Excellent:** Eats most of every meal. Never refuses a meal. Usually eats a total of 4 or more servings of meat and dairy products. Occasionally eats between meals. Does not require supplements.

Instructions: Score client in each of the six subscales. Maximum score is 23, indicating little or no risk. A score of ≤16 indicates "at risk"; ≤9 indicates high risk.

Continued

Braden Scale for Predicting Pressure Sore Risk—cont'd			Table 34-1
	1 Point	2 Points	3 Points	4 Points

	1 Point	2 Points	3 Points
Friction and Shear	**Problem:** Requires moderate to maximal assistance in moving. Complete lifting without sliding against sheets is impossible. Frequently slides down in bed or chair, requiring frequent repositioning with maximal assistance. Spasticity, contractions, or agitation leads to almost constant friction.	**Potential problem:** Moves feebly or requires minimal assistance. During a move skin probably slides to some extent against sheets, chair, restraints, or other devices. Maintains relatively good position in chair or bed most of the time but occasionally slides down.	**No apparent problem:** Moves in bed and in chair independently and has sufficient muscle strength to sit up completely during move. Maintains good position in bed or chair at all times.

tools. Knowing normal physiology and the impact of pressure on the skin enables you to practice preventive nursing measures. In addition, knowledge of the normal healing pattern helps you to recognize alterations requiring intervention. In choosing interventions, consider the type of wound, the pain associated with it, conditions that affect healing, and the client's psychological well-being.

EXPERIENCE.   By observing the normal characteristics of a healing wound, you can assess how the client's wound is healing. This is especially important when the client has some factors that may impede wound healing, such as peripheral vascular disease, poor nutrition, or reduced mobility.

You are better able to assess a client's wound by being able to draw from experience and recognize normal characteristics of wound healing. When caring for a client who develops problems with wound healing, learn the clinical signs of complications. This is especially important when caring for a client with darkly pigmented skin (Box 34-2). Reflecting on such experience prepares you to assess wounds more accurately.

ATTITUDES.   Be observant when caring for an acutely ill client; at times assessment for skin breakdown may be overlooked because of other perceived priorities, such as respiratory or cardiac status. As a client advocate, you must ensure that meticulous skin assessment and pressure ulcer prevention measures are incorporated into the plan of care. Skin assessment is important whenever a client's health status changes (AHCPR, 1992, 1994).

In the immediate postoperative period, clients may require well-thought-out modifications of wound care techniques. The dressing may not be changed, but you are responsible for ensuring that the dressing remains dry and intact. With knowledge about pressure ulcers, wounds, and normal wound healing, you can find creative measures to reduce the risks of impaired skin integrity and promote wound healing.

STANDARDS.   The 1992 and 1994 clinical guidelines written by the AHCPR are the standards of care for clients with pres-

Assessment Tips for Examining Intact Dark Skin	Box 34-2

ASSESS SKIN COLOR
Appears darker than surrounding skin
May have a purplish/bluish hue

IMPORTANCE OF LIGHTING SOURCE
Use natural or halogen light
Avoid fluorescent lamps

ASSESS SKIN TEMPERATURE
When first touched, skin will feel warm, compared to surrounding area
Later this will be replaced by an area of coolness, which is a sign of tissue devitalization

ASSESS FOR EDEMA/FLUID
May be taut, shiny, or indurated; edema may occur with induration of more than 15 mm in diameter

Data from Bennett MA: Report of the Taskforce on the implications for darkly pigmented intact skin in the prediction and prevention of pressure ulcers, *Adv Wound Care* 8(6):34, 1998.

sure ulcers (Murphy, 1996). A summary of the AHCPR prevention points compiled by NPUAP can be found in Box 34-3.

Wound care protocols vary by agency policy. It is important that you know agency policy regarding the use of skin care products, dressing materials, and frequency of dressing change.

▋ NURSING PROCESS

 Assessment

Baseline and continual focused assessment data provide critical information about the client's skin integrity and the increased risk for pressure ulcer development or impaired wound healing (see Table 34-2).

PRESSURE ULCERS.   Assessment for pressure ulcers is not limited to the skin but must also include the underlying tis-

Pressure Ulcer Prevention Points

Box 34-3

RISK ASSESSMENT

1. Consider all bed- or chair-bound persons, or those whose ability to reposition is impaired, to be at risk for pressure ulcers.
2. Select and use a method of risk assessment, such as the Norton scale or the Braden Scale, that ensures systematic evaluation of individual risk factors.
3. Assess all at-risk clients at the time of admission to health care facilities and at regular intervals thereafter.
4. Identify all individual risk factors (decreased mental status, moisture, incontinence, nutritional deficits) to direct specific preventive treatments. Modify care according to the individual factors.

SKIN CARE AND EARLY TREATMENT

1. Inspect the skin at least daily, and document assessment results.
2. Individualize bathing frequency. Use a mild cleansing agent. Avoid hot water and excessive friction.
3. Assess and treat incontinence. When incontinence cannot be controlled, cleanse skin at time of soiling, use a topical moisture barrier, and select underpads or briefs that are absorbent and provide a quick-drying surface to the skin.
4. Use moisturizers for dry skin. Minimize environmental factors leading to dry skin, such as low humidity and cold air.
5. Avoid massage over bony prominences.
6. Use proper positioning, transferring, and turning techniques to minimize skin injury due to friction and shear.
7. Use dry lubricants (cornstarch) or protective coverings to reduce friction injury.
8. Identify and correct factors compromising protein/calorie intake, and consider nutritional supplementation/support for nutritionally compromised persons.
9. Institute a rehabilitation program to maintain or improve mobility/activity status.
10. Monitor and document interventions and outcomes.

MECHANICAL LOADING AND SUPPORT SURFACES

1. Reposition bed-bound persons at least every 2 hours, chair-bound persons at least every hour.
2. Use a written repositioning schedule.
3. Place at-risk persons on a pressure-reducing mattress/chair cushion. Do not use donut type of devices.
4. Consider postural alignment, distribution of weight, balance, and stability, and pressure relief when positioning persons in chairs or wheelchairs.
5. Teach chair-bound persons, who are able, to shift weight every 15 minutes.
6. Use lifting devices (e.g., trapeze, bed linen) to move rather than drag persons during transfer and position changes.
7. Use pillows or foam wedges to keep bony prominences such as knees and ankles from direct contact with each other.
8. Use devices that totally relieve pressure on the heels (e.g., place pillows under the calf to raise the heels off the bed).
9. Avoid positioning directly on the trochanter when using the side-lying position (use the 30-degree lateral inclined position).
10. Elevate the head of the bed as little (maximum 30-degree angle) and for as short a time as possible.

EDUCATION

1. Implement educational programs for the prevention of pressure ulcers that are structured, organized, comprehensive and directed at all levels of health care providers, clients, family, and caregivers.
2. Include information on:
   a. Etiology of and risk factors for pressure ulcers
   b. Risk assessment tools and their application
   c. Skin assessment
   d. Selection/use of support surfaces
   e. Development with implementation of individualized programs of skin care
   f. Demonstration of positioning to decrease risk of tissue breakdown
   g. Accurate documentation of pertinent data

Data from National Pressure Ulcer Advisory Panel: Pressure ulcers incidence, economics, risk assessment, Consensus Development Conference Statement, *Decubitus* 2(2):24, 1989.

sue and muscle. Assessment of the client for risk of development of pressure ulcers should be done using one of the established predictive tools, such as the Braden Scale, on admission to the agency, 24 to 48 hours after admission, and at regular intervals. It is important that assessment be ongoing because the client's condition may change; continual assessments may identify changes that increase the client's risk for pressure ulcer development. In addition to assessing the client for potential risk factors, a skin assessment should be done on a daily basis. The skin assessment can provide for prompt problem identification and development of individualized interventions (Skill 34-1).

PREDICTIVE MEASURES. Predictive instruments increase early detection of clients at greatest risk for ulcer development. Prompt identification of such clients enables nurses to individualize costly resources to appropriate clients and reduce their risk.

SKIN. Assessment for tissue pressure indicators includes visual and tactile inspection of the skin (Pires and Muller, 1991). Baseline assessment determines the client's normal skin characteristics and any actual or potential areas of breakdown. This is especially important with high-risk clients. The skin of an older adult client is more fragile and has an increased risk for skin breakdown (Box 34-4). Pay particular attention to areas exposed to casts, traction, or splints. Systematic skin assessment should occur at least once a day on those clients at greater risk for pressure ulcer development (AHCPR, 1992).

Assess all areas of the skin, from head to toe, paying attention to any reddened areas or breaks in skin integrity. The assessment should be documented. When hyperemia is noted, document its location, size, and color and reassess the area after 1 hour. If you suspect nonblanching reactive hyperemia, outlining the affected area with a marker makes reassessment easier. Nonblanching reactive hyperemia can be

		Table 34-2
Example of a Focused Client Assessment		
Factors to Assess	**Questions and Approaches**	**Physical Assessment Strategies**
Adequacy of the client's sensory perception	• Ask client to respond to verbal commands; observe whether client follows commands. • Reposition a bed-bound client and determine whether client responds verbally, by moaning, or not at all.	• Observe whether client responds to verbal commands (no impairment). • Apply painful stimuli to various body locations; if client cannot respond except by moaning, the client is very limited in sensory perception.
Moisture	• Observe client's bed linens on a routine basis to assess for the presence of moisture. • Determine client's ability to use toileting facilities when needed.	• Observe client's skin, noting if it is dry (rarely moist) or seldom damp (occasionally moist) or if skin is often but not always wet (moist). • Check whether the client is incontinent of urine and stool; if almost constantly moist by fecal or urinary incontinence, this client is constantly moist.
Activity	• Ask client/family about the client's level of physical activity.	• Assess client's ability to walk at least once every 2 hours while awake (walks frequently), or whether client can only ambulate short distance (walks occasionally). • Observe if client's ability to ambulate is limited to assistance to the chair (chairfast) or is confined to bed (bedfast).
Nutrition	• Ask client and family about level of appetite and ability to eat a complete meal.	• Observe client eating: determine if most of meal is taken and if intake is balanced (excellent nutrition). • Assess the amount of food the client eats at meals; if over half of meals are finished (or whether client is on tube feeds or TPN), this is adequate nutrition. • Determine if the client rarely eats a complete meal or eats about half of the food offered. This is probably inadequate nutrition. • Observe whether client is eating less than one third of meal, taking fluids poorly, or NPO or on clear liquids for >3 days. This is very poor nutrition.
Friction and shear	• Place client in bed with head of bed in semi-Fowler's position; watch for sliding toward the foot of the bed. • Ask client if assistance is needed in moving up in bed or chair.	• Assess if client moves in bed and chair independently and if client maintains a good position at all times (no apparent problem). • Observe client in bed and in a chair; if client moves feebly or requires minimum assistance, this may indicate a potential problem. • Determine if client requires moderate to maximum assistance in moving, and if the client slides down in the bed and/or chair, which would indicate a problem.

TPN, Total parenteral nutrition.

Skill 34-1

ASSESSMENT OF CLIENT FOR PRESSURE ULCER DEVELOPMENT: RISK ASSESSMENT AND SKIN ASSESSMENT

DELEGATION CONSIDERATIONS

Assessment of adults for risk of pressure ulcers requires problem solving and knowledge application unique to professional nursing. For this procedure delegation is not appropriate. Instruct assistive personnel to report any changes in skin integrity or client's mobility, sensation, or continence. The frequency of risk and skin assessments will depend upon agency policy.

EQUIPMENT

■ Risk assessment tool
■ Documentation record
■ Gloves

STEPS	RATIONALE
1. Identify client's risk for pressure ulcer formation using the Braden Scale; assign a score for each of the subscales:	Identifies clients at risk for developing pressure ulcers, allowing you to initiate individualized preventive interventions.

STEPS	RATIONALE
a. Sensory perception	Determines client's ability to respond meaningfully to pressure-related discomfort, thus indicating if client will be able to sense the need to reposition on a frequent basis.
b. Moisture	Determines degree to which the skin is exposed to moisture. Moisture softens skin and reduces skin's resistance to trauma; thus client who is incontinent is at high risk for skin breakdown.
c. Activity	Assesses client's degree of physical activity. Bedfast clients will be susceptible to skin breakdown because of the inability to reposition off pressure points.
d. Mobility	Determines client's ability to change and control body position. A client who is completely immobile or is very limited in mobility cannot make position changes necessary to prevent skin breakdown.
e. Nutrition	Assesses client's usual food intake. A malnourished client produces protein deficiency, making tissue susceptible to skin breakdown.
f. Friction and shear	Friction causes skin damage to the top layers of skin, often reported as "sheet burn." Shear stretches and angulates blood vessels, causing deep tissue damage.
2. Use the risk score and evaluate based upon client's overall condition.	The score will predict the need for interventions to prevent skin breakdown.
3. If any of the risk factors are found to receive low scores on the risk assessment tool, consider one or more of the interventions listed in Box 34-3, p. 851.	The identified risk factors can be eliminated or reduced by instituting appropriate interventions.
4. Perform a systematic skin assessment of bony prominences. If open areas are noted, wear examination gloves. Look for areas of skin breakdown in the following locations (see Figure 34-6, p. 855):	Bony prominences are at high risk of skin breakdown because of high pressures exerted on these areas when client is immobile. A finding of redness or impairment in skin integrity necessitates planning appropriate interventions.
a. Back of head	
b. Shoulders	
c. Ribs	
d. Hips	
e. Sacral area	
f. Ischiums	
g. Inner and outer knees	
h. Inner and outer ankles	
i. Heels	
j. Feet	
5. Assess the following potential areas of skin breakdown:	
a. Ears and nares	Cartilage that is compressed by nasal cannulas or tubing can develop pressure necrosis.
b. Lips	Oral airway and endotracheal tubes can exert pressure if left in for prolonged time periods.
c. Tube sites	Foley tubes and Jackson-Pratt drain tubes can exert pressure if taped snugly against skin or if there is stress at the insertion site. If moisture is present around tube insertion sites, leakage of bodily fluids can denude skin.
6. When a reddened area is noted, check for the following:	
a. Blanching erythema	Indicates pressure damage that should resolve (Pieper, 2000).
b. Nonblanching erythema	Indicates damage to blood vessels and tissue damage (Pieper, 2000).
7. Assess all skin surfaces for the following:	
a. Absence of superficial skin layers	Damage of superficial skin layers is indicative of injury from friction or moisture.

STEPS	RATIONALE
b. Blisters	Suggests skin damage from friction and/or inappropriate tape removal.
c. Any loss of epidermis and dermis	Indicates damage to skin. Cause of this damage must be determined, and interventions to prevent further damage must be instituted.

UNEXPECTED OUTCOMES AND RELATED INTERVENTIONS

- Skin becomes mottled, reddened, or blistered.
  - Document and communicate interval for reevaluation of skin assessment score.
  - Obtain physician's order for skin care or supportive mattresses.
- Pressure areas become discolored or indurated or exhibit temperature changes.
  - Document findings.
  - Consult nurse specialist to revise skin care regimen for client.
  - Consider supportive mattresses.

REPORTING AND RECORDING

- Record risk score and frequency of risk assessment.
- Record appearance of skin, especially pressure points.
- Describe positioning and turning schedule.
- Report changes in skin care protocol.
- Document consultation from skin/wound care specialists.

Gerontological Nursing Practice   Box 34-4

- The older adult's skin is less tolerant to pressure, friction, and shear because of decreased elasticity from normal aging.
- The older adult's skin loses the ability to retain moisture within the dermis, resulting in less pliable tissue vulnerable to minor trauma.
- With aging the capacity for epidermal proliferation is decreased, so more time is required for healing.
- The major change in aging skin is dryness, which affects as many as 59% to 85% of clients over the age of 64.
- The thinning of the dermis and flattening of the dermal-epidermal junction that occur in aging predispose the older adult's skin to tearing.
- Risk factors for skin tears include sensory loss, impaired nutritional status, impaired cognition, dependency on staff for activities of daily living and the need for mechanical devices (e.g., lifts, wheelchairs).

Data from Bryant RA, Rolstad BS: Examining threats to skin integrity, *Ostomy/Wound Management* 47(6):18, 2001.

an early indicator of impaired skin integrity, but damage to the underlying tissue may be more progressive. Palpate the tissues adjacent to the observed area to acquire further data about **induration** and the damage to the skin and underlying tissues.

Assess clients with lightly pigmented skin for blanching with return to normal skin tones. Also note changes in color, temperature, and hardness of the surrounding skin and tissues. Use visual and tactile inspection over the body areas most frequently at risk for pressure ulcer development (Figure 34-6). When a client lies in bed or sits in a chair, body weight is heavily placed on certain bony prominences.

Body surfaces subjected to the greatest weight or pressure are at greatest risk for pressure ulcer formation.

MOBILITY.   Assessment includes documenting level of mobility, the potential effects of impaired mobility on skin integrity, and data regarding the quality of muscle tone and strength. For example, determine whether the client can lift the weight off the ischial tuberosities and can roll the body to a side-lying position. The client may have adequate range of motion (ROM) to independently move into a more protective position. Finally, assess the client's activity tolerance (see Chapter 24).

NUTRITIONAL STATUS.   An assessment of the client's nutritional status should be done at least every 3 months as an integral part of the initial assessment data for clients at risk for impaired skin integrity (AHCPR, 1994) (Box 34-5; see Chapter 30). Total protein levels are correlated with pressure ulcer development. Total protein levels below 5.4 g/100 ml decrease colloid osmotic pressure, which leads to interstitial edema and decreased oxygen to the tissues. Edema decreases the skin and underlying tissue's tolerance to pressure, friction, and shear.

WOUNDS.   The assessment of a client's wound varies from one health care setting to another. It is important that you be thorough in this assessment and accurately collect pertinent data. Accurate and regular assessments of the client's wounds drive treatment decisions and provide a baseline to evaluate the wounds' status (Cooper, 2000).

EMERGENCY SETTING.   In an emergency the type of wound determines the criteria for inspection. After a client's car-

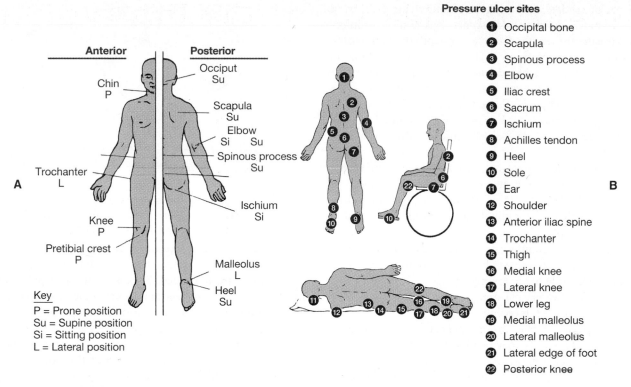

Pressure ulcer sites

❶ Occipital bone
❷ Scapula
❸ Spinous process
❹ Elbow
❺ Iliac crest
❻ Sacrum
❼ Ischium
❽ Achilles tendon
❾ Heel
❿ Sole
⓫ Ear
⓬ Shoulder
⓭ Anterior iliac spine
⓮ Trochanter
⓯ Thigh
⓰ Medial knee
⓱ Lateral knee
⓲ Lower leg
⓳ Medial malleolus
⓴ Lateral malleolus
㉑ Lateral edge of foot
㉒ Posterior knee

Anterior   **Posterior**

Chin
P
Occiput
Su

Scapula
Su

Elbow
Si   Su

Spinous process
Su

Trochanter
A   L

Ischium
Si

Knee
P

Pretibial crest
P

Malleolus
L

Heel
Su

Key
P = Prone position
Su = Supine position
Si = Sitting position
L = Lateral position

B

FIGURE **34-6**   **A,** Bony prominences most frequently underlying pressure ulcers. **B,** Pressure ulcer sites. (From Trelease CC: Developing standards for wound care, *Ostomy/Wound Manage* 20:46, 1988.)

diopulmonary status is stabilized (see Chapter 27), inspect the wound for bleeding. An **abrasion,** or loss of the dermis, is usually superficial with little bleeding but some weeping (plasma leakage from damaged capillaries). A **laceration** is damage to the dermis and epidermis and is a torn, jagged wound. The depth and location of the laceration affect the extent of bleeding, with serious bleeding possible in lacerations greater than 5 cm (2 inches) long or 2.5 cm (1 inch) deep.

Puncture wounds bleed in relation to the depth and size of the wound; internal bleeding and infection are the primary dangers. Inspect the wound for contaminant material such as soil, broken glass, shreds of cloth, and foreign substances clinging to penetrating objects. Next assess the size of the wound and the need for suturing or surface protection. When the injury is the result of trauma from a dirty penetrating object, determine if the client has received a tetanus toxoid injection within the last year.

STABLE SETTING.   Once an acute wound is stable after surgery or treatment, assess its progress toward healing. If the wound is covered by a dressing and there are written orders not to change it, inspect only the dressing and any external drains. Should a dressing appear saturated with drainage, you may reinforce the secondary dressing pending a definitive response and orders from the physician. Saturated dressings provide an excellent environment for bacterial growth, and the physician will need to be informed of the color, odor, and estimate of drainage amount.

When a dressing change is planned, it may help to administer an analgesic at least 30 minutes before exposing a wound. You must avoid accidentally removing or displacing underlying drains.

First inspect the appearance of the wound, noting the anatomic location, size, approximation of wound edges, the presence of exudate, the condition of underlying tissue in an open wound, and signs of dehiscence, evisceration, or infection. Measure the length, diameter, or depth of wound using a centimeter ruler. Note any **ecchymosis,** skin discoloration or bruising caused by blood leakage into subcutaneous tissues after trauma to underlying vessels. The outer edges of a wound normally appear inflamed for the first 2 to 3 days, but this slowly disappears. When an infection develops, the wound edges are usually brightly inflamed, warm, tender, and swollen.

Next assess the character of wound drainage by noting the amount, color, odor, and consistency. The amount of drainage depends on the location and extent of the wound. A simple method for estimating the volume of wound drainage is to report the number and type of dressings used and saturated over an interval of time. The color and consistency of drainage vary, depending on its components. Types of drainage include the following:

1. Serous: clear, watery plasma
2. Sanguineous: fresh bleeding
3. Serosanguineous: pale, more watery, a combination of plasma and red cells, may be blood-streaked
4. Purulent: thick, yellow, green, or brown, indicating the presence of dead or living organisms and white blood cells

If the drainage has a pungent or strong odor, an infection is likely. Objectively document the integrity of the wound and the character of drainage, describing the appearance by observable characteristics.

The presence of drains is another important assessment. A drain is used in surgical wound if a large amount of drainage is expected and if keeping wound layers closed is especially important, because accumulated fluid under the tissues prevents closure. A drain may lie under a dressing, extend through a dressing, or be connected to a drainage bag or suction apparatus. A pin or clip through a Penrose drain prevents it from slipping farther into a wound (Figure 34-7). As wound drainage decreases, the physician slowly withdraws the drain or leaves orders for you to withdraw the drain a specified length over several days. First observe the security of the drain and its location with respect to the wound. Next note the character and amount of drainage if there is a collecting device. You need to pay particular attention to the flow of drainage through the tubing and notify the physician of any sudden decrease that might indicate a blocked drain or an increase indicating bleeding or infection.

In the case of a surgical wound, inspect the staples, sutures, or wound closures for irritation and note whether the closures are intact. You may choose to count sutures when the physician has removed a portion of them. After the first few days when normal swelling around closures usually has subsided, continued swelling may indicate overly tight closures, which can cause wound separation or dehiscence. Early suture removal reduces formation of defects along the suture line and minimizes chances of unattractive scar formation.

When a wound exhibits swelling, separation of its edges, or redness in the periwound area, it is important to evaluate

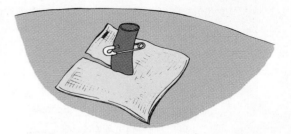

FIGURE **34-7**   Penrose drain.

for the presence of cellulitis. Use light palpation to detect localized areas of tenderness or collection of drainage. Wearing sterile gloves, gently place your fingertips along the wound edges. If pressure causes fluid to be expressed from the wound, note the character of the drainage and collect a wound culture if needed. Sensitivity to such palpation is normal, but extreme tenderness may indicate infection.

Pain assessment is an important component of wound assessment for detecting complications and planning future wound care (Rook, 1996) (see Chapter 29). Serious discomfort during inspection or palpation of the wound suggests underlying problems, whereas discomfort related to dressing removal or application calls for administration of analgesics before future dressing changes.

WOUND CULTURES.   If you detect purulent or suspicious-looking drainage, a **wound culture** may be indicated. You should never collect a wound culture sample from old drainage, because resident colonies of bacteria grow in exudate. First clean the wound to remove skin flora. Aerobic organisms grow in superficial wounds exposed to the air, and anaerobic organisms tend to grow within body cavities. To collect an aerobic specimen, wipe a sterile swab from a culturette tube onto clean, healthy-looking tissue, return the swab to the culturette tube, cap the tube, and crush the inner ampule so that the medium for organism growth coats the swab tip (Stotts, 2000). Label the specimen appropriately, and send the labeled specimen to the laboratory immediately.

To collect an anaerobic specimen deep in a body cavity, use a sterile syringe tip to aspirate visible drainage from the inner wound, expel any air from the syringe, and inject contents into a special vacuum container with culture medium. In some institutions, you may place a cork over the needle to prevent entrance of air and send the syringe to the lab. The AHCPR (1994) guidelines recommend using the needle aspiration technique rather than the quantitative swab technique (Box 34-6).

CLIENT EXPECTATIONS.   When clients have a pressure ulcer or a chronic wound, their course of treatment is usually costly and lengthy. Because the client must be involved with the wound care management, it is important to know the client's expectations. A client who unrealistically expects rapid wound healing may be easily discouraged and not adhere to the treatment regimen. Likewise, a client who knows

Recommendations for Standardized Techniques for Wound Cultures
Box 34-6

NEEDLE ASPIRATION PROCEDURE

- Use a 10-ml syringe with a 22-gauge needle.
- Aspirate 5 ml of air into the syringe.
- Clean intact skin with a disinfectant. Allow to dry.
- Insert needle adjacent to the wound.
- Aspirate wound drainage.
- Repeat in two to four areas of the wound.

QUANTITATIVE SWAB PROCEDURE

- Obtain a sterile swab, sterile normal saline, and antiseptic solution.
- Clean wound surface with an antiseptic solution, and allow to dry.
- Moisten swab with normal saline.
- Swab wound in a 1×1 cm (4 cm²) area of clean tissue.
- Apply pressure to express fluid from wound onto the sterile swab.

Modified from Stotts NS: Wound infection: diagnosis and management. In Bryant RA, editor: *Acute and chronic wounds: nursing management,* ed 2, St. Louis, 2000, Mosby.

Case Study SYNTHESIS IN PRACTICE

When Lynda returns the next day, she finds that Mr. Ahmed has a small 1×2 inch (2.5 × 5 cm) × ⅛ inch deep shallow wound on his sacrum. There is no necrotic tissue, and the wound bed has beefy red tissue. When Lynda prepares to conduct a skin assessment on Mr. Ahmed, she recalls information about the pathogenesis of pressure ulcers and guidelines for skin assessment for clients with darkly pigmented skin. She will focus on determining changes in Mr. Ahmed's skin integrity.

Lynda observed care of a stage IV pressure ulcer during an experience in an extended care facility. From that experience she increased her knowledge about the debilitating effects of pressure ulcers. In addition, she was able to practice skin assessment techniques during her clinical experience in the extended care facility.

---

that the process is lengthy may unrealistically expect the area to heal without scarring. Knowing these expectations assists you in providing individualized care and helping the client modify expectations when needed.

Nursing Diagnosis

A client with actual or high risk for *impaired skin integrity* may also have one or more nursing diagnoses related to the condition. Assessment reveals clusters of data that indicate whether an actual or a risk for *impaired skin integrity* exists. After gathering appropriate assessment data, cluster defining characteristics to establish nursing diagnoses. For example, the destruction of the skin's surface clearly allows you to diagnose *impaired skin integrity.* The identification of nursing

Nursing Diagnoses for
CLIENTS WITH IMPAIRED SKIN INTEGRITY
Box 34-7

- Infection, risk for
- Mobility, impaired physical
- Nutrition, imbalanced: less than body requirements
- Pain, acute
- Pain, chronic
- Self-esteem, situational low
- Skin integrity, impaired
- Skin integrity, risk for impaired
- Tissue perfusion, ineffective

diagnoses related to wound healing helps you to anticipate the need for supportive or preventive care (Box 34-7).

Assess related factors contributing to each diagnostic statement. These related factors become the focus of your interventions. For example, the client with *impaired skin integrity related to a surgical incision* requires a different set of interventions than the client with *impaired skin integrity related to pressure and nutritional deficiency.* The client whose surgical incision has increased drainage will require different and perhaps more frequent skin cleansing and dressings chosen to contain additional drainage.

Planning

Plan therapeutic interventions for clients with actual or potential risks to skin integrity (see care plan). These therapies are designed according to severity of risks to the client, and the plan is individualized according to developmental stage and level of health.

GOALS AND OUTCOMES.   You must also develop client-centered goals aimed at preventing or reducing impaired skin integrity or promoting wound healing. Care planning is individualized to the client, taking into consideration the client's most immediate needs. All clients should be assessed for risk of skin breakdown and have skin and wound assessments performed on a routine basis. The information from the pressure ulcer risk and skin assessments are integrated into the plan of care and reasonable goals, such as "Client will not develop further skin breakdown" and "Client's wounds will demonstrate healing," are written.

SETTING PRIORITIES.   When planning care, priorities must be established based on comprehensive assessments and goals and expected outcomes. Acute needs are immediate; however, preventive interventions should also be prioritized and instituted in a timely manner. Maintenance of skin integrity and promotion of wound healing prevent additional health care issues and are major nursing priorities. Skin and wound priorities include ongoing assessment of pressure ulcer risk, wound assessment, and

Case Study Nursing Care Plan SKIN INTEGRITY AND WOUND CARE

ASSESSMENT

Mr. Ahmed **has limited activity tolerance.** He does not **tolerate position changes or sitting out of bed;** he **wants to stay in a semi-Fowler's position** at all times. He complains of a **painful, burning sensation** in his **sacral** region. A 1 × 2 inch **open area** with a depth of $^{1}/_{8}$ inch **is present.** The base of the **wound is red and moist,** and the **surrounding tissue is slightly reddened.** On palpation, **underlying skin is soft and indurated.**

*Defining characteristics are shown in bold type.

NURSING DIAGNOSIS

Impaired skin integrity related to pressure over bony prominence in sacral region.

PLANNING

GOAL	EXPECTED OUTCOMES
Pressure will be reduced to the sacral area, and the wound will show significant movement toward healing in 1 week.	Wound will decrease in diameter in 7 days. There will be no evidence of further wound formation in 3 days.

IMPLEMENTATION

STEPS	RATIONALE
1. Post and implement a turning schedule.	Repositioning removes pressure.
2. Cleanse wound and periwound skin; dry periwound skin.	Removes debris and old drainage from wound site, preventing further wound progression and/or skin breakdown (Rolstad and others, 2000a).
3. Measure wound diameter, assess the quality of the wound tissue, noting the condition of the periwound skin, and determine the presence of wound exudate at dressing change.	Wounds should be cleansed at every wound dressing change Wound assessment will provide a basis for determining effectiveness of wound treatment interventions (Cooper, 2000).
4. Apply a hydrocolloid dressing to wound, as per order, extend the dressing $1^{1}/_{2}$ inches beyond the wound edges.	The use of hydrocolloid dressing will support moist wound healing and protect the wound.

EVALUATION

- Compare wound assessment to determine progress (e.g., measure wound size at dressing change, observe the color and amount of drainage with each dressing change).
- Observe all bony prominences when repositioning client.

---

providing interventions to control or eliminate contributing factors of pressure, shear, friction, moisture, and infection.

Other client factors to be considered when setting priorities include everyday activities and family factors. You may need the help of another health care team member, such as a physical or occupational therapist, when considering mobility needs. These factors are important for clients in institutional and home settings.

CONTINUITY OF CARE. With the trend toward earlier discharge from health care settings, it is important to consider the client's plan for discharge. Discharge planning begins when a client enters the health care system. Anticipating the client's discharge from an institution, a referral to a skilled nursing care facility or home health agency may be necessary to help the client remain or regain mobility at home.

Clients and their families may need to continue the objectives of wound management after discharge. Thus they may need to discuss the likelihood of the client returning home, returning home with the assistance of home nursing, or transferring to a skilled nursing facility for more care and observation.

Implementation

HEALTH PROMOTION. Early identification of high-risk clients and their risk factors aids you in preventing pressure ulcers. Prevention minimizes the impact that risk factors or contributing factors may have on pressure ulcer development. Table 34-3 outlines some nursing interventions for the prevention of pressure ulcers. Three major areas of nursing interventions for prevention of pressure ulcers are topical skin care, positioning and use of the 30-degree lateral position, and the use of support surfaces.

TOPICAL SKIN CARE. Skin assessment should be done daily, paying special attention to the bony prominences. Reddened areas should not be massaged because reddened areas may be indicative of tissue injury (Olson, 1989). Massage to these areas further injures the tissue by causing breaks in the tissue capillaries. Skin should be examined for signs of dryness, cracking, edema, or excessive moisture. When skin is cleansed, a mild cleansing agent should be used. Soaps can alter the skin's acid mantle, causing dryness and increasing the risk of skin infection. Skin lubrication will maintain intact skin; consider using a moisturizer on a routine basis (Pieper, 2000). Keep the client's skin clean and dry because this is an initial

A Quick Guide to Prevention of Pressure Ulcers   Table 34-3

Risk Factor	Intervention
Sensory perception	Develop and post a turning schedule. Use a pressure-reducing device. Assess pressure points daily.
Moisture related to incontinence	After each incontinent episode use a no-rinse cleanser and protect skin with a moisture barrier cream or ointment.
Activity/mobility	Frequent position changes per schedule. Limit chair sitting to 1 hour at a time. Use a pressure-reducing device. Consult with dietary staff.
Nutrition	Ensure adequate caloric and fluid intake. Monitor intake and output.
Friction/shear	If appropriate, use a trapeze. Keep skin moisturized. Protect friction-prone areas with a liquid skin barrier or thin hydrocolloid.

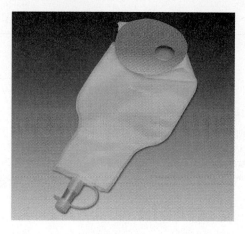

FIGURE **34-8**   Hollister® Fecal Incontinence Collector. (Permission to use and/or reproduce this copyrighted material has been granted by the owner, Hollister Incorporated.)

line of defense for preventing skin breakdown. The types of products available for skin care are numerous, and their uses need to be matched to the specific needs of the client.

For a client who is incontinent of stool or urine, use a specialized incontinence cleanser. To protect the skin a moisture-barrier product (generally petrolatum or dimethicone based) is liberally applied to the exposed area. The moisture barrier will provide skin protection from the irritating effects of stool or urine and will allow the next incontinent episode to be easily cleansed. The moisture-barrier ointment is applied after each cleansing. For skin that has become denuded from incontinence, a barrier paste (zinc oxide based) should be used that will adhere to the irritated area and not be removed with each cleansing. Fecal incontinence can be collected using a fecal incontinence collector (Figure 34-8), an adhesive skin barrier attached to a drainable pouch applied around the anus to collect liquid stool. A fecal incontinence collector is used when the client is experiencing frequent liquid bowel movements and has intact perirectal skin. Other external collection devices include male external catheters applied to the shaft of the penis to collect urine. Underpads and briefs can be used to protect skin in clients incontinent of stool and urine. Most underpads and briefs have a plastic outer lining that can hold moisture against skin. The occlusive nature of diapers and underpads can irritate skin if left under clients for prolonged periods of time. When providing skin care to the incontinent client, the health care team must first assess and treat the cause of the incontinence, then decide upon protection and/or collection interventions.

POSITIONING.   Positioning interventions are designed to reduce pressure and shear to the skin. The immobilized client's position should be changed according to activity level, perceptual ability, and daily routines (Bergstrom and others, 1987a, 1987b). Therefore a standard turning interval of 1 to 2 hours may not prevent pressure sore development in some clients. The Wound, Ostomy and Continence Nurses Society (WOCN) and AHCPR recommend reducing shear by keeping the client's head of bed below the 30-degree angle, using assistive devices when turning or transferring clients, using the bed gatch or footboard, and using the 30-degree lateral position (Figure 34-9) (Bryant and others, 2000).

When the client can sit in the chair, the client should be repositioned every hour. In the sitting position, the pressure on the ischial tuberosities is greater than when in the supine position. In addition, clients with the ability should be taught or assisted to shift weight every 15 minutes. A client should also sit on gel or an air cushion to redistribute weight, decreasing the amount of weight on the ischial tuberosities. Donut-shaped cushions are contraindicated because they can reduce blood supply to the area, resulting in wider areas of ischemia (AHCPR, 1992).

An area of concern because of the small surface area is the client's heels (Figure 34-10). Heels should be kept off the bed with a pillow under the lower leg or by the use of a heel protector (AHCPR, 1992).

SUPPORT SURFACES.   Support surfaces are used to decrease the amount of pressure exerted over the bony prominences by maximizing contact (allowing the body to touch the entire surface) and thereby redistributing weight over a large area. Support surfaces include mattresses, overlays, framed special beds, chair pads, table pads, and crib mattresses or pads. In addition to reducing or relieving pressure, many of the support surfaces reduce shear and friction and decrease moisture. When selecting a support surface, thoroughly assess the client's needs (Box 34-8). A flow diagram (Figure 34-11) can assist you in clinical decision making. When using a support surface, minimal layers should be between the

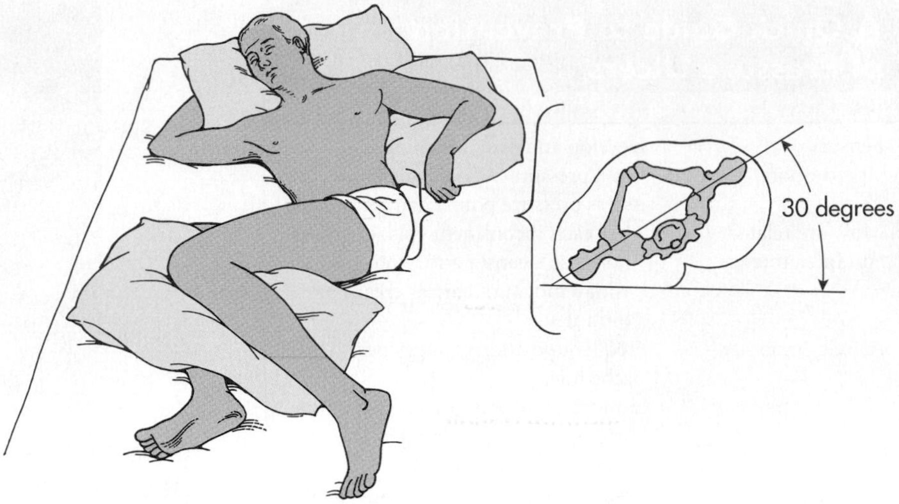

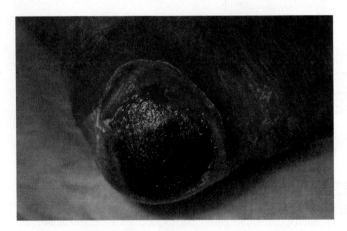

FIGURE **34-9** Thirty-degree lateral position to avoid pressure points. (From Bryant RA, and others: Pressure ulcer. In Bryant RA, editor: *Acute and chronic wounds: nursing management*, ed 2, St. Louis, 2000, Mosby.)

30 degrees

FIGURE **34-10** Formation of pressure ulcer on heel resulting from external pressure from mattress of bed. (Courtesy Tom Colwell, RN, MS, CWOCN, clinical nurse specialist, University of Chicago Hospitals, Chicago.)

AHCPR 1994 Support Surface Recommendations   Box 34-8

Assess all clients with existing pressure ulcers to determine their risk for developing additional pressure ulcers. If the client remains at risk, use a pressure-reducing surface.

Use a static support surface if a client can assume a variety of positions without bearing weight on a pressure ulcer and without "bottoming out."

Use a dynamic support surface if the client cannot assume a variety of positions without bearing weight on a pressure ulcer, if the client fully compresses the static support surface, or if the pressure ulcer does not show evidence of healing.

If a client has large stage III or stage IV pressure ulcers on multiple turning surfaces, a low–air-loss bed or an air-fluidized bed may be indicated.

When excess moisture on intact skin is a potential source of maceration and skin breakdown, a support surface that provides air flow can be important in drying skin and preventing additional pressure ulcers.

client and the surface. The client must be as close as possible to the surface for it to be effective. **Remember that the client must still be repositioned even when a support surface is used.** Once a support surface is in use, reevaluate the client on a frequent basis to determine the continued need and the effectiveness of the product. Client and caregiver education on the importance and use of the support products is essential (Box 34-9).

ACUTE CARE

PRESSURE ULCERS. Wound management principles must be addressed in an orderly fashion (Box 34-10). The etiology, pressure, shear, friction, and/or moisture must be managed as part of wound management (Skill 34-2).

The client must receive systemic support to move toward wound healing. Concurrent cardiovascular or pulmonary disease can decrease the amount of oxygen-rich hemoglobin available to be delivered to injured tissue. Oxygen is an essential element in angiogenesis, epithelialization, and resistance to infection. Interventions to maximize oxygen levels include use of pulmonary hygiene interventions, assessment and monitoring of tissue oxygen levels, and low-flow supplemental oxygen (Bates-Jensen and Wethe, 1998).

Wound healing depends on adequate nutrition. Protein intake is necessary to support new blood vessels and collagen synthesis. Carbohydrates, fats, and vitamins provide energy for cellular function. Interventions to support adequate nutritional intake are a nutritional referral, dietary supplements, and assessment of intake and output levels.

Certain medications (e.g., steroids) and medical conditions (e.g., diabetes) can influence wound healing. Because hyperglycemia can cause problems with wound healing, blood glucose control is essential.

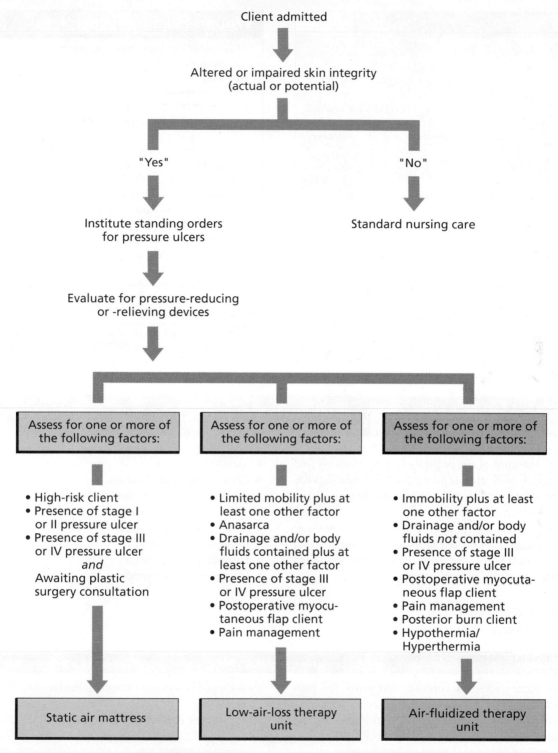

FIGURE **34-11**   Flow diagram for ordering specialty beds. (From Thomas C: Specialty beds: decision-making made easy, *Ostomy/Wound Manage* 23:51, 1989.)

A stable wound environment is necessary to promote healing. To maintain a stable environment it is important to control infection and promote cleansing, debridement, exudate management, control of dead space, and wound protection. The client with a pressure ulcer should be assessed for signs and symptoms of a wound infection: redness, warmth of sur-

rounding tissue, odor, and the presence of exudate. Should any of these signs be present, a consultation with the health care team must be made to determine if the wound should be cultured and if systemic or topical antibiotics are indicated.

Pressure ulcers should be cleansed at each dressing change to promote removal of wound debris and bacteria

	Box 34-9
Client Teaching	

THERAPEUTIC BEDS AND MATTRESSES

- Explain the rationale for utilization of support surfaces.
- Teach client and family the importance of minimal layers between the client and the surface.
- Instruct in the importance of frequent position changes, demonstrating small shifts of weight.
- Demonstrate to client and caregiver the procedure for lateral positioning at a 30-degree angle.
- If the support surface is dynamic (motorized), demonstrate to the client and the family how to set the device to achieve maximum comfort and effectiveness.

Wound Healing Principles	Box 34-10

1. Control or eliminate causative factors
   a. Pressure
   b. Shear
   c. Friction
   d. Moisture
   e. Circulatory impairment
   f. Neuropathy
2. Provide systemic support to reduce existing and potential cofactors
   a. Nutritional and fluid support
   b. Control of systemic conditions affecting wound healing
3. Maintain physiological wound environment
   a. Prevent and manage infection
   b. Cleanse wound
   c. Remove nonviable tissue (debridement)
   d. Manage exudate
   e. Eliminate dead space
   f. Control odor
   g. Protect wound

From Bryant RA and others, editors: *Acute and chronic wounds: nursing management,* ed 2, St. Louis, 2000, Mosby, p. 87.

from the wound surface (WOCN, 1992). Dirty wounds can be cleansed with irrigation; clean wounds require only gentle flushing with normal saline solution.

Necrotic tissue slows wound healing because it can become a source for infection and a barrier for epithelialization. If consistent with the client's overall plan of care, a method for removal of the necrotic tissue (**debridement**)

Skill 34-2
TREATING PRESSURE ULCERS

DELEGATION CONSIDERATIONS

Treatment of pressure ulcers requires problem solving and knowledge application unique to professional nursing. For this procedure delegation is not appropriate. Instruct assistive personnel to report changes in skin integrity to you immediately. In some states and practice settings, *nonsterile* dressing application may be delegated to others for chronic, established wounds where the protocol has been evaluated and designated by a professional nurse.

EQUIPMENT

- Disposable gloves (clean) (2 pairs)
- Goggles and cover gown, if risk of splash
- Plastic bag for dressing disposal
- Measuring device
- Cotton-tipped applicators
- Camera and tracing film (optional)
- Topical cleansing agent
- Sterile solution container
- Dressing of choice
- Hypoallergenic tape (if needed)
- Documentation records

STEPS	RATIONALE
1. Assess client's level of comfort and need for pain medication.	Pain should be under control while ulcer care is provided.
2. Determine if client has allergies to latex and/or topical agents.	May cause local or systemic allergic reactions.
3. Review order for topical agent and/or dressing.	Ensures that proper medication and treatments are delivered.
4. Assemble all supplies.	Allows you to stay at bedside while providing care.
5. Provide privacy for client. Wash hands, and apply clean gloves.	Reduces transmission of microorganisms and prevents accidental exposure to body fluids.
6. Position client to allow dressing removal.	Area should be accessible.
7. Remove dressings; discard.	Removes soiled dressings from work area.
8. Remove gloves, and replace with clean gloves.	
9. Cleanse ulcer per treatment order.	Removes surface bacteria from wound (Rolstad and others, 2000a).
10. Assess pressure ulcer:	Determines the effectiveness of treatment plan and provides a baseline for wound healing (Cooper, 2000).

STEPS	RATIONALE
a. Measure two dimensions: length and width (per facility's protocol).	Decrease or increase in wound size, length, width, or depth may indicate progress or lack of progress.
b. Measure depth using a cotton-tipped applicator (see illustration).	
c. Determine tissue type in wound bed: estimate the percentage of viable tissue (red, moist) and nonviable tissue.	The higher the percentage of red, moist tissue, the closer the wound is toward healing; the presence of necrotic tissue may indicate the need for debridement.
d. Presence of exudate, volume, color, consistency, and odor.	Excessive exudate may indicate a wound infection or the need for a change in the treatment plan.
e. Evaluate condition of surrounding skin; note integrity, presence of redness or moisture.	If the periwound skin is macerated, skin protection must be planned.
11. Apply topical agents per treatment order. Options include:	
a. Moist saline gauze	Provides moisture to granulation tissue, fills dead space, and will absorb some wound fluid.
b. Hydrogel	Provides a moist environment, used in dry to minimally draining wounds, available in sheets or gels.
c. Hydrocolloid	The adhesive and absorbent dressing maintains a moist wound environment, available in sheets.
d. Alginate dressings	Absorb moderate to heavy wound exudate, available in sheets and ropes.
e. Enzymes	Break down necrotic tissue.
f. Topical antimicrobials	Treat wound infections based on matching infection with specific antimicrobial (Stotts, 2000).
12. Reposition client.	Provides for client comfort.
13. Remove gloves, dispose of soiled supplies, and wash hands.	Reduces transmission of microorganisms.
14. Compare wound measurements.	Wound diameter should begin to decrease in size if the wound is beginning to show evidence of healing. The only exception will be a wound that had been significantly debrided at the start of the treatment. (A wound covered with avascular tissue can not always be assessed for size until the dead tissue is removed.) A clean pressure ulcer should show signs of healing in 2 to 4 weeks (AHCPR, 1994).

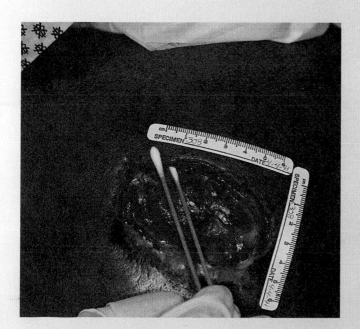

STEP 10A, B   Measuring length, width, and depth of pressure ulcer.

STEPS	RATIONALE
15. Determine the amount of red granular tissue versus slough or necrotic tissue, and compare this percentage of tissue with previous assessments.	The wound base needs to be covered with granulation tissue to facilitate contraction and epithelialization.

• *Critical Decision Point*
A reevaluation of the wound care treatment plan is warranted if the wound is not progressing toward healing in 4 weeks. The external causative factors of pressure, shear, friction, and moisture and the systemic factors of nutrition, medications, and medical conditions should be reevaluated and a new treatment plan instituted.

UNEXPECTED OUTCOMES AND RELATED INTERVENTIONS
■ Skin surrounding ulcer becomes macerated.
  • Reduce exposure of surrounding to moisture.
  • Select a dressing that has increased moisture-absorbing properties.
■ Ulcer does not heal or worsens.
  • Reevaluate current wound management.
  • Determine need for a more aggressive turning and positioning schedule.
  • Obtain wound culture to determine the presence of an infection.

RECORDING AND REPORTING
■ Record the wound assessments on a routine basis (check agency policy).
■ Describe the wound treatment plan and the therapy delivered.
■ Report any deterioration in wound appearance.
■ Report the pain assessment, the intervention planned to reduce and/or relieve the client's pain, and the client's response to the intervention.

should be planned. Types of debridement include mechanical, chemical, and autolytic (Singhal and others, 2001).

A moist wound environment supports wound healing; however, excessive wound moisture can macerate the wound edges and interfere with wound healing. A dressing must be selected that absorbs excessive moisture while providing the wound with the necessary hydration.

Dead space should be eliminated by loosely filling all cavities with dressings. Wound cavities need to be filled so that areas do not "wall off" and become abscessed (AHCPR, 1994).

WOUNDS

First Aid for Wounds.   In an emergency setting use first aid measures for wound care. Under more stable conditions you are able to use a variety of interventions for wound healing. When a client suffers a traumatic wound, first aid interventions include promoting **hemostasis,** cleansing the wound, and protecting the wound from further injury.

Hemostasis.   After assessing the type and extent of the wound, control bleeding from a laceration with application of direct pressure to the wound with a sterile or clean dressing. After bleeding subsides, an adhesive bandage strip or gauze dressing taped over the laceration allows skin edges to close and a blood clot to form. If a dressing becomes saturated with blood, add another layer of dressing, continue to apply pressure, and elevate the affected part. Serious lacerations should be sutured by a physician in an emergency clinic or hospital.

A puncture wound is allowed to bleed to remove dirt and other contaminants. If a penetrating object such as a knife blade is in a client's body, do not remove the object. Removal could cause massive, uncontrolled bleeding. You may apply pressure around the object but not on it or on adjacent tissues.

Cleansing.   Gentle cleansing of a wound removes contaminants that serve as sources of infection. However, vigorous cleaning can cause bleeding or further injury. For abrasions, minor lacerations, and small puncture wounds rinse the wound in running water, gently cleanse with mild soap and water, and apply an over-the-counter antiseptic. When a laceration is bleeding profusely, you should only brush away surface contaminants and concentrate on hemostasis until the client can be cared for in a clinic or hospital.

Protection.   Regardless of whether bleeding has stopped, protect the wound by applying sterile or clean dressing, and immobilize the body part. A light dressing applied over minor wounds prevents entrance of microorganisms. In the case of small abrasions, it is acceptable to leave the wound open to air so that a scab can form.

The more extensive the wound, the larger the bandage required. In the home a clean towel or diaper may be the best dressing. A bulky dressing applied with pressure minimizes movement of underlying tissues and helps to immobilize the entire body part. A bandage or cloth wrapped around a penetrating object should immobilize it adequately.

DRESSINGS.   The use of dressings requires an understanding of wound healing and factors influencing healing. A variety of dressing materials are commercially available. Unless a dressing is suited to the characteristics of a wound, the dressing can hinder wound repair.

The choice of dressing and the method of dressing a wound influence healing. The proper dressing should not allow a full-thickness wound to become overly dry with extensive scab formation. When this occurs, the dermis dehydrates and crusts. As a result, a barrier forms against normal epidermal cell growth, slowing wound healing. Furthermore, dryness may increase discomfort. Ideally a dressing provides a moist environment to promote normal epidermal cell migration. The dressing should also absorb drainage to prevent pooling of exudate that may promote bacterial growth and to prevent wound drainage from coming into contact with intact skin.

For surgical wounds that heal by primary intention, dressings are commonly removed as soon as drainage stops. The primary dressing placed in the operating room is frequently removed by the physician 24 to 48 hours postoperatively. This coincides with initial epithelialization, so when the primary dressing is removed, the risk of infection is reduced.

Purposes.   A dressing may serve several purposes. It discourages wound exposure to microorganisms. However, if a wound has minimal drainage, the natural formation of a fibrin seal eliminates the need for a dressing. A pressure dressing promotes hemostasis by exerting localized, downward pressure over an actual or potential bleeding site and fosters normal healing by eliminating dead space in underlying tissues. You must assess skin color, pulses in distal extremities, client comfort, and any changes in sensation to ensure pressure dressings do not interfere with circulation.

A dry dressing promotes healing by protecting a wound healing by primary intention and absorbing minimal oozing of wound drainage. In some instances, when a wound is healing by secondary intention a dressing is used to provide a moist environment. When this is needed, it is moistened with a solution, usually normal saline, wrung out, unfolded, and lightly packed into the wound. The purpose of a moist dressing is to act as a sponge, absorbing excessive wound drainage, while providing a moist environment. A moist dressing is always covered with a dry, secondary dressing.

A firmly taped or wrapped dressing supports or immobilizes a body part, minimizing movement of the underlying incision and traumatized tissues. Finally, a dressing promotes thermal insulation to the wound surface and protects it from the dehydrating effects of air.

Types.   Dressings vary by type of material and mode of application (dry, wet to dry, and moist). They should be easy to apply, comfortable, and made of materials that promote wound healing.

Gauze is the most common dressing type. Gauze does not interact with wound tissues and thus causes little wound irritation. Gauze is available in different textures and in squares, rectangles, and rolls of various lengths and widths. Gauze dressings are best used for wounds with moderate drainage, deep wounds, undermining, and tunnels (Rolstad and others, 2000b).

For wounds requiring debridement, a wet-to-dry dressing may be effective. However, this type of debridement is not selective and can remove viable as well as nonviable tissue. Moisten the gauze with normal saline and wring it out until it is slightly damp. The damp gauze is fluffed and applied to the wound bed and then covered with a dry dressing. The entire dressing is removed when the contact layer is almost dry. The wound debris will adhere to the gauze when it is removed. Because of the potential for tissue trauma and pain to the client, this type of dressing is not often used (Singhal and others, 2001).

Increasing awareness and acceptance of moist wound healing encourages the use of a moist dressing that must remain damp along the wound surface. It is critical that the first layer remain damp because moist wounds heal more quickly and autolytic debridement is enhanced in a moist environment. Autolysis involves the breakdown of necrotic tissue provided by the body's own white blood cells. If a moist dressing begins to dry, it must be changed.

Transparent film dressings are clear sheets coated on one side with an adhesive. The adhesive side will not stick to the wound because of the moisture and will trap moisture over the wound bed. The film is impermeable to fluid but semipermeable to oxygen. This type of dressing can be used as a primary dressing in wounds with minimal tissue loss that have very little wound drainage.

Hydrocolloid dressings are made of gelling agents and have an adhesive wound surface. They come in a variety of sizes and shapes and are used to cover wounds, extending the hydrocolloid dressing at least $1\frac{1}{2}$ inches beyond the wound margin. Hydrocolloids form a gel as they interact with the wound surface. Because hydrocolloids are occlusive, they protect the wound from surface contaminants and can be left over a wound for several days. When removed, a gel is noted over the wound base; the gel has maintained a moist environment to support healing.

Hydrogel dressings are available in sheets or in gels. They contain a high percentage of water and are indicated for wounds that require moisture, either a wound with granulation (maintaining the moist wound environment needed for healing) or a wound that has a high percentage of necrotic tissue (the hydrogel can facilitate debridement by softening the dead tissue). Hydrogels can maintain moisture in some wounds for 1 to 3 days.

Alginate dressings, available in sheets or ropes, are highly absorbent dressings created from a seaweed derivative. They are used in wounds with significant drainage and are lightly packed to fill the wound. A secondary dressing is applied. Because of the absorptive nature of the dressing, a moist environment is maintained while preventing **maceration.**

A new treatment modality for chronic wounds is the wound vacuum-assisted closure (known as a wound VAC). Assisted wound closure uses negative pressure to the wound to promote and accelerate healing. An open foam sponge is placed in the wound bed and sealed with a transparent dressing. A tube is placed on the wound, within the foam dressing, and the tube is connected to a prescribed amount of negative pressure, which creates a suction. This therapy is thought to provide removal of excess wound fluid, to stimulate granulation tissue, and to decrease wound bacteria. This therapy has been shown to reduce healing time in chronic wounds and has resulted in early grafting of wounds (Broussard and others, 2000).

Changing Dressings. To prepare for changing a dressing, you must know the type of dressing, any underlying drains used, and the type of supplies needed for wound care. You can adjust the type and amount of dressings if the amount of drainage changes or if a wound becomes deeper. Notifying the physician of any change is essential.

The order for changing a dressing should indicate the dressing type, frequency of changing, and solutions or ointments to be applied. An order to "reinforce dressing prn." (add dressings without removing existing ones as needed) is common immediately after surgery, when the physician does not want accidental disruption of the suture line or loss of hemostasis. A client's medical or operating room record usually reveals whether drains are present. After the initial dressing change, communicate on the care plan the type of dressing materials and solutions to use and the type and location of drains.

Use aseptic technique during dressing change procedures (see Chapter 10). Also essential is ensuring that the client understands the steps of the procedure beforehand so less anxiety is experienced. Describe normal signs of the healing process, and offer to answer questions about the procedure or wound.

If wound care is needed in the home, you must demonstrate dressing changes to the client and family and then provide an opportunity for practice. In the home, wound healing stabilizes so that sterile technique is usually unnecessary. However, clients must learn clean technique. The client should be able to change a dressing independently or with assistance from a family member before discharge unless home health care is to be provided. Skill 34-3 outlines the steps for applying moist saline dressings.

Skill 34-3

APPLYING DRESSINGS: WET-TO-DRY, HYDROCOLLOID, AND TRANSPARENT

DELEGATION CONSIDERATIONS
Controversy about delegating wound care to other personnel exists. All nurses should check their specific state practice act as to what interventions are considered within the scope of nursing practice and which can be delegated to others, including assistive personnel. In some states, aspects of wound care such as dressing change can be delegated. This may include the changing of dressings using *clean* technique for chronic wounds. The care of acute new wounds and those that require sterile technique for dressing change generally remain within the domain of professional nursing practice. The *assessment* of the wound remains within the scope of the professional nurse even if the dressing change is delegated to others.

EQUIPMENT
- Sterile gloves (optional for transparent and hydrocolloid dressings)
- Dressing set (scissors and forceps)
- Sterile saline or other cleansing agents, as prescribed
- Clean, disposable gloves
- Tape, ties, or bandage as needed

- Waterproof bag
- Bath blanket, waterproof pad
- Adhesive remover (optional)
- Disposable mask (optional)
- Moisture proof gown (optional)
- Goggles (optional)

DRESSING SUPPLIES
Wet-to-dry dressing
- Thin, fine mesh gauze or packing strip
- Gauze dressings and pads
Transparent Dressing
- Cotton swabs
- Mineral oil (optional)
- Transparent dressing
- Sterile gauze 4 × 4's
Hydrocolloid Dressing
- Hydrocolloid dressing
- Sterile gauze 4 × 4s

STEPS	RATIONALE
1. Assess size and location of wound to be dressed.	Assists you in planning for proper type and amount of supplies needed. Alerts you when assistance is needed to hold dressings in place.
2. Assess client's level of comfort. Offer analgesic 30 minutes before if appropriate.	Removal of dry dressing can be painful; client may require pain medication (Rook, 1996).
3. Review medical orders for frequency and type of dressing change. Obtain all equipment.	Indicates type of dressing or applications to use.
4. Explain procedure to client, and instruct client not to touch wound area or sterile supplies.	Decreases anxiety. Sudden, unexpected movement on client's part could result in contamination of wound and supplies.
5. Close room or cubicle curtains and windows.	Provides privacy and reduces airborne microorganisms.

STEPS	RATIONALE
6. Position client comfortably, and drape with bath blanket to expose only wound site. Place waterproof pad under client where dressing is to be changed.	Provides access to the wound, yet minimizes unnecessary exposure. Prevents soiling of bed linen.
7. Place disposable waterproof bag within reach of work area. Fold top of bag to make cuff.	Ensures easy disposal of soiled dressings. Prevents soiling of bag's outer surface.
8. Wash hands and apply clean disposable gloves. Face mask, protective eyewear, and waterproof gown are worn when risk of spray exists.	Reduces transmission of pathogens to exposed tissues. Protects nurse from splashes.
9. Remove old dressing including tape, bandage, or ties. For easier removal of tape use adhesive remover. Pull dressing back slowly across direction of hair growth, parallel to skin.	Pulling tape toward dressing reduces stress on suture line. Removal of dressing in direction of hair growth reduces discomfort.
10. Change dressing.	Removal of one layer at a time reduces the chance of accidental removal of underlying drains. Careful removal of dressing reduces client discomfort and prevents accidental removal of drains.

A. Wet to Dry

(1) With gloved hand or forceps, lift outer secondary layer of dressing. Then remove inner dressing. Take care not to dislodge drains or tubes.

- *Critical Decision Point*

Inner dressing should have dried and adhered to underlying tissue. Do not moisten to remove. This is a common error.

B. Hydrocolloid

(1) Hydrocolloid interacts with wound fluids and forms a soft whitish-yellow gel that may have a faint odor. This is normal.

C. Transparent

(1) Ease off with cotton swabs soaked in mineral oil.

11. Observe character and amount of drainage on dressing and appearance of wound.	Provides estimate of drainage amount and assessment of wound's condition.
12. Dispose of soiled dressings in disposable bag. Avoid having client see drainage.	Reduces transmission of microorganisms. Appearance can upset client.
13. Remove gloves by pulling them inside out. Discard in bag.	Prevents contact of your hands with material on gloves.
14. Open sterile dressing tray or individually wrapped sterile supplies. Place on bedside table (see illustration).	Sterile dressings remain sterile while on or within sterile surface. Preparation of supplies prevents break in technique during dressing change.

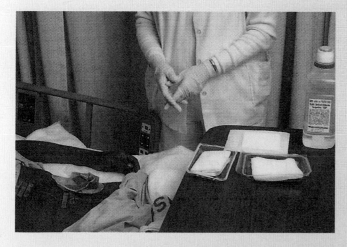

STEP 14   Sterile supplies on bedside table.

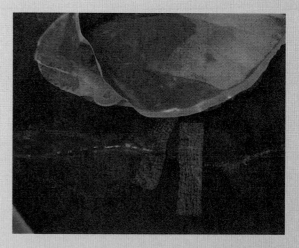

STEP 15A(2)   Large, open abdominal wound.

STEPS	RATIONALE

15. Apply new dressing
    A. Wet to Dry

(1) Apply sterile gloves.	Allows handling of sterile supplies without contamination.
(2) Inspect wound for tissue appearance, presence of drainage, and size (see illustration). Note condition of periwound skin.	Provides assessment of wound healing.
(3) Cleanse wound with prescribed solution. Clean from least to most contaminated area.	Assists in debridement and cleanses wound of debris.
(4) Remove excess moisture from gauze. Unfold and apply moist fluffed mesh gauze or packing strip directly into wound surface. Continue with additional gauze until wound is filled (see illustration).	Wound should be loosely packed to facilitate wicking of drainage into absorbent outer layer of dressing. Gauze acts as a sponge to absorb wound debris while providing a moist surface to the healing wound.
(5) Make sure any dead space from sinus tracts are filled.	Prevents accumulation of debris into dead space or tracts, which delays wound healing.
(6) Apply dry, sterile 4 × 4 gauze over moist gauze.	Acts as an absorbent layer.
(7) Cover with ABD pad, Surgipad, or gauze.	Protects wound from entrance of microorganisms.
(8) Apply tape over dressing, Kling roll (for circumferential dressings), or Montgomery ties. For application of Montgomery ties (see Figure 34-12, p. 870).	Secures dressing in place.
a. Expose adhesive surface of tape on end of each tie. Apply adhesive surface to skin perpendicular to the wound. Position gauze over wound and secure ties to hold dressing in place.	Montgomery ties allow for frequent dressing changes without repeated removal of adhesive tape.

    B. Hydrocolloid

(1) Pour saline or prescribed solution over 4 × 4s.	Maintains sterility of dressing.
(2) Apply gloves (sterile or clean, check agency policy).	Allows nurse to handle dressings.
(3) Cleanse area gently with moist 4 × 4s, swabbing exudate away from wound.	Reduces introduction of organisms into wound.
(4) Thoroughly pat area dry with 4 × 4 gauze.	

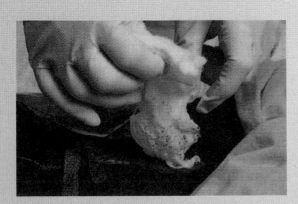 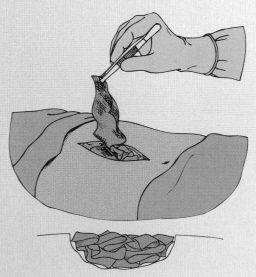

STEP 15A(4)   Packing wound with gauze one layer at a time, until wound bed is filled.

STEPS	RATIONALE
(5) Inspect wound for tissue type, color, odor, and drainage. Measure wound size and depth.	Appearance indicates state of wound healing.

- **Critical Decision Point**
  For some brands of hydrocolloid wafers, the size of the dressing used should be larger in comparison to the wound size to leave a 1 to 1¹/₂ inch margin of dressing beyond the wound end.

STEPS	RATIONALE
(6) Apply hydrocolloid dressings according to manufacturer's directions. Apply granules or paste before wafer dressing in deeper wounds.	Dressing should not be stretched during applications. Avoid wrinkles that would provide tunnel for exudate drainage. Hydrocolloid granules assist in absorbing drainage to increase wearing time of dressing.
C. **Transparent**	
(1) Pour saline or prescribed solution over 4 × 4s.	Maintains sterility of dressing.
(2) Apply gloves (sterile or clean, check agency policy).	Allows nurse to handle dressing.
(3) Cleanse gently with moist 4 × 4s, swabbing exudate away from wound.	
(4) Thoroughly pat dry skin around wound.	Transparent dressings with adhesive backing does not adhere to damp surface.
(5) Inspect wound for tissue type, color, odor, and drainage. Measure if indicated.	Appearance indicates state of wound healing.

- **Critical Decision Point**
  If wound has a large amount of drainage, choose anointed dressing that has increased absorptive properties.

STEPS	RATIONALE
(6) Apply transparent dressing (see illustration) according to manufacturer. Film should not be stretched during application. Avoid wrinkles in film.	Wrinkles provide tunnel for exudate drainage.
16. Remove gloves and discard in bag. Remove mask and gown and eyewear.	Reduces transmission of infection.
17. Assist client to comfortable position.	Promotes client's sense of well-being. Enhances comfort.
18. Dispose of supplies and wash hands.	Reduces transmission of infection.

UNEXPECTED OUTCOMES AND RELATED INTERVENTIONS

- Character of wound drainage changes (e.g., increases, becomes purulent).
  - Monitor for signs of infection (e.g., fever, local tenderness).
  - Obtain wound culture if ordered.
  - Notify physician.
- Skin around wound margins becomes red and excoriated.
  - Dressings are too moist.
  - Modify dressings to decrease moisture.

RECORDING AND REPORTING

- Report brisk, bright red bleeding or evidence of wound dehiscence or evisceration to physician immediately.
- Report wound appearance and characteristics of drainage at shift change.
- Record wound appearance, color, presence, and characteristics of exudate, type and amount of dressings used, and tolerance of client to procedure.
- Write date and time dressing applied on tape in ink (not marker).

Securing Dressings.   Use tape, ties, or bandages and cloth binders to secure a dressing over a wound site. The choice of anchoring depends on the wound size, location, drainage, frequency of dressing changes, and the client's level of activity. You most often use tape strips to secure dressings if the client is not allergic to them. Nonallergenic paper, plastic, and woven fabric tapes minimize skin reactions. More skin tears occur with silk tape compared with soft cloth tape. Adhesive tape, the most likely anchor to cause skin irritation, adheres well to the skin's surface, whereas elastic adhesive tape compresses closely around pressure bandages and permits more movement of a body part (O'Brien and Reilly, 1995).

Tape is available in various widths; choose a size that sufficiently secures the dressing. The tape should cross the dressing and adhere to several inches of skin on each side. When securing the dressing, press the tape gently, exerting pressure

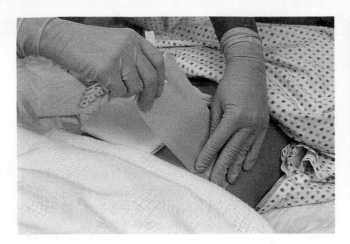
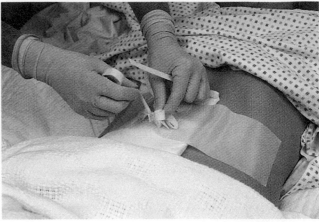

FIGURE **34-12** Montgomery ties.

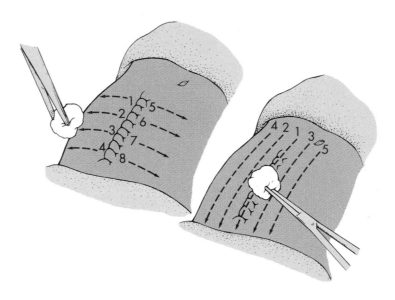

FIGURE **34-13** Methods for cleansing wound site.

away from the wound. Tape is never applied over irritated skin. An adhesive skin barrier wafer may be applied to the skin around the wound so that the tape is secured to the skin barrier wafer rather than to sensitive skin. To remove tape safely, loosen the tape ends and gently release the tape from the client's skin by pressing the skin away from the tape.

To avoid repeated removal of tape from sensitive skin, you can secure dressings with reusable Montgomery ties (Figure 34-12). Each tie consists of a long strip; half contains an adhesive backing to apply to the skin, and the other half folds back and contains a cloth tie to be tied across a dressing and untied at dressing changes. A large, bulky dressing may require two or more sets of Montgomery ties. To provide even support to a wound and immobilize a body part, you may apply elastic gauze or cloth bandages and binders over a dressing.

Comfort Measures. Any wound can be painful, depending on the extent of tissue injury. You can use several techniques to minimize discomfort. Careful removal of tape, gentle cleansing of wound edges, and gentle manipulation of dressings and drains minimize stress on sensitive tissues. Proper turning and positioning of the client also reduce strain on the wound. Administration of analgesic medications 30 to 60 minutes before dressing changes (depending on a drug's time of peak action) also reduces discomfort (Rook, 1996) (see Chapter 29).

WOUND CLEANSING. Wound cleansing removes surface bacteria preventing the invasion of healthy tissue. Normal saline is an effective cleansing agent when delivered to the wound site with adequate force to agitate and wash away bacteria (Rolstad and others, 2000b). Solutions that should not be used to irrigate a clean, granular wound include povidone-iodine (e.g., Betadine), hydrogen peroxide, or acetic acid. These solutions are toxic to fibroblasts, a key component in wound healing. When cleaning around an incision or drain, begin at the least contaminated area and

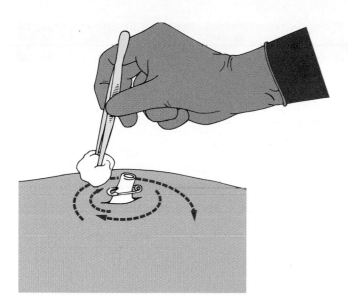

FIGURE **34-14**   Cleansing of drain site.

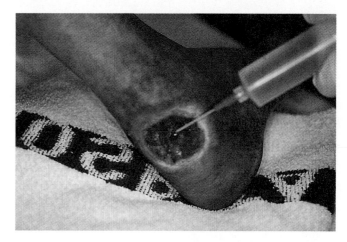

FIGURE **34-15**   Wound irrigation by 35-ml syringe and 19-gauge catheter to facilitate removal of necrotic slough.

move to the most contaminated area. This will protect the clean areas.

1. Cleanse in a direction from the least contaminated area to the most contaminated, such as from the wound or incision to the surrounding skin or drain site (Figure 34-13) or from an isolated drain site to the surrounding skin (Figure 34-14).
2. Use friction when applying antiseptics locally to the skin.
3. When irrigating, allow the solution to flow from the least contaminated to the most contaminated area.

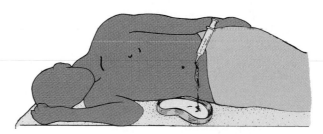

FIGURE **34-16**   Position of client for abdominal wound irrigation.

Wound Irrigation.   Irrigation is a way of cleansing wounds of exudate and debris. You use an irrigating syringe to flush the area with a constant flow of solution. Irrigations are useful for cleaning open deep wounds or sensitive or inaccessible body parts. Administer the prescribed solution (usually normal saline) at body temperature to enhance comfort and provide local cleansing application.

When irrigating clean proliferative wounds, use sterile technique and an irrigation system with a safe pressure (4 to 15 psi) to prevent trauma to the newly formed granulation tissue (AHCPR, 1994). An example of a safe wound cleansing and irrigation system is a 35-ml syringe and a 19-gauge needle, which has a psi of 8. This method provides an ideal solution pressure for cleansing wounds while minimizing tissue trauma (Figure 34-15). The syringe tip should be over but not sticking into the wound (Figure 34-16). Skill 34-4 lists steps for wound irrigation.

Suture Care.   A surgeon closes a wound by bringing the edges as close together as possible to reduce the formation of scar tissue while minimizing trauma and tension and controlling bleeding. Sutures are threads or wires made of silk, steel, cotton, nylon, and polyester (Dacron) and are used to sew

body tissues together. Dacron sutures minimize scar formation. Steel staples, a type of outer skin closure, are frequently used because they result in less tissue trauma while providing extra strength (Figure 34-17). It is also common to see wounds closed with Steri-strips, a sterile tape applied along both sides of a wound to keep the edges closed (Figure 34-18).

Policies vary at institutions as to who may remove sutures. If you remove sutures, a physician's order is required. You must be familiar with the types of suture methods (Figure 34-19). Never pull the visible contaminated portion of the suture through underlying tissue because infection could result.

Drainage Evacuation.   When drainage interferes with healing, drainage evacuation can be achieved by using a drain or a drainage tube with continuous suction. **Drainage evacuators** are convenient, portable units that connect to tubular drains within a wound bed and exert a safe, constant, low-pressure vacuum to remove and collect drainage (Figure 34-20). Ensure that suction is exerted and that all connection points between the evacuator and tubing are intact. The evacuator collects drainage that you assess for volume and character. When the evacuator fills, measure output by emptying the contents into a graduated cylinder, and immediately reset the evacuator to apply suction. Special skin

Skill 34-4
PERFORMING WOUND IRRIGATION

DELEGATION CONSIDERATIONS

Check institutional policy and the state's Nurse Practice Act regarding which wound care interventions can be delegated to assistive personnel. The skill of wound irrigation requires problem solving and knowledge application unique to a professional nurse, particularly regarding the assessment of any wounds and care of acute new wounds. However, cleansing of chronic wounds using *clean* technique can be delegated to assistive personnel. In this situation, instruct staff on what to report when a wound is cleansed. Assistive personnel must also know how to use clean technique to avoid cross contamination from irrigation syringes and equipment.

EQUIPMENT

- Irrigant/cleansing solution (volume 1.2 to 2 times the estimated wound volume)
- Irrigation delivery system depending on amount of pressure desired:
  Sterile irrigation 35-ml syringe with sterile soft angiocath or 19-gauge needle (AHCPR, 1994) *or*
  Hand-held shower or whirlpool
- Clean gloves
- Sterile gloves
- Waterproof underpad, if needed
- Dressing supplies
- Disposable waterproof bag
- Gown, if risk of spray
- Goggles, if risk of spray

STEPS	RATIONALE
1. Review physician's order for irrigation of open wound and type of solution to be used.	Open wound irrigation requires medical order including type of solution(s) to use (Waldrop and Doughty, 2000).
2. Review recent recorded assessments related to client's open wound:	
a. Extent of impairment of skin integrity, including size of wound (measure length, width, and depth). Wounds should be measured in cm and in the following order: length, width, and depth (Cooper, 2000).	This asseses volume of irrigation solution needed. Data also used as baseline to indicate change in condition of wound.
b. Elevation of body temperature.	May indicate response to infection.
c. Drainage from wound (amount, color and consistency). Amount can be measured by part of dressing saturated or in terms of quantity (e.g., scant, moderate, copious).	Expect amount to decrease as healing takes place. Serous drainage is clear; sanguineous or bright red drainage indicates fresh bleeding; serosanguineous drainage is pink; purulent drainage is thick and yellow, pale green, or white (Cuzzell, 1997).
d. Odor. Must state that there is no odor if none is present. More frequent cleansing is needed if wound has a foul odor (AHCPR, 1994).	Strong odor indicates infectious process.
e. Wound color.	Color represents a balance between necrotic tissue and new scar tissue. Proper selection of wound products, based on the color of the wound, facilitates removal of necrotic tissue and promotes new tissue growth (Cuzzell, 1997).
f. Culture reports.	Remember that chronic wounds healing by secondary intention are often colonized.
g. Stage of healing of the client's wound.	Client's wound characteristics determine type and amount of pressure to use during irrigation.
h. Dressing: dry and clean; evidence of bleeding, profuse drainage.	Provides an initial assessment of present wound drainage.
3. Assess comfort level or pain, and identify symptoms of anxiety. Administer prescribed analgesic 30 to 45 minutes before starting wound irrigation.	Discomfort may be related directly to wound or indirectly to muscle tension or immobility. Anxiety results from multiple factors (e.g., surgery, diagnosis, awaiting pathology reports) and anticipation of unknown nursing interventions (e.g., first wound irrigation).
4. Assess client for history of allergies to antiseptics, tapes, or dressing material.	Known allergies suggest application of a sample of prescribed antiseptic as skin test before flushing wound with large volume of solution.

STEPS	RATIONALE
5. Explain procedure of wound irrigation and cleansing.	Information will reduce client's anxiety.
6. Position client.	
a. Position client comfortably to permit gravitational flow of irrigating solution through wound and into collection receptacle (see Figure 34-16, p. 871).	Directing solution from top to bottom of wound and from clean to contaminated area prevents further infection. Positioning client during planning stage provides bed surfaces for later preparation of equipment.
b. Position client so that wound is vertical to collection basin.	
c. Place padding or extra towels.	Protects bedding.
d. Expose wound only.	Prevents chilling of client.
7. Warm irrigation solution to approximate body temperature. Place container in basin of hot water.	Warmed solution increases comfort and reduces vascular constriction response in tissues.
8. Form cuff on waterproof bag, and place it near bed.	Cuffing helps to maintain large opening, thereby permitting placement of contaminated dressing without touching refuse bag itself.
9. Wash hands.	Reduces transmission of microorganisms.
10. Close room door or bed curtains.	Maintains privacy.
11. Apply gown and goggles if needed.	Protects nurse from splashes or sprays of blood and body fluids.
12. Put on clean gloves, remove soiled dressing, and discard in waterproof bag. Discard gloves.	Reduces transmission of microorganisms.
13. Prepare equipment; open sterile supplies.	
14. Put on sterile gloves.	
15. To irrigate wound with moderate pressure:	
a. Fill 35-ml syringe with irrigation solution.	Moderate irrigant pressure helps remove debris and facilitates healing by secondary intention.
b. Attach 19-gauge needle or angiocath (see Figure 34-15, p. 871).	Provides ideal pressure for cleansing and removal of debris.
c. Hold syringe tip 2.5 cm (1 inch) above upper end of wound and over area being cleansed.	Prevents syringe contamination. Careful placement of the syringe prevents unsafe pressure of the flowing solution.
d. Using continuous pressure, flush wound; repeat Steps 15a, b, and c until solution draining into basin is clear.	Clear solution indicates all loose debris has been removed.
16. To irrigate deep wound with minimal pressure:	Minimal pressure to wounds with very little debris.
a. Attach soft angiocatheter to piston syringe filled with irrigation solution.	Catheter permits direct flow of irrigant into wound. Expect wound to take longer to empty when opening is small.
b. Using slow, continuous pressure, flush wound.	Slow continuous pressure prevents injury to wound bed.

• *Critical Decision Point*
CAUTION: *Splashing may occur during this step.*

c. Refill syringe, and repeat until solution draining into basin is clear.	
17. To cleanse wound with hand-held shower:	Useful for clients able to shower with assistance or independently. May be accomplished at home. A shower table is helpful for bed-bound or acutely ill clients.
a. With client seated comfortably in shower chair, adjust spray in gentle flow; water temperature should be warm.	
b. Cover shower head with clean washcloth if needed.	
c. Shower for 5 to 10 minutes with shower head 12 inches (30 cm) from wound.	
18. To cleanse wound with whirlpool:	
a. Adjust water level and temperature; add prescribed cleansing agent.	Wound is hypersensitive to hot temperature.

• *Critical Decision Point*
To avoid tissue damage, position client so that water jets are not directly over clean granulating wound tissue.

b.	Assist client into whirlpool, or place extremity into whirlpool.	
c.	Allow client to remain in whirlpool for prescribed interval.	Ensures thorough wound cleansing.

- **Critical Decision Point**
  Clients who are confused, have poor activity tolerance, or have impaired mobility should never be left alone in the whirlpool.

19.	When indicated, obtain cultures after cleansing with nonbacteriostatic saline.	Routine culturing of open wounds is not recommended by AHCPR (1994). AHCPR (1994) recommends using quantitative bacterial cultures (tissue biopsy or wound fluid by needle aspiration) rather than swab cultures, which often detect only surface bacterial contaminants.

- **Critical Decision Point**
  Consider culturing a wound if it has a foul, purulent odor; inflammation surrounds the wound; a nondraining wound begins to drain; or client is febrile.

20.	Dry wound edges with gauze; dry client if shower or whirlpool is used.	Prevents maceration of surrounding tissue from excess moisture.
21.	Observe type of tissue in wound bed and wound diameter.	Identifies wound healing progress.
22.	Apply appropriate dressing.	Maintains protective barrier and healing environment for wound.
23.	Remove gloves, mask, goggles, and gown.	Prevents transfer of microorganisms.
24.	Assist client to comfortable position.	
25.	Dispose of equipment and soiled supplies, and wash hands.	Reduces transmission of microorganisms.
26.	Inspect dressing periodically.	Determines client's response to wound irrigation and need to modify plan of care.
27.	Evaluate skin integrity.	Determines if extension of wound has occurred.
28.	Observe client for signs of discomfort.	Client's pain should not increase as a result of wound irrigation.
29.	Observe for presence of retained irrigant.	Retained irrigant is a medium for bacterial growth and subsequent infection.

UNEXPECTED OUTCOMES AND RELATED INTERVENTIONS

- Bleeding or serosanguineous drainage appears.
  - Flush wound during next irrigation using less pressure.
  - Notify physician of bleeding.
- Suture line opening extends.
  - Notify physician.
  - Reevaluate amount of pressure to use for next wound irrigation.
- Retained fluid and debris appear.
  - Increase amount of fluid used during irrigation.
  - Increase amount of pressure when flushing wound.
  - Make sure wound is clear of retained fluid and debris before applying dressing.

RECORDING AND REPORTING

- Record wound irrigation and client response in progress notes.
- Immediately report any evidence of fresh bleeding, sharp increase in pain, retention of irrigant, or signs of shock to attending physician.
- Record and report expected and unexpected outcomes that have actually occurred.

---

barriers, similar to those used with ostomies (Chapter 32), may be applied around drain sites. The soft, waferlike, plastic barriers are applied to the skin with adhesive. If drain sites are leaking, drainage flows on the barrier but not directly onto the client's skin.

BANDAGES AND BINDERS.   A simple gauze dressing is often not enough to immobilize or provide support to a wound. **Bandages** and **binders** applied over or around dressings can provide extra protection and therapeutic benefits by creating pressure over a body part, immobilizing a body part, sup-

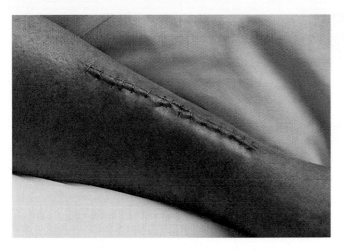

FIGURE **34-17**   Wound closed with staples.

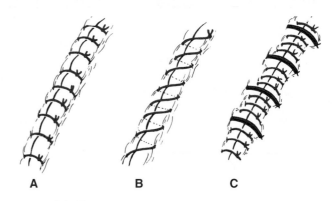

FIGURE **34-19**   Examples of suturing methods. **A,** Intermittent. **B,** Continuous. **C,** Retention.

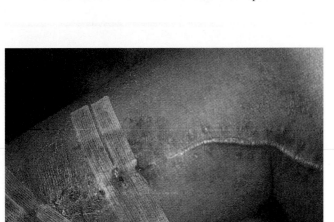

FIGURE **34-18**   Steri-strips placed over incision for closure.

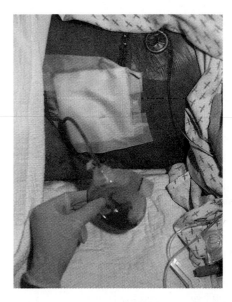

FIGURE **34-20**   Jackson-Pratt drainage tube and reservoir.

porting a wound, reducing or preventing edema, securing a splint, or securing dressings.

Bandages are available in rolls of various widths and materials including gauze, elasticized knit, elastic webbing, flannel, and muslin. Gauze bandages are lightweight and inexpensive, mold easily around contours of the body, and permit air circulation to underlying skin to prevent maceration. Elastic bandages conform well to body parts but can also be used to exert pressure over a body part.

Binders are bandages made of large pieces of material to fit a specific body part. An arm sling and a breast binder are two examples of binders. A binder can reduce stress on a wound.

Principles for Application of Bandages and Binders.
Correctly applied bandages and binders do not cause injury to underlying or nearby body parts or create discomfort for the client. Before applying a bandage or binder, perform the following steps:

1. Inspect the skin for abrasions, edema, discoloration, or exposed wound edges.

2. Cover exposed wounds or open abrasions with a sterile dressing.
3. Assess the condition of underlying dressings, and change if they are soiled.
4. Assess the skin of underlying body parts and parts that will be distal to the bandage for signs of circulatory impairment (coolness, pallor or cyanosis, diminished or absent pulses, swelling, numbness, and tingling) to provide a means for comparing changes in circulation after bandage application.

Table 34-4 outlines the principles of bandage and binder application. After a bandage is applied, you assess, document, and immediately report any changes in circulation, comfort level, body function such as ventilation, and skin integrity. After you apply a bandage you can loosen or readjust it as necessary, but you should seek an order before loosen-

Principles for Bandage and Binder Application

Table 34-4

Principle	Rationale
Position body part to be bandaged in comfortable position of normal anatomical alignment.	Bandages cause restriction in movement. Immobilization in normal functioning position reduces risks of deformity or injury.
Prevent friction between and against skin surfaces by applying gauze or cotton padding.	Skin surfaces in contact with each other (e.g., between toes, under breasts) can rub against each other to cause abrasion or chafing. Bandages over bony prominences may rub against skin to cause breakdown.
Apply bandages securely to prevent slippage during movement.	Friction between bandage and skin can cause skin breakdown.
When bandaging extremities, apply bandage first at distal end and progress toward trunk.	Gradual application of pressure from distal toward proximal portion of extremity promotes venous return and minimizes risk of edema or circulatory impairment.
Apply bandages firmly, with equal tension exerted over each turn or layer. Avoid excess overlapping of bandage layers.	Equal tension prevents unequal pressure distribution over bandaged body part. Localized pressure causes circulatory impairment.
Position pins, knots, or ties away from wound or sensitive skin areas.	Pins and ties used to secure bandages and binders can exert localized pressure and irritation.

ing or removing a bandage applied by the physician. Explain to the client that any bandage or binder will feel relatively firm or tight, assesses the bandage carefully to be sure it is applied properly and is providing therapeutic benefit, and replace bandages when they become soiled.

Binder Application. Binders are especially designed for the body part to be supported. The most common types of binders are the breast binder, abdominal binder, and sling (Box 34-11).

Breast Binder. A breast binder looks like a tight-fitting sleeveless vest. It conforms to the shape of the chest wall and is available in different sizes. Breast binders can provide support after breast surgery or exert pressure to reduce lactation after childbirth. Chest expansion should be unimpaired, but if pulmonary secretions increase, you must encourage active pulmonary hygiene exercises.

Abdominal Binder. An abdominal binder supports large incisions that are vulnerable to stress when the client moves or coughs. It is a rectangular piece of cotton or elasticized material with many tails attached to the two longer sides or long extensions on each side to surround the abdomen (Figure 34-21).

Slings. Slings support arms with muscular sprains or fractures. A commercially made sling consists of a long sleeve that extends to the elbow and a strap that fits around the neck. In the home a large triangular piece of cloth can be used as a sling. The client may sit or lie supine for a sling application (Figure 34-22). Instruct the client to bend the affected arm, bringing the forearm straight across the chest. The open sling fits under the client's arm and over the chest, with the base of the triangle under the wrist and the triangle's point at the elbow. One end of the sling fits around the back of the neck. Bring the other end up over the affected arm while supporting the extremity. Tie the two ends at the side of the neck so that the knot does not press against the cervical spine. The loose fold at the elbow can be folded

evenly around the elbow and pinned. The lower arm should always be supported at a level above the elbow to prevent the formation of dependent edema.

Bandage Application. Rolls of bandage can secure or support dressings over irregularly shaped body parts. Each roll has a free outer end and a terminal end at the center. The rolled portion of the bandage is its body, and its outer surface is placed against the client's skin or dressing. Box 34-12 describes essential points when applying an elastic bandage.

HEAT AND COLD THERAPY. The local application of heat and cold to an injured body part provides therapeutic benefits. Before using these therapies, however, you must understand normal body responses to local temperature variations, assess the integrity of the body part, determine the client's ability to sense temperature variations, and ensure proper operation of equipment. You are legally responsible for the safe administration of all heat and cold applications.

Body Responses to Heat and Cold. Exposure to heat and cold can cause systemic and local responses. Systemic responses occur through heat loss mechanisms (sweating or vasodilation) or mechanisms promoting heat conservation (vasoconstriction or piloerection) and heat production (shivering) (Chapter 11). Local responses to heat and cold occur through stimulation of temperature-sensitive nerve endings within the skin.

The body's adaptive ability creates the major problem in protecting clients from injury resulting from temperature extremes. A person initially feels an extreme change in temperature but within a short time hardly notices the temperature variation. This phenomenon can be dangerous because a person insensitive to heat and cold extremes can suffer serious tissue injury. You must recognize clients most at risk for injuries from heat and cold applications (Table 34-5).

Procedural Guidelines for
Applying Abdominal or Breast Binders

Box 34-11

1. Observe client with need for support of thorax or abdomen. Observe ability to breathe deeply and cough effectively.
2. Review medical record if medical prescription for particular binder is required and reasons for application.
3. Inspect skin for actual or potential alterations in integrity. Observe for irritation, abrasion, skin surfaces that rub against each other, or allergic response to adhesive tape used to secure dressing.
4. Inspect any surgical dressing.
5. Assess client's comfort level, using analog scale of 0 to 10 (see Chapter 29) and noting any objective signs and symptoms.
6. Gather necessary data regarding size of client and appropriate binder.
7. Explain procedure to client.
8. Wash hands, and apply gloves (if likely to contact wound drainage).
9. Close curtains or room door.
10. Apply binder.

    A. **ABDOMINAL BINDER:**

       (1) Position client in supine position with head slightly elevated and knees slightly flexed.

       (2) Fanfold far side of binder toward midline of binder.

       (3) Instruct and assist client in rolling away from you toward raised side rail while firmly supporting abdominal incision and dressing with hands.

       (4) Place fanfolded ends of binder under client.

       (5) Instruct or assist client in rolling over folded ends toward you.

       (6) Unfold and stretch ends out smoothly on far side of bed.

       (7) Instruct client to roll back into supine position.

       (8) Adjust binder so that supine client is centered over binder using symphysis pubis and costal margins as lower and upper landmarks.

       (9) Close binder. Pull one end of binder over center of client's abdomen. While maintaining tension on that end of binder, pull opposite end of binder over center and secure with Velcro closure tabs, metal fasteners, or horizontally placed safety pins (see Figure 34-21).

      (10) Assess client's comfort level.

      (11) Adjust binder as necessary.

    B. **BREAST BINDER:**

       (1) Assist client in placing arms through binder's armholes.

       (2) Assist client to supine position in bed.

       (3) Pad area under breasts if necessary.

       (4) Using Velcro closure tabs or horizontally placed safety pins, secure binder at nipple level first. Continue closure process above and then below nipple line until entire binder is closed.

       (5) Make appropriate adjustments, including individualizing fit of shoulder straps and pinning waistline darts to reduce binder size.

       (6) Instruct and observe skill development in self-care related to reapplying breast binder.

11. Remove gloves, and wash hands.
12. Observe site for skin integrity, circulation, and characteristics of the wound. (Periodically remove binder and surgical dressing to assess wound characteristics.)
13. Assess comfort level of client, using analog scale of 0 to 10 and noting any objective signs and symptoms.
14. Assess client's ability to ventilate properly, including deep breathing and coughing.

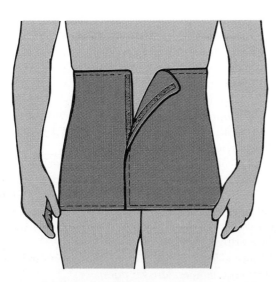

FIGURE **34-21**   Abdominal binder secured with Velcro.

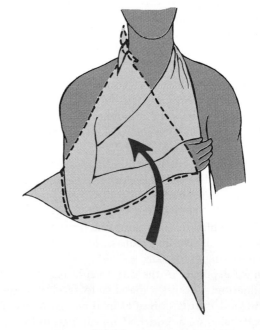

FIGURE **34-22**   Application of a sling.

Procedural Guidelines for
APPLYING ELASTIC BANDAGES

Box 34-12

1. Review client's medical record and order for application of elastic bandage.
2. Inspect areas to be bandaged for
   a. Intact skin
   b. Abrasions
   c. Draining wounds
   d. Skin discoloration
3. Note circulation to the area requiring an elastic bandage.
   a. Palpate skin, noting temperature.
   b. Palpate pulse, noting pulse quality.
   c. Observe extremity for edema or dehydration.
4. Determine level of function of affected extremity.
5. Gather equipment:
   a. Correct width and number of elastic bandages
   b. Clips, adhesive tape, or mesh dressing to secure elastic bandage
   c. Gloves if wound drainage is present
6. Explain procedure to client.
7. Wash hands, and apply gloves, if indicated.
8. Close curtains or room door.
9. Hold roll of elastic bandage in dominant hand, and use other hand to tightly hold the beginning of bandage at distal body part.

10. Apply bandage from distal point toward proximal boundary, stretching the bandage slightly, using a variety of bandage turns to cover various body shapes. Prevent uneven bandage tension or circulatory impairment by overlapping turns by one-half to two-thirds width of bandage roll. NOTE: Be sure bandage is smooth (without creases.)
11. Secure each roll with clip or tape before applying additional roll(s).
12. When finished with application, secure last elastic roll with clip, adhesive tape, or mesh to prevent wrap from becoming dislodged and thus decreasing extremity support.
13. Remove gloves, and wash hands.
14. Assess circulation to bandaged area every 4 hours.
   a. Palpate distal pulse.
   b. Palpate skin, noting temperature every 4 hours.
   c. Observe skin color.
15. Determine client's level of comfort, using analog scale of 0 to 10 and noting any objective signs and symptoms.
16. Observe for changes from baseline assessment in level of extremity function.

Conditions That Increase Risk of Injury From Heat and Cold Application

Table 34-5

Condition	Risk Factors
Very young; older adults	Thinner skin layers in children and older adults increase risk of burns; older adults have reduced sensitivity to pain.
Open wounds, broken skin, stomas	Subcutaneous and mucosal tissues are more sensitive to temperature variations; they also contain no temperature and fewer pain receptors.
Areas of edema or scar formation	There is reduced sensation to temperature stimuli because of scar formation.
Peripheral vascular disease (e.g., diabetes, arteriosclerosis)	Body's extremities are less sensitive to temperature and pain stimuli because of circulatory impairment and local tissue injury; cold application would further compromise blood flow.
Confusion or unconsciousness	There is reduced perception of sensory or painful stimuli.
Spinal cord injury	Alterations in nerve pathways prevent reception of sensory or painful stimuli.

Local Effects of Heat and Cold. Heat and cold stimuli create different physiological responses. The choice of heat or cold therapy depends on the local responses desired for wound healing (Table 34-6).

Heat generally is therapeutic. If heat is applied for 1 hour or more, however, blood flow is reduced by a reflex vasoconstriction as the body attempts to control heat loss from the area. The periodic removal and reapplication of local heat will restore vasodilation. Continuous exposure to heat damages epithelial cells, causing redness, localized tenderness, and even blistering of the skin.

Prolonged exposure of the skin to cold results in a reflex vasodilation. The cell's inability to receive adequate blood flow and nutrients results in tissue ischemia. The skin initially takes on a reddened appearance, followed by a bluish-purple mottling with numbness and a burning type of pain. Tissues can actually freeze from exposure to extreme cold.

Factors Influencing Heat and Cold Tolerance. The body's response to heat and cold therapies depends on the following factors:

1. *Duration of application.* A person is better able to tolerate short exposures to any temperature extremes.
2. *Body part.* The neck, inner aspect of the wrist and forearm, and perineal regions are more sensitive to temperature variations. The foot and the palm of the hand are less sensitive.
3. *Damage to body surface.* Exposed skin layers are more sensitive to temperature variations.

Therapeutic Effects of Heat and Cold Applications — Table 34-6

Physiological Response	Therapeutic Benefit	Examples of Conditions Treated
Heat Therapy		
Vasodilation	Improves blood flow to injured body part	Arthritis or degenerative joint disease
Reduced blood viscosity	Promotes delivery of nutrients and removal of wastes	Localized joint pain or muscle strains
Reduced muscle tension	Improves delivery of leukocytes and antibiotics to wound site	Low back pain
Increased tissue metabolism	Promotes muscle relaxation	Menstrual cramping
Increased capillary permeability	Reduces pain from spasm or stiffness	Hemorrhoidal, perianal, and vaginal inflammation
	Increases blood flow	Local abscesses
	Provides local warmth	
	Promotes movement of waste products and nutrients	
Cold Therapy		
Vasoconstriction	Reduces blood flow to injured site, preventing edema formation	Immediately after direct trauma (e.g., sprains, strains, fractures, muscle spasms)
Local anesthesia	Reduces inflammation	Superficial laceration or puncture wound
Reduced cell metabolism	Reduces localized pain	Minor burn
Increased blood viscosity	Reduces oxygen needs of tissues	After injections
Decreased muscle tension	Promotes blood coagulation at injury site	Arthritis or joint trauma
	Relieves pain	

4. *Prior skin temperature.* The body responds best to minor temperature adjustments.
5. *Body surface area.* A person is less tolerant of temperature changes over a large area of the body.
6. *Age and physical condition.* The very young and old are most sensitive to heat and cold. If a client's physical condition reduces the reception or perception of sensory stimuli, the tolerance to temperature extremes is high, but the risk of injury is also high.

Assessment for Temperature Tolerance. Before applying heat or cold therapies, first observe the area to be treated so that therapy-related skin changes can later be evaluated. Alterations in skin integrity, such as abrasions, open wounds, edema, bruising, bleeding, or localized areas of inflammation, increase the risk of thermal injury. Identify conditions that contraindicate heat or cold therapy. Heat should not be applied over an active area of bleeding (risk of continued bleeding) or an acute localized inflammation such as appendicitis (risk of rupture). If the client has cardiovascular problems, it is unwise to apply heat to large portions of the body because massive vasodilation may disrupt blood supply to vital organs. Cold is contraindicated if the site of injury is edematous or the client has impaired circulation or is shivering (may intensify shivering and reduce blood flow).

Also assess the client's sensory function and ability to recognize when heat or cold becomes excessive. If a client has peripheral vascular disease, observe circulation to the extremities. If a client is confused or unresponsive, observe skin temperature, circulation, and integrity frequently after therapy begins.

Finally, assess the condition of all equipment used, checking for cracked cords, frayed wires, damaged insulation, exposed heating components, leaks, and evenness of temperature distribution.

Client Education and Safety. Before application of heat or cold therapy, the client should understand its purpose, the symptoms of temperature exposure, and the precautions taken to prevent injury. Box 34-13 provides hints for safely applying heat and cold therapy.

Applying Heat and Cold. A prerequisite to using heat or cold application is a physician's order, which should include the body site to be treated and the type, frequency, and duration of application. The correct temperature to use for heat and cold applications varies according to agency policy.

Choice of Moist or Dry. Heat and cold applications can be administered in dry or moist forms. The type of wound or injury, location of the body part, and presence of drainage or inflammation are considered when selecting dry or moist applications.

Warm Moist Compresses. A warm, moist compress improves circulation, relieves edema, and promotes concentration of pus and drainage. A **compress** is a piece of gauze dressing moistened in a prescribed warmed solution. A pack is a larger cloth or dressing applied to a larger body area.

Explain to the client the sensations to be felt during the procedure.

Instruct the client to report changes in sensation or discomfort immediately.

Provide a timer, clock, or watch so that the client can help you to time the application.

Keep the call light within the client's reach.

Refer to the institution's policy and procedure manual for safe temperatures.

Do not allow the client to adjust temperature settings.

Do not allow the client to move an application or place his or her hands on the wound site.

Do not place the client in a position that prevents movement away from the temperature source.

Do not leave unattended a client who is unable to sense temperature changes or move from the temperature source.

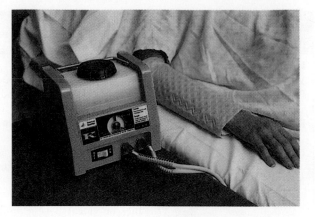

FIGURE **34-23** Aquathermia pad.

Heat from warm compresses evaporates quickly. To maintain a constant temperature, you must change the compress frequently or apply a warm aquathermic pad or waterproof heating pad over the compress. Because moisture conducts heat, any device's temperature setting should be lower for a moist compress than for a dry application. A layer of plastic wrap or a dry towel can also be used to insulate the compress and retain heat. Moist heat promotes vasodilation and evaporation of heat from the skin's surface. For this reason a client may feel chilly. Control drafts, and keep the client covered with a blanket or robe.

Warm Soaks. Immersion of a body part in a warmed solution promotes circulation, lessens edema, increases muscle relaxation, and can apply medicated solution. A soak can also be accomplished by wrapping the body part in dressings and saturating them with the warmed solution.

Position the client comfortably, place waterproof pads under the area to be treated, and heat the solution to the client's tolerance. Check the temperature by placing a small amount of solution on the inside of the forearm. After immersing the body part, cover the container and extremity with a towel to reduce heat loss. It is usually necessary to remove the cooled solution and the body part and add heated solution after about 10 minutes. The problem is to keep the solution at a constant temperature. Never add a hotter solution while the body part remains immersed. After any soak, dry the body part thoroughly to prevent maceration.

Sitz Bath. The client who has had rectal surgery or an episiotomy during childbirth or who has painful hemorrhoids or vaginal inflammation may benefit from a **sitz bath,** a bath in which only the pelvic area is immersed in warm fluid. The client sits in a special tub or chair or in a basin that fits on the toilet so that the legs and feet remain out of the water. Immersing the entire body causes wide-

spread vasodilation and negates the effect of local heat to the pelvic area.

The desired temperature for a sitz bath depends on whether the purpose is to promote relaxation or to clean a wound. It may be necessary to carefully add warm water during the procedure, which usually lasts 20 minutes. A disposable basin contains an attachment that resembles an enema bag and allows the gradual introduction of warmer water.

Prevent overexposure by draping bath blankets around the client's shoulders and thighs and controlling drafts. The client should be able to sit in the basin or tub with feet flat on the floor and without pressure on the sacrum or thighs. Because exposure of a large portion of the body to heat causes extensive vasodilation, assess the client's pulse and facial color and ask whether the client feels light-headed or nauseated.

Aquathermia (Water-Flow) Pads. The aquathermia pad is useful for treating muscle sprains and areas of mild inflammation or edema (Figure 34-23). The unit consists of a waterproof plastic or rubber pad connected by two hoses to an electrical control unit that has a heating element and motor. Distilled water circulates through hollowed channels within the pad to the control unit where water is heated or cooled (depending on temperature setting). Although the units are safer than the conventional heating pad, you should still check for equipment malfunctions. The temperature setting is fixed by inserting a plastic key into the temperature regulator. If the water in the unit runs low, simply add distilled water to the reservoir at the top of the control unit.

To avoid burning the client's skin, fold a thin cloth or pillowcase over the heating pad; use tape, ties, or a gauze roll to hold the pad in place. Pins are never used. Observe the skin frequently for signs of burning. An application should last only 20 to 30 minutes, and the client must not lie on the pad.

Commercial Hot Packs. Commercially prepared, disposable hot packs apply warm, dry heat to an injured area.

Striking, kneading, or squeezing the pack mixes chemicals that release heat. Package directions recommend the time for heat application.

Hot-Water Bottles. The hot-water bottle is an economical means of applying heat to an injured body part. Many clients use them in the home. Give clients and family members the following instructions about the safe use of water bottles:

1. Ensure that there are no leaks. Fill the bottle with warm tap water, secure the cap, and turn the bottle upside down.
2. Fill the bag only two-thirds full, expel air at the top, and secure the cap. The bag is then easier to mold over a body part.
3. Wipe off moisture on the outside of the bag.
4. Never apply a water bottle directly to the skin surface. Cover it with a towel or pillowcase.
5. Keep the bottle in place for 20 to 30 minutes.

Electric Heating Pads. Another conventional form of heat therapy is the heating pad, an electric coil enclosed within a waterproof pad covered with cotton or flannel cloth. The pad is connected to an electric cord that has a temperature-regulating unit for a high, medium, or low setting. Advise clients to avoid using the high setting and to never lie on the pad. Another precaution to note is that a safety pin inserted through a pad can result in an electrical shock.

Cold Moist Compresses. The procedure for applying cold moist compresses is the same as that for warm compresses. Cold compresses should be applied for 20 minutes at a temperature of 15° C (59° F) to relieve inflammation and swelling. They may be clean or sterile. Observe for adverse reactions such as burning or numbness, mottling of the skin, redness, extreme paleness, or a bluish skin discoloration.

Cold Soaks. The procedure for preparing cold soaks and immersing a body part is the same as for warm soaks. The desired temperature for a 20-minute soak is 15° C (59° F). Take precautions to protect the client from chilling.

Ice Bag or Collar. For a client who has a muscle sprain, localized hemorrhage, or hematoma or has undergone dental surgery, an ice bag is ideal to prevent edema formation, control bleeding, and anesthetize the body part. Proper use of the bag requires the following:

1. Fill the bag with water, secure the cap, invert to check for leaks, and pour out the water.
2. Fill the bag two-thirds full with crushed ice so that the bag can mold easily over a body part.
3. Release air from the bag by squeezing its sides before securing the cap (because excess air interferes with conduction of cold).
4. Wipe off excess moisture.
5. Cover the bag with a flannel cover, towel, or pillowcase.

6. Apply the bag to the injury site for 30 minutes; the bag can be reapplied in an hour.

Commercial Cold Packs. Commercially prepared single-use ice packs come in various sizes and shapes. When the pack is squeezed or kneaded, an alcohol-based solution is released inside to create the cold temperature. The soft outer coverings can usually be safely applied directly to the skin surface.

RESTORATIVE AND CONTINUING CARE. Healing for a pressure ulcer or a chronic wound is lengthy and requires continuity of care from the acute care setting to the restorative care setting. In this setting many of the principles and interventions detailed in the acute care section are used. Continue diligent assessment to identify those clients at risk for impaired skin integrity, and institute preventive measures as needed.

Despite efforts with wound care, wound healing will not occur if the client is malnourished. Tissue repair requires more protein, carbohydrates, fats, vitamins, minerals, water, and oxygen than normal tissue metabolism (see Chapter 30). In addition, the delivery of nutritional substances to tissues depends on a healthy circulatory system. Malnutrition causes an insufficient supply of the necessary nutritional elements and alterations in blood vessel integrity. Therefore work closely with dietitians to provide a well-balanced diet, and educate the client about the importance of good dietary habits. For clients weakened or debilitated by illness, supportive nutritional therapies may become necessary. The surgical client who is well nourished and has no complications requires at least 0.8 g of protein per kilogram daily for nutritional maintenance. Supplemental tube feedings (enteral feedings) introduce nutrients directly into the gastrointestinal tract. If a client is unable to tolerate enteral feedings, the physician may order parenteral (intravenously administered) nutrition.

The client with a wound that restricts mobility or has the potential to compromise the function of a joint may require additional physical and/or occupational therapy. Work closely with the physical therapist in monitoring the client's activity and tolerance for exercise. It is important to optimize activity within the client's physical limitations and return function as rapidly as possible.

Some chronic wounds are the result of underlying pathologic conditions that may continue long after wound healing occurs.

 Evaluation

CLIENT CARE. Nursing interventions for reducing and treating pressure ulcers are evaluated by determining the client's response to nursing therapies and by determining whether each goal was achieved (Box 34-14). The optimal goals are to prevent injury to the skin and tissues, to reduce injury to the skin and underlying tissues, and to restore skin integrity. Also evaluate specific interventions designed to

Outcome Evaluation for MR. AHMED

Box 34-14

Nursing Action	Client Response/Finding	Achievement of Outcome
Measure wound size.	Ulcer is 1×1.5 inches.	Wound diameter is decreasing.
Observe wound and any drainage, noting color, amount, and type of drainage.	Serous drainage present. Wound color remains beefy red.	Ulcer remains present, but signs of healing are present.
Palpate underlying skin around wound.	Underlying skin around wound remains intact with no palpable tissue change.	No evidence of advancing pressure ulcer or tissue damage.
Ask Mr. Ahmed about any discomfort or new sensations of burning or tingling at wound site.	Mr. Ahmed does not notice any decrease in level of comfort or any new "pain or burning."	No evidence of new tissue damage.
Ask Mr. Ahmed about his food intake.	Mr. Ahmed reports that his appetite is increasing, and he eats most of his meals. Review of caloric count for the last week documents that Mr. Ahmed's nutritional intake has improved.	He is improving nutritional intake.

Client Teaching

Box 34-15

SKIN INTEGRITY IN THE HOME SETTING

ASSESSMENT

- Assessment and documentation (of the pressure ulcer) should be carried out at least weekly, unless there is evidence of deterioration, in which case both the pressure ulcer and the client's overall management must be reassessed immediately. In the home setting, this may require the assistance of the client and family because weekly assessment by health care providers is not always feasible.

ULCER CARE—DRESSINGS

- Consider caregiver ability and frequency of any nursing visits when selecting a dressing.

  In the home setting, caregivers may choose extended-wear dressing to reduce the frequency of dressing changes and the need for nursing visits.

INFECTION CONTROL

- Clean dressing may be used in the home setting. Disposal of contaminated dressings in the home should be done in a manner consistent with local regulations.

  The "no-touch" technique can be used for dressing changes. This technique is a method of changing dressings without touching the wound or the surface of any dressing that might be in contact with the wound. Adherent dressings should be grasped by the corner and removed slowly, whereas gauze dressings can be pinched in the center and lifted off.

  The Environmental Protection Agency recommends that soiled dressings be placed in securely fastened plastic bags before being added to other household trash. Have client or family member check local regulations.

Modified from Agency for Health Care Policy and Research Panel for the Treatment of Pressure Ulcers in Adults: *Treatment of pressure ulcers: clinical practice guidelines,* No. 15, Pub. No. 95-0653, Rockville, Md, 1994, U.S. Department of Health and Human Services, Public Health Service.

Case Study   EVALUATION

Lynda Abraham has completed her clinical experience with Mr. Ahmed. His pressure ulcer is still present, but it is reduced in size and is healing. No other sites of abnormal reactive hyperemia were assessed, and the rest of his skin remains intact. He is going to be discharged to his home in 2 days. Lynda has taught Mr. Ahmed's wife how to do the dressing changes and how to assess her husband's skin for signs of increased risk for or actual further skin breakdown. On her last day of this clinical experience, Lynda has prepared to refer her client to a home care agency. Lynda, with the help of her instructor, has devised a plan of care for the home; Lynda and her instructor are meeting with the home care nurse today when she visits Mr. and Mrs. Ahmed in the hospital.

Documentation Note
Small amount of serous drainage from stage II pressure ulcer on his sacrum. Wound is 1 × 1 inch (2.5 × 2.5 cm) × $\frac{1}{8}$ inch deep, with beefy red tissue. Mrs. Ahmed cleansed the wound with normal saline and applied a hydrocolloid dressing. She maintained aseptic technique. During the dressing change she correctly assessed her husband's skin. She reminds her husband to change his position every $1\frac{1}{2}$ to 2 hours. Awaiting visit from home care nurse.

promote skin integrity and to teach the client and family to reduce future threats to skin integrity (Box 34-15). In addition, evaluate the client's and family's need for additional support services, and initiate the referral process.

CLIENT EXPECTATIONS.   The client and caregiver must understand how to prevent or treat pressure ulcers. Helping them understand the content in the AHCPR consumer version of the prevention and treatment guidelines is beneficial. Clients may enter into the wound-healing phase with unrealistic expectations regarding duration of care. Collect evaluation data about the client's perception of wound care management. Clients with chronic wounds are often cared for in their home settings and have certain expectations about their level of comfort, lifestyle, independence, and privacy. Therefore you must determine from the client whether his or her expectations were respected and met.

Key Terms

abrasion, p. 855
approximate, p.845 — *nearness*
bandages, p. 874
binders, p. 874
cachexia, p. 844 — *wasting*
compress, p. 879
debridement, p. 862
dehiscence, p. 848 — *sep of tissue layers in wound not healing*
drainage evacuators, p. 871

ecchymosis, p. 856 — *skin tissue or wasting death or wasting*
edema, p. 844
evisceration, p. 848 — *protruding organs*
fistula, p. 848
friction, p. 843
granulation tissue, p. 845
hematoma, p. 848
hemostasis, p. 864
induration, p. 854
laceration, p. 855
maceration, p. 865

nonblanching reactive hyperemia, p. 843
pressure ulcer, p. 843
primary intention, p. 845
reactive blanching hyperemia, p. 843
secondary intention, p. 845
shear, p. 843
sitz bath, p. 880
tissue ischemia, p. 843 — *wasting*
wound culture, p. 856

Key Concepts

- Wounds with partial-thickness tissue loss heal by epidermal repair, and full-thickness wounds heal by forming scar tissue.
- A clean surgical incision with little tissue loss heals by primary intention.
- Wounds healing by secondary intention proceed through three overlapping phases: inflammation, proliferation, and remodeling.
- When there is extensive tissue loss, a wound heals by secondary intention.
- The chances of wound infection are greater when the wound contains dead or necrotic tissue, when foreign bodies lie on or near the wound, and when blood supply and tissue defenses are reduced.
- Physical stress from vomiting, coughing, or sudden muscular contraction can cause separation of wound edges, dehiscence.
- Wound assessment must include anatomical location, size (dimensions and depth of wound), type and percentage of wound tissue, volume and color of wound drainage, and condition of surrounding skin.

- Wound drains remove secretions within tissue layers to promote wound closure.
- Never collect a wound culture from old drainage.
- Principles of wound management include controlling or eliminating the cause, providing systemic support to reduce existing and potential cofactors, and maintaining a physiological local wound environment.
- A moist environment supports wound healing.
- The wet-to-dry dressing mechanically removes dead tissue to debride the wound.
- When cleaning wounds or drain sites, cleans from the least to most contaminated area, away from wound edges.
- A bandage or binder should be applied in a manner that does not impair circulation or irritate the skin.
- The safe use of heat or cold therapy requires an assessment of the client's sensory function, identification of risk factors, and understanding of the physiological effects of heat and cold.
- An acute sprain, fracture, or bruise responds best to cold applications.
- Warm applications are effective for improving circulation to wound sites and promoting muscle relaxation.

Critical Thinking Activities

1. You are teaching a client's family how to irrigate the mid-abdominal wound that is healing by secondary intention. The spouse states, "I always thought it was best to paint the wound with povidone-iodine to prevent infection." How should you respond to the spouse? What is the rationale behind your response? What does the spouse need to know about irrigating the wound?
2. A client has two Jackson-Pratt drainage collectors on the right side of the abdomen. What nursing assessments should be made to ensure proper functioning of this system? Can any aspects of care for this type of drain collector be delegated? Explain the rationale for your answer.
3. Your 85-year-old black male client is admitted to the hospital with a diagnosis of left cerebral vascular accident. He has right-sided weakness, and he cannot turn or walk without assistance. He also has difficulty swallowing, and he is incontinent of urine and stool. What risk factors, if any, for pressure ulcers does this client have? What characteristics would you assess this client for to monitor for a stage I pressure ulcer? How should this be accomplished?

Review Questions

1. When repositioning an immobile client, you notice redness over a bony prominence. When the area is assessed, the red spot blanches with fingertip pressure, indicating:
   1. a local skin infection requiring antibiotics.
   2. this client has sensitive skin and requires special bed linen.
   3. a stage III pressure ulcer, needing the appropriate dressing.
   4. blanching hyperemia, a reaction that causes the blood vessels to dilate in the injured area.

2. Pressure injury to the skin results from:
   1. blood vessel damage from repeated injections.
   2. continual exposure of the skin to fecal or urinary incontinence.
   3. skin compressed by two surfaces for a prolonged period of time.
   4. excessive dryness of the epidermis, allowing damage to the dermis.

3. The topical management of a clean, granular wound healing by secondary intention requires:
   1. a moist wound dressing.
   2. an antibiotic cream applied twice a day.
   3. whirlpool treatments to stimulate granulation tissue.
   4. a treatment plan that allows the wound to be exposed to air for 15 minutes twice a day.

4. When obtaining a wound culture to determine the presence of a wound infection, the specimen should be taken from:
   1. the necrotic tissue.
   2. the wound drainage.
   3. the drainage on the dressing.
   4. clean, healthy-looking tissue.

5. Postoperatively the client with a closed abdominal wound reports a sudden "pop" after coughing. When you examine the surgical wound site, the sutures are open and pieces of small bowel are noted at the bottom of the now opened wound. The correct intervention would be:
   1. to allow the area to be exposed to air until all drainage has stopped.
   2. to place several cold packs over the area, protecting the skin around the wound.
   3. to cover the area with sterile saline-soaked towels and immediately notify the surgical team; this is likely to indicate a wound evisceration.
   4. to cover the area with sterile gauze, place a tight binder over the area, and ask the client to remain in bed for 30 minutes because this is a minor opening in the surgical wound and should reseal quickly.

6. Serous drainage from a wound is defined as:
   1. fresh bleeding.
   2. thick and yellow.
   3. clear, watery plasma.
   4. beige to brown and foul smelling.

7. Interventions to manage a client who is experiencing fecal and urinary incontinence include:
   1. use of a large absorbent diaper, changing when saturated.
   2. keeping the buttocks exposed to air at all times.
   3. utilization of an incontinence cleanser, followed by application of a moisture-barrier ointment.
   4. frequent cleansing, application of an ointment, and covering the area with a thick absorbent towel.

8. The best description of a hydrocolloid dressing is:
   1. a seaweed derivative that is highly absorptive.
   2. premoistened gauze, placed over a granulating wound.
   3. a debriding enzyme that is used to remove necrotic tissue.
   4. a dressing that forms a gel that interacts with the wound surface.

9. A binder placed around a surgical client with a new abdominal wound is indicated for:
   1. collection of wound drainage.
   2. reduction of abdominal swelling.
   3. reduction of stress on the abdominal incision.
   4. stimulation of peristalsis (return of bowel function) from direct pressure.

10. Application of a warm compress is indicated:
    1. to relieve edema.
    2. for a client who is shivering.
    3. to promote healing by stimulating blood flow.
    4. to protect bony prominences from pressure ulcers.

References

Agency for Health Care Policy and Research: Panel for Prediction and Prevention of Pressure Ulcers in Adults: *Pressure ulcers in adults: prediction and prevention,* Clinical practice guideline No. 3, AHCPR Pub. No. 92-0047, Rockville, Md, May 1992, Agency for Health Care Policy and Research, Public Health Service, U.S. Department of Health and Human Services.

Agency for Health Care Policy and Research Panel for the Treatment of Pressure Ulcers in Adults: *Treatment of pressure ulcers: clinical practice guidelines,* No. 15, Pub. No. 95-0653, Rockville, Md. 1994, U.S. Department of Health and Human Services, Public Health Service.

Bates-Jensen BM: Pressure ulcers: pathophysiology and prevention. In Sussman C, Bates-Jensen BM: *Wound care: a collaborative practice manual for physical therapists and nurses,* Gaithersburg, Md, 1998, Aspen Publishers.

Bates-Jensen BM, Wethe J: Acute surgical wound management. In Sussman C, Bates-Jensen BM: *Wound care: a collaborative practice manual for physical therapists and nurses,* Gaithersburg, Md, 1998, Aspen Publishers.

Bennett MA: Report of the Task Force on the implications for darkly pigmented intact skin in the prediction and prevention of pressure ulcers, *Adv Wound Care* 8(6):34, 1995.

Bergstrom N and others: A clinical trial of the Braden Scale for predicting pressure sore risk, *Nurs Clin North Am* 22(2):417, 1987a.

Bergstrom N and others: The Braden Scale for predicting pressure sore risk, *Nur Res* 36:205, 1987b.

Bergstrom NL and others: Predicting pressure ulcer risk: a multisite study of the predictive validity of the Braden Scale, *Nurs Res* 47(5):261, 1998.

Boynton PR and others: Meeting the challenges of healing chronic wounds in older adults, *Nurs Clin North Am* 34(4):921, 1999.

Breslow RA and others: The importance of dietary protein in healing pressure ulcers, *J Am Geriatr Soc* 41:357, 1993.

Broussard CL and others: Adjuvant wound therapies. In Bryant RA, editor: *Acute and chronic wounds: nursing management,* ed 2, St. Louis, 2000, Mosby.

Bryant RA, Rolstad BS: Examining threats to skin integrity, *Ostomy/Wound Manage* 47(6):18, 2001.

Bryant RA and others: Pressure ulcer. In Bryant RA, editor: *Acute and chronic wounds: nursing management,* ed 2, St. Louis, 2000, Mosby.

Cooper DM: Assessment, measurement and evaluation. their pivotal roles in wound healing. In Bryant RA, editor: *Acute and chronic wounds: nursing management,* ed 2, St. Louis, 2000, Mosby.

Jeter KF, Lutz JB: Skin care in the frail, elderly, dependent, and incontinent patient, *Adv Wound Care* 9(1):29, 1996.

Landis EM: Micro-injection studies of capillary blood pressure in human skin, *Heart* 15:209, 1930.

Murphy RN: Legal and practical impact of clinical practice guidelines on nursing and medical practice, *Adv Wound Care* 9(5):31, 1996.

National Pressure Ulcer Advisory Panel: Pressure ulcers incidence, economics, risk assessment, Consensus Development Conference Statement, *Decubitus* 2(2):24, 1989.

National Pressure Ulcer Advisory Panel: *Pressure ulcer staging,* August 1999, www.npuap.org.postin4.html.

O'Brien JM, Reilly NJ: Comparison of tape products on skin integrity, *Adv Wound Care* 8(6):26, 1995.

Olson B: The effects of massage for prevention of pressure ulcers, *Decubitus* 2(4):32, 1989.

Pieper B: Mechanical forces: pressure, shear and friction. In Bryant RA, editor: *Acute and chronic wounds: nursing management,* ed 2, St. Louis, 2000, Mosby.

Pires M, Muller A: Detection and management of early tissue pressure indicators: a pictorial essay, *Progressions* 3(3):3, 1991.

Ramundo JM: Reliability and validity of the Braden Scale in the home care setting, *J Wound Ostomy Continence Nurs* 22(3):128, 1995.

Rolstad BS and others: Principles of wound management. In Bryant RA, editor: *Acute and chronic wounds: nursing management,* ed 2, St. Louis, 2000a, Mosby.

Rolstad, BS and others: Wound care product formulary. In Bryant RA, editors: *Acute and chronic wounds: nursing management,* ed 2, St. Louis, 2000b, Mosby.

Rook JL: Wound care pain management, *Adv Wound Care* 9(6):24, 1996.

Singhal A and others: Options for nonsurgical debridement of necrotic wounds, *Adv Skin Wound Care* 14:96, 2001.

Stotts NA: Wound infection: diagnosis and management. In Bryant RA, editor: *Acute and chronic wounds: nursing management,* ed 2, St. Louis, 2000, Mosby.

Sussman C: Wound healing biology and chronic wound healing. In Sussman C, Bates-Jensen BM: *Wound care: a collaborative practice manual for physical therapists and nurses,* Gaithersburg, Md, 1998, Aspen Publishers.

Thomas C: Specialty beds: decision-making made easy, *Ostomy/Wound Manage* 23:51, 1989.

Trelease CC: Developing standards for wound care, *Ostomy/Wound Manage* 20:46, 1988.

Waldrop J, Doughty D: Wound healing physiology in acute and chronic wounds in Bryant RA, editor: *Acute and chronic wounds: nursing management,* ed 2, St. Louis, 2000, Mosby.

Wound, Ostomy and Continence Nurses Society: *Standards of care, patient with dermal wound: pressure ulcers,* Laguna Beach, Calif, 1992, The Society.

35

Sensory Alterations

Objectives

- Define key terms.
- Differentiate among the processes of reception, perception, and reaction to sensory stimuli.
- Discuss common causes and effects of sensory alterations.
- Discuss common sensory changes that occur with aging.
- Identify factors to assess in determining a client's sensory status.
- Describe behaviors indicating sensory alterations.
- Develop a care plan for clients with visual, auditory, tactile, speech, gustatory, and olfactory alterations.
- Describe nursing interventions that promote effective communication with clients who have sensory alterations.
- Describe conditions in the health care agency or client's home that can be adjusted to promote meaningful sensory stimulation.
- Discuss ways to maintain a safe environment for clients with sensory alterations.

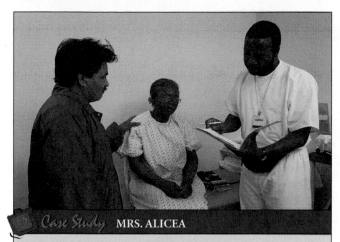

Case Study MRS. ALICEA

Mrs. Alicea is a 73-year-old woman who is at the senior health center for her routine 6-month checkup. She has been visiting the senior center on a regular basis for the past 8 years. Mrs. Alicea has lived alone since her husband died 1 year ago. She lives in a small, single-story, four-room home a few miles away from the health center. Her son, Rico, lives 5 minutes away. Rico drives Mrs. Alicea to her health care visits. Six months ago Mrs. Alicea reported a progressive hearing loss. Today when she enters the clinic she reports "having trouble seeing."

Peter Morris is a 33-year-old junior nursing student assigned to the senior health center. He is learning to conduct assessments and to develop health promotion plans for visiting clients. Peter is married and has two children. For the past month, Peter has been attending his clinical rotation at the center and participating in teaching health promotion activities. He is enjoying this rotation because he is learning more about geriatric clients and is recognizing that they are very independent and capable of productive lifestyles.

*P*eople are unique because they can sense a variety of stimuli from changes in their environment. The sense organs of sight (**visual**), hearing (**auditory**), touch (**tactile**), smell (**olfactory**), taste (**gustatory**), balance, and the body's ability to sense its position and movement in space (**proprioception**) produce special senses and initiate reflexes important for homeostasis. People learn about the environment from healthy sensory organs. When sensory function is altered, the client's ability to relate to and function within the environment changes. As a nurse, you must understand and help to meet the needs of clients with sensory alterations and recognize clients who are most at risk for developing sensory problems. Your nursing care will help clients learn to react safely and effectively in their environment.

SCIENTIFIC KNOWLEDGE BASE
Normal Sensation

When a person's nervous system is intact, he or she can feel and react to sensations. Perception or awareness of sensations depends on a region of the cerebral cortex where specialized brain cells interpret the quality and nature of each sensory stimulus. Sensory experiences include reception,

perception, and reaction. People react to stimuli that are most meaningful to them. When a person attempts to react to every stimulus within their environment or when stimuli are lacking, sensory alterations can occur.

Types of Sensory Alterations

Many factors influence the capacity to receive or perceive sensations (Box 35-1). In your nursing experience you will care for clients with **sensory deficits, sensory deprivation,** and **sensory overload.** When clients suffer from more than one sensory alteration, their ability to function and relate within the environment is seriously impaired.

SENSORY DEFICITS. A sensory deficit happens when a problem with sensory reception or perception occurs (Box 35-2). Clients may not be able to receive certain stimuli (e.g., blindness and deafness) or stimuli are distorted (e.g., blurred vision from cataracts and abnormal taste sensation from xerostomia). A sudden sensory loss caused by injury or as a side effect to medications (Box 35-3) can cause fear, anger, and feelings of helplessness. Clients may withdraw socially to cope with that loss. The client's safety is threatened because the person is unable to respond normally to stimuli. When a deficit is chronic or develops gradually, the client learns to rely on unaffected senses. Some senses may even become more acute to compensate for an alteration. For example, a blind client often develops an acute sense of hearing. Changes in sensory deficits may cause clients to change their behaviors in adaptive or maladaptive ways.

SENSORY DEPRIVATION. Sensory deprivation occurs when inadequate quality or quantity of stimuli impairs perception. Reduced sensory input (hearing loss), confusion, and a restricted environment (bed rest) are three types of sensory deprivation. These effects can produce cognitive changes such as the inability to solve problems, poor task performance, and disorientation. Second, affective changes, which may include boredom, restlessness, increased anxiety, or emotional lability occur. Last, perceptual changes such as reduced attention span, disorganized visual and motor coordination, and confusion of sleeping and waking states also occur.

Behaviors in children are often demonstrated by a higher-than-normal level of anxiety that causes restlessness, difficulty with problem solving, and depression (Wong and others, 1999). In adults the symptoms of sensory deprivation can be similar to psychological illness, confusion, symptoms of severe electrolyte imbalance, or the influence of psychotropic drugs. Accurate diagnosis of a problem is crucial.

SENSORY OVERLOAD. When a person receives multiple sensory stimuli, the brain can have difficulty distinguishing the stimuli that cause a sensory overload to occur. The person no longer perceives the environment in a way that makes sense. Overload prevents a meaningful response to a stimulus by the brain. As a result, thoughts race, attention moves in many directions, and restlessness occurs. The client can demonstrate

Factors That Influence Sensory Function   Box 35-1

AGE
Infants

Binocular vision begins at 6 weeks and is well established by 4 months. During the second year of life, infants can discriminate shapes, objects, and colors.

Neonates will initially respond generally to loud noises. Within a year the infant can visually locate the source of the noise.

Newborns react to strong odors such as alcohol and vinegar by turning their heads. Newborns are able to discriminate their own mother's milk.

Children

Refractive errors are the most common types of visual disorders in children and can be treated with corrective lenses. Serious visual impairment affects a child's ability to play and socialize. The senses of hearing, smell, taste, and touch develop and become coordinated with each other. A toddler will visually inspect an object, turn it over, taste it, smell it and touch it several times while investigating it (Wong and others, 1999).

Adults

Visual changes during adulthood include presbyopia (inability to focus on near objects) and the need for glasses for reading (ages 40 to 50).

Older Adults

Hearing changes include decreased hearing acuity, speech intelligibility, and pitch discrimination, which is referred to as *presbycusis*. Low-pitched sounds are heard the best, but it is difficult to hear conversation over background noise. It is also difficult to discriminate consonants (*f, z, s, th, ch, p, k, t,* and *g*). Vowels that have a low pitch are easier to hear. Speech sounds are garbled, and there is a delayed reception and reaction to speech. A decrease in active sebaceous glands causes the cerumen to become dry and completely obstruct the external auditory canal (Wilson and Giddens, 2001).

Visual changes include reduced visual fields, increased glare sensitivity, impaired night vision, reduced accommodation, reduced depth perception, and reduced color discrimination. Older adults require 3 times as much light to see objects as they did when they were in their 20s (Ebersole and Hess, 1998).

Older Adults—cont'd

Olfactory changes begin around age 50 and include a loss of cells in the olfactory bulb of the brain and a decrease in the number of sensory cells in the nasal lining (Ebersole and Hess, 1998). Reduced sensitivity to odors is common.

Aging causes taste buds to atrophy, to lose efficiency in relaying flavor, and to reduce in number (Ebersole and Hess, 1998). Reduced taste discrimination is common.

Proprioceptive changes include an increased difficulty with balance and coordination. Older adults cannot avoid obstacles as quickly, nor are they able to prevent an accident from happening to themselves when fast action is needed. The automatic response to protect and brace oneself when falling is slower (Ebersole and Hess, 1998).

Older adults experience tactile changes, including declining sensitivity to pain, pressure, and temperature.

MEDICATIONS

Ototoxic medications may affect hearing, balance, or both, with the most common symptom being **tinnitus.** Ototoxicity causes a progressive or continuing hearing loss that in many clients goes unnoticed (Wilson and Giddens, 2001).

ENVIRONMENT

Excessive environmental stimuli can result in sensory overload, marked by confusion, disorientation, and inability to make decisions. Restricted environmental stimulation can lead to sensory deprivation. Poor quality of environment can worsen sensory impairment.

PREEXISTING ILLNESSES

Peripheral vascular disease causes reduced sensation in the extremities and impaired cognition. Chronic diabetes can cause reduced vision or blindness or peripheral neuropathy. Some neurological disorders such as stroke impair sensory reception.

SMOKING

Chronic tobacco use can atrophy the taste buds and affect olfactory function.

NOISE LEVELS

Constant exposure to high noise levels can cause hearing loss.

---

panic, confusion, and aggressiveness. Sleep loss is common. Overload causes a state similar to sensory deprivation.

Acutely ill clients may easily develop sensory overload because of noise in the health care environment. The constant monitoring of clients, noise from equipment, and the nursing activities of turning, repositioning, and administering treatments bombard clients with stimuli. Some clients are more sensitive to sensory overload than others. Behavioral changes can easily be confused with mood swings or disorientation.

▌NURSING KNOWLEDGE BASE

The population of the United States is growing old. Between the years 2010 and 2030, the baby boomer generation will reach 65 years old. The American Association of Retired Persons (AARP) (1998) estimated that 39 million people will reach 65 years of age by 2010. As a nurse, you must stay informed of new nursing knowledge as it pertains to the older adult population and the effects of diverse sensory changes.

Nursing research has demonstrated that there is a relationship between hearing loss, self-esteem, and communication (Jones, 1998). Hearing impairments can cause a person to experience loss and fear. A client's sense of loss is experienced as a loss of control, independence, or self-esteem. Feelings of grief, anger, isolation, depression, and loneliness are also common. Knowledge regarding the effects of sensory loss is important for you to assess how a sensory impairment can influence a client's self-concept and ability to communicate and function in the everyday world.

Older adults who experience sensory deficits often withdraw from social activities. The risk of social isolation, depression, and low self-esteem interferes with their ability to care for themselves and interact with others. These clients

Common Sensory Deficits
Box 35-2

VISUAL

Presbyopia—Gradual decline in ability of the lens to accommodate or to focus on close objects. Reduces ability to see near objects clearly.

Cataract—Cloudy or opaque areas in part or all of the lens. Interferes with passage of light through the lens. Cataracts usually develop gradually, without pain, redness, or tearing in the eye.

Dry eyes—Result when tear glands produce too few tears. Common in older adults and results in itching, burning, or even reduced vision.

Open-angle glaucoma—An increase in intraocular pressure that causes progressive pressure against the optic nerve, resulting in visual field loss, decreased visual acuity, and a halo effect around the eyes, if untreated.

Diabetic retinopathy—Pathological changes in the blood vessels of the retina result in decreased vision or vision loss.

Senile macular degeneration—The macula (specialized portion of the retina responsible for central vision) loses its ability to function efficiently. First signs may include blurring of reading matter, distortion or loss of central vision, and distortion of vertical lines.

HEARING

Presbycusis—A common progressive hearing disorder in older adults.

Cerumen accumulation—Buildup and hardening of earwax in the external auditory canal causes a conduction deafness.

BALANCE

Dizziness and disequilibrium—Common condition in older adulthood, usually resulting from vestibular dysfunction and precipitated by change in position of the head to the rest of the body.

TASTE

Xerostomia—Decrease in salivary production that leads to thicker mucus and a dry mouth. Can interfere with the ability to eat and leads to appetite and nutritional problems.

NEUROLOGICAL

Peripheral neuropathy—Commonly caused in older adults by diabetes, Guillain-Barré syndrome, and neoplasms (Ebersole and Hess, 1998). Symptoms include numbness and tingling of the affected area and stumbling gait.

Stroke—Cerebrovascular accident caused by clot, hemorrhage, or emboli affecting blood vessel leading to or within the brain. Creates altered proprioception with marked incoordination and imbalance. Loss of sensation and motor function in extremities controlled by the affected area of the brain also occurs.

Medications Reported to Cause Ototoxicity
Box 35-3

ANTIBIOTICS
Aminoglycosides
Minocycline
Vancomycin
Polymixin B
Polymixin C
Erythromycin

DIURETICS
Ethacrynic acid
Furosemide
Bumetanide
Torsemide

CARDIAC DRUGS
Class Ia antidysrhythmics
Quinidine

CARDIAC DRUGS—cont'd
Procainamide
Disopyramide

ANALGESICS/NSAIDS
Aspirin
Ibuprofen
Naproxen

ANTINEOPLASTIC AGENTS
Bleomycin
Cisplatin
Dactinomycin
Mechlorethamine

From: Lilley LL, Auker R: *Pharmacology and the nursing process,* ed 3, St. Louis, 2001, Mosby.

often tend to become dependent on family members and experience changes in their activities of daily living (ADLs) (Lueckenotte, 2000).

Managing clients with sensory alterations challenges you to apply nursing research and information from your practice to assist clients in remaining socially interactive and productive. In addition, your application of critical thinking principles will help you to promote clients' sensory function and to protect them from possible injury.

CRITICAL THINKING
Synthesis

As you apply the nursing process for clients with sensory alterations, information from a variety of sources needs to be analyzed and integrated. Learn to anticipate the kind of information necessary to form good clinical judgments. A combination of past client care experiences and the application of scientific and nursing knowledge assists you in selecting an individualized plan of care for the client.

KNOWLEDGE.   A number of factors can cause sensory alterations. Knowledge of those factors, the normal components of a sensory experience, and anatomy and physiology help you to understand how a particular alteration affects a client's function. Knowledge of the pathophysiologic changes of sensory organ disorders can also help you to anticipate how a client will be affected by a sensory change. When you are able to identify characteristics of sensory alterations and the interventions to minimize them, a comprehensive plan of care can be implemented.

Depending on the client's problem, use your knowledge of communication principles (see Chapter 8) to select the best method to communicate with clients. Clients with hearing impairment require different communication approaches to obtain a complete and accurate nursing assessment and to deliver interventions effectively. You also need to have a good knowledge of pharmacology because a variety of medications can affect sensory function. Being able to anticipate the side effects of medications allows you to prepare clients for possible sensory changes.

EXPERIENCE.   Many of us have had an alteration in sensory function or encountered this experience while interacting with family and friends. A previous personal or clinical experience with sensory changes allows you to anticipate the type of care clients will require. How do individuals adapt to hearing aids and glasses? What adjustments do they make to function safely in their homes? What communication techniques are necessary when speaking to individuals with hearing impairment? Such experiences will help you to choose successful nursing interventions when caring for clients in a variety of health care settings.

ATTITUDES.   Critical thinking attitudes make you a more disciplined thinker. Creativity is often necessary to find the right solutions for a client's problems. For example, living in a nonstimulating home environment may be a cause of a client's sensory deprivation. Working with a client, you may suggest changes to the environment that would improve the quality of stimulation and reduce the client's risk for injury. Curiosity applies when a client shows unexplained behavioral changes. Asking why and being curious may help you to assess a less obvious sensory problem.

STANDARDS.   An important ethical standard to follow when assisting clients with sensory alterations is preservation of autonomy (see Chapter 4). For the client to regain independence, you must not override autonomy with the principle of beneficence. You need to remember that although professionals believe they know what is best, clients have to live with the sensory alteration and adapt to the consequences of their own choices.

NURSING PROCESS

 ## Assessment

When assessing clients with sensory alterations or those who are at risk for them, consider age and other factors that influence sensory function. Collect a complete nursing history by examining how a sensory deficit affects a client's lifestyle, self-care ability, psychosocial adjustment, health promotion habits, and safety. This assessment also focuses on the quality and quantity of stimuli within the client's environment.

CLIENTS AT RISK.   Learn to conduct a sensory assessment for any client at risk for sensory alteration. The older adult is obviously in a high-risk group because of normal physiological changes associated with aging. Older clients often underreport certain sensory changes, assuming the change is a part of aging (Ebersole and Hess, 1998). Clients who are immobilized by bed rest, physical impediments (e.g., casts or traction), or chronic disability are unable to experience all the normal sensations of free movement. Such conditions can lead to sensory deprivation. Always remain alert for any behavioral changes common to sensory deprivation. Clients isolated in a health care setting or at home

due to conditions such as active tuberculosis are often restricted to a private room and unable to enjoy normal interactions with visitors.

A hospital environment is full of sensory stimuli. When ill or hospitalized, a client is often confined to an unfamiliar and unresponsive environment. This does not mean that all hospitalized clients experience sensory overload. You must assess carefully those clients subjected to high stress levels (e.g., intensive care unit [ICU] environment, long-term hospitalization, and multiple therapies).

SENSORY STATUS.   The nursing history is a tool for assessing the nature and characteristics of sensory alterations. Assessment categories include the type and extent of sensory impairment, the onset and duration of symptoms, and whether there are factors that aggravate or relieve symptoms. Often you can observe such characteristics by watching the client perform routine activities of daily living in the home or health care setting. Table 35-1 provides examples of factors to assess and relevant questions to address with your client.

CLIENT'S LIFESTYLE.   You need to fully explore a client's perception of a sensory loss to find out how the client's quality of life has been influenced. Ask clients to describe any problems the sensory alteration creates for their normal daily routines and lifestyle. Does a sensory alteration change a client's ability to retain social relationships, continue performing at work or school, or function within the home?

SOCIALIZATION.   The amount and quality of contact with family members or significant others determines whether a client with sensory alterations becomes isolated. Assess if a client lives alone and whether family, friends, or neighbors frequently visit. The absence of visitors to a health care setting creates a sense of monotony that contributes to social isolation. Also assess the client's social skills and level of satisfaction in the support given by family and friends.

SELF-CARE MANAGEMENT.   A client's functional ability incorporates ADLs (e.g., grooming, bathing, and toileting) and instrumental activities of daily living (IADLs) (e.g., grocery shopping, writing a check, and using a phone). If a sensory alteration impairs a client's functional ability, planning for discharge from a health care setting and providing resources within the home become necessary. You need to consider the activities clients normally can do for themselves and how the sensory alteration impairs their functioning (see Table 35-1, p. 891).

PSYCHOSOCIAL ADJUSTMENT.   Because sensory changes can alter a client's behavior, family and friends are often the best resources for this information. The client may be unaware of or unwilling to discuss such changes. Assess if the client has shown any recent mood swings (e.g., outbursts of anger, depression, fear, or irritability). Sensory alterations may also cause changes in the client's orientation and ability to concentrate.

Example of a Focused Client Assessment		Table 35-1
Factors to Assess	**Questions and Approaches**	**Physical Assessment Strategies**
Sensory status	Ask if client has difficulty seeing, hearing, sensing touch, or maintaining balance. Ask when the difficulty started.	Assess client's vision, hearing, balance, and sense of touch. Observe client behaviors during conversation and while watching the client perform IADLs and ADLs. Observe home for factors that hinder or support vision changes.
Self-care management in home and community care settings	Ask if the client with a visual alteration can prepare a meal. Write a check? Ask if the client with decreased tactile sensation can button a shirt. A dress? Bathe safely using hot water?	Observe client in the home, in the kitchen while preparing a meal. Observe client during dressing and bathing.
Health promotion practices	Ask the client to explain how he or she practices ear/eye hygiene. Ask if the client has difficulty with routine care of glasses, hearing aids, contact lenses. Ask clients about activity/work where eye injuries are possible. Are they wearing safety glasses? Eye shields?	Find out when the client last had an eye or ear screening. Observe routine care. Check for appropriate eye protection.

HEALTH PROMOTION PRACTICES.   Assess the daily routines clients follow in maintaining sensory function. The information will determine the client's need for education or referral to appropriate resources (see Table 35-1).

HAZARDS.   The home environment should be healthy, comfortable, and safe. A thorough assessment of the home will help you provide options for ways to make the home safe. First assess the home setting for any hazards that increase the risk for injury (e.g., poorly lit stairs). A home safety checklist is usually available in most home care agencies. The type of sensory alteration makes certain home features more hazardous than others. Clients with visual problems will require more changes in lighting. Clients with hearing deficits may require safety alarms with visual signals.

In a health care setting, assess for any factors that can be dangerous to the client. A client's hospital room should be assessed for clutter, unnecessary equipment, and obstacles in the path leading to the bathroom. Also ask the client about barriers or obstacles the client perceives as potentially dangerous.

MEANINGFUL STIMULI.   Meaningful stimuli reduce the incidence of sensory deprivation. In the home, check for the use of bright colors, comfortable furnishings, adequate lighting, good ventilation, and clean surroundings. Also observe for presence of pets, family pictures, television, a clock, or calendar. In a health care setting, note if clients have roommates, visitors, or any personal items such as pictures. A client can become disoriented in a barren environment that gives few signals for normal sensory perception. Meaningful stimuli influence the client's alertness and the ability to participate in self-care.

ENVIRONMENT.   Excessive environmental stimuli can cause sensory overload. In an acute care setting, the frequency of observations, tests, and procedures may be stressful to the client. The location of a client's room near repetitive or loud noises (e.g., nurses' station or supply room) may contribute to sensory overload. In addition, a loud television or roommate or a bright room light should be explored as possible contributing factors. Clients who are in pain, traction, or restricted by a cast may also be at risk for excessive stimulation. Your responsibility as a nurse is to reduce or eliminate excessive stimuli.

COMMUNICATION METHODS.   To understand the quality of clients' communication, you must assess whether they have trouble speaking, understanding, reading, or writing. Clients with existing sensory deficits often develop alternative ways of communicating. A hearing-impaired client may read lips, use sign language, wear a hearing aid, or read and write notes. The visually impaired learn to detect voice tones and inflections to identify the emotional tone of a conversation. To assess communication methods, sit facing the client, speaking in a normal tone. Disorganized speech, long periods of silence, or a client who continually asks you to repeat your sentence indicates a sensory deficit in the client.

PHYSICAL EXAMINATION.   Clients with known or suspected sensory deficits resulting from visual and hearing losses, spinal cord injury, or peripheral neuropathies will require complete and detailed sensory examinations. Table 35-2 summarizes sensory deficits in adults and children and associated behavioral changes. If you suspect the client has a sensory deprivation, observation during history taking, physical examination, or care can provide information

Behaviors Indicating Sensory Deficits

Table 35-2

Behavior Indicating Deficit (Children)	Behavior Indicating Deficit (Adults)
Vision	
Self-stimulation, including eye rubbing, body rocking, sniffing, arm twirling; hitching (using legs to propel while in sitting position) instead of crawling	Poor coordination, squinting, underreaching or overreaching for objects, persistent repositioning of objects, impaired night vision, accidental falls
Hearing	
Frightened when unfamiliar people approach, no reflex or purposeful response to sounds, failure to be awakened by loud noise, slow or absent development of speech, greater response to movement than to sound, avoidance of social interaction with others	Blank looks, decreased attention span, lack of reaction to loud noises, increased volume of speech, positioning of head toward sound, smiling and nodding of head in approval when someone speaks, use of other means of communication such as lip reading or writing, complaints of ringing in ears
Touch	
Inability to perform developmental tasks related to grasping objects or drawing, repeated injury from handling of harmful objects (e.g., hot stove, sharp knife)	Clumsiness, overreaction or underreaction to painful stimulus, failure to respond when touched, avoidance of touch, sensation of pins and needles, numbness
Smell	
Difficult to assess until child is 6 or 7 years old, difficulty discriminating noxious odors	Failure to react to noxious or strong odors, increased body odor, decreased sensitivity to odors
Taste	
Inability to tell whether food is salty or sweet, possible ingestion of strange-tasting things	Change in appetite, excessive use of seasoning and sugar, complaints about taste of food, weight change
Position Sense	
Clumsiness, extraneous movement, excessive arm swinging in those with hyperactivity or learning difficulty	Poor balance and spatial orientation, shuffling gait, reduced response to brace self when falling, more precise and deliberate movements

 Case Study **SYNTHESIS IN PRACTICE**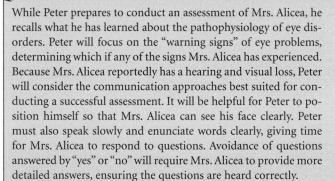

While Peter prepares to conduct an assessment of Mrs. Alicea, he recalls what he has learned about the pathophysiology of eye disorders. Peter will focus on the "warning signs" of eye problems, determining which if any of the signs Mrs. Alicea has experienced. Because Mrs. Alicea reportedly has a hearing and visual loss, Peter will consider the communication approaches best suited for conducting a successful assessment. It will be helpful for Peter to position himself so that Mrs. Alicea can see his face clearly. Peter must also speak slowly and enunciate words clearly, giving time for Mrs. Alicea to respond to questions. Avoidance of questions answered by "yes" or "no" will require Mrs. Alicea to provide more detailed answers, ensuring the questions are heard correctly.

Peter also recognizes the need to respect Mrs. Alicea's cultural background and to explore the role Rico plays in supporting his mother. Is Rico the primary individual who offers assistance with IADLs or other activities? Geissler's research (1999) on the Hispanic culture finds that the traditional clients of all socioeconomic and educational levels use biomedical and folk health systems. Family interdependence takes precedence over independence. Rico may play

a key role in Mrs. Alicea's ability to maintain self-care. Hispanic clients value health practitioners who are informal and friendly and who include family members in the interactions. Taking time to listen is also important. Giger and Davidhizar (1999) note that when being interviewed, Mexican-Americans may engage in "small talk" before discussing the serious aspect of the interview. Providing time for small talk will help you to gather a complete assessment. Finally, Mexican-Americans tend to use diplomacy and tactfulness when communicating with others. Self-disclosure is reserved for those whom the individual knows well. It will thus be important for Peter to spend time in conveying a sense of caring and respect for Mrs. Alicea to be successful with the assessment.

Peter's own grandmother has bilateral cataracts. Peter has witnessed how his grandmother has made adaptations around her home to continue activities she enjoys. Similarly, Peter has learned in class that a variety of adaptations can be made to maximize the sensory functions a client still has. Peter will plan to discover if Mrs. Alicea has made any adaptations in her home environment. Creativity will be an important attitude to exercise.

about the person's condition. Also observe the client's physical appearance and behavior, measure cognitive ability, and assess emotional stability. At this time, also remember that factors other than sensory deprivation or overload may cause impaired perception (e.g., medications, pain, or electrolyte imbalances).

CLIENT EXPECTATIONS. When conducting an assessment, review the client's expectations. Some clients enter the health care system willingly, whereas others experience confusion or unfamiliarity in that environment. Many clients have a definite plan as to how they want their care delivered. Clients may expect you to either perform care or provide

Nursing Diagnoses for

CLIENTS WITH SENSORY ALTERATIONS

Box 35-4

- Body image, disturbed
- Fear
- Hopelessness
- Injury, risk for
- Powerlessness
- Self-care deficit, bathing/ hygiene
- Self-care deficit, dressing/ grooming
- Self-esteem, risk for situational low
- Sensory/perception, disturbed
- Social interaction, impaired
- Social isolation
- Thought processes, disturbed

equipment for them so their sensory aids (glasses or hearing aids) can be properly cared for. Asking clients what they expect helps you to know if special communication methods are needed. Clients may request that family members or friends help with their care. You can begin by asking, "What do you expect from the nursing staff to feel you are being well cared for?" "Now that I better understand what affects your ability to see/hear, what do you expect in the care we will be providing you?"

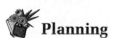

Nursing Diagnosis

After assessment, review all available data and look for patterns of defining characteristics that represent nursing diagnoses relating to sensory alterations (Box 35-4). For example, asking others to repeat spoken words, inappropriate response to questions, head tilting, social avoidance, irritability, ear pain, and withdrawal are defining characteristics for the nursing diagnosis *disturbed sensory perception: auditory* (Gulanick and others, 1998). Validate your findings by collaborating with a colleague or asking the client to self-rate his or her hearing on a scale of 1 to 10, 1 representing perfect hearing and 10 representing deafness.

Next determine the likely related factor for the nursing diagnosis to ensure appropriate interventions will be selected. For example, impacted cerumen can be the cause of the client's hearing alteration. In this case, regular ear canal irrigation can improve auditory perception (Wilson and Giddens, 2001). If the client's auditory alteration is related to hearing loss from nerve deafness, nursing interventions of alternative communication methods will be more successful in minimizing the client's hearing impairment.

Planning

The client's plan of care depends on your assessment of the client's perception and acceptance of the sensory alteration and how well the client has adjusted to the loss (see care plan).

GOALS AND OUTCOMES.   The client can work with you in adapting to the environment and remaining safe and productive if the plan includes clear goals and attainable out-

comes. Goals should not only meet the immediate needs of the client, but also strive towards rehabilitation. Some sensory alterations are short term, requiring only temporary interventions. Permanent sensory alterations require long-term goals, with a series of outcomes that can be reached over time. For example, if a client suffers an injury causing blindness, the long-term goal of "managing self-care within the home" will require numerous short-term outcomes and outcomes that require progressive advancement. Examples of outcomes include "Client will learn to ambulate within the home in 2 weeks" and "Client will perform ADLs within 4 weeks."

SETTING PRIORITIES.   After selecting nursing diagnoses and setting mutually agreed-upon goals and outcomes, work with the client in setting priorities. Generally you will rank diagnoses in order of importance based on the client's safety, personal desires, and needs. When setting priorities, safety is a top priority. However, the client may prefer to learn about ways to communicate more effectively or about adaptive methods that will enable participation in a favorite hobby. Sometimes the client needs to make major changes in the way self-care activities, communication, and socialization are performed.

CONTINUITY OF CARE.   Review all resources available to clients when you develop a plan of care. The family can play a key role in providing meaningful stimulation and learning ways to help a client adjust to any limitations once the client returns home. Hospitalized clients and their families are taught how to adapt interventions to their lifestyles. Clients should be encouraged to participate in family and social activities. Referral to resources such as occupational therapists, social service, and speech therapists ensures a multidisciplinary approach. Community resources such as the American Foundation for the Blind, American National Red Cross, Lions Club, and National Association for Speech and Hearing provide information to assist clients and family with discharge planning and potential home needs.

Implementation

Nursing interventions involve the client and family so that a safe, pleasant, and stimulating sensory environment can be maintained. Effective interventions help the client with sensory alterations to function safely with existing deficits and to continue a normal lifestyle.

HEALTH PROMOTION.   Good sensory function begins with prevention. When a client seeks health care, provide interventions that reduce risk for sensory losses.

SCREENING AND PREVENTION.   Children need appropriate visual screenings to prevent visual impairment (Wong and others, 1999). Three common interventions include screening women considering pregnancy for rubella and syphilis; advocating adequate prenatal care to prevent premature

Case Study Nursing Care Plan SENSORY ALTERATION

ASSESSMENT

Mrs. Alicea comes to the clinic reporting **"having trouble seeing,"** especially with **"having a hard time judging distances between objects, which seems worse at night."** Peter spends 20 minutes speaking with Mrs. Alicea and finds the client needs to have questions repeated several times. Mrs. Alicea **cannot judge steps clearly** and has also noticed **a sensitivity to glare.** In addition, when the client tries to read or sew, her **vision is blurred even with glasses.** On physical examination, Mrs. Alicea's corneas appear opaque and there is a **reduction in accommodation.** Her external auditory canals are free from cerumen. Motor function and peripheral sensation appear intact. Mrs. Alicea reports that it has been about 2 years since she has been to an eye doctor. Peter also speaks with Rico, Mrs. Alicea's son. Peter recalls the importance of inspecting the home of a client with a sensory alteration for safety hazards. Rico has made a safety environmental check but asks Peter for any tips he has, considering Mrs. Alicea's condition.

*Defining characteristics are shown in bold type.

NURSING DIAGNOSIS Risk for injury related to visual alterations from cataracts.

PLANNING

GOAL	EXPECTED OUTCOMES
Client's home environment is safe and free of hazards within 4 weeks.	Client will report a decreased difficulty with depth perception within 4 weeks.
	Client and son will make recommended changes to home environment within 4 weeks.

IMPLEMENTATION

STEPS	RATIONALE
1. Recommend son installs a nonglare work surface in the kitchen area.	Sensitivity to glare increases markedly because of the clouding of lens and vitreous that results in scattering of light that passes through the lens (Ebersole and Hess, 1998).
2. Explain use of a pocket magnifier, and offer list of locations where one can be purchased.	Magnifier can enlarge visual images when reading or doing close work.
3. Recommend son install incandescent lights in the home.	The intensity of lighting needs to be 3 times as powerful for older adults to produce the same results (Ebersole and Hess, 1998).
4. Have client make appointment with ophthalmologist within the next 4 weeks.	Older adults should have routine eye examination at least annually. Client is presenting symptoms of cataracts.
5. Teach son methods to improve environmental safety such as installation of handrails along stairs, securing carpeting, removal of throw rugs, and painting of stairs.	A decrease in visual acuity and depth perception can place the client at risk for falls in the presence of environmental hazards.

EVALUATION

- Have client describe positive changes in her vision.
- Have client describe perception of risk for accidents in the home.
- Ask client and son to discuss changes made in the home to reduce environmental hazards.

---

birth, which results in infants' being exposed to excessive oxygen during care; and periodic screening of all children for congenital blindness and visual impairment caused by **refractive errors** and strabismus. Children should also receive immunizations for rubella (see Chapter 10).

Nearsightedness is common during childhood. School nurses usually conduct routine vision testing of school-age and adolescent children. Your role as a nurse is one of detection, education, and referral. Parents need to know the signs of visual impairment (e.g., failure to react to light and reduced eye contact from the infant). Any signs should be reported to their health care provider.

Trauma is a common cause of blindness in children. Examples include injury from flying objects or penetrating wounds. Parents and children need to be educated on ways to avoid eye trauma (e.g., wearing safety devices and buying only "safe" toys). Safety equipment can be found in sport and department stores.

Adults need routine visual screenings. If left undetected and untreated, glaucoma can lead to permanent visual loss. The American Academy of Ophthalmology (2000) recommends regular medical eye examinations every 2 to 4 years for those over 40 years old. Clients 65 years and older need examinations every 1 to 2 years, especially those who are of African descent, have a family history of glaucoma, have a serious eye injury, or are taking steroid medications.

Adults are at risk for eye injury when playing sports and working in jobs involving exposure to chemicals or flying objects. The Occupational Safety and Health Administration (OSHA) has guidelines for workplace safety. Employers must have employees wear eye goggles and/or use equipment that reduces risk of injury. Nurses play a role in reinforcing eye safety.

In the United States hearing impairment is common. At-risk children include those with a family history of childhood hearing impairment, perinatal infection (rubella, herpes, or cytomegalovirus), low birth weight, chronic ear infection, and Down syndrome. Advise pregnant women to seek early prenatal care, avoid ototoxic drugs, and undergo testing for syphilis and rubella.

Chronic middle ear infections are a common cause of hearing impairment in children. These children need periodic auditory testing. Exposure to loud or high-intensity noise are risk factors for hearing loss. Advise both children and parents to take precautions and use earplugs or earphones to block high-decibel sound.

In adults guidelines for hearing screening are variable. If a client works or lives in a high noise level environment, an annual screening is recommended. The most important concept for adults to understand is hearing loss is not a natural part of aging. Once a client reports a hearing loss, regular testing becomes necessary.

USE OF ASSISTIVE AIDS.   Clients with sensory deficits often require use of assistive aids. Clients who wear corrective lenses, eyeglasses, or hearing aids should keep them accessible, functional, and clean (see Chapter 26). A family member or friend should also know how to clean these aids. Contact lens wearers are subject to serious eye infections, caused by infrequent lens disinfection, contamination of lens storage cases or contact lens solutions, and use of homemade saline. You need to reinforce proper lens care in any health maintenance discussions.

A wide variety of cosmetically acceptable hearing aids that enhance a person's hearing ability are currently available. Chapter 26 summarizes the care of hearing aids. A person who sees the need for good hearing will likely be influenced to wear hearing aids (Ebersole and Hess, 1998). You can give clients information on the benefits of hearing aid use. Family members or friends who support the use of the aid can improve client adherence. Wilson and Giddens (2001) warn that older persons who use hearing aids often do not use them in social situations because of the extraneous noise emitted or batteries that can become nonfunctional.

PROMOTING MEANINGFUL STIMULATION.   You can help clients make their environments more stimulating by considering the normal physiological changes that accompany sensory deficits (Box 35-5). When the client ages, the pupil loses the ability to adjust to light. This sensitivity to glare can be decreased by reducing the amount of bright light in the person's living environment. Cerumen impaction is a reversible cause of hearing loss in older adults. Impacted earwax can be softened and loosened with alternating instillation of glycerin (to soften) and hydrogen peroxide (to loosen) followed by irrigations of warm water (Phipps and others, 1999). Irrigation of the canal with tepid water in a 60-ml syringe will remove cerumen.

Some clients experience reduced tactile sensations in a limited portion of their body. Touch therapy helps to stimulate existing function. If the client is willing, your brushing and combing the client's hair, giving a back rub, and touching of the arms or shoulders increase tactile contact. Turning and positioning also improves the quality of tactile sensation.

Box 35-5

PROMOTING SENSORY STIMULATION
- Reduce glare by eliminating waxed floors and shiny surfaces exposed to bright sunlight, installing tinted glass or sheer curtains over large windows, and using soft and diffused lighting
- Teach use of assistive devices to improve visual acuity (e.g., pocket magnifiers, telescopic lens eyeglasses, large-print books, clocks, watches).
- Recommend introducing brighter colors (e.g., red, orange, yellow) into the home environment so that differentiations can be made in surfaces and room objects.
- Explain how to maximize hearing reception or minimize effects of hearing loss by increasing amplification on TVs or radios and using recorded music in low-frequency sound.
- Promote sense of taste through good oral hygiene, serving well-seasoned and differently textured foods, avoiding blending or mixing foods, and chewing food thoroughly.
- Enhance the sense of smell by removing unpleasant odors from the environment and introducing pleasant smells such as mild room deodorizers or fragrant flowers.

CREATING A SAFE ENVIRONMENT.   Clients become less secure within their home and workplace when they have a sensory alteration. An actual or potential sensory loss determines the type of safety precautions necessary. Security is necessary for a person to feel independent. You can make recommendations for improving safety within a client's living environment without restricting the client's independence. Be sure the client participates in choosing any changes to be made in the home.

Visual Adaptations.   When a client experiences a decrease in visual acuity, peripheral vision, adaptation to the dark, or depth perception, safety is a concern. With reduced peripheral vision a client cannot see panoramically. Older adults with reduced adaptation to the dark require 3 times as much light to see objects (Ebersole and Hess, 1998). With reduced depth perception, a person cannot judge how far away objects are located. The home safety assessment helps you identify hazards in the client's living environment. Clutter such as footstools or electrical cords should be removed. Furniture needs to be arranged so that a client can move about easily without fear of tripping or running into objects. All flooring should be kept in good repair, and throw rugs should be removed. Stairwells should be well lighted and have securely fastened handrails extending the full length of the stairs.

Front and back entrances to the home and work areas need good lighting. Light fixtures need high wattage bulbs with wider illumination. A light switch located at the top and bottom of stairwells adds an additional safety element. Fluorescent lighting should be replaced with incandescent lights.

Driving can be a safety hazard for older adults. A sensitivity to glare creates a problem for driving at night with headlights. Reduced peripheral vision may prevent a driver from seeing cars in the next lane. Reduced vision, complicated by a decrease in reaction time, reduced hearing, and decreased strength in the legs and arms, can seriously limit an older adult's driving skills. To minimize clients' risk, encourage them to drive only in familiar areas and not during rush hour. Urge clients to drive defensively and to avoid driving at night or at dusk. Older adults should drive slowly but not so slowly that they create a safety problem for other drivers.

Clients may have problems seeing dials or controls on electrical appliances and equipment when they cannot contrast colors. Color contrasts (e.g., tape, paint, or nail enamel) can be used to highlight dials. You can tour the client's home to find opportunities for color coding.

Hearing Adaptations. Individuals need to hear environmental sounds such as fire alarms, alarm clocks, phones, or doorbells. The sound of these devices can be amplified or changed to a more low-pitched, buzzerlike quality. Signaling devices, such as a flashing light on a phone, allow the hearing impaired greater independence. Sound lamps that respond with light to the sounds of babies crying, smoke detectors, and burglar alarms are also available. Advise family and friends who call the client regularly to let the phone ring for a longer period.

Smell and Tactile Adaptations. The client with a reduced sensitivity to odors may be unable to smell leaking gas, a smoldering cigarette, fire, or tainted food. The client should use smoke detectors and take precautions such as checking ashtrays or placing cigarette butts in water. Also advise the client to check food package dates and inspect the appearance of food. Clients with reduced tactile sensation need to use water bottles or heating pads cautiously and never use the high setting. The temperature on the home water heater should be no higher than 120° F.

COMMUNICATION. Individuals need to interact with people around them. The type of sensory loss influences the methods and styles of communication you use during interactions with clients. A client with a hearing impairment may be able to speak normally. To more clearly hear what a person communicates, family and friends may need to learn to move away from background noise, rephrase rather than repeat sentences, be positive, and have patience. On the other hand, a deaf client can have serious speech alterations. Deaf clients may use sign language, use lip reading, write with pad and pencil, or learn to use a computer for communication (Box 35-6).

Effective client education depends on clear communication. Large-print teaching booklets are available for the visually impaired. A blind client may require more frequent and detailed verbal explanations. The visually impaired can also learn by listening to audiotapes or by reading booklets printed in Braille. Clients with hearing impairment may benefit from written instructional materials and visual teaching aids (e.g., posters and graphs). Your demonstrations can also be helpful.

ACUTE CARE. Some clients are admitted for the therapeutic management of sensory deficits (e.g., acute eye infection) and some have preexisting sensory problems. You need to know the client's health history to appropriately support self-care activities while promoting a safe environment.

ORIENTATION TO THE ENVIRONMENT. It is important to completely orient clients with sensory impairments to a care setting. Always keep your name tag visible, address the client by name, explain the client's location, and frequently include the time and date in conversations. Repeating explanations in short and simple terms helps to reduce confusion. You can encourage family and friends not to argue with or contradict a confused client but to explain calmly their location, identify, and time of day.

Clients with serious visual impairments must feel comfortable in knowing the boundaries of their environment. The client needs to walk through a room and feel the walls to establish a sense of direction. Remember to approach the blind client from the front. Explain the location of objects within the room, such as chairs or equipment. It is important to keep all objects in the same place and position. Moving an object, even a short distance can create a safety hazard. You may need to reorient the client frequently by describing the location of key items. Necessary objects such as the call light, patient-controlled analgesia (PCA) button,

---

Communication Methods for the Hearing Impaired — Box 35-6

Get the client's attention. Do not startle the client when entering the room. Approach a client from the front. Be sure the client knows you wish to speak.

Face the client, and stand or sit on the same level. Be sure your face and lips are illuminated to promote lip reading. Avoid glare and shadows. Do not speak with something in your mouth. Keep your hands away from your mouth.

If the client wears glasses, be sure they are clean so that your gestures and face can be seen. If the client wears a hearing aid, make sure it is in place and working.

Speak slowly and articulate clearly. Older adults may take longer to process verbal messages. Use a normal tone of voice and inflections of speech.

Avoid eating, chewing, or smoking while speaking.

When you are not understood, rephrase rather than repeat the conversation.

Use visible expressions. Speak with your hands, your face, and your eyes.

Do not shout. Loud sounds are usually higher pitched and may impede hearing by accentuating vowel sounds and concealing consonants. If speaking loudly is necessary, speak in lower tones.

Talk toward the client's best or normal ear.

Avoid speaking from another room or while walking away. Reduce or eliminate background noise.

Use written information to enhance the spoken word.

Do not restrict a deaf client's hands. Never have intravenous lines in both of the client's hands if the preferred method of communication is sign language.

glasses, water, or facial tissue should be placed in front of clients to prevent falls caused by reaching. A night-light in the bathroom can help reduce falls by decreasing the time required for the eyes to adapt to the dark. You may also ask the client how to arrange objects so ambulation can be easier. Remove clutter and unnecessary equipment. Always keep the path to the bathroom clear.

SAFETY MEASURES.   To ensure the safety of clients with an acute visual impairment, you may need to help them with walking. Stand at the client's nondominant side, approximately one step in front, as you describe the course of movement (Figure 35-1). The client uses the nondominant hand to grasp your elbow or upper arm. You then walk one-half step ahead and slightly to the client's side. The client's shoulder should be directly behind your shoulder. Relax and walk at a comfortable pace. Warn the client when approaching doorways or narrow spaces. A client with visual impairment should not be left alone in an unfamiliar area.

A client with a hearing impairment may have difficulty hearing typical hospital sounds such as an intravenous pump alarm, nurse intercom system, or nurse instructions. Always visit the client's bedside more frequently. Never restrict both arms of deaf or hearing-impaired clients with intravenous lines or restraints. Always alert the entire multidisciplinary team when a client has a sensory alteration.

CONTROLLING SENSORY STIMULI.   You can reduce sensory overload by organizing the client's care to control for excessive stimuli. Combining activities such as dressing changes, bathing, and vital sign assessment in one visit prevents the client from becoming overly fatigued. Coordination with other departments can reduce the time needed for tests and examinations. The client needs time for rest and quiet. Routine nursing procedures should be performed as quietly as possible. Encourage a family member to sit quietly with a client or involve the client in an undemanding repetitive activity such as combing hair.

Try to control extraneous noise in and around a client's room, such as television volume and visitors. Bedside equipment not in use should be turned off. Close the client's room door if necessary. Hospital staff need to control loud laughter or conversation at the nurses' station. In addition to controlling excess stimuli, try to introduce meaningful stimulation (Box 35-7) that makes the environment pleasing and comfortable.

RESTORATIVE AND CONTINUING CARE.   After clients have experienced a sensory loss, they need to make adjustments to continue a normal lifestyle. Many of the interventions previously discussed under health promotion can be adapted in the home setting. The home environment should be healthy, comfortable, and safe. You may need to suggest changes in a person's home environment after you assess the home setting for any hazards that increase the risk for injury.

PROMOTING SELF-CARE.   Clients who have had surgery related to a sensory deficit need a plan of care that allows them to return safely to their home environment. Most clients have same-day surgical procedures (see Chapter 36). Family members or friends need to understand how the client's sensory impairment will affect the ability to perform normal ADLs and IADLs and the factors that lessen or worsen sensory problems. Community resources discussed in the planning section can be useful.

Sensorially impaired clients can continue independent self-care activities. In the case of eating meals, you can

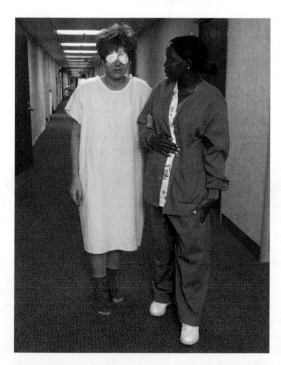

FIGURE **35-1**   Nurse assists visually impaired client with ambulation.

Introducing Stimuli Into the Care Setting   Box 35-7

VISUAL
Open the drapes to the client's room.
Raise the head of the bed, and draw back dividing curtains or partitions.
Provide attractive decorations on tables or cabinets, such as fresh flowers, plants, a picture, or greeting cards.
Provide talking books and large-print reading material.

AUDITORY
Sit down and speak with the client. Make the conversation meaningful.
Turn on a radio with the type of music the client enjoys.
A favorite radio or television program can be stimulating.

TASTE AND SMELL
Provide attractive, taste-appealing meals. Be sure tableware and glasses are clean. Foods meant to be served warm should be warm, and cold foods should be cold.
Provide a variety of textures, aromas, and flavors to enhance the client's appetite.

arrange food on the plate and condiments, salad, or drinks around the plate according to numbers on the face of a clock (Figure 35-2). The client can become oriented to the items after the family member explains each item's location. Clients may need assistance in arranging self-care items, such as clothing, hygiene, food supplies, and utensils in a consistent location to continue managing daily care activities.

The visually impaired client may also need assistance in reaching the bathroom safely. Safety bars need to be installed near the toilet. A bar that is a different color from the wall is easier to see. Towels should never be placed on safety bars to interfere with a person's grasp.

If tactile sense is decreased, the client can dress more easily with zippers or Velcro strips, pullover sweaters or blouses, and elasticized waists. If the client has a partial paralysis, the affected side should be dressed first. A client may also need assistance with basic grooming such as brushing, combing, shaving, and shampooing hair.

SOCIALIZATION.   Interacting with others can be difficult for many clients. A client with a hearing loss can become embarrassed and exhausted after asking people to continuously repeat what they say. Clients often lose the motivation to engage in social activities and withdraw from interaction. You can introduce therapies to reduce loneliness, particularly for older adult clients (Box 35-8). Family members must learn to focus on a person's ability rather than his or her disability. You should never assume that a hearing impaired person does not wish to speak.

Evaluation

CLIENT CARE.   It is important to evaluate whether care measures maintain or improve a client's ability to interact and function within the environment. Adapt evaluation measures to determine whether actual outcomes are the same as expected outcomes (Box 35-9). Be sure a client with a hearing deficit can hear your questions about responses to treatment. When expected outcomes have not been achieved, there may be a need to change interventions or add new ones.

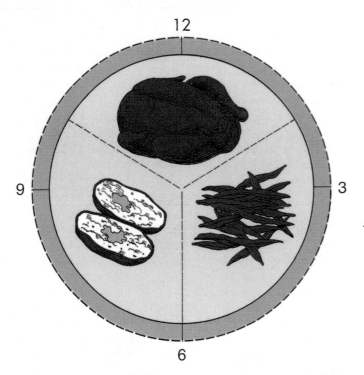

FIGURE **35-2**   Arrange food on a plate and orient client to placement based on numbers on a clock face.

Gerontological Nursing Practice   Box 35-8

- Recommend alterations in living arrangements if physical isolation is a factor.
- Give older adults extra time to communicate.
- Assist clients in keeping contact with people important to them.
- Encourage and facilitate some socialization (Ebersole and Hess, 1998).
- Help clients acquire information about mutual help groups.
- Arrange for security escort services as needed.
- Link clients with religious organizations attuned to the social needs of older adults.
- Bring a pet into the home.

Outcome Evaluation for MRS. ALICEA   Box 35-9

Nursing Action	Client Response/Finding	Achievement of Outcome
Ask Mrs. Alicea to describe her ability to see the edge of stairs and to discern other objects in the distance. Have her read a portion of the newspaper.	Mrs. Alicea states she is able to see objects in the distance a bit more clearly and feels less hesitant to ambulate through hallways of home. She is using pocket magnifier less often for near objects.	Outcome met.
Ask Mrs. Alicea if she visited ophthalmologist.	She visited ophthalmologist; new eyeglass prescription was written.	Outcome met. Encourage annual eye examinations in the future.
Observe Mrs. Alicea walk through home and down stairs.	She is able to walk with steady, purposeful gait.	Outcome met.
Conduct a home visit, and reassess the home environment.	Son has changed all lightbulbs and removed all throw rugs. He also painted edges of stairs and installed handrails to the downstairs.	Home environment has improved. Recommend that son change the work surface in the kitchen.

Case Study EVALUATION

One month has passed since Mrs. Alicea's last visit to the senior health care center. Today Peter sits down and talks with both the client and her son Rico. He learns that Mrs. Alicea is no longer having difficulty with glare because Rico changed the lights in the house to incandescent bulbs. Rico also reports that he plans to install some sheer curtains Mrs. Alicea chose last week, to hang over the large window in the living room. Mrs. Alicea also tells Peter that Rico has made a "few changes around the house," including rearranging furniture, securing the rugs, installing a handrail to the basement, and removing extension cords. After purchasing a magnifier at a local drug store, Mrs. Alicea is able to read the newspaper more easily.

On examination, Mrs. Alicea's visual acuity continues to reveal blurring when she tried to read an informational pamphlet. Her pupils continue to respond slowly to accommodation. Peter in-quires as to whether Mrs. Alicea has made an appointment with her ophthalmologist. She confirms that the appointment is scheduled within the next 2 weeks.

Overall, Mrs. Alicea confides, "I think I have been helped with the ideas we talked about last time. I feel a little better about getting around the house and doing the things I like to do." When asked if he has noticed any changes in his mother's actions, Rico states, "She seems less fearful of possibly falling."

Documentation Note

Client visited clinic this morning as scheduled. Has implemented measures at home to improve her visual acuity and sensitivity to glare. Son has been very supportive in making necessary home environment changes and plans to make additional ones. Client has set an appointment with ophthalmologist within next 2 weeks.

If nursing care has been directed at improving or maintaining sensory acuity, evaluate the integrity of the sensory organs and the client's ability to perceive stimuli. This may involve a simple vision or hearing assessment by asking the client to perform a self-care skill. When client teaching is done to improve a client's sensory function, you need to know if the client is following recommended therapies. Asking the client to explain or demonstrate a newly learned self-care skill is an effective evaluative measure.

CLIENT EXPECTATIONS.   It is important to learn if clients think they are receiving appropriate care. A sensory deficit can be embarrassing and threaten a person's self-image. Does the client feel comfortable relating to you? Was the client able to maintain a plan of care for assistive devices? Did the client think you were exhibiting a caring, professional approach? Asking clients if nursing care successfully met their expectations will provide valuable knowledge when you care for other clients with similar sensory problems.

Key Terms

auditory, *p. 887*
gustatory, *p. 887*
olfactory, *p. 887*

ototoxic, *p. 888*
proprioception, *p. 887*
refractive errors, *p. 894*
sensory deficits, *p. 887*
sensory deprivation, *p. 887*

sensory overload, *p. 887*
tactile, *p. 887*
visual, *p. 887*

Key Concepts

- Sensory perception depends on a region in the cerebral cortex where specialized brain cells interpret the quality and nature of sensory stimuli.
- Because a client learns to rely on unaffected senses after a sensory loss, you design interventions to preserve function of these senses.
- Sensory deprivation results from an inadequate quality or quantity of sensory stimuli.
- Aging results in a gradual decline of acuity in all senses.
- Environmental stimuli in a hospital, such as an intensive care unit, place a client at risk for sensory overload.
- The extent of support from family members and significant others can influence the quality of sensory experiences.
- Assessment of sensory function includes a physical examination and measurement of functional abilities.
- The presence of cerumen in the external auditory canal is a common cause of hearing loss in older adults.

- A client's self-rating of hearing is an important defining characteristic for disturbed sensory perception (auditory).
- Sensory losses can create loneliness and impair the ability to socialize.
- An assessment of environment includes identifying hazards, sources of meaningful stimulation, and the amount of stimuli.
- Prenatal screening and childhood immunizations are critical in preventing sensory alterations in the newborn and child.
- The care plan for clients with sensory alterations should include participation by family members.
- Clients with visual impairments must learn boundaries within the environment to ambulate safely.
- Clients with existing hearing deficits can learn alternative ways to communicate.
- Nursing care for clients with sensory alterations includes using stronger sensory stimuli, compensating with other senses, and modifying the environment to maximize remaining sensory function.

Continued

Key Concepts —cont'd

- To prevent sensory overload you control stimuli, orient the client to the environment, and promote rest by minimizing interruptions.

- Medications, electrolyte imbalance, or pain may also contribute to a sensory deprivation or overload.
- Safety is a top concern when setting priorities for clients who experience sensory deprivation.

Critical Thinking Activities

1. Mrs. Wilson, 72 years of age, attends the clinic for regular checkups every 6 months. During a routine conversation, she states, "I am not seeing as well these days." Discuss three symptoms clients experience with aging. What strategies can you use to assist Mrs. Wilson to see better?

2. Mr. Thomas is a 72-year-old client who exhibits a blank, dull affect; a hesitancy to communicate; and a tendency to speak loudly when spoken to. Physical examination should be focused on what potential problem area for this client?

3. Mrs. Tillis lives in a two-room apartment on the second floor. During your home visit you notice there is a single light over the stairwell. The client's apartment is painted in a dull gray, with throw rugs throughout. Mrs. Tillis is 80 years of age and lives alone. What recommendations might you make to improve the safety of Mrs. Tillis's environment?

4. An eighth-grade teacher reports to you, the school nurse, that 13-year-old Sarah has been having difficulty following simple directions with homework assignments and seems disinterested when assigned to surf the web for in-class assignments. In the school health care clinic you identify that Sarah has decreased visual acuity. What nursing actions are important to assure her safety?

Review Questions

1. Based on an understanding of physiology, normal physiological changes the older adult client experiences include:
   1. decreased sensitivity to glare.
   2. increased number of taste buds.
   3. increased peripheral neuropathy.
   4. difficulty discriminating vowel sounds.

2. When assessing a client whose regimen includes use of nonsteroidal antiinflammatory drugs (NSAIDs), you should be aware that a common side effect includes:
   1. ototoxicity.
   2. loss of taste.
   3. optic irritation.
   4. alteration in perception.

3. For a hearing-impaired client to better hear a spoken conversation, you should:
   1. approach a client quietly from behind.
   2. use a louder than normal tone of voice.
   3. select a public area to have a spoken conversation.
   4. use your hands and eyes as visual aids while speaking.

4. When obtaining a history of the client's hearing loss, you should ask:
   1. How long have you been deaf?
   2. Do you also have vision problems?
   3. Why don't you pay attention to me while I speak?
   4. How does your hearing loss compare to a year ago?

5. A confused hospitalized patient is disoriented. An intervention to properly introduce stimuli would be to:
   1. keep the room darkened.
   2. introduce an all-talk radio program.
   3. speak with the client in muted tones.
   4. draw back dividing curtains or partitions.

6. You are caring for an older adult hearing- and vision-impaired client in a nursing home. The assessment data that best indicates signs of sensory deprivation include:
   1. diminished anxiety.
   2. altered spatial perception.
   3. improved completion of tasks.
   4. decreased need for physical stimulation.

7. When you are performing a home assessment, the observation that would be most significant for the safety of a client with peripheral neuropathy includes:
   1. cluttered walkways.
   2. absence of smoke detectors.
   3. lack of bathroom safety bars.
   4. improper water heater setting.

8. A realistic goal for an older adult driving client is:
   1. drive very, very slowly all of the time.
   2. keep the car in good working condition.
   3. always drive at night to prevent sun glare.
   4. drive during rush hours when others are on the road.

9. Because hearing impairment is one of the most common disabilities among children, an intervention you teach parents is to:
   1. avoid activities in which crowds and loud noises occur.
   2. delay childhood immunizations until hearing can be verified.
   3. take precautions when involved in activities associated with high-intensity noises.
   4. prophylactically administer antibiotics to reduce the incidence of infections.

10. During a home visit you notice that your client's environment is poorly illuminated. An intervention you will make includes:
    1. using fluorescent lightening.
    2. recommending muted colors.
    3. doubling the amount of light fixtures throughout the house.
    4. placing incandescent, higher wattage lightbulbs into light fixtures.

11. A high-priority home assessment for a client with diminished olfaction is the inclusion of:
    1. low water heater setting.
    2. extra lighting in hallways.
    3. smoke detectors on all levels.
    4. amplified telephone receivers.

12. Sensory deficits happen when a problem with sensory reception or perception occurs. As a result clients may:
    1. rely solely on one sense.
    2. respond normally to stimuli.
    3. withdraw socially to cope with the loss.
    4. function safely within their environment.

13. When assessing for the effects of a sensory deprivation, you should be aware that the client will demonstrate:
    1. calm demeanor.
    2. normal behavior.
    3. diminished level of anxiety.
    4. difficulty with problem solving.

References

American Academy of Ophthalmology: *Comprehensive adult medical eye evaluation,* San Francisco, 2000, American Academy of Ophthalmology.

American Association of Retired Persons: *A profile of older Americans,* Washington, DC, 1998, The Association.

Ebersole P, Hess P: *Toward healthy aging,* ed 5, St. Louis, 1998, Mosby.

Geissler E: *Pocket guide to cultural assessment,* ed 2, St. Louis, 1999, Mosby.

Giger JN, Davidhizar RE: *Transcultural nursing: assessment and intervention,* ed 3, St. Louis, 1999, Mosby.

Gulanick M and others: *Nursing care plans: nursing diagnosis and interventions,* ed 4, St. Louis, 1998.

Lilley LL, Auker R: *Pharmacology and the nursing process,* ed 3, St. Louis, 2001, Mosby.

Lueckenotte A: *Gerontologic nursing,* ed 2, St. Louis, 2000, Mosby.

Jones B: Integrating hearing loss was a complex and dynamic process for patients (a commentary on Herth K: Integrating hearing loss into one's life, *Qual Health Res* 8(2):207, 1998, *Evid Based Nurs* 1(4):131, 1998.

Phipps W and others: *Medical-surgical concepts and clinical practice,* ed 6, St. Louis, 1999, Mosby.

Wilson S, Giddens J: *Health assessments for nursing practice,* ed 2, St. Louis, 2001, Mosby.

Wong DL and others: *Whaley and Wong's nursing care of infants and children,* ed 6, St. Louis, 1999, Mosby.

36

Surgical Client

Objectives

- Define key terms.
- Explain the concept of perioperative nursing care.
- Differentiate among classifications of surgery and types of anesthesia.
- List factors to include in the preoperative assessment of a surgical client.
- Design a preoperative teaching plan.
- Prepare a client for surgery.
- Explain the differences in caring for the client undergoing outpatient surgery versus the client undergoing inpatient surgery.
- Describe intraoperative factors that can affect a client's postoperative course.
- Identify factors to include in the assessment of a client in postoperative recovery.
- Describe the rationale for nursing interventions designed to prevent postoperative complications.

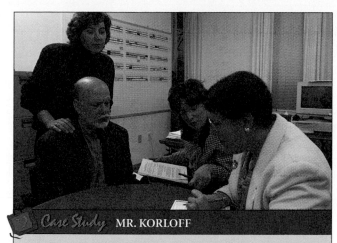

Case Study **MR. KORLOFF**

Mr. Korloff is a 53-year-old man who has been experiencing abdominal pain for 2 months. Following a series of diagnostic tests, he is now scheduled for an elective laparoscopic cholecystectomy. Mr. Korloff is originally from Russia and has lived in the United States for 20 years. He speaks English quite well but still has a Russian accent. He is a vice president for an international business firm. He is widowed and has two adult daughters, both of whom were born in Russia before coming to the United States. The daughters are married and live in the same neighborhood as Mr. Korloff.

Sue Collins is a nursing student assigned to the preadmission center at the local hospital where she has been working for 2 weeks. She is completing her last clinical rotation and will be graduating in 1 month. Sue is 30 years old, is married, and has no children. She plans to seek employment in a hospital on a general surgery floor after graduation. Sue's father recently had surgery for prostate cancer.

*T*his chapter synthesizes many concepts and skills previously presented in this text. You should recognize these previously learned areas and be able to apply this information to the surgical client in the preoperative and postoperative phases.

Perioperative nursing care includes nursing care given before (preoperative), during (intraoperative), and after (postoperative) surgery. Today surgery is performed in a variety of settings, including hospitals, ambulatory surgery centers, clinics, physicians' offices, and even mobile units. Minor surgeries are performed on an **outpatient** basis, with the client entering the setting, undergoing surgery, and being discharged the same day. Most clients undergoing major surgery enter the setting as outpatients for preoperative screening and testing and are admitted to the hospital after surgery. Only clients requiring extensive preoperative care are admitted to the hospital before surgery. You must understand the principles of caring for perioperative clients regardless of the setting in which you find them.

▮ SCIENTIFIC KNOWLEDGE BASE

Classification of Surgery

Surgical procedures are classified according to the seriousness, urgency, and purpose of surgery (Table 36-1). For example, a breast biopsy, done for diagnostic purposes, would be classified as urgent and done on an outpatient basis. Knowing the classification will help you to plan appropriate preoperative and postoperative care for each client.

Surgical Risk Factors

Knowledge regarding the physiology of stress (see Chapter 21) and risk factors that may affect how a client responds to the stress of surgery is necessary to anticipate client needs for preoperative preparation, teaching, and postoperative care. A study by Brooks-Brunn (1997) identified six risk factors that have a significant association with postoperative pulmonary complications, specifically pneumonia and **atelectasis.** These factors include the following: age 60 years or older, impaired preoperative cognitive function, smoking history within the past 8 weeks, body mass index of 27 or greater indicating obesity, history of cancer, and a midline abdominal incision site that is either above the umbilicus or both above and below the umbilicus.

AGE. Very young and older clients are at greater surgical risk as a result of an immature or a declining physiological status. Maintaining the client's normal body temperature is a concern during surgery. When compared with an adult, an infant has a proportionately greater surface area and less subcutaneous fat, placing these clients at risk for wide temperature variations. In addition, general anesthetics can inhibit shivering, a protective reflex to maintain body temperature, and can cause vasodilation, which results in heat loss. During surgery an infant also has difficulty in maintaining a normal circulatory blood volume. The total blood volume of infants is considerably less than that of older children and adults, creating a risk for both dehydration and overhydration. With advancing age a client's physical capacity to adapt to the stress of surgery is hampered because of deterioration of certain body functions. Table 36-2 summarizes physiological factors that place older adult clients at risk for surgery.

NUTRITION. Normal tissue repair and resistance to infection depend on adequate nutrition. Surgery intensifies the need for nutrients. Postoperatively a client requires at least 1500 kilocalories per day to maintain energy reserves. Additional protein, carbohydrates, zinc, and vitamins A, B, C, and K are needed for proper wound healing (see Chapters 30 and 34). A malnourished client is prone to poor tolerance of anesthesia, negative nitrogen balance, delayed blood-clotting mechanisms, infection, poor wound healing, and the potential for multiple organ failure after surgery (Fortunato, 2000).

OBESITY. An obese client usually has reduced ventilatory capacity because of upward pressure against the diaphragm by an enlarged abdomen. The recumbent and supine positions required on the **operating bed** (table) for surgery may further limit the obese client's ventilation. Cardiovascular function is often compromised because of the increased workload of the heart and atherosclerotic blood vessels. Because of these physiological changes, obese clients often have difficulty in resuming normal physical activity after surgery. Hypertension, coronary artery disease, type 2 dia-

Classification for Surgical Procedures

Table 36-1

Type	Description	Example
Seriousness		
Major	Involves extensive reconstruction or alteration in body parts; poses great risks to well-being	Coronary artery bypass, colon resection, removal of larynx, resection of lung lobe
Minor	Involves minimal alteration in body parts; often designed to correct deformities; involves minimal risks compared with major procedures	Cataract extraction, facial plastic surgery, skin graft, tooth extraction
Urgency		
Elective	Performed on basis of client's choice; not essential and may not be necessary for health	Bunionectomy, facial plastic surgery, hernia repair, breast reconstruction
Urgent	Necessary for client's health, may prevent additional problems from developing (e.g., tissue destruction, impaired organ function); not necessarily emergency	Excision of cancerous tumor, removal of gallbladder for stones, vascular repair for obstructed artery (e.g., coronary artery bypass)
Emergency	Must be done immediately to save life or preserve function of body part	Repair of perforated appendix, repair of traumatic amputation, control of internal hemorrhaging
Purpose		
Diagnostic	Surgical exploration that allows physician to confirm diagnosis; may involve removal of tissue for further diagnostic testing	Exploratory laparotomy (incision into peritoneal cavity to inspect abdominal organs), breast mass biopsy
Ablative	Excision or removal of diseased body part	Amputation, removal of appendix, cholecystectomy
Palliative	Relieves or reduces intensity of disease symptoms; will not produce cure	Colostomy, debridement of necrotic tissue, resection of nerve roots
Reconstructive/restorative	Restores function or appearance to traumatized or malfunctioning tissues	Internal fixation of fractures, scar revision
Procurement for transplant	Removal of organs and/or tissues from a person pronounced brain dead for transplantation into another person	Kidney, cornea, or liver transplant
Constructive	Restores function lost or reduced as result of congenital anomalies	Repair of cleft palate, closure of atrial septal defect in heart
Cosmetic	Performed to improve personal appearance	Blepharoplasty to correct eyelid deformities; rhinoplasty to reshape nose

betes mellitus, and congestive heart failure are common in this population. Obese clients also develop **embolism,** atelectasis, and pneumonia more frequently postoperatively than nonobese clients (Brooks-Brunn, 1997).

In addition, excess weight placed on skin over bony prominences may restrict blood flow and result in skin impairment. The obese client is susceptible to poor wound healing and wound infection because fatty tissue contains a poor blood supply and slows the delivery of essential nutrients and antibodies needed for healing. It is often difficult to close the surgical wound of an obese client because of the thick adipose layer. The risk for **dehiscence** and **evisceration** is increased because of these factors (see Chapter 34).

IMMUNOCOMPETENCE.   The client with cancer may often undergo radiotherapy before surgery to reduce the size of the cancerous tumor so it can be removed surgically. Radiation causes fibrosis and vascular scarring in the radiated area. This causes tissues to become fragile and poorly oxygenated. Ideally surgery is delayed 4 to 6 weeks after the completion of radiation treatments to avoid wound-healing problems. Radiation and chemotherapeutic drugs used for cancer therapy, immunosuppressive agents used to prevent rejection after organ transplantation, and steroids such as

prednisone used to treat a variety of inflammatory conditions all render the body vulnerable to infection.

FLUID AND ELECTROLYTE BALANCE.   The body responds to surgery as a form of trauma. As a result of the adrenocortical stress response, hormonal reactions cause sodium and water retention and potassium loss within the first 2 to 5 days after surgery. Severe protein breakdown creates a negative nitrogen balance. The severity of the stress response influences the degree of fluid and electrolyte imbalance. The more extensive the surgery, the more severe is the physiological stress. Clients with preexisting renal, gastrointestinal, respiratory, or cardiovascular problems are at greatest risk for operative complications. For example, a client who is dehydrated from vomiting preoperatively is at greater risk for hypovolemic shock (see Chapter 14).

PREGNANCY.   When dealing with a pregnant client, be prepared to consider the needs of both the pregnant woman and her unborn fetus. For this reason surgery is only considered for urgent or emergent reasons, such as appendicitis or trauma. The gravid uterus displaces abdominal organs and distorts landmarks, making surgery more complex.

Anesthetics and medication may cause fetal abnormalities during the first trimester. During pregnancy the following

Physiological Factors That Place the Older Adult at Risk During Surgery   Table 36-2

Alterations	Risks	Nursing Implications
Cardiovascular System		
Degeneration of myocardium and valves	Change reduces cardiac reserve.	Assess baseline vital signs.
Rigid arteries and reduction in sympathetic and parasympathetic innervation to heart	Alterations predispose client to postoperative hemorrhage and hypertension.	Instruct client in techniques for performing leg exercises and proper turning.
Increase in calcium and cholesterol deposits within small arteries; thickened arterial walls	Problems predispose client to clot formation in lower extremities.	Apply elastic stockings; sequential compression devices (SCDs).
Integumentary System		
Decreased subcutaneous tissue and increased fragility of skin	Client is prone to pressure ulcers and tears.	Assess skin every 2 hr or more often; pad all bony prominences during surgery. Turn or reposition.
Pulmonary System		
Rib cage stiffened and reduced in size	Complication reduces vital capacity.	Instruct client in proper technique for coughing, deep breathing, and use of spirometers.
Reduced range of movement in diaphragm	Greater residual capacity or volume of air left in lung after normal breath, reducing amount of new air brought into lungs with each inspiration.	When possible, have client ambulate and sit in chair frequently.
Stiffened lung tissue and enlarged air spaces	Alteration reduces blood oxygenation.	
Renal System		
Reduced blood flow to kidneys	Reduced flow increases danger of shock when blood loss occurs.	For clients hospitalized before surgery, determine baseline urinary output for 24 hr.
Reduced glomerular filtration rate and excretory times	Problem limits ability to eliminate drugs or toxic substances.	
Reduced bladder capacity	Voiding frequency increases, and larger amount of urine stays in bladder after voiding.	Instruct client to notify nurse immediately when sensation of bladder fullness develops.
	Sensation of need to void may not occur until bladder is filled.	Keep call light and bedpan within easy reach.
Neurological System		
Sensory losses, including reduced tactile sense and increased pain tolerance	Client is less able to respond to early warning signs of surgical complications.	Orient client to surrounding environment. Observe for nonverbal signs of pain.
Decreased reaction time	Client becomes easily confused after anesthesia.	
Metabolic System		
Reduced number of red blood cells and hemoglobin levels	Ability to carry adequate oxygen to tissues is reduced.	Administer necessary blood products. Monitor blood test results.
Change in total amounts of body potassium and water volume	Greater risk for fluid or electrolyte imbalance occurs.	Monitor electrolyte levels.

maternal physiological changes occur that make monitoring this surgical client very difficult (Fortunato, 2000):

1. Cardiac output and respiratory tidal volume increase to keep up with the increase in metabolic rate and blood pressure decreases, making interpretation of vital signs more difficult.
2. The high level of progesterone relaxes the lower esophageal sphincter (LES) and decreases gastrointestinal motility, which slows gastric emptying, resulting in an increased risk for aspiration of stomach contents.
3. Normal laboratory values change during pregnancy and include a decrease in hemoglobin and hematocrit, blood urea nitrogen (BUN), and albumin because of hemodilution from an increase in plasma volume at the beginning of the third trimester. Blood loss must exceed 1000 ml for signs and symptoms of hypovolemia to be manifested.

4. Near term there is an increase in white blood cells beyond the normal range for that of nonpregnant women who have no infection.

5. Fibrinogen levels are increased and clotting time is decreased, making deep vein thrombosis a real possibility.

In addition, the pregnant client and her family experience increased psychological stress because of fear of fetal loss or deformity. The perioperative team must address these concerns.

NURSING KNOWLEDGE BASE

The concept of perioperative nursing stresses the importance of providing continuity of care for the surgical client using the nursing process. In some hospitals, perioperative nurses assess a client's health status preoperatively, identify specific client needs, teach and counsel, attend to the client's needs in the operating room, and then follow the client's recovery. However, in other institutions, different nurses care for the surgical client during each phase of the surgical experience. Therefore adequate verbal and written information from each perioperative nurse is essential to ensure continuity of care. Your major responsibility as a perioperative nurse is safe, consistent, and effective nursing care during each phase of the perioperative experience.

CRITICAL THINKING
Synthesis

It is important that you synthesize knowledge, experience, attitudes, and standards when developing care for a client having surgery. Doing so will help you prevent complications, promote rehabilitation, and promote a timely return of clients to their home.

KNOWLEDGE. It is essential that you have a strong knowledge base in anatomy and physiology, principles of aseptic technique (see Chapter 10), pharmacology, and teaching-learning principles (see Chapter 9). In addition, you must understand the effect on body systems that the procedure and drugs will have, as well as the normal stress response, in order to anticipate potential complications during the perioperative experience. Your role as the perioperative nurse in infection control is based on knowledge of microbiology, the immune system, and aseptic technique. Effective **preoperative teaching** starts when you first assess the client's and family's readiness and ability to learn and requires a knowledge base of teaching and communication principles and the planned surgical procedure.

EXPERIENCE. Any personal experience with surgery helps you to understand the anxiety of the client and family, as well as to explain some of the physical sensations that the client may experience. Previous experiences with surgical clients enable you to anticipate questions that may be asked by the client and family and to help focus preoperative teaching. In addition, past experiences will help you to recognize physiological changes in clients more quickly so that preventive and/or corrective measures can be initiated early.

ATTITUDES. One of your principal roles as perioperative nurse is that of client advocate. When a client consents to surgery and receives an anesthetic agent that alters the level of consciousness, health care providers have the responsibility for protecting the client. You are accountable to the client for maintaining the rights of the client when the client cannot speak on his or her own behalf.

Perioperative nurses must also be creative in developing plans of care that incorporate the clients' individual differences. For example, pregnant clients must be positioned on the operating bed in a way that promotes venous return. Placing a wedge under the right hip to displace the uterus to the left corrects the problem. Assess each client and use the most appropriate padding and positioning techniques possible to prevent injury.

Your attitude about the discipline of nursing is also important when caring for surgical clients. The surgical client will experience numerous routines necessary both for preparation for surgery and for an efficient and optimal recovery. You must systematically adhere to the current standards of practice to ensure high-quality care for each client.

STANDARDS. The application of critical thinking intellectual standards is important for the surgical client, particularly if the client has preexisting physical or psychological factors that might influence the outcomes of surgery. Be very precise, accurate, and complete in gathering assessment data, and use a logical, relevant, and well-thought-out approach in making clinical decisions because the client's condition can change quickly.

The Association of Perioperative Registered Nurses (AORN) has established standards of practice for nurses practicing in the surgical suite. The standards cover practices that ensure safety of the client, appropriate monitoring and evaluation, infection-control practices, and timely and effective nursing interventions. As the perioperative nurse, you are responsible for adhering to these standards (AORN, 1997).

PREOPERATIVE SURGICAL PHASE

Surgical clients enter the health care setting in different stages of health. A client may enter the facility feeling relatively healthy while awaiting elective surgery or may be in great distress when facing emergency surgery. Many tests and procedures may be needed to ensure that surgery is indicated and that the client is in optimum condition for surgery. During these tests and procedures the client meets many health care personnel, all of whom play a role in care and recovery. Family members or friends also play an important role by providing support through their presence, but they also face many of the same stressors as the client.

Clients may undergo preoperative preparation several days before the day of surgery. Preadmission testing may be done in the hospital, physician's office, or outpatient laboratory. With this testing completed, the client usually enters the hospital the day surgery is performed. Many hospitals have special outpatient or "ambulatory" surgery units for elective surgery, where clients come to the hospital, undergo surgery, and return home on the same day. Outpatient surgery is also performed in freestanding clinics and ambulatory surgery centers. The more traditional preoperative routine involves the client entering the hospital the day before surgery. You must be able to properly prepare the client for surgery regardless of the method of entry into the health care setting.

NURSING PROCESS

 ## Assessment

Your assessment of the surgical client establishes a normal baseline for the client and alerts you to special needs and potential intraoperative and postoperative complications.

NURSING HISTORY.   The preoperative history includes key elements that pertain to the surgical client's risks and needs. In the ambulatory surgical setting the history may be less detailed than that collected when the client is hospitalized the evening before surgery; however, the basic information outlined below is necessary for competent care in each setting. If a client is unable to relate all the necessary information, interview family members or significant others. As with any admission to a health care facility, you must include information concerning advance directives. Ask if the client has a durable power of attorney for health care and a living will (see Chapter 3), and include a copy in the chart. The law requires that this be done no matter what the client's age or how serious the condition or surgical procedure.

MEDICAL HISTORY.   A review of the client's medical history includes past illnesses and the primary reason for seeking medical care. Candidates for ambulatory surgery should also be screened for major medical conditions that may increase the risk for complications (Table 36-3). If a client is at increased risk, surgery as an outpatient may not be advisable. Women of childbearing age are asked about the date of their last menstrual period (LMP), if their last period was "typical" for them, and if they have had unprotected sex in the last month. Because many women do not know that they are pregnant early in the first trimester, a pregnancy test should be considered when a client of childbearing age is scheduled for surgery and has not had surgical sterilization.

PREVIOUS SURGERIES.   Past experience with surgery can reveal potential physical and psychological responses to a procedure and alert you to special needs and risk factors. Complications such as anaphylaxis or **malignant hyperthermia** (see Chapter 11) during previous surgery should alert you to the need for preventive measures and availability of emergency equipment. A history of postoperative complica-

tions, such as persistent vomiting or excessive pain, should also alert you to the possible need for different medications. Reports of severe anxiety before a previous surgery may identify the need for additional emotional support and preoperative teaching.

MEDICATION HISTORY.   Review whether the client is taking any medications that might predispose him or her to surgical complications (Table 36-4). If a client regularly uses prescription or over-the-counter (OTC) medications, or herbal supplements, the physician may decide to temporarily discontinue the drugs before surgery or adjust the dosages. Instruct clients to ask the physician if they should take their usual medications the morning of surgery. If the client is undergoing inpatient surgery, all prescription drugs taken before surgery are automatically discontinued after surgery unless reordered. Be vigilant in reviewing the surgeon's postoperative orders so that any needed medication taken preoperatively is not forgotten.

ALLERGIES.   Allergies to medications, topical agents used to prepare the skin for surgery, and latex can create significant risks for the surgical client. An allergic response to any agent can be potentially fatal, depending on its severity. Latex allergies are on the rise (see Chapter 10). A latex allergy may be manifested as contact dermatitis with redness, inflammation, and blisters; as contact urticaria with pruritus, redness, and swelling; or as hay fever–like symptoms and anaphylaxis.

If one or more allergies exist, the client receives an allergy identification band to be worn during the surgery and until the client is discharged. Also be sure that the front of the client's chart has an allergy alert label listing all allergies.

SMOKING HABITS.   The client who smokes is at a greater risk for postoperative pulmonary complications than a nonsmoker. Smoking decreases ciliary movement of mucus from the lower airways upward, increases mucus production, and causes bronchial constriction, increasing airway obstruction. After surgery this client will have greater difficulty clearing the airways of mucous secretions and is at increased risk for **bronchospasm** and **laryngospasm.** Use this information to plan aggressive postoperative **pulmonary hygiene,** including more frequent turning, deep breathing, coughing, use of incentive spirometry, and chest physical therapy (PT) if ordered.

ALCOHOL AND CONTROLLED SUBSTANCE USE AND ABUSE.   The surgical team must be aware of the use of alcohol and controlled substances by clients to be prepared for adverse reactions, such as withdrawal, that may occur during surgery. The physician and nurse must also be alert for an increased need for postoperative analgesics.

CLIENT EXPECTATIONS.   It is important to identify the client's and family's perceptions and expectations regarding surgery, recovery, and health care providers. This information provides you with information to plan interventions for

Medical Conditions That Increase the Risks of Surgery

Table 36-3

Type of Condition	Reason for Risk
Bleeding disorders (thrombocytopenia, hemophilia)	Disorders increase risk of hemorrhaging during and after surgery.
Diabetes mellitus	Diabetes increases susceptibility to infection and may impair wound healing from altered glucose metabolism and associated circulatory impairment. Fluctuating blood levels may cause central nervous system (CNS) malfunction during anesthesia. Stress of surgery may cause increases in blood glucose levels.
Heart disease (recent myocardial infarction, dysrhythmias, congestive heart failure) and peripheral vascular disease	Stress of surgery causes increased demands on myocardium to maintain cardiac output. General anesthetic agents depress cardiac function.
Upper respiratory infection	Infection increases risk of respiratory complications during anesthesia (e.g., pneumonia, spasm of laryngeal muscles).
Liver disease	Liver disease alters metabolism and elimination of drugs administered during surgery and impairs wound healing and clotting time because of alterations in protein metabolism.
Fever	Fever predisposes client to fluid and electrolyte imbalances and may indicate underlying infection.
Chronic respiratory disease (emphysema, bronchitis, asthma)	Respiratory disease reduces client's means to compensate for acid-base alterations. Anesthetic agents reduce respiratory function, increasing risk for severe hypoventilation.
Immunological disorders (leukemia, acquired immunodeficiency syndrome [AIDS], bone marrow depression, use of chemotherapeutic drugs)	Immunological disorders increase risk of infection and delay wound healing after surgery.
Abuse of street drugs	Persons abusing drugs may have underlying disease (human immunodeficiency virus [HIV], hepatitis) and altered wellness, which affect healing.
Chronic pain	Regular use of pain medications may result in higher tolerance. Increased doses of narcotics or analgesics may be required to achieve postoperative pain control.

Drugs With Special Implications for the Surgical Client

Table 36-4

Drug Class	Effects During Surgery
Antibiotics	Antibiotics potentiate action of anesthetic agents. If taken within 2 wk before surgery, aminoglycosides (gentamicin, tobramycin, neomycin) may cause mild respiratory depression from depressed neuromuscular transmission.
Antidysrhythmics	Antidysrhythmics can reduce cardiac contractility and impair cardiac conduction during anesthesia.
Anticoagulants	Anticoagulants alter normal clotting factors and thus increase risk of hemorrhaging. They should be discontinued at least 48 hr before surgery. Aspirin is a commonly used medication that can alter clotting mechanisms.
Anticonvulsants	Long-term use of certain anticonvulsants (e.g., phenytoin [Dilantin], phenobarbital) can alter metabolism of anesthetic agents.
Antihypertensives	Antihypertensives interact with anesthetic agents to cause bradycardia, hypotension, and impaired circulation. They inhibit synthesis and storage of norepinehrine in sympathetic nerve endings.
Corticosteroids	With prolonged use, corticosteroids cause adrenal atrophy, which reduces body's ability to withstand stress. Before and during surgery, dosages may be temporarily increased.
Insulin	Diabetic client's need for insulin after surgery is reduced because client's nutritional intake is decreased. Stress response and intravenous (IV) administration of glucose solutions can increase dosage requirements after surgery.
Diuretics	Diuretics potentiate electrolyte imbalances (particularly potassium) after surgery.
Nonsteroidal antiinflammatory drugs (NSAIDs)	NSAIDs inhibit platelet aggregation and may prolong bleeding time, increasing susceptibility to postoperative bleeding.

teaching and emotional preparation, as well as provides the basis for evaluation of care. For example, clients may have expectations regarding pain control and the use of pain medications that are unrealistic. Clients prepared to experience pain and taught the proper use of pharmacological and nonpharmacological pain-relief measures tend to require less medication (Gammon and Mulholland, 1996; Meeker and Rothrock, 1999).

Clients and family members may often have misconceptions about surgery. It is important to discuss with them their understanding of the purpose of the tests, the possible outcomes, and the persons responsible for informing them of results and providing follow-up care.

You may face an ethical dilemma when a client is unaware of the real reason for surgery. In such a case, confer with the physician before revealing specific information related to the medical diagnosis to prevent confusion and to alert the physician that clarification may be needed. When a client is well prepared and knows what to expect, you can reinforce the client's knowledge.

FAMILY SUPPORT.   Determine the extent of the client's support from family members or friends. Surgery often results in temporary disability that often requires direct care and assistance from significant others during recovery. The client cannot always immediately assume the same level of physical activity and often returns home with dressings to change or exercises to perform. You can ask questions to determine the condition of the client's home environment and factors that may interfere with postoperative restrictions or care activities.

OCCUPATION.   Surgery may result in physical alterations that hinder or prevent a person from returning to work. Assess the client's occupational history to anticipate the effects surgery might have on convalescence and eventual work performance. This prepares you to explain any restrictions the client may have when returning to work.

FEELINGS.   Surgery causes anxiety and a feeling of loss of control for most clients. The family may be concerned about the ability of the client to return to a productive life and the impact recovery will have on the family. You may be able to detect the client's feelings about having surgery from both verbal and nonverbal cues. A client who is fearful may ask many questions or be very quiet, may seem uneasy when strangers enter the room, or may actively seek the company of friends and relatives.

It is often difficult to assess feelings thoroughly when ambulatory surgery is scheduled because of limited time spent with the client. As the nurse in an outpatient surgical program, you can telephone the client at home before surgery or interview the client during a preadmission testing visit. For hospital inpatients, choose a time for discussion after preliminary admitting or diagnostic tests have been completed. The client's ability to share feelings depends in part on your willingness to ask questions, listen, be supportive, and clarify misconceptions.

CULTURAL AND SPIRITUAL FACTORS.   Cultural differences in the use of both verbal and nonverbal communication require you to validate interpretation of cues with the client and family. This is especially important after you conduct the initial preoperative assessment and then look for changes in the client's status after surgery. For example, clients from Asian cultures may remain silent out of respect, not fear, and individuals from Central America prefer to have many family members and friends surrounding them and helping to express their needs. Some cultures believe that women must follow what the significant male member of their family dictates; therefore it is very important to explain everything to your female client's husband, father, or brother in order that she be allowed to participate in the plan of care (Geissler, 1998). Many cultural and religious taboos exist concerning the body, who cares for the physical needs of others, and treatments appropriate for healing, so it is important to explore these issues with the client and/or family. Although it is important to recognize and plan for differences based on culture, remember that each member may not hold the beliefs of a particular religion or culture. Asking pertinent questions of each client concerning cultural and spiritual beliefs and expectations will further individualize your nursing care (see Chapter 16 and 17).

COPING RESOURCES.   Assessment of a client's feelings and self-concept helps to reveal whether the client has the ability to cope with the stress of surgery. It is also valuable to ask the client about stress management. If the client has had previous surgery, you can discuss with the client the behaviors that helped to resolve past tension or nervousness. You may need to instruct the client on relaxation exercises (see Chapter 29), which can help to control anxiety.

BODY IMAGE.   Surgical removal of a diseased tissue often leaves permanent disfigurement or alteration in body function. Concern over mutilation, change in sexuality, or loss of a body part compounds a client's fears. Individuals react differently, depending on age, culture, occupation, self-image, and degree of self-esteem. Encourage clients to express these concerns. The client facing even temporary disability or sexual dysfunction requires understanding and support (see Chapter 19).

PHYSICAL EXAMINATION.   You will conduct a partial or complete physical examination (see Chapter 12), depending on the setting and nature of the surgery. The assessment focuses on findings related to the client's medical history and on body systems that will be affected by anesthesia and surgery (Table 36-5).

GENERAL SURVEY.   Gestures and body movements may reflect decreased energy or weakness caused by illness. Height and body weight are important indicators of nutritional status and are used to calculate medication dosages. Preoperative vital signs provide a baseline with which to compare alterations that occur during and after surgery. Anesthetic agents and medications can produce vital sign changes. Preoperative as-

Example of a Focused Client Assessment   Table 36-5

Factors to Assess	Questions and Approaches	Physical Assessment Strategies
Significant medical history and previous surgeries	Ask client about condition requiring surgery and expectations derived from having surgery. Ask if client experiences conditions that increase risk of surgery (see Table 36-3) and how each is being treated. Ask client for list of past surgeries with approximate dates. Ask client about family history of cardiac, renal, liver, and endocrine diseases.	Monitor vital signs, and note any abnormalities. Inspect neck for jugular vein distention (cardiac disease, fluid overload). Inspect skin for turgor, dryness, surgical scars, rashes, skin breakdown. Auscultate heart, lungs, vascular system, and abdomen for abnormal sounds (murmurs, congestion, bruits, absence of bowel sounds). Palpate heart, vascular system, abdomen for abnormalities (thrill, masses). Assess extremities for decreased sensation, hair loss, clubbed fingers, deformed nails, sluggish capillary reflex, color.
Medication history and allergies	Ask client for detailed list of all prescription, OTC, and herbal medications. Ask client about instructions from surgeon concerning taking or omitting any medications preoperatively. Ask client and/or family about any personal and/or family history of allergic responses to medications (including anesthetics), environmental factors (e.g., latex, foods). Ask client about manifestations of allergic reactions.	Inspect any medication containers brought in by client or family. Monitor laboratory values for any evidence of side effects of medications or drug levels, if ordered. Observe skin and mucous membranes for any evidence of allergic response.
Diet history	Ask client about any medical, cultural, religious, or personal dietary restrictions.	Assess for evidence of nutritional alterations (rash, dry skin, hair loss, decreased muscle mass, obesity).

sessment of vital signs is also important in ruling out fluid and electrolyte abnormalities (see Chapter 14).

An elevated temperature is cause for concern. If the client has an underlying infection, surgery may be postponed until the infection has been treated. An elevated body temperature also alters drug metabolism and increases the risk of fluid and electrolyte imbalances.

HEAD AND NECK.   The condition of oral mucous membranes reveals the level of hydration. Dehydration increases the risk for the development of serious fluid and electrolyte imbalances during surgery. During the oral examination, loose or capped teeth must be identified because they can become dislodged during endotracheal intubation. Dentures must be noted so that they can be protected from loss or damage.

Inspection of the soft palate and nasal sinuses can reveal sinus drainage indicative of respiratory or sinus infection. To rule out the possibility of local or systemic infection, palpate for cervical lymph node enlargement. Also inspect the jugular veins for distention. Excess fluid within the circulatory system or failure of the heart to contract efficiently may lead to jugular vein distention. A client with heart disease or fluid overload is at risk for cardiovascular complications during surgery.

SKIN.   Conduct a thorough inspection of the client's skin overlying all body parts, especially bony prominences.

During surgery a client must lie in a fixed position, often for several hours. Avoid positioning a client over an area where the skin shows signs of pressure over bony prominences. A client is susceptible to skin breakdown if the skin is thin or dry or has poor turgor (see Chapter 34).

THORAX AND LUNGS.   A decline in ventilatory function, assessed through breathing pattern and chest excursion, may indicate a client's risk for respiratory complications. Serious pulmonary congestion may cause postponement of surgery. Narrowing of the airways, as occurs with chronic lung disease (CLD, formerly known as chronic obstructive pulmonary disease [COPD]) and identified by the presence of wheezing on auscultation of the lungs, would increase the risk of airway obstruction because of bronchospasm related to endotracheal intubation and anesthesia.

HEART AND VASCULAR SYSTEM.   If the client has heart disease, assess the apical pulse. After surgery compare the rate and rhythm of the pulse with preoperative baseline values.

Assessment of peripheral pulses, color, and temperature of extremities is particularly important for the client undergoing vascular surgery, the client undergoing surgery on an extremity using a tourniquet, or when constricting bandages or casts will be applied to an extremity after surgery. Postoperative color changes, change in sensation, or development

As Sue prepares to conduct the preadmission assessment of Mr. Korloff, she will recall what she has learned regarding risk factors for clients undergoing surgery. Mr. Korloff has had a history of heart disease in the past, according to the referral note. Five years ago he was treated for a cardiac dysrhythmia but has had no further problems. Sue will plan to question Mr. Korloff thoroughly about any potential cardiac symptoms.

Sue's knowledge of laparoscopic surgery will help her anticipate the types of postoperative problems Mr. Korloff is likely to develop, such as food intolerance and abdominal or referred pain from the carbon dioxide gas used during laparoscopy. Sue's knowledge regarding family dynamics, particularly within the Russian culture, will assist her in assessing the level of involvement of Mr. Korloff's daughters in his preparation and care. Russian-Americans typically have strong family ties and values. The father usually plays a primary role in the function of the family. It will be important to assess Mr. Korloff's opinions about surgery first and then work to include the family.

Sue's experience with her own father after surgery will help her to explain some of the sensations that Mr. Korloff can expect, such as a sore throat from the endotracheal tube used for administering anesthesia. She will also need to draw on her experiences with clients she cared for after laparoscopic cholecystectomies during her previous rotation on a general surgery floor. She will be able to inform Mr. Korloff and his daughters that he will have IV fluids infusing until he is able to tolerate oral fluids and that he will likely experience only mild discomfort. Mr. Korloff will be able to get out of bed the evening of surgery, and if all goes well he will likely be discharged the next day.

of a weak or absent pulse in a client who had adequate circulation before surgery indicates impaired circulation.

ABDOMEN. Alteration in gastrointestinal function after surgery may result in decreased or absent bowel sounds and distention. You need to recognize whether the client is simply obese or the abdomen has become distended. Assessment of preoperative bowel sounds and normal elimination pattern is useful as a baseline. If surgery requires manipulation of portions of the gastrointestinal tract of if a general anesthetic is used, normal peristalsis may not return and bowel sounds will be absent or diminished for up to several days.

NEUROLOGICAL STATUS. A client's level of consciousness will change as a result of general anesthesia. However, after the effects of anesthesia disappear, the client should return to the preoperative level of responsiveness.

Spinal or epidural anesthesia causes temporary paralysis of the lower extremities. Be aware of preexisting weakness or impaired mobility of the lower extremities to avoid becoming alarmed when full motor function does not return immediately after the procedure.

RISK FACTORS. Knowledge of preoperative risk factors discussed earlier will enable you to take necessary precautions in planning care.

DIAGNOSTIC SCREENING. Before a client has surgery, diagnostic tests are ordered to screen for preexisting abnormalities. Clients scheduled for elective surgery undergo these tests as an outpatient on or before the morning of surgery. If tests reveal severe problems, the surgeon or anesthesiologist may cancel surgery until the condition is stabilized. As the preoperative nurse, you are responsible for coordinating the completion of tests and for verifying that the client is prepared properly. You must also review diagnostic results as they become available, alerting the surgeon and/or anesthesiologist of findings and planning appropriate therapy.

Screening tests depend on the condition of the client and the nature of the surgery. Routine screening tests are summarized in Table 36-6. In addition, a blood type and screen may be needed if transfusions are necessary; a urinalysis screens for urinary tract infections, renal disease, or diabetes mellitus; and a 12-lead electrocardiogram determines the normality of the heart rate and rhythm. A chest x-ray study to assess the size and shape of the heart, presence of lung lesions and chest wall abnormalities, and position of the diaphragm and the aorta may also be ordered.

Nursing Diagnosis

Cluster defining characteristics gathered during assessment to identify appropriate nursing diagnoses and related factors (Box 36-1). The nature and type of surgery, as well as the client's age and health status, suggest defining characteristics for many nursing diagnoses. The diagnoses establish direction for care that will be provided during one or all of the surgical phases. For example, a client's restlessness, poor eye contact, and expressed concern about the results of surgery point to the diagnosis of *anxiety.* However, the assessment must be validated to avoid misdiagnosis. In the assessment above, restlessness may also indicate pain.

A diagnosis and its related factors offer direction to the most effective nursing interventions. The related factors must be accurate to avoid inappropriate interventions. For example, *anxiety related to deficient knowledge of perioperative routines* will require you to offer thorough instruction preoperatively and immediately postoperatively. However, *anxiety related to threat of ineffective role performance* will require counseling and coaching during the postoperative recovery. If the threat is real, it may be necessary to notify social services.

Preoperatively, nursing diagnoses may focus on the intraoperative and postoperative risks a client may face. Preventive care is essential to manage the surgical client effectively.

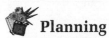

Planning

It is essential to include the client, family, and primary caregiver in any discussions before surgery. Involving the client early minimizes surgical risks and postoperative complications. Structured preoperative teaching reduces the amount of anesthesia and postoperative pain medication needed, decreases the occurrence of postoperative uri-

Common Laboratory Blood Tests

Table 36-6

Test	Normal Values*	Significance	
		Low	High
Complete Blood Count (CBC)			
Hemoglobin (Hgb)	Female: 12-16 g/dl; male: 14-18 g/dl	Anemia	Polycythemia
Hematocrit (Hct)	Female: 37%-47%; male: 42%-52%	Fluid overload	Dehydration
Platelet count	150,000-400,000/mm³	Decreased clothing	Increased thrombosis
White blood cell count	5000-10,000/mm³	Immunosuppression	Infection
Blood Chemistry (SMA 7 or CHEM 7)			
Sodium (Na)	136-145 mEq/L	Hyponatremia/fluid overload	Hypernatremia/dehydration
Potassium (K)	3.5-5.0 mEq/L	Cardiac dysrhythmias	
Chloride (Cl)	90-110 mEq/L	Follows shifts in sodium blood levels	
Carbon dioxide (CO_2)	23-30 mEq/L	Indirect measurement of bicarbonate (HCO_3^-)	
Blood urea nitrogen (BUN)	10-20 mg/dl	Liver disease/fluid overload	Renal disease/dehydration
Glucose	70-105 mg/dl fasting	Hypoglycemia/insulin reaction	Hyperglycemia/diabetes mellitus
Creatinine	Female: 0.5-1.1 mg/dl; male: 0.6-1.2 mg/dl	Malnutrition	Renal disease
Coagulation Studies			
Prothrombin time (PT)	11.0-12.5 sec	Risk of thrombosis	Risk of hemorrhage Coumadin response
Partial thromboplastin time (PTT)	60-70 sec	Risk of thrombosis	Risk of hemorrhage Heparin response
Activated PTT (APTT)	30-40 sec	Activators added to PTT reagent to shorten time	

From Pagana KD, Pagana TJ: *Diagnostic testing and nursing implications: a case study approach,* ed 5, St. Louis, 1999, Mosby.
*Normal ranges vary slightly among laboratories.

Nursing Diagnoses for THE PREOPERATIVE CLIENT

Box 36-1

- Anxiety
- Conflict, decisional
- Coping, compromised family
- Coping, ineffective
- Fear
- Fluid volume, risk for imbalanced
- Hopelessness
- Knowledge, deficient
- Nutrition, imbalanced: less than body requirements
- Nutrition, imbalanced: more than body requirements
- Powerlessness
- Role performance, ineffective
- Skin integrity, risk for impaired
- Sleep pattern, disturbed
- Spiritual distress, risk for

nary retention, promotes an earlier return to normal oral intake, and decreases length of hospital stay (Meeker and Rothrock, 1999). Clients informed about the surgical experience are less likely to be fearful and are able to prepare for expected outcomes.

GOALS AND OUTCOMES. The plan of care begins in the preoperative phase and is modified during the intraoperative and postoperative phases (see care plan). The goals of care for the surgical client include the following:
Understanding the physiological and psychological responses to surgery
Understanding intraoperative and postoperative events
Achieving emotional and physiological comfort and rest
Achieving return of normal physiological function after surgery (e.g., return of normal vital signs, fluid and electrolyte balance, muscle function)
Remaining free of surgical wound infection
Remaining safe from harm during the perioperative period
Outcomes established for each goal of care provide measurable behavioral evidence to gauge the client's progress toward meeting stated goals.

Care Study Nursing Care Plan SURGERY

ASSESSMENT

As Mr. Korloff enters the preadmission center for his testing, Sue greets him and his daughters. She explains the need to gather a history and asks Mr. Korloff if he wishes to have his daughters join him. He smiles and says, "Yes, my daughters will be my nurses for a few days." Sue asks Mr. Korloff what he has been told regarding the preoperative procedures and postoperative recovery. Mr. Korloff **states that he knows very little about the surgery.** His physician explained that the procedure is safe, **but he knows few specifics. He asks if he will have an IV line, where his daughters can wait, and if he will be awake during the surgery.** The nursing staff report that **Mr. Korloff's daughters have been calling on the phone and asking many questions about intraoperative and postoperative events.**

*Defining characteristics are shown in bold type.

NURSING DIAGNOSIS

Deficient knowledge regarding implications of surgery (cholecystectomy) related to first surgical experience and inadequate preparation.

PLANNING

GOAL	EXPECTED OUTCOMES
Client will understand intraoperative and postoperative events before the day of surgery.	Client and his daughters will describe events that commonly occur in the holding area and operating room on the day before surgery. Client and his daughters will describe routine postoperative nursing procedures on the day of admission. Client and his daughters will describe ways to participate in postoperative care on the day of admission.

IMPLEMENTATION

STEPS	RATIONALE
1. Send Mr. Korloff a copy of the teaching booklet *Your Surgical Experience*. Arrange time to call at home and answer any questions on booklet's content.	Clients who are prepared for surgery experience less anxiety and report a greater sense of psychological well-being (Shuldham, 1999).
2. Provide planned teaching session for Mr. Korloff and his daughters after preadmission testing. Explain events that will occur in holding area (e.g., insertion of IV line, vital sign check) and in operating room (e.g., positioning, anesthesia). Use visual aids to assist Mr. Korloff's understanding of the laparoscopic procedure.	Teaching focused on information client will need to know on morning of admission will decrease anxiety and allow client and family to better participate in care (Dunn, 1998; Shuldham, 1999).
3. Provide planned teaching session on day of admission with Mr. Korloff and his daughters to explain common events that occur after surgery and demonstrate postoperative exercises included in the teaching booklet.	Preoperative teaching improves client's ability to ambulate, participate in care activities, and resume activities of daily living after surgery. Demonstration is an effective method in teaching psychomotor skills.

EVALUATION

- Ask Mr. Korloff and his daughters to identify the basic purpose of the surgery and changes to expect afterward.
- Ask Mr. Korloff and his daughters to identify routine types of postoperative monitoring and treatment.
- Ask Mr. Korloff to state the most frightening aspect of surgery for him.
- Have Mr. Korloff perform postoperative exercises.

SETTING PRIORITIES.   You must establish individualized care by prioritizing nursing diagnoses and interventions based on the assessed needs of each client. Setting priorities requires clinical judgment. For example, if a client is diagnosed as having *anxiety* and *deficient knowledge,* the client's priority may be deficient knowledge, wherein instruction is needed to improve the client's knowledge, which will then relieve the anxiety. Your approach to each client must be thorough and reflect your understanding of the implications of the client's age, physical and psychological health, educational level, cultural and religious practices, and stated and/or written wishes concerning advance medical directives.

CONTINUITY OF CARE.   For the ambulatory surgical client the preoperative planning phase usually occurs in the outpatient surgery setting before or on the morning of surgery. Ideally, it begins in the surgeon's office and continues in the home. This gives the client time to think about the surgical experience, make necessary physical preparations, and ask questions about postoperative procedures. Well-planned preoperative care ensures that the client is well informed and able to actively participate during recovery. The family or significant others may also play an active supportive role for the client.

Planning may also require referral to other members of the health care team. Clients who will require aggressive pulmonary rehabilitation, such as those undergoing thoracic surgery, may be referred to a respiratory therapist. Many clients and their families benefit from referral to pastoral care, especially if the procedure is an emergency or is life threatening.

Implementation

Preoperative nursing interventions provide the client with an understanding of the physical and psychological aspects of surgical intervention.

INFORMED CONSENT.   A surgeon cannot legally perform surgery nor can an anesthesia care provider administer an anesthetic until a client understands the need for the procedure and the steps involved, risks, expected results, and alternative treatments. Chapter 3 summarizes issues and guidelines for informed consent. All consent forms must be signed before you administer preoperative medications that will sedate the client. The primary responsibility for informing the client rests with the surgeon and anesthesia care personnel (Dunn, 1999). However, if the client is confused or uncertain about the procedure, you have an ethical obligation to contact the surgeon and/or anesthesia care provider so that further discussion and clarification are provided to meet the client's information and emotional needs. The client always has the right to refuse surgery or treatment even after written consent is given (Iocono, 2000).

HEALTH PROMOTION.   Health promotion activities during the preoperative phase focus on prevention of complications, health maintenance, and support of possible rehabilitation needs postoperatively.

PREOPERATIVE TEACHING.   Client education relieves anxiety, increases self-esteem, speeds up the recovery process, reduces medical costs, decreases the amount of perceived pain, and facilitates a more rapid return to work or normal functioning (Fox, 1998). Preoperative teaching provided in a systematic and structured format has a positive influence on clients' recovery (Gammon and Mulholland, 1996). Structured teaching can influence the following postoperative factors:

1. *Ventilatory function:* Teaching improves the ability and willingness to deep breathe and cough effectively.
2. *Physical functional capacity:* Teaching increases understanding and willingness to ambulate and resume activities of daily living.
3. *Sense of well-being:* Clients who are prepared for surgery experience less anxiety and report a greater sense of psychological well-being (Shuldham, 1999).
4. *Length of hospital stay:* Teaching can reduce the client's length of hospital stay by preventing or minimizing postoperative complications.
5. *Anxiety about pain and amount of pain medication needed for comfort:* Clients who learn about pain and ways to relieve it are less anxious about the pain, ask for what they need, and actually require less pain medication.

Box 36-2

PERIOPERATIVE PREPARATION

1. Preoperative procedures
   - State time to arrive at facility (if not already admitted).
   - State time of surgery (approximate time or to follow).
   - Explain extent and purpose of food and fluid restrictions.
   - Explain or review informed consent.
   - Teach about physical preparation required (bowel or skin preparation).
   - Explain about procedures just before transport to operating room (OR) (IV line, catheterization or void, preoperative medications). These may be done as part of preanesthesia care unit activities.
2. Intraoperative procedures
   - Describe preanesthesia care environment and activities.
   - Describe operating room environment.
   - Explain about the roles of circulating nurse, scrub nurse, anesthesia care provider.
3. Postoperative procedures
   - Describe postanesthesia care environment and activities.
   - Teach about pain control and other comfort measures.
   - Explain purpose of any anticipated tubes, drains, or IV lines.
   - Emphasize importance of deep breathing, coughing, turning, and leg exercises.
   - Teach or review above exercises.
   - Demonstrate exercises, and have client return demonstration.
   - Encourage client and family to verbalize any concerns.
   - Assess client's and family's understanding of perioperative preparation, and respond appropriately.

The most effective type of teaching program for surgical clients is planned to cover the entire surgical experience. Box 36-2 outlines the parameters for perioperative preparation. Today, because many clients are not admitted to the hospital before surgery, preoperative teaching may occur in the home, physician's office, or preadmission unit. Offer printed literature and videotapes to clients. Preoperatively, you may call clients the evening before surgery to clarify questions (Lancaster, 1997).

Always include family members and significant others in preoperative preparation. They are frequently the coaches for postoperative exercises when the client returns from surgery. If family members and significant others do not understand routine postoperative events, their anxiety can heighten the client's fears or concerns. Their misunderstanding and anxiety can be reduced with thoughtful preparation. However, if the client does not wish them to be included, respect the request for privacy.

Timing.   Preoperative teaching is most useful when started the week before admission and reinforced immediately before surgery (Shuldham, 1999). Teaching performed when the client is less anxious will result in more effective learning. Anxiety and fear are barriers to learning. Assess the surgical client's readiness and ability to learn (see Chapter 9). Always present information in a logical sequence beginning with preoperative events and advancing to intraoperative and postoperative routines. Preoperative teaching checklists offer helpful guidelines for presenting clients with a comprehensives set of instructions.

Content.   Preoperative teaching should include information to assist the client, family, and significant others in preparing for the surgical experience and participating in the plan of care (Dunn, 1998). Always assess their level of understanding about the surgery, perioperative routines, and expectations first, and then reinforce or teach, based on their prior knowledge, the information discussed in the following sections.

Surgical Procedure.   After the surgeon has explained the basic purpose of the surgical procedure and its steps, the client may ask you additional questions. Be careful to avoid saying anything that contradicts the surgeon's explanation. One way to avoid contradictions is to first ask what the client has been told. If the client has little or no understanding about the surgery, you must refer the client back to the surgeon for additional information.

Preoperative Routines.   Certain preoperative routines are expected and should be explained. For example, the client may need to have a chest x-ray examination. Knowing what tests are planned and why will increase the client's sense of control.

The anesthesiologist may visit with the client to complete a preanesthesia assessment either during the preoperative admission process or when the client is in the presurgical care unit. The client and family need to know about this visit, so they can ask any questions they have or provide necessary information.

The client and family must understand that the client can have no oral intake (either food or liquids) for approximately 2 hours (clear liquids) to 8 hours (meat or fried foods) before surgery, unless explicitly specified by the anesthesiologist or surgeon (American Society of Anesthesiologists Task Force on Perioperative Fast, 1999). During the use of general anesthesia, the muscles relax and gastric contents can reflux into the esophagus. The anesthetic eliminates the client's ability to gag. Therefore the client is at risk for aspiration of food or fluids from the stomach into the lungs. The physician's orders provide additional guidance for routines to be explained to the client (e.g., intravenous [IV] therapy, preoperative medications, or insertion of a urinary catheter or a nasogastric tube).

Intraoperative Routines.   The scheduled operative time is only an anticipated time, because other surgeries may be scheduled first. Unanticipated delays may occur for many reasons that have nothing to do with your client. Emphasize that this time is a rough estimate and the actual time could be much longer. Tell family members where to wait, and inform them that the surgeon will speak to them when the surgery has been completed. Communicate excessive delays to the family if they occur.

Postoperative Routines.   The client and family want to know about postoperative events. If they understand routine postoperative vital sign monitoring, they are less likely to worry when nurses perform these assessments. You can also explain if the client is to have IV lines, dressings, or drainage tubes. It is important to neither overprepare nor underprepare the client and family. You cannot predict all the client's requirements, and a client may be misinformed about a therapy that may not be initiated. Contradictions between your explanations and reality can cause anxiety.

Sensory Preparation.   Provide the client with information about sensations typically experienced before, during, and after surgery. Preparatory information helps clients anticipate the steps of a procedure and form a realistic image of the surgical experience. When events occur as predicted, the client is better able to cope with the experiences. For example, the operating room is very bright. Explain that a cuff for a noninvasive blood pressure monitor will be applied to the client's arm. This monitor may make a hum and a beep, and the cuff tightens around the client's arm. Informing the client about these and other sensations in the operating room will reduce anxiety before the client is anesthetized, which will help to decrease the amount of anesthetic needed for induction. Other postoperative sensations to describe include blurred vision from ophthalmic ointment, dryness of the mouth or the sensation of a sore throat resulting from an endotracheal tube, pain at the incision site, tightness of the dressings, and feeling cold.

Pain Relief.   One of the surgical client's greatest fears is pain. The family is also concerned for the client's comfort. Preoperative preparation regarding pain and pain control can help the client to cope with the pain. Patient-controlled analgesia (PCA) is commonly used and provides the client with control over pain. Explain to the client how to operate the pump and the importance of administering medication as soon as pain becomes persistent (see Chapter 29). Analgesics will not provide adequate pain relief if the client waits until the pain becomes excruciating before using or requesting an analgesic. Encourage the client to use analgesics as needed and not be fearful of any dependence.

If epidural, intramuscular, or oral analgesics will be used, the client needs to know the schedule for these drugs. Encourage the client to inform nurses as soon as pain becomes a persistent discomfort. The client should also know it takes time for a drug to act and that all the discomfort will rarely be eliminated. In addition, inform the client and family of other therapies available for pain relief, such as focused breathing and relaxation, distraction, and the use of a K-pad or an ice pack.

POSTOPERATIVE EXERCISES.   Every preoperative teaching program includes explanation and demonstration of the five postoperative exercises: diaphragmatic breathing, incentive spirometry, controlled coughing, turning, and leg exercises (Skill 36-1).

Diaphragmatic breathing improves lung expansion and oxygen delivery without using excess energy. The client learns to use the diaphragm during deep breathing to take slow, deep, and relaxed breaths. Eventually the client's lung volume improves. Deep breathing also helps to clear any anesthetic gases from the airways.

Text continued on p. 921

Skill 36-1
Teaching Postoperative Exercises

DELEGATION CONSIDERATIONS

The skill of teaching postoperative exercises requires problem solving and knowledge application unique to a nurse. Assistive personnel can reinforce and assist clients in performing postoperative exercises.

EQUIPMENT

- Pillow (optional; used to splint surgical incision when coughing)
- Incentive spirometer
- Elastic stockings or sequential compression stockings

STEPS	RATIONALE
1. Assess client's risk for postoperative respiratory complications: review medical history to identify presence of chronic pulmonary condition (e.g., emphysema, asthma), any condition that affects chest wall movement, history of smoking, and presence of reduced hemoglobin (low red blood cell [RBC] count).	General anesthesia predisposes client to respiratory problems because lungs are not fully inflated during surgery, cough reflex is suppressed, and mucus collects within airway passages. After surgery client may have reduced lung volume and require greater efforts to deep breathe and cough; inadequate lung expansion can lead to atelectasis and pneumonia. Client is at greater risk for developing respiratory complications if chronic lung conditions are present. Smoking damages ciliary clearance and increases mucus secretion. A reduced hemoglobin level can lead to inadequate oxygenation.
2. Assess client's ability to cough and deep breathe by having client take a deep breath and observing movement of shoulders, chest wall, and abdomen. Measure chest excursion during a deep breath. Ask client to cough after taking a deep breath.	Reveals maximum potential for chest expansion and ability to cough forcefully; serves as baseline to measure client's ability to perform exercises postoperatively. Diaphragmatic breathing allows for greater lung expansion, improved ventilation, and increased blood oxygenation. Coughing loosens and removes secretions from the pulmonary alveoli.
3. Assess client's risk for postoperative thrombus formation (older clients, immobilized clients, clients with personal or family history of clots, women over 35 years who smoke and are taking oral contraceptives). Observe for a positive Homans' sign (which may or may not be present) by monitoring calf pain when dorsiflexing the client's foot with the knee flexed. Observe for calf pain, redness, swelling, or vein distention, usually unilaterally.	Venous stasis, hypercoagulability, and vein trauma must exist simultaneously for a thrombus to form (Lewis and others, 2000). Following general anesthesia circulation is slowed, resulting in a greater tendency for clot formation. Immobilization results in decreased muscular contraction in lower extremities, which promotes venous stasis. The physical stress of surgery creates a hypercoagulable state in most individuals. Manipulation and positioning during surgery may inadvertently cause trauma to leg veins.

- *Critical Decision Point*
  If calf tenderness is present, notify the physician and do not manipulate the extremity any further. Antiembolism stockings or pneumatic compression cuffs may be ordered for clients at risk for thrombus formation (Box 36-2).

STEPS	RATIONALE
4. Assess client's ability to move independently while in bed.	Clients confined to bed rest, even for limited periods, will need to turn regularly. Determines existence of any mobility restrictions.
5. Assess client's willingness and capability to learn exercises; note attention span, anxiety, level of consciousness, and language level.	Ability to learn depends on readiness, ability, and learning environment.
6. Assess family members' or significant other's willingness to learn and to support client postoperatively.	Family member or significant other can coach clients on exercise performance.
7. Assess client's medical orders preoperatively and postoperatively.	May require adaptations in way exercises are performed.
8. Teach importance of postoperative exercises to recovery and physiological benefits.	Adults learn new skills when they understand the benefits derived.
A. **Diaphragmatic Breathing**	
(1) Assist client to a comfortable sitting or standing position with knees flexed. If client chooses to sit, assist to side of bed or to upright position in chair.	Upright position facilitates diaphragmatic excursion.

STEPS	RATIONALE
(2) Stand or sit facing client.	Allows client to observe breathing exercises performed by nurse.
(3) Instruct client to place palms of hands across from each other, down, and along lower borders of anterior rib cage; place tips of third fingers lightly together (see illustration). Demonstrate for client.	Position of hands allows client to feel movement of chest and abdomen as diaphragm descends and lungs expand.
(4) Have client take slow, deep breaths, inhaling through nose, and pushing abdomen against hands. Tell client to feel middle fingers separate as client inhales. Explain that client will feel normal downward movement of diaphragm during inspiration.	Slow, deep breaths prevent panting or hyperventilation. Inhaling through nose warms, humidifies, and filters air. Diaphragmatic breathing allow air to pass by partially obstructing mucous plug, thus increasing the force with which to expel the mucus.
(5) Explain that abdominal organs descend and chest wall expands. Demonstrate for client.	Explanation and demonstration focus on normal ventilatory movement of chest wall. Client learns to understand how diaphragmatic breathing feels.
(6) Avoid using chest and shoulders while inhaling, and instruct client in same manner.	Using auxillary chest and shoulder muscles during breathing increases useless energy expenditures and does not promote full lung expansion.
(7) Have client hold a slow, deep breath, hold for count of three, and then slowly exhale through mouth as if blowing out a candle (pursed lips). Tell client middle fingertips will touch as chest wall contracts.	Allows for gradual expulsion of air.
(8) Repeat breathing exercise 3 to 5 times.	Allows client to observe slow, rhythmical breathing pattern.
(9) Have client practice exercise. Instruct client to take 10 slow, deep breaths every hour while awake.	Repetition of exercise reinforces learning. Regular deep breathing prevents postoperative complications.

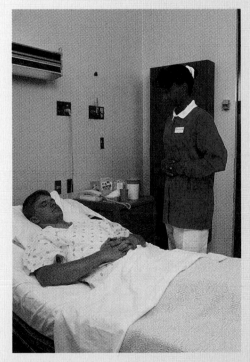

STEP 8A(3)   Deep breathing exercise: placement of hands during inhalation. (From *Mosby's medical, nursing, and allied health dictionary*, ed 5, St. Louis, 1998, Mosby.)

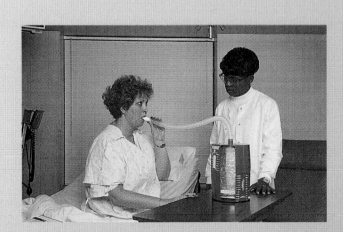

STEP 8B(4)   Client demonstrating incentive spirometry.

STEPS	RATIONALE
B. Incentive Spirometry	
(1) Wash hands.	Reduces transmission of microorganisms.
(2) Instruct client to assume semi-Fowler's or high Fowler's position.	Promotes optimal lung expansion during respiratory maneuver.
(3) Indicate on the device the volume level to be obtained with each inhalation.	Establishes goal of volume level necessary for adequate lung expansion.
(4) Demonstrate to client how to place mouthpiece so that lips completely cover mouthpiece (see illustration).	Demonstration is a reliable technique for teaching psychomotor skill and enables client to ask questions.
(5) Instruct client to inhale slowly and maintain constant flow through unit. When maximal inspiration is reached, client should hold breath for 2 to 3 seconds (see illustration) and then exhale slowly. Number of breaths should not exceed 10 to 12 per minute.	Maintains maximal inspiration and reduces risk of progressive collapse of individual alveoli. Slow breathing (<12 breaths per minute) prevents or minimizes pain from sudden pressure changes in chest.
(6) Instruct client to breathe normally for short period.	Prevents hyperventilation and fatigue.
(7) Have client repeat maneuver until goals are achieved.	Ensures correct use of spirometer.
(8) Wash hands.	Reduces transmission of microorganisms.
C. Positive Expiratory Pressure Therapy and "Huff" Coughing	
(1) Wash hands.	Reduces transmission of microorganisms.
(2) Set positive expiratory pressure (PEP) device for setting ordered.	The higher the setting, the more effort will be required by the client.
(3) Instruct client to assume semi-Fowler's or high Fowler's position, and place nose clip on client's nose (see illustration).	Promotes optimum lung expansion and expectoration of mucus.
(4) Have client place lips around mouthpiece. Client should take a full breath and then exhale 2 or 3 times longer than inhalation. Pattern should be repeated for 10 to 20 breaths.	Ensures that all breathing is done through mouth and that the device is used properly.

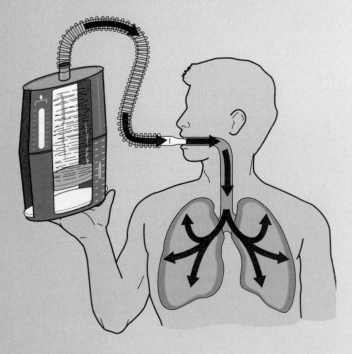

STEP 8B(5)   Diagram of use of incentive spirometer.

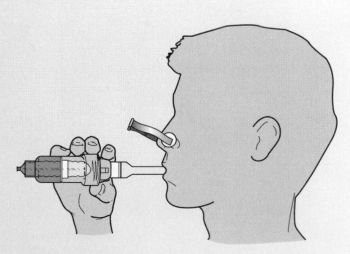

STEP 8C(3)   Diagram of use of positive expiratory pressure device.

(5) Remove device from mouth, and have client take a slow, deep breath and hold for 3 seconds.	Promotes lung expansion before coughing.
(6) Instruct client to exhale in quick, short, forced "huffs."	"Huff" coughing, or forced expiratory technique, promotes bronchial hygiene by increasing expectoration of secretions.

D. Controlled Coughing

(1) Explain importance of maintaining an upright position.	Position facilitates diaphragm excursion and enhances thorax expansion.
(2) Demonstrate coughing. Take two slow, deep breaths, inhaling through nose and exhaling through mouth.	Deep breaths expand lungs fully so that air moves behind mucus and facilitates effects of coughing.
(3) Inhale deeply a third time, and hold breath to count of three. Cough fully for two or three consecutive coughs without inhaling between coughs. (Tell client to push all air out of lungs.)	Consecutive coughs help remove mucus more effectively and completely than one forceful cough.

- **Critical Decision Point**

Coughing may be contraindicated after brain, spinal, head, neck, or eye surgery.

(4) Caution client against just clearing throat instead of coughing. Explain that coughing will not cause injury to incision.	Clearing throat does not remove mucus from deeper airways. Postoperative incisional pain makes it harder to cough effectively.
(5) If surgical incision is to be either abdominal or thoracic, teach client to place pillow or bath blanket over incisional area and place hands over pillow to splint incision. During breathing and coughing exercises, press gently against incisional area for splitting or support. This can be done with hands (see illustrations).	Surgical incision cuts through muscles, tissues, and nerve endings. Deep breathing and coughing exercises place additional stress on suture line and cause discomfort. Splinting incision with hands or pillow provides firm support and reduces incisional pulling.
(6) Client continues to practice coughing exercises, splinting imaginary incision. The client is instructed to cough 2 or 3 times while awake.	Value of deep coughing with splinting is stressed to effectively expectorate mucus with minimal discomfort.
(7) Instruct client to examine sputum for consistency, odor, amount, and color changes.	Sputum consistency, odor, amount, and color changes may indicate the presence of a pulmonary complication, such as pneumonia.

E. Turning

(1) Instruct client to assume supine position and move toward left side of bed by bending knees and pressing heels against the mattress to raise and move buttocks (see illustration).	Positioning begins on right side of bed so that turning to left side will not cause client to roll toward bed's edge. Buttocks lift prevents shearing force from body movement against sheets.

- **Critical Decision Point**

If client has decreased strength or mobility on the right side, have client assume position on the left side of the bed. Pull sheet can also be used to turn client.

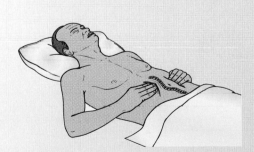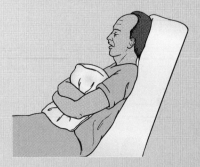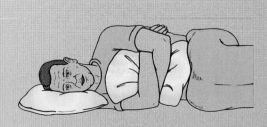

STEP 8D(5)   Techniques for splinting incision. (From Lewis S and others: *Medical-surgical nursing: assessment and management of clinical problems,* ed 5, St. Louis, 2000, Mosby.)

(2) Instruct client to place the right hand over incisional area to splint it.

Splinting incision supports and minimizes pulling on suture line during turning.

(3) Instruct client to keep right leg straight and flex left knee up (see illustration).

Straight leg stabilizes the client's position. Flexed left leg shifts weight for easier turning.

- **Critical Decision Point**

Clients who have had back surgery or vascular repair may be restricted from flexing their legs or turning or may need assistance for positioning.

(4) Have client grab right side rail with left hand, pull toward right, and roll onto right side.

Pulling toward side rail reduces effort needed for turning.

(5) Instruct client to turn every 2 hours while awake.

Reduces risk of vascular and pulmonary complications.

F.   Leg Exercises

(1) Have client assume supine position in bed. Demonstrate leg exercises by performing passive range-of-motion exercises and simultaneously explaining exercise.

Provides normal anatomical position of lower extremities.

- **Critical Decision Point**

If client's surgery involve one or both extremities or if vascular alteration is present, surgeon must order leg exercises in postoperative period.

(2) Rotate each ankle in complete circle. Instruct client to draw imaginary circles with big toe. Repeat 5 times (see illustration).

Maintains joint mobility and promotes venous return.

Desirable
Foot circles

Essential
Alternate dorsiflexion and plantar flexion

Quadriceps (thigh) setting

Hip and knee movements

STEP 8E(1)   Buttocks lift. (From Lowdermilk D and others: *Maternity nursing*, ed 5, St. Louis, 1999, Mosby.)

STEP 8E(3)   Leg position for turning. (From Lowdermilk D and others: *Maternity nursing*, ed 5, St. Louis, 1999, Mosby.)

STEP 8F(2-5)   Leg exercises. (From Lewis S and others: *Medical-surgical nursing: assessment and management of clinical problems*, ed 5, St. Louis, 2000, Mosby.)

Steps	Rationale
(3) Alternate dorsiflexion and plantar flexion of both feet. Direct client to feel calf muscles contract and relax alternately (see illustration).	Stretches and contracts gastrocnemius muscles, improving venous return.
(4) Perform quadricepts setting by tightening thigh and bringing knee down toward mattress, then relaxing (see illustration). Repeat 5 times.	Contracts muscles of upper legs, maintains knee mobility, and enhances venous return.
(5) Have client alternately raise each leg up from bed surface, keeping legs straight and then have client bend leg at hip and knee (see illustration). Repeat 5 times.	Contracts and relaxes quadriceps muscles and prevents venous pooling. Bending leg reduces strain on back.
9. Have client continue to practice exercises at least every 2 hours while awake. Instruct client to coordinate turning and leg exercises with diaphragmatic breathing, incentive spirometry, and coughing exercises.	Repetition of exercise sequence reinforces learning. Establishes routine for exercises that develops habit for performance. Sequence of exercises should be leg exercises, turning, breathing, and coughing.
10. Observe client performing all four exercises independently.	Provides opportunity for practice and return demonstration of exercises. Ensures client has learned correct technique.

UNEXPECTED OUTCOMES AND RELATED INTERVENTIONS

- Client is unable to perform exercises correctly.
  - Assess for the presence of anxiety, pain, and fatigue.
  - Teach client stress reduction techniques and/or pain management strategies.
  - Repeat teaching using more demonstration or re-demonstration at time when family member is present.
- Client is unwilling to perform exercises because of incisional pain of thorax or abdomen (deep breathing and coughing, turning) or because of surgery in lower abdomen, groin, buttocks, or legs (leg exercises).
  - Instruct client to ask for pain medication 30 minutes before performing postoperative exercises or to use patient-controlled analgesia (PCA) immediately before exercising.
  - Report to surgeon inadequate pain relief and need to change analgesic or increase dose.

- Client develops pulmonary complications postoperatively.
  - Assess breath sounds in all lobes, and compare bilaterally.
  - Place client in upright position.
  - Notify physician of findings.
  - Be prepared to start oxygen or IV antibiotics as ordered.
- Client develops circulatory complications, such as venous stasis or thrombophlebitis, postoperatively.
  - Assess calves for redness, warmth, edema, and pain on dorsiflexion, and compare bilaterally.
  - Place client on bed rest with affected leg elevated.
  - Notify physician of findings.
  - Continue to have client do exercises with unaffected leg.

RECORDING AND REPORTING

- Record which exercises have been demonstrated to client and whether client can perform exercises independently.
- Report any problems client has in practicing exercises to nurse assigned to client on next shift for follow-up.

To facilitate deep breathing the physician often orders an incentive spirometer for the client (see Chapter 27). Incentive spirometry encourages forced inspiration. The therapy is effective in preventing atelectasis postoperatively.

Coughing assists in removing retained mucus in the airways. A deep, productive cough is more beneficial than merely clearing the throat. The client must anticipate postoperative discomfort and understand the importance of coughing, even when it is difficult. Teach the client to splint an abdominal incision to minimize pain during coughing.

Leg exercises and turning improve blood flow to the extremities and thus reduce venous stasis, reducing the risk for clot formation and subsequent pulmonary emboli. Contractions of lower leg muscles promote venous return, making it difficult for clots to form. Turning also helps to mobilize pulmonary secretions and increases ventilation and

perfusion of the lungs. After explaining each exercise, demonstrate it. Then, while acting as a coach, ask the client to redemonstrate each exercise.

ACTIVITY RESUMPTION.   The type of surgery a client undergoes affects the speed with which normal physical activity and regular eating habits can be resumed. Explain that it is normal for the client to progress gradually in activity and eating. If the client tolerates activity and diet well, activity levels will progress more quickly.

PROMOTION OF NUTRITION.   The surgical client is vulnerable to fluid and electrolyte imbalances as a result of inadequate preoperative intake, excessive fluid loss during surgery, and the stress response. A client usually takes nothing by mouth after midnight before the morning of surgery to reduce risks of vomiting and aspirating emesis during surgery. Instruct the client to eat and drink sufficient amounts before fasting to ensure adequate fluid and nutrition intake. The client's diet should include foods high in protein, with sufficient amounts of carbohydrates, fat, and vitamins. Instruct the client and family members regarding preoperative fasting requirements and oral medication use. Notify the surgeon and anesthesiologist as soon as possible if the client eats or drinks during the fasting period.

For hospitalized clients, remove all fluids and solid foods from the bedside and post a sign over the bed to alert hospital personnel and family members about fasting restrictions. Instruct the client to rinse the mouth with water or mouthwash and brush the teeth as long as nothing is swallowed. Oral medications may be taken with sips of water if ordered by the physician. Notify the dietary department to cancel meals.

A client who is at home the evening before surgery must understand the importance of not taking food or fluids and be willing to follow restrictions.

PROMOTION OF REST.   Rest is essential for normal healing. Anxiety about surgery can interfere with the ability to relax or sleep. The underlying condition necessitating surgery may be painful, further impairing rest. Frequent visits by staff members, diagnostic testing, and physical preparation for surgery consume a large amount of time, and the client has few opportunities to reflect on events. Make sure that the client feels like an individual. The client and family need time to express feelings about surgery, either together or separately. The client's level of anxiety influences the frequency of discussions, and you may need to encourage expression of these concerns.

Attempt to make the client's environment quiet and comfortable. The surgeon may order a sedative-hypnotic or antianxiety agent for the night before surgery. Sedative-hypnotics affect and promote sleep. Antianxiety agents act on the cerebral cortex and limbic system to relieve anxiety. An advantage to ambulatory surgery or same-day surgical admissions is that the client is able to sleep at home the night before surgery.

ACUTE CARE.   The degree of preoperative physical preparation depends on the client's health status, the surgery to be performed, and the surgeon's preferences. A seriously ill client will receive more supportive care than the client facing a less serious elective procedure.

MINIMIZE RISK OF SURGICAL WOUND INFECTION.   The risk of developing a surgical wound infection is determined by the amount and type of microorganisms contaminating a wound, the susceptibility of the host, and the condition of the wound at the end of the operation. All three factors interact, determining the risk for infection (see Chapter 10).

The skin is a favorite site for microorganisms to grow and multiply. Without proper skin preparation, the risk of postoperative wound infection is high. Many surgeons have clients bathe or shower with an antimicrobial soap the

evening before surgery. Some physicians may order clients to bathe or shower more than once, whereas others may have clients give special attention to cleansing the proposed operative site. If the surgical procedure involves the head, neck, or upper chest area, the client may also be required to shampoo the hair. Hair removal is ordered only if the hair has the potential to interfere with exposure, closure, or dressing of the surgical site. This is done as close to the time of surgery as possible (AORN, 1999).

PREVENTION OF BOWEL INCONTINENCE AND CONTAMINATION. The client may receive a bowel preparation (e.g., a cathartic or an enema) if surgery involves the lower gastrointestinal system. Manipulation of portions of the gastrointestinal tract during surgery results in absence of peristalsis for 24 hours and sometimes longer. Enemas and cathartics, such as GoLYTELY, cleanse the gastrointestinal tract to prevent problems with incontinence or constipation. An empty bowel reduces risk of injury to the intestines and minimizes contamination of the operative wound in case a portion of the bowel is incised or opened. Chapter 32 summarizes enema administration.

INTERVENTIONS ON DAY OF SURGERY.   On the morning of surgery, complete the routine procedures discussed in the following sections before releasing the client for surgery.

Documentation.   Before the client goes to the operating room, check the medical record to be sure all pertinent laboratory and test results are present. Check all consent forms for completeness and accuracy of information. A preoperative checklist (Figure 36-1) provides guidelines for ensuring completion of all nursing interventions. Also check the nurses' notes to be sure documentation is current. This is especially important if the client experienced unpredicted problems the night before surgery.

Assessment of Vital Signs.   Make a final assessment of vital signs, and document them on the preoperative checklist and in the nurse's notes. If the preoperative vital signs are abnormal, notify the surgeon because surgery may need to be postponed:

Hygiene.   Basic hygiene measures remove skin contamination and increase the client's comfort. If the client is unwilling or unable to take a complete bath, a partial bath is refreshing and removes irritating secretions or drainage from the skin. Because the client cannot wear personal nightwear to the operating room, provide a clean hospital gown and instruct the client to remove all other articles of clothing, including undergarments. After having nothing by mouth throughout the night, the client usually has a very dry mouth. You may offer mouthwash and toothpaste, again cautioning the client not to swallow anything.

Preparation of Hair and Removal of Cosmetics.   During surgery the anesthesiologist positions the client's head to put

A-1c PREOPERATIVE/PREPROCEDURAL CHECKLIST

• File with other A-1c's of same date. •

PROCEDURE: _____

DATE OF PROCEDURE: _____

1. Place initials in appropriate box: YES, NO, N/A (not applicable, or was not ordered). Each item must have an entry.
2. Explain any "No." This can be done in the space after the item or in the "Comments" section. Use back of form, if needed.
3. To give more information on any item, use the space after the item. If more space is needed, use the "Comments" section or back of form.

DATE

HOSP. NO.

NAME

BIRTHDATE

ADDRESS

IF NOT IMPRINTED, PLEASE PRINT DATE, HOSP. NO., NAME AND LOCATION.

YES	NO	N/A	
			Special information (e.g., blind, O₂, combative)
			Preoperative orders written.
			(If "NO", Dr. _____ notified at _____ date/time.)
			Consent complete and in medical record.
			Allergies (or NKA) labelled on cover of medical record.
			Specify Allergies:
			Isolation label on cover of medical record. Specify type.
			Ordered lab results in medical record.
			Urinalysis results in medical record.
			Chest x-ray completed. (Report in medical record: Yes____ No____)
			EKG in medical record.
			Type and cross/screen (circle) done. Date drawn:
			History and physical in medical record.
			Forms complete and in medical record:
			1. Nursing documentation with assessment, VS, and wt./ht.
			2. IV Solution Administration Cardex.
			3. Medication Administration Cardex.
			Addressograph plate on cover of medical record. All volumes to procedure, if required.

COMMENTS:

			Blood band on patient and legible. Specify location _____ and blood band #_____
			Identification band on patient and legible. Specify location:
			Bathed and in proper attire.
			Nail polish, makeup, and hairpins removed.
			Jewelry removed. Specify item(s) removed and disposition:
			Prosthesis removed: hearing aid, dentures, eye glasses, contact lenses (circle).
			Other: _____ Disposition: _____
			Anti-embolism stockings on.
			Sequential compression device sleeves on and controller to OR.
			NPO since:
			Teaching completed and documented.
			Preps/tests completed as ordered. Specify:
			Voided/catheterized (circle). Time:
			Medication(s) given.
			Medication(s)/article(s) sent with patient. Specify:

COMMENTS:

Date	Initials	Signature and Title of Individuals Filling Out Form
Date	Initials	Signature of RN Sending Patient to Procedure

41006/4-93/H7528   THE UNIVERSITY OF IOWA HOSPITALS AND CLINICS

FIGURE **36-1**   Preoperative/preprocedural checklist. (Courtesy University of Iowa Hospitals and Clinics.)

an endotracheal tube into the airway (see Chapter 27). This may involve manipulation of the hair and scalp. To avoid injury, ask the client to remove hairpins or clips. Clients should also remove hairpieces or wigs. Long hair can be braided. The client will be asked to wear a disposable hat to contain hair before entering the operating room.

During and after surgery the anesthesia care provider and nurses assess skin and mucous membranes to determine the client's level of oxygenation, circulation, and fluid balance. A pulse oximeter is usually applied to a finger to monitor oxygen saturation of the blood. For these reasons all makeup (lipstick, powder, blush, nail polish) and artificial fingernails should be removed to expose normal skin and nail coloring. Anything in or around the eye may irritate or injure the eye during surgery. Therefore contact lenses, false eyelashes, and eye makeup must also be removed. Glasses usually remain in the room or are given to the family immediately before the client enters the operating room.

Removal of Prostheses. It is easy for any type of prosthetic device to become lost or damaged during surgery. The client must remove all removable prosthetics for safekeeping. If the client has a brace or splint, check with the surgeon to determine whether it should remain with the client, to be reapplied after surgery.

Although hearing aids, dentures, and eyeglasses must be removed, this should not be done until immediately before the client is taken to surgery. Allowing the client to wear these aids facilitates communication and increases the client's sense of control. Refer to the institution's policies for clarification.

Having dentures in place provides a better seal for ventilation during intubation in the operating room. Therefore in some settings dentures are left in place until after the first stages of anesthesia. For many clients, removing dentures is embarrassing. If the dentures are to be removed before surgery, provide privacy. Place dentures in special containers and label with the client's name for safekeeping to prevent breakage. Assess the client for loose teeth. A broken tooth can become dislodged during insertion of an endotracheal tube and obstruct the airway.

You may need to inventory and secure all prosthetic devices, give prosthetics to family members or significant others, or keep the devices at the client's bedside. Follow agency policy, and document where these devices are located.

Preparation of Bowel and Bladder. The client may receive an enema or cathartic the morning of surgery. If so, it should be given at least 1 hour before the client is scheduled to leave, allowing time for the client to defecate without rushing.

The bladder is not prepared until the morning of surgery. Instruct the client to void just before leaving for the operating room. If the client is unable to void, enter a notation on the preoperative checklist. An empty bladder minimizes incontinence and injury to the bladder during surgery. An empty bladder also makes abdominal organs more accessible during surgery. An indwelling catheter may be ordered if the surgery is long or the incision is in the lower abdomen (see Chapter 31).

Application of Antiembolism Devices. Many physicians order **antiembolism stockings** for wear during surgery. They maintain compression of small veins and capillaries of the lower extremities. The constant compression forces blood into larger vessels, thus promoting venous return and preventing venous stasis (see Box 33-7, p. 838). When correctly sized and properly applied, antiembolism stockings can reduce the risk of thrombi (see Chapter 33). **Sequential compression stockings** are also used for promoting venous return. These stockings are attached to an air pump that inflates and deflates the stockings, applying intermittent pressure sequentially from the ankle to the knee.

Promotion of Client's Dignity. During preoperative preparations, care can become depersonalized unless you maintain the client's privacy and reduce sources of anxiety. Ambulatory and same-day surgical admission clients often must sit in a waiting room before surgery. To protect clients' modesty, allow clients to wear underclothes when possible and provide cover robes. Ensure hospitalized clients their privacy by closing room curtains or doors during preoperative preparation. Allow family to stay until the client is transported to the operating room.

Performing Special Procedures. A client's condition may warrant special interventions before surgery. The surgeon's orders state the need to start IV infusions, to insert a Foley catheter or **nasogastric (NG) tube** (see Box 13-11, p. 307), or to administer medications.

Safeguarding Valuables. If a client has valuables, turn them over to family members or secure them for safekeeping in a designated location. Many facilities require clients to sign a release to free the institution of responsibility for lost valuables. Prepare a list with a description of items, place a copy with the client's chart, and give a copy to a designated family member. Clients are often reluctant to remove wedding rings or religious medals. A wedding band can be taped in place; however, care should be taken not to create a tourniquet with the tape. If there is a risk that the client will experience swelling of the hand or fingers, the band should be removed. Many hospitals allow clients to pin religious medals to their gowns, although the risk of loss increases (Fortunato, 2000).

Administering Preoperative Medications. Typically, the physician orders preoperative drugs to be given before the client leaves for the operating room. You must provide all nursing care measures before giving the medication. Because these drugs cause sedation, keep the side rails in the up position, the bed in the low position, and the call bell within easy reach for the client. Instruct the client to remain in bed until the surgical nursing assistant or transporter arrives to

Case Study — EVALUATION

It is the morning of Mr. Korloff's surgery, and Sue is admitting him to the hospital with the assistance of one of his daughters. She checks that the informed consent has been signed and witnessed and completes his physical assessment, which focuses on assessing breath sounds, condition of his skin, and vital signs. Sue also completes the preoperative checklist. She asks Mr. Korloff is he has any questions about the nature or purpose of the surgery. Sue also reviews with Mr. Korloff and his daughter the events that will occur in the holding area and the postanesthesia care unit (PACU). She asks if they are frightened or anxious about any aspect of the procedure or routine, and she addresses their concerns. Sue then reviews with Mr. Korloff the exercises that were in the booklet he received in the mail. Sue has Mr. Korloff demonstrate coughing and deep breathing, while reinforcing its importance once surgery is over. Mr. Korloff is then provided with a hospital gown and cover-up and shown to the changing area. After he has removed his clothes and put on the hospital gown, Mr. Korloff and his daughter are accompanied to the holding area.

Documentation Note

Client admitted for scheduled laparoscopic cholecystectomy. BP 142/84, P 88, R 18, T 98.9° F. Lungs are clear to auscultation bilaterally with normal excursion. Skin warm and dry; no evidence of lesions. Client remained NPO during the night. Reviewed instructions on postoperative exercises, and client is able to demonstrate coughing and deep breathing. Daughters will be in waiting area during procedure.

---

take the client to the operating room and to call for assistance if there is a need to get out of bed. Warn the client to anticipate dry mouth and drowsiness, although the drugs administered, such as benzodiazepines, opioids, antiemetics, and anticholinergics, usually do not induce sleep.

Evaluation

Evaluation of the preoperative goals and outcomes of the plan of care begins before surgery and extends into the postoperative period, providing direction for future interventions. The client's surgery may be an emergency, or procedures may be required up until the time the client is taken to surgery. This leaves little time for evaluation. For some measures, such as those to prevent infection, evaluation is done postoperatively when the outcome can be determined.

CLIENT CARE. Determine if the client and family have adequate preoperative preparation by asking the client to describe the surgical procedure, its purpose, and the postoperative care that will be performed. By having the client and family describe the reasons for postoperative exercises and spirometry you can evaluate the client's understanding of the physiological and psychological responses to surgery. Evaluate adequacy of preoperative teaching by asking the client to demonstrate exercises. Evaluate anxiety by monitoring pulse and blood pressure, facial expressions, and verbal interactions. In addition, ask the client if he or she remains anxious or fearful of any aspect of the surgery.

CLIENT EXPECTATIONS. Determine if the client's and family's expectations have been met up to this point. Spend time talking with the client and family to learn if they are satisfied with their preparation and the approach used by the nursing staff. Knowing this information assists you in helping the client to redefine expectations that can be realistically met. In emergency situations this may become more difficult to evaluate. The family may become the focus of the evaluation if the client is unable to respond or is in a condition that prevents a meaningful discussion.

Transport to the Operating Room

Personnel in the **operating room** notify the nursing unit when it is time for surgery. In many hospitals a nursing assistant or a transporter brings a stretcher for transporting the client. The transporter checks the client's identification bracelet against the client's medical record to be sure the correct person is going to surgery. When a client is to be transported by a stretcher, the nurses and transporter assist the client to safely transfer from bed to stretcher. The ambulatory surgery client, if able and not medicated, may walk to the operating room, providing more control over the event.

Provide the family with an opportunity to visit before the client is transported to the operating room. Then direct the family to the appropriate waiting area. If the client has been hospitalized before surgery and will be returning to the same nursing unit, prepare the bed and room for the client's return. You will be better prepared for postoperative care if the room is readied before the client's return.

Include the following in a postoperative bedside unit:

1. Sphygmomanometer, stethoscope, and thermometer
2. Emesis basin
3. Clean gown
4. Washcloth, towel, and fascial tissues
5. IV pole and pump
6. Suction equipment (if needed)
7. Oxygen equipment if ordered
8. Extra pillows for positioning the client comfortably
9. Bed pads to protect bed linen from drainage
10. PCA pump and tubing if ordered
11. Bed raised to stretcher height with bed linen turned back and furniture moved to accommodate the stretcher

INTRAOPERATIVE SURGICAL PHASE

Care of the client during surgery requires careful preparation and knowledge of the events that will occur during the surgical procedure.

Nurse's Role During Surgery

A nurse usually assumes one of two roles in the operating room: **circulating nurse** or **scrub nurse.** The circulating

Example of a Focused Client Assessment		Table 36-7
Factors to Assess	**Questions and Approaches**	**Physical Assessment Strategies**
The right client	Ask client to state full name.	Inspect client identification band.
The right surgical procedure on the right body part	Ask client to state in his or her own words what has to be done in surgery and where, and compare with operative permit.	Inspect and palpate body part to add any physical evidence of need for surgery (redness, edema, pain). There may be none depending on the nature of the surgery.
The right set of data in chart	Verify and clarify with client any medical, surgical, medication, and allergy history found in preoperative assessment. Review findings from laboratory reports, diagnostic tests, x-ray films, and electrocardiogram (ECG) ordered.	Inspect skin for stated surgical scars. Observe for the presence and patency of ordered tubes and lines (NG, Foley, IV).
The right frame of mind of client	Discuss with client expected outcomes of surgery. Ask client how he or she feels about surgery. If client changes mind about surgery, notify surgeon. Surgery may need to be canceled or postponed.	Observe for signs of fear and anxiety. Monitor vital signs for indications of excessive anxiety. Compare vital signs to baseline.

nurse, who must be a licensed registered nurse (RN), cares for the client while in the operating room by completing another preoperative assessment, establishing and implementing the intraoperative plan of care, evaluating the care, and providing for the continuity of care postoperatively. The circulating nurse assists the anesthesiologist or nurse anesthetist with endotracheal intubation, calculating blood loss and urinary output, and administering blood. This nurse monitors sterile technique and a safe operating room environment, assists the surgeon and scrub nurse by operating nonsterile equipment and providing additional instruments and supplies, and maintains accurate and complete written records.

The scrub nurse, who may be an RN, a licensed practical nurse (LPN), or a surgical technician, is responsible for maintaining a sterile field during the surgical procedure and adhering to strict surgical asepsis. This nurse assists with applying surgical drapes and hands the surgeon instruments, sponges, sutures, and other supplies.

PREANESTHESIA CARE UNIT. In most hospitals the client enters a **preanesthesia care unit** or **presurgical care unit (PSCU)** (sometimes called a holding area) outside the operating room, where preoperative preparations are completed. Nurses in the PSCU are usually part of the operating room staff and wear surgical scrub suits.

In the PSCU a nurse, nurse anesthetist, or anesthesiologist will insert an IV catheter into the client's vein to establish a route for fluid replacement, IV drugs, and blood or blood products if needed. Preoperative medications and/or conscious sedation may be administered at this time.

If hair around the surgical site needs to be removed, this is done in a private area near the operating room immediately before surgery. AORN-recommended practices include the use of clippers for preoperative hair removal when needed. Clippers minimize the risk of irritation and small cuts, which predispose the client to infection (AORN, 1999). Consult the physician's order sheet and the institution's policy and procedure manual.

Admission to the Operating Room

The circulating nurse transfers the client to the operating room. The client is usually still awake and will notice nurses and physicians wearing surgical masks, protective eye wear, and gowns. The staff members carefully transfer the client to the operating bed, being sure the stretcher and bed are locked in place. After the client is on the operating bed, a safety strap is fastened across the client's thighs and the client's arms are secured on padded arm boards with Kling wrap.

NURSING PROCESS

 Assessment

As a nurse in the PSCU, you will conduct a special preoperative assessment to verify the client is ready for surgery and to plan intraoperative care. Ask the client his or her name, and compare the response with the identification band and chart. Then review consent forms, allergies, medical history, physical assessment findings, and test results, and verify with the client what surgery is to be performed and the surgical site (Table 36-7). Pay special attention to the psychological comfort of the client. Also perform a brief assessment of key body systems (Table 36-5, p. 910).

 Nursing Diagnosis

Review preoperative nursing diagnoses, and modify them to individualize the care plan in the operating room. Additional diagnoses and related factors are added based on the client's condition, specific surgical intervention, and method and type of anesthesia used (Box 36-3). Additional diagnoses typical in the intraoperative phase may include *risk for aspiration, ineffective thermoregulation,* and *risk for infection related to the surgical incision.* Nursing care in the operating room must also include monitoring for *latex allergy response* and prevention of *perioperative-positioning injury.* These di-

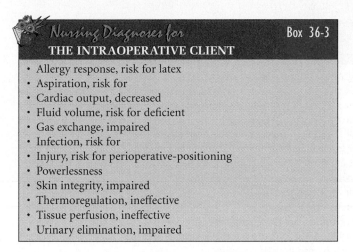

- Allergy response, risk for latex
- Aspiration, risk for
- Cardiac output, decreased
- Fluid volume, risk for deficient
- Gas exchange, impaired
- Infection, risk for
- Injury, risk for perioperative-positioning
- Powerlessness
- Skin integrity, impaired
- Thermoregulation, ineffective
- Tissue perfusion, ineffective
- Urinary elimination, impaired

Examples of Complications of Anesthesia	Table 36-8
Type	Complications
General anesthesia	Aspiration of vomitus
	Cardiac irregularities
	Decreased cardiac output
	Hypotension
	Hypothermia
	Hypoxia
	Laryngospasm
	Malignant hyperthermia
	Nephrotoxicity
	Respiratory depression
Regional anesthesia	Hypotension
Epidural	Hypothermia
Spinal	Injury to spinal cord
	Injury to numb legs
	Respiratory paralysis
	Spinal headache
Local anesthesia	Anaphylactic shock
	Hives
	Rash
Conscious sedation	Aspiration
	Decreased level of consciousness
	Hypoxemia
	Respiratory depression

agnoses provide direction for both intraoperative and postoperative care for this client.

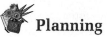

Planning

GOALS AND OUTCOMES.   Some client-centered outcomes of preoperative care extend into the intraoperative phase. These include remaining free of infection and achieving psychological and physical comfort. Additional goals include maintaining skin integrity, therapeutic body temperature, and fluid and electrolyte balance. Achievement of the goals will be measured through outcome criteria, such as the presence of intact skin, without redness or irritation; body temperature within the client's normal range; stable vital signs and adequate urinary output.

Priority setting and continuity of care flow from the plan of care and any additional information from oral and written reports of the preadmission area and/or the presurgical care unit.

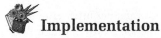

Implementation

A major focus of intraoperative care is to prevent injury and complications related to anesthesia, surgery, positioning, and equipment used. As the perioperative nurse you must act as an advocate for the client during surgery. Protect the client's dignity and rights at all times.

ACUTE CARE
PHYSICAL PREPARATION.   After securing the client safely first apply small plastic electrodes on the chest and extremities for continuous electrocardiographic monitoring during surgery. A monitor displays the heart's electrical activity. Next, apply a blood pressure cuff around the client's arm for the anesthesiologist to measure the blood pressure. Attach a pulse oximeter probe to the client's finger or earlobe, which allows measurement of the oxygen saturation of the blood and an evaluation of ventilation.

PSYCHOLOGICAL SUPPORT.   Entering the operating room is stressful for most clients. Reassure the client and remain at the client's side until after anesthesia is induced. Offering a hand to hold is often helpful. If the client is awake during surgery, this support is given throughout the surgical procedure.

INTRODUCTION OF ANESTHESIA.   The nature and extent of a client's surgery and the client's current physical status influence the type of anesthesia administered in surgery. It is especially important postoperatively that you know the complications to watch for after anesthesia has been administered to a client (Table 36-8).

General Anesthesia.   Under **general anesthesia** all sensation and consciousness are lost, muscles relax, reflexes including gag and blink reflexes are lost, and amnesia is experienced. General anesthesia is used for major procedures requiring extensive tissue manipulation or anytime analgesia, muscle relaxation, immobility, and control of autonomic nervous system are desired. This may include minor procedures, especially with children (Burden, 2000).

Regional Anesthesia.   **Regional anesthesia** results in loss of sensation in an area of the body by anesthetizing sensory pathways. This type of anesthesia is given by infiltration and local application. Administration techniques include peripheral nerve blocks and spinal, epidural, and caudal blocks. There are risks involved with infiltrative anesthetics, particularly in the case of spinal and epidural anesthesia. The client requires careful monitoring during and immediately after regional anesthesia.

Intraoperative Nursing Care	Table 36-9
Outcomes	**Interventions**
Client will be free of infection.	Maintain standard precautions.
	Monitor surgical asepsis.
	Perform surgical skin scrub.
	Apply sterile surgical drapes.
Client will be free of injury.	Perform accurate sponge, needle, and instrument counts.
	Provide grounding for electrosurgical cautery.
	Provide eye protection when laser is used.
Client will maintain body temperature.	Warm room.
	Monitor body temperature.
	Warm irrigating solutions.
	Apply warming blanket immediately after surgery.
Client will maintain fluid and electrolyte balance.	Monitor blood loss, NG drainage, and urinary output.
	Provide blood products as ordered.
	Monitor type and flow rate of IV fluids.

Local Anesthesia.   Local anesthesia involves loss of sensation at the desired site by inhibiting peripheral nerve conduction. Local anesthesia is commonly used for minor procedures performed in ambulatory surgery. Local anesthetics are also administered to clients receiving general or regional anesthesia. Long-acting local anesthetics are sometimes injected into the incision at the end of the client's surgery for postoperative pain relief.

Conscious Sedation.   IV **conscious sedation** is routinely used for procedures that do not require complete anesthesia but simply a decreased level of consciousness. The client must be able to maintain respirations and respond appropriately to physical and verbal stimuli. Advantages to IV conscious sedation include adequate sedation, diminished anxiety, amnesia, pain relief, mood alteration, enhanced client cooperation, stable vital signs, and the rapid recovery with minimal risk (Litwack, 1999).

As the nurse assisting with the administration of conscious sedation, you must be certified in the care of these clients. You must also be able to assess, diagnose, and intervene if a complication arises. Skill in airway management, oxygen delivery, and use of resuscitation equipment is essential (Litwack, 1999). Document vital signs, oxygen saturation, auscultation of breath sounds and heart rhythm, and level of consciousness every 15 minutes during the procedure and the immediate recovery period (American Society of Anesthesiologists, 1996).

Support any client who remains awake by explaining procedures, encouraging questions, and warning the client when unpleasant sensations will be experienced. In some settings music is provided to mask unpleasant sounds and to promote relaxation.

POSITIONING.   Ideally the client's position during surgery provides good access to and exposure of the operative site and sustains adequate circulatory and respiratory function. It should not impair neuromuscular structures or skin in-

tegrity. When using general anesthesia, the nursing personnel and surgeon usually do not position the client until the anesthesia care provider notifies them that the stage of complete relaxation and intubation have been achieved.

The client's comfort and safety must be considered. It is sometimes difficult to understand why clients may feel the range of discomfort after surgery. The alert person maintains normal range of motion by pain and pressure receptors. If a joint is extended too far, pain stimuli warn that muscle and joint strain is too great. In a client who is anesthetized, normal defense mechanisms cannot guard against joint damage and muscle stretch and strain. The client's muscles are so relaxed that it is relatively easy to place the client in a position he or she normally could not assume while awake. The client often remains in a given position for several hours. Once the client awakens, musculoskeletal pain can be significant.

Intraoperative nursing care also includes interventions to prevent infection and injury to the client, to maintain fluid and electrolyte balance, and to control the client's temperature (Table 36-9).

DOCUMENTATION OF INTRAOPERATIVE CARE.   During the intraoperative phase, the nursing staff continues the established plan of care and modifies it as needed. Throughout the surgical procedure you must keep an accurate record of client care activities and procedures performed by operating room personnel. This record provides useful data for the nurse who cares for the client postoperatively.

 Evaluation

Many interventions implemented during the intraoperative phase are evaluated postoperatively, because complications (e.g., infection) can arise days after surgery.

CLIENT CARE.   After surgery, perform a postoperative evaluation of the client. Inspect the skin under the ground-

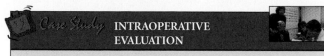

Mr. Korloff's surgery is completed, and he is being transferred to the PACU. Sue has requested that she accompany Mr. Korloff into the PACU. He received general anesthesia, and the procedure was uneventful. Mr. Korloff did not receive any blood or blood products. He did receive Ringer's lactate solution intravenously via a catheter in the left lower forearm. Small gauze dressings were applied to the four small abdominal puncture wounds. At this time the priorities are to maintain Mr. Korloff's vital signs and airway, which is established with an oral airway, and to protect him from injury during transport to the PACU.

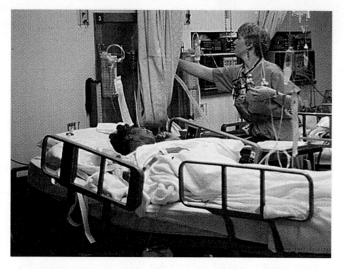

FIGURE **36-2**   Nurse in postanesthesia care unit (PACU).

ing pad and areas of the skin where pressure may have been exerted by equipment or because of positioning. Monitor body temperature during the procedure and immediately postoperatively to assess thermoregulation. Obtain vital signs and auscultate lung sounds to assess pulmonary and fluid and electrolyte status.

CLIENT EXPECTATIONS.   Question a client who is not receiving general anesthesia frequently during the procedure regarding pain, numbness, and perceived room temperature. This determines if adequate analgesia is being maintained and if the client is comfortable in regard to position and temperature.

When the client is undergoing major surgery, it is very important to keep the family informed. Typically, family members want to know if surgery is progressing without problems. Many hospitals provide phones within waiting areas that allow nursing staff to reach families and to explain the progress of the surgery. Nursing staff on the surgical nursing unit can also step by the waiting area to give the families additional information and support.

POSTOPERATIVE SURGICAL PHASE

Following surgery, a client's postoperative course involves two phases: the immediate **recovery** period and **convalescence.** For an ambulatory surgical client the immediate recovery period normally lasts only 1 to 2 hours, and convalescence will occur at home. For a hospitalized client the immediate postoperative period may last a few hours, with convalescence taking 1 or more days, depending on the extent of surgery and the client's response.

Recovery

During recovery it is important for you to be very conscientious in monitoring the surgical client and making the clinical judgments necessary to determine if the client is progressing as expected. This is a time when the client's condition can change very quickly. Immediately after surgery the client is transferred to the **postanesthesia care unit (PACU)** for close monitoring (Figure 36-2). Before the client arrives, you, as the PACU nurse, will receive a report from the surgical team in the operating room to determine

the client's most current status, nursing care priorities, and the need for special equipment. The report will include information about anesthetic agents given during surgery, IV fluids and blood products administered, status of the wound including the presence of drainage devices, and whether the client has had any surgical complications, such as excessive blood loss. The information from the report will allow you to monitor the client, assess for change, and take appropriate preventive action. While the client is in the PACU, conduct ongoing assessments every 15 minutes or more often.

POSTANESTHESIA CARE IN AMBULATORY SURGERY. The postanesthesia care of ambulatory surgery clients occurs in two phases. Phase 1 is essentially the same as described for hospitalized clients in the PACU. Phase 2, however, prepares the client for discharge and self-care. The client receiving only local anesthesia may be admitted directly to the phase 2 area. In phase 2, encourage the client to gradually sit up on the stretcher or recliner and begin to take ice chips or sips of water after regaining full alertness.

Phase 2 postanesthesia care occurs in a room equipped with medical recliner chairs, side tables, and footrests. Kitchen facilities for preparing light snacks and beverages are located in the area, along with bathrooms. The phase 2 environment promotes the client's and family's comfort and well-being until discharge. Continue to monitor the client but not at the same intensity as in phase 1. In phase 2 initiate postoperative teaching with the client and family members (Box 36-4). After the client's condition becomes stable, he or she is discharged.

Convalescence

Once it has been determined a client is stable, usually within 2 to 3 hours, the anesthesia provider or surgeon transfers the hospitalized client to a postoperative nursing unit, whereas the ambulatory surgical client will return home. Unstable clients may remain in the PACU or be transferred to an intensive care unit for more intense monitoring and care.

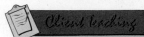

Box 36-4

AMBULATORY SURGICAL CLIENTS
- Physician's office telephone number (24-hour answer)
- Surgery center's telephone number
- Follow-up appointment, date, time
- Review of prescribed medications
- Guidelines related to specific surgery and physician's preference: dressing and wound care, activity restrictions
- Guidelines related to anesthesia: diet resumption, activity restrictions
- Warning signs of complications

During **convalescence** you will consider the goals of care established during the preoperative and intraoperative phases, because your aim is to support the client in returning to normal physiological function. In addition, your nursing care will be directed toward facilitating a client's smooth transition home. This is a time to encourage family participation in the client's plan of care. The family can provide coaching during postoperative exercises and important psychosocial support to the client.

NURSING PROCESS

Assessment

The parameters that you assess for a surgical client are basically the same during recovery and convalescence. When the client enters the PACU, perform a rapid assessment of the respiratory and circulatory status of the client and attach electronic monitors. Assessments must be made while considering the client's surgical risks and the type of surgery performed. For example, if a client has a history of smoking and abdominal surgery involving a high abdominal incision, you will be concerned about the status of respirations. The client's pain could potentially reduce ventilation, potentiating the development of atelectasis.

Once a client reaches a postoperative nursing unit, the measurements and observations are performed less often, usually every 15 to 30 minutes initially, then hourly, and then less often per physician's orders. Table 36-10 summarizes a focused assessment to be performed postoperatively.

RESPIRATION.   Assess the quality of the client's respirations and the patency of the airway. A client receiving a general anesthetic may have an artificial airway still in place when arriving in the PACU. Certain anesthetic agents and opioids may continue to cause respiratory depression. Thus you must be especially alert for slow, shallow breathing. Assess respiratory rate, rhythm, and depth and quality of ventilatory movement. Auscultate lung sounds to identify any abnormalities such as rales, which might be caused by retained secretions, or wheezing, resulting from laryngospasm. If breathing is unusually shallow, place your hand over the client's face or mouth to feel exhaled air. Pulse oximetry reflecting 92% to 100% saturation is within normal limits unless the physician orders other limits (see Chapter 11).

Once a client is on a surgical nursing unit, respirations have usually stabilized. Frequent monitoring of lung sounds is still important because the client is still at risk for developing pneumonia unless postoperative exercises are routinely followed. Remember that pain control will be important during convalescense so that the client can cough and deep breathe with relative ease.

CIRCULATION.   The client is at risk for cardiovascular complications from actual or potential blood loss at the surgical site, side effects of anesthesia, electrolyte imbalances, and depression of normal circulatory regulating mechanisms. Continuous electrocardiographic (ECG) monitoring is routine in the PACU to detect rhythm and rate disturbances. Assessment of heart rate and rhythm and blood pressure reveals the client's cardiovascular status. Compare preoperative vital signs with postoperative values to determine the client's status.

Assess circulatory perfusion, especially for clients who have undergone procedures that impair circulation, such as vascular surgery, use of a tourniquet, or application of casts or tight dressings. Always be alert to the amount of bleeding that occurs after surgery and the possibility of hemorrhage. The risk for hemorrhage continues for several days postoperatively. Blood loss may occur externally through a drain or incision or internally within the surgical wound. Either type of hemorrhage may manifest itself by a fall in blood pressure; elevated heart and respiratory rates; thready pulse; and cool, clammy, pale skin and restlessness.

TEMPERATURE CONTROL.   The operating room environment is cool, and the client's depressed level of body function results in a lowering of metabolism and fall in body temperature. When clients begin to awaken in the PACU, they may complain of feeling cold and uncomfortable. Shivering may not be a sign of hypothermia but rather a side effect of certain anesthetic agents. Measure body temperature to provide direction for interventions. On a surgical unit, monitoring of body temperature is important for detecting early occurrence of wound infection. If a client develops a fever, report it to the surgeon immediately.

NEUROLOGICAL FUNCTION.   In the PACU the client is usually drowsy and reacting to verbal commands. However, drugs, electrolyte and metabolic changes, pain, oxygen saturation, and emotional factors influence level of consciousness. Normally as anesthetic agents are metabolized, the client's reflexes return, muscle strength is regained, and a normal level of orientation returns. Check for pupillary and gag reflexes, hand grasp, and movements of the extremities (see Chapter 12). If a client has had surgery involving a portion of the neurological system, conduct a more thorough neurological assessment.

Example of a Focused Client Assessment

Table 36-10

Factors to Assess	Questions and Approaches	Physical Assessment Strategies
Respirations	Review baseline vital signs for current comparison. Review history for medical conditions involving respiratory system, medications taken, and any allergies. Review report of type of anesthesia and agents used. Review report of any medications given during surgery or after that affect respiratory function (analgesics, antianxiety agents). Ask client to breathe deeply and cough when awake.	Monitor respiratory rate, rhythm, and depth every 15 min × 4 or until stable, then every 30 min × 2, and then every hour × 4. Observe for symmetry of chest wall movements, color of skin and mucous membrane. Auscultate breath sounds for rales, wheezing, decreased or absent sounds. Apply pulse oximeter to detect O_2 saturation.
Circulation	Review baseline vital signs for current comparison. Review report of amount of blood loss and any replacement blood or blood products. Review intake of IV fluids as to type and amount to date. Review current IV orders as to type of fluid and infusion rate. Ask if client experiences dizziness and/or visual disturbances when changing positions. Ask client if extremities are cold and clammy.	Monitor pulse rate and rhythm as well as blood pressure every 15 min × 4 or until stable, then every 30 min × 2, and then every hour × 4 or more often as client's condition warrants. Observe skin and mucous membranes for color and hydration. Observe nail beds for color and capillary refill. Palpate peripheral pulses distal to surgical site, tight dressing, tourniquet, or cast if present. Inspect for amount of bleeding on dressing, in drainage systems (NG suction, Hemovac, Jackson-Pratt drain, Foley catheter) and underneath client. Assess level of consciousness and symptoms of restlessness or altered mental status. Monitor ECG if ordered.
Infection control	Review client history for risk factors for infection (contaminated surgical site, history of diabetes mellitus, human immunodeficiency virus [HIV], or use of immunosuppressing drugs [Prednisone]). Ask client about symptoms of urinary tract or respiratory tract infections.	Monitor client temperature and white blood cell count as indicated. Observe surgical wound for redness, edema, warmth, purulent drainage, and dehiscence. Inspect any output (urine, wound drainage) for color, consistency, and odor. Auscultate lungs for signs of congestion.
Gastrointestinal function	Review report for history of problems with gastrointestinal function. Ask client about symptoms of nausea, cramping, anorexia. Ask client about symptoms of return of bowel function (passing flatus, having bowel movement).	Inspect for abdominal distention caused by gas or bleeding. Auscultate for bowel sounds in all four quadrants at least every shift until discharge. Palpate abdomen for firmness caused by gas, fluid, or mass. Monitor NG tube for patency and NG tube output for color and amount of drainage if present. Observe client's ability and willingness to tolerate fluids and food. Advance diet only with return of active bowel sounds.
Comfort	Review symptoms of pain before surgery, type of anesthesia, location of surgery, and expected level of pain associated with this type of surgery (large incision or laparoscopic procedure). Review history of pain medication use before surgery and since. Review any history of alcohol or illicit drug use. Ask client to rate pain on a 0-10 scale before and after each administration of pain medication. Assess previous pain management techniques.	Observe for signs and symptoms of discomfort (restlessness; elevated pulse, respirations, blood pressure; grimaces; guarding). Observe client for individualized manner of dealing with pain and discomfort. Assess for any side effects of pain medication (altered mental status, depressed respirations, bradycardia, orthostatic hypotension, nausea or vomiting, urinary retention, constipation).

Once a client returns to a surgical nursing unit, a sudden change in consciousness is not normal. However, routine neurological assessment is unnecessary unless a client is slow to awaken fully or has had surgery involving the neurological system.

FLUID AND ELECTROLYTE BALANCE.   Because of the surgical client's risk for fluid and electrolyte abnormalities, assess hydration status and monitor cardiac and neurological function for signs of electrolyte alterations (see Chapter 14). Routinely inspect the IV catheter and insertion site to be sure it is patent, no signs of infiltration are present, and the IV fluids are infusing properly. It is important that a good venous access is available in case the client requires fluid and/or blood replacement. IV fluids will continue on the surgical nursing unit, sometimes for several days. If the IV catheter is in place for over 24 hours, routinely assess for the presence of phlebitis. An IV catheter will remain in place depending on the type of surgery, the medications the client receives, and how well the client tolerates continuation of oral fluids and food.

Monitoring and accurate recording of intake and output help to assess fluid balance, as well as renal and cardiac function. Measure all sources of output, and consult with the physician if appropriate.

SKIN INTEGRITY AND CONDITION OF THE WOUND. Thoroughly assess the condition of the client's skin. A rash may indicate a drug sensitivity or allergy. Abrasions or petechiae may result from inadequate padding during positioning or restraining on the operating bed. If a client has burns or serious injury to the skin, communicate this information by completing an incident report (see Chapter 3).

The surgical wound may have no dressing, or it may be covered with a gauze or transparent dressing that protects the wound site. For open wounds or during the changing of a dressing, observe the appearance of the suture line and note the color, odor, and consistency of any drainage (see Chapter 34). Estimate the amount of drainage by noting the extent and area of the dressing covered (example: lower half of dressing saturated with sanguineous drainage). If a client has a wound drainage system, monitor the output routinely and note the character of drainage. Keep the drainage tubes patent. A sudden increase in drainage can indicate hemorrhage.

A critical time for wound healing is 24 to 72 hours after surgery (see Chapter 34). A client can exert physical stress on a wound from coughing, vomiting, or movement. Inadequate nutrition, impaired circulation, and metabolic alterations can further impair healing. Observe the incision for signs of dehiscence and evisceration. Notify the surgeon of any area of dehiscence. Evisceration is a medical emergency. In the event of evisceration, cover any exposed abdominal contents with a gauze soaked with sterile normal saline. Prepare an IV infusion set for rapid infusion of IV fluids.

If a wound becomes infected, it usually occurs 3 to 6 days after surgery, so it often may develop in the home. Ongoing observation of the wound includes inspection for redness, increased warmth, edema, and purulent drainage.

GENITOURINARY FUNCTION.   Spinal anesthesia may prevent the client from feeling bladder fullness or distention and cause urinary retention for up to 6 to 8 hours. Palpate the lower abdomen just above the symphysis pubis for bladder distention. A full bladder can be painful and is often the cause of a client's restlessness, agitation, or high blood pressure. If the client has a Foley catheter (see Chapter 31), there should be a continuous flow of urine of at least 30 ml/hr in adults. Observe the color and odor of urine. Surgery involving portions of the urinary tract normally causes bloody urine for at least 12 to 24 hours.

GASTROINTESTINAL FUNCTION.   Anesthetic agents slow gastrointestinal motility and may cause nausea. In addition, manipulation of the intestines during abdominal surgery further impairs peristalsis. You will normally hear faint or absent bowel sounds in all four quadrants during the immediate recovery phase. Normal bowel sounds should return in about 24 hours, unless major abdominal surgery was performed. **Paralytic ileus** is always a possibility after abdominal surgery. On the surgical nursing unit ask whether the client is passing flatus, an important sign indicating return of normal bowel function. Inspection of the abdomen rules out distention that may be caused by the accumulation of gas. Distention may also develop if internal bleeding occurs in a client who has had abdominal surgery. If an NG tube is in place, assess the patency of the tube (see Chapter 30) and the color and amount of any drainage.

COMFORT.   As a client awakens from general anesthesia, the sensation of discomfort can become prominent. Pain can be perceived before full consciousness is regained. Acute incisional pain causes the client to become restless and may cause changes in vital signs. Pain management is perhaps one of the most important priorities in postoperative care. If a client has a PCA device, have the client begin using it as soon as possible. It is difficult for clients to begin deep breathing and coughing exercises and to eventually begin turning and ambulation when they have pain, particularly if there is an abdominal or chest incision.

The client who had regional or local anesthesia usually does not experience pain initially, because the incisional area is still anesthetized. You must be skilled at assessing levels of pain and be alert to the client's need for pain medication. Pain scales are an effective method to assess pain, evaluate the response to analgesics, and objectively document the severity of a client's pain (see Chapter 29).

 Nursing Diagnosis

Based on your assessment and information gathered from the reports of members of the surgical team, you will identify nursing diagnoses that apply to your client. These diagnoses give direction to the continuing care of the client in the PACU and on the surgical nursing unit (Box 36-5).

Be sure to analyze and validate assessment data and cluster findings to identify correct nursing diagnoses. For exam-

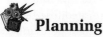

Nursing Diagnoses for
THE POSTOPERATIVE CLIENT   Box 36-5

- Activity intolerance
- Airway clearance, ineffective
- Anxiety
- Body image, disturbed
- Breathing pattern, ineffective
- Communication, impaired verbal
- Constipation, risk for
- Fluid volume, risk for deficient
- Infection, risk for
- Mobility, impaired physical
- Nausea
- Nutrition, imbalanced: less than body requirements
- Pain, acute
- Sleep pattern, disturbed
- Surgical recovery, delayed
- Therapeutic regimen management, ineffective
- Tissue perfusion, ineffective
- Urinary elimination, impaired
- Ventilation, impaired spontaneous

Case Study   POSTOPERATIVE ASSESSMENT AND PLANNING

Mr. Korloff's stay in the PACU is uneventful except for pain in the right shoulder. Air is insufflated into the abdominal cavity during a laparoscopy. The air can cause referred pain. In the PACU Mr. Korloff's pain was a 7 on a 10-point scale.

It is the evening of the day of Mr. Korloff's surgery. Mr. Korloff has been transferred to the nursing division for an overnight stay because of his previous cardiac history. He performs deep breathing and coughing exercises and uses the incentive spirometer as ordered. Because he is ambulating frequently in the hall, with the assistance of his daughters, he is not performing postoperative leg exercises. The IV fluids were discontinued just before he left the PACU. Mr. Korloff was able to tolerate a clear liquid diet and had adequate bowel sounds. He rates his pain as 5 on a 10-point scale, continuing to note some discomfort in the shoulder area. His pain has been controlled with an oral pain medication, acetaminophen, which he receives every 3 to 4 hours. His vital signs are within normal limits compared to preoperative values, and his lungs are clear on auscultation. The four small abdominal puncture wounds are without drainage or redness.

ple, a finding of *anxiety* manifested by restlessness could be related to *acute pain, urinary retention,* or *ineffective tissue perfusion.* Further assessment and clustering of findings will lead to the correct diagnosis.

Planning

Because of the critical nature of the immediate postoperative period, the plan of care in the PACU always involves close monitoring of the client and frequent assessments to ensure stable physiological function. On the surgical nursing unit, your care will become more focused on facilitating the client's recovery. Nursing care will be based on your nursing assessment and the surgeon's postoperative orders. Typical postoperative orders include the following:

1. Frequency of vital signs monitoring and special assessments
2. Types of IV fluids and rate of infusion
3. Postoperative medications (especially those for pain and nausea)
4. Oxygen therapy or incentive spirometry
5. Fluids and food allowed by mouth
6. Level of activity the client is allowed to resume
7. Position that client is to maintain while in bed
8. Intake and output measures
9. Laboratory tests and x-ray studies

GOALS AND OUTCOMES. During recovery in the PACU, goals of care include returning the client to normal physiological functioning without complications and maintaining physical and psychological comfort. Examples of outcomes include stable vital signs within the client's normal range, patent airway, palpable peripheral pulses, oxygen saturation over 95%, an intact incision with minimal wound drainage, and balanced intake and output. The client should also be awake and oriented to the PACU environment with the ability to move all extremities and to verbalize pain relief and decreased anxiety.

Once the client is on the surgical nursing unit, goals are more long term. Maintenance of pain control with improvement in physiological function is still a priority. Adequate wound healing without the presence of infection, restoration of nutrition, the client's return to a functional state of health, and maintenance of self-concept and body image are additional goals. Examples of measurable outcomes include the following: client states level of pain relief is acceptable, appetite and nutritional intake return to previous or improved state, and client states willingness to participate in discharge instruction.

SETTING PRIORITIES. While in the PACU, a client's priorities usually center on physiological needs. As you review preoperative and intraoperative data, as well as your ongoing assessments in the PACU, you will determine how a client is progressing and set priorities on developing needs. For example, if a client begins to awaken without complications but urinary output is less than normal, you may consult with the physician to determine if IV fluids need to be increased to prevent dehydration. Data indicating any immediate postoperative complications such as hemorrhage will require you to alter your plan of care and to take necessary emergency measures.

The client's physical status can still change on the surgical nursing unit, so it remains important to be alert for developing complications. However, management of acute pain will often be the priority of postoperative nursing care. If a surgical client's pain is properly managed, ambulation will begin earlier, deep breathing and coughing will be less difficult, and the client will have a better sense of well-being. In addition, you will begin to prepare the client for discharge by providing the client and family necessary instruction and ensuring that adequate resources are available in the home. Monitoring the client for any psychosocial problems such as body image disturbance or altered coping will also be important during convalescence.

CONTINUITY OF CARE.   Continuity of nursing care between the operating room (OR), the PACU, and the surgical nursing unit depends on good communication among all members of the nursing and surgical team. Nursing staff within each area must be able to convey clear and accurate information about the client's status to the next nurse who assumes care for the client. For example, the condition of a wound must be thoroughly described so that each nurse knows what to anticipate during wound assessment and care. In that way any signs of poor wound healing will be detected early.

The ambulatory surgical client will likely be discharged home with family members or friends. It is essential that the client and family understand continuing care needs of the client. Usually the ambulatory surgery nursing staff has discharge instruction sheets available. When you care for clients on surgical nursing units, be sure that the client's continuing care needs in the home are considered. Referral to home care services or a clinical nurse specialist in wound care or ostomy care, for example, can provide valuable assistance.

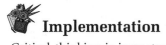 **Implementation**

Critical thinking is important in the postoperative care of the surgical client because you must consider the interrelationship of all body system, and the effect of therapies that are provided. The client remains at risk for a variety of postoperative complications (Table 36-11) unless you provide aggressive care and unless the client becomes actively involved in recovery and convalescence. Review the client's perioperative teaching, and reinforce as needed (Box 36-6). If the client is an older adult, the gerontological nursing practice guidelines in Box 36-7 can be helpful.

RESPIRATION.   Following general anesthesia, a client in the PACU often has an oral or nasal airway inserted to maintain a patent airway until regular breathing at a normal rate resumes. This airway is not taped in place. As respiratory function returns, ask the client to expel the airway. The client's ability to do so signifies a return of a normal gag reflex.

One of your greatest concerns should be airway obstruction resulting from weakness of pharyngeal or laryngeal muscle tone (from the effects of anesthetics), aspiration of emesis, accumulation of secretions in the pharynx or trachea or bronchial tree, or laryngeal or subglottic edema (Litwack, 1999). Often the tongue causes airway obstructions. The following measures maintain airway patency:

1. *Position the client on one side with the face downward and the neck slightly extended.* A small, folded towel supports the head. Neck extension prevents occlusion of the air-

way at the pharynx. When the face is kept turned downward, the tongue moves forward and mucous secretions flow out of the mouth instead of accumulating in the pharynx. If the nature of the surgery prevents turning the client on one side, the head of the bed is slightly elevated and the client's neck slightly extended, with the head turned to the side. Never position the client with arms over or across the chest, because this reduces maximum chest expansion.
2. *Suction the artificial airway and oral cavity for mucous secretions as necessary* (see Chapter 27). Care must be taken to avoid continually eliciting the gag reflex, which might cause vomiting. Before removing an airway, suction the back of the airway to remove any mucous plugs or secretions.
3. *Begin deep breathing and coughing exercises* as soon as the client can respond to instructions.
4. *Administer oxygen as ordered,* and monitor oxygen saturation with a pulse oximeter.

Once a client reaches a surgical nursing unit, begin aggressive pulmonary hygiene. The client should be able to participate actively if your preoperative instruction was effective. Remember, the family can help to coach clients in completing their exercises. Encourage diaphragmatic breathing exercises every hour while the client is awake. Follow diaphragmatic breathing by having the client use the incentive spirometer. The client should try to reach the inspiratory volume achieved preoperatively on the spirometer. Proper use of the spirometer will ensure a maximum inspiration. Encourage regular turning and early ambulation. Walking causes the client to assume a position that does not restrict chest wall expansion, stimulates an increased respiratory rate, and improves circulation. Assist clients who are restricted to bed to turn side-to-side every 1 to 2 hours while awake and to sit when possible. If a client develops pulmonary secretions, encourage coughing exercises followed by deep breathing at least once an hour. Be sure to maintain pain control so that the client can achieve a full, productive cough. Provide frequent oral hygiene to help the client expectorate mucus easily. If the client is not allowed anything by mouth (NPO) or is on a limited fluid intake, the mouth easily becomes dry. Finally, initiate postural drainage and suctioning if the client is too weak or unable to cough secretions (see Chapter 27).

CIRCULATION.   In the PACU it is important to monitor for changes in blood pressure or heart rate. The surgeon may have written an order indicating which changes are to be reported. However, you must use critical thinking and notify the surgeon when there is a significant change or a continuous negative trend in vital signs. If hemorrhage is external, observe for increased bloody drainage on dressings or through drains. If a dressing becomes saturated, the blood will ooze down the client's sides and collect in a pool under bedclothes. Always check under the client for drainage whether or not the dressing is saturated. When hemorrhage is internal, the operative site becomes swollen and tight, and

Common Postoperative Complications

Table 36-11

Complication	Cause

Respiratory System

Atelectasis   Collapse of alveoli with retained mucous secretions. Signs and symptoms: elevated respiratory rate, dyspnea, fever, crackles over involved lobes of lungs, productive cough.

Caused by inadequate lung expansion. Greater risk in clients with upper abdominal surgery who have pain during inspiration and repress deep breathing.

Pneumonia   Inflammation of alveoli caused by infectious process. Usually develops in lower dependent lobes of lung if client is immobilized. Signs and symptoms: fever, chills, productive cough, chest pain, purulent mucus, dyspnea.

Caused by poor lung expansion with retained secretions. *Diplococcus pneumoniae*, a resident bacterium in the respiratory tract, causes most cases of pneumonia.

Hypoxia   Inadequate concentration of oxygen in arterial blood. Signs and symptoms: restlessness, dyspnea, hypertension, tachycardia, diaphoresis, cyanosis.

Respirations depressed by anesthetics or analgesics. Increased retention of mucus with impaired ventilation occurs from pain, poor positioning, or poor coughing and deep breathing.

Pulmonary embolism   Clot blocking pulmonary artery and disrupting blood flow to one or more lobes of lung. Signs and symptoms: dyspnea, sudden chest pain, cyanosis, tachycardia, hypotension.

Immobilized surgical client with preexisting circulatory or coagulation disorders is at risk.

Circulatory System

Hemorrhage   Loss of large amount of blood externally or internally in short period of time. Signs and symptoms: same as for hypovolemic shock.

Caused by slipping of suture or dislodged clot at incisional site. Clients with coagulation disorders are at greater risk.

Hypovolemic shock   Reduced perfusion of tissues and cells from loss of circulatory fluid volume. Signs and symptoms: hypotension, weak and rapid pulse, cool and clammy skin, rapid breathing, restlessness, reduced urine output.

In surgical client, hypovolemic shock is usually caused by hemorrhage.

Thrombophlebitis   Inflammation of vein (usually in leg), often accompanied by clot formation. Signs and symptoms: swelling and inflammation of involved site, aching or cramping pain, positive Homans' sign. Vein feels hard, cordlike, and sensitive to touch.

Venous stasis, trauma to vessel wall, and hypercoagulability of blood increase risk of vessel inflammation.

Embolus   Piece of thrombus that has dislodged and circulates in bloodstream until it lodges in another vessel, commonly lungs, heart, or brain.

Thrombi also form from increased coagulability of blood.

Gastrointestinal System

Abdominal distention   Retention of air within intestines. Signs and symptoms: increased abdominal girth, complaint of fullness and "gas pains."

Caused by slowed peristalsis from anesthesia, bowel manipulation, or immobilization.

Nausea and vomiting   Symptoms of improper gastric emptying or chemical stimulation of vomiting center. Client complains of gagging or feeling full or sick to stomach.

Caused by severe pain, abdominal distention, fear, medications, eating or drinking before peristalsis returns, and initiation of gag reflex.

Genitourinary System

Urinary retention   Involuntary accumulation of urine in bladder as result of loss of muscle tone. Signs and symptoms: inability to void, restlessness, and bladder distention occurring 6-8 hr postoperatively.

Caused by effects of anesthesia, narcotic analgesics, local manipulation of tissues surrounding bladder, and poor positioning of client, which impairs voiding reflex.

Integumentary System

Wound infection   An invasion of deep or superficial wound tissues by pathogenic microorganisms. Signs and symptoms: warm, red, and tender skin around incision, fever and chills, purulent drainage. It appears 3-6 days postoperatively.

Caused by poor aseptic technique and contaminated wound before surgical exploration.

Wound dehiscence   Separation of wound edges at suture line. Signs and symptoms: increased drainage and appearance of underlying tissues occurring 6-8 days after surgery.

Caused by malnutrition, obesity, preoperative radiation to surgical site, old age, poor circulation to tissues, and unusual strain on suture line from coughing.

Wound evisceration   Protrusion of internal organs and tissues through incision. It usually occurs 6-8 days after surgery.

See Wound dehiscence. Client with dehiscence is at risk for developing dehiscence.

THE POSTOPERATIVE PHASE
- Encourage client to practice postoperative exercises every 1 to 2 hours.
- Review rationale for exercise because adults participate more when they know how participation will benefit them.
- Reinforce the need for the client to ask for pain medication before pain becomes severe.
- Encourage client to avoid smoking because nicotine accelerates the metabolism of pain medication, resulting in shorter duration of effect.
- Teach nonpharmacological means of pain control, such as slow deep breathing, progressive relaxation, and use of tactile stimulation, such as back rubs (see Chapter 29).
- Teach the names, purpose, and timing of medications that client will continue at home.
- Teach signs and symptoms of hemorrhage, wound infection, and dehiscence.
- Instruct in proper hand washing and wound care techniques that may be necessary after discharge (see Chapter 34).
- Teach the need for adequate nutrition, rest, and recuperation to optimize wound healing.

- If older client is to be on bed rest for more than 24 hours, an order for subcutaneous heparin may be needed to prevent deep vein thrombosis.
- Intake and output should be maintained longer postoperatively because perfusion of kidneys may be compromised in older adults and they may decrease fluids to minimize voiding frequency.
- Any fluid, electrolyte, or acid-base imbalance will quickly alter mental status. Older adults may need to be placed closer to the nurse's station and be monitored more frequently for confusion, disorientation, or decreased level of consciousness. Fall precautions are a must.
- Clients with increased pain tolerance must be appropriately medicated when they indicate the need. Clients should be asked often to rate their pain and should be given treatment options from which to choose.
- Pain medication is more likely to cause altered mental status in older adults, increasing the need to monitor for confusion and disorientation.
- Metabolism of drugs is slowed in older clients, so the effects of medication may persist for a longer period of time.
- Nutritional deficits are common, and diets high in protein, calcium, and vitamins B and C are needed for wound healing and positive nitrogen balance. Carbohydrate intake is needed for energy and to spare protein use for wound healing. Iron intake should be increased if the client is anemic.
- Older adults have more difficulty with constipation because of decreased peristalsis, decreased activity and abdominal muscles, and decreased neurological stimulation. Orders for a stool softener and/or extra fiber must be accompanied by increased fluid intake despite the resulting increased need to void.

a hematoma may develop. The first signs of suspected hemorrhaging should be reported to the surgeon immediately. Maintain the IV infusion, monitor vital signs continuously, continue oxygen, and raise the client's legs in a modified Trendelenburg's position to promote venous return until the client's condition stabilizes.

Early measures directed at preventing venous stasis will prevent deep vein thrombosis during convalescence. On the surgical nursing unit, begin the following interventions as soon as possible:

1. *Encourage a client to perform leg exercises at least every hour while awake unless contraindicated by surgery.*
2. *Apply elastic antiembolism stockings or pneumatic compression stockings as ordered by the physician (see Chapter 33).* Often these devices are placed on the client in the operating room. The stockings should be removed every 8 hours and left off for 1 hour. Do a thorough assessment of the skin of the legs at this time.
3. *Encourage early ambulation.* Most clients are ordered to ambulate the evening of surgery, depending on the severity of surgery and the client's condition. The degree of activity allowed progresses as the client's condition improves. Before ambulation, assess vital signs.

Abnormalities may contraindicate ambulation. If vital signs are normal, first assist the client to sit on the side of the bed. Dizziness is a sign of postural hypotension (see Chapter 11). A recheck of blood pressure determines whether ambulation is safe. Assist with ambulation by standing at the client's side and helping to either hold or move equipment. During the first few times out of bed, the client may be able to walk only a few feet. Tolerance should improve each time. Evaluate the client's tolerance to activity by periodically assessing pulse rate.

4. *Avoid positioning the client in a manner that interrupts blood flow to the extremities.* While in bed the client should not have pillows or rolled blankets placed directly under the knees. Compression of the popliteal vessels can cause a thrombus to form. When sitting in a chair, the client should elevate the legs on a footstool, avoiding hyperextension of the knee. Never allow the client to sit with one leg crossed over the other.
5. *Administer anticoagulant drugs if ordered.* Small doses of anticoagulants, such as heparin given subcutaneously, reduce risk for thrombus formation. Orthopedic clients often receive low doses of aspirin for anticoagulation.
6. *Promote adequate fluid intake orally or intravenously.* Adequate hydration prevents the concentration of platelets and red blood cells and thus prevents formation of small clots within blood vessels. Adequate hydration also promotes tissue healing and liquefies respiratory secretions.

TEMPERATURE CONTROL.   The client is usually cool when arriving in the PACU. Provide specially warmed blankets or other warming devices (e.g., warming mattress). Increasing body warmth causes the client's metabolism to rise and circulatory and respiratory functions to improve.

A client may still feel cold when reaching a surgical nursing unit. Offer extra blankets or apply a loose-fitting pair of socks to the feet.

NEUROLOGICAL FUNCTION.

Deep breathing and coughing help to expel retained anesthetic gases and increase the client's level of consciousness. Try to arouse the client by calling his or her name in a moderate tone of voice, noting whether the client responds appropriately. If the client remains asleep or is unresponsive, attempt to arouse through touch or by gently moving a body part. If a painful stimulus is needed to arouse the client, then notify the anesthesia care provider. Orientation to the environment is important in maintaining alertness. Explain that surgery is completed, and describe all procedures and nursing measures performed.

FLUID AND ELECTROLYTE BALANCE.

The client's only source of fluid intake immediately after surgery is intravenously; therefore it is important to maintain patency of the IV catheter (see Chapter 14). Once an ambulatory surgical client awakens and is able to tolerate water without gastrointestinal upset, the IV line is usually removed. A more seriously ill client may require an IV line to receive blood products, depending on the amount of blood lost during surgery. The physician orders a prescribed solution and rate for each IV infusion. Most often IV solutions are infused through a pump to ensure the correct volume is delivered hourly.

GENITOURINARY FUNCTION.

A full bladder is painful and can cause a client awakening from surgery to become restless or agitated. Clients who undergo abdominal surgery or surgery of the urinary system frequently have indwelling catheters inserted until voluntary control of urination returns. If a catheter is in place and urinary output is less than 30 ml/hr in an adult client, check for catheter occlusion or kinking and notify the surgeon if measured output does not improve.

During convalescence the following measures promote normal urinary elimination (see Chapter 31):

1. *Assist the client in assuming normal positions for voiding.*
2. *Check the client frequently for the need to void when a catheter is not in place.* The feeling of bladder fullness and urgency to void is often sudden, and you must respond promptly when the client calls for assistance.
3. *Assess for bladder distention.* It may be necessary to insert a straight urinary catheter if a client does not void within 8 hours of surgery or sooner if the bladder is distended. Even if the client has been NPO for hours, IV fluids have been infusing, giving the renal system sufficient fluid to excrete urine. Continued difficulty in voiding may require an indwelling catheter, although the risk for urinary tract infection increases.
4. *Monitor intake and output.* If the client's urine is dark and concentrated, notify the surgeon. A client can easily become dehydrated. Remember, if the output is less than 30 ml/hour, the client may be experiencing acute renal insufficiency or failure, and immediate notification of the surgeon is imperative.

GASTROINTESTINAL FUNCTION.

Minimize a client's nausea during recovery in the PACU by avoiding sudden movement of the client. If the client has an NG tube, maintain tube patency with normal saline irrigations as ordered (skill 36-2). Occlusion of an NG tube causes the accumulation of gastric contents in the stomach. Because stomach emptying slows under anesthesia, the accumulated contents cannot escape, and nausea and vomiting develop. Normally a client does not receive fluids to drink in the PACU because of the risk of vomiting and altered mental status from general anesthesia. You can use a moist cloth or swab to relieve dryness of the client's lips and mouth. If the client is nauseated, give prescribed medication to prevent vomiting and aspiration.

Interventions for preventing gastrointestinal complications during convalescence promote the return of normal elimination and faster resumption of normal nutritional intake. It takes several days for a client who has had surgery on gastrointestinal structures to resume a normal dietary intake. Normal peristalsis may not return for 24 to 48 hours. In contrast, the client whose gastrointestinal tract is unaffected directly by surgery must simply endure the effects of anesthesia before resuming dietary intake. Follow these guidelines:

1. *Maintain a gradual progression in dietary intake.* Immediately after surgery, a client receives only IV fluids. Once the surgeon orders a resumption of oral intake, you will first provide clear liquids, such as water, apple juice, gelatin, or tea, after nausea subsides. Overloading with large amounts of fluids may lead to distention and vomiting. If the client tolerates liquids without nausea, advance the diet to full liquids, followed by a light diet of solid foods, and finally a regular diet, stressing the importance of foods that are high in protein and vitamin C. Clients who have had abdominal surgery are usually NPO the first 24 hours or until the return of bowel sounds.
2. *Promote ambulation and exercise.* Physical activity stimulates a return of peristalsis. The client who suffers abdominal distention and "gas pain" will often obtain relief while walking.
3. *Maintain an adequate fluid intake.* Fluids keep fecal material soft for easy passage.
4. *Administer fiber supplements, stool softeners, enemas, and rectal suppositories as ordered.* Constipation or distention can develop postoperatively related to side effects of anesthetic agents and pain medication.
5. *Stimulate the client's appetite* by removing sources of noxious odors and providing small servings of nonspicy foods.
6. *Assist the client to sit* (if possible) during mealtime to minimize pressure on the abdomen.
7. *Provide frequent oral hygiene.*
8. *Provide meals when the client is rested and free from pain.* A client will often lose interest in eating if mealtime has been preceded by exhausting activities such as ambulation.

Skill 36-2
INSERTING AND MAINTAINING A NASOGASTRIC TUBE

DELEGATION CONSIDERATIONS

The skill of inserting and maintaining the NG tube requires problem solving and knowledge application unique to a professional nurse. Assistive personnel may measure and record the drainage from the NG tube and provide oral and nasal hygiene and comfort measures.

EQUIPMENT

- No. 14 or no. 16 Fr NG tube (smaller-lumen catheters are not used for decompression in adults because they must be able to remove thick secretions)
- Water-soluble lubricating jelly
- pH test strips (measure gastric aspirate acidity)
- Tongue blade

- Flashlight
- Asepto bulb or catheter-tipped syringe
- 1-in (2.5-cm) wide hypoallergenic tape
- Safety pin and rubber band
- Clamp, drainage bag, or suction machine or pressure gauge if wall suction is to be used
- Bath towel
- Glass of water with straw
- Facial tissues
- Normal saline
- Tincture of benzoin (optional)
- Disposable gloves

STEPS	RATIONALE
1. Inspect condition of client's nasal and oral cavity.	Baseline condition of nasal and oral cavity determines need for special nursing measures for oral hygiene after tube placement.
2. Ask if client has had history of nasal surgery and note if deviated nasal septum is present.	Nurse should insert tube into uninvolved nasal passage. Procedure may be contraindicated if surgery is recent.
3. Palpate client's abdomen for distention, pain, and rigidity. Auscultate for bowel sounds.	Baseline determination of level of abdominal distention later serves as comparison once tube is inserted.
4. Assess client's level of consciousness and ability to follow instructions.	Determines client's ability to assist in procedure.

• *Critical Decision Point*
  If client is confused, disoriented, or unable to follow commands, obtain assistance from another staff member to insert the tube.

STEPS	RATIONALE
5. Check medical record for surgeon's order, type of NG tube to be placed, and whether tube is to be attached to suction or drainage bag.	Procedure requires physician's order. Adequate decompression depends on NG suction.
6. Prepare equipment at the bedside. Have a 2- to 3-in piece of tape ready with one end split in half.	
7. Identify client and explain procedure.	Identification prevents error of placing tube in wrong client. Explanation gains client's cooperation and lessens possibility that client will remove tube.
8. Wash hands and apply disposable gloves.	Reduces transmission of microorganisms.
9. Position client in high Fowler's position with pillows behind head and shoulders. Raise bed to a horizontal level comfortable for the nurse.	Promotes client's ability to swallow during procedure. Good body mechanics prevent injury to nurse or client.
10. Pull curtain around the bed or close room door.	Provides privacy.
11. Stand on client's right side if right-handed, left side if left-handed.	Allows easiest manipulation of tubing.
12. Place bath towel over client's chest; give facial tissues to client.	Prevents soiling of client's gown. Tube insertion through nasal passages may cause tearing and coughing with increased salivation.
13. Instruct client to relax and breathe normally while occluding one naris. Then repeat this action for other naris. Select nostril with greater air flow.	Tube passes more easily through naris that is more patent.

14. Measure distance to insert tube:
    A. **Traditional method:** Measure distance from tip of nose to earlobe to xiphoid process (see illustration).

    B. **Hanson method:** First mark 50-cm point on tube, then do traditional measurement. Tube insertion should be to midway point between 50 cm (20 in) and traditional mark.

    Tube should extend from nares to stomach; distance varies with each client.

15. Mark length of tube to be inserted with small piece of tape placed so it can easily be removed.

    Marks amount of tube to be inserted from nares to stomach.

16. Cut a 10-cm (4-in) piece of tape. Split one end down the middle lengthwise 5 cm (2 in). Place on bed rail or bedside table.

    Tape will be used after tube insertion to anchor the tube securely.

17. Curve 10 to 15 cm (4 to 6 in) of end of tube tightly around index finger, then release.

    Curving tube tip aids insertion and decreases stiffness of tube.

18. Lubricate 7.5 to 10 cm (3 to 4 in) of end of tube with water-soluble lubricating jelly.

    Minimizes friction against nasal mucosa and aids insertion of tube.

19. Alert client that procedure is to begin.

    Decreases client anxiety and increases client cooperation.

20. Initially instruct client to extend neck back against pillow; insert tube slowly through naris with curved end pointing downward (see illustration).

    Facilitates initial passage of tube through naris and maintains clear airway for open naris.

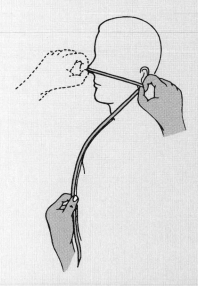

STEP 14A

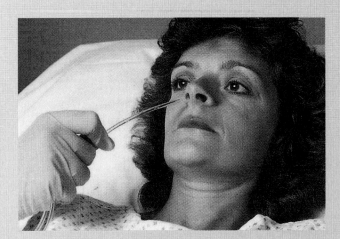

STEP 20

21. Continue to pass tube along floor of nasal passage, aiming down toward ear. When resistance is felt, apply gentle downward pressure to advance tube (do not force past resistance).

    Minimizes discomfort of tube rubbing against upper nasal turbinates. Resistance is caused by posterior nasopharynx. Downward pressure helps tube curl around corner of nasopharynx

22. If resistance is met, try to rotate the tube and see if it advances. If still resistant, withdraw tube, allow client to rest, relubricate tube, and insert into other naris.

    Forcing against resistance can cause trauma to mucosa. Helps relieve client's anxiety.

• **Critical Decision Point**
If unable to insert tube in either naris, stop procedure and notify physician.

STEPS	RATIONALE
23. Continue insertion of tube until just past nasopharynx by gently rotating tube toward opposite naris.	
a. Stop tube advancement, allow client to relax, and provide tissues.	Relieves client's anxiety; tearing is natural response to mucosal irritation, and excessive salivation may occur because of oral stimulation.
b. Explain to client that next step requires that client swallow. Give client glass of water unless contraindicated.	Sipping of water aids passage of NG tube into esophagus.
24. With tube just above oropharynx, instruct client to flex head forward, take a small sip of water, and swallow. Advance tube 2.5 to 5 cm (1 to 2 in) with each swallow of water. If client is not allowed fluids, instruct to dry swallow or suck air through straw. Advance tube with each swallow.	Flexed position closes off upper airway to trachea and opens esophagus. Swallowing closes epiglottis over trachea and helps move the tube into the esophagus. Swallowing water reduces gagging or choking. Water can be removed later from stomach by suction.
25. If client begins to cough, gag, or choke, withdraw slightly and stop tube advancement. Instruct client to breathe easily and take sips of water.	Tubing may accidentally enter larynx and initiate cough reflex. Gaging is eased by swallowing water. Risk for aspiration increases if vomiting occurs.

• *Critical Decision Point*

If vomiting occurs, assist client in clearing airway; oral suctioning may be needed. Do not proceed until airway is cleared.

STEPS	RATIONALE
26. If client continues to cough during insertion, pull tube back slightly.	Tube may enter larynx and obstruct airway.
27. If client continues to gag, check back of pharynx using flashlight and tongue blade.	Tube may coil around itself in back of throat and stimulate gag reflex.
28. After client relaxes, continue to advance tube desired distance.	Tip of tube should be within stomach to decompress properly.
29. Once tube is correctly advanced, remove tape used to mark length of tube and place the prepared split tape with nonsplit side on nose. Anchor with one of split ends while checking tube placement.	Tube should be partially anchored before placement is checked.
30. Checking tube placement: check institutional policy for preferred methods for checking tube placement.	
a. Ask client to talk.	Client is unable to talk if NG tube has passed through vocal cords.
b. Inspect posterior pharynx for presence of coiled tube.	Tube is pliable and can coil up in back of pharynx instead of advancing into esophagus.
c. Aspirate gently back on syringe to obtain gastric contents, observing color (see illustration).	Gastric contents are usually cloudy and green, but may be off-white, tan, bloody, or brown in color. Aspiration of contents provides means to measure fluid pH and thus determine tube tip placement in gastrointestinal tract. Other common aspirate colors include the following: Duodenal placement (yellow or bile stained), esophagus (may or may not have saliva-appearing aspirate).
d. Measure pH of aspirate with color-coded pH paper with range of whole numbers 1 to 11 (see illustration).	Gastric aspirates have decidedly acidic pH values, preferably 4 or less, compared with intestinal aspirates, which are usually greater than 4, or respiratory secretions, which are usually greater than 5.5 (Metheny and others, 1993, 1994, 1998).

• *Critical Decision Point*

Be sure to use gastric (Gastrocult) pH test and not Hemoccult test.

STEPS	RATIONALE
e. If tube is not in stomach, advance another 2.5 to 5 cm (1 to 2 in) and repeat steps, 30C, D, and E to check tube position.	Tube must be in stomach to provide decompression.

STEPS	RATIONALE
31. Anchoring tube: a. After tube is properly inserted and positioned, either clamp end or connect it to drainage bag or suction machine.	Drainage bag is used for gravity drainage. Intermittent suction is most effective for decompression. Client going to the operating room often has tube clamped.
b. Tape tube to nose; avoid putting pressure on nares.	Prevents tissue necrosis. Tape anchors tube securely. Benzoin prevents loosening of tape if client perspires.
(1) Before taping tube to nose, apply small amount of tincture of benzoin to lower end of nose and allow to dry (optional). Be sure top end of tape over nose is secure.	
(2) Carefully wrap two split ends of tape around tube (see illustration).	
(3) Alternative: Apply tube fixation device using shaped adhesive patch (see illustration).	
c. Fasten end of NG tube to client's gown by looping rubber band around tube in slip knot. Pin rubber band to gown (provides slack for movement).	Reduces pressure on the nares if tube moves.
d. Unless physician orders otherwise, head of bed should be elevated 30 degrees.	Helps prevent esophageal reflux and minimizes irritation of tube against posterior pharynx.
e. Explain to client that sensation of tube should decrease somewhat with time.	Adaptation to continued sensory stimulus.
f. Remove gloves and wash hands.	Reduces transmission of microorganisms.

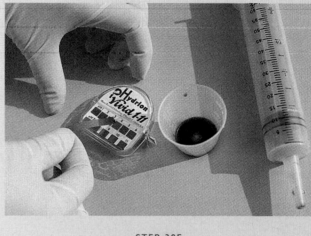

STEP 30E

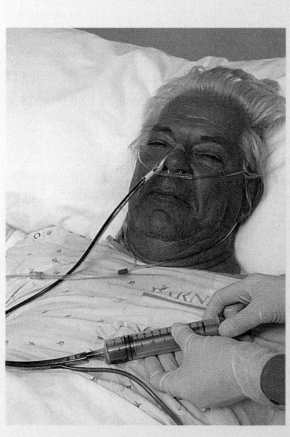

STEP 30C

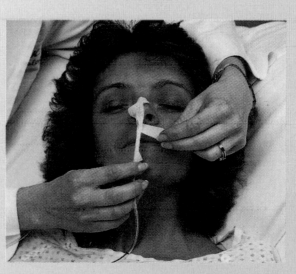

STEP 31B(2)

STEPS	RATIONALE

32. Safety:
    a. Once placement is confirmed, place a mark, either a red mark or tape, on the tube to indicate where the tube exits the nose. — The mark or tube length is to be used as a guide to indicate whether displacement may have occurred.
    b. Measurement of the tube length from nares to connector is an alternate method. If tube length is the method used, document the tube length in the client record.

33. Tube irrigation:
    a. Wash hands and apply gloves. — Reduces transmission of microorganisms.
    b. Check for tube placement in stomach (see Step 30). Reconnect NG tube to connecting tube. — Prevents accidental entrance of irrigating solution into lungs.
    c. Draw up 30 ml of normal saline into Asepto or catheter-tipped syringe. — Use of saline minimizes loss of electrolytes from stomach fluids.
    d. Clamp NG tube. Disconnect from connection tubing and lay end of connection tubing on towel. — Reduces soiling of client's gown and bed linen.
    e. Insert tip of irrigating syringe into end of NG tube. Remove clamp. Hold syringe with tip pointed at floor and inject saline slowly and evenly. Do not force solution. — Position of syringe prevents introduction of air into vent tubing, which could cause gastric distention. Solution introduced under pressure can cause gastric trauma.

• **Critical Decision Point**
Do not introduce saline through blue colored "pigtail" air vent of Salem sump tube.

    f. If resistance occurs, check for kinks in tubing. Turn client onto left side. Repeated resistance should be reported to surgeon. — Tip of tube may lie against stomach lining. Repositioning on left side may dislodge tube away from the stomach lining. Buildup of secretions will cause distention.
    g. After instilling saline, immediately aspirate or pull back slowly on syringe to withdraw fluid. If amount aspirated is greater than amount instilled, record the difference as output. If amount aspirated is less than amount instilled, record the difference as intake. — Irrigation clears tubing, so stomach should remain empty. Fluid remaining in stomach is measured as intake.
    h. Reconnect NG tube to drainage or suction. (If solution does not return, repeat irrigation.) — Reestablishes drainage collection; may repeat irrigation or repositioning of tube until NG tube drains properly.
    i. Remove gloves and wash hands. — Reduces transmission of microorganisms.

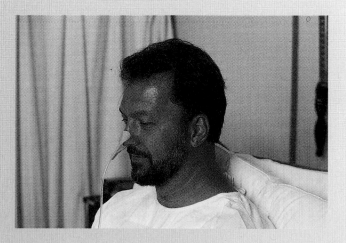

STEP 31B(3)

STEPS	RATIONALE
34. Discontinuation of NG tube:	
a. Verify order to discontinue NG tube.	Physician's order required for procedure.
b. Explain procedure to client and reassure that removal is less distressing than insertion.	Minimizes anxiety and increases cooperation. Tube passes out smoothly.
c. Wash hands and apply disposable gloves.	Reduces transmission of microorganisms.
d. Turn off suction and disconnect NG tube from drainage bag or suction. Remove tape from bridge of nose and unpin tube from gown.	Have tube free of connections before removal.
e. Stand on client's right side if right-handed, left side if left-handed.	Allows easiest manipulation of tube.
f. Hand the client facial tissue; place clean towel across chest. Instruct client to take and hold a deep breath.	Client may wish to blow nose after tube is removed. Towel may keep gown from getting soiled. Airway will be temporarily obstructed during tube removal.
g. Clamp or kink tubing securely and then pull tube out steadily and smoothly into towel held in other hand while client holds breath.	Clamping prevents tube contents from draining into oropharynx. Reduces trauma to mucosa and minimizes client's discomfort. Towel covers tube, which can be an unpleasant sight. Holding breath helps to prevent aspiration.
h. Measure amount of drainage and note character of content. Dispose of tube and drainage equipment.	Provides accurate measure of fluid output. Reduces transfer of microorganisms.
i. Clean nares and provide mouth care.	Promotes comfort.
j. Position client comfortably and explain procedure for drinking fluids, if not contraindicated.	Depends on physician's order. Sometimes clients are allowed nothing by mouth (NPO) for up to 24 hours. When fluids are allowed, the order usually begins with a small amount of ice chips each hour and increases as client is able to tolerate more.
35. Clean equipment and return to proper place. Place soiled linen in utility room or proper receptacle.	Proper disposal of equipment prevents spread of microorganisms and ensures proper exchange procedures.
36. Remove gloves and wash hands.	Reduces transmission of microorganisms.
37. Observe amount and character of contents draining from NG tube. Ask if client feels nauseated.	Determines if tube is decompressing stomach of contents.
38. Palpate client's abdomen periodically, noting any distention, pain, and rigidity and auscultate for the presence of bowel sounds. Turn off suction while auscultating.	Determines success of abdominal decompression and the return of peristalsis. The sound of the suction apparatus may be transmitted to abdomen and be misinterpreted as bowel sounds.
39. Inspect condition of nares and nose.	Evaluates onset of skin and tissue irritation.
40. Observe position of tubing.	Determines if tension is being applied to nasal structures.
41. Ask if client feels sore throat or irritation in pharynx.	Evaluates level of client's discomfort.

UNEXPECTED OUTCOMES AND RELATED INTERVENTIONS

- Client develops abdominal distention, vomiting, or absence of drainage from NG tube.
  - Assess patency of tube and irrigate as needed.
  - If tube remains clogged or obsructed notify physician.
- Persistent gagging leads to vomiting with aspiration of GI contents.
  - Position client on side, remove tube if gagging continues, and suction airway as needed.
  - Notify physician.
- Nasal mucosa becomes inflamed, tender and/or eroded.
  - Retape tube to relieve pressure on mucosa.
  - Consider removal of tube, and reinsert in opposite naris (Physician order required).

- Client complains of sore throat from dry, irritated mucous membranes.
  - Perform oral hygiene more frequently.
  - Ask physician whether client can suck on ice chips or throat lozenges or chew gum.

RECORDING AND REPORTING

- Record in nurses' notes time and type of NG tube inserted, client's tolerance of procedure, confirmation of placement, character of gastric contents, pH value, and whether tube is clamped or connected to drainage device.
- Record in nurses' notes and/or flow sheet amount and character of contents draining from NG tube every shift, unless ordered more frequently by physician.

COMFORT. The anesthesiologist or nurse anesthetist orders medications for pain management in the PACU. IV opioid analgesics, such as morphine sulfate, are the drugs of choice for the immediate postoperative period. Administer morphine intravenously, titrating it as ordered until pain relief is achieved. Morphine may depress vital signs and level of consciousness, but at appropriate doses this is rare. However, a low blood pressure may be caused by acute pain. In such a situation an analgesic may improve vital sign values. You must be skilled at determining the proper dose of an analgesic and knowing possible side effects. Once a client is awake, a PCA pump may be ordered.

A client's pain increases as the effects of anesthesia wear off once the client reaches the surgical nursing unit. The client becomes more aware of surroundings and more perceptive of discomfort. The incisional area may be only one source of pain. Irritation from drainage tubes, tight dressings, or casts and the muscular strains caused from positioning on the operating bed can cause discomfort.

Pain can significantly slow recovery. The client becomes reluctant to perform necessary postoperative exercises. Assess the client's pain thoroughly. Do not assume that the pain is incisional in origin. When the client requests pain medication, determine the nature and character of the pain. Clients have the most surgical pain during the first 24 to 48 hours after surgery. Provide analgesics as often as allowed during this time. IV or epidural PCA systems allow the client to administer analgesics from specially prepared pumps (see Chapter 29). A PCA device is attached to the IV line, or the analgesic is given via an epidural catheter, as with fentanyl or morphine. The client controls the amount of analgesia received within set parameters ordered by the surgeon or anesthesia care provider and programmed into the pump. PCA medication can be delivered at a preprogrammed basal rate, a specific bolus dose at specified intervals as needed, or both. When a client is on a PCA, document respirations and level of consciousness. Documentation of frequent objective pain assessment using a pain scale, appropriate nursing interventions, and evaluation of the client's response must be in every client's medical record as of January 2001 according to the Joint Commission on Accreditation of Healthcare Organizations (JCAHO) 2000 Standards (Sandlin, 2000).

PROMOTING WOUND HEALING. Surgical dressings should be left in place to reduce the risk of infection. During the first 24 hours you may simply add an extra layer of gauze on top of the original dressing if drainage develops. Notify the physician if bleeding is excessive. In certain types of surgery the surgeon may choose to use no dressing at all.

During convalescence continue close observation of the surgical wound. If a wound becomes infected, it usually occurs 3 to 6 days after surgery. Always use aseptic technique during dressing changes and wound care. Surgical drains must remain patent so that accumulated secretions are removed from the incision site. Observation of the wound identifies early signs and symptoms of infection such as redness, increased warmth, edema, odor, and purulent drainage (see Chapter 34).

To ensure continuity of care be sure that all staff are aware of the proper materials to use in a dressing change. It is not uncommon for clients to feel discomfort during an extensive dressing change, so offer a pain medication 30 minutes before the procedure. If you anticipate that the client will need to continue dressing changes in the home, plan instruction at a time when the client is alert and comfortable, and family caregivers are present. Be sure at the time of discharge that a client knows how to obtain the materials needed for the dressing change.

MAINTAINING SELF-CONCEPT. During a client's convalescence, the appearance of wounds, bulky dressings, and extruding drains and tubes threatens a client's self-concept. The nature of the surgery may also create a permanent change in body image. If surgery leads to impairment in body function, the client's role within the family and community can change significantly. Observe the client for alterations in self-concept (see Chapter 19). Clients may show revulsion toward their appearance by refusing to look at an incision or carefully covering dressings with bedclothes. The fear of not being able to return to a functional role in the family or at a previously held job may even cause the client to avoid participating in the care plan.

The family can play an important role in efforts to improve the client's self-concept. Help the family to accept the client's needs and still encourage independence. The following measures maintain the clients' self-concept:

1. *Provide privacy* during dressing changes or wound inspection by closing room curtains and draping the client so that only the dressing and incisional area are exposed.
2. *Maintain the client's hygiene.* A complete bath the first day after surgery can make the client feel renewed. Offer a clean gown and washcloth when the gown become soiled. Keep the client's hair neatly combed, and offer frequent oral hygiene, especially for the client who is allowed nothing by mouth.
3. *Prevent drainage sets from overflowing.* Typically the drainage sets are measured every 8 hours for output recording, but they may need to be emptied and measured more often.
4. *Maintain a pleasant environment.* Store or remove all unused supplies, and keep the bedside orderly and clean.
5. *Offer opportunities for the client to discuss feelings about appearance.* Clients worry about permanent scarring. When the client chooses to look at an incision for the first time, the area should be clean. Eventually the client should be able to care for the incision site by applying simple dressings or bathing.
6. *Give the family opportunities to discuss ways to promote the client's self-concept.* Encouraging independence can be difficult for a family member who has a strong desire to assist the client in any way. By knowing about the appearance of a wound or incision, family members can be supportive during dressing changes.

RESTORATIVE AND CONTINUING CARE. Other activities that are involved in postoperative care are to promote return to a functional state of health. Throughout the postoperative convalescent period promote the client's independence and active participation in care. When a client is in pain or suffers from postoperative complications, there is little motivation for self-care. The goals you set for a client's involvement must be realistic. It is unrealistic to involve the client if movement is highly restricted or if participation increases the client's discomfort.

Keep the client and family informed of progress made toward recovery. Many clients become depressed if they think recovery is slow. Explain the length of time expected to reach a level of maximal recovery. Surgery may also cause permanent physical limitations that will require time for the client to accept.

You should plan care daily, keeping in mind the ultimate goals for recovery. From the moment the client enters the hospital, anticipate and plan for the client's return home.

Involvement of family members in the care plan can facilitate early discharge and adequate care at home. Instruct family members in care activities. If family members are unable to assist the client, work with the surgeon, social worker, and/or discharge planner for referrals to home care agencies to provide services that may be needed at home.

Evaluation

CLIENT CARE.   As a PACU nurse, you continuously evaluate the effectiveness of interventions and the client's response. The client's condition can change quickly. Your evaluation of the client's status involves ongoing measurement of vital signs, pulse oximetry, wound drainage, intake and output, and other physical assessments. The Glascow Coma Scale (see Chapter 12) evaluates the client's level of consciousness

and return of motor function. You may need to increase frequency of interventions based on the client's response. If evaluation reveals the client is recovering from anesthesia, the surgeon will discharge the client from the PACU.

On the surgical nursing unit evaluate the effectiveness of care on the basis of expected outcomes resulting from nursing interventions (Box 36-8). Your evaluation will occur over several days. It is important to evaluate the client's clinical progress by observing the client's participation in

---

Case Study   EVALUATION

Mr. Korloff progressed well and is ready for discharge the day after surgery. He expresses relief that everything went well so that he will be able to return to work, hopefully by next week. Sue continues to care for him on the surgical division. Sue explains how to remove the gauze on the puncture sites and to bathe and shower tomorrow. Symptoms the client and family should be observant for are redness, swelling, bile-colored drainage or pus from the abdominal wounds, severe abdominal pain, nausea, vomiting, and fever or chills. Any of these symptoms should be reported to Mr. Korloff's physician immediately. His daughters observed the puncture sites and are able to identify symptoms of complications. Mr. Korloff is ready for discharge and plans to stay with one of his daughters over the weekend. Sue makes a follow-up surgical appointment for Mr. Korloff.

Documentation Note
Sue documents Mr. Korloff's readiness for discharge as follows: Abdominal puncture sites dry and intact, without redness. Discharge teaching provided to client and daughters. Repeated signs and symptoms of complications; wound care instructions; activity restrictions; and follow-up appointment time, date, and place.

Outcome Evaluation for   MR. KORLOFF   Box 36-8

Nursing Action	Client Response/Finding	Achievement of Outcome
Observe Mr. Korloff's willingness and ability to turn, deep breathe with incentive spirometer, and to cough every 1 to 2 hours while awake.	He is able and willing to turn, deep breathe, and cough every 2 hours without assistance. He is able to use incentive spirometer to 1500 ml.	Breath sounds clear in all lobes and equal bilaterally.
Observe Mr. Korloff performing leg exercises every 1 to 2 hours while awake until he is ambulating.	He is able to perform ankle circles and calf pumping every 2 hours without difficulty. He refused to do quadriceps setting and leg lift exercises.	Lower extremities warm and pink with brisk capillary refill.
Ambulate Mr. Korloff progressively starting first morning postoperatively as ordered.	He is able to ambulate in room and in hall by postoperative day 2 without assistance.	No redness, edema, excessive warmth, or pain in either calf noted.
Monitor intake and output every shift.	Intake: IV 1000 ml Output: Foley 950 ml PO 400 ml Void 300 ml Total 1400 ml Total 1250 ml	Intake and output within normal limits.
Monitor infusion of IV solutions via pump as ordered.	IV solution of D5NS infusing via pump at 125 ml/hr without signs of redness or edema.	
Ask Mr. Korloff if nausea is experienced.	He is taking clear fluids PO without nausea.	Mr. Korloff is able to resume oral fluid intake and normal urinary elimination without difficulty.
Encourage early voiding postoperatively or after catheter removal.	He is able to void 300 ml in bathroom without difficulty within 2 hours after surgery or Foley catheter removed.	
Monitor for bladder distention and urinary retention with overflow.	No bladder distention noted.	

postoperative exercises, self-care activities, and ambulation. Evaluate the ambulatory surgical client's outcomes by making a postoperative telephone call to the client's home. The call, usually placed 24 hours after surgery, reassures the client that you are concerned and allows you to evaluate the progress of recovery and to answer any questions the client or family may have.

CLIENT EXPECTATIONS. In the PACU the client may not be able to voice expectations. However, evaluation of pain is critical. Because pain is subjective, it must be validated by frequently asking the client how he or she feels. If possible, use a pain assessment scale. Note the client's movement and positioning, because nonverbal behaviors can indicate

whether comfort is achieved. If pain is not adequately relieved, the dosage or type of medication may need to be changed. Also evaluate the client's level of anxiety by assessing presence of any concerns or fears. Further explanation of postoperative progress and procedures can reduce anxiety.

As a client progresses through convalescence, physical and psychological comfort continue to be typical expectations of clients and families. Also evaluate if the client feels prepared for discharge from the acute care facility. Is the client able to explain the care that must continue following discharge? Have the client demonstrate any procedures such as wound care or medication administration. Give the client and family numerous opportunities to ask questions about what to anticipate once the client returns home.

Key Terms

antiembolism stockings, *p. 924*
atelectasis, *p. 903*
bronchospasm, *p. 907*
circulating nurse, *p. 925*
conscious sedation, *p. 928*
convalescence, *p. 929*
dehiscence, *p. 904*
embolism, *p. 904*

evisceration, *p. 904*
general anesthesia, *p. 927*
laryngospasm, *p. 907*
malignant hyperthermia, *p. 907*
nasogastric (NG) tube, *p. 924*
operating bed, *p. 903*
operating room, *p. 925*
outpatient, *p. 903*
paralytic ileus, *p. 932*
perioperative nursing, *p. 903*

postanesthesia care unit (PACU), *p. 929*
preanesthesia care unit, *p. 926*
preoperative teaching, *p. 906*
presurgical care unit (PSCU), *p. 926*
pulmonary hygiene, *p. 907*
recovery, *p. 929*
regional anesthesia, *p. 927*
scrub nurse, *p. 925*
sequential compression stockings, *p. 924*

Key Concepts

- Perioperative nursing is professional nursing care given to the surgical client before, during, and after surgery.
- Previous illnesses and past surgeries influence the ability to tolerate surgery.
- Older adult clients are at surgical risk because of their declining physiological status.
- All medications taken before surgery are automatically discontinued after surgery unless a physician reorders the drugs.
- Family members are important in assisting clients with physical limitations and in providing emotional support postoperatively.
- Preoperative assessment of vital signs and physical findings provides an important baseline with which to compare postoperative assessment data.
- A client's feelings about surgery can influence relationships with nursing staff and the client's ability to participate in care.
- Nursing diagnoses of the surgical client may pose implications for nursing care during one or all phases of surgery.
- Primary responsibility for informed consent rests with the surgeon.

- Structured preoperative teaching positively influences postoperative recovery.
- If hair around the incision must be removed, it should be clipped as close as possible to the time of surgery to minimize infection.
- In ambulatory surgery, nurses use the limited time available to assess, prepare, and educate clients for surgery.
- The responsibility of nurses within the operating room focuses on protecting the client from potential harm.
- Assessment of the postoperative client centers on the body systems most likely to be affected.
- Because a surgical client's condition may change rapidly during recovery, the nurse monitors the client's status at least every 15 minutes until stable.
- The PACU nurse reports to the nurse on the postoperative unit information pertaining to the client's current physical status and risk for postoperative complications.
- Nursing interventions postoperatively focus on prevention of complications.
- Failure of the client to become actively involved in recovery adds to the risk of complications developing.
- From the time of admission the nurse plans for the surgical client's discharge.

Critical Thinking Activities

1. Mr. Wilson is a 76-year-old client admitted for a fractured hip. He has a history of emphysema. What risk does Mr. Wilson face as a result of surgery, and why? What additional questions should be asked of Mr. Wilson concerning this risk?

2. Mary is the nurse working in the preadmission center for surgical services. She is interviewing Mrs. Rice, who states that she has been taking one baby aspirin every day to help with her circulation. Why is this important for Mary to document?

3. Angie is a nursing student assigned to Mrs. Lyons, a 45-year-old woman who is recovering from surgery for a colon resection. It is the third day after surgery, and Mrs. Lyons's NG tube was removed yesterday afternoon. During her morning rounds Angie is assessing Mrs. Lyons and finds that her abdomen is distended. What might this indicate? What additional assessment data should be gathered?

4. Mr. Pulley had a colon resection yesterday and has a midline incision that extends from the xiphoid process to the symphysis pubis. Carmen has been assigned as his nurse and assesses rales when auscultating his lungs. What information regarding Mr. Pulley's incision must Carmen consider in planning interventions to address the nursing diagnosis of *ineffective airway clearance*?

5. A postoperative client with an IV infusion of 5% dextrose in 0.45% solution chloride has an order to discontinue the IV infusion. What client parameters must the nurse consider before following this order?

Review Questions

1. An obese client is at risk for poor wound healing postoperatively because:
   1. ventilatory capacity is reduced.
   2. fatty tissue has a poor blood supply.
   3. risk for dehiscence is increased.
   4. resuming normal physical activity is delayed.

2. Because an older adult is at increased risk for respiratory complications after surgery, you must:
   1. ambulate client every 2 hours.
   2. monitor fluid and electrolyte status every shift.
   3. orient the client to surrounding environment frequently.
   4. encourage the client to turn, deep breathe, and cough frequently.

3. You must ask each client preoperatively for the name and dose of all prescription and over-the-counter medications taken before surgery because they:
   1. may cause allergies to develop.
   2. may interact with anesthetic agents.
   3. will need to be reordered after surgery.
   4. should be taken the morning of surgery with sips of water.

4. A client with a prothrombin time (PT) or an activated partial thromboplastin time (APTT) greater than normal is at risk postoperatively for:
   1. anemia.
   2. bleeding.
   3. infection.
   4. cardiac dysrhythmias.

5. A client who smokes two packs of cigarettes per day is most at risk postoperatively for:
   1. infection.
   2. pneumonia.
   3. hypotension.
   4. drug withdrawal.

6. When monitoring pain postoperatively you must ask each client if he or she is experiencing pain and document:
   1. the client's pain scale rating.
   2. the client's level of consciousness.
   3. what the client wants for treatment.
   4. how often the client asks for pain medication.

7. Fluid balance is best monitored by:
   1. skin turgor.
   2. daily weights.
   3. capillary refill.
   4. intake and output.

8. A client on the first postoperative day is at risk for hemorrhage. You should always:
   1. turn the client to check underneath.
   2. reinforce a dry dressing to add more padding.
   3. have the client use a pillow to splint the incision.
   4. remove the dressing to look directly at the incision.

9. In the PACU you note that the client is having difficulty breathing because of an obstruction. You would first:
   1. suction the pharynx and bronchial tree.
   2. give oxygen through a mask at 10 L/min.
   3. position the client so that the tongue falls forward.
   4. ask the client to use an incentive spirometer.

10. Early ambulation is ordered postoperatively to prevent the postoperative complication of:
    1. pain.
    2. nausea.
    3. wound dehiscence.
    4. deep vein thrombosis.

11. Family members should be included when you teach the client preoperative exercises so that they can:
    1. supervise the client at home.
    2. coach the client postoperatively.
    3. practice with the client while waiting to be taken to the operating room.
    4. relieve the nurse by getting the client to do exercises every 2 hours.

12. When the client is deep breathing and coughing it is important to have the client sitting because this position:
    1. is more comfortable.
    2. facilitates expansion of the thorax.
    3. increases the client's view of the room.
    4. helps the client to splint with a pillow.

13. The most important reason for the client to do postoperative leg exercises is in order to:
    1. decrease leg fatigue.
    2. increase muscle tone.
    3. increase venous return.
    4. maintain blood pressure.

References

American Society of Anesthesiologists: Practice guidelines for sedation and analgesia by nonanesthesiologists, *Anesthesiology* 84:459,1996.

American Society of Anesthesiologists Task Force on Perioperative Fast: Practice guidelines for preoperative fasting and the use of pharmacologic agents to reduce the risk of pulmonary aspiration: application to healthy patients undergoing elective procedures, *Anesthesiology* 90(3):896, 1999.

Association of Operating Room Nurses: *Standards and recommended practices for perioperative nursing,* Denver, 1997, The Association.

Association of Operating Room Nurses: *Standards, recommended practices, and guidelines,* Denver, 1999, The Association.

Brooks-Brunn J: Surgery: protecting the lungs, *Reflections* 23(1):16, 1997.

Burden N: *Ambulatory surgical nursing,* ed 2, London, 2000, WB Saunders.

Dunn D: Preoperative assessment criteria and patient teaching for ambulatory surgery patients, *J Perianesth Nurs* 13(5):274, 1998.

Dunn D: Exploring the gray areas of informed consent, *Nursing 99* 29(7):41, 1999.

Fortunato N: *Berry & Kohn's operating room techniques,* ed 9, St. Louis, 2000, Mosby.

Fox V: Postoperative education that works, *AORN J* 67:1010, 1998.

Gammon J, Mulholland C: Effects of preparatory information prior to elective total hip replacement on post-operative physical coping outcomes, *Int J Nurs Stud* 33(6):589, 1996.

Geissler E: *Pocket guide to cultural assessment,* St. Louis, 1998, Mosby.

Iocono M: Informed consent, *J Perianesth Nurs* 15(3):180, 2000.

Lancaster K: Patient teaching in ambulatory surgery, *Nurs Clin North Am* 32(2):417, 1997.

Lewis S and others: *Medical-surgical nursing: assessment and management of clinical problems,* ed 5, St. Louis, 2000, Mosby.

Litner M, Zilling T: Pre- and postoperative information needs, *Patient Educ Couns* 40:29, 2000.

Litwack K: *Core curriculum for perianesthesia nursing practice,* ed 4, Philadelphia, 1999, WB Saunders.

Lowdermilk D and others: *Maternity nursing,* ed 5, St. Louis, 1999, Mosby.

Meeker M, Rothrock J: *Alexander's care of the patient in surgery,* ed 11, St. Louis, 1999, Mosby.

Mosby's medical, nursing, and allied health dictionary, ed 5, St. Louis, 1998, Mosby.

Pagana K, Pagana T: *Diagnostic testing and nursing implications: a case study approach,* ed 5, St. Louis, 1999, Mosby.

Sandlin D: The new Joint Commission Accreditation of Healthcare Organization's requirements for pain assessment and treatment: a pain in the assessment? *J Perianesth Nurs* 15(3):182, 2000.

Shuldham C: A review of the impact of pre-operative education on the recovery from surgery, *Int J Nurs Stud* 36:171, 1999.

Glossary

abduction Movement of a limb away from the body.

abrasion Scraping or rubbing away of epidermis; may result in localized bleeding and later weeping of serous fluid.

absorption Passage of drug molecules into the blood. Factors influencing drug absorption include route of administration, ability of the drug to dissolve, and conditions at the site of absorption.

acceptance Fifth stage of Kübler-Ross's stages of dying. An individual comes to terms with a loss rather than submitting to resignation and hopelessness.

accessory muscles Muscles in the thoracic cage that assist with respiration.

accommodation Process of responding to the environment through new activity and thinking and changing the existing schema or developing a new schema to deal with the new information. For example, a toddler whose parent consistently corrected him when he called a horse a "doggie" accommodates and forms a new schema for horses.

accountability State of being answerable for one's actions—a nurse answers to herself, the client, the profession, the employing institution such as a hospital, and society for the effectiveness of nursing care performed.

accreditation Process whereby a professional association or nongovernmental agency grants recognition to a school or institution for demonstrated ability to meet predetermined criteria.

acne Inflammatory, papulopustular skin eruption, usually occurring on the face, neck, shoulders, and upper back.

acromegaly Chronic metabolic condition caused by overproduction of growth hormone and characterized by gradual, marked enlargement and elongation of bones of the face, jaw, and extremities.

active listening Listening attentively with the whole person—mind, body, and spirit. It includes listening for main and supportive ideas, acknowledging and responding, giving appropriate feedback, and paying attention to the other person's total communication, including the content, the intent, and the feelings expressed.

active range-of-motion (ROM) exercise Completion of exercise to the joint by the client, while doing activities of daily living, or during joint assessment.

active strategies of health promotion Activities that depend on the client being motivated to adopt a specific health program.

active transport Movement of materials across the cell membrane by means of chemical activity that allows the cell to admit larger molecules than would otherwise be possible.

activities of daily living (ADLs) Activities usually performed in the course of a normal day in the client's life, such as eating, dressing, bathing, brushing the teeth, or grooming.

activity tolerance Kind and amount of exercise or work that a person is able to perform.

actual loss Loss of an object, person, body part or function, or emotion that is overt and easily identifiable.

actual nursing diagnosis A judgment that is clinically validated by the presence of major defining characteristics.

acuity charting Mechanism by which entries describing client care activities are made over a 24-hour period. The activities are then translated into a rating score, or acuity score, that allows for a comparison of clients who vary by severity of illness.

acute care Pattern of health care in which a client is treated for an acute episode of illness, for the sequelae of an accident or other trauma, or during recovery from surgery.

acute illness Illness characterized by symptoms that are of relatively short duration, are usually severe, and affect the functioning of the client in all dimensions.

adduction Movement of a limb toward the body.

adolescence The period in development between the onset of puberty and adulthood. It usually begins between 11 and 13 years of age.

adult day care centers Facility for the supervised care of older adults, providing activities such as meals and socialization during specified day hours.

advanced sleep phase syndrome Common in older adults, a disturbance in sleep manifested as early waking in the morning with an inability to get back to sleep. It is believed that this syndrome is caused by advancing of the body's circadian rhythm.

adventitious sounds Abnormal lung sounds heard with auscultation.

adverse effect Harmful or unintended effect of a medication, diagnostic test, or therapeutic intervention.

adverse reaction Any harmful, unintended effect of a medication, diagnostic test, or therapeutic intervention.

advocacy Process whereby a nurse objectively provides clients with the information they need to make decisions and supports the clients in whatever decisions they make.

afebrile Without fever.

affective learning Acquisition of behaviors involved in expressing feelings in attitudes, appreciation, and values.

afterload Resistance to left ventricular ejection; the work the heart must overcome to fully eject blood from the left ventricle.

agnostic Individual who believes that any ultimate reality is unknown or unknowable.

airborne precautions Safeguards designed to reduce the risk of transmission of infectious agents through the air a person breathes.

alarm reaction Mobilization of the defense mechanisms of the body and mind to cope with a stressor. The initial stage of the general adaptation syndrome.

aldosterone Mineralocorticoid steroid hormone produced by the adrenal cortex with action in the renal tubule to regulate sodium and potassium balance in the blood.

allergic reactions Unfavorable physiological response to an allergen to which a person has previously been exposed and to which the person has developed antibodies.

alopecia Partial or complete loss of hair; baldness.

Alzheimer's disease Disease of the brain parenchyma that causes a gradual and progressive decline in cognitive functioning.

AMBULARM Device used for the client who climbs out of bed unassisted and is in danger of falling. This device is worn on the leg and signals when the leg is in a dependent position such as over the side rail or on the floor.

amino acid Organic compound of one or more basic groups and one or more carboxyl groups. Amino acids are the building blocks that construct proteins and the end products of protein digestion.

anabolism Constructive metabolism characterized by conversion of simple substances into more complex compounds of living matter.

analgesic Relieving pain; drug that relieves pain.

analogies Resemblances made between things otherwise unlike.

anaphylactic reactions Hypersensitive condition induced by contact with certain antigens.

aneurysms Localized dilations of the wall of a blood vessel, usually caused by atherosclerosis, hypertension, or a congenital weakness in a vessel wall.

anger Second stage of Kübler-Ross's stages of dying. During this stage an individual resists loss by expressing extreme displeasure, indignation, or hostility.

angiotensin Polypeptide occurring in the blood, causing vasoconstriction, increased blood pressure, and the release of aldosterone from the adrenal cortex.

anion gap Difference between the concentrations of serum cations and anions, determined by measuring the concentrations of sodium cations and chloride and bicarbonate anions.

anions Negatively charged electrolytes.

anorexia Lack or loss of appetite resulting in the inability to eat.

anthropometric measurements Body measures of height, weight, and skinfolds to evaluate muscle atrophy.

anthropometry Measurement of various body parts to determine nutritional and caloric status, muscular development, brain growth, and other parameters.

antibodies (antibody) Immunoglobulins, essential to the immune system, that are produced by lymphoid tissue in response to bacteria, viruses, or other antigens.

anticipatory grief Grief response in which the person begins the grieving process before an actual loss.

antidiuretic hormone (ADH) Hormone that decreases the production of urine by increasing the reabsorption of water by the renal tubules. ADH is secreted by cells of the hypothalamus and stored in the posterior lobe of the pituitary gland.

antiembolic stockings Elasticized stockings that prevent formation of emboli and thrombi, especially after surgery or during bed rest.

antigen Substance, usually a protein, that causes the formation of an antibody and reacts specifically with that antibody.

antipyretic Substance or procedure that reduces fever.

anxiolytics Drugs used primarily to treat episodes of anxiety.

aphasia Abnormal neurological condition in which language function is defective or absent; related to injury to speech center in cerebral cortex, causing receptive or expressive aphasia.

apical pulse Heartbeat as listened to with the bell or diaphragm of a stethoscope placed on the apex of the heart.

apnea Cessation of airflow through the nose and mouth.

apothecary system System of measurement. The basic unit of weight is a grain. Weights derived from the grain are the gram, ounce, and pound. The basic measure for fluid is the minim. The fluidram, fluid ounce, pint, quart, and gallon are measures derived from the minim.

approximate To come close together, as in the edges of a wound.

arcus senilis Opaque ring, gray to white in color, that surrounds the periphery of the cornea. The condition is caused by deposits of fat granules in the cornea. Occurs primarily in older adults.

asepsis Absence of germs or microorganisms.

aseptic technique Any health care procedure in which added precautions are used to prevent contamination of a person, object, or area by microorganisms.

assault Unlawful threatening or inflicting of harm on another.

assertive communication Type of communication based on a philosophy of protecting individual rights and responsibilities. It includes the ability to be self-directive in acting to accomplish goals and advocate for others.

assessment First step of the nursing process; activities required in the first step are data collection, data validation, data sorting, and data documentation. The purpose is to gather information for health problem identification.

assimilation To become absorbed into another culture and to adopt its characteristics.

assisted living Residential living facilities in which each resident has his or her own room and shares dining and social activity areas.

associative play Form of play in which a group of children participates in similar or identical activities without formal organization, direction, interaction, or goals.

atelectasis Collapse of alveoli, preventing the normal respiratory exchange of oxygen and carbon dioxide.

atheist Individual who does not believe in the existence of God.

atherosclerosis Common arterial disorder characterized by yellowish plaques of cholesterol, lipids, and cellular debris in the inner layers of the walls of the large- and medium-size arteries.

atrioventricular (AV) node A portion of the cardiac conduction system located on the floor of the right atrium; it receives electrical impulses from the atrium and transmits them to the bundle of His.

atrophied Wasted or reduced size or physiological activity of a part of the body caused by disease or other influences.

attachment Initial psychosocial relationship that develops between parents and the neonate.

attentional set Internal state of the learner that allows focusing and comprehension.

auditory Related to, or experienced through, hearing.

auscultation Method of physical examination; listening to the sounds produced by the body, usually with a stethoscope.

auscultatory gap Disappearance of sound when obtaining a blood pressure; typically occurs between the first and second Korotkoff's sounds.

authority The right to act in areas in which an individual has been given and accepts responsibility.

autologous transfusion Procedure in which blood is removed from a donor and stored for a variable period before it is returned to the donor's own circulation.

autonomy Ability or tendency to function independently.

bacteremia Presence of bacteria in the blood.

bacteriuria Presence of bacteria in the urine.

balance Position when the person's center of gravity is correctly positioned so that falling does not occur.

bandages Available in rolls of various widths and materials including gauze, elasticized knit, elastic webbing, flannel, and muslin. Gauze bandages are lightweight and inexpensive, mold easily around contours of the body, and permit air circulation to underlying skin to prevent maceration. Elastic bandages conform well to body parts but can also be used to exert pressure over a body part.

bargaining Third stage of Kübler-Ross's stages of dying. A person postpones the reality of a loss by attempting to make deals in a subtle or overt manner with others or with a higher being.

basal cell carcinoma Malignant epithelial cell tumor that begins as a papule and enlarges peripherally, developing a central crater that erodes, crusts, and bleeds. Metastasis is rare.

basal metabolic rate (BMR) Amount of energy used in a unit of time by a fasting, resting subject to maintain vital functions.

battery Legal term for touching of another's body without consent.

bed boards Boards placed under the mattress of a bed that provide extra support to the mattress surface.

bed rest Placement of the client in bed for therapeutic reasons for a prescribed period.

beneficence Doing good or active promotion of doing good. One of the four principles of the ethical theory of deontology.

bereavement Response to loss through death; a subjective experience that a person suffers after losing a person with whom there has been a significant relationship.

binders Bandages made of large pieces of material to fit specific body parts.

bioethics Branch of ethics within the field of health care.

biological clocks Cyclical nature of body functions; functions controlled from within the body are synchronized with environmental factors; same meaning as biorhythm.

biotransformation The chemical changes that a substance undergoes in the body, such as by the action of enzymes.

body image Persons' subjective concept of their physical appearance.

body mechanics Coordinated efforts of the musculoskeletal and nervous systems to maintain proper balance, posture, and body alignment.

bone resorption Destruction of bone cells and release of calcium into the blood.

borborygmi Audible abdominal sounds produced by hyperactive intestinal peristalsis.

bradycardia Slower-than-normal heart rate; heart contracts fewer than 60 times per minute.

bradypnea Abnormally slow rate of breathing.

bronchospasm An excessive and prolonged contraction of the smooth muscle of the bronchi and bronchioles resulting in an acute narrowing and obstruction of the respiratory airway.

bruit Abnormal sound or murmur heard while auscultating an organ, gland, or artery.

bruxism Grinding of teeth during sleep.

buccal Of or pertaining to the inside of the cheek or the gum next to the cheek.

buccal cavity Consists of the lips surrounding the opening of the mouth, the cheeks running along the side walls of the cavity, the tongue and its muscles, and the hard and soft palate.

buffer Substance or group of substances that can absorb or release hydrogen ions to correct an acid-base imbalance.

bulbar synchronizing region (BSR) Area in the pons and medial forebrain region releasing serotonin from specialized cells believed to aid in sleep.

bundle of His A portion of the cardiac conduction system that arises from the distal portion of the atrioventricular (AV) node and extends across the AV groove to the top of the intraventricular septum, where it divides into right and left bundle branches.

cachexia Malnutrition marked by weakness and emaciation, usually associated with severe illness.

capitation Payment mechanism in which a provider (e.g., health care network) receives a fixed amount of payment per enrollee.

carbohydrates Dietary classification of foods comprising sugars, starches, cellulose, and gum.

carbon monoxide Colorless, odorless, poisonous gas produced by the combustion of carbon or organic fuels.

cardiac index The adequacy of the cardiac output for an individual. It takes into account the body surface area (BSA) of the client.

cardiac output Volume of blood expelled by the ventricles of the heart, equal to the amount of blood ejected at each beat, multiplied by the number of beats in the period of time used for computation (usually 1 minute).

cardiopulmonary rehabilitation Actively assisting the client to achieve and maintain an optimal level of health through controlled physical exercise, nutrition counseling, relaxation and stress management techniques, prescribed medications and oxygen, and compliance.

cardiopulmonary resuscitation (CPR) Basic emergency procedures for life support consisting of artificial respiration and manual external cardiac massage.

care To feel concern or interest in one who has sorrow or difficulties.

care management Care delivery model that structures accountability for client outcomes within a unit or area of care. Typically one caregiver coordinates care from admission through discharge within an acute care setting.

caring Universal phenomenon that influences the way we think, feel, and behave in relation to one another.

carriers Person or animal who harbors and spreads an organism that causes disease in others but does not become ill.

case management Organized system for delivering health care to an individual client or group of clients across an episode of illness and/or a continuum of care; includes assessment and development of a plan of care, coordination of all services, referral, and follow-up; usually assigned to one professional.

catabolism Breakdown of body tissue into simpler substances.

cataplexy Condition characterized by sudden muscular weakness and loss of muscle tone.

cathartics Drugs that act to promote bowel evacuation.

catheterization Introduction of a catheter into a body cavity or organ to inject or remove fluid.

cations Positively charged electrolytes.

center of gravity Midpoint or center of the weight of a body or object.

centigrade Denotes temperature scale in which 0 degrees is the freezing point of water and 100 degrees is the boiling point of water at sea level; also called Celsius.

cerumen Yellowish or brownish waxy secretion produced by sweat glands in the external ear.

change-of-shift reports Reports that occur between two scheduled nursing work shifts. Nurses communicate information about their assigned clients to nurses working on the next shift of duty.

chancres Skin lesion or venereal sore (usually primary syphilis) that begins at the site of infection as a papule and develops into a red, bloodless, painless ulcer with a scooped-out appearance.

channel Method used in the teaching-learning process to present content: visual, auditory, taste, smell. In the communication process, a method used to transmit a message: visual, auditory, touch.

charting by exception (CBE) Charting methodology in which data are entered only when there is an exception from what is normal or expected. Reduces time spent documenting in charting. It is a shorthand method for documenting normal findings and routine care.

chest percussion Striking of the chest wall with a cupped hand to promote mobilization and drainage of pulmonary secretions.

chest physiotherapy (CPT) Group of therapies used to mobilize pulmonary secretions for expectoration.

chest tube A catheter inserted through the thorax into the chest cavity for removing air or fluid, used after chest or heart surgery or pneumothorax.

chronic illness Illness that persists over a long time and affects physical, emotional, intellectual, social, and spiritual functioning.

chyme Viscous, semifluid contents of the stomach present during digestion of a meal, which eventually pass into the intestines.

circadian rhythm Repetition of certain physiological phenomena within a 24-hour cycle.

circulating nurse Assistant to the scrub nurse and surgeon whose role is to provide necessary supplies, dispose of soiled instruments and supplies, and keep an accurate count of instruments, needles, and sponges used.

circumduction Movement of the arm in full circle; includes all movements of the shoulder ball-and-socket joint.

civil law Statutes concerned with protecting a person's rights.

client-centered goal Specific measurable objective designed to reflect the client's highest level of wellness and independence in function.

climacteric Physiological, developmental change that occurs in the male reproductive system between the ages of 45 and 60.

clinical criteria Objective or subjective signs and symptoms, clusters of signs and symptoms, or risk factors.

clubbing Bulging of the tissues at the nail base that is caused by insufficient oxygenation at the periphery, resulting from conditions such as chronic emphysema and congenital heart disease.

code of ethics Formal statement that delineates a profession's guidelines for ethical behavior; a code of ethics sets standards or expectations for the professional to achieve.

cognitive learning Acquisition of intellectual skills that encompass behaviors such as thinking, understanding, and evaluating.

collaboration Process in which a nurse works with other health care providers and the client to develop a plan of care to address the client-identified care needs, as well as those identified by the professional team.

collaborative interventions Therapies that require the knowledge, skill, and expertise of multiple health care professionals.

colloid osmotic pressure Abnormal condition of the kidney caused by the pressure of concentrations of large particles, such as protein molecules, that will pass through a membrane.

colon Portion of the large intestine from the cecum to the rectum.

colonization The presence and multiplication of microorganisms without tissue invasion or damage.

comforting Acts toward another individual that display both an emotional and physical calm. The use of touch, establishing presence, the therapeutic use of silence, and the skillful and gentle performance of a procedure are examples of comforting nursing measures.

common law One source for law that is created by judicial decisions as opposed to those created by legislative bodies (statutory law).

communicable disease Any disease that can be transmitted from one person or animal to another by direct or indirect contact, or by vectors.

communication Ongoing, dynamic series of events that involves the transmission of meaning from sender to receiver.

community-based nursing Involves the acute and chronic care of individuals and families in community settings that enhances their capacity for self-care and promotes autonomy in decision making.

community health nursing Field of nursing that is a blend of primary health care and nursing practice with public health nursing.

competence Specific range of skills necessary to perform a task.

complete bed bath Bath in which the entire body of a client is washed in bed.

compliance Person's fulfillment of the prescribed course of treatment.

compress Soft pad of gauze or cloth used to apply heat, cold, or medications to the surface of a body part.

computer-based client record (CBCR) Comprehensive computerized system used by all health care practitioners to permanently store information pertaining to a client's health status, clinical problems, and functional abilities.

concentration Relative content of a component within a substance or solution.

concentration gradient Gradient that exists across a membrane separating a high concentration of a particular ion from a low concentration of the same ion.

conjunctivitis Highly contagious eye infection. The crusty drainage that collects on eyelid margins can easily spread from one eye to the other.

connotative meaning The shade or interpretation of a word's meaning influenced by the thoughts, feelings, or ideas people have about the word.

conscious sedation Administration of central nervous system depressant drugs and or analgesics to provide analgesia, relieve anxiety, and or provide amnesia during surgical, diagnostic, or interventional procedures.

constipation Condition characterized by difficulty in passing stool or an infrequent passage of hard stool.

consultation Process in which the help of a specialist is sought to identify ways to handle problems in client management or in the planning and implementing of programs.

contact precautions Safeguards designed to reduce the risk of transmission of epidemiologically important microorganisms by direct or indirect contact.

convalescence Period of recovery after an illness, injury, or surgery.

coping Making an effort to manage psychological stress.

core temperature Temperature of deep structures of the body.

cough Sudden, audible expulsion of air from the lungs. The person breathes in, the glottis is partially closed, and the accessory muscles of expiration contract to expel the air forcibly.

crackles Fine bubbling sounds heard on auscultation of the lung; produced by air entering distal airways and alveoli, which contain serous secretions.

crime Act that violates a law and that may include criminal intent.

criminal law Concerned with acts that threaten society but may involve only an individual.

crisis Transition for better or worse in the course of a disease, usually indicated by a marked change in the intensity of signs and symptoms.

crisis intervention Use of therapeutic techniques directed toward helping a client resolve a particular and immediate problem.

critical pathways Tools used in managed care that incorporate the treatment interventions of caregivers from all disciplines who normally care for a client. Designed for a specific care type, a pathway is used to manage the care of a client throughout a projected length of stay.

critical period of development Specific time period when the environment has its greatest effect on a specific aspect of an individual's development.

critical thinking The active, purposeful, organized, cognitive process used to carefully examine one's thinking and the thinking of other individuals.

crutch gate A gait achieved by a person using crutches.

cultural values Values adopted as a result of the social setting in which a person lives.

culturally competent care Nursing care provided to clients from various ethnic and cultural backgrounds, incorporating cultural preferences of the client in all aspects of care.

culture Nonphysical traits, such as values, beliefs, attitudes, and customs, that are shared by a group of people and passed from one generation to the next.

cutaneous stimulation Stimulation of a person's skin to prevent or reduce pain perception. A massage, warm bath, hot and cold therapies, and transcutaneous electric nerve stimulation are some ways to reduce pain perception.

cyanosis Bluish discoloration of the skin and mucous membranes caused by an excess of deoxygenated hemoglobin in the blood or a structural defect in the hemoglobin molecule.

data, actions, client response (DAR) The format used in focus charting for recording client information.

data analysis Logical examination of and professional judgment about client assessment data; used in the diagnostic process to derive a nursing diagnosis.

data clustering Categorizing of related data into groups.

data collection Part of the assessment step of the nursing process when all pertinent subjective and objective information about the client is gathered. Data collection includes the nursing history, physical examination, laboratory data and diagnostic tests, and information from health team members and the client's family and significant others.

data documentation A thorough and accurate documentation of facts is necessary when recording client data. If an item is not recorded, it is lost and unavailable to anyone researching the client's medical record. If specific information is not given, the reader is left with only general impressions.

database Store or bank of information, especially in a form that can be processed by computer.

death Cessation of life as indicated by the absence of heartbeat or respiration. Legally, death is total absence of activity in the brain and central nervous, cardiovascular, and respiratory systems.

debridement Removal of dead tissue from a wound.

decentralized management An organizational philosophy that brings decisions down to the level of the staff. Individuals best informed about a problem or issue participate in the decision-making process.

decision making Process involving critical appraisal of information that results from recognition of a problem and ends with the generation, testing, and evaluation of a conclusion. Comes at the end of critical thinking.

defecation Passage of feces from the digestive tract through the rectum.

defendant Individual or organization against whom legal charges are brought forth in a court of law.

defining characteristics Related signs and symptoms or clusters of data that support the nursing diagnosis.

dehiscence Separation of a wound's edges, revealing underlying tissues.

dehydration Excessive loss of water from the body tissues, accompanied by a disturbance of body electrolytes.

delegation Process of assigning another member of the health care team to be responsible for aspects of client care; for example, assigning nurse assistants to bathe a client.

dementia Irreversible mental state characterized by decreased intellectual function, changes in personality, impaired judgment, and often changes in affect as a result of permanently altered cerebral metabolism.

denial Unconscious refusal to admit an unacceptable idea.

denotative meaning Is shared by individuals who use a common language. The word "baseball" has the same meaning for all individuals who speak English, but the word "code" denotes cardiac arrest primarily to health-care providers.

dental caries Abnormal destructive condition in a tooth caused by a complex interaction of food, especially starches and sugars, with bacteria that form dental plaque.

deontology Traditional theory of ethics that proposes to define actions as right or wrong based on the characteristics of fidelity to promises, truthfulness, and justice. The conventional use of ethical terms such as justice, autonomy, beneficence, and nonmaleficence constitutes the practice of deontology.

depression Mood disturbance characterized by feelings of sadness, despair, and discouragement resulting from and normally proportionate to some personal loss or tragedy.

dermis Sensitive vascular layer of the skin directly below the epidermis composed of collagenous and elastic fibrous connective tissues that give the dermis strength and elasticity.

determinants of health The many variables that influence the health status of individuals or communities.

detoxify To remove the toxic quality of a substance; the liver acts to detoxify chemicals in drug compounds.

development Qualitative or observable aspects of the progressive changes one makes in adapting to the environment.

developmental crises Crises associated with normal and expected phases of growth and development, for example, the response to menopause; same as maturational crises.

diagnostic process Mental steps (data clustering and analysis, problem identification) that follow assessment and lead directly to the formulation of a diagnosis.

diagnostic reasoning Process that enables an observer to assign meaning and to classify phenomena in clinical situations by integrating observations and critical thinking.

diagnosis-related group (DRG) Group of clients classified to establish a mechanism for health care reimbursement based on length of stay; classification is based on the following variables: primary and secondary diagnosis, comorbidities, primary and secondary procedures, and age.

diaphoresis Secretion of sweat, especially profuse secretion associated with an elevated body temperature, physical exertion, or emotional stress.

diaphragmatic breathing Respiration in which the abdomen moves out while the diaphragm descends on inspiration.

diarrhea Increase in the number of stools and the passage of liquid, unformed feces.

diastolic Pertaining to diastole, or the blood pressure at the instant of maximum cardiac relaxation.

dietary referenced intake Information on each vitamin or mineral to reflect a range of minimum to maximum amounts that avert deficiency or toxicity.

diffusion Movement of molecules from an area of high concentration to an area of lower concentration.

digestion Breakdown of nutrients by chewing, churning, mixing with fluid, and chemical reactions.

discharge planning Activities directed toward identifying future proposed therapy and the need for additional resources before and after returning home.

disinfection Process of destroying all pathogenic organisms, except spores.

distress Damaging stress; one of the two types of stress identified by Selye.

disuse osteoporosis Reductions in skeletal mass routinely accompanying immobility or paralysis.

diuresis Increased rate of formation and excretion of urine.

documentation Written entry into the client's medical record of all pertinent information about the client. These entries validate the client's problems and care and exist as a legal record.

dorsiflexion Flexion toward the back.

drainage evacuators Convenient portable units that connect to tubular drains lying within a wound bed and exert a safe, constant, low-pressure vacuum to remove and collect drainage.

droplet precautions Safeguards designed to reduce the risk of droplet transmission of infectious agents.

durable power of attorney Document that designates an agent or proxy to make health care decisions if the patient is no longer able to make them.

dysmenorrhea Painful menstruation.

dyspnea Sensation of shortness of breath.

dysrhythmias Deviation from the normal pattern of the heartbeat.

dysuria Painful urination resulting from bacterial infection of the bladder and obstructive conditions of the urethra.

ecchymosis Discoloration of the skin or bruise caused by leakage of blood into subcutaneous tissues as a result of trauma to underlying tissues.

ectropion Eversion of the eyelid, exposing the conjunctival membrane and part of the eyeball.

eczema Superficial dermatitis of unknown cause.

edema Abnormal accumulation of fluid in interstitial spaces of tissues.

egocentric Developmental characteristic wherein a toddler is only able to assume the view of his or her own activities and needs.

electrocardiogram (ECG) Graphic record of the electrical activity of the myocardium.

electrolyte Element or compound that, when melted or dissolved in water or other solvent, dissociates into ions and can carry an electrical current.

embolism Abnormal condition in which an a blood clot (embolus) travels through the bloodstream and becomes lodged in a blood vessel.

empathy Understanding and acceptance of a person's feelings and the ability to sense the person's private world.

empowerment Management technique that fosters the growth and development of individual staff members so that they become less and less dependent on their work leader. Empowerment helps staff make decisions confidently on their own.

endogenous infections Infections produced within a cell or organism.

endorphins Hormones that act on the mind like morphine and opiates, producing a sense of well-being and reducing pain.

enema Procedure involving introduction of a solution into the rectum for cleansing or therapeutic purposes.

enteral nutrition (EN) Provision of nutrients through the gastrointestinal tract when the client cannot ingest, chew, or swallow food but can digest and absorb nutrients.

entropion Condition in which the eyelid turns inward toward the eye.

environment All of the many factors, such as physical and psychological, that influence or affect the life and survival of a person.

epidermis Outer layer of the skin that has several thin layers of skin in different stages of maturation; shields and protects the underlying tissues from water loss, mechanical or chemical injury, and penetration by disease-causing microorganisms.

epidural infusion Type of nerve block anesthesia in which an anesthetic is intermittently or continuously injected into the lumbosacral region of the spinal cord.

erythema Redness or inflammation of the skin or mucous membranes that is a result of dilation and congestion of superficial capillaries; sunburn is an example.

ethics of care Delivery of health care based on ethical principles and standards of care.

ethical dilemma Dilemma existing when the right thing to do is not clear. Resolution requires the negotiation of differing values among those involved in the dilemma.

ethical principles Set of guidelines for a profession's expectations and standards of behavior for its members.

ethics Principles or standards that govern proper conduct.

ethnicity Cultural group's sense of identification associated with the group's common social and cultural heritage.

etiology Study of all factors that may be involved in the development of a disease.

eupnea Normal respirations that are quiet, effortless, and rhythmical.

eustress Stress that protects health; one of the two types of stress identified by Selye.

evaluation Determination of the extent to which established client goals have been achieved.

evisceration Protrusion of visceral organs through a surgical wound.

exacerbations Increases in the seriousness of a disease or disorder as marked by greater intensity in signs or symptoms.

excoriation Injury to the skin's surface caused by abrasion.

exhaustion stage Phase that occurs when the body can no longer resist the stress; when the energy necessary to maintain adaptation is depleted.

exogenous infection Infection originating outside an organ or part.

exostosis An abnormal benign growth on the surface of a bone.

expected outcomes Expected conditions of a client at the end of therapy or of a disease process, including the degree of wellness and the need for continuing care, medications, support, counseling, or education.

extended care facility An institution devoted to providing medical, nursing, or custodial care for an individual over a prolonged period, such as during the course of a chronic disease or during the rehabilitation phase after an acute illness.

extension Movement by certain joints that increases the angle between two adjoining bones.

extracellular fluids Portion of body fluids composed of the interstitial fluid and blood plasma.

exudate Fluid, cells, or other substances that have been slowly discharged from cells or blood vessels through small pores or breaks in cell membranes.

Fahrenheit Denotes temperature scale in which 32 degrees is the freezing point of water and 212 degrees is the boiling point of water at sea level.

faith Set of beliefs and a way of relating to self, others, and a Supreme Being.

family Group of interacting individuals composing a basic unit of society.

family as client Nursing perspective in which the family is viewed as a unit of interacting members having attributes, functions, and goals separate from those of the individual family members.

family as context Nursing perspective in which the primary focus of care is on an individual within a family.

family as system Based on a systems theory framework whereby the family is viewed as an open system with boundaries, self-regulating mechanisms, subsystems, and suprasystems all affecting the family unit.

family forms Patterns of people considered by family members to be included in the family.

family functioning Processes families use to achieve their goals.

family hardiness Internal strengths and durability of the family unit; characterized by a sense of control over the outcome of life events and hardships, a view of change as beneficial and growth-producing, and an active rather than passive orientation in responding to stressful life events.

family health Determined by the effectiveness of the family's structure, the processes that the family uses to meet its goals, and internal and external resources.

family structure Based on organization (i.e., ongoing membership) of the family and the pattern of relationships.

febrile Pertaining to or characterized by an elevated body temperature.

fecal impaction Accumulation of hardened fecal material in the rectum or sigmoid colon.

fecal incontinence Inability to control passage of feces and gas from the anus.

fecal occult blood test Measures microscopic amounts of blood in the feces.

feces Waste or excrement from the gastrointestinal tract.

feedback Process in which the output of a given system is returned to the system.

felony Crime of a serious nature that carries a penalty of imprisonment or death.

feminist ethic Ethical approach that focuses on relationships of those involved in an ethical dilemma rather than traditional abstract principles of deontology.

fever Elevation in the hypothalamic set-point, so that body temperature is regulated at a higher level.

fibrocystic breast disease A benign condition characterized by lumpy, painful breasts and sometimes nipple discharge. Symptoms are more apparent before the menstrual period. Known to be a risk factor for breast cancer.

fidelity The agreement to keep a promise.

fight-or-flight response The total physiological response to stress that occurs during the alarm reaction stage of the general adaptation syndrome. Massive changes in all body systems prepare a human being to choose to flee or to remain and fight the stressor.

filtration The straining of fluid through a membrane.

fistula Abnormal passage from an internal organ to the body surface or between two internal organs.

flashback A recollection so strong that the individual thinks he or she is actually experiencing the trauma again or seeing it unfold before his or her eyes.

flatus Intestinal gas.

flora Microorganisms that live on or within a body to compete with disease-producing microorganisms and provide a natural immunity against certain infections.

flow sheets Documents on which frequent observations or specific measurements are recorded.

fluid volume deficit (FVD) A fluid and electrolyte disorder caused by failure of the body's homeostatic mechanisms to regulate the retention and excretion of body fluids. The condition is characterized by decreased output of urine, high specific gravity of urine, output of urine that is greater than the intake of fluid in the body, hemoconcentration, and increased serum levels of sodium.

fluid volume excess (FVE) A fluid and electrolyte disorder characterized by an increase in fluid retention and edema, resulting from failure of the body's homeostatic mechanisms to regulate the retention and excretion of body fluids.

focus charting A charting methodology for structuring progress notes according to the focus of the note, for example, symptoms and nursing diagnosis. Each note includes data, actions, and client response.

folk medicine The use of herbs, plants, minerals, and animal substances to prevent and treat illnesses. The treatments may be passed from one generation to the next.

food poisoning Toxic processes resulting from the ingestion of a food contaminated by toxic substances or by bacteria-containing toxins.

foot boots Soft, foot-shaped devices designed to reduce the risk of footdrop, by maintaining the foot in dorsiflexion.

footdrop An abnormal neuromuscular condition of the lower leg and foot, characterized by an inability to dorsiflex, or evert, the foot.

friction Effects of rubbing or the resistance that a moving body meets from the surface on which it moves; a force that occurs in a direction to oppose movement.

functional health patterns Method for organizing assessment data based on the level of client function in specific areas, for example, mobility.

functional illiteracy Inability to read or comprehend above a fifth-grade level.

functional nursing Method of client care delivery in which each staff member is assigned a task that is completed for all clients on the unit.

gait Manner or style of walking, including rhythm, cadence, and speed.

gastrostomy feeding tube The insertion of a feeding tube, through a stoma, into the stomach for the purpose of providing enteral nutrition.

general adaptation syndrome (GAS) Generalized defense response of the body to stress, consisting of three stages: alarm, resistance, and exhaustion.

general anesthesia Intravenous or inhaled medications that cause the client to lose all sensation and consciousness.

geriatrics Branch of health care dealing with the physiology and psychology of aging and with the diagnosis and treatment of diseases affecting older adults.

gerontology The study of all aspects of the aging process and its consequences.

gingivae Gum of the mouth; a mucous membrane with supporting fibrous tissue that overlies the crowns of unerupted teeth and encircles the necks of those teeth that have erupted.

glomerulus Cluster or collection of capillary vessels within the kidney involved in the initial formation of urine.

gluconeogenesis Formation of glucose or glycogen from substances that are not carbohydrates, such as protein or lipid.

glucose The primary fuel for the body, needed to carry out major physiological functions.

glycogen Polysaccharide that is the major carbohydrate stored in animal cells.

glycogenesis The process for storage of glucose in the form of glycogen in the liver.

goals Desired results of nursing actions, set realistically by the nurse and client as part of the planning stage of the nursing process.

Good Samaritan laws Legislation enacted in some states to protect health care professionals from liability in rendering emergency aid, unless there is proven willful wrong or gross negligence.

graduated measuring container Receptacle for volume measurement.

granulation tissue Soft, pink, fleshy projections of tissue that form during the healing process in a wound not healing by primary intention.

graphic record Charting mechanism that allows for the recording of vital signs and weight in such a manner that caregivers can quickly note changes in the client's status.

grief Form of sorrow involving the person's thoughts, feelings, and behaviors, occurring as a response to an actual or perceived loss.

grieving process Sequence of affective, cognitive, and physiological states through which the person responds to and finally accepts an irretrievable loss.

grounded Connection between the electric circuit and the ground, which becomes part of the circuit.

growth Measurable or quantitative aspect of an individual's increase in physical dimensions as a result of an increase in cell number. Indicators of growth include changes in height, weight, and sexual characteristics.

guided imagery Method of pain control in which the client creates a mental image, concentrates on that image, and gradually becomes less aware of pain.

gustatory Pertaining to the sense of taste.

hand rolls Roll of cloth that keeps the thumb slightly adducted and in opposition to the fingers.

hand-wrist splints Splints individually molded for the client to maintain proper alignment of the thumb, slight adduction of the wrist, and slight dorsiflexion.

health Dynamic state in which individuals adapt to their internal and external environments so that there is a state of physical, emotional, intellectual, social, and spiritual well-being.

health beliefs Client's personal beliefs about levels of wellness, which can motivate or impede participation in changing risk factors, participating in care, and selecting care options.

health belief model Conceptual framework that describes a person's health behavior as an expression of the person's health beliefs.

health care problems Any conditions or dysfunctions that the client experiences as a result of illness or treatment of an illness.

health care team All those people, departments, and ancillary services that collectively render care and services to the client.

health maintenance organization Type of group health care practice that provides basic and supplemental health maintenance and treatment services to voluntary enrollees who prepay a fixed periodic fee that is set without regard to the amount or kind of services received.

health promotion Activities such as routine exercise and good nutrition that help clients maintain or enhance their present levels of health and reduce their risk of developing certain diseases.

health promotion model Defines health as a positive, dynamic state, not merely the absence of disease. The health promotion model emphasizes well-being, personal fulfillment, and self-actualization rather than reacting to the threat of illness.

health status Description of health of an individual or community.

health-illness continuum model Scale by means of which a person's level of health can be described, ranging from high-level wellness to severe illness. The scale takes into account the presence of risk factors.

heat exhaustion Abnormal condition caused by depletion of body fluid and electrolytes resulting from exposure to intense heat or the inability to acclimatize to heat.

heat stroke Continued exposure to extreme heat raising the core body temperature to 47° C (105° F) or higher.

hematemesis Vomiting of blood, indicating upper gastrointestinal bleeding.

hematoma Collection of blood trapped in the tissues of the skin or an organ.

hematuria Abnormal presence of blood in the urine.

hemolysis Breakdown of red blood cells and release of hemoglobin that may occur after administration of hypotonic intravenous solutions, causing swelling and rupture of erythrocytes.

hemoptysis Coughing up blood from the respiratory tract.

hemorrhoids Permanent dilation and engorgement of veins within the lining of the rectum.

hemostasis Termination of bleeding by mechanical or chemical means or by the coagulation process of the body.

hemothorax Accumulation of blood and fluid in the pleural cavity between the parietal and visceral pleurae.

hernia Protrusion of an organ through an abnormal opening in the muscle wall of the cavity that surrounds it.

holistic Of or pertaining to the whole; considering all factors.

holistic health model Comprehensive view of the person as a biopsychosocial and spiritual being.

home health care Health service provided in the client's place of residence for the purpose of promoting, maintaining, or restoring health or minimizing the effects of illness and disability.

homeostasis State of relative constancy in the internal environment of the body, maintained naturally by physiological adaptive mechanisms.

homophobia Fear of or prejudice against homosexuals.

hope Confident, yet uncertain, expectation of achieving a future goal.

hospice System of family-centered care designed to help terminally ill persons be comfortable and maintain a satisfactory lifestyle throughout the terminal phase of their illness.

Hoyer lift A mechanical device that uses a canvas sling to easily lift dependent clients for transfer.

humidification Process of adding water to gas.

humor Coping strategy based on an individual's cognitive appraisal of a stimulus that results in behavior such as smiling, laughing, or feelings of amusement that lessen emotional distress.

hydrocephalus Abnormal accumulation of cerebrospinal fluid in the ventricles of the brain.

hydrostatic pressure Pressure caused by a liquid.

hypercalcemia Greater-than-normal amount of calcium in the blood.

hypercapnia Greater-than-normal amounts of carbon dioxide in the blood; also called hypercarbia.

hyperextension Position of maximal extension of a joint.

hyperglycemia Elevated serum glucose levels.

hypertension Disorder characterized by an elevated blood pressure persistently exceeding 120/80 mm Hg.

hyperthermia Situation in which body temperature exceeds the setpoint.

hypertonic Situation in which one solution has a greater concentration of solute than another solution; therefore the first solution exerts greater osmotic pressure.

hypertonicity Excessive tension of the arterial walls or muscles.

hyperventilation Respiratory rate in excess of that required to maintain normal carbon dioxide levels in the body tissues.

hypnotics Class of drug that causes insensibility to pain and induces sleep.

hypostatic pneumonia Pneumonia that results from fluid accumulation as a result of inactivity.

hypotension Abnormal lowering of blood pressure that is inadequate for normal perfusion and oxygenation of tissues.

hypothermia Abnormal lowering of body temperature below 35° C, or 93° F, usually caused by prolonged exposure to cold.

hypotonic Situation in which one solution has a smaller concentration of solute than another solution; therefore the first solution exerts less osmotic pressure.

hypotonicity Reduced tension of the arterial walls or muscles.

hypoventilation Respiratory rate insufficient to prevent carbon dioxide retention.

hypovolemia Abnormally low circulating blood volume.

hypoxemia Arterial blood oxygen level less than 60 mm Hg; low oxygen level in the blood.

hypoxia Inadequate cellular oxygenation that may result from a deficiency in the delivery or use of oxygen at the cellular level.

iatrogenic infection Infection caused by a treatment or diagnostic procedure.

identity Component of self-concept characterized by one's persisting consciousness of being oneself, separate and distinct from others.

idiosyncratic reaction Individual sensitivity to effects of a drug caused by inherited or other bodily constitution factors.

illness Abnormal process in which any aspect of a person's functioning is diminished or impaired compared with that person's previous condition.

illness behavior Ways in which people monitor their bodies, define and interpret their symptoms, take remedial actions, and use the health care system.

illness prevention Health education programs or activities directed toward protecting clients from threats or potential threats to health and toward minimizing risk factors.

immobility Inability to move about freely, caused by any condition in which movement is impaired or therapeutically restricted.

immunity The quality of being insusceptible to or unaffected by a particular disease or condition.

immunocompromised Clients who have damage to the integumentary system (wounds) or are infected or colonized with epidemiologically significant organisms. Clients whose immune systems are impaired.

implementation Initiation and completion of the nursing actions necessary to help the client achieve health care goals.

incentive spirometry Method of encouraging voluntary deep breathing by providing visual feedback to clients of the inspiratory volume they have achieved.

incident report Confidential document that describes any client accident while the person is on the premises of a health care agency.

independent practice association Managed care organization that contracts with physicians who usually are members of groups and whose practices include fee-for-service and capitated clients.

induration Hardening of a tissue, particularly the skin, because of edema or inflammation.

infection The invasion of the body by pathogenic microorganisms that reproduce and multiply.

inferences Taking one proposition as a given and guessing that another proposition follows.

infiltration Dislodging an intravenous catheter or needle from a vein into the subcutaneous space.

inflammation Protective response of body tissues to irritation or injury.

informed consent Process of obtaining permission from a client to perform a specific test or procedure, after describing all risks, side effects, and benefits.

infusions Introduction of fluid into the vein, giving intravenous fluid over time.

infusion pump Device that delivers a measured amount of fluid over a period of time.

inhalation Method of medication delivery through the client's respiratory tract. The respiratory tract provides a large surface area for drug absorption. Inhalation can be through the nasal or oral route.

injections Parenteral administration of medication; four major sites of injection: subcutaneous, intramuscular, intravenous, and intradermal.

insensible water loss Water loss that is continuous and is not perceived by the person.

insomnia Condition characterized by chronic inability to sleep or remain asleep through the night.

inspection Method of physical examination by which the client is visually systematically examined for appearance, structure, function, and behavior.

instillation To cause to enter drop by drop, or very slowly.

instrumental activities of daily living (IADLs) Activities that are necessary to be independent in society beyond eating, grooming, transferring, and toileting and include such skills as shopping, preparing meals, banking, and taking medications.

integrated delivery network (IDN) Set of providers and services organized to deliver a coordinated continuum of care to the population of clients served at a capitated cost.

interdisciplinary Representation of the various professional disciplines that are involved in a particular work issue or clinical practice problem.

interpersonal communication Exchange of information between two persons or among persons in a small group.

interstitial fluid Fluid that fills the spaces between most of the cells of the body and provides a substantial portion of the liquid environment of the body.

interview Organized, systematic conversation with the client designed to obtain pertinent health-related subjective information.

intracellular fluid Liquid within the cell membrane.

intractable pain Pain not easily relieved, such as that occurring with some types of cancer.

intradermal (ID) Injection given between layers of the skin, into the dermis. Injections are given at a 5- to 15-degree angle.

intramuscular (IM) Injections given into muscle tissue. The intramuscular route provides a fast rate of absorption that is related to the muscle's greater vascularity. Injections are given at a 90-degree angle.

intraocular Method of medication delivery that involves inserting a medication disk, similar to a contact lens, into the client's eye.

intrapersonal communication Communication that occurs within an individual; that is, persons "talk with themselves" silently or form an idea in their own mind.

intravascular fluid Pertaining to fluids circulating within blood vessels of the body.

intravenous Injection directly into the bloodstream. Action of the drug begins immediately when given intravenously.

intubation Insertion of a breathing tube through the mouth or nose into the trachea to ensure a patent airway.

intuition The inner sensing that something is so.

ions Electrically charged particles including anions and cations.

irrigation Process of washing out a body cavity or wounded area with a stream of fluid.

ischemia Decreased blood supply to a body part, such as skin tissue, or to an organ, such as the heart.

isolation Separation of a seriously ill patient from others to prevent the spread of an infection or to protect the patient from irritating environmental factors.

isometric exercises Activities that involve muscle tension without muscle shortening, do not have any beneficial effect on preventing orthostatic hypotension, but may improve activity tolerance.

isotonic Situation in which two solutions have the same concentration of solute; therefore both solutions exert the same osmotic pressure.

jaundice Yellow discoloration of the skin, mucous membranes, and sclera, caused by greater-than-normal amounts of bilirubin in the blood.

jejunostomy tube Hollow tube inserted into the jejunum thru the abdominal wall for administration of liquefied foods to patients who have a high risk of aspiration.

joint contracture Abnormality that may result in permanent condition of a joint, is characterized by flexion and fixation, and is caused by disuse, atrophy, and shortening of muscle fibers and surrounding joint tissues.

joints Connections between bones; classified according to structure and degree of mobility.

judgment Ability to form an opinion or draw sound conclusions.

justice The ethical standard of fairness.

Kardex Trade name for card-filing system that allows quick reference to the particular need of the client for certain aspects of nursing care.

Korotkoff sound Sound heard during the taking of blood pressure using a sphygmomanometer and stethoscope.

kyphosis Exaggeration of the posterior curvature of the thoracic spine.

laceration Torn, jagged wound.

language Code that conveys specific meaning as words are combined.

laryngospasm Sudden uncontrolled contraction of the laryngeal muscles, which in turn decreases airway size.

law Rule, standard, or principle that states a fact or a relationship between factors.

laxative Drug that acts to promote bowel evacuation.

learning Acquisition of new knowledge and skills as a result of reinforcement, practice, and experience.

learning objective Written statement that describes the behavior a teacher expects from an individual after a learning activity.

left-sided heart failure Abnormal condition characterized by impaired functioning of the left ventricle due to elevated pressures and pulmonary congestion.

leukoplakia Thick, white patches observed on oral mucous membranes.

licensed practical nurse (LPN) Also known as the licensed vocational nurse (LVN), or in Canada, registered nurse's assistant (RNA); trained in basic nursing skills and the provision of direct patient care.

licensed vocational nurse (LVN) The LVN is the same as a Licensed Practical Nurse (LPN), an individual trained in the United States in basic nursing techniques and direct client care who practices under the supervision of a registered nurse. The LVN is licensed by a board after completing what is usually a 12-month educational program and passing a licensure examination. In Canada an LVN is called a certified nursing assistant.

life-saving measure Independent, dependent, or interdependent nursing intervention that is implemented when a client's physiological or psychological status is threatened.

lipids Compounds that are insoluble in water but soluble in organic solvents.

lipogenesis Process during which fatty acids are synthesized.

living wills Instruments by which a dying person makes wishes known.

local anesthesia Loss of sensation at the desired site of action.

logroll Maneuver used to turn a reclining patient from one side to the other or completely over without moving the spinal column out of alignment.

lordosis Increased lumbar curvature.

loss Absence of a significant other, object, or state of health to which the person must adapt through the grieving process.

lymphocyte One type of leukocyte developing in the bone marrow; responsible for synthesizing antibodies and T cells that attack antigens.

maceration Softening and breaking down of skin from prolonged exposure to moisture.

malignant hyperthermia Autosomal dominant trait characterized by often fatal hyperthermia in affected people exposed to certain anesthetic agents.

malpractice Injurious or unprofessional actions that harm another.

malpractice insurance Type of insurance to protect the health care professional. In case of a malpractice claim, the insurance pays the award to the plaintiff.

managed care Health care system in which there is administrative control over primary health care services. Redundant facilities and services are eliminated, and costs are reduced. Preventive care and health education are emphasized.

management The process that involves planning, organizing, directing, and controlling of work activities to achieve a functional and productive work group.

masticate To chew or tear food with the teeth while it becomes mixed with saliva.

maturation The genetically determined biological plan for growth and development. Physical growth and motor development are a function of maturation.

maturational crises Same as developmental crises. Those crises associated with normal and expected phases of growth and development, for example, the response to menopause.

maturational loss Loss, usually of an aspect of self, resulting from the normal changes of growth and development.

Medicaid State medical assistance to people with low incomes, based on Title XIX of the Social Security Act. States receive matching federal funds to provide medical care and services to people meeting categorical and income requirements.

medical asepsis Procedures used to reduce the number of microorganisms and prevent their spread.

medical diagnosis Formal statement of the disease entity or illness made by the physician.

medical record Client's chart; a legal document.

Medicare Federally funded national health insurance program in the United States for people over 65 years of age. The program is administered in two parts. Part A provides basic protection against costs of medical, surgical, and psychiatric hospital care. Part B is a voluntary medical insurance program financed in part from federal funds and in part from premiums contributed by people enrolled in the program.

medication abuse Maladaptive pattern of recurrent medication use.

medication allergy Adverse reaction to a medication such as rash, chills, or gastrointestinal disturbances. Once a drug allergy occurs, the client can no longer receive that particular medication.

medication dependence Maladaptive pattern of medication use in the following patterns: using excessive amounts of the medication, increased activities directed toward obtaining the medication, withdrawal from professional or recreational activities, and so on.

medication error Any event that could cause or lead to a client's receiving inappropriate drug therapy or failing to receive appropriate drug therapy.

medication interaction The response when one drug modifies the action of another drug. The interaction can potentiate or diminish the actions of another drug, or it may alter the way a drug is metabolized, absorbed, or excreted.

melanoma Group of malignant neoplasms, primarily of the skin, that are composed of melanocytes. Common in fair-skinned people having light-colored eyes and in persons who have had a sunburn.

melena Abnormal black, sticky stool containing digested blood, indicative of gastrointestinal bleeding.

menarche Onset of a girl's first menstruation.

menopause Physiological cessation of ovulation and menstruation that typically occurs during middle adulthood in women.

message Information sent or expressed by sender in the communication process.

metabolic acidosis Abnormal condition of high hydrogen ion concentration in the extracellular fluid caused by either a primary increase in hydrogen ions or a decrease in bicarbonate.

metabolic alkalosis Abnormal condition characterized by the significant loss of acid from the body or by increased levels of bicarbonate.

metabolism Aggregate of all chemical processes that take place in living organisms, resulting in growth, generation of energy, elimination of wastes, and other functions concerned with the distribution of nutrients in the blood after digestion.

metacommunication Dependent not only on what is said but also on the relationship to the other person involved in the interaction. It is a message that conveys the sender's attitude toward the self and the message and the attitudes, feelings, and intentions toward the listener.

metastasize Spread of tumor cells to distant parts of the body from a primary site, for example, lung, breast, or bowel.

metered dose inhaler (MDI) Device designed to deliver a measured dose of an inhalation drug.

metric system Logically organized decimal system of measurement; metric units can easily be converted and computed through simple multiplication and division. Each basic unit of measurement is organized into units of 10.

microorganisms Microscopic entities, such as bacteria, viruses, and fungi, capable of carrying on living processes.

micturition Urination; act of passing or expelling urine voluntarily through the urethra.

milliequivalent per liter (mEq/L) Number of grams of a specific electrolyte dissolved in 1 liter of plasma.

minerals Inorganic elements essential to the body because of their role as catalysts in biochemical reactions.

minimum data set (MDS) Required by the Omnibus Reconciliation Act of 1987, the MDS is a uniform data set established by the Department of Health and Human Services. The MDS serves as the framework for any state-specified assessment instruments used to develop a written and comprehensive plan of care for newly admitted residents of nursing facilities.

misdemeanor Lesser crime than a felony; the penalty is usually a fine or imprisonment for less than 1 year.

mobility Person's ability to move about freely.

morals Personal conviction that something is absolutely right or wrong in all situations.

motivation Internal impulse that causes a person to take action.

mourning The process of grieving.

murmurs Blowing or whooshing sounds created by changes in blood flow through the heart or by abnormalities in valve closure.

muscle tone Normal state of balanced muscle tension.

myocardial contractility Measure of stretch of the cardiac muscle fiber. It can also affect stroke volume and cardiac output. Poor contraction decreases the amount of blood ejected by the ventricles during each contraction.

myocardial infarction Necrosis of a portion of cardiac muscle caused by obstruction in a coronary artery.

myocardial ischemia Condition that results when the supply of blood to the myocardium from the coronary arteries is insufficient to meet the oxygen demands of the organ.

NANDA North American Nursing Diagnosis Association, organized in 1973, which formally identifies, develops, and classifies nursing diagnoses.

narcolepsy Syndrome involving sudden sleep attacks that a person cannot inhibit; uncontrollable desire to sleep may occur several times during a day.

narcotic Drug substance, derived from opium or produced synthetically, that alters perception of pain and that with repeated use may result in physical and psychological dependence.

nasogastric (NG) tube Tube passed into the stomach through the nose for the purpose of emptying the stomach of its contents or for delivering medication and/or nourishment.

nebulization Process of adding moisture to inspired air by the addition of water droplets.

necrotic Of or pertaining to the death of tissue in response to disease or injury.

negative health behaviors Practices actually or potentially harmful to health, such as smoking, drug or alcohol abuse, poor diet, and refusal to take necessary medications.

negative nitrogen balance Condition occurring when the body excretes more nitrogen than it takes in.

negligence Careless act of omission or commission that results in injury to another.

neonate Stage of life from birth to 1 month of age.

nephrons Structural and functional units of the kidney containing renal glomeruli and tubules.

neuromodulator Substance that alters transmission of nerve impulses.

neurotransmitter Chemical that transfers the electrical impulse from the nerve fiber to the muscle fiber.

nitrogen balance Relationship between the nitrogen taken into the body, usually as food, and the nitrogen excreted from the body in urine and feces. Most of the body's nitrogen is incorporated into protein.

nociceptors Somatic and visceral free nerve endings of thinly myelinated and unmyelinated fibers. They usually react to tissue injury but may also be excited by endogenous chemical substances.

nocturia Urination at night; can be a symptom of renal disease or may occur in persons who drink excessive amounts of fluids before bedtime.

nonblanching reactive hyperemia Common symptom of the skin after a person has laid in a dependent position. When a finger is pressed against the red or purple area of the skin it does not turn lighter in color, indicating tissue damage.

nonmaleficence The fundamental ethical agreement to do no harm. Closely related to the ethical standard of beneficence.

nonrapid eye movement (NREM) sleep Sleep that occurs during the first four stages of normal sleep.

nonshivering thermogenesis Occurs primarily in neonates. Because neonates cannot shiver, a limited amount of vascular brown adipose tissue present at birth can be metabolized for heat production.

nonverbal communication Communication using expressions, gestures, body posture, and positioning rather than words.

normal sinus rhythm (NSR) The wave pattern on an electrocardiogram that indicates normal conduction of an electrical impulse through the myocardium.

nosocomial infection Infections acquired during hospitalization or stay in a health care facility.

nurse practice acts Statutes enacted by the legislature of any of the states or by the appropriate officers of the districts or possessions that describe and define the scope of nursing practice.

nurse-initiated interventions The response of the nurse to the client's health care needs and nursing diagnoses. This type of intervention is an autonomous action based on scientific rationale that is executed to benefit the client in a predicted way related to the nursing diagnosis and client-centered goals.

nursing diagnosis Formal statement of an actual or potential health problem that nurses can legally and independently treat. The second step of the nursing process, during which the client's actual and potential unhealthy responses to an illness or condition are identified.

nursing health history Data collected about a client's present level of wellness, changes in life patterns, sociocultural role, and mental and emotional reactions to illness.

nursing intervention Nursing action performed to prevent harm from occurring to a client or to improve the mental, emotional, physical, or social function of a client.

nursing process Systematic problem-solving method by which nurses individualize care for each client. The five steps of the nursing process are assessment, diagnosis, planning, implementation, and evaluation.

nutrients Foods that contain elements necessary for body function, including water, carbohydrates, proteins, fats, vitamins, and minerals.

nurturant Behavior that involves caring for or fostering the well-being of another individual.

nystagmus Involuntary, rhythmical movements of the eyes; the oscillations may be horizontal, vertical, rotatory, or mixed. May be indicative of vestibular, neurological, or vascular disease.

obesity Abnormal increase in the proportion of fat cells, mainly in the viscera and subcutaneous tissues of the body.

objective data Information that can be observed by others; free of feelings, perceptions, prejudices.

olfactory Pertaining to the sense of smell.

oncotic pressure The total influence of the protein on the osmotic activity of plasma fluid.

operating bed Table for surgery.

operating room (1) Room in a health care facility in which surgical procedures requiring anesthesia are performed. (2) Informal: a suite of rooms or an area in a health care facility in which patients are prepared for surgery, undergo surgical procedures, and recover from the anesthetic procedures required for the surgery.

ophthalmic Drugs given into the eye, in the form of either eye drops or ointments.

ophthalmoscope Instrument used to illuminate the structures of the eye in order to examine the fundus, which includes the retina, choroid, optic nerve disk, macula, fovea centralis, and retinal vessels.

oral hygiene Condition or practice of maintaining the tissues and structures of the mouth.

orthopnea Abnormal condition in which a person must sit or stand up to breathe comfortably.

orthostatic hypotension Abnormally low blood pressure occurring when a person stands up.

osmolality Concentration or osmotic pressure of a solution expressed in osmoles or milliosmoles per kilogram of water.

osmolarity Osmotic pressure of a solution expressed in osmoles or milliosmoles per kilogram of the solution.

osmoreceptors Neuron in the hypothalamus that is sensitive to the fluid concentration in the blood plasma and regulates the secretion of antidiuretic hormone.

osmosis Movement of a pure solvent through a semipermeable membrane from a solution with a lower solute concentration to one with a higher solute concentration.

osmotic pressure Drawing power for water, which depends on the number of molecules in the solution.

osteoporosis Disorder characterized by abnormal rarefaction of bone, occurring most frequently in postmenopausal women, in sedentary or immobilized individuals, and in clients on long-term steroid therapy.

ostomy Surgical procedure in which an opening is made into the abdominal wall to allow the passage of intestinal contents from the bowel (colostomy) or urine from the bladder (urostomy).

otoscope Instrument, with a special ear speculum, used to examine the deeper structures of the external and middle ear.

ototoxic Having a harmful effect on the eighth cranial (auditory) nerve or the organs of hearing and balance.

ototoxicity Having a harmful effect on the eighth cranial (auditory) nerve or the organs of hearing and balance.

outcome Condition of a client at the end of treatment, including the degree of wellness and the need for continuing care, medication, support, counseling, or education.

outliers Clients with extended lengths of stay beyond allowable inpatient days or costs.

outpatient Client who has not been admitted to a hospital but receives treatments in a clinic or facility associated with the hospital.

oxygen saturation The amount of hemoglobin fully saturated with oxygen, given as a percent value.

oxygen therapy Procedure in which oxygen is administered to a client to relieve or prevent hypoxia.

pain Subjective, unpleasant sensation caused by noxious stimulation of sensory nerve endings.

palliative care A level of care that is designed to relieve or reduce intensity of uncomfortable symptoms but not to produce a cure. Palliative care relies on comfort measures and use of alternative therapies to help individuals become more at peace during end of life.

pallor Unnatural paleness or absence of color in the skin.

palpation Method of physical examination whereby the fingers or hands of the examiner are applied to the client's body for the purpose of feeling body parts underlying the skin.

palpitations Bounding or racing of the heart associated with normal emotions or a heart disorder.

Papanicolaou (Pap) smear Painless screening test for cervical cancer. Specimens are taken of squamous and columnar cells of the cervix.

parallel play Form of play among a group of children, primarily toddlers, in which each one engages in an independent activity that is similar but not influenced by or shared with the others.

paralytic ileus Usually temporary paralysis of intestinal wall that may occur after abdominal surgery or peritoneal injury and that causes cessation of peristalsis. Leads to abdominal distention and symptoms of obstruction.

parenteral administration Giving medication by a route other than the gastrointestinal tract.

parenteral nutrition (PN) The administration of a nutritional solution into the vascular system.

partial bed bath Bath in which body parts that might cause the client discomfort if left unbathed (i.e., face, hands, axillary areas, back, and perineum) are washed in bed.

passive range-of-motion (PROM) exercises Range of movement through which a joint is moved with assistance.

passive strategies of health promotion Activities that involve the client as the recipient of actions by health care professionals.

pathogenicity Ability of a pathogenic agent to produce a disease.

pathogens Microorganisms capable of producing disease.

pathological fractures Fractures resulting from weakened bone tissue; frequently caused by osteoporosis or neoplasms.

patient-centered care Concept to improve work efficiency by changing the way client care is delivered.

patient-controlled analgesia (PCA) Drug delivery system that allows clients to self-administer analgesic medications when they want.

perceived loss Loss that is less obvious to the individual experiencing it. Although easily overlooked or misunderstood, a perceived loss results in the same grief process as an actual loss.

perception Persons' mental image or concept of elements in their environment, including information gained through the senses.

perceptual biases Human tendencies that interfere with accurately perceiving and interpreting messages from others.

percussion Method of physical examination whereby the location, size, and density of a body part is determined by the tone obtained from the striking of short, sharp taps of the fingers.

perfusion (1) Passage of a fluid through a specific organ or an area of the body. (2) Therapeutic measure whereby a drug intended for an isolated part of the body is introduced via the bloodstream.

perineal care Procedure prescribed for cleaning the genital and anal areas as part of the daily bath or after various obstetrical and gynecological procedures.

perioperative nursing Refers to the role of the operating room nurse during the preoperative, intraoperative, and postoperative phases of surgery.

peripherally inserted central catheter (PICC) Alternative intravenous access when the client requires intermediate-length venous access greater than 7 days to 3 months. Intravenous access is achieved by inserting a catheter into a central vein by way of a peripheral vein.

peristalsis Rhythmical contractions of the intestine that propel gastric contents through the length of the gastrointestinal tract.

peritonitis Inflammation of the peritoneum produced by bacteria or irritating substances introduced into the abdominal cavity by a penetrating wound or perforation of an organ in the gastrointestinal tract or the reproductive tract.

PERRLA Acronym for "pupils equal, round, reactive to light, accommodative"; the acronym is recorded in the physical examination if eye and pupil assessments are normal.

petechiae Tiny purple or red spots that appear on skin as minute hemorrhages within dermal layers.

pharmacokinetics Study of how drugs enter the body, reach their site of action, are metabolized, and exit from the body.

phlebitis Inflammation of a vein.

physical examination Assessment of the client's body using the techniques of inspection, auscultation, palpation, and percussion for the purpose of determining physical abnormalities.

physician-initiated interventions Based on the physician's response to a medical diagnosis, the nurse responds to the physician's written orders.

PIE note Problem-oriented medical record; the four interdisciplinary sections are the database, problem list, care plan, and progress notes.

placebos Dosage form that contains no pharmacologically active ingredients but may relieve pain through psychological effects.

plaintiff Individual who files formal charges against an individual or organization for a legal offense.

planning Process of designing interventions to achieve the goals and outcomes of health care delivery.

plantar flexion Toe-down motion of the foot at the ankle.

pleural friction rub Adventitious lung sound caused by inflamed parietal and visceral pleura rubbing together on inspiration.

pneumothorax Collection of air or gas in the pleural space.

point of maximal impulse (PMI) Point where the heartbeat can most easily be palpated through the chest wall. This is usually the fourth intercostal space at the midclavicular line.

poison Any substance that impairs health or destroys life when ingested, inhaled, or absorbed by the body in relatively small amounts.

poison control center One of a network of facilities that provides information regarding all aspects of poisoning or intoxication, maintains records of their occurrence, and refers clients to treatment centers.

polypharmacy Use of a number of different drugs by a client who may have one or several health problems.

polyunsaturated fatty acid Fatty acid that has two or more carbon double bonds.

positive health behaviors Activities related to maintaining, attaining, or regaining good health and preventing illness. Common positive health behaviors include immunizations, proper sleep patterns, adequate exercise, and nutrition.

postanesthesia care unit (PACU) Area adjoining the operating room to which surgical clients are taken while still under anesthesia.

postmortem After death.

postmortem care Care of a client's body after death.

postural drainage Use of positioning along with percussion and vibration to drain secretions from specific segments of the lungs and bronchi into the trachea.

postural hypotension Abnormally low blood pressure occurring when an individual assumes the standing posture; also called orthostatic hypotension.

posture Position of the body in relation to the surrounding space.

preadolescence Transitional developmental stage that occurs between childhood and adolescence.

preanesthesia care unit Area outside the operating room where preoperative preparations are completed.

preload Volume of blood in the ventricles at the end of diastole, immediately before ventricular contraction.

preoperative teaching Instruction regarding a client's anticipated surgery and recovery given before surgery. Instruction includes, but is not limited to, dietary and activity restrictions, anticipated assessment activities, postoperative procedures, and pain relief measures.

prescriptions Written directions for a therapeutic agent (e.g., medication, drugs).

pressure ulcer Inflammation, sore, or ulcer in the skin over a bony prominence.

presurgical care unit (PSCU) Area outside the operating room where preoperative preparations are completed.

preventive nursing actions Nursing actions directed toward preventing illness and promoting health to avoid the need for primary, secondary, or tertiary health care.

primary appraisal Evaluating an event for its personal meaning related to stress.

primary care First contact in a given episode of illness that leads to a decision regarding a course of action to resolve the health problem.

primary intention Primary union of the edges of a wound, progressing to complete scar formation without granulation.

primary nursing Method of nursing practice in which the client's care is managed, for the duration, by one nurse, who directs and coordinates other nurses and health care personnel. When on duty, the primary nurse cares for the client directly.

primary prevention First contact in a given episode of illness that leads to a decision regarding a course of action to prevent worsening of the health problem.

problem identification One of the steps of the diagnostic process in which the client's health care problem is recognized as a result of data analysis based on professional knowledge and experience.

problem solving Methodical, systematic approach to explore conditions and develop solutions, including analysis of data, determination of causative factors, and selection of appropriate actions to reverse or eliminate the problem.

problem-oriented medical record (POMR) Method of recording data about the health status of a client that fosters a collaborative problem-solving approach by all members of the health care team.

productive cough Sudden expulsion of air from the lungs that effectively removes sputum from the respiratory tract and helps clear the airways.

professional registered nurse See Registered nurse.

professional standards review organization (PSRO) Focuses on evaluation of nursing care provided in a health care setting. The quality, effectiveness, and appropriateness of nursing care for the client is the focus of evaluation.

prone Position of the client lying face-down.

proprioception The body's ability to sense its position and movement in space.

Prospective payment system (PPS) Payment mechanism for reimbursing hospitals for inpatient health care services in which predetermined rate is set for treatment of specific illnesses.

prostaglandins Potent hormone-like substances that act in exceedingly low doses on target organs. They can be used to treat asthma and gastric hyperacidity.

proteins Any of a large group of naturally occurring, complex, organic nitrogenous compounds. Each is composed of large combinations of amino acids containing the elements carbon, hydrogen, nitrogen, oxygen, usually sulfur, and occasionally phosphorus, iron, iodine, or other essential constituents of living cells. Protein is the major source of building material for muscles, blood, skin, hair, nails, and the internal organs.

proteinuria Presence in the urine of abnormally large quantities of protein, usually albumin. Persistent proteinuria is usually a sign of renal disease or renal complications of another disease, or hypertension or heart failure.

protocol Written and approved plan specifying the procedures to be followed during an assessment or in providing treatment.

pruritus Symptom of itching; an uncomfortable sensation leading to the urge to scratch.

psychomotor learning Acquisition of ability to perform motor skills.

ptosis Abnormal condition of one or both upper eyelids in which the eyelid droops, caused by weakness of the levator muscle or paralysis of the third cranial nerve.

puberty Developmental period of emotional and physical changes, including the development of secondary sex characteristics and the onset of menstruation and ejaculation.

public communication Interaction of one individual with large groups of people.

pulmonary hygiene More frequent turning, deep breathing, coughing, use of incentive spirometry, and chest physical therapy (PT) if ordered.

pulse deficit Condition that exists when the radial pulse is less than the ventricular rate as auscultated at the apex or seen on an electrocardiogram. The condition indicates a lack of peripheral perfusion for some of the heart contractions.

pulse pressure Difference between the systolic and diastolic pressures, normally 30 to 40 mm Hg.

Purkinje network Complex network of muscle fibers that spread through the right and left ventricles of the heart and carry the impulses that contract those chambers almost simultaneously.

pursed-lip breathing Deep inspiration followed by prolonged expiration through pursed lips.

pyrexia Abnormal elevation of the temperature of the body above 37° C (98.6° F) because of disease; same as fever.

pyrogens Substances that cause a rise in body temperature, as in the case of bacterial toxins.

quality improvement Monitoring and evaluation of processes and outcomes in health care or any other business to identify opportunities for improvement.

quality indicator Quantitative measure of an important aspect of care that determines whether quality of service conforms to requirements or standards of care.

race Vague, unscientific term for a group of genetically related people who share certain physical characteristics.

range of motion Range of movement of a joint, from maximum extension to maximum flexion, as measured in degrees of a circle.

rapid eye movement (REM) sleep Stage of sleep in which dreaming and rapid eye movements are prominent; important for mental restoration.

reaction Component of the pain experience that may include both physiological responses, such as in the general adaptation syndrome, and behavioral responses.

reactive blanching hyperemia Mechanism that causes the blood vessels to dilate in the area of injury.

reality orientation Therapeutic modality for restoring an individual's sense of the present.

receiver Person to whom message is sent during the communication process.

reception Neurophysiological components of the pain experience, in which nervous system receptors receive painful stimuli and transmit them through peripheral nerves to the spinal cord and brain.

record Written form of communication that permanently documents information relevant to health care management.

recovery A period of time immediately postoperative when the client is closely observed for effects of anesthesia, changes in vital signs, and bleeding. The area is usually in the postanesthesia care unit.

referent Factor that motivates a person to communicate with another individual.

reflection Process of thinking back or recalling an event to discover the meaning and purpose of that event. Useful in critical thinking.

refractive error Defect in the ability of the lens of the eye to focus light, such as occurs in nearsightedness and farsightedness.

regional anesthesia Loss of sensation in an area of the body supplied by sensory nerve pathways.

registered nurse (RN) In the United States a nurse who has completed a course of study at a state-approved accredited school of nursing and has passed the National Council Licensure Examination (NCLEX-RN).

regression Return to an earlier developmental stage or behavior.

regulatory agencies Local, state, provincial, or national agencies that inspect and certify health care agencies as meeting specified standards. These agencies can also determine the amount of reimbursement for health care delivered.

rehabilitation Restoration of an individual to normal or near-normal function after a physical or mental illness, injury, or chemical addiction.

reinforcement Provision of a contingent response to a learner's behavior that increases the probability of the behavior's recurring.

related factor Any condition or event that accompanies or is linked with the client's health care problem.

relaxation Act of being relaxed or less tense.

reminiscence Recalling the past for the purpose of assigning new meaning to past experiences.

remissions Partial or complete disappearances of the clinical and subjective characteristics of chronic or malignant disease; remission may be spontaneous or the result of therapy.

renal calculi Calcium stones in the renal pelvis.

renin Proteolytic enzyme, produced by and stored in the juxtaglomerular apparatus that surrounds each arteriole as it enters a glomerulus. The enzyme affects the blood pressure by catalyzing the change of angiotensinogen to angiotensin, a strong repressor.

reports Transfer of information from the nurses on one shift to the nurses on the following shift. Report may also be given by one of the members of the nursing team to another health care provider, for example, a physician or therapist.

resident flora Microorganisms that reside on the surface and deep layers of skin, the saliva, the mucosa, and the GI tract. Flora do not normally cause disease.

residual urine Volume of urine remaining in the bladder after a normal voiding; the bladder normally is almost completely empty after micturition.

resistance stage Third stage of the stress response, when the person attempts to adapt to the stressor. The body stabilizes, hormone levels stabilize, and heart rate, blood pressure, and cardiac output return to normal.

resource utilization group (RUG) Method of classification for health care reimbursement for long-term care facilities.

respiratory acidosis Abnormal condition characterized by increased arterial carbon dioxide concentration, excess carbonic acid, and increased hydrogen ion concentration.

respiratory alkalosis Abnormal condition characterized by decreased arterial carbon dioxide concentration and decreased hydrogen ion concentration.

respite care Short-term health services to dependent older adults either in their home or in an institutional setting.

responsibility Carrying out duties associated with a particular role.

restorative care Health care settings and services where clients who are recovering from illness or disability receive rehabilitation and supportive care.

restraint Device to aid in the immobilization of a client or client's extremity.

reticular activating system (RAS) Group of specialized nerve cells located in the brainstem, upper spinal cord, and cerebral cortex.

return demonstration Demonstration after the client has first observed the teacher and then practiced the skill in mock or real situations.

rhonchi Abnormal lung sound auscultated when the client's airways are obstructed with thick secretions.

right-sided heart failure Abnormal condition that results from impaired functioning of the right ventricle characterized by venous congestion in the systemic circulation.

risk factor Any internal or external variable that makes a person or group more vulnerable to illness or an unhealthy event.

risk nursing diagnosis Describes human responses to health conditions/life processes that may develop in a vulnerable, individual, family, or community.

role Set of behaviors by means of which a person participates in a social group.

sandbags Sand-filled plastic tubes that can be shaped to body contours. They can immobilize an extremity or maintain body alignment.

saturated fatty acid Fatty acid in which each carbon in the chain has an attached hydrogen atom.

scientific method Codified sequence of steps used in the formulation, testing, evaluation, and reporting of scientific ideas.

scientific rationale Reason, based on supporting literature, why a specific nursing action was chosen.

scoliosis Lateral spinal curvature.

scrub nurse Registered nurse or operating room technician who assists surgeons during operations.

secondary appraisal Evaluating one's possible coping strategies when confronted with a stressor.

secondary intention Wound closure in which the edges are separated, granulation tissue develops to fill the gap, and, finally, epithelium grows in over the granulation, producing a larger scar than results with primary intention.

secondary prevention Level of preventive medicine that focuses on early diagnosis, use of referral services, and rapid initiation of treatment to stop the progress of disease processes.

sedatives Medications that produce a calming effect by decreasing functional activity, diminishing irritability, and allaying excitement.

segmentation Alternating contraction and relaxation of gastrointestinal mucosa.

self-concept Complex, dynamic integration of conscious and unconscious feelings, attitudes, and perceptions about one's identity, physical being, worth, and roles; how a person perceives and defines self.

self-esteem Feeling of self-worth characterized by feelings of achievement, adequacy, self-confidence, and usefulness.

sender Person who initiates interpersonal communication by conveying a message.

sensible water loss Loss of fluid from the body through the secretory activity of the sweat glands and the exhalation of humidified air from the lungs.

sensory deficits Defects in the function of one or more of the senses, resulting in visual, auditory, or olfactory impairments.

sensory deprivation State in which stimulation to one or more of the senses is lacking, resulting in impaired sensory perception.

sensory overload State in which stimulation to one or more of the senses is so excessive that the brain disregards or does not meaningfully respond to stimuli.

sequential compression stockings Plastic stockings attached to an air pump that inflates and deflates the stockings, applying intermittent pressure sequentially from the ankle to the knee.

serum half-life Time needed for excretion processes to lower the serum drug concentration by half.

sexual dysfunction Inability or difficulty in sexual functioning caused by physiological or psychological factors or both.

sexual orientation Clear, persistent erotic preference for a person of one sex or the other.

sexuality "A function of the total personality . . . concerned with the biological, psychological, sociological, spiritual and culture variables of life . . ." (Sex Information and Education Council of the United States, 1980).

sexually transmitted disease Infectious process spread through sexual contact, including oral, genital, or anal sexual activity.

shear Force exerted against the skin while the skin remains stationary and the bony structures move.

side effect Any reaction or consequence that results from medication or therapy.

side rails Bars positioned along the sides of the length of the bed or stretcher to reduce the client's risk of falling.

sinoatrial (SA) node Called the "pacemaker of the heart" because the origin of the normal heartbeat begins at the SA node. The SA node is in the right atrium next to the entrance of the superior vena cava.

situational crisis Unexpected crisis that arises suddenly in response to an external event or a conflict concerning a specific circumstance.

situational loss Loss of a person, thing, or quality resulting from a change in a life situation, including changes related to illness, body image, environment, and death.

sitz bath Bath in which only the hips or buttocks are immersed in fluid.

skilled nursing facility Institution or part of an institution that meets criteria for accreditation established by the sections of the Social Security Act that determine the basis for Medicaid and Medicare reimbursement for skilled nursing care, including rehabilitation and various medical and nursing procedures.

sleep State marked by reduced consciousness, diminished activity of the skeletal muscles, and depressed metabolism.

sleep apnea Cessation of breathing for a time during sleep.

sleep deprivation Condition resulting from a decrease in the amount, quality, and consistency of sleep.

SOAP note Progress notes that focus on a single client problem and include subjective and objective data, analysis, and planning; most often used in the POMR.

solute Substance dissolved in a solution.

solution Mixture of one or more substances dissolved in another substance. The molecules of each of the substances disperse homogeneously and do not change chemically. A solution may be a liquid, gas, or solid.

solvent Any liquid in which another substance can be dissolved.

source record Organization of a client's chart so that each discipline (e.g., nursing, medicine, social work, or respiratory therapy) has a separate section in which to record data. Unlike POMR, the information is not organized by client problems. The advantage of a source record is that caregivers can easily locate the proper section of the record in which to make entries.

sphygmomanometer Device for measuring the arterial blood pressure that consists of an arm or leg cuff with an air bladder connected to a tube and a bulb for pumping air into the bladder and a gauge for indicating the amount of air pressure being exerted against the artery.

spiritual distress State of being out of harmony with a system of beliefs, a Supreme Being, or God.

spiritual well-being Individual's spirituality that enables a person to love, have faith and hope, seek meaning in life, and nurture relationships with others.

spirituality Spiritual dimension of a person, including the relationship with humanity, nature, and a Supreme Being.

standardized care plans Written care plans used for groups of clients that have similar health care problems.

standard of care Minimum level of care accepted to ensure high-quality care to clients. Standards of care define the types of therapies typically administered to clients with defined problems or needs.

standard of practice Provide clients with assurance that they are receiving high-quality nursing care, the nurses know how to provide the care, and there are measures to determine if the care meets the established standards and expected outcomes.

standard precautions Guidelines recommended by the Centers for Disease Control and Prevention (CDC) to reduce the risk of transmission of blood-borne and other pathogens in hospitals.

standing order Written and approved documents containing rules, policies, procedures, regulations, and orders for the conduct of client care in various stipulated clinical settings.

statutory law Of or related to laws enacted by a legislative branch of the government.

stenosis Abnormal condition characterized by the constriction or narrowing of an opening or passageway in a body structure.

sterilization (1) Rendering a person unable to produce children; accomplished by surgical, chemical, or other means. (2) A technique for destroying microorganisms using heat, water, chemicals, or gases.

stereotyping Generalization about a form of behavior, an individual, or a group.

stoma Artificially created opening between a body cavity and the body's surface; for example, a colostomy, formed from a portion of the colon pulled through the abdominal wall.

stress Physiological or psychological tension that threatens homeostasis or a person's psychological equilibrium.

stressor Any event, situation, or other stimulus encountered in a person's external or internal environment that necessitates change or adaptation by the person.

striae Streaks or linear scars that result from rapid development of tension in the skin.

stroke volume Amount of blood ejected by the ventricles with each contraction. It can be affected by the amount of blood in the left ventricle at the end of diastole (preload), the resistance to left ventricular ejection (afterload), and myocardial contractility.

subacute care Level of medical specialty care provided to clients who need a greater intensity of care than that provided in a skilled nursing facility but who do not require acute care.

subcutaneous Injection given into the connective tissue, under the dermis. The subcutaneous tissue absorbs drugs more slowly than those injected into muscle. Injections are usually given at an angle of 45 degrees.

subcutaneous layer Continuous layer of connective tissue over the entire body between the skin and the deep fascia.

subjective data Information gathered from client statements; the client's feelings and perceptions. Not verifiable by another except by inference.

sublingual Route of medication administration in which the medication is placed underneath the client's tongue.

supine Position of the client in which the client is resting on his or her back.

suprainfection Secondary infection usually caused by an opportunistic pathogen.

suprapubic catheter Catheter surgically inserted through abdomen into bladder.

surfactant Chemical produced in the lung by alveolar type 2 cells that maintains the surface tension of the alveoli and keeps them from collapsing.

surgical asepsis Procedures used to eliminate any microorganisms from an area. Also called sterile technique.

symbolic communication Use of an image, object, or action to represent something else and to help convey meaning, which is established by the symbol's association, resemblance, or conventional or personal use.

sympathy Concern, sorrow, or pity felt by the nurse for the client in which the nurse personally identifies with the client's needs. Sympathy is a subjective look at another person's world that prevents a clear perspective of all sides of the issues confronting that person.

synapse Region surrounding the point of contact between two neurons or between a neuron and an effector organ.

syncope A brief lapse in consciousness caused by transient cerebral hypoxia.

synergistic effect Effect resulting from two drugs acting synergistically; the effect of the two drugs combined is greater than the effect that would be expected if the individual effects of the two drugs acting alone were added together.

systolic Pertaining to or resulting from ventricular contraction.

tachycardia Rapid regular heart rate ranging between 100 and 150 beats per minute.

tachypnea Abnormally rapid rate of breathing.

tactile Relating to the sense of touch.

tactile fremitus Tremulous vibration of the chest wall during breathing that is palpable on physical examination.

teaching Implementation method used to present correct principles, procedures, and techniques of health care; to inform clients about their health status; and to refer clients and family to appropriate health or social resources in the community.

team nursing Decentralized system in which the care of a client is distributed among the members of a team. The charge nurse delegates authority to a team leader, who must be a professional nurse.

teratogens Chemical or physiological agents that may produce adverse effects in the embryo or fetus.

tertiary prevention Activities directed toward rehabilitation rather than diagnosis and treatment.

therapeutic communication Process in which the nurse consciously influences a client or helps the client to a better understanding through verbal and/or nonverbal communication.

therapeutic effect Desired benefit of a medication, treatment, or procedure.

thermoregulation Internal control of body temperature.

threshold Point at which a person first perceives a painful stimulus as being painful.

thrill Continuous palpable sensation like the purring of a cat.

thrombus Accumulation of platelets, fibrin, clotting factors, and the cellular elements of the blood attached to the interior wall of a vein or artery, sometimes occluding the lumen of the vessel.

tinnitus Ringing heard in one or both ears.

tissue ischemia Point at which tissues receive insufficient oxygen and perfusion.

tolerance Point at which a person is not willing to accept pain of greater severity or duration.

tort Act that causes injury for which the injured party can bring civil action.

total parenteral nutrition (TPN) Administration of a nutritionally adequate hypertonic solution consisting of glucose, protein hydrolysates, minerals, and vitamins through an indwelling catheter into the superior vena cava or other main vein.

total patient care A nursing delivery of care model originally developed during Florence Nightingale's time. In the model a registered nurse (RN) is responsible for all aspects of care for one or more clients. The nurse works directly with the client, family, physician, and health care team members. The model typically has a shift-based focus.

toxic effect Effect of a medication that results in an adverse response.

transcultural Concept of care as the essence and dominant domain that distinguishes nursing from other health disciplines.

transcendence An awareness of that which cannot be seen or known in ordinary physical ways.

transcultural nursing Individualized nursing care provided to clients of various ethnic and cultural backgrounds.

transcutaneous electrical nerve stimulation (TENS) Technique in which a battery-powered device blocks pain impulses from reaching the spinal cord by delivering weak electrical impulses directly to the skin's surface.

transdermal disk Medication delivery device in which the medication is saturated on a waferlike disk, which is affixed to the client's skin. This method ensures that the client receives a continuous level of medication.

transfer report Verbal exchange of information between caregivers when a client is moved from one nursing unit or health care setting to another. The report includes information necessary to maintain a consistent level of care from one setting to another.

transfusion reaction Systemic response by the body to the administration of blood incompatible with that of the recipient.

transient flora Flora not commonly found in a particular area of the body.

trapeze bar Metal triangular-shaped bar that can be suspended over a client's bed from an overhanging frame; permits clients to move up and down in bed while in traction or some other encumbrance.

triangulation Complaining to a third party rather than confronting the problem or expressing concerns directly to the source. It lowers team morale and is often contagious.

trimester Referring to one of the three phases of pregnancy.

trochanter roll Rolled towel support placed against the hips and upper leg to prevent external rotation of the legs.

turgor Normal resiliency of the skin caused by the outward pressure of the cells and interstitial fluid.

unsaturated fatty acid Fatty acid in which an unequal number of hydrogen atoms are attached and the carbon atoms attach to each other with a double bond.

ureterostomy Diversion of urine away from a diseased or defective bladder through an artificial opening in the skin.

urinal Receptacle for collecting urine.

urinary diversion Surgical diversion of the drainage of urine from a diseased or dysfunctional bladder.

urinary incontinence Inability to control urination.

urinary reflux Abnormal, backward flow of urine.

urinary retention Retention of urine in the bladder; condition frequently caused by a temporary loss of muscle function.

urine hat Receptacle for collecting urine that fits toilet.

urometer Device for measuring frequent and small amounts of urine from an indwelling urinary catheter system.

urosepsis Organisms in the bloodstream.

utilitarianism Ethic that proposes that the value of something is determined by its usefulness. The greatest good for the greatest number of people constitutes the guiding principle for action in a utilitarian model of ethics.

utilization review (UR) committees Physician-supervised committee to review admissions, diagnostic testing, and treatments provided by physicians to clients.

validation Act of confirming, verifying, or corroborating the accuracy of assessment data or the appropriateness of the care plan.

Valsalva maneuver Any forced expiratory effort against a closed airway, such as when an individual holds the breath and tightens the muscles in a concerted, strenuous effort to move a heavy object or to change positions in bed.

value Personal belief about the worth of a given idea or behavior.

valvular heart disease Acquired or congenital disorder of a cardiac valve characterized by stenosis and obstructed blood flow or valvular degeneration and regurgitation of blood.

variances The unexpected event that occurs during client care and that is different from what is predicted on a CareMap. Variance or exceptions are interventions or outcomes that are not achieved as anticipated. Variance may be positive or negative.

vascular access devices Catheters, cannulas, or infusion ports designed for long-term, repeated access to the vascular system.

vasoconstriction Narrowing of the lumen of any blood vessel, especially the arterioles and the veins in the blood reservoirs of the skin and abdominal viscera.

vasodilation Increase in the diameter of a blood vessel caused by inhibition of its vasoconstrictor nerves or stimulation of dilator nerves.

venipuncture Technique in which a vein is punctured transcutaneously by a sharp rigid stylet (e.g., a butterfly needle), a cannula (e.g., an angiocatheter that contains a flexible plastic catheter), or a needle attached to a syringe.

ventilation Respiratory process by which gases are moved into and out of the lungs.

ventricular gallop Abnormal, low-pitched extra heart sound (S_4) heard in early diastole.

verbal communication The sending of messages from one individual to another or to a group of individuals through the spoken word.

vertigo Sensation of dizziness or spinning.

vibration Fine, shaking pressure applied by hands to the chest wall only during exhalation.

virulence Very pathogenic or rapidly progressive condition.

visual Related to, or experienced through, vision.

vital signs Temperature, pulse, respirations, and blood pressure.

vitamins Organic compound essential in small quantities for normal physiological and metabolic functioning of the body. With few exceptions, vitamins cannot be synthesized by the body and must be obtained from the diet or dietary supplements.

vocal fremitus Vibration of the chest wall as the person speaks or sings

that allows the person's voice to be heard by the examiner during auscultation of the chest with a stethoscope.

voiding The process of urinating.

vulnerable population Clients who are more likely to develop health problems as a result of excess risks, who have limits in access to health care services, or who are dependent on others for care.

wellness Dynamic state of health in which an individual progresses toward a higher level of functioning, achieving an optimum balance between internal and external environments.

wellness education Activities that teach people how to care for themselves in a healthy manner.

wellness nursing diagnosis Clinical judgment about an individual, group, or community in transition from a specific level of wellness to a higher level of wellness.

wheezes, wheezing Adventitious lung sound caused by a severely narrowed bronchus.

work redesign Formal process used to analyze the work of a certain work group and to change the actual structure of the jobs performed.

wound culture Specimen collected from a wound to determine the specific organism that is causing an infectious process.

Z-track injection Technique for injecting irritating preparations into muscle without tracking residual medication through sensitive tissues.

Appendix A

Common Abbreviations

NOTE: Abbreviations in common use can vary widely from place to place. Each institution's list of acceptable abbreviations is the best authority for its records.

°C	degrees centigrade
°F	degrees Fahrenheit
μg	microgram
μm	micrometer
ʒ	dram

A

aa	of each
ABG	arterial blood gas
ac	before meals
ad lib	freely as desired
ADL	activities of daily living
Ag	silver, antigen
AIDS	acquired immuno-deficiency syndrome
ALS	amyotrophic lateral sclerosis
AM	morning
ama	against medical advice
AMI	acute myocardial infarction
amp	ampule
ARC	AIDS-related complex
ARDS	adult respiratory distress syndrome
AS	aortic stenosis
ASD	atrial septal defect

B

Ba	barium
BE	barium enema
bid	two times a day
BM, bm	bowel movement
BMR	basal metabolic rate
BP	blood pressure
BPH	benign prostatic hypertrophy
BRP	bathroom privileges
BSA	body surface area
BUN	blood urea nitrogen

C

c̄	with
c/o	complains of
Ca	calcium, cancer, carcinoma
CAD	coronary artery disease
cap	capsule
CAT	computed axial tomography
cath	catheter, catheterize

CBC	complete blood count
CBR	complete bed rest
CC	chief complaint
cc	cubic centimeter
CCU	coronary care unit, critical care unit
CDC	Centers for Disease Control and Prevention
CEA	carcinoembryonic antigen
CFT	complement-fixation test
cg	centigram
CHF	congestive heart failure
CHO	carbohydrate
Cl	chlorine
cm	centimeter
cm³	cubic centimeter
CNS	central nervous system
CO	carbon monoxide
CO_2	carbon dioxide
COPD	chronic obstructive pulmonary disease
CPK	creatine phosphokinase
CPR	cardiopulmonary resuscitation
CSF	cerebrospinal fluid
CT	computed tomography
CVA	cerebrovascular accident, costovertebral angle
CVP	central venous pressure

D

D&C	dilation and curettage
D_5W	5% dextrose in water
db, dB	decibels
dc	discontinue
DIC	disseminated intravascular coagulation
diff	differential blood count
dil	dilute
DJD	degenerative joint disease
dl	deciliter
DM	diastolic murmur
DNR	do not resuscitate
DOE	dyspnea on exertion
dx, Dx	diagnosis

E

EBV	Epstein-Barr virus
ECF	extracellular fluid
ECG	electrocardiogram

ECHO	echocardiography
ECT	electroconvulsive therapy
EDC	estimated date of confinement
EDD	estimated date of delivery
EEG	electroencephalogram
EKG	electrocardiogram
elix	elixir
EMG	electromyogram
ENG	electronystagmography
ER	emergency room
ERG	electroretinogram
ESRD	end-stage renal disease
EST	electroshock therapy

F

ʒ	fluid ounce
FANA	fluorescent antinuclear antibody test
FBS	fasting blood sugar
Fe	iron
FEV	forced expiratory volume
FHR	fetal heart rate
FRC	functional residual capacity
FSH	follicle-stimulating hormone
FUO	fever of unknown origin
Fx, fx	fracture, fractional urine test

G

g, gm, Gm	gram
Gc, GC	gonococcus
GI	gastrointestinal
gr	grain
grav I, II, III, etc.	pregnancy one, two, three, etc.
gt, gtt	drop, drops
GTT	glucose tolerance test
GU	genitourinary
GYN, Gyn	gynecological

H

H_2O	water
h, hr	hour
H^+	hydrogen ion
h/o	history of
H&P	history and physical examination

HAV	hepatitis A virus
Hb	hemoglobin
HBAg	hepatitis B antigen
HBV	hepatitis B virus
Hct, HCT	hematocrit
HDL	high-density lipoprotein
Hg	mercury
Hgb	hemoglobin
HIV	human immuno-deficiency (AIDS) virus
HLA	human lymphocyte antigen
HSV2	herpes simplex virus, type 2

I

I&O	intake and output
IC	inspiratory capacity
ICP	intracranial pressure
ICU	intensive care unit
IDDM	insulin-dependent diabetes mellitus
IE	immunoelectrophoresis
Ig	immunoglobulin
IgA, etc.	immunoglobulin A, etc.
IM	intramuscular
IOP	intraocular pressure
IPPB	intermittent positive pressure breathing
IV	intravenous
IVP	intravenous push; intravenous pyelogram
IVU	intravenous urogram

J

JRA	juvenile rheumatoid arthritis

K

K	potassium
kg	kilogram
KUB	kidney, ureters, and bladder (radiograph)
KVO	keep vein open

L

L	liter
L&A	light and accommodation
LBBB	left bundle branch block
LE	lupus erythematosus
LGV	lymphogranuloma venereum
LLL	left lower lobe
LLQ	left lower quadrant
LMP	last menstrual period
LNMP	last normal menstrual period
LP	lumbar puncture
LUL	left upper lobe
LUQ	left upper quadrant
LVH	left ventricular hypertrophy

M

m	meter
m, min, ℳ	minum
MAP	mean arterial pressure
mcg	microgram
MCH	mean corpuscular hemoglobin
MCHC	mean corpuscular hemo-globin concentration
MCV	mean cell volume; mean corpuscular volume
mg	milligram
Mg	magnesium
MG	myasthenia gravis
MI	myocardial infarction
MICU	medical intensive care unit
ml	milliliter
mm	millimeter
mm³	cubic millimeter
mm Hg	millimeters of mercury
MRI	magnetic resonance imaging
MS	multiple sclerosis
MW	molecular weight

N

N	nitrogen
Na	sodium
NICU	neonatal intensive care unit
NIH	National Institutes of Health
nm	nanometer
NMR	nuclear magnetic reso-nance
NPO	nothing by mouth
NS	normal saline

O

O_2	oxygen
OD	right eye; optical density; overdose
OL	left eye
OOB	out of bed
ORIF	open reduction and internal fixation
OS	left eye
OT	occupational therapy
OTC	over-the-counter
ou	both eyes
oz, ℥	ounce

P

P&A	percussion and auscultation
$PaCO_2$	partial pressure of carbon dioxide (arterial blood)
PaO_2	partial pressure of oxygen (arterial blood)
para I, II, etc.	unipara, bipara, etc.

PAT	paroxysmal atrial tachycardia
pc	after meals
PCG	phonocardiogram
PCO_2	partial pressure of carbon dioxide
PCP	pulmonary capillary pressure, phencyclidine
PCV	packed cell volume
PCWP	pulmonary capillary wedge pressure
PD	interpupillary distance; postural drainage
PE	pulmonary embolism, physical examination
PEEP	positive end-expiratory pressure
PEG	pneumoencephalography
per	through, by way of
PERRLA	pupils equal, round, and reactive to light and accommodation
PET	positron emission tomography
PG	prostaglandin
pH	hydrogen ion concentra-tion (acidity and alkalinity)
PID	pelvic inflammatory disease
PKU	phenylketonuria
PM	postmortem
PM	evening
PMS	premenstrual syndrome
PND	paroxysmal nocturnal dyspnea, postnasal drip
PO_2	partial pressure of oxygen
PO, po	orally
PPD	purified protein derivative
ppm	parts per million
prn	when required, as often as necessary
PT	physical therapy; prothrombin time
PTT	partial thromboplastin time
PUO	pyrexia of unknown origin
PVC	premature ventricular contraction

Q

q	every
q2h	every 2 hours
q3h	every 3 hours
q4h	every 4 hours
qd	every day
qh	every hour
qid	four times a day
qn	every night
qod	every other day
qns	quantity not sufficient

R

R/O	rule out
RBBB	right bundle branch block
RBC	red blood cell
RDS	respiratory distress syndrome
Rh+	positive Rh factor
Rh−	negative Rh factor
RHD	rheumatic heart disease
RLL	right lower lobe
RLQ	right lower quadrant
RML	right middle lobe
ROM	range of motion
ROS	review of systems
RS	Reiter's syndrome
RSV	Rous sarcoma virus
RUL	right upper lobe
RUQ	right upper quadrant
Rx	take; treatment

S

s̄	without
SB	sternal border
SC	subcutaneous
sib	sibling
SICU	surgical intensive care unit
SIDS	sudden infant death syndrome
Sig	write on label
SLE	systemic lupus erythematosus
sol	solution, dissolved
sos	if necessary
sp gr, SG, sg	specific gravity
SQ, subq	subcutaneous
SR	sedimentation rate
ss	half
SSS	sick sinus syndrome; specific soluble substance; short-stay surgery
stat	immediately
STD	sexually transmitted disease
STS	serologic test for syphilis
susp	suspension
SV	stroke volume

T

T_3	triiodothyronine
T_4	tetraiodothyronine
T&A	tonsillectomy and adenoidectomy
TAB	typhoid and paratyphoid A and B
TAH	total abdominal hysterectomy
TAT	tetanus antitoxin; thematic apperception test
TB, TBC	tuberculosis
TBG	thyroxin-binding globulin
TG	triglyceride
TIA	transient ischemic attack
TIBC	total iron-binding capacity
tid	three times a day
TKO	to keep open
TLC	total lung capacity; thin layer chromatography
TPN	total parenteral nutrition
TPR	temperature, pulse, and respirations
tr, tinct	tincture
TST	triple sugar iron test
TSH	thyroid-stimulating hormone

U

UA	urinalysis
UGI series	upper gastrointestinal series
UIBC	unsaturated iron-binding capacity
URI	upper respiratory infection
US	ultrasound
UTI	urinary tract infection

V

V&T	volume and tension
VC	vital capacity
VD	venereal disease
VDA	visual discriminatory acuity
VDH	valvular disease of the heart
VDRL	Venereal Disease Research Laboratory
VLDL	very low-density lipoprotein
VS	vital signs
VSD	ventricular septal defect
V_T	tidal volume

W

W/V	weight/volume
WBC	white blood cell, white blood count
WNL	within normal limits
WR	Wassermann reaction

Appendix B

OVERVIEW OF CDC HAND HYGIENE GUIDELINES

The Centers for Disease Control and Prevention recently released new recommendations for hand hygiene in health care settings. Hand hygiene is a term that applies to either handwashing, use of an antiseptic hand rub, or surgical hand antisepsis. Evidence suggests that hand antisepsis, the cleansing of hands with an antiseptic hand rub is more effective in reducing nosocomial infections than plain handwashing.

Follow these guidelines in the care of all patients

- Continue to wash hands with either a non-antimicrobial or an antimicrobial soap and water whenever the hands are visibly soiled.
- Use an alcohol-based hand rub to routinely decontaminate the hands in the following clinical situations: (Note: if alcohol-based hand rubs are not available, the alternative is hand washing)
  - Before and after client contact.
  - Before donning sterile gloves when inserting central intravascular catheters.
  - Before performing non-surgical invasive procedures (e.g. urinary catheter insertion, nasotracheal suctioning).
  - After contact with body fluids or excretions, mucous membranes, nonintact skin, and wound dressings.
  - If moving from a contaminated-body site (rectal area or mouth) to a clean-body site (surgical wound, urinary meatus) during client care.
  - After contact with inanimate objects (including medical equipment) in the immediate vicinity of the client).
  - After removing gloves.
- Before eating and after using a restroom, wash hands with a non-antimicrobial or an antimicrobial soap and water.
- Antimicrobial-impregnated wipes (i.e., towelettes) are not a substitute for using an alcohol-based hand rub or antimicrobial soap.
- If exposure to Bacillus anthracis is suspected or proven, wash hands with a non-antimicrobial or an antimicrobial soap and water. The physical action of washing and rinsing hands is recommended because alcohols, chlorhexidine, iodophors, and other antiseptic agents have poor activity against spores.

Method for decontaminating hands

When using an alcohol-based hand rub, apply product to palm of one hand and rub hands together, covering all surfaces of hands and fingers, until hands are dry. Follow the manufacturer's recommendations regarding the volume of product to use.

Follow these guidelines for surgical hand antisepsis

- Surgical hand antisepsis reduces the resident microbial count on the hands to a minimum.
  - The CDC recommends using an antimicrobial soap, and to scrub hands and forearms for the length of time recommended by the manufacturer, usually 2–6 minutes. The Association of Operating Room Nurses recommends 5 to 10 minutes. Refer to agency policy for time required.
  - When using an alcohol-based surgical hand-scrub product with persistent activity, follow the manufacturer's instructions. Before applying the alcohol solution, prewash hands and forearms with a non-antimicrobial soap and dry hands and forearms completely. After application of the alcohol-based product as recommended, allow hands and forearms to dry thoroughly before donning sterile gloves.

General Recommendations for Hand Hygiene

- Use hand lotions or creams to minimize the occurrence of irritant contact dermatitis associated with hand antisepsis or handwashing.
- Do not wear artificial fingernails or extenders when having direct contact with clients at high risk (e.g., those in intensive-care units or operating rooms).
- Keep natural nails tips less than 1/4-inch long.
- Wear gloves when contact with blood or other potentially infectious materials, mucous membranes, and nonintact skin could occur.
- Remove gloves after caring for a client. Do not wear the same pair of gloves for the care of more than one client, and do not wash gloves between uses with different clients.
- Change gloves during client care if moving from a contaminated body site to a clean body site.

(From Centers for Disease Control and Prevention (Morbidity and Mortality Weekly Report [MMWR], October 25, 2002 51 (RR16): 1-44 www.cdc.gov/handhygiene)

Answers for Chapter Review Questions

Chapter 1
1. 4
2. 4
3. 3
4. 3
5. 4
6. 3
7. 1
8. 4
9. 3
10. 4
11. 3
12. 4
13. 3
14. 4

Chapter 2
1. 4
2. 1
3. 3
4. 1
5. 2
6. 3
7. 2

Chapter 3
1. 4
2. 3
3. 2
4. 4
5. 4
6. 4
7. 3

Chapter 4
1. 2
2. 4
3. 2
4. 3
5. 1
6. 1
7. 3
8. 3

Chapter 5
1. 1
2. 3
3. 1
4. 3
5. 3

Chapter 6
1. 3
2. 2
3. 4
4. 4
5. 1
6. 1
7. 3
8. 4

Chapter 7
1. 4
2. 4
3. 3
4. 3
5. 2
6. 3
7. 4
8. 1
9. 3
10. 2
11. 2
12. 3

Chapter 8
1. 4
2. 3
3. 3
4. 4
5. 4
6. 4
7. 2
8. 3

Chapter 9
1. 3
2. 2
3. 3
4. 3
5. 3
6. 1
7. 3
8. 4
9. 2
10. 3

Chapter 10
1. 1
2. 3
3. 2
4. 3
5. 2
6. 4
7. 3
8. 4

Chapter 11
1. 3
2. 1
3. 2
4. 2
5. 3
6. 3
7. 1
8. 4
9. 1

Chapter 12
1. 2
2. 3
3. 2
4. 3
5. 4
6. 4
7. 1
8. 3
9. 2
10. 3
11. 4
12. 4
13. 4
14. 4
15. 1
16. 1
17. 3
18. 4
19. 1
20. 4
21. 2
22. 3
23. 2
24. 1
25. 4

Chapter 13
1. 1
2. 2
3. 3
4. 2
5. 4
6. 1
7. 4
8. 2
9. 2
10. 3
11. 4

Chapter 14
1. 1
2. 3
3. 3
4. 4
5. 3
6. 4
7. 1
8. 3

Chapter 15
1. 2
2. 1
3. 4
4. 3
5. 4

Chapter 16
1. 3
2. 1
3. 2
4. 1
5. 2

Chapter 17
1. 2
2. 3
3. 3
4. 3
5. 4
6. 1

Chapter 18
1. 3
2. 4
3. 2
4. 1
5. 4
6. 3
7. 3
8. 2

Chapter 19
1. 2
2. 3
3. 4
4. 4
5. 3

Chapter 20
1. 1
2. 3
3. 4
4. 4
5. 3

Chapter 21
1. 4
2. 4
3. 2
4. 4
5. 3
6. 4
7. 2
8. 3
9. 4

Chapter 22
1. 2
2. 4
3. 3
4. 2
5. 3
6. 2

Chapter 23
1. 3
2. 2
3. 2
4. 4
5. 3
6. 1

Chapter 24
1. 2
2. 2
3. 1
4. 2
5. 1
6. 2
7. 1
8. 1

Chapter 25
1. 4
2. 2
3. 4
4. 4
5. 3
6. 4
7. 3
8. 1
9. 2
10. 1

Chapter 26
1. 4
2. 1
3. 1
4. 1
5. 2
6. 1

Chapter 27
1. 3
2. 2
3. 3
4. 4
5. 3
6. 3
7. 3
8. 4
9. 2
10. 1
11. 3
12. 4
13. 4

Chapter 28
1. 4
2. 3
3. 4
4. 4
5. 1
6. 3
7. 4
8. 2
9. 4
10. 4

Chapter 29
1. 3
2. 4
3. 4
4. 3
5. 4
6. 3
7. 3

Chapter 30
1. 4
2. 4
3. 2
4. 2
5. 3
6. 4
7. 4
8. 1

Chapter 31
1. 3
2. 3
3. 2
4. 4
5. 4
6. 1
7. 3
8. 4
9. 4

Chapter 32
1. 4
2. 3
3. 4
4. 3
5. 4
6. 4
7. 3

Chapter 33
1. 2
2. 3
3. 2
4. 2
5. 4
6. 3
7. 4
8. 3
9. 3
10. 2

Chapter 34
1. 4
2. 3
3. 1
4. 4
5. 3
6. 3
7. 3
8. 4
9. 3
10. 1

Chapter 35
1. 3
2. 1
3. 4
4. 4
5. 4
6. 2
7. 4
8. 2
9. 3
10. 4
11. 3
12. 3
13. 4

Chapter 36
1. 2
2. 4
3. 2
4. 2
5. 2
6. 1
7. 2
8. 1
9. 3
10. 4
11. 2
12. 2
13. 3

Index

t denotes table; f denotes figure; b denotes box.